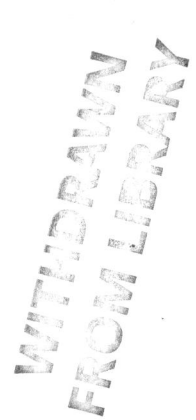

DIAGNOSTIC PATHOLOGY

NEOPLASTIC DERMATOPATHOLOGY

AMIRSYS®

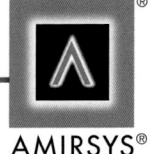

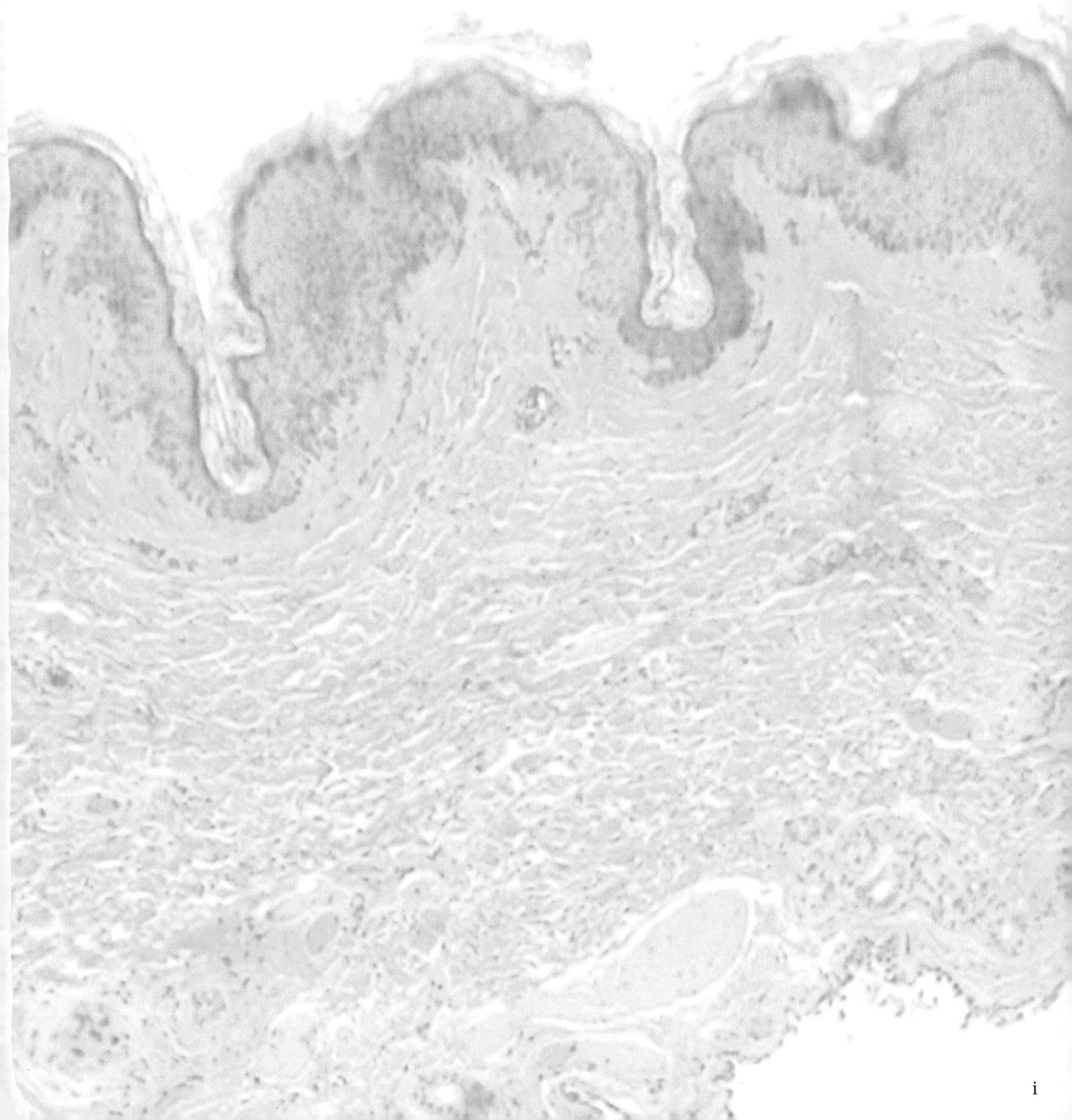

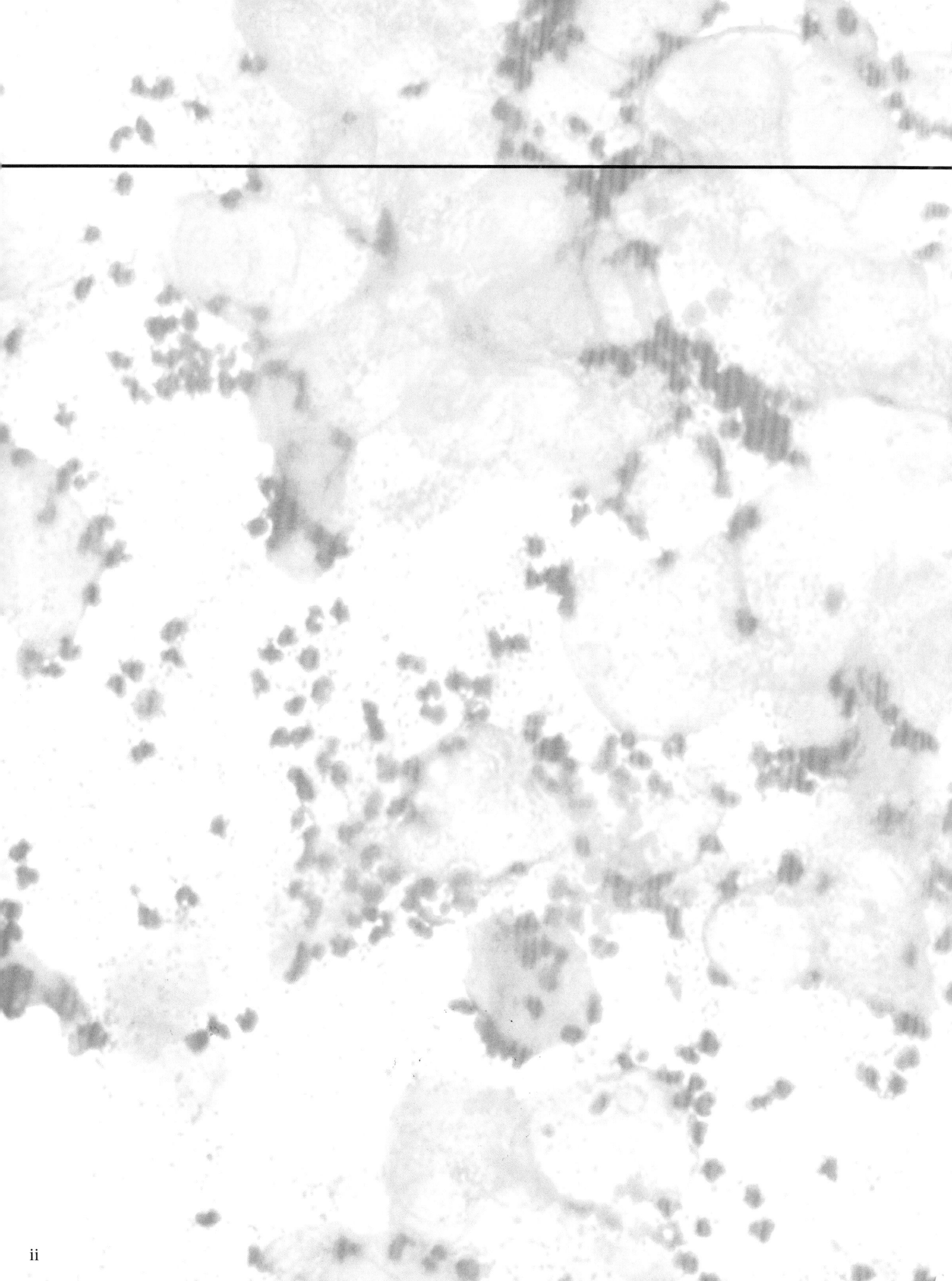

DIAGNOSTIC PATHOLOGY
NEOPLASTIC DERMATOPATHOLOGY

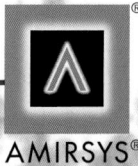

AMIRSYS®

David Cassarino, MD, PhD
Consultant Dermatopathologist
Southern California Permanente Medical Group
Los Angeles, CA
Clinical Professor of Dermatopathology
University of California, Irvine
Irvine, CA

Aaron Auerbach, MD, PhD
Pathologist
The Joint Pathology Center (JPC)
Silver Spring, MD

Christine J. Ko, MD
Associate Professor of Pathology
Yale University School of Medicine
New Haven, CT

Elizabeth A. Montgomery, MD
Professor of Pathology, Oncology, and Orthopedic
Surgery
John Hopkins Medical Institutions
Baltimore, MD

Steven D. Billings, MD
Staff Pathologist
Cleveland Clinic
Cleveland, OH

Cyril Fisher, MD, DSc, FRCPath
Consultant Histopathologist
Royal Marsden NHS Foundation Trust
Professor of Tumor Pathology
Institute of Cancer Research
University of London
London, United Kingdom

Elsa F. Velazquez, MD
Dermatopathologist
Caris Diagnostics
Clinical Assistant Professor Dermatology
Tufts University School of Medicine
Boston, MA

Soheil Sam Dadras, MD, PhD
Pathologist
Department of Dermatopathology and
Genetics/Developmental Biology
Farmington, CT

Senait W. Dyson, MD
Pathologist
Dyson Dermatopathology Lab
Tuscon, AZ

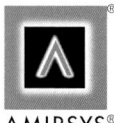

First Edition

© 2012 Amirsys, Inc.

Compilation © 2012 Amirsys Publishing, Inc.

Published in Salt Lake City, Utah

Printed in Canada by Friesens, Altona, Manitoba, Canada

ISBN: 978-1-931884-64-8

Notice and Disclaimer

Library of Congress Cataloging-in-Publication Data

Diagnostic pathology. Neoplastic dermatopathology / [edited by] David Cassarino. -- 1st ed.
    p. ; cm.
  Neoplastic dermatopathology
  Includes bibliographical references.
  ISBN 978-1-931884-64-8
  I. Cassarino, David. II. Title: Neoplastic dermatopathology.
  [DNLM: 1. Skin Neoplasms--pathology--Atlases. 2. Skin Neoplasms--diagnosis--Atlases.
  WR 17]

  616.99'477--dc23
                 2011043605

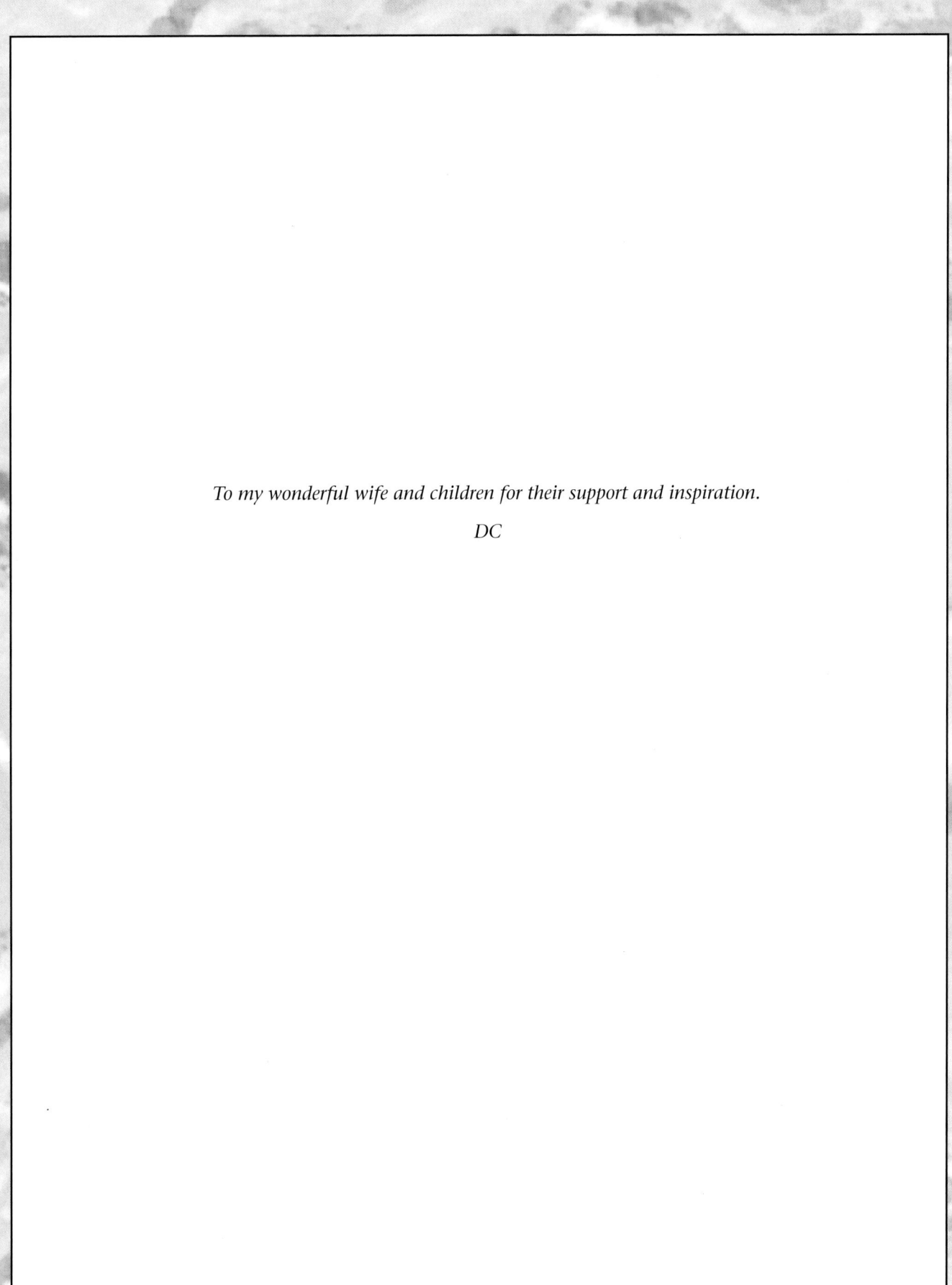

To my wonderful wife and children for their support and inspiration.

DC

CONTRIBUTORS

Lester D. R. Thompson, MD
Consultant Pathologist
Department of Pathology and Laboratory
Medicine
Southern California Permanente Medical Group
Woodland Hills, CA

Amitabh Srivastava, MD
Assistant Professor
Harvard Medical School
Pathologist
Brigham and Women's Hospital
Boston, MA

Sa A. Wang, MD
Associate Professor
Department of Hematopathology
The University of Texas M. D. Anderson
Cancer Center
Houston, TX

Jessica M. Comstock, MD
Assistant Professor
Division of Pediatric Pathology
University of Utah Hospital
Salt Lake City, UT

Francisco Vega, MD, PhD
Assistant Professor
Department of Hematopathology
The University of Texas M. D. Anderson
Cancer Center
Houston, TX

Khin Thway, BSc, MBBS, FRCPath
Consultant Histopathologist
Royal Marsden NHS Foundation Trust
London, United Kingdom

Jeremy C. Wallentine, MD
Pathologist
Intermountain Healthcare and Utah Pathology
Services, Inc.
LDS Hospital
Salt Lake City, UT

David R. Lucas, MD
Director of Surgical Pathology
Professor of Pathology
University of Michigan Medical School
Ann Arbor, MI

**Alexandros D. Polydorides,
MD, PhD**
Assistant Professor
Mount Sinai School of Medicine
Attending Pathologist
Mount Sinai Medical Center
New York, NY

DIAGNOSTIC PATHOLOGY
NEOPLASTIC DERMATOPATHOLOGY

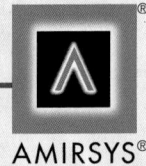

AMIRSYS®

Amirsys, creators of the highly acclaimed radiology series Diagnostic Imaging, proudly introduces its new Diagnostic Pathology series, designed as easy-to-use reference texts for the busy practicing surgical pathologist. Written by world-renowned experts, the series will consist of 15 titles in all the crucial diagnostic areas of surgical pathology.

The newest book in this series, *Diagnostic Pathology: Neoplastic Dermatopathology*, contains approximately 850 pages of comprehensive, yet concise, descriptions of more than 230 specific diagnoses. Amirsys's pioneering bulleted format distills pertinent information to the essentials. Each chapter has the same organization providing an easy-to-read reference for making rapid, efficient, and accurate diagnoses in a busy surgical pathology practice. A highlighted Key Facts box provides the essential features of each diagnosis. Detailed sections on Terminology, Etiology/Pathogenesis, Clinical Issues, Macroscopic and Microscopic Findings, and the all important Differential Diagnoses follow so you can find the information you need in the exact same place every time.

Most importantly, every diagnosis features numerous high-quality images, including gross pathology, H&E and immunohistochemical stains, correlative radiographic images, and richly colored graphics, all of which are fully annotated to maximize their illustrative potential.

We believe that this lavishly illustrated series, with its up-to-date information and practical focus, will become the core of your reference collection. Enjoy!

Elizabeth H. Hammond, MD
Executive Editor, Pathology
Amirsys, Inc.

Paula J. Woodward, MD
President
Amirsys Publishing, Inc.

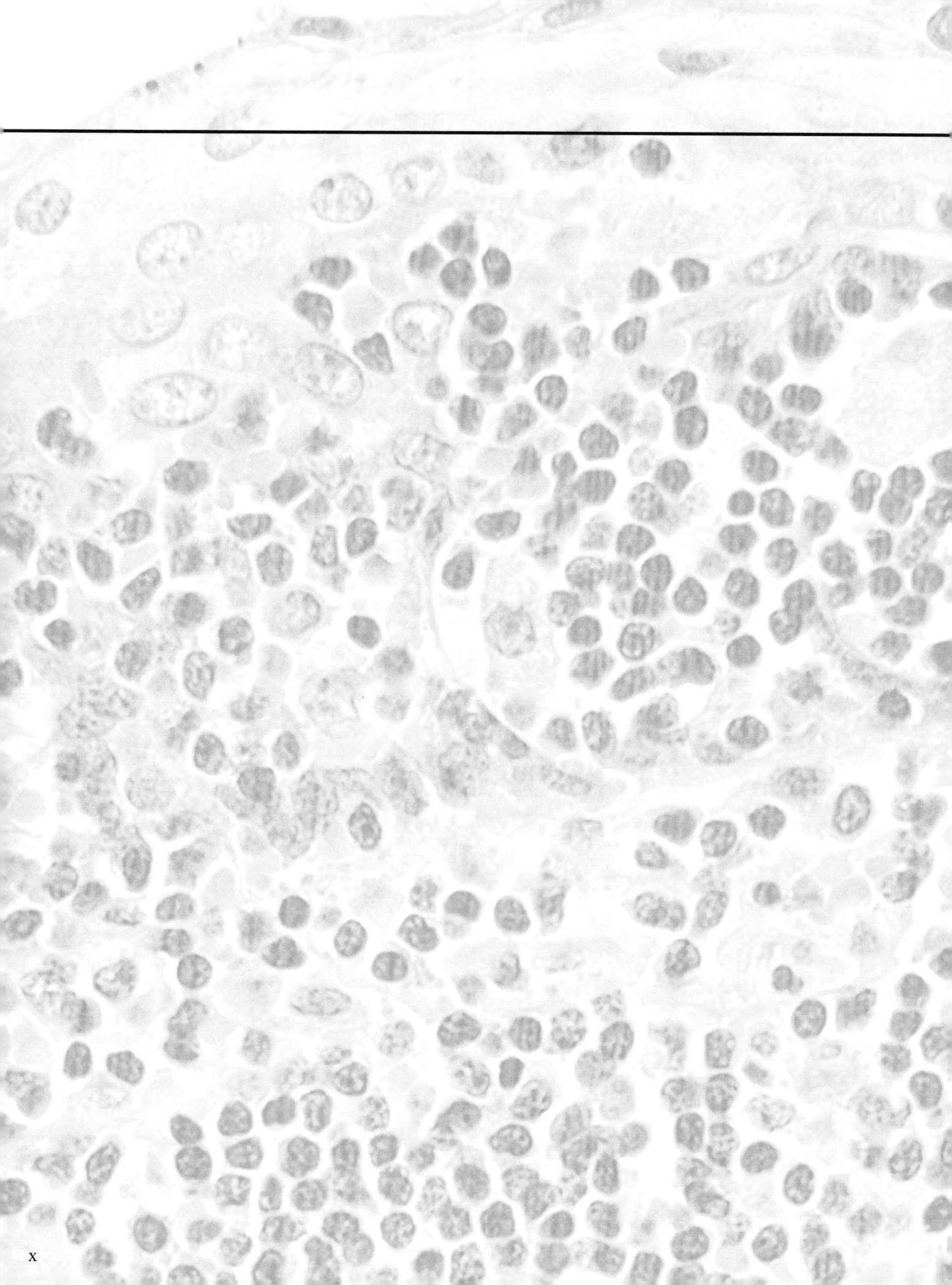

x

PREFACE

Cutaneous neoplasms include a wide array of benign and malignant proliferations with diverse etiology and differentiation. Many unusual and rare tumors unique to the skin have been described. These can be difficult to identify, as they may show overlapping features with other tumors in the differential, and can prove challenging for general pathologists, dermatologists, and dermatopathologists. *Diagnostic Pathology: Neoplastic Dermatopathology* is designed as a concise, practical, richly illustrated reference covering cutaneous neoplasms and their differential diagnosis to allow for accurate interpretation and diagnosis.

Although there are many dermatopathology textbooks currently available, these are mostly traditional textbooks in a paragraph-based format with relatively few clinical and histologic photographs. In contrast, this book is lavishly illustrated and written in a detailed yet concise bulleted format that facilitates the reader's ability to quickly find relevant information. Each chapter includes information such as Definitions, Etiology/Pathogenesis, Epidemiology, Clinical Presentation, Prognosis and Treatment, Histologic Findings, Ancillary Techniques including Immunohistochemistry and Molecular Pathology, Differential Diagnosis, and Pathologic Interpretation Pearls. Current CAP-approved Staging Protocols for tumors including melanoma, squamous cell carcinoma, and Merkel cell carcinoma are also included for reference.

As in other subspecialities of pathology, there is a rapidly growing body of knowledge in dermatopathology, including new diagnostic immunohistochemical, molecular, and genetic techniques, making it difficult for any textbook to remain fully up to date. To that end, this book includes the Amirsys eBook Advantage™, which provides users access to timely updates on relevant topics, as well as a fully searchable text and complete listing of antibodies.

We hope that *Diagnostic Pathology: Neoplastic Dermatopathology* will be a useful and valuable reference for practicing pathologists, dermatologists, and dermatopathologists.

David Cassarino, MD, PhD
Consultant Dermatopathologist
Southern California Permanente Medical Group
Los Angeles, CA
Clinical Professor of Dermatopathology
University of California, Irvine
Irvine, CA

ACKNOWLEDGMENTS

Text Editing

Arthur G. Gelsinger, MA

Matthew R. Connelly, MA

Lorna Morring, MS

Rebecca L. Hutchinson, BA

Angela M. Green, BA

Image Editing

Jeffrey J. Marmorstone, BS

Lisa A. Magar, BS

Medical Text Editing

Sara Cuadra Acree, MD

Illustrations

Laura C. Sesto, MA

Lane R. Bennion, MS

Richard Coombs, MS

Art Direction and Design

Laura C. Sesto, MA

Mirjam Ravneng, BA

Assistant Editor

Dave L. Chance, MA

Publishing Lead

Katherine L. Riser, MA

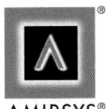

AMIRSYS®

Names you know. Content you trust.®

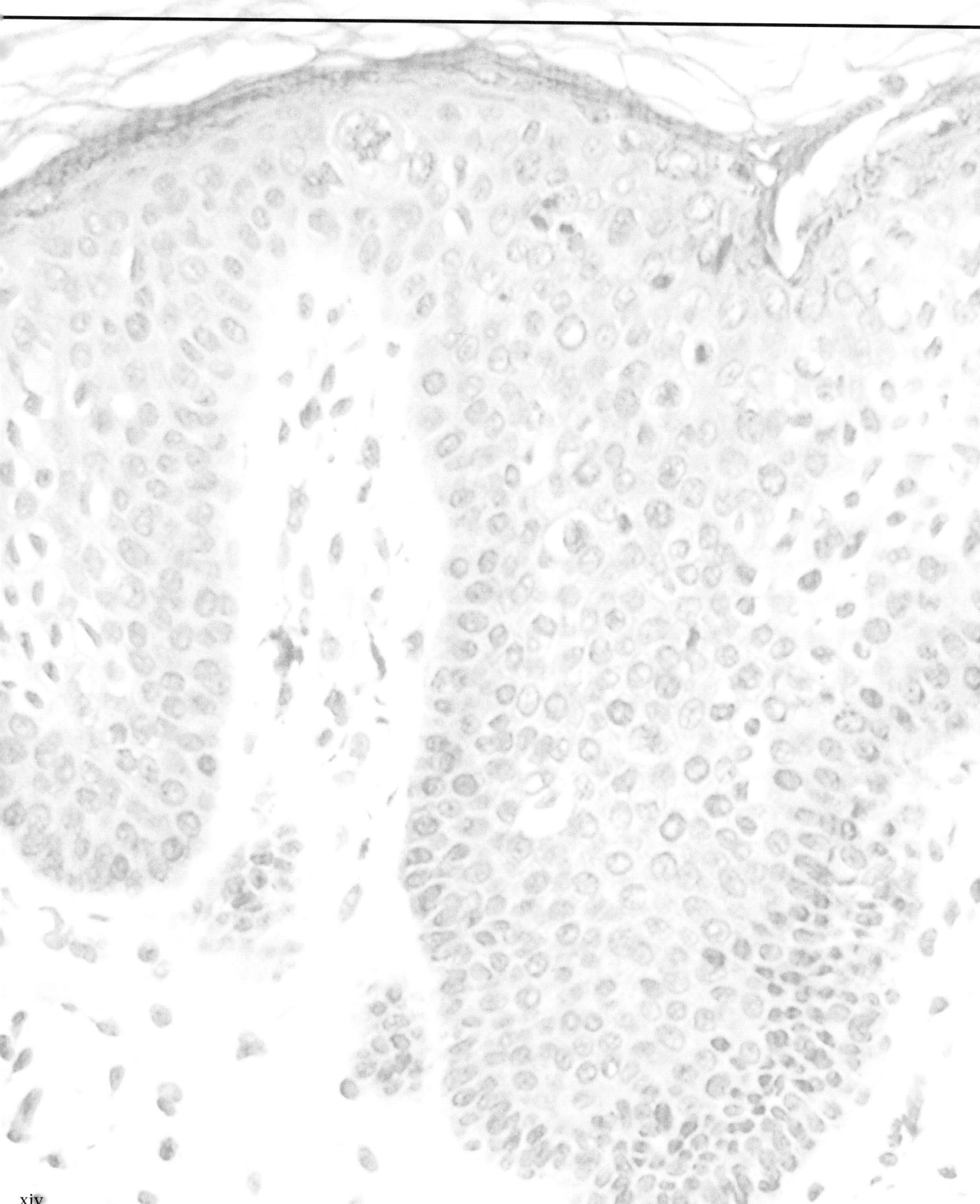

SECTIONS

Nonmelanocytic Tumors of the Skin

Epithelial Cysts

Epidermal Tumors

Tumors and Tumor-like Conditions of the Hair Follicle

Tumors and Tumor-like Conditions with Sebaceous Differentiation

Neoplasms and Proliferations of Eccrine and Apocrine Sweat Glands

Metastatic Tumors

Fibrous and "Fibrohistiocytic" Tissue Tumors

Vascular and Perivascular Tumors and Pseudotumors

Tumors and Tumor-like Conditions with Neural, Nerve Sheath, and Neuroendocrine Differentiation

Tumors of Muscle, Fat, Cartilage, and Bone

Histiocytic Proliferations

Lymphomas and Hematopoietic Proliferations

Melanocytic Tumors of the Skin

Benign Melanocytic Tumors (Nevi)

Malignant Tumors (Melanomas and Related Lesions)

Reference

TABLE OF CONTENTS

SECTION 3
Tumors and Tumor-like Conditions of the Hair Follicle

SECTION 4
Tumors and Tumor-like Conditions with Sebaceous Differentiation

SECTION 5
Neoplasms and Proliferations of Eccrine and Apocrine Sweat Glands

SECTION 10
Tumors of Muscle, Fat, Cartilage, and Bone

SECTION 11
Histiocytic Proliferations

SECTION 12
Lymphomas and Hematopoietic Proliferations

B-cell Neoplasms

T-cell and NK-cell Neoplasms

PART II
Melanocytic Tumors of the Skin

SECTION 1
Benign Melanocytic Tumors (Nevi)

SECTION 2
Malignant Tumors (Melanomas and Related Lesions)

Melanoma In Situ

Invasive Melanoma

PART III
Reference

SECTION 1
Reference Indices

DIAGNOSTIC PATHOLOGY
NEOPLASTIC DERMATOPATHOLOGY

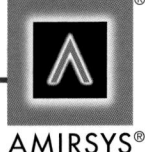

Epithelial Cysts

EPIDERMOID/EPIDERMAL INCLUSION CYST

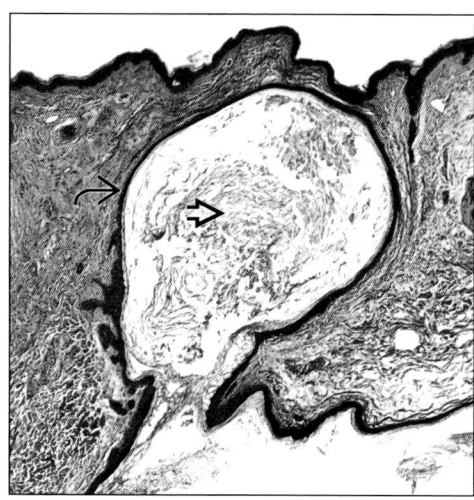

A solitary epidermoid cyst is appreciated in the dermis. Note the thin squamous epithelium ⇗ and abundant keratin contents ⇘. The punctum is not represented in this section.

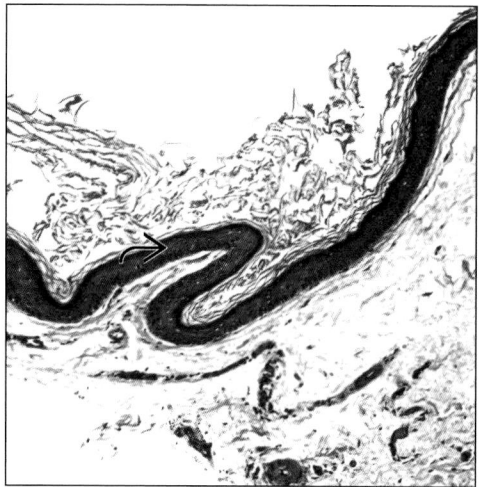

The contents of the epidermoid cyst consist of laminated orthokeratotic material. The cyst lining is composed of a bland squamous epithelium ⇗ similar to the epidermis.

TERMINOLOGY

Abbreviations
- Epidermoid/epidermal inclusion cyst (EIC)

Synonyms
- Infundibular cyst

Definitions
- Unilocular cysts lined by epidermis-like epithelium

ETIOLOGY/PATHOGENESIS

Etiology
- Damage to the pilosebaceous unit
  - Infundibular cyst variant
    - Cystically dilated follicular infundibulum
    - Shows connection to the surface (punctum)
  - Implantation (inclusion) cyst variant
    - Secondary to trauma (e.g., surgery, sewing needle)
    - No connection to the epidermis
- Cyclosporin treatment in transplant recipients
- Multiple lesions may be associated with Gardner syndrome

CLINICAL ISSUES

Epidemiology
- Incidence
  - Very common
- Age
  - Young and middle-aged adults
- Gender
  - Both genders equally affected

Site
- Preferentially face, neck, and trunk
- Scrotum and labia majora are also common

Presentation
- Dome-shaped lesions with smooth surface
  - May show dark dot-like punctum on the surface
- A few millimeters to a few centimeters in diameter

Prognosis
- Can rupture and become inflamed &/or infected
- Benign lesions with excellent prognosis
- Malignant transformation is exceptional

MACROSCOPIC FEATURES

General Features
- Cut sections show dermal &/or subcutaneous unilocular cystic structure
  - Thin white smooth wall and "cheesy" contents

MICROSCOPIC PATHOLOGY

Histologic Features
- Unilocular cyst
- Lined by squamous epithelium with granular layer
- Contains laminated ("basket weave") keratin
- Ruptured lesions are surrounded by acute/suppurative and granulomatous inflammation with giant cells
  - In older ruptured lesions, epithelial lining may disappear
    - Fibrosis and foreign body giant cell reaction with variable amounts of keratin material (keratin granuloma)
    - Most common cause of granulomatous inflammation in dermis and subcutis is ruptured epidermoid cyst
- Hybrid cysts show mixed features of epidermoid and pilar cysts (rare)
  - Pilomatrixoma-like features (presence of basaloid cells and ghost cells) should raise suspicion for Gardner syndrome

EPIDERMOID/EPIDERMAL INCLUSION CYST

Key Facts

Etiology/Pathogenesis
- Infundibular cyst variant
- Implantation (inclusion) cyst variant

Clinical Issues
- Very common lesions
- Usually affecting face, neck, and trunk

Microscopic Pathology
- Unilocular cyst

- Lined by squamous epithelium with granular layer
- Contains laminated ("basket weave") keratin
- May rupture and become inflamed
  - Keratin granuloma

Top Differential Diagnoses
- Tricholemmal (pilar) cyst
- Vellus hair cyst
- Dermoid cyst
- HPV-related epidermoid cyst

- EIC may coexist with melanocytic nevi (common)
  - May explain an increase in size of the mole
- Exceptionally, malignant tumors may arise in association with epidermoid cysts
  - Squamous cell carcinoma (in situ and invasive)
  - Basal cell carcinoma
  - Paget disease and neuroendocrine carcinoma

Cytologic Features
- Epidermis-like lining with granular layer

DIFFERENTIAL DIAGNOSIS

Tricholemmal (Pilar) Cyst
- Absence of granular layer
- Eosinophilic compact (not laminated) keratin

Vellus Hair Cyst
- Thin squamous epithelium with granular layer
- Laminated keratin contents with numerous small hair shafts

Dermoid Cyst
- Stratified squamous epithelium with granular layer and laminated keratin contents
- Associated hair follicles and sebaceous glands

Verrucous Cyst
- Epidermoid cyst variant associated with HPV (koilocytosis may be present)

- Papillomatous acanthotic epithelium with prominent hypergranulosis (enlarged keratohyalin granules)

Epidermoid Cyst of the Sole
- HPV-associated (mainly seen in Japanese)
- Eosinophilic intracytoplasmic inclusions in the cyst wall

DIAGNOSTIC CHECKLIST

Pathologic Interpretation Pearls
- In older ruptured epidermoid cysts, wall may disappear
  - Residual keratin material admixed with granulomatous inflammation is a clue to the diagnosis

SELECTED REFERENCES

1. Urabe K et al: Pilomatricoma-like changes in the epidermoid cysts of Gardner syndrome with an APC gene mutation. J Dermatol. 31(3):255-7, 2004
2. Schoendorff C et al: Multiple epidermoid cysts in a renal transplant recipient taking cyclosporine A. Cutis. 50(1):36-8, 1992
3. Perse RM et al: Trabecular (Merkel cell) carcinoma arising in the wall of an epidermal cyst. Am J Dermatopathol. 9(5):423-7, 1987
4. McGavran MH et al: Keratinous cysts of the skin. Identification and differentiation of pilar cysts from epidermal cysts. Arch Dermatol. 94(4):499-508, 1966

IMAGE GALLERY

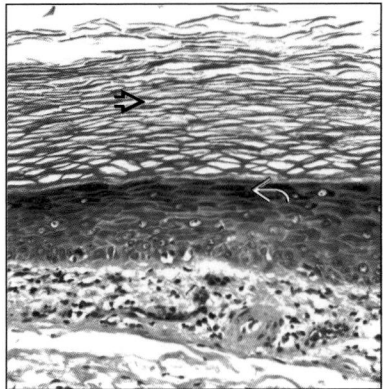 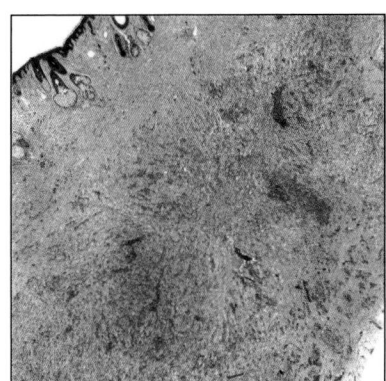 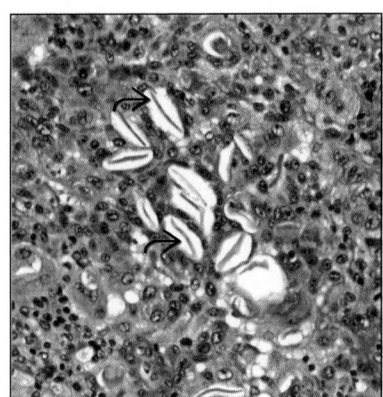

(Left) The cyst wall is composed of squamous epithelium with a granular layer ➡, and the contents consist of laminated keratin ➤. (Center) This ruptured epidermoid cyst is characterized by a diffuse infiltrate of histiocytes, lymphoid cells, and neutrophils in the dermis. The cyst wall is no longer present. (Right) Even when the epithelium is not identified, the presence of a foreign body giant cell reaction to keratin material ➔ is characteristic of a ruptured epidermoid cyst.

PILAR (TRICHOLEMMAL) CYST

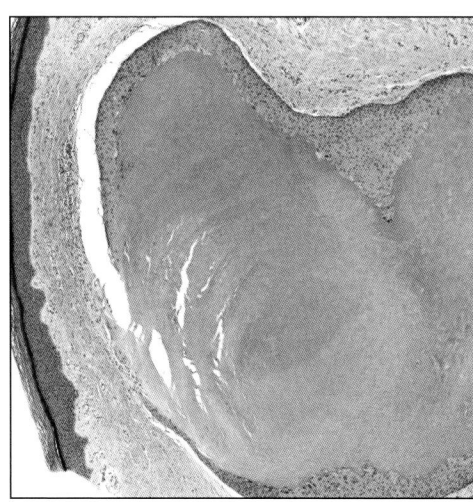

Scanning magnification shows a dermal-based benign cystic lesion with dense eosinophilic tricholemmal keratinization, characteristic of a pilar cyst.

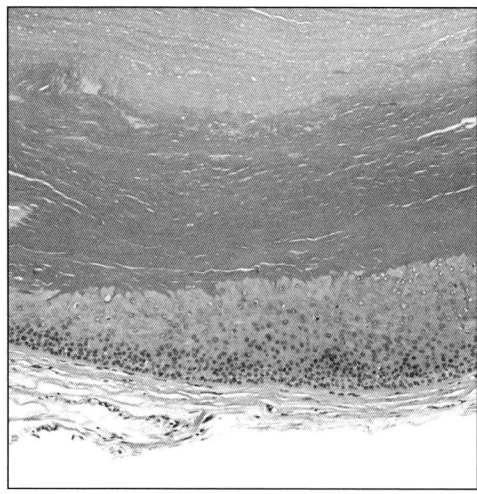

The lining is composed of stratified squamous epithelium with an abrupt transition to dense eosinophilic keratin.

TERMINOLOGY

Synonyms
- Pilar cyst
- Trichilemmal cyst
- Isthmus-catagen cyst

Definitions
- Benign unilocular cyst lined by squamous epithelium lacking a granular layer and containing abundant dense keratin material

CLINICAL ISSUES

Epidemiology
- Incidence
  - 2nd most common type of cutaneous cyst
- Age
  - Most common in adults
- Gender
  - More common in women than men

Site
- 90% of pilar cysts present on scalp

Presentation
- Autosomal dominant inheritance common
- Multiple lesions common
- Usually present as asymptomatic lesion on scalp as dermal or subcutaneous nodule

Treatment
- Surgical approaches
  - Simple excision

Prognosis
- Benign lesions
- Proliferating pilar (tricholemmal) cysts or malignant pilar (tricholemmal) cysts may rarely arise in longstanding pilar cysts

MACROSCOPIC FEATURES

General Features
- Dermal or subcutaneous cystic structure

Sections to Be Submitted
- Representative sections appropriate

Size
- Wide range, can be less than 0.5 cm to several cm in size

MICROSCOPIC PATHOLOGY

Histologic Features
- Circumscribed simple cyst located in dermis &/or subcutaneous tissue
- Filled with dense laminated eosinophilic keratin
- Stratified squamous epithelium lining the cyst
- Abrupt keratinization from large polygonal keratinocytes
  - So-called tricholemmal keratinization
- Granular layer generally absent
  - Occasionally, cells with a few keratohyaline granules may be seen
- Rupture with associated granulomatous response common

DIFFERENTIAL DIAGNOSIS

Proliferating Pilar Cyst/Tumor
- Multiloculated cystic neoplasm
- Nodules of proliferating squamous cells
- Squamous eddies
- Mitotic activity present, especially in peripheral cells
- At least focal abrupt tricholemmal keratinization

PILAR (TRICHOLEMMAL) CYST

Key Facts

Clinical Issues
- 90% of pilar cysts present on scalp

Microscopic Pathology
- Circumscribed simple cyst
- Filled with dense eosinophilic keratin
- Stratified squamous epithelium
- Abrupt keratinization from large polygonal keratinocytes
- Granular layer generally absent

- Rupture with associated granulomatous response common

Diagnostic Checklist
- Abrupt tricholemmal keratinization is a key diagnostic feature
- Simple unilocular cyst
  - If architectural complexity is present, consider proliferating pilar cyst or malignant pilar cyst

Malignant Proliferating Pilar Cyst/Tumor
- Similar to proliferating pilar tumor but with at least focal areas of
  - Infiltrative growth
  - Cytologic atypia
  - Mitotic activity ± atypical mitotic figures

Epidermoid Cyst/Epidermal Inclusion Cyst
- Unilocular cyst
- Squamous epithelial lining
- Intact granular layer
- Epidermal keratinization with loose layers of keratin, not dense eosinophilic tricholemmal keratinization as in pilar cyst

DIAGNOSTIC CHECKLIST

Pathologic Interpretation Pearls
- Abrupt tricholemmal keratinization is a key diagnostic feature
- Simple unilocular cyst
  - If architectural complexity present, consider proliferating pilar cyst or malignant proliferating pilar cyst
- Rupture is common
  - Granulomatous inflammation can partially obscure histologic features

SELECTED REFERENCES

1. Eskander A et al: Squamous cell carcinoma arising in a proliferating pilar (trichilemmal) cyst with nodal and distant metastases. J Otolaryngol Head Neck Surg. 39(5):E63-7, 2010
2. Karaman E et al: Giant trichilemmal cyst at the neck region. J Craniofac Surg. 20(3):961-2, 2009
3. Anolik R et al: Proliferating trichilemmal cyst with focal calcification. Dermatol Online J. 14(10):25, 2008
4. Berk DR et al: Milia: a review and classification. J Am Acad Dermatol. 59(6):1050-63, 2008
5. González-Vela MC et al: Proliferating trichilemmal cyst associated with an epidermal nevus. J Dermatol. 35(1):52-4, 2008
6. Takeda H et al: Hybrid cyst: case reports and review of 15 cases in Japan. J Eur Acad Dermatol Venereol. 17(1):83-6, 2003
7. Vandeweyer E et al: Cutaneous cysts: a plea for systematic analysis. Acta Chir Belg. 103(5):507-10, 2003
8. Leppard BJ et al: The natural history of trichilemmal cysts. Br J Dermatol. 94(4):379-90, 1976
9. McGavran MH et al: Keratinous cysts of the skin. Identification and differentiation of pilar cysts from epidermal cysts. Arch Dermatol. 94(4):499-508, 1966

IMAGE GALLERY

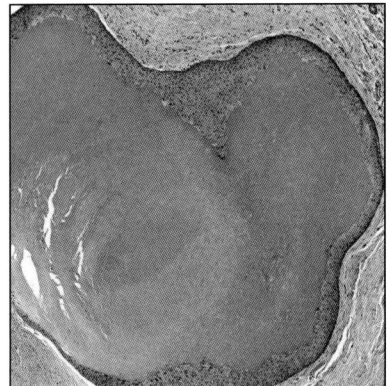
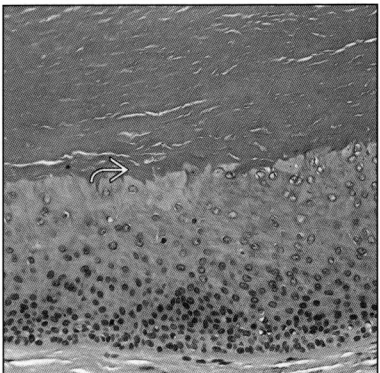
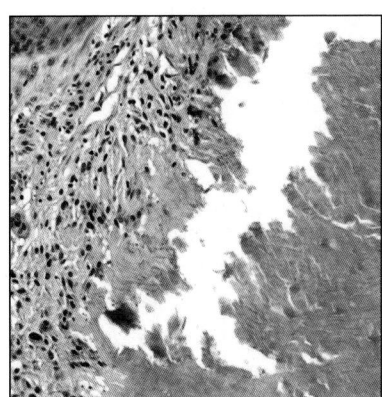

(Left) Pilar cysts are well-circumscribed simple cysts involving the dermis &/or subcutis. *(Center)* The epithelium at the interface with the keratin is composed of large polygonal keratinocytes with abundant eosinophilic cytoplasm. There is abrupt keratinization ➜ without a granular layer, but scattered keratohyaline granules may be seen. *(Right)* Pilar cysts often rupture, resulting in granulomatous inflammation. Recognition of cyst remnants help make the diagnosis.

PROLIFERATING PILAR (TRICHOLEMMAL) CYST/TUMOR

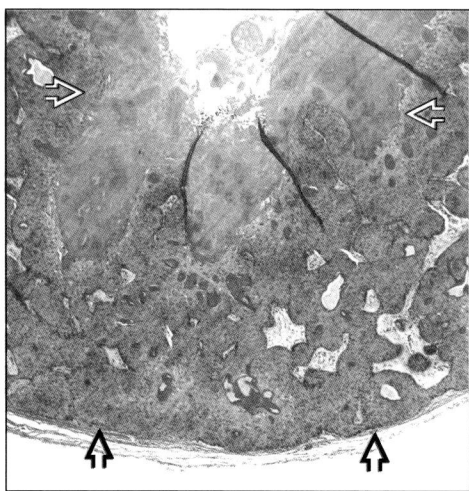

Scanning magnification of PPT shows a smooth-bordered ➡, circumscribed tumor composed of thickened cords of squamous cells surrounding a large cystic cavity ➡ containing abundant keratin material.

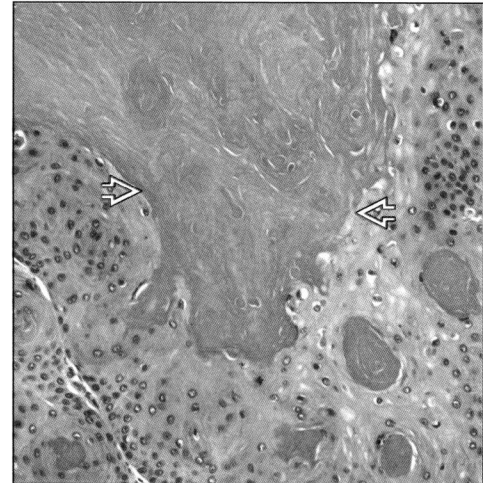

High-magnification examination of a benign PPT shows bland squamous keratinocytes with abundant eosinophilic cytoplasm surrounding keratin-filled spaces. Note the lack of an intervening granular layer ➡.

TERMINOLOGY

Abbreviations
- Proliferating pilar tumor (PPT)
- Proliferating pilar cyst (PPC)

Synonyms
- Proliferating trichilemmal cyst/tumor

Definitions
- Multicystic squamous neoplasm composed of mature keratinocytes lining keratin-filled spaces

ETIOLOGY/PATHOGENESIS

Unknown
- Postulated that most cases arise in preexisting pilar (tricholemmal) cyst; may be related to chronic inflammation or trauma

CLINICAL ISSUES

Epidemiology
- Incidence
  - Uncommon tumors
- Age
  - Typically occur in older adults
- Gender
  - Much more common in females than males

Site
- Typically occur on scalp (90%); also may occur on face, trunk, and extremities

Treatment
- Surgical approaches
  - Complete surgical excision is recommended in order to prevent recurrence and malignant transformation

Prognosis
- PPTs behave in benign fashion, but malignant PPTs are aggressive tumors that have a high rate of metastasis

MACROSCOPIC FEATURES

General Features
- Often multicystic dermal-based tumors that may involve subcutis

Size
- Large tumors, 6 cm or greater in diameter

MICROSCOPIC PATHOLOGY

Histologic Features
- Large, multicystic, dermal-based tumor with squamous lining and spaces containing dense keratin
  - Typically symmetric and well circumscribed at low-power examination
  - Cystic spaces are irregularly formed and anastomosing
    - Cysts are filled with abundant, dense, eosinophilic keratin (similar to pilar/tricholemmal cysts)
    - Cells lining cyst show keratinization without granular layer (tricholemmal/pilar-type keratinization), unlike proliferating epidermoid cyst (PEC), which shows a granular layer
  - Squamous eddies may be seen in cyst lining
  - Peripheral palisading of basilar layer is typically present, and there may be thickened basement membrane
  - Squamous epithelial cells show mild enlargement and nuclear hyperchromasia
  - Occasional mitotic figures are present, but no high-grade atypia or increased mitotic activity should be present

PROLIFERATING PILAR (TRICHOLEMMAL) CYST/TUMOR

Key Facts

Terminology

- Proliferating pilar tumor (PPT), proliferating pilar cyst (PPC), proliferating trichilemmal cyst/tumor
  - Multicystic squamous neoplasm composed of mature keratinocytes lining keratin-filled spaces

Clinical Issues

- Typically occur on scalp (90% of cases)
- Most cases of PPT behave in benign fashion, but malignant PPTs are aggressive tumors that have a high rate of metastasis

Microscopic Pathology

- Cystic spaces are irregularly formed and anastomosing
- Cysts show keratinization without granular layer (unlike PEC)

- Large, multicystic, dermal-based tumor with squamous lining and spaces containing dense keratin
- Peripheral palisading of basilar layer is typically present, and there may be thickened basement membrane
- Occasional mitotic figures are present, but no high-grade atypia or increased mitotic activity should be present

Top Differential Diagnoses

- Pilar/tricholemmal cyst
- Proliferating epidermoid cyst (PEC)
- Malignant PPT (squamous cell carcinoma arising in PPT)

- Focal epidermal connections may be present in a minority (about 25%) of cases

Cytologic Features

- Squamous cells demonstrate abundant eosinophilic cytoplasm and mildly enlarged and hyperchromatic-staining nuclei

DIFFERENTIAL DIAGNOSIS

Pilar/Tricholemmal Cyst

- Unicystic structure lined by mature squamous cells that keratinize without granular layer
- Cyst contains abundant, dense, laminated keratin and may show focal calcifications
- May be found in association with a PPT, as most PPTs likely arise in preexisting pilar cysts

Proliferating Epidermoid Cyst (PEC)

- Shows overlapping features with PPT but exhibits granular layer and loose tiers of laminated keratin (similar to epidermoid/epidermal inclusion cysts)
- Occurs more frequently in anogenital region and on extremities than PPT (which typically occurs on scalp)
- Hybrid lesions that show features of both PPT and PEC may be encountered
- Malignant change occurs in a significant minority of cases; characterized by infiltrative component resembling invasive squamous cell carcinoma

Malignant PPT (Squamous Cell Carcinoma Arising in PPT)

- Tumors are usually larger than benign PPTs and clinically often present as rapidly enlarging nodular mass lesion, may be ulcerated or bleeding
- May arise in a PPT but shows greater cytologic atypia and mitotic activity, with infiltrative features
  - Typically resembles conventional SCC but may also show features of spindle cell/sarcomatoid carcinoma in some cases

- Malignant PPTs are aggressive carcinomas with high incidence of both local recurrence and metastasis (up to 30% reported)

DIAGNOSTIC CHECKLIST

Pathologic Interpretation Pearls

- Large, multicystic, dermal-based tumor with squamous epithelium lacking granular layer lining cystic spaces containing abundant keratin debris

SELECTED REFERENCES

1. Cassarino DS et al: Cutaneous squamous cell carcinoma: a comprehensive clinicopathologic classification--part two. J Cutan Pathol. 33(4):261-79, 2006
2. Ye J et al: Proliferating pilar tumors: a clinicopathologic study of 76 cases with a proposal for definition of benign and malignant variants. Am J Clin Pathol. 122(4):566-74, 2004
3. Haas N et al: Carcinoma arising in a proliferating trichilemmal cyst expresses fetal and trichilemmal hair phenotype. Am J Dermatopathol. 24(4):340-4, 2002
4. Mathis ED et al: Malignant proliferating trichilemmal tumor. Am J Clin Oncol. 24(4):351-3, 2001
5. Sau P et al: Proliferating epithelial cysts. Clinicopathological analysis of 96 cases. J Cutan Pathol. 22(5):394-406, 1995
6. Rutty GN et al: Malignant change in trichilemmal cysts: a study of cell proliferation and DNA content. Histopathology. 21(5):465-8, 1992
7. Mehregan AH et al: Malignant proliferating trichilemmal tumors--report of three cases. J Dermatol Surg Oncol. 13(12):1339-42, 1987
8. Amaral AL et al: Proliferating pilar (trichilemmal) cyst. Report of two cases, one with carcinomatous transformation and one with distant metastases. Arch Pathol Lab Med. 108(10):808-10, 1984
9. Jones EW: Proliferating epidermoid cysts. Arch Dermatol. 94(1):11-9, 1966

PROLIFERATING PILAR (TRICHOLEMMAL) CYST/TUMOR

Microscopic Features

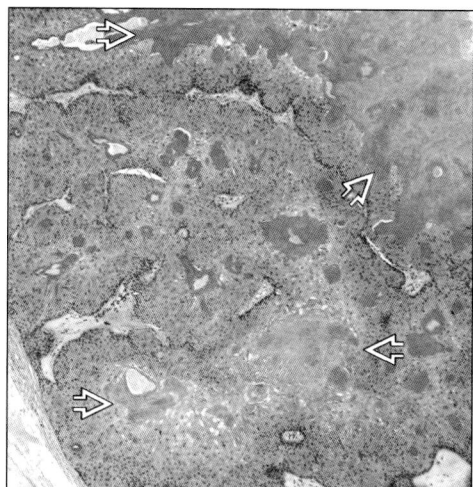

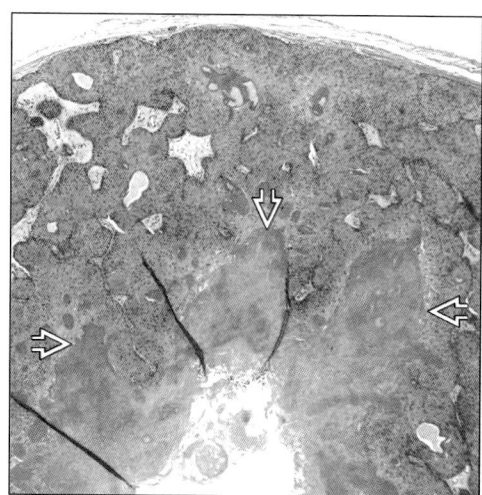

(Left) Low magnification of a PPT shows multiple thickened, anastomosing cords of squamous keratinocytes surrounding several cystic cavities ⊟ that contain abundant keratin material. (Right) Scanning magnification view of a PPT shows a smooth-bordered tumor composed of thickened cords of squamous keratinocytes surrounding a large cystic cavity ⊟ that contains abundant keratin material.

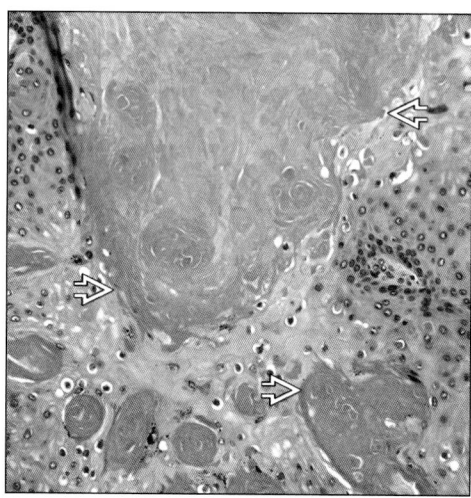

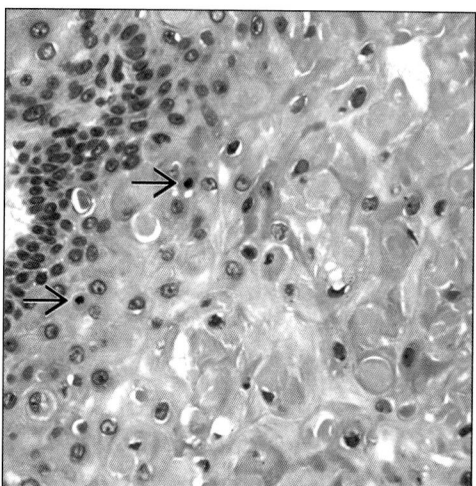

(Left) High-magnification examination of a PPT shows bland squamous keratinocytes with abundant eosinophilic cytoplasm surrounding multiple keratin-filled spaces that lack an intervening granular layer ⊟. (Right) High-magnification examination shows the bland cytologic features of the squamous cells, which show uniform nuclei, small nucleoli, and abundant amounts of dense eosinophilic cytoplasm. Scattered dyskeratotic keratinocytes are present →.

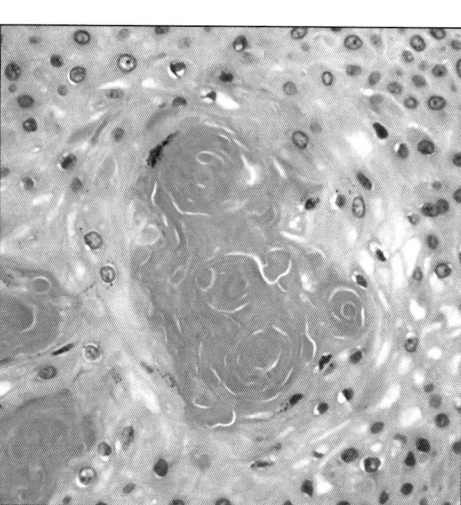

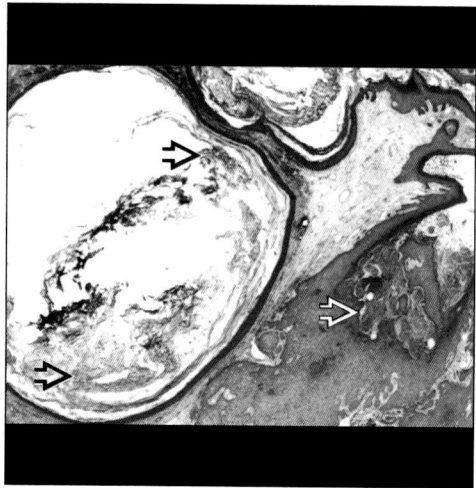

(Left) High-magnification examination shows several small foci of dense keratin material surrounded by bland-appearing squamous cells. (Right) Scanning magnification shows a proliferating cystic neoplasm with combined features of a proliferating epidermoid cyst (showing a granular layer and loose, laminated keratin ⊟) and a proliferating pilar cyst (lacking a granular layer and showing dense eosinophilic keratin ⊟).

PROLIFERATING PILAR (TRICHOLEMMAL) CYST/TUMOR

Differential Diagnosis

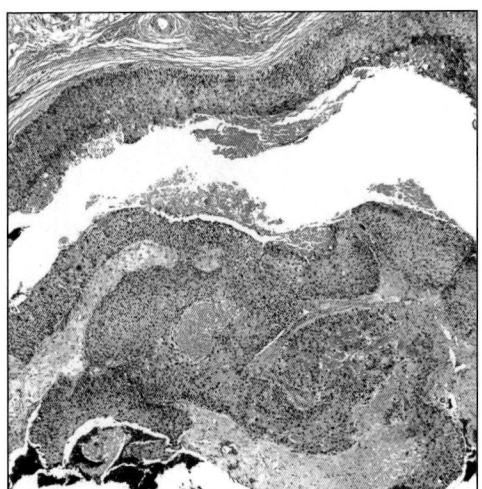

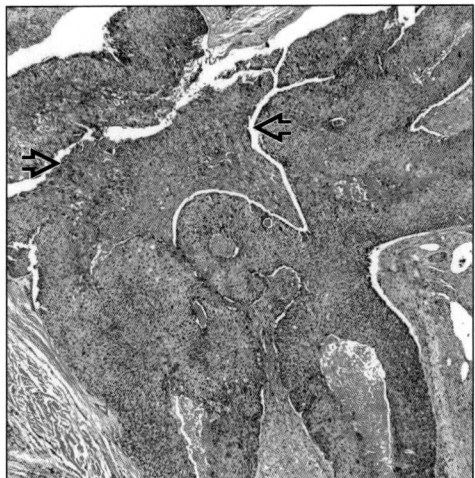

(Left) Low-magnification view of a malignant PPT shows cystic spaces lined by enlarged, atypical squamous cells. *(Right)* Malignant proliferating pilar tumor composed of irregular, anastomosing cords of enlarged, atypical squamous cells with areas of keratinization and necrotic cellular debris ➡ is seen.

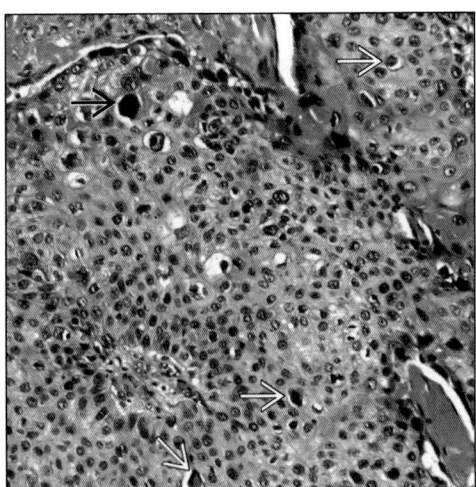

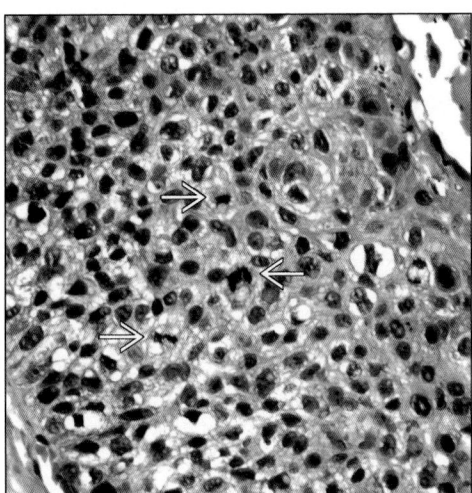

(Left) High-magnification view of a malignant PPT demonstrates nuclear pleomorphism with marked nuclear enlargement ➡ and atypia, along with scattered mitotic figures and dyskeratotic cells ➡. *(Right)* High magnification of a malignant PPT shows nuclear hyperchromasia, irregular nuclear borders, and multiple mitotic figures ➡ in a single high-power field.

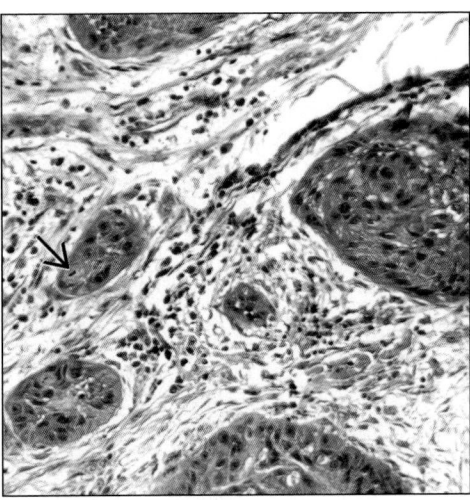

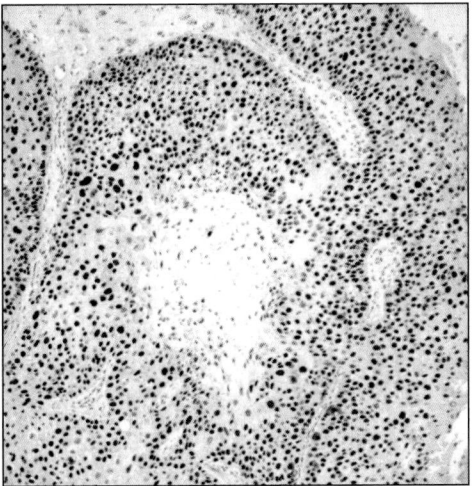

(Left) Another example of a malignant proliferating pilar tumor shows infiltrating small islands of atypical squamous cells in an inflamed, edematous stroma. Scattered mitotic figures are present ➡. *(Right)* Immunohistochemical stain for p63 in a malignant PPT shows strong and diffuse nuclear staining. p63 is not a specific marker for PPT, but it is positive in most adnexal tumors and thus favors a primary cutaneous carcinoma over a metastatic tumor to the skin.

HPV-RELATED EPIDERMAL CYST

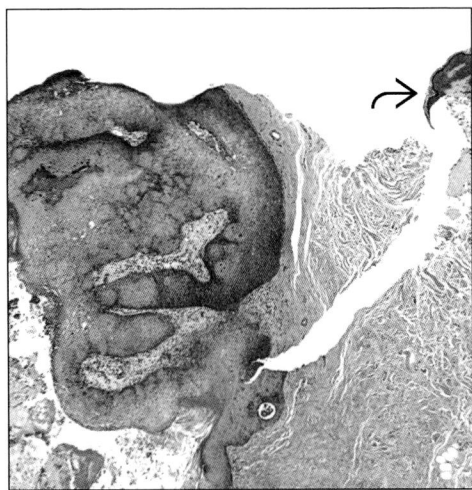

Verrucous epidermal cyst shows an acanthotic and papillated epithelial structure in the dermis. Note the separation from the epidermis ⮕.

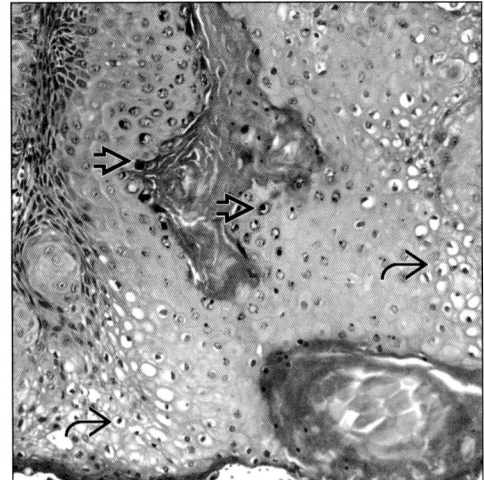

High magnification shows the acanthotic epithelium of an HPV-related verrucous epidermal cyst showing prominent keratohyaline granules ⮕ and koilocytosis ⮕.

TERMINOLOGY

Synonyms
- Verrucous cyst, epidermoid cyst of the palm and sole

Definitions
- Epidermoid cysts associated with human papillomavirus (HPV) infection

ETIOLOGY/PATHOGENESIS

Infectious Agents
- Human papillomaviruses (HPV)
  - Verrucous cysts have been reported to be associated with HPV-20 and -34 (epidermodysplasia verruciformis strains)
  - Epidermoid cyst of the palm and sole mainly associated with HPV-60 and -57
    - Traumatic implantation of HPV-infected epidermis (or perhaps eccrine ducts) into dermis

CLINICAL ISSUES

Epidemiology
- Incidence
  - Rare
- Age
  - Adults
- Gender
  - Both genders equally affected
- Ethnicity
  - HPV-related cysts of soles and palms mainly affect Japanese

Site
- Verrucous cysts
  - Face, neck, trunk
- Cysts of palms and soles
  - Palms and soles

Presentation
- Dome-shaped lesion

Prognosis
- Cosmetic problems
- May rupture and become inflamed or infected
- Benign lesions with excellent prognosis

MACROSCOPIC FEATURES

General Features
- Dome-shaped lesion sometimes showing a dark punctum on the surface
- Cut sections show dermal &/or subcutaneous unilocular round cyst
  - Thin to slightly papillary white wall and cheesy yellowish contents

MICROSCOPIC PATHOLOGY

Histologic Features
- Verrucous cysts
  - Papillary and acanthotic squamous epithelium with hypergranulosis and hyperkeratosis (focal parakeratosis)
    - Keratohyalin granules and koilocytic changes
  - Part of the cyst shows classical features of epidermoid cyst, or less often, pilar cyst
  - May or may not show connection to overlying epidermis
- Epidermoid cyst of the palm and sole
  - Epidermis-like lining as in a classical epidermoid cyst
    - Eosinophilic intracytoplasmic inclusions in wall
    - Vacuolated cells in keratin contents
  - Electron microscopy
    - Viral inclusions

HPV-RELATED EPIDERMAL CYST

Key Facts

Etiology/Pathogenesis
- HPV-related cysts
  - Verrucous cysts have been reported to be associated with HPV-20 and -34
  - Epidermoid cyst of the palm and sole is associated with HPV-60 and -57 (affects Japanese)

Microscopic Pathology
- Verrucous epidermal cyst

- Papillary and acanthotic squamous epithelium with hypergranulosis and hyperkeratosis (focal parakeratosis)
  - Keratohyalin granules
  - Koilocytic change
- Epidermoid cyst of the palm and sole
  - Epidermis-like lining
  - Eosinophilic intracytoplasmic inclusions in wall
  - Vacuolated cells in keratin contents

- Less well-characterized variant of HPV-related cyst with molluscum-like inclusions has also been described
  - Usually affects big toe and is associated with HPV-1

Cytologic Features
- Verrucous cyst
  - Prominent keratohyalin granules and koilocytosis
- Epidermoid cyst of the sole
  - Intracytoplasmic eosinophilic inclusions

ANCILLARY TESTS

Immunohistochemistry
- May confirm presence of HPV

DIFFERENTIAL DIAGNOSIS

Epidermoid (Epidermal Inclusion) Cyst
- Epidermis-like smooth lining without papillary surface
- Presence of a granular layer and abundant laminated keratin
- No viral cytopathic changes

Tricholemmal (Pilar) Cyst
- Squamous epithelium without granular layer
- Compact (tricholemmal) keratinization
- Absence of viral cytopathic changes

DIAGNOSTIC CHECKLIST

Pathologic Interpretation Pearls
- Papillary surface with hypergranulosis and koilocytic changes in verrucous cysts
- Intracytoplasmic eosinophilic inclusions in HPV-related cysts of soles and palms

SELECTED REFERENCES

1. Kohno M et al: Human papillomavirus 1 induced epidermoid cystic structure mimicking molluscum bodies. J Eur Acad Dermatol Venereol. 22(10):1242-4, 2008
2. Egawa K et al: Human papillomavirus-associated plantar epidermoid cyst related to epidermoid metaplasia of the eccrine duct epithelium: a combined histological, immunohistochemical, DNA-DNA in situ hybridization and three-dimensional reconstruction analysis. Br J Dermatol. 152(5):961-7, 2005
3. Misago N et al: Verrucous trichilemmal cyst containing human papillomavirus. Clin Exp Dermatol. 30(1):38-9, 2005
4. Egawa K et al: Human papillomavirus 57 identified in a plantar epidermoid cyst. Br J Dermatol. 138(3):510-4, 1998
5. Reis MD et al: Verrucous cyst. Eur J Dermatol. 8(3):186-8, 1998
6. Aloi F et al: HPV-related follicular cysts. Am J Dermatopathol. 14(1):37-41, 1992
7. Kato N et al: Two cases of plantar epidermal cyst associated with human papillomavirus. Clin Exp Dermatol. 17(4):252-6, 1992

IMAGE GALLERY

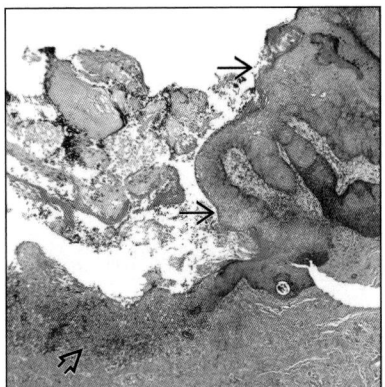 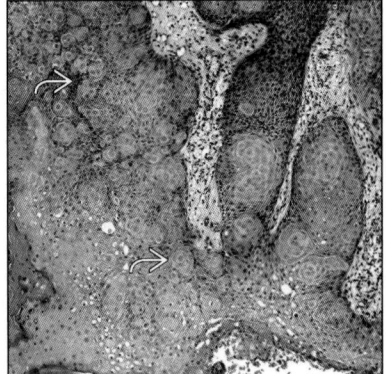 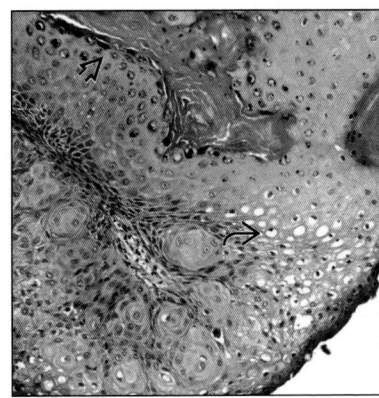

(Left) HPV-related cysts may also rupture and elicit an inflammatory response ➡. Note the acanthotic and papillary squamous lining ➡ of this verrucous cyst. *(Center)* Acanthotic squamous epithelium of a verrucous cyst shows areas of koilocytosis and prominent squamous whorls ➡, similar to an irritated seborrheic keratosis. *(Right)* Hypergranulosis ➡ and koilocytosis ➡ are characteristic features of HPV-related verrucous epidermal cysts.

VELLUS HAIR CYST

Multiple, slightly brownish small follicular papules are seen on the chest. This is a classic presentation of eruptive vellus hair cysts. (Courtesy J. Wu, MD.)

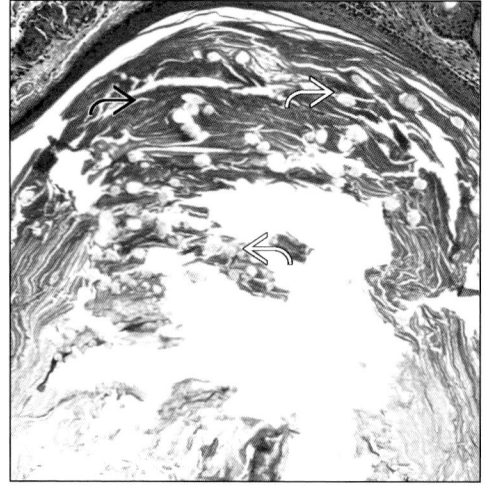

Low magnification shows a cyst lined by a keratinizing squamous epithelium. The cyst contents include laminated keratin ⇗ and numerous transversely sectioned hair shafts ⇗.

TERMINOLOGY

Abbreviations
- Vellus hair cyst (VHC)

Synonyms
- Eruptive vellus hair cyst (EVHC)

Definitions
- Similar histology to epidermoid (follicular, infundibular type) cyst with the addition of intraluminal vellus hairs

ETIOLOGY/PATHOGENESIS

Genetics
- Rare cases reported to be autosomal dominant
  - Rarely associated with the following diseases
    - Ectodermal dysplasia (anhidrotic and hidrotic)
    - Lowe syndrome (oculocerebrorenal syndrome)
    - Pachyonychia congenita

Associations
- Can present concomitantly with steatocystoma multiplex (SM) and milial cysts
  - Some consider VHC and SM to be a variation of the same entity
    - Considered to arise from 1 pilosebaceous duct
    - Designation as multiple pilosebaceous cysts has been used to define these 2 entities together
  - Cytokeratin (CK) studies, however, have suggested that VHC and SM are distinct entities
    - Vellus hair cysts express CK17
    - Steatocystoma multiplex expresses CK10 and -17

CLINICAL ISSUES

Epidemiology
- Incidence
  - Uncommon
- Age
  - Children and young adults
- Gender
  - No gender predilection
- Ethnicity
  - No race predilection

Site
- Commonly on the chest
- Upper extremities and other sites can be affected

Presentation
- Small (1-4 mm), discrete, asymptomatic papules
  - Skin-colored, erythematous, yellowish, brown, or bluish-gray
  - Occasional central umbilication
- Usually multiple (up to a few hundred lesions)

Treatment
- Not necessary
  - If cosmetically bothersome: Mechanical dermabrasion, retinoids, needle evacuation, simple excision, or laser treatment are some options
  - May spontaneously resolve

Prognosis
- Excellent, no malignant potential

MACROSCOPIC FEATURES

General Features
- Usually small, skin-colored papule

MICROSCOPIC PATHOLOGY

Histologic Features
- Dermal cyst lined by bland stratified squamous epithelium with granular layer

VELLUS HAIR CYST

Key Facts

Terminology
- Similar histology to epidermoid cyst with the addition of intraluminal vellus hairs

Clinical Issues
- Small, discrete, follicular papules; often on the chest

Microscopic Pathology
- Dermal cyst lined by bland stratified squamous epithelium with granular layer
- Intraluminal laminated keratin and numerous vellus hair shafts

Top Differential Diagnoses
- Epidermoid (epidermal inclusion, follicular infundibular) cyst
- Milial cyst
- Steatocystoma
- Trichofolliculoma

- Intraluminal laminated keratin and numerous transversely and obliquely sectioned vellus hair shafts
  - Hair shafts are doubly refractile with polarized light
- Small hair follicle may be seen attached to the wall
- Cyst can rupture and show surrounding granulomatous inflammation

Cytologic Features
- Bland squamous cells with uniform nuclei, small nucleoli, and eosinophilic cytoplasm

DIFFERENTIAL DIAGNOSIS

Epidermoid (Epidermal Inclusion, Follicular Infundibular) Cyst
- Typically larger in size
- Lacks intraluminal vellus hairs

Milial Cyst
- Small follicular cyst that lacks intraluminal vellus hairs

Steatocystoma
- Corrugated, eosinophilic cuticle lines inside of cyst wall
- Cyst lacks keratin and granular layer in cyst wall
- Associated sebaceous glands and small follicles usually present

Trichofolliculoma
- Usually solitary lesion
- Multiple primitive hair follicles open into a larger follicle

DIAGNOSTIC CHECKLIST

Pathologic Interpretation Pearls
- Small epidermoid (follicular infundibular) cyst with intraluminal vellus hairs

SELECTED REFERENCES

1. Fernández-Torres R et al: Treatment of multiple eruptive vellus hair cysts with carbon dioxide laser vaporization and manual lateral pressure. Clin Exp Dermatol. 34(8):e716-8, 2009
2. Patrizi A et al: Persistent milia, steatocystoma multiplex and eruptive vellus hair cysts: variable expression of multiple pilosebaceous cysts within an affected family. Dermatology. 196(4):392-6, 1998
3. Tomková H et al: Expression of keratins (K10 and K17) in steatocystoma multiplex, eruptive vellus hair cysts, and epidermoid and trichilemmal cysts. Am J Dermatopathol. 19(3):250-3, 1997
4. Kiene P et al: Eruptive vellus hair cysts and steatocystoma multiplex. variants of one entity? Br J Dermatol. 134(2):365-7, 1996
5. Sexton M et al: Eruptive vellus hair cysts. A follicular cyst of the sebaceous duct (sometimes). Am J Dermatopathol. 11(4):364-8, 1989

IMAGE GALLERY

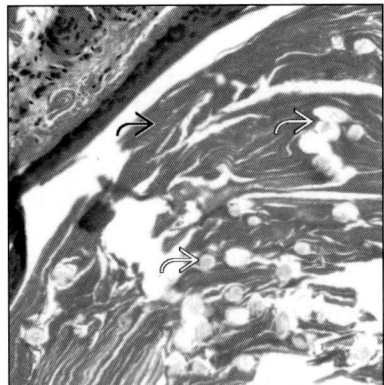 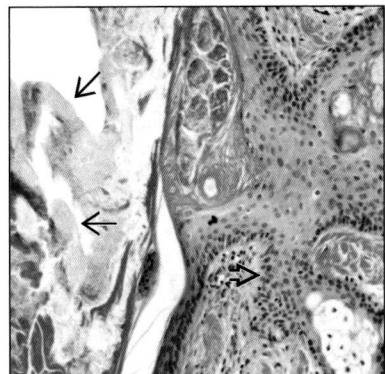 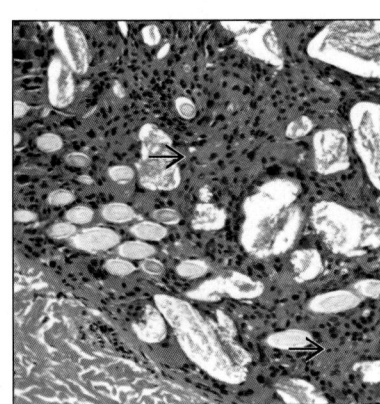

(Left) The cyst is lined by keratinizing squamous epithelium with a granular layer. The cyst lumen contains abundant laminated keratin ⊅ and numerous transversely sectioned hair shafts ⊒. *(Center)* Some cysts have a pilosebaceous unit attached to the cyst wall ⊵. Fragments of hair shafts are present within the cyst ⊡. *(Right)* Ruptured vellus hair cysts are often accompanied by an exuberant foreign body granulomatous response ⊐.

STEATOCYSTOMA (MULTIPLEX)

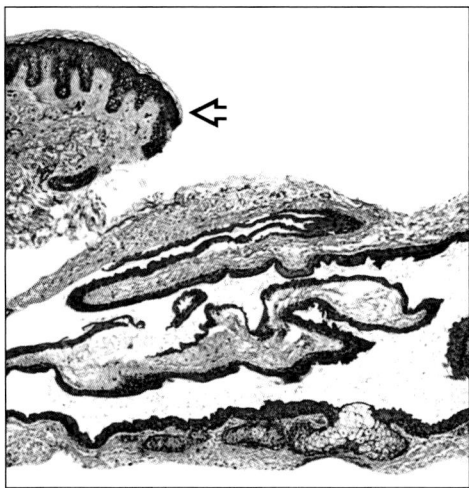

Steatocystomas present as thin-walled dermal cysts. Note the normal epidermis in the upper left corner ⊳.

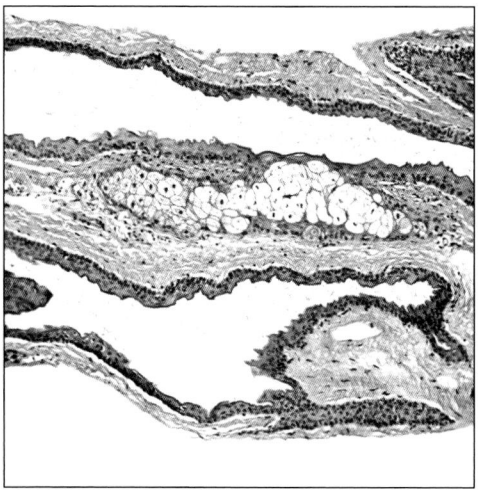

The cyst is lined by a thin squamous epithelial lining that has an eosinophilic cuticle and is associated with sebaceous glands.

TERMINOLOGY

Definitions
- Benign cyst derived from the sebaceous duct that may present as multiple lesions (steatocystoma multiplex) or as a single lesion (steatocystoma simplex)

CLINICAL ISSUES

Epidemiology
- Incidence
  - Uncommon
- Age
  - Steatocystoma multiplex usually presents in adolescents
  - Steatocystoma simplex usually presents in adults

Site
- May occur at any site, but trunk is most common location for steatocystoma multiplex
  - Axillae and groin commonly affected in females
- Steatocystoma simplex most common on face, neck, chest, and axillae

Presentation
- Steatocystoma multiplex
  - Autosomal dominant inheritance or sporadic
  - Multiple translucent flesh-colored to yellow dome-shaped papules or nodules
- Steatocystoma simplex
  - Sporadic; no mode of inheritance
  - Solitary translucent flesh-colored to yellow dome-shaped papule or nodule

Treatment
- For steatocystoma multiplex, no treatment is necessary, as lesions are often too numerous to excise
- Excision is option for specific bothersome lesions or lesions that have ruptured, resulting in inflammatory response
- Simple excision can be offered for solitary lesions of steatocystoma simplex

Prognosis
- Benign lesions with no malignant potential

MACROSCOPIC FEATURES

General Features
- Dermal-based cystic lesion; sectioning often releases dark, oily fluid

Size
- Usually between 3 mm and 3 cm

MICROSCOPIC PATHOLOGY

Histologic Features
- Thin-walled multiloculated cyst located in dermis
- Stratified squamous epithelial lining
- Undulating, densely eosinophilic cuticle forms the inner lining of the cyst wall
- Absent granular layer
- Sebaceous lobules usually identified within cyst wall
- Associated primitive follicle may be seen
- Cystic space is usually empty except for occasional presence of vellus hairs

DIFFERENTIAL DIAGNOSIS

Vellus Hair Cyst
- Dermal cyst lined by bland squamous epithelium
- Contains numerous vellus hairs
- Lining epithelium has a granular layer, unlike steatocystoma
- Rare hybrid cysts may show combined features of vellus hair cyst and steatocystoma

STEATOCYSTOMA (MULTIPLEX)

Key Facts

Terminology
- Benign cyst derived from the sebaceous duct that may present as multiple lesions (steatocystoma multiplex) or as a single lesion (simplex)

Clinical Issues
- Steatocystoma multiplex usually presents in adolescents, simplex in adults
- May occur at any site, but trunk most common location overall

Microscopic Pathology
- Thin-walled multiloculated cyst located in dermis
- Undulating, eosinophilic cuticle forms the inner lining of the cyst
- Sebaceous lobules usually identified within cyst wall

Top Differential Diagnoses
- Vellus hair cyst
- Dermoid cyst
- Epidermoid cyst/epidermal inclusion cyst

Dermoid Cyst
- Presents at birth or in infancy
- Head and neck location, most common around eyes
- Cyst lined by stratified squamous epithelium with granular layer
- Sebaceous lobules and follicular structures often present in wall of cyst
- Multiple hair shafts often present

Epidermoid Cyst/Epidermal Inclusion Cyst
- Simple cyst lined by squamous epithelium
- Shows prominent granular layer and contains loose keratin
- Lacks follicular structures and vellus hairs

Pilar (Tricholemmal) Cyst
- Simple cyst lined by squamous epithelium
- Solitary or multiple
- Lacks a granular layer and contains dense laminated keratin, often with calcifications

Cutaneous Keratocyst
- Usually associated with Gorlin-Goltz syndrome (nevoid basal cell carcinoma syndrome), but rare cases are sporadic
- Shows identical epithelial lining, with eosinophilic cuticle, as in steatocystoma
- Lacks associated sebaceous glands, vellus hairs, and primitive hair follicles

DIAGNOSTIC CHECKLIST

Pathologic Interpretation Pearls
- Undulating, eosinophilic cuticle is the key microscopic feature
- Sebaceous glands in or closely associated with the cyst wall should prompt consideration of steatocystoma
  - Sebaceous glands sometimes sparse or even absent

SELECTED REFERENCES

1. Marzano AV et al: Familial syringoma: report of two cases with a published work review and the unique association with steatocystoma multiplex. J Dermatol. 36(3):154-8, 2009
2. Cassarino DS et al: Cutaneous keratocyst arising independently of the nevoid basal cell carcinoma syndrome. Am J Dermatopathol. 27(2):177-8, 2005
3. Cambiaghi S et al: Steatocystoma multiplex and leuconychia in a child with Alagille syndrome. Br J Dermatol. 138(1):150-4, 1998
4. Covello SP et al: Keratin 17 mutations cause either steatocystoma multiplex or pachyonychia congenita type 2. Br J Dermatol. 139(3):475-80, 1998
5. Requena L et al: A facial variant of steatocystoma multiplex. Cutis. 51(6):449-52, 1993
6. Olsen DB et al: Steatocystoma simplex in the oral cavity: a previously undescribed condition. Oral Surg Oral Med Oral Pathol. 66(5):605-7, 1988
7. Leppard B et al: Gardner's syndrome and steatocystoma multiplex. Two unusual genetically determined conditions occurring in same patient. J Med Genet. 13(5):407-11, 1976

IMAGE GALLERY

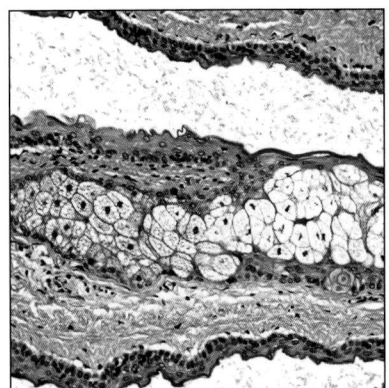 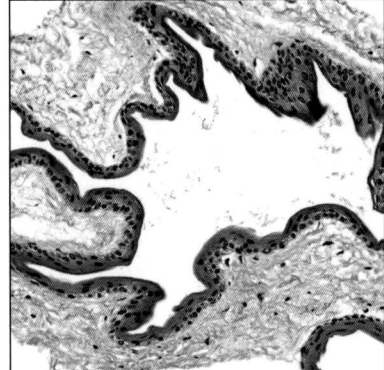 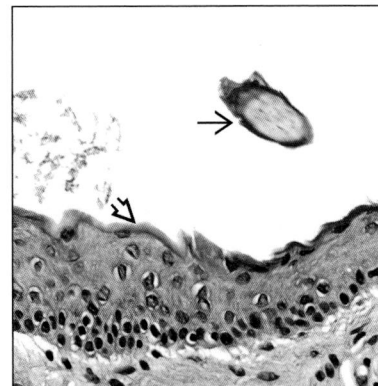

(Left) Steatocystoma is characterized by a thin-walled squamous-lined cyst with associated sebaceous glands in the wall or adjacent to the wall of the cyst. *(Center)* In some cases of steatocystoma, sebaceous glands may not be evident in a given histologic section. *(Right)* The eosinophilic cuticle ⊵ with its undulating, crenulated appearance is a key diagnostic feature. This cyst also has a vellus hair ⊵, a feature sometimes seen in steatocystomas.

CUTANEOUS KERATOCYST

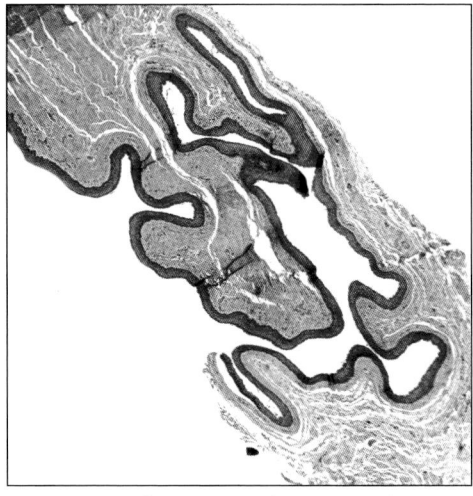

Scanning magnification view of a cutaneous keratocyst shows an undulating squamous epithelium lining the irregularly shaped cystic spaces.

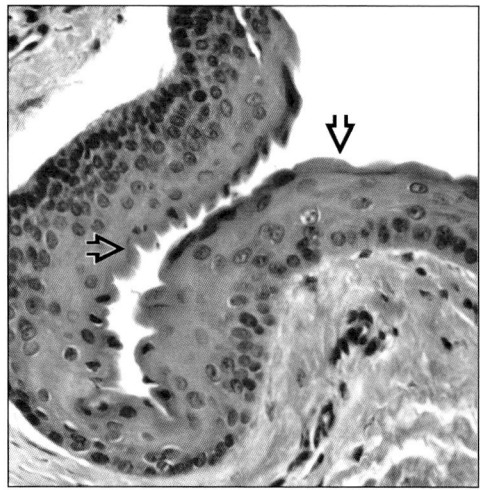

High magnification of a cutaneous keratocyst shows a bland squamous epithelium with a dense eosinophilic cuticle ⊵ lining the cystic space.

TERMINOLOGY

Synonyms
- Nevoid basal cell carcinoma syndrome (NBCCS)/ Gorlin-Goltz syndrome-associated cutaneous cyst

Definitions
- Rare cutaneous cyst showing features identical to oral keratocysts, often associated with NBCCS

ETIOLOGY/PATHOGENESIS

Genetic
- Most cases are associated with NBCCS (Gorlin-Goltz syndrome: Multiple cutaneous basal cell carcinomas, odontogenic keratocysts of the jaw, palmar and plantar pits, rare medulloblastomas, and skeletal abnormalities)
  - Mutations for NBCCS in *PTCH1* gene on chromosome 9q22.3-q31, which encodes a receptor for the Sonic Hedgehog signaling pathway
- Rare cases not associated with NBCCS also reported

CLINICAL ISSUES

Epidemiology
- Incidence
  - Extremely rare lesions
- Age
  - Typically occur in older adults

Site
- Variable, but typically on head and neck region

Presentation
- Dermal cyst, usually multiple lesions, but may be single

Treatment
- Surgical approaches
  - Incision and drainage
  - Not necessary, but complete conservative excision may be performed to prevent recurrence

Prognosis
- Excellent; no malignant potential, but diagnosis should prompt clinical examination for other tumors (e.g., basal cell carcinomas, odontogenic keratocysts, medulloblastomas), as well as genetic studies for NBCCS

MACROSCOPIC FEATURES

General Features
- Dark, oily fluid contents seen on gross sectioning

Size
- Typically small cystic lesion

MICROSCOPIC PATHOLOGY

Histologic Features
- Dermal-based cystic proliferation lined by 2-5 cell layers of bland squamous cells
  - Typically shows corrugated eosinophilic lining (cuticle) on luminal surface, lacking a granular layer, very similar to steatocystoma
- Clear proteinaceous cystic contents
- No evidence of follicular or sebaceous differentiation (unlike steatocystoma)

Cytologic Features
- Bland squamous cells with abundant eosinophilic cytoplasm

CUTANEOUS KERATOCYST

Key Facts

Terminology

- NBCCS cutaneous cyst/Gorlin-Goltz syndrome
- Rare cutaneous cyst showing features identical to oral keratocysts

Etiology/Pathogenesis

- Most cases are associated with NBCCS
- Rare cases not associated with NBCCS also reported

Microscopic Pathology

- Dermal-based cystic proliferation lined by 2-5 cell layers of bland squamous cells
- Typically shows corrugated eosinophilic lining (cuticle) on luminal surface
- No evidence of follicular or sebaceous differentiation (unlike steatocystoma)

Top Differential Diagnoses

- Steatocystoma, epidermoid (epidermal inclusion) cyst

DIFFERENTIAL DIAGNOSIS

Steatocystoma

- Often multiple (steatocystoma multiplex)
- Similar cyst lining, lacking a granular layer, but connections to sebaceous glands or primitive follicles, by definition, should be present (especially if multiple deeper level sections examined)

Epidermoid (Epidermal Inclusion) Cyst

- Keratinizing squamous lining with granular layer and lacking eosinophilic cuticle
- Usually shows abundant laminated keratin contents; may show hair fragments
- Often rupture and are associated with mixed acute and granulomatous inflammatory infiltrate

Pilar (Tricholemmal) Cyst

- Keratinizing squamous lining without granular layer and lacking eosinophilic cuticle
- Abundant dense hyalinized keratin contents, often with calcifications

Vellus Hair Cyst

- Large cystic follicular structure demonstrating numerous intraluminal miniaturized hairs
- Lacks classic eosinophilic corrugated lining of keratocyst and steatocystoma

Hidrocystoma

- Thin (1-2 cell layer thick) cyst lining composed of cuboidal epithelial cells, often with apocrine features

- Lacks corrugated lining of keratocyst

DIAGNOSTIC CHECKLIST

Pathologic Interpretation Pearls

- Bland squamous-lined cyst, which typically shows prominent corrugated eosinophilic lining (cuticle)

SELECTED REFERENCES

1. Peñaranda JM et al: Cutaneous keratocyst not associated to gorlin syndrome: an incidental finding in a healthy male. Am J Dermatopathol. 29(6):584-5, 2007
2. Cassarino DS et al: Cutaneous keratocyst arising independently of the nevoid basal cell carcinoma syndrome. Am J Dermatopathol. 27(2):177-8, 2005
3. Manfredi M et al: Nevoid basal cell carcinoma syndrome: a review of the literature. Int J Oral Maxillofac Surg. 33(2):117-24, 2004
4. Hamel AF et al: The cutaneous keratocyst: a rare hallmark of the nevoid basal cell carcinoma syndrome. Int J Surg Pathol. 11(1):36, 2003
5. Barr RJ et al: Cutaneous keratocysts of nevoid basal cell carcinoma syndrome. J Am Acad Dermatol. 14(4):572-6, 1986
6. Gorlin RJ et al: Multiple nevoid basal-cell epithelioma, jaw cysts and bifid rib. A syndrome. N Engl J Med. 262:908-12, 1960

IMAGE GALLERY

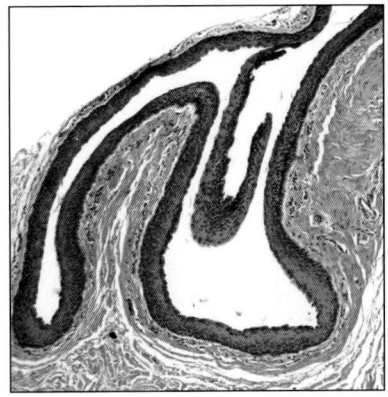 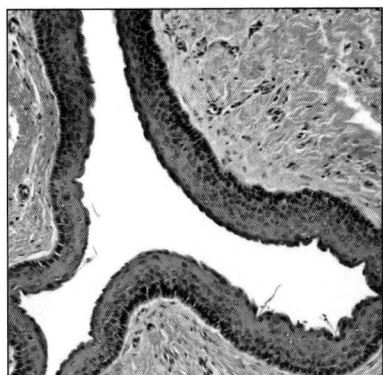 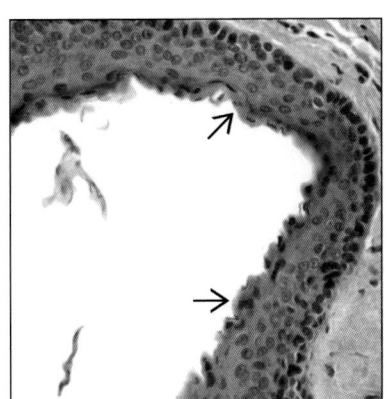

(Left) Low magnification of a cutaneous keratocyst shows an undulating squamous epithelium lining irregular cystic spaces. Note the absence of associated sebaceous or follicular structures (present in steatocystomas). *(Center)* The cyst shows a bland, multilayered squamous lining surrounding an irregular cystic space. *(Right)* High-magnification view of the lining of the cyst shows a bland, multilayered squamous epithelium with a dense eosinophilic cuticle ➡ and parakeratosis lining the cystic space.

MILIAL CYSTS

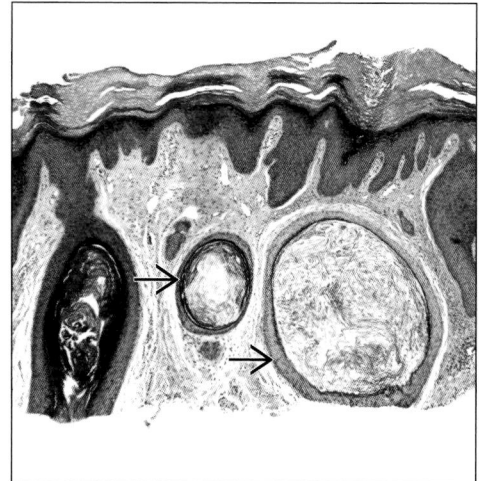

Low magnification shows multiple small dermal cysts ⮕, which appear essentially identical to miniature epidermoid/follicular, infundibular-type cysts.

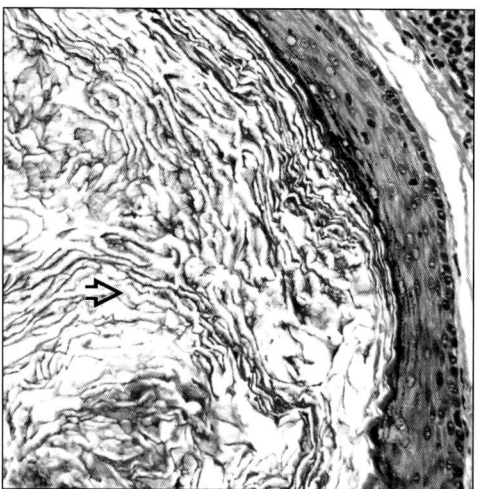

The cyst contains abundant loose keratin flakes ⮕.

TERMINOLOGY

Synonyms
- Milia

Definitions
- Small epidermoid (follicular, infundibular-type) cysts

CLINICAL ISSUES

Epidemiology
- Incidence
  - Very common
- Age
  - Any age
    - Newborns, children, and adults
- Gender
  - No gender predilection
- Ethnicity
  - No race predilection

Site
- Primary milial cysts
  - Face
- Secondary milial cysts
  - Any site

Presentation
- Primary milial cysts
  - Occur spontaneously
  - Typically seen on the face
    - Rarely on mucosa (Epstein pearls) and palate (Bohn nodules)
  - Common in newborns
- Secondary milial cysts
  - Sites of trauma
    - After surgery, dermabrasion, burns, laser resurfacing
  - Sites of subepidermal blistering diseases such as
    - Bullous pemphigoid

- Porphyria cutanea tarda
- Epidermolysis bullosa
- Bullous lichen planus
- Eruptive milia are very rare
  - Idiopathic
  - Familial, autosomal dominant inheritance
  - Rarely associated with genodermatoses, including
    - Basaloid follicular hamartoma syndrome
    - Bazex syndrome
    - Rombo syndrome
    - Gardner syndrome
    - Orofaciodigital syndrome
- Milia en plaque
  - Very rare
  - Multiple milia on erythematous and edematous plaque
  - Head and neck

Treatment
- Not necessary
  - If cosmetically bothersome: Needle evacuation, mechanical dermabrasion, retinoids, and laser treatment are some options

Prognosis
- Excellent, no malignant potential

MACROSCOPIC FEATURES

General Features
- Small, skin-colored to whitish, firm papules

Size
- 1-2 mm

MICROSCOPIC PATHOLOGY

Histologic Features
- Dermal-based, small cystic structures

MILIAL CYSTS

Key Facts

Terminology
- Small epidermoid/infundibular cyst

Clinical Issues
- Very common
- Primary milial cysts
  - Occur spontaneously and typically seen on the face
- Secondary milial cysts
  - Occur at sites of trauma or subepidermal blistering diseases

Microscopic Pathology
- Dermal cyst lined by squamous epithelium with granular layer
- Intraluminal laminated keratin

Top Differential Diagnoses
- Epidermoid (epidermal inclusion, follicular infundibular) cyst
- Vellus hair cyst

- Lined by stratified squamous epithelium with granular layer
- Abundant intraluminal laminated keratin debris

Cytologic Features
- Bland squamous cells with small uniform nuclei and eosinophilic cytoplasm
- No mitoses

DIFFERENTIAL DIAGNOSIS

Epidermoid (Epidermal Inclusion, Follicular Infundibular) Cyst
- Larger; otherwise shows the same histology, with abundant luminal keratin and granular layer

Vellus Hair Cyst
- Larger, similar to epidermoid cysts
- Shows numerous intraluminal vellus hairs

Steatocystoma
- Shows an eosinophilic corrugated lining
- Lacks intraluminal keratin

DIAGNOSTIC CHECKLIST

Pathologic Interpretation Pearls
- Small cyst with squamous epithelium and keratin cyst content

SELECTED REFERENCES

1. Hallaji Z et al: Bilateral retro-auricular milia en plaque: a case report and review of the literature. Dermatol Online J. 16(1):12, 2010
2. Leong T et al: Pronounced secondary milia precipitated by a superficial traumatic abrasion in a 4-year-old boy. J Pediatr. 156(5):854, 2010
3. Pozo J et al: Variants of milia successfully treated with CO(2) laser vaporization. J Cosmet Laser Ther. 12(4):191-4, 2010
4. Berk DR et al: Milia: a review and classification. J Am Acad Dermatol. 59(6):1050-63, 2008
5. Dogra S et al: Milia en plaque. J Eur Acad Dermatol Venereol. 19(2):263-4, 2005
6. Langley RG et al: Multiple eruptive milia: report of a case, review of the literature, and a classification. J Am Acad Dermatol. 37(2 Pt 2):353-6, 1997
7. Wolfe SF et al: Eruptive milia. Cutis. 60(4):183-4, 1997
8. Inman P: Milia following bullous dermatitis. Br J Dermatol. 81(2):132-3, 1969

IMAGE GALLERY

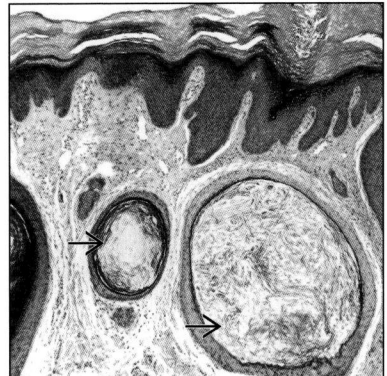 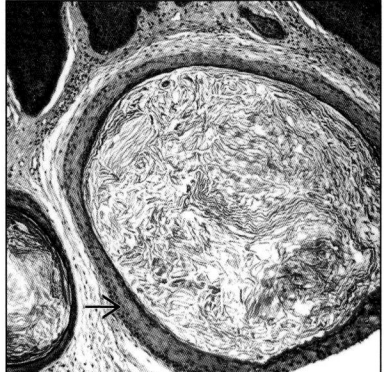 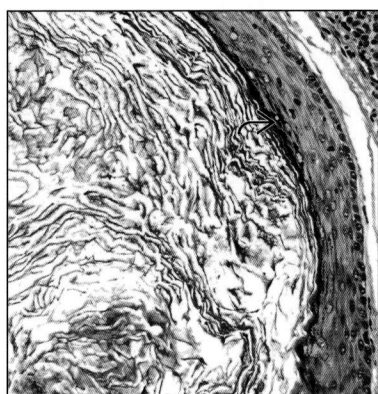

(Left) More than 1 milial cyst ⊟ often can be seen in a single biopsy. *(Center)* Cyst is lined by squamous epithelium ⊟. *(Right)* Granular layer ⊟ is present within the stratified squamous epithelium.

HIDROCYSTOMA (APOCRINE AND ECCRINE)

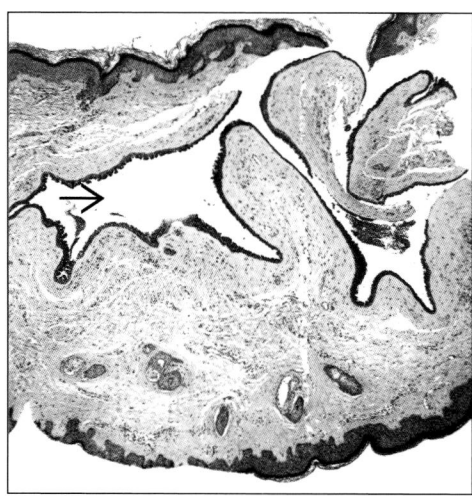

Hidrocystoma on low magnification shows characteristic thin-walled, dermal-based, empty cystic spaces ➔.

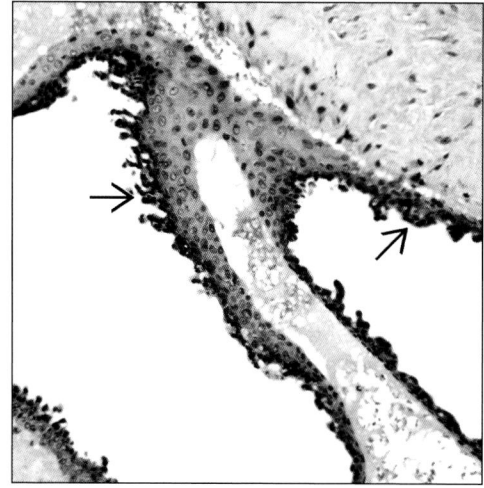

Hidrocystomas can be multilocular. A thin layer of bland-appearing apocrine epithelium ➔ lines the cystic lumina.

TERMINOLOGY

Synonyms
- Cystadenoma (apocrine and eccrine)
- Apocrine gland cyst
- Sudoriferous cyst
- Moll gland cyst
- Papillary apocrine gland cyst

Definitions
- Cystic, dome-shaped, translucent papules with bluish hue commonly found on the eyelids

ETIOLOGY/PATHOGENESIS

Eccrine vs. Apocrine Hidrocystomas
- Most, if not all, hidrocystomas are now considered to be of apocrine origin
- Apocrine hidrocystoma
  - Usually multiloculate
  - Cytoplasmic projections into cyst cavity: "Decapitation" secretion present
- Eccrine hidrocystoma
  - Usually unilocular
  - No "decapitation" secretion
  - Considered to be retention of dilated eccrine duct or gland, and not a true cyst

Associated Disease
- Schöpf-Schulz-Passarge syndrome (SSPS): Rare ectodermal dysplasia
  - Multiple apocrine hidrocystomas on the eyelids

CLINICAL ISSUES

Epidemiology
- Incidence
  - Relatively common
- Age

- Adults, no particular age group
- Gender
  - Females slightly more than males
- Ethnicity
  - No race predilection

Site
- Commonly on the face
  - Predominately in periorbital region
  - May occur on scalp, neck, trunk, extremities, and genitalia

Presentation
- Translucent to bluish, dome-shaped papule
- Solitary or multiple

Treatment
- Not necessary
  - If cosmetically bothersome, needle evacuation or simple excision are some options

Prognosis
- Excellent, no malignant potential

MACROSCOPIC FEATURES

General Features
- During sectioning, clear, brownish, or blackish fluid is released, and the cyst collapses

Size
- Commonly 1-15 mm
  - Can be larger than 20 mm ("giant" hidrocystomas)

MICROSCOPIC PATHOLOGY

Histologic Features
- Dermal-based unilocular or multilocular cyst
- Often, no cyst contents: Appears empty

HIDROCYSTOMA (APOCRINE AND ECCRINE)

Key Facts

Terminology
- Cystic, dome-shaped, translucent papules with bluish hue commonly found on the eyelids

Etiology/Pathogenesis
- Most, if not all, hidrocystomas are now considered to be of apocrine origin

Clinical Issues
- Relatively common

- Predominately in periorbital region

Microscopic Pathology
- Dermal unilocular or multilocular cyst
- Often, no cyst content and appears empty
- Cystic spaces lined by 1-2 layers of cuboidal or columnar epithelium
- Papillary projection into cyst cavity: "Decapitation" secretion present

---

  o Cyst contents often leak during incision or during sectioning of tissue
- Cystic spaces lined by 1-2 layers of cuboidal or columnar epithelium
  o Secretory cells have abundant eosinophilic cytoplasm with basally located nucleus
  o Foci of hyperplasia and papillomatous areas of secretory cells
   ■ Occasionally with papillary projections into cyst space
   ■ Cytoplasmic projections consistent with "decapitation" secretion
   ■ If prominent hyperplasia and connective tissue core are present, considered to be a cystadenoma
  o PAS-positive, diastase-resistant granules are seen in the secretory cells
- Secretory cells occasionally contain pigment granules
  o Cause brownish-blue color of cystic fluid
  o This pigment is neither melanin nor hemosiderin
- Beneath secretory cells are elongated myoepithelial cells

Cytologic Features
- Secretory cells are bland cuboidal or columnar epithelium

DIFFERENTIAL DIAGNOSIS

Apocrine (Papillary) Cystadenoma
- Some consider this entity to be a type of apocrine hidrocystoma

- Studies, however, have shown this to be a proliferative tumor and not a simple cyst like hidrocystoma
  o Papillary projections with fibrous core
  o Increased mitotic rate within secretory cells
   ■ Increased Ki-67 staining

Median Raphe Cysts
- Located on ventral penis, scrotum, or perineum
- Cyst is lined by pseudostratified columnar epithelium
  o Occasional mucin-containing cells present
  o Rarely, ciliated cells present

Cutaneous Ciliated Cyst
- Lower extremities of women
- Cyst is lined by ciliated cuboidal to columnar epithelium
  o Foci of pseudostratified epithelium common

DIAGNOSTIC CHECKLIST

Pathologic Interpretation Pearls
- Dermal, empty unilocular or multilocular cyst
- Cyst lined by 1-2 layers of cuboidal or columnar epithelium

SELECTED REFERENCES

1. Jakobiec FA et al: A reappraisal of eyelid eccrine and apocrine hidrocystomas: microanatomic and immunohistochemical studies of 40 lesions. Am J Ophthalmol. 151(2):358-74, 2011

IMAGE GALLERY

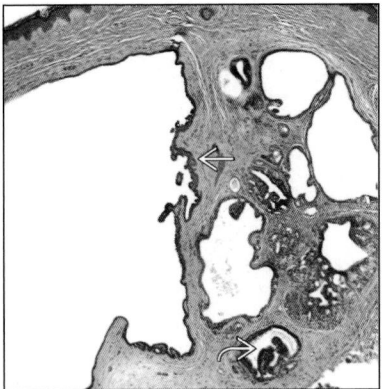 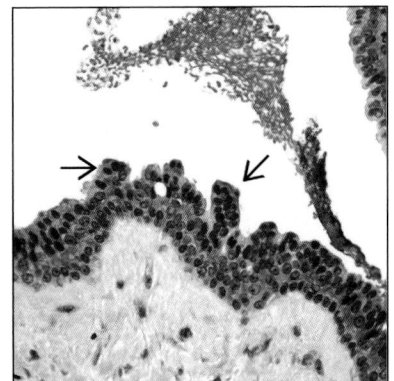 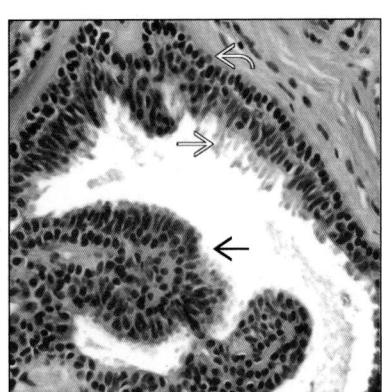

(Left) A multilocular hidrocystoma is seen with areas of hyperplastic epithelium ➡ and papillary projections into a cystic space ➘. *(Center)* Hyperplastic epithelial lining with small, thin papillary projections ➡ can be seen in some cases. *(Right)* Two or more layers of cuboidal-columnar epithelium ➡ line the cyst. An outer layer of myoepithelial cells ➘ is present. Prominent "decapitation" secretion ➡ (indicative of apocrine differentiation) is seen.

DIGITAL MUCOUS CYST

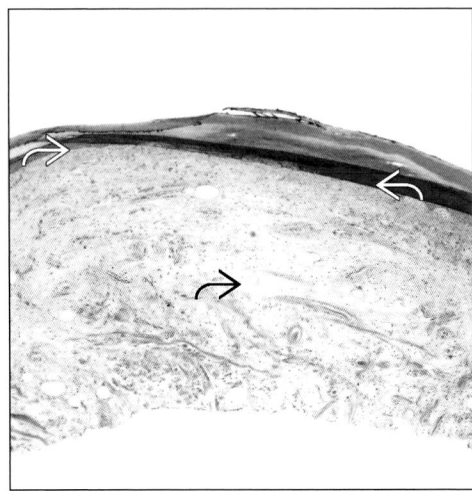

Earlier lesions show pools of mucin infiltrating between collagen bundles ➰. Prominent effacement of the overlying epidermal rete ridges is present ➤.

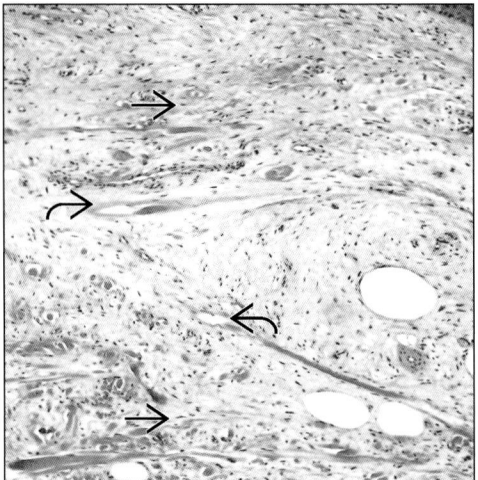

Within a mucinous matrix, an increased number of small vessels ➰ and stromal fibroblasts ➤ are seen.

TERMINOLOGY

Abbreviations
- Digital mucous cyst (DMC)

Synonyms
- Digital myxoid cyst
- Digital myxoid pseudocyst
- Digital synovial cyst
- Nail cysts
- Periungual ganglions
- Myxomatous degenerative cysts
- Myxomatous cutaneous cysts
- Cystomata

Definitions
- Solitary, dome-shaped, skin-colored to translucent papule

ETIOLOGY/PATHOGENESIS

Unclear
- There are 2 views as to possible etiology
  - Lesions near the proximal nail are from local synthesis of mucin by fibroblasts
    - Identical to focal mucinosis of skin and are termed digital mucous cyst
  - Lesions on the distal interphalangeal joint are herniation of joint lining
    - Identical to ganglion and are termed myxoid cyst
- Most view digital mucous cyst and digital myxoid cyst to be synonymous

CLINICAL ISSUES

Epidemiology
- Incidence
  - Relatively common
- Age
  - Adults
- Gender
  - Slight female predilection
- Ethnicity
  - No ethnic predilection

Site
- Dorsum of fingers
  - Occasionally dorsum of toes

Presentation
- Solitary papule
- Dorsum of fingers, typically at base of nail
- Can cause deformity of involved nail

Treatment
- Not necessary
- For symptoms such as pain or if cosmetically bothersome
  - Steroid injection
  - Electrocautery
  - Chemical cautery
  - Lesions tend to recur and often require multiple treatments

Prognosis
- Excellent, no malignant potential

MACROSCOPIC FEATURES

General Features
- Gelatinous fluid contents released during gross sectioning

Size
- Commonly 3-7 mm

DIGITAL MUCOUS CYST

Key Facts

Terminology
- Solitary, dome-shaped, skin-colored to translucent papule
- Synonyms: Digital myxoid cyst, digital synovial cyst

Etiology/Pathogenesis
- Most view digital mucous cyst and digital myxoid cyst to be synonymous

Microscopic Pathology
- Subepidermal cystic space or clefts with collection of mucin and stellate fibroblasts
- No epithelial lining
- Mucin is positive with colloidal iron and Alcian blue stains

Top Differential Diagnoses
- Ganglion cyst
- Focal mucinosis

MICROSCOPIC PATHOLOGY

Histologic Features
- Subepidermal cystic space or clefts with collection of mucin and stellate fibroblasts
  - Overlying acral skin with stratum lucidum is diagnostic clue
- No epithelial lining
- Overlying epidermis is often thinned
- Surrounding collagen is often compressed
- Often show increased numbers of small blood vessels
- Mucin is positive with colloidal iron and Alcian blue stains

Cytologic Features
- Bland-appearing, small stromal fibroblasts

DIFFERENTIAL DIAGNOSIS

Ganglion Cyst
- DMC may be considered a superficial variant of a ganglion cyst
  - Ganglion cysts are larger and more deeply located; usually located around the wrists

Focal Mucinosis
- Histologically identical findings
- Location distinguishes from DMC (not on fingers)

Cutaneous Myxoma (Superficial Angiomyxoma)
- Solitary or multiple (associated with Carney complex)
- Prominent myxoid stroma with increased numbers of fibroblasts
- Differs from DMC by increased vascularity

DIAGNOSTIC CHECKLIST

Clinically Relevant Pathologic Features
- Cystic space with mucin on finger is characteristic for DMC

Pathologic Interpretation Pearls
- Subepidermal collection of mucin with stellate fibroblasts
- No epithelial lining, and overlying thin acral skin with stratum lucidum

SELECTED REFERENCES

1. Li K et al: Digital mucous cysts. J Cutan Med Surg. 14(5):199-206, 2010
2. Misago N et al: Digital superficial angiomyxoma. Clin Exp Dermatol. 32(5):536-8, 2007
3. Lawrence C: Skin excision and osteophyte removal is not required in the surgical treatment of digital myxoid cysts. Arch Dermatol. 141(12):1560-4, 2005
4. Sonnex TS: Digital myxoid cysts: a review. Cutis. 37(2):89-94, 1986

IMAGE GALLERY

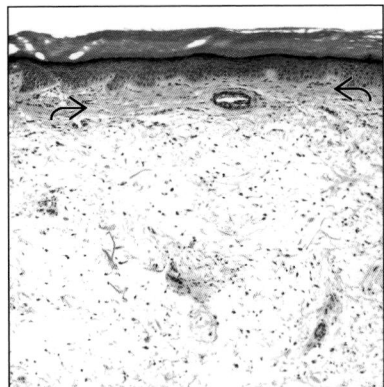 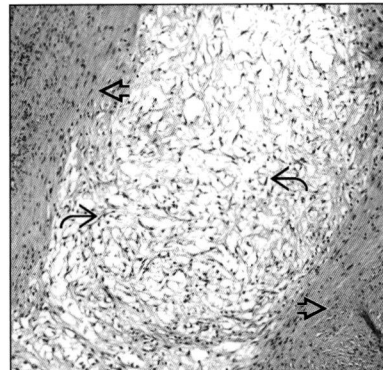 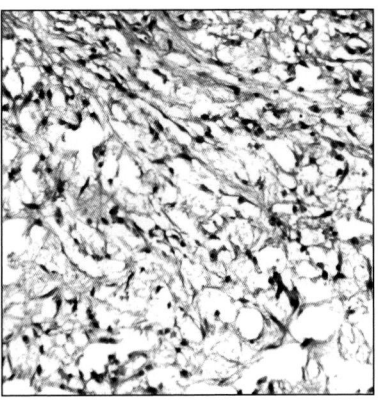

(Left) Digital mucous cyst at low magnification shows that the epidermis is separated from the mucinous deposits by a thin grenz zone ➡. *(Center)* Deep dermal area involved by digital mucous cyst shows a central collection of prominent mucinous material with increased numbers of small, spindle-shaped fibroblasts ➡ surrounded by compressed stroma ➤. *(Right)* High magnification of a digital mucous cyst shows small, bland-appearing fibroblasts in a prominent myxoid matrix.

BRONCHOGENIC CYST

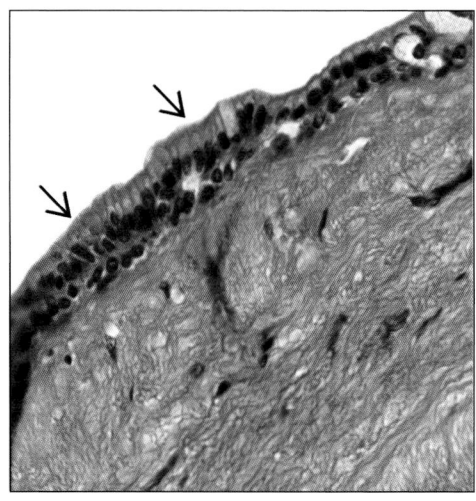

A cervical bronchogenic cyst is shown from the lateral neck of a 2-month-old male. Clinically it was thought to be a branchial cleft cyst. Note the ciliated respiratory epithelium →.

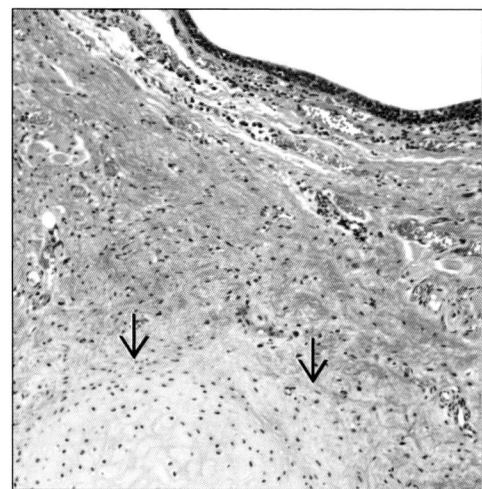

Although hyaline cartilage ⇒ is readily seen in intrathoracic bronchogenic cysts, it may be more difficult to identify the cervical variant. Multiple recuts may be required.

TERMINOLOGY

Synonyms
• Bronchial cyst

Definitions
• Rare congenital malformation of ventral foregut

ETIOLOGY/PATHOGENESIS

Embryogenesis
• Derived from diverticula buds that separate from foregut during formation of tracheobronchial tree

CLINICAL ISSUES

Epidemiology
• Incidence
  ○ Rare cystic lesion within the anterior neck
• Age
  ○ Pediatric population, rare in adults
• Gender
  ○ Male > > female (4:1)

Site
• **Cervical**
  ○ Most commonly identified in the midline
    ▪ Superficial to the presternal region or suprasternal
  ○ Much less commonly will affect lateral neck, thyroid, or subcutaneous tissues
• **Noncervical**
  ○ Anterior mediastinum
  ○ Adjacent to the hilum

Presentation
• Compression or compromise of the airway
  ○ Respiratory distress, cough, dyspnea
• Dysphagia
• Infection is uncommon development
  ○ Drainage associated with sinus tract
  ○ Patient may be febrile
• Asymptomatic presentation is uncommon

Endoscopic Findings
• May show compression of laryngotracheal axis

Treatment
• Options, risks, complications
  ○ Fistula with drainage and infection are possible complications
• Surgical approaches
  ○ Complete surgical excision is treatment of choice
    ▪ Neck exploration and selective dissection via transcervical approach
    ▪ Great vessels and recurrent laryngeal nerve are at risk
    ▪ If sinus tract is present, it should be removed with cyst
  ○ Incision, drainage, and ablation
    ▪ Indicated for only high-risk adults

Prognosis
• Excellent long-term clinical prognosis
• Recurrence develops if incompletely excised
• Rare cases of carcinoma arising from bronchogenic cyst

IMAGE FINDINGS

Radiographic Findings
• Best study: Contrast-enhanced T1WI or T2WI MR to show homogeneously increased signal
• Well-defined, solitary, smooth-bordered mass

MACROSCOPIC FEATURES

General Features
• Grossly tubular

BRONCHOGENIC CYST

Key Facts

Terminology
- Rare congenital malformation of ventral foregut

Clinical Issues
- Pediatric population, rare in adults
- Midline superficial presternal or suprasternal is most common neck location
- Male > > female (4:1)
- Presents with airway compression, dysphagia, infection, or may be asymptomatic

- Complete surgical excision is treatment of choice

Image Findings
- Best study: Contrast-enhanced T1WI or T2WI MR to show well-defined, solitary, smooth-bordered mass

Microscopic Pathology
- Cyst lined by respiratory-type epithelium
- Cyst wall with mucoserous glands, hyaline cartilage, and smooth muscle

---

  o May be altered by infection
- Cut sections show clear serous to mucoid material

MICROSCOPIC PATHOLOGY

Histologic Features
- Cyst lined by respiratory-type epithelium
  o Ciliated, pseudostratified, columnar epithelium
- Epithelium may be altered by infection
  o Usually results in a stratified squamous epithelium
- Cyst wall contains various "bronchial tree" elements
  o Mucoserous glands
  o Hyaline cartilage
  o Haphazardly distributed smooth muscle
  o Scant lymphoid tissue

ANCILLARY TESTS

Cytology
- Normal ciliated columnar cells
- Serous or mucinous material

DIFFERENTIAL DIAGNOSIS

Teratoma
- All 3 germ cell layers must be present: Ectoderm, endoderm, mesoderm
- Tissues will include respiratory epithelium but will have neural tissue as well

Dermoid Cyst
- Squamous epithelium associated with hair and skin appendages
  o Sebocytes, adnexal structures, follicles

Branchial Cleft Cyst
- Clinically, usually found laterally
- Typically has stratified squamous epithelium
- Lymphoid tissue arranged in germinal centers surrounding epithelium
- Lacks smooth muscle and cartilage

Thyroglossal Duct Cyst
- Midline lesion, usually associated with hyoid bone
- Thyroid follicles with colloid should be present
- Lacks smooth muscle and cartilage

Cystic Hygroma (Lymphangioma)
- Variably sized lymphatic vessels
- Lymphocytes and smooth muscle in the wall of vascular spaces

SELECTED REFERENCES

1. Moz U et al: Bronchogenic cysts of the neck: a rare localization and review of the literature. Acta Otorhinolaryngol Ital. 29(1):36-40, 2009
2. Teissier N et al: Cervical bronchogenic cysts: usual and unusual clinical presentations. Arch Otolaryngol Head Neck Surg. 134(11):1165-9, 2008
3. Newkirk KA et al: Bronchogenic cysts of the neck in adults. Ann Otol Rhinol Laryngol. 113(9):691-5, 2004

IMAGE GALLERY

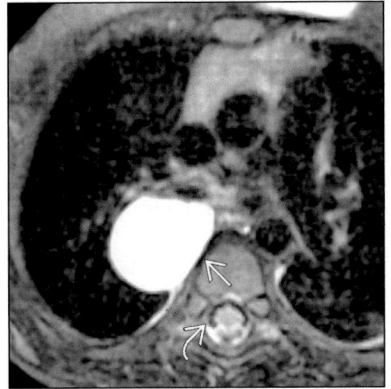 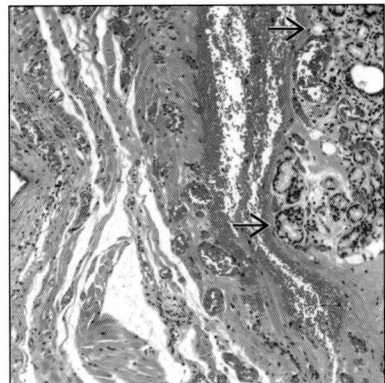 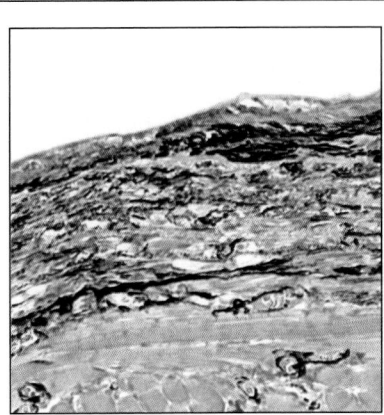

(Left) Axial T2WI MR shows a homogeneous, well-circumscribed ovoid mass ➡ with signal greater than CSF ➡. This lesion extended into the lower neck. (Center) Low magnification shows the fibrous wall of a bronchogenic cyst. Seromucinous glands ➡ are found throughout the wall and may contribute to the mucoid material found within the cyst. (Right) Smooth muscle, highlighted with a smooth muscle actin immunostain, is characteristic within the wall of a bronchogenic cyst.

BRANCHIAL CLEFT CYST

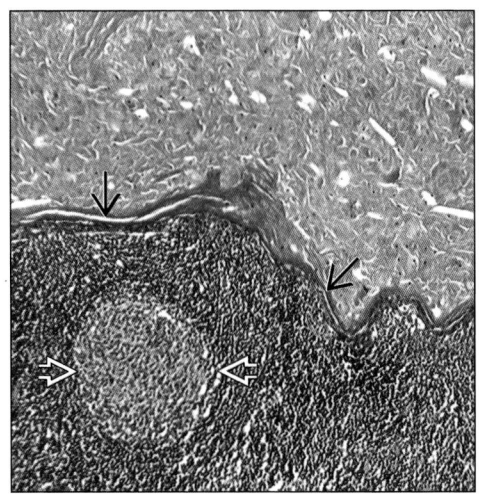

The lumen of this BrCC is filled with keratinaceous debris. There is a thin, squamous epithelium ➡ without any atypia. There is a germinal center ⧁ within the associated lymphoid tissue.

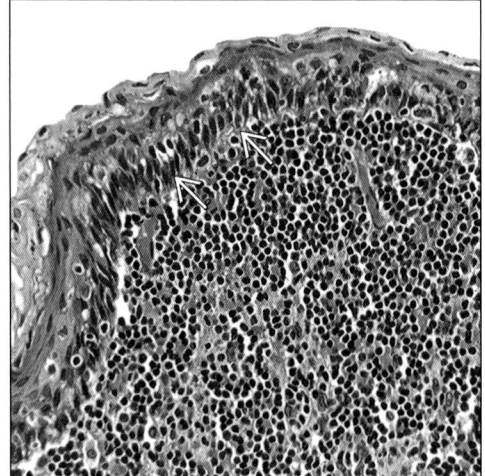

The cyst is lined by metaplastic squamous epithelium although a residuum of columnar epithelium is still present ➡. There is a very thin basement membrane between the epithelium and lymphoid tissue.

TERMINOLOGY

Abbreviations
- Branchial cleft cyst (BrCC)

Definitions
- By convention, "branchial cleft cyst" refers to congenital developmental lateral cervical cyst derived from remnants of 2nd branchial apparatus
  - Encompasses branchial cyst, sinus, or fistula

ETIOLOGY/PATHOGENESIS

Branchial Apparatus
- Precursor of many head and neck structures
- 2nd branchial arch overgrows 2nd, 3rd, and 4th clefts
- This overgrowth forms "cervical sinus"
- Embryogenesis is usually complete by 6-7 weeks of gestation
- Failure of obliteration of cervical sinus results in 2nd branchial cleft remnant (cyst, sinus, or fistula)
- 2nd branchial cleft fistula extends from skin anterior to sternocleidomastoid muscle (SCM), through carotid artery bifurcation to terminate in tonsillar fossa
- 3rd and 4th branchial cleft cysts are very uncommon (< 5%)
  - Recurrent neck abscess or acute suppurative thyroiditis
  - Vast majority on left side (90-95%)
- Some posit cystic transformation of cervical lymph nodes
  - Especially in adults

CLINICAL ISSUES

Epidemiology
- Incidence
  - Uncommon

- Still, BrCC is one of the most commonly encountered congenital anomalies in pediatric otolaryngic practice
    - Thyroglossal duct cysts are most common
  - BrCC accounts for ~ 20% of all congenital cervical cysts
    - Cysts > > sinuses (3:1)
  - About 80-90% of all branchial cleft anomalies are 2nd branchial cleft cysts
- Age
  - Bimodal presentation
    - < 5 years old (25%)
    - 20-40 years old (75%)
    - ~ 1% in patients > 50 years old
- Gender
  - Equal sex distribution

Site
- Lateral neck near mandibular angle
- Along anterior border of SCM
  - Anywhere from hyoid bone to suprasternal notch
- Curiously, left-sided predominance for 4th branchial anomalies (> 90%)

Presentation
- Painless cervical swelling
  - Along anterior border of SCM
  - Often present for long duration
  - May be painful (if infected)
- Waxing and waning lesion
  - Frequently enlarges in concert with upper respiratory tract infection
  - Patients present during phase of recent enlargement
  - May lie dormant (clinically silent) for years
- Compressible, fluctuant
- Mucoid or pus-like secretions from sinus tract skin opening (when opening is present)
- Clinically, some lesions may mimic parotid mass or odontogenic infection

BRANCHIAL CLEFT CYST

Key Facts

Terminology
- Branchial cleft cyst refers to congenital developmental lateral cervical cyst derived from remnants of 2nd branchial apparatus

Etiology/Pathogenesis
- Failure of obliteration of cervical sinus results in 2nd branchial cleft remnant (cyst, sinus, or fistula)

Clinical Issues
- Comprises ~ 20% of all congenital cervical cysts
- Bimodal presentation (< 5 years; 20-40 years)
- Waxing and waning, painless, compressible, cervical swelling
  - Enlarges after upper respiratory tract infection
- Along anterior border of sternocleidomastoid muscle

- Initial work-up of suspected branchial cleft anomaly (in order)
  - Intravenous or oral antibiotics (if infected), FNA, endoscopy &/or radiographic studies, surgery
- Complete surgical excision yields a low recurrence risk

Microscopic Pathology
- Usually a unilocular cyst
- Cyst lined by various types of epithelium (90% stratified squamous)
- Lymphoid aggregates in cyst wall

Top Differential Diagnoses
- Epidermal inclusion cyst, metastatic cystic squamous cell carcinoma, bronchogenic cyst, metastatic thyroid papillary carcinoma, cervical thymic cyst

---

- Bilateral lesions are usually identified in syndromic or familial association
- Clinically, 1st or 4th BrCC more likely to have incision and drainage procedures, resulting in "recurrence"
- **Important**: Must consider metastatic cystic squamous cell carcinoma in adults

Endoscopic Findings
- Advocated as part of initial assessment of neck cyst
  - Assess internal opening or draining sinus/fistula

Treatment
- Options, risks, complications
  - Initial work-up of suspected branchial cleft anomaly (in order)
    - Intravenous or oral antibiotics (if infected)
    - Fine needle aspiration
    - Endoscopy (concurrent with surgery in some cases)
    - Radiographic studies
    - Surgery in nonresolving cases
  - Avoid repeated incision and drainage
    - Yields high recurrence rate
  - Noninfected lesions are more easily removed than infected lesions
  - Entire fistula tract must be removed to prevent recurrence
- Surgical approaches
  - Combined, simultaneous endoscopic identification of sinus tract with lateral external cervical dissection
    - Cauterization of fistula used by some
    - Endoscopic placement of catheter into sinus lumen before surgical exploration
  - Complete surgical excision
    - Excision performed during quiescent phase (no active infection; 6-8 weeks after antibiotics)
  - Must dissect around cyst bed to exclude fistula
    - If superomedial tract: Usually ends in faucial tonsil
    - If inferior tract: Travels down carotid space, exiting in supraclavicular-area skin

Prognosis
- Lesions are benign without malignant potential
- Recurrence rate is variable
  - < 3% if not infected before surgery
  - ~ 20% if infected or previously incised/drained or incompletely removed

IMAGE FINDINGS

Radiographic Findings
- Combination of radiographic studies and endoscopy greatly improve surgical management and outcome
- Contrast CT (or MR) will easily suggest this diagnosis and differentiate it from a solid mass
- Well-circumscribed nonenhancing low-density cystic mass with smooth cavity and thin wall (unless infected)

MACROSCOPIC FEATURES

General Features
- Unilocular, with clear to grumous material

Size
- Wide range, up to 10 cm

MICROSCOPIC PATHOLOGY

Histologic Features
- Usually a unilocular cyst
- Cyst lined by various types of epithelium
  - Stratified squamous (90%)
  - Respiratory epithelium (~ 8%)
    - Considered native lining in uninflamed cyst
  - Transitional or both (2%)
- Lumen filled with keratinaceous debris
- Lymphoid aggregates usually subtend epithelial lining
  - Basement membrane frequently seen between epithelium and lymphoid elements
- Reactive germinal centers commonly present (~ 80%)

BRANCHIAL CLEFT CYST

- Lymph node architecture is not present
  - No subcapsular sinus formation
  - No medullary region
  - No interfollicular zone
- Acute and chronic inflammation frequently present
- Foreign body giant cell reaction within wall of cyst
- Fibrosis is frequently seen
  - Not heavy, thick "capsule" formation seen in metastatic cystic squamous cell carcinoma (SCC)
- Salivary gland tissue may be detected in wall
- Adnexa and cartilage are not seen in this type of BrCC
  - Only seen in 1st branchial cleft cysts/sinuses
- Absence of dysplasia, pleomorphism, carcinoma

ANCILLARY TESTS

Cytology
- Composed of anucleate squames and mature squamous epithelium
  - Columnar respiratory-type cells are less common
- Amorphous debris often associated with macrophages
- Lymphoid infiltrate, including plasma cells

Immunohistochemistry
- Variety of keratins are positive, depending on type of lining
  - Pseudostratified respiratory, transitional, stratified keratinizing, or nonkeratinizing squamous epithelium
- Glucose transporter 1 (*GLUT-1*) negative in BrCC but positive in metastatic cystic SCC

DIFFERENTIAL DIAGNOSIS

Epidermal Inclusion Cyst
- Specific anatomic site may be a clue (preauricular, postauricular)
- Lacks lymphoid stroma, adnexal structures, and cartilage (specifically when excluding Work type II)

Metastatic Cystic Squamous Cell Carcinoma
- Jugulodigastric lymph node most commonly affected
- Unilocular cyst
- Very thick and well-developed capsule
- Subcapsular sinus, medullary zone, and interfollicular zones usually identified
- Ribbon-like distribution of atypical epithelium
- Lack of maturation; cellular enlargement, mitoses
- Pleomorphism is often limited and subtle
- Primary usually identified in Waldeyer ring area
  - Tonsil
  - Base of tongue
  - Nasopharynx
- For practical purposes: Primary branchiogenic carcinoma does not exist!

Bronchogenic Cyst (Bronchial Cyst)
- Identified in subcutaneous tissue of supraclavicular region
- Radiographic appearance is different from BrCC: Low in neck

- Cyst is lined by respiratory mucosa
- Cyst wall contains smooth muscle, bronchial glands, and hyaline cartilage

Metastatic Cystic Thyroid Papillary Carcinoma
- Lymph node architecture is easily identified
- May be unilocular lesion, with only serum or clear fluid in lumen
- Lining shows characteristic features of thyroid papillary carcinoma
  - Cellular crowding and overlapping, with cells having high nuclear to cytoplasmic ratio
  - Nuclear features of papillary carcinoma
    - Nuclear grooves, nuclear contour irregularities, intranuclear cytoplasmic inclusions, nuclear chromatin clearing
  - Papillary architecture is frequently absent

Cervical Thymic Cyst
- Often develops in children
- Affects lateral cervical region
  - Angle of mandible to sternum, although usually lower neck
- Thymic tissue is present in cyst wall
  - Hassall corpuscles (squamous eddies), calcifications, lymphoid elements

Lymphangioma (Cystic Hygroma)
- Generally a clinical consideration
- Usually involves posterior cervical space
- Endothelial-lined spaces with serum, lymphocytes, and wall smooth muscle

Thyroglossal Duct Cyst
- Midline location
- Associated with thyroid tissue and involves hyoid bone

Dermoid Cyst
- Squamous lining with adnexal structures, without lymphoid elements
- **No** other components (muscle, nerve, cartilage)

SELECTED REFERENCES

1. Ozolek JA: Selective pathologies of the head and neck in children: a developmental perspective. Adv Anat Pathol. 16(5):332-58, 2009
2. Kadhim AL et al: Pearls and pitfalls in the management of branchial cyst. J Laryngol Otol. 118(12):946-50, 2004
3. Thompson LD: Branchial cleft cyst. Ear Nose Throat J. 83(11):740, 2004
4. Glosser JW et al: Branchial cleft or cervical lymphoepithelial cysts: etiology and management. J Am Dent Assoc. 134(1):81-6, 2003
5. Choi SS et al: Branchial anomalies: a review of 52 cases. Laryngoscope. 105(9 Pt 1):909-13, 1995
6. Takimoto T et al: Branchial cleft (pouch) anomalies: a review of 42 cases. Auris Nasus Larynx. 18(1):87-92, 1991
7. Kenealy JF et al: Branchial cleft anomalies: a five-year retrospective review. Trans Pa Acad Ophthalmol Otolaryngol. 42:1022-5, 1990
8. Doi O et al: Branchial remnants: a review of 58 cases. J Pediatr Surg. 23(9):789-92, 1988

BRANCHIAL CLEFT CYST

Clinical, Radiologic, Gross, and Microscopic Features

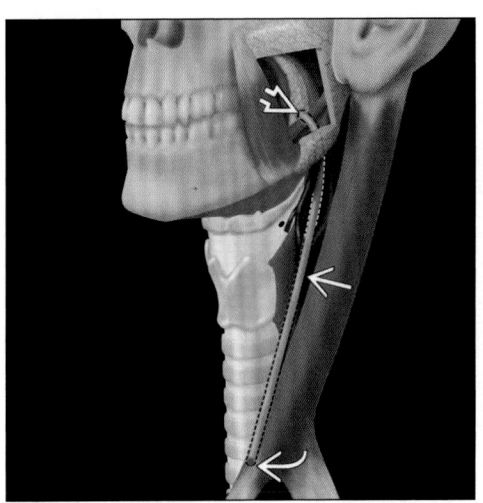

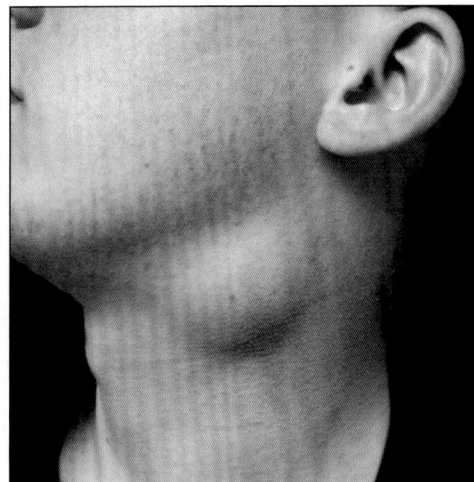

(Left) A 2nd branchial cleft cyst/sinus/fistula can develop anywhere along the normal development of the branchial pouches and arches. The tonsillar opening ⇥ may be associated with a tract ➔ along the anterior border of the SCM, extending to a supraclavicular skin opening ⇥. (Right) This clinical photograph shows a compressible lateral neck mass in a young adult male, quite characteristic for a 2nd branchial cleft cyst.

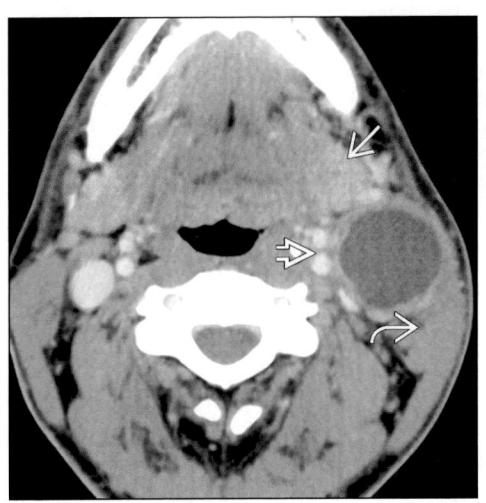

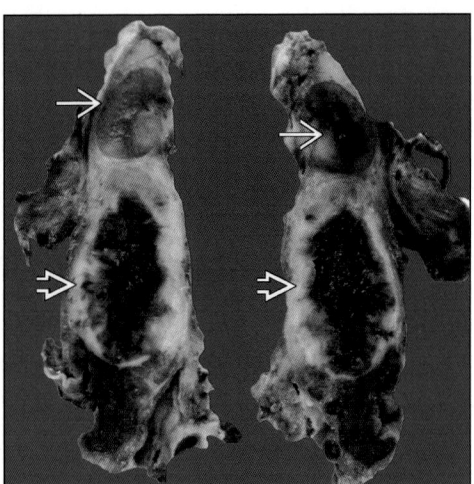

(Left) Axial contrast CT reveals a typical 2nd branchial cleft cyst located posterior to the submandibular gland ⇥, lateral to the carotid space ⇥, and anterior to the sternomastoid muscle ➔. (Right) The resection specimen includes a benign lymph node ➔ completely separate from the cyst immediately below. Note the thick, fibrous connective tissue wall ⇥ surrounding the cyst, which is filled with hemorrhagic and keratinaceous material.

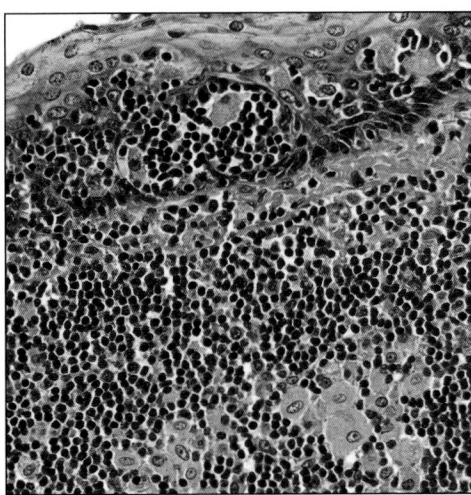

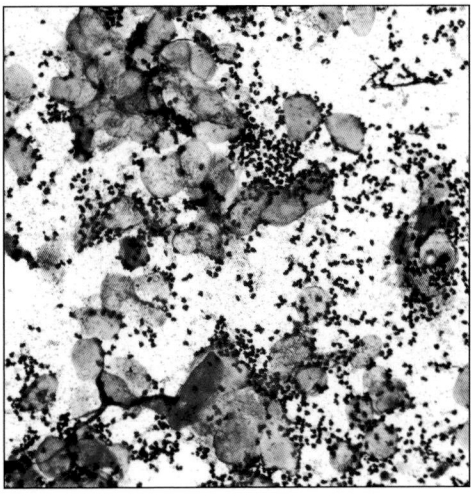

(Left) The squamous epithelium is mature and lacks cytologic atypia. A well-developed basement membrane is seen, separating the epithelium from the stroma. Histiocytes are also present within the lymphoid background. (Right) There are many neutrophils intimately associated with squamous and anucleated squames in this smear from a BrCC. There are no irregular shapes, no mitotic figures, and no pleomorphism. Necrosis is absent although debris is present.

MEDIAN RAPHE CYST

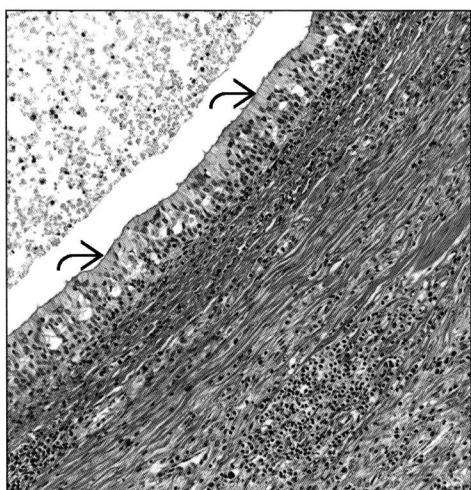

This median raphe cyst is lined by pseudostratified columnar epithelium with mucin-containing cells on the surface ⟶.

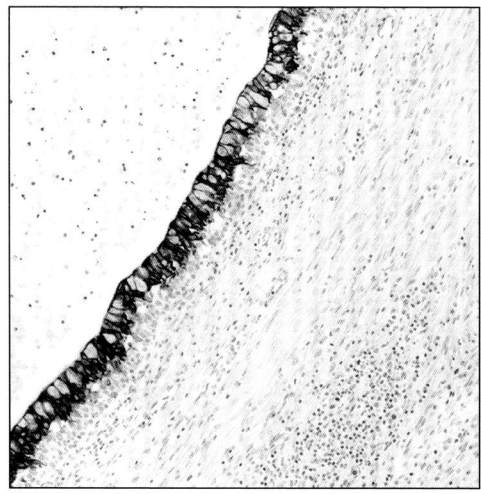

Immunostain for CK7 shows that the upper layers of the pseudostratified columnar epithelial lining are positive.

TERMINOLOGY

Definitions
- Midline developmental cyst found at any point from external urethral meatus to anus
  - Commonly located on ventral aspect of penis with predilection for glans

ETIOLOGY/PATHOGENESIS

Developmental Anomaly
- Thought to arise from defective embryological closure of median raphe
- Some may result from anomalous budding and separation of columnar epithelium from urethra

CLINICAL ISSUES

Epidemiology
- Incidence
  - Rare
- Age
  - Congenital cyst that becomes apparent in young adults
    - First 3 decades of life
- Gender
  - Males

Presentation
- Solitary cyst
  - Less frequently multiple
  - Multiple lesions in linear arrangement have been described
- Usually located on ventral aspect of penis
  - Predilection for glans
  - May be located at any point between meatus urethralis and anus
  - Perineal and scrotal lesions may occur

- Usually present as papule/nodule
  - Polypoid lesions have been described
- Usually measure < 1 cm
- Spontaneous regression is rare
- Median raphe canal is probably closely related to median raphe cyst
  - Presents as elongated canal in ventral portion of penis

Treatment
- Surgical approaches
  - Simple excision

Prognosis
- Excellent

MACROSCOPIC FEATURES

General Features
- Solitary cyst
- Clear contents
  - Turbid when mucous cells are prominent
- Asymptomatic

Size
- A few millimeters

Sections to Be Submitted
- Specimen usually consists of entire cyst
  - Easily entirely submitted in 1 or a few sections

MICROSCOPIC PATHOLOGY

Histologic Features
- Lined by pseudostratified columnar epithelium
  - 1-4 cells in thickness
  - Similar to penile urethral epithelium
  - Epithelium may be flattened in areas
- May contain mucin-secreting columnar cells
- Squamous lining may be seen

MEDIAN RAPHE CYST

Key Facts

Etiology/Pathogenesis
- Defective embryological closure of median raphe
- Anomalous separation of columnar epithelium from urethra

Clinical Issues
- Solitary cyst
- Typically < 1 cm in size
- Ventral portion of glans

Microscopic Pathology
- Located in dermis
- Lined by pseudostratified columnar epithelium
  - Focal to extensive mucinous, squamous, ciliated, and apocrine lining

Top Differential Diagnoses
- Epidermoid inclusion cyst
- Dermoid cyst
- Apocrine hidrocystoma/cystadenoma

  - Especially near meatus
  - Focal or extensive
- Ciliated lining is exceptional
- Apocrine cells have been described but are exceptional
- Epithelium may be pigmented
  - Melanocytes may be present in epithelial lining

Cytologic Features
- Columnar cells

ANCILLARY TESTS

Immunohistochemistry
- Epithelial lining positive for AE1/AE3, CAM5.2, CK13, CK7, and p63
  - CK7 stains upper portion of the epithelium
  - p63 stains lower portion of the epithelium
- Negative for CK20 and human milk fat globule 1

DIFFERENTIAL DIAGNOSIS

Epidermoid/Epidermal Inclusion Cyst
- Lacks pseudostratified columnar/mucous lining
- Different (variable) anatomical location

Dermoid Cyst
- Squamous lining with associated adnexal structures (hair follicles and sebaceous glands)

Apocrine Hidrocystoma/Cystadenoma
- Apocrine lining

- Positive for human milk fat globule 1

DIAGNOSTIC CHECKLIST

Pathologic Interpretation Pearls
- Median raphe cyst shows no connection to overlying epidermis and is lined by pseudostratified columnar epithelium similar to penile urethral epithelium

SELECTED REFERENCES

1. LaCarrubba F et al: Canal versus cysts of the penile median raphe: advancing diagnostic methods using videodermatoscopy. Pediatr Dermatol. 27(6):667-9, 2010
2. Colmenero I et al: [Pigmented cyst of the median raphe of the scrotum in a boy.] Actas Dermosifiliogr. 100(7):633-4, 2009
3. Krauel L et al: Median raphe cysts of the perineum in children. Urology. 71(5):830-1, 2008
4. Sagar J et al: Ciliated median raphe cyst of perineum presenting as perianal polyp: a case report with immunohistochemical study, review of literature, and pathogenesis. ScientificWorldJournal. 6:2339-44, 2006
5. Aceñero MJ et al: Median raphe cyst with ciliated cells: report of a case. Am J Dermatopathol. 25(2):175-6, 2003
6. Dini M et al: Median raphe cyst of the penis: a report of two cases with immunohistochemical investigation. Am J Dermatopathol. 23(4):320-4, 2001
7. Ohnishi T et al: Immunohistochemical analysis of human milk fat globulin 1 and cytokeratin expression in median raphe cyst of the penis. Clin Exp Dermatol. 26(1):88-92, 2001

IMAGE GALLERY

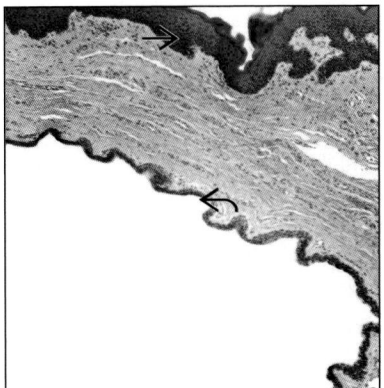 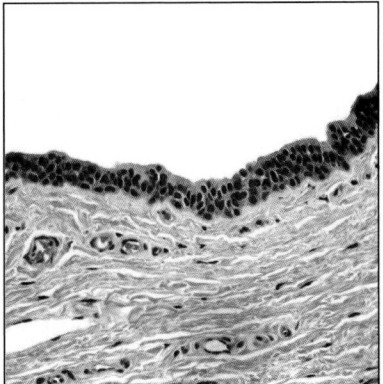 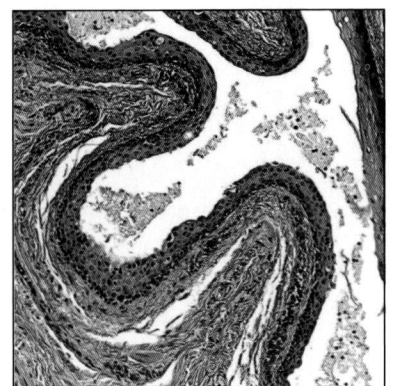

(Left) This median raphe cyst ➲ is located in the dermis without connection with the overlying surface epidermis ➲. *(Center)* Pseudostratified columnar epithelium is the characteristic lining of median raphe cysts. *(Right)* Occasionally, the epithelium of median raphe cyst is stratified squamous, especially when the cyst is located near the meatus.

CUTANEOUS CILIATED CYST

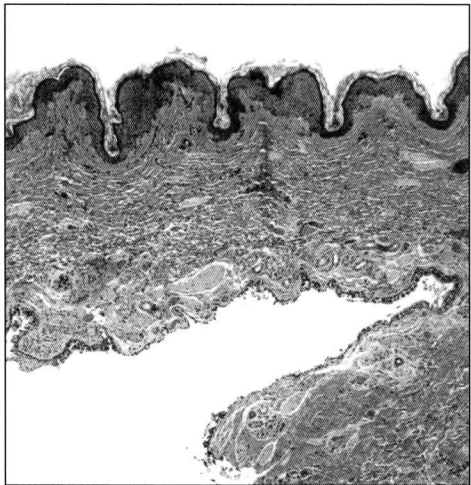

Cutaneous ciliated cyst presented as an unilocular cavity within the dermis. Occasionally, they may be located in the subcutis.

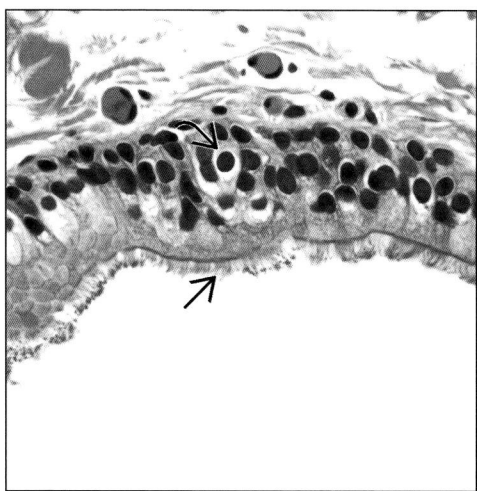

High magnification shows a cutaneous ciliated cyst. The epithelial lining is pseudostratified columnar with a prominent ciliated surface ➔. There are intercalated dark nuclei ➔.

TERMINOLOGY

Synonyms
- Cutaneous müllerian cyst

Definitions
- Solitary cyst with ciliated epithelium, usually affecting lower extremities of young females

ETIOLOGY/PATHOGENESIS

Developmental Anomaly
- Limbs of young females
  - Müllerian (paramesonephric) heterotopia
    - Migration abnormality during fetal development

Metaplasia of Preexisting Cyst
- e.g., sweat gland cyst
- Cysts affecting other sites &/or males
  - These cysts may represent completely separate entities

CLINICAL ISSUES

Epidemiology
- Incidence
  - Very rare
- Age
  - Young women (2nd to 3rd decades)
- Gender
  - Female predilection
    - Exceptional in males (may represent a separate entity)

Site
- Lower extremities
  - Thigh > buttock > calf > foot
- Unusual sites include
  - Back, shoulder, scalp, chest, abdominal wall

Presentation
- Solitary cyst affecting limbs of females shortly after menarche

Treatment
- Surgical excision is curative

Prognosis
- Excellent

MACROSCOPIC FEATURES

General Features
- Solitary cyst
  - Deep dermis
  - Subcutaneous tissue

Size
- Up to several centimeters

MICROSCOPIC PATHOLOGY

Histologic Features
- Unilocular in most cases
  - May be multilocular
- Intraluminal papillae
- Pseudostratified cuboidal or columnar epithelium with ciliated surface
  - Similar to epithelium of fallopian tubes
  - Intercalated dark cells may be present
  - Squamous metaplasia is common
  - Mucin secreting cells are rare
  - Apocrine metaplasia is exceptional
- Fibrovascular stroma without smooth-muscle bundles
  - May show variable degree of inflammation

Cytologic Features
- Bland ciliated cuboidal or columnar cells

CUTANEOUS CILIATED CYST

Key Facts

Terminology
- Cutaneous müllerian cyst
- Solitary cyst with ciliated epithelium, usually affecting lower extremities of young females

Etiology/Pathogenesis
- Müllerian (paramesonephric) heterotopia

Clinical Issues
- Solitary cysts typically affecting limbs of females

Microscopic Pathology
- Pseudostratified cuboidal or columnar epithelium with ciliated surface
  - Similar to fallopian tubes

Top Differential Diagnoses
- Bronchogenic cyst
- Thyroglossal duct cyst
- Branchial cyst
- Thymic cyst

ANCILLARY TESTS

Immunohistochemistry
- Positive: CAM5.2, CK7, EMA
- Negative: CEA, GCDFP-15, CK20

DIFFERENTIAL DIAGNOSIS

Bronchogenic Cyst
- Male predilection
- Precordial location
- Pseudostratified ciliated cuboidal/columnar epithelium
- Adjacent tissue may show lymphoid follicles

Branchial Cyst
- Near jaw angle
- Stratified squamous epithelium
  - Occasionally cuboidal/columnar ciliated epithelium
- Adjacent tissue shows prominent lymphoid follicles

Thyroglossal Duct Cyst
- Midline of neck (hyoid bone proximity)
- Clinically, moves with swallowing
- Pseudostratified cuboidal/columnar epithelium
  - Often ciliated
- Adjacent tissue often shows thyroid follicles

Thymic Cyst
- Anterior neck
- Variable lining epithelium
  - Stratified squamous
  - Ciliated cuboidal/columnar
- Adjacent tissue shows thymic remnants

Mature Cystic Teratoma
- Face, neck, scalp
- Usually lined by stratified squamous epithelium
- Associated hair follicles and sebaceous glands
- Adjacent tissue often contains smooth-muscle bundles

DIAGNOSTIC CHECKLIST

Pathologic Interpretation Pearls
- Epithelial lining similar to that of fallopian tubes

SELECTED REFERENCES

1. Bivin WW Jr et al: Cutaneous ciliated cyst: a case report with focus on mullerian heterotopia and comparison with eccrine sweat glands. Am J Dermatopathol. 32(7):731-4, 2010
2. Lee JS et al: Cutaneous ciliated cyst of the inguinal area in a man. J Dermatol. 33(2):146-9, 2006
3. Lee MT et al: Cutaneous ciliated cyst with interspersed apocrine features presenting as a pilonidal cyst in a child. Pediatr Dev Pathol. 4(3):310-2, 2001
4. al-Nafussi AI et al: Cutaneous ciliated cyst: a case report and immunohistochemical comparison with fallopian tube. Histopathology. 16(6):595-8, 1990
5. Park CH et al: Cutaneous ciliated cyst case report and discussion of pathogenesis. J Pediatr Surg. 17(4):410-1, 1982

IMAGE GALLERY

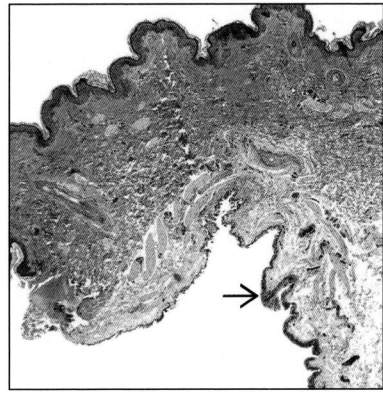 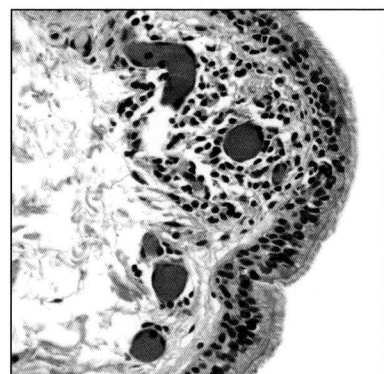 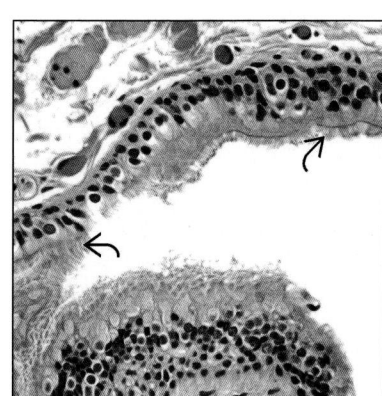

(Left) Low magnification shows a cutaneous ciliated cyst with slightly papillary surface ➡. *(Center)* The fibroconnective stromal tissue underlying the cyst wall shows small blood vessels with variable amount of inflammatory cells, which consist mostly of lymphocytes. Smooth muscle bundles are usually absent. *(Right)* The epithelium is pseudostratified columnar with prominent cilia ➡. The epithelial lining appears very similar to that of the fallopian tubes.

Epidermal Tumors

EPIDERMAL NEVUS

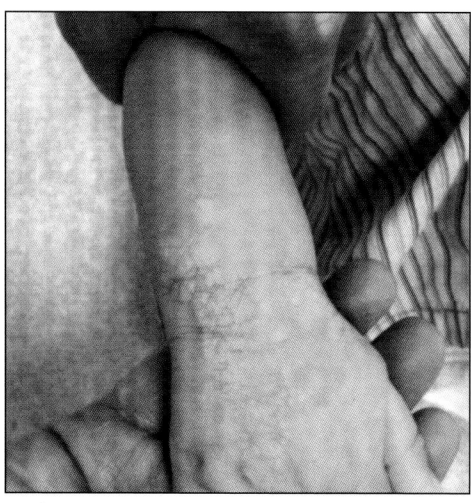

Epidermal nevus is shown presenting as a warty, broad band of hypopigmented growth over the dorsal forearm and extensor wrist, extending onto the back of this child's hand. (Courtesy Univ. of Utah Dept. of Dermatology.)

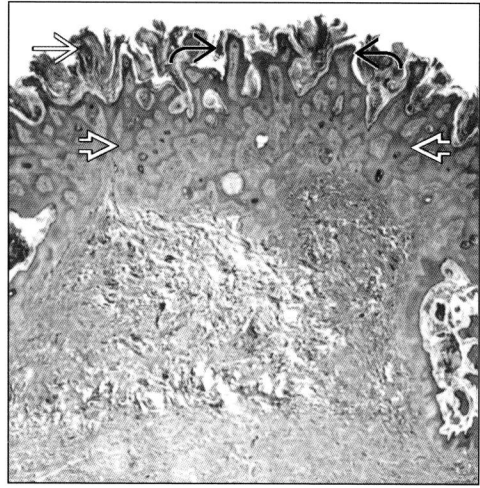

Low magnification shows a common type of epidermal nevus with prominent hyperkeratosis ➡, papillomatosis ➤, and acanthosis ➡.

TERMINOLOGY

Synonyms
- Nevus verrucosus
  - Localized wart-like variants
- Nevus unius lateris
  - Long linear lesions on extremities
- Ichthyosis hystrix
  - Large bilateral lesions on trunk

Definitions
- Developmental malformation of epidermis with hyperplasia of keratinocytes
- Specific entity that does not include adnexal malformations or appendageal tumors such as organoid/sebaceous nevus

ETIOLOGY/PATHOGENESIS

Epidermal Nevus Syndrome
- Epidermal nevi (usually extensive) with
  - Neurological abnormalities (epilepsy, mental retardation)
  - Ocular abnormalities (cataracts)
  - Skeletal anomalies (kyphoscoliosis, limb hypertrophy)
- Various systemic cancers at young age

Other Associations
- Polyostotic fibrous dysplasia
- Proteus syndrome
- Phakomatosis pigmentokeratotica

CLINICAL ISSUES

Epidemiology
- Age
  - Usually early onset but can be seen in adulthood

Site
- Neck, trunk, extremities

Treatment
- Excision if lesion small
- Larger lesions can be treated by laser or cryotherapy
  - Frequently recur

Prognosis
- Benign
- Very rarely, tumors can arise within epidermal nevi
  - Basal cell carcinoma
  - Squamous cell carcinoma and keratoacanthoma

MACROSCOPIC FEATURES

General Features
- Single or multiple
- Warty plaque
- May be linear or zosteriform
- Scaly discoloration

MICROSCOPIC PATHOLOGY

Histologic Features
- At least 10 different patterns
  - > 1 pattern can exist in single nevus
- Common patterns
  - Hyperkeratosis with acanthosis and broad papillomatosis
  - Thickened granular layer
  - Increased basal melanin pigment
- Less common patterns resemble
  - Acrokeratosis verruciformis
  - Epidermolytic hyperkeratosis
  - Seborrheic keratosis
    - Elongated rete ridges with flat bottoms
- Rare patterns include
  - Verrucoid

EPIDERMAL NEVUS

Key Facts

Terminology
- Developmental malformation of epidermis with keratinocytic hyperplasia

Etiology/Pathogenesis
- Epidermal nevus syndrome includes neurological, ocular, and skeletal abnormalities

Clinical Issues
- Common sites include neck, trunk, and extremities

Microscopic Pathology
- At least 10 different patterns
- > 1 pattern can exist in single lesion
- Common pattern includes hyperkeratosis with papillomatosis and acanthosis
- ILVEN is considered a subtype of epidermal nevus

Top Differential Diagnoses
- Seborrheic keratosis
- Acanthosis nigricans

---

o Porokeratotic
o Focal acantholytic dyskeratotic
o Acanthosis nigricans-like
o Hailey-Hailey disease-like

Inflammatory Linear Verrucous Epidermal Nevus (ILVEN)
- Subtype of epidermal nevus
- Pruritic linear eruption on lower extremities
- May resemble linear psoriasis
  o Psoriasiform epidermal hyperplasia
  o Overlying parakeratosis alternating with orthokeratosis
  o Mild dermal lymphocytic infiltrate

Nevus Comedonicus
- Distinct entity, though sometimes grouped as a histologic pattern of epidermal nevus
- Grouped or linear comedonal papules
- Dilated keratin-filled invaginations of the epidermis

DIFFERENTIAL DIAGNOSIS

Seborrheic Keratosis
- Clinically distinctive, well-demarcated "stuck-on" lesions occurring in older patients
- Pseudohorn cysts are more common
- Epidermal nevi show rete ridges with flat bottoms

Acanthosis Nigricans
- Symmetric, velvety-appearing plaques in axillae and neck region
- Mild epidermal acanthosis with hyperkeratosis and papillomatosis

Confluent and Reticulated Papillomatosis of Gougerot and Carteaud
- Clinical appearance more diffuse and reticulated
- Undulating papillomatosis with mild acanthosis

Organoid Nevus (Nevus Sebaceous)
- Sebaceous hyperplasia underlying epidermal component
- Loss or hypoplasia of hair follicles

SELECTED REFERENCES

1. Happle R: The group of epidermal nevus syndromes Part I. Well defined phenotypes. J Am Acad Dermatol. 63(1):1-22; quiz 23-4, 2010
2. Happle R: The group of epidermal nevus syndromes Part II. Less well defined phenotypes. J Am Acad Dermatol. 63(1):25-30; quiz 31-2, 2010
3. García-Vargas A et al: An epidermal nevus syndrome with cerebral involvement caused by a mosaic FGFR3 mutation. Am J Med Genet A. 146A(17):2275-9, 2008
4. Paley K et al: Delayed diagnosis of epidermal nevus syndrome associated with substantial brain malformations: a case report and review of the literature. Cutis. 81(3):274-6, 2008

IMAGE GALLERY

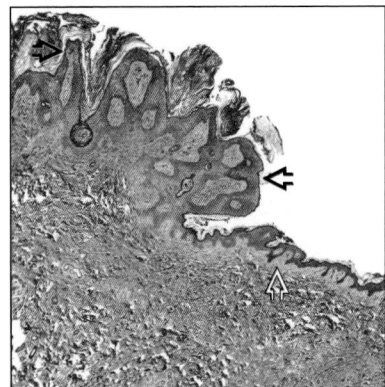 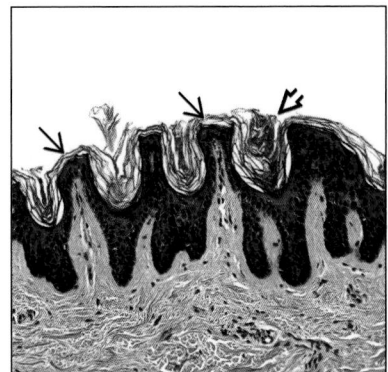 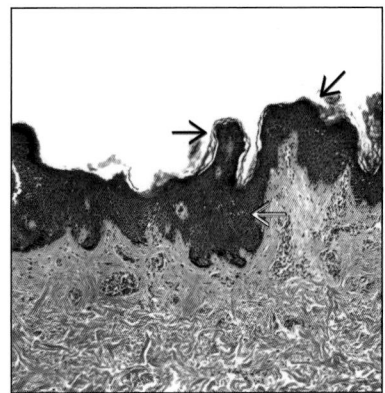

(Left) Epidermal nevus ⊵ is sharply demarcated from the adjacent normal epidermis ⊳. *(Center)* Epidermal nevus shows papillomatosis ⊡, acanthosis, hyperkeratosis ⊡, and minimal dermal perivascular lymphocytes. *(Courtesy C. Cockerell, MD.)* *(Right)* Confluent and reticulated papillomatosis is shown. Note the acanthosis ➡ present in the valley between papillomatous projections ⊡. *(Courtesy G. Fraga, MD.)*

SEBORRHEIC KERATOSIS (AND VARIANTS)

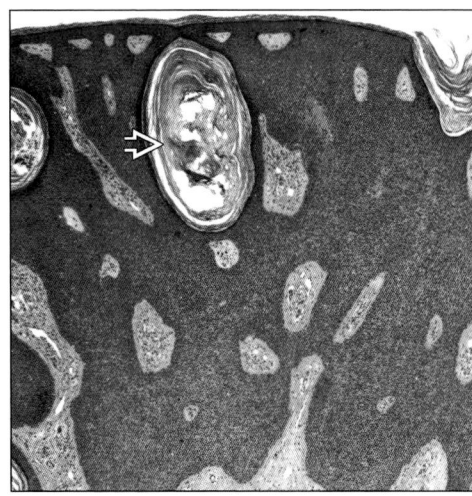

Seborrheic keratosis, acanthotic/endophytic variant. Note the smooth, rounded surface and thickened epithelium. The lesion is predominantly composed of basaloid cells with a prominent horn cyst ➡.

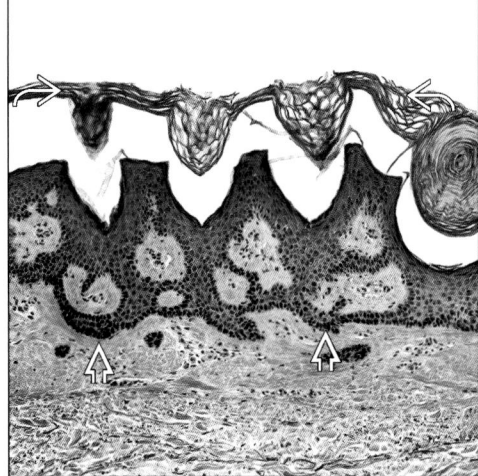

Adenoid seborrheic keratosis composed of narrow and hyperpigmented trabeculae ➡. This variant of SK often evolves from a solar lentigo. Note the "basket weave," orthokeratotic surface ➡.

TERMINOLOGY

Abbreviations
- Seborrheic keratosis (SK)

Definitions
- Benign epidermal proliferation

ETIOLOGY/PATHOGENESIS

Benign Epidermal Tumor
- Monoclonal
- Likely neoplasm rather than hyperplasia

CLINICAL ISSUES

Epidemiology
- Incidence
  - Very common lesions
- Age
  - Middle-aged and elderly
    - Affect approximately 20% of elderly population

Site
- Most common on face, chest, and back
  - Unusual locations: Conjunctiva, areola, areas of cleavage
  - May be found anywhere except palms and soles

Presentation
- Sharply delineated plaques with greasy appearance
- Solitary or multiple
- Measuring a few mm to a few cm
- Verruciform or flat surface
  - Surface shows characteristic keratotic plugs
- Soft and friable
- Round or oval
- From flesh-colored to brown-black

- Darkly pigmented lesions may be clinically mistaken for melanoma
- Often appearing as stuck on skin surface
- Inverted follicular keratosis variant presents as warty papulonodule
- Leser-Trélat sign
  - Sudden onset of multiple seborrheic keratoses
    - Usually associated with internal malignancies (most commonly gastric adenocarcinoma)

Prognosis
- Excellent

MACROSCOPIC FEATURES

General Features
- Exophytic tumors
  - Verruciform/warty or smooth surface

Size
- A few mm to a few cm in diameter

Sections to Be Submitted
- As lesions are small, they tend to be almost entirely sampled in most biopsies
- Specimens may be bisected or serially sectioned before submission
- Curettage specimens are received as multiple fragments

MICROSCOPIC PATHOLOGY

Histologic Features
- Sharply defined tumors
- Exophytic or endophytic or combination of both
- Ortho-hyperkeratosis ("Van Gogh sky")
  - Heavily inflamed, irritated, or infarcted SK may show foci of parakeratosis

SEBORRHEIC KERATOSIS (AND VARIANTS)

Key Facts

Macroscopic Features

- Sharply delineated plaques with greasy appearance
- Verruciform or flat surface
  - Surface shows characteristic keratotic plugs
- From flesh-colored to brown-black
  - Darkly pigmented lesions may be clinically mistaken for melanoma

Microscopic Pathology

- Exophytic/endophytic
- Ortho-hyperkeratosis typically present
- Composed of basaloid and squamoid cells
- Horn cysts/pseudocysts
- Squamous eddies may be present
- Often pigmented
- Stromal amyloid deposition may be seen
- Variable degree of inflammation

- Several variants have been described
  - Acanthotic
  - Papillomatous (hyperkeratotic)
  - Adenoid (reticulated)
  - Clonal (Borst-Jadassohn epithelioma)
  - Inverted follicular keratosis (irritated SK)
  - Lichenoid SK
  - Inflammatory
  - Desmoplastic
  - Adamantinoid
  - Overlapping features are common

Top Differential Diagnoses

- Verruca vulgaris
- Hidroacanthoma simplex
- Hypertrophic actinic keratosis
- Squamous cell carcinoma in situ

- Composed of bland-appearing basaloid and squamoid cells (variable amounts of each)
- Keratin-filled invaginations and small pseudocysts (pseudohorn cysts) are characteristic
- Nests of keratinocytes (squamous eddies) may be seen
  - Usually seen in irritated SK
  - Apparently related to acrotrichia
- Frequently hyperpigmented
  - Pigmentation in SK has been linked to increased expression of keratinocyte-derived endothelin 1
  - Melanocytes may be increased in number and size
    - Melanoacanthomas are SKs with marked melanocytic proliferation and pigmentation
- Tricholemmal differentiation (glycogen-rich) may be focally present
- Sebaceous differentiation is uncommon and focal finding
- Acantholysis &/or dyskeratosis may be rarely seen
- Many different variants of SK have been described
  - **Acanthotic SK**
    - Smooth, rounded and ortho-hyperkeratotic surface
    - Acanthotic epithelium
    - Basaloid cells predominate over squamoid cells
    - Often pigmented
    - Horn cysts tend to be prominent
  - **Papillomatous (keratotic) SK**
    - Ortho-hyperkeratosis
    - Papillomatosis
    - Acanthosis
    - Squamoid cells predominate over basaloid cells
    - Prominent horn cysts
  - **Adenoid (reticulated) SK**
    - Ortho-hyperkeratosis
    - Flat or papillomatous surface
    - Thin proliferating strands emanating from epidermis
    - Basaloid cells predominate over squamoid cells
    - Often pigmented
    - Horn cysts are absent or sparse
  - **Clonal SK (type of irritated SK)**

- Borst-Jadassohn phenomenon: Oval to round aggregates of intraepidermal keratinocytes
  - **Inverted follicular keratosis (type of irritated SK)**
    - Endophytic growth pattern
    - Prominent squamous eddies
  - **Lichenoid SK**
    - Prominent lymphoid infiltrate
    - Apoptotic cells (Civatte bodies)
    - Some cases probably evolve to lichenoid keratosis (lichen planus-like keratosis)
    - Any of the variants of SK may show lichenoid features
  - **Inflammatory SK**
    - Any variant of SK may be heavily inflamed
    - Rarely, neutrophils may be abundant in inflammatory infiltrate
    - Overlapping features with lichenoid SK
  - **Desmoplastic SK**
    - Irregular cords and strands of squamous cells surrounded by desmoplastic stroma
    - These trapped strands and cords may mimic infiltrative squamous cell carcinoma (SCC)
    - Bulk of lesion is typical SK
    - Analogous to desmoplastic tricholemmoma
  - **Adamantinoid SK**
    - Very unusual
    - Small basaloid keratinocytes with spindled cytoplasm
    - Intercellular mucin
  - **SK with pseudorosettes**
    - Very rare
    - Basaloid cells arranged around central small spaces
- Overlapping features of different variants is common finding
- SKs are benign tumors
  - Malignant transformation is exceptional but may rarely occur
    - Cases of SCC in situ arising in SK have been described
  - Collision of SK with benign and malignant neoplasms may very rarely occur (e.g., melanoma and SK)

Cytologic Features

- Basaloid and squamoid cells

DIFFERENTIAL DIAGNOSIS

Verruca Vulgaris

- Hypergranulosis and usually dense compact hyperkeratosis with tiers of parakeratosis (not "Van Gogh sky" of SK)
- Koilocytosis typically present
- Intracorneal hemorrhage

Condyloma Acuminatum (CA)

- SK-like lesions in genital areas usually represent old CAs
- They may show horn pseudocysts and basaloid cells

Stucco Keratosis

- Extremities of elderly people
- Multiple tiny lesions
- Microscopically indistinguishable from early SK (may be considered SK variant)
- Acanthosis with church spire appearance
- Ortho-hyperkeratosis

Epidermal Nevus

- Often present at birth or appear during childhood
- Microscopically may be indistinguishable from SK

Acanthosis Nigricans

- Associated with internal malignancies and other systemic conditions
- Symmetrical, pigmented plaques in flexural areas
- Mild acanthosis with papillomatosis and hyperkeratosis
- Horn cysts are not present
- Histologically may be indistinguishable from SK

Confluent and Reticulated Papillomatosis

- Mild acanthosis with papillomatosis and hyperkeratosis
- Horn cysts are not present
- Histologically may be indistinguishable from early SK

Arsenical and Tar Keratosis

- Mild acanthosis with papillomatosis and hyperkeratosis
- Histologically may be indistinguishable from early seborrheic keratosis

Clear Cell Acanthoma

- Psoriasiform hyperplasia and parakeratosis containing neutrophils
- Sharp demarcation from adjacent epidermis
- Lesional keratinocytes have abundant pale cytoplasm

Poroma and Hidroacanthoma Simplex (HS)

- Nests of basaloid adnexal cells attached to (poroma) or in epidermis (HS)
- Cells are smaller than basaloid cells of SK
- Poromatous cells often contain glycogen
- Scattered ductal structures may be present

Hypertrophic Actinic Keratosis (AK)

- Alternating foci of ortho- and parakeratosis
- Atypical (dysplastic) keratinocytes usually underneath the parakeratotic foci

Squamous Cell Carcinoma In Situ (SCCis)

- Full thickness keratinocytic atypia
- Often hyperchromatic nuclei
- Numerous mitoses including in upper levels of the epidermis
- Abnormal keratinization (usually confluent parakeratosis)

DIAGNOSTIC CHECKLIST

Pathologic Interpretation Pearls

- In superficial biopsies, presence of orthokeratosis with appearance of "Van Gogh sky" is a hint to underlying SK
- Infarcted and inflamed SKs may show reactive keratinocytic atypia
  - Entire infarcted papillae are often seen on top of atypical foci
- Many different variants of SK have been described
  - Overlapping features are common
- SK-like lesions in genital areas often represent old condyloma acuminata

SELECTED REFERENCES

1. Battistella M et al: From hidroacanthoma simplex to poroid hidradenoma: clinicopathologic and immunohistochemic study of poroid neoplasms and reappraisal of their histogenesis. Am J Dermatopathol. 32(5):459-68, 2010
2. Choi HJ et al: Squamous eddies in irritated seborrheic keratosis. Am J Dermatopathol. 2007 Feb;29(1):28-31. Erratum in: Am J Dermatopathol. 29(2):229, 2007
3. Requena L et al: Seborrheic keratosis with pseudorosettes and adamantinoid seborrheic keratosis: two new histopathologic variants. J Cutan Pathol. 33 Suppl 2:42-5, 2006
4. Sharma P et al: Seborrheic keratosis with in-situ squamous cell carcinoma changes. Dermatol Online J. 12(7):19, 2006
5. Vun Y et al: Seborrhoeic keratosis and malignancy: collision tumour or malignant transformation? Australas J Dermatol. 47(2):106-8, 2006
6. King R et al: Desmoplastic seborrheic keratosis. Am J Dermatopathol. 25(3):210-4, 2003
7. Manaka L et al: The mechanism of hyperpigmentation in seborrhoeic keratosis involves the high expression of endothelin-converting enzyme-1alpha and TNF-alpha, which stimulate secretion of endothelin 1. Br J Dermatol. 145(6):895-903, 2001
8. Baer RL et al: Papillated squamous cell carcinoma in situ arising in a seborrheic keratosis. J Am Acad Dermatol. 5(5):561-5, 1981
9. Nakayasu K et al: Trichilemmal differentiation in seborrheic keratosis. J Cutan Pathol. 8(3):256-62, 1981
10. Wade TR et al: The many faces of seborrheic keratoses. J Dermatol Surg Oncol. 5(5):378-82, 1979

SEBORRHEIC KERATOSIS (AND VARIANTS)

Variant Microscopic Features

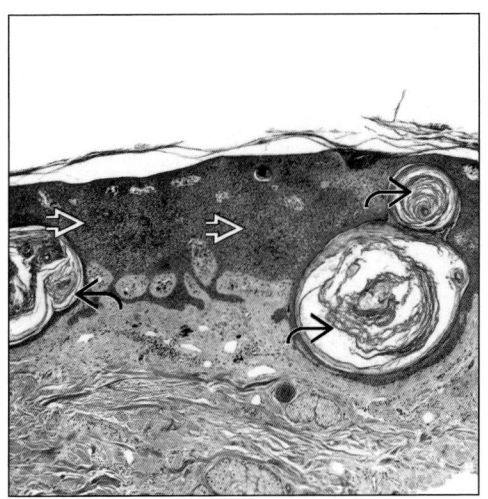

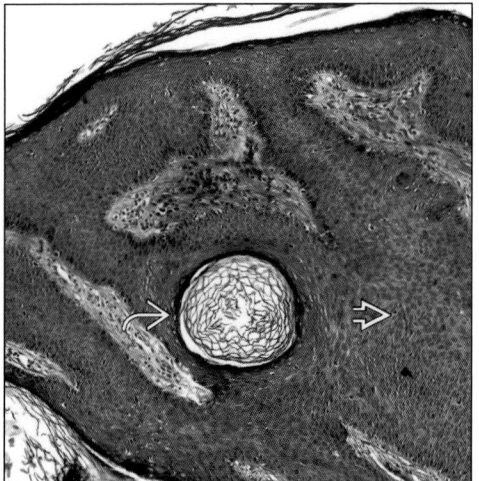

(Left) Acanthotic and pigmented SK characterized by a flat surface and marked acanthosis and prominent horn cysts ➪. Note the presence of abundant melanin within the basaloid keratinocytes ➪. (Right) Acanthotic variant of SK characterized by broad columns of bland and uniform basaloid cells shows intervening horn cysts ➪ and areas with early clonal features ➪.

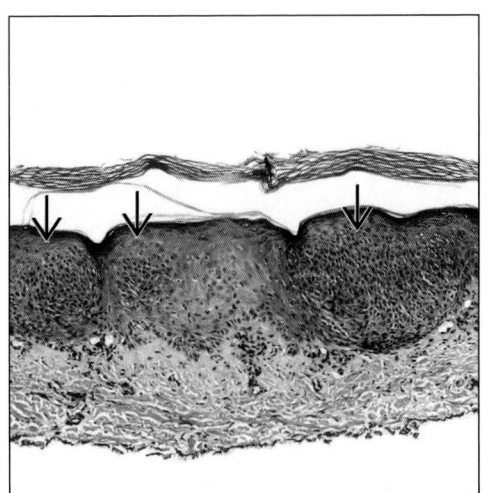

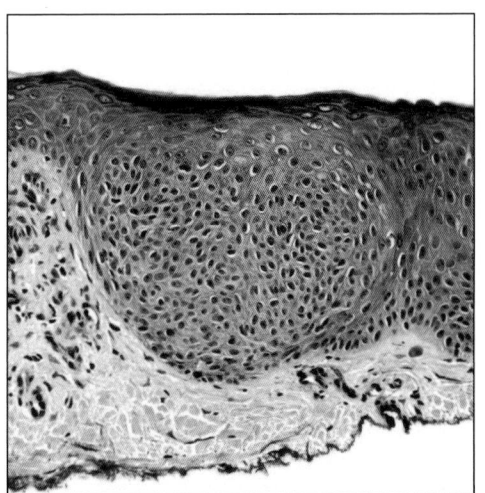

(Left) Clonal SK with round to oval, intraepidermal aggregates of keratinocytes shows the so-called Borst-Jadassohn phenomenon ➪. (Right) Nests of bland-appearing neoplastic keratinocytes surrounded by normal epidermis are characteristic of clonal SK. Borst-Jadassohn phenomenon (epithelioma) likely refers more to a histopathological pattern rather than a precise clinical-pathological entity, as clonal SKs & hidroacanthoma simplex both show this pattern.

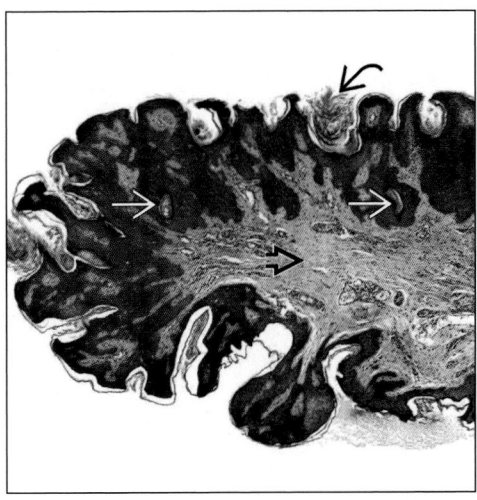

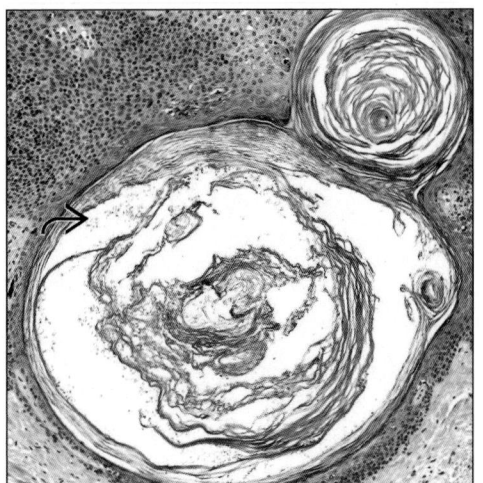

(Left) Papillomatous SK shows hyperkeratosis ➪, papillomatosis, acanthosis, and horn cysts ➪. This lesion is from the axilla, where SKs can share some features with acrochordons. Note the prominent stromal core ➪ without adnexal structures. (Right) Horn cysts may be absent or numerous, tiny to large. Note the large horn cyst ➪ in this SK. These horn cysts may rupture and be associated with a dermal granulomatous foreign body giant cell reaction in some cases.

SEBORRHEIC KERATOSIS (AND VARIANTS)

Variant Microscopic Features

(Left) Horn cysts are absent or sparse in nearly macular (early) SK. Because of their flat surface, these lesions may clinically mimic lentigo or dysplastic nevi. **(Right)** Early SK characterized by orthokeratosis, early papillomatosis, mild acanthosis, and predominance of basaloid cells. Horn cysts are not present in this area. The lesion has mixed features of a hyperkeratotic (papillomatous) and adenoid (reticulated) SK.

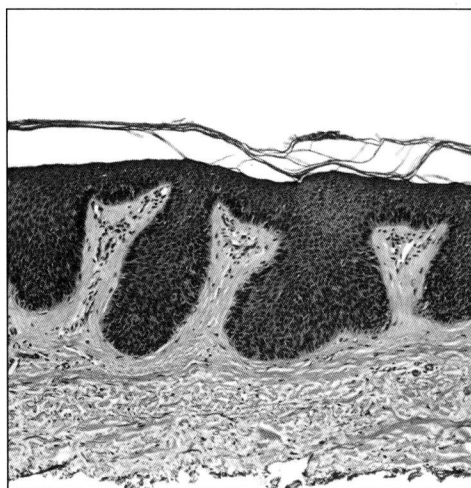
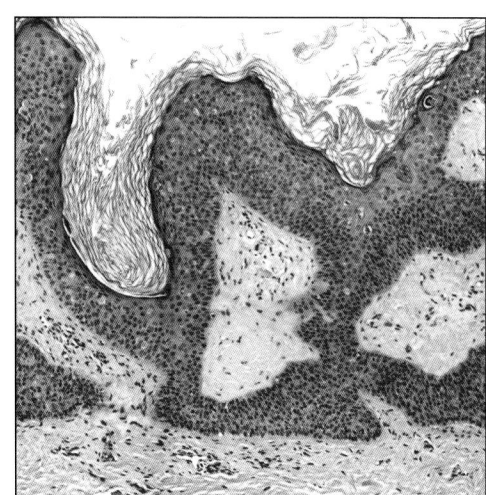

(Left) Irritated seborrheic keratosis with endophytic pattern and numerous squamous eddies ⊳. These types of SK are also known as inverted follicular keratosis. **(Right)** Note the conspicuous squamous eddies ➜ in this irritated SK with features of an inverted follicular keratosis. Squamoid cells predominate over basaloid cells.

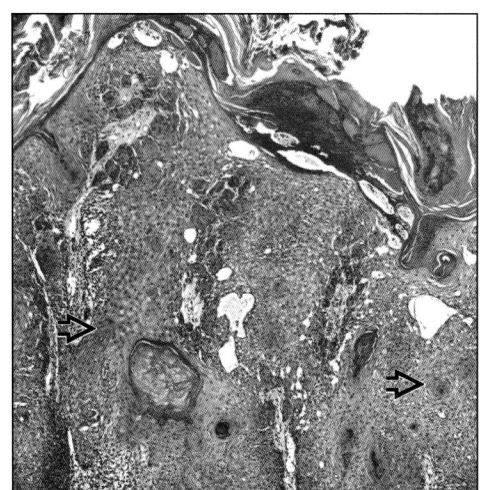
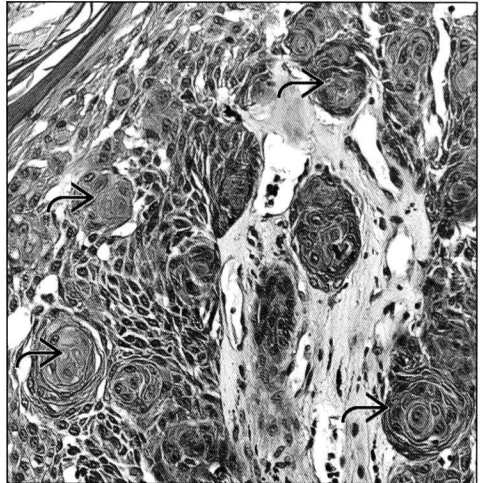

(Left) Partially infarcted SK. Entire papillae with their epithelium ➜ and stromal cores ➡ are infarcted. The viable portion ➜ may show a variable degree of reactive keratinocytic atypia. **(Right)** Partially infarcted SK ➡ shows reactive atypia and prominent squamous eddies ➡. The atypical keratinocytes are enlarged and show nuclear atypia and a few mitoses. However, markedly pleomorphic nuclei, mitoses in the upper epithelium, and atypical mitoses are usually not seen.

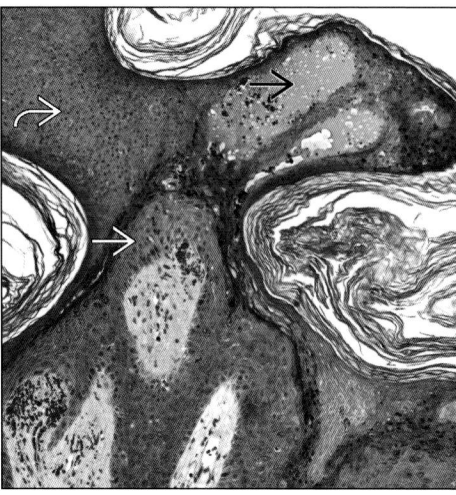
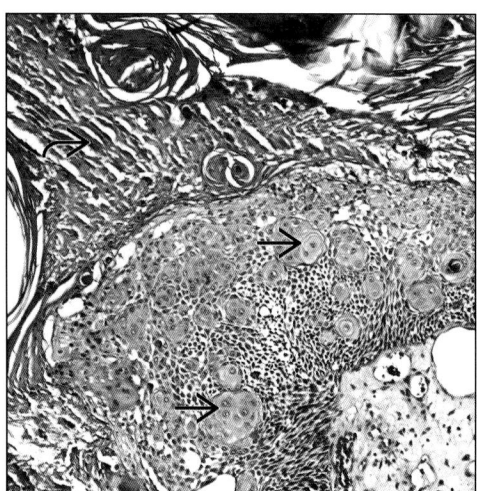

SEBORRHEIC KERATOSIS (AND VARIANTS)

Variant Microscopic Features and Differential Diagnosis

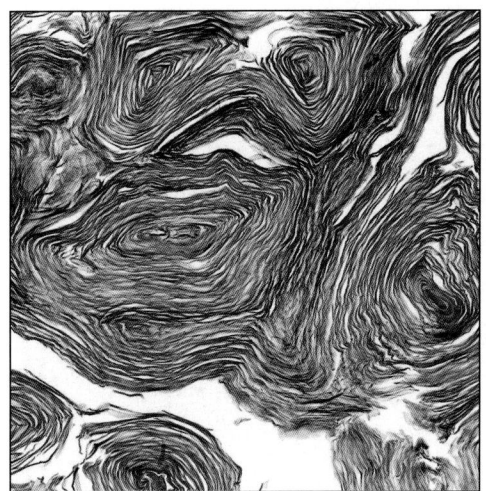 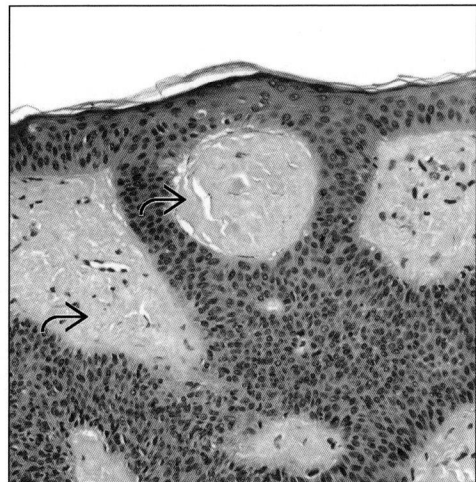

(Left) Characteristic keratin layer of a SK. Unless the lesion is irritated, inflamed, or infarcted, the keratin layer is orthokeratotic. Some authors describe this pattern as "Van Gogh sky" for the resemblance with the artist's paintings. (Right) Stromal amyloid deposition is occasionally seen in SKs. Note the homogeneous eosinophilic and globular dermal deposits ➡. This is keratin-derived amyloid (the same as in macular and lichen amyloidosis) and has no clinical significance.

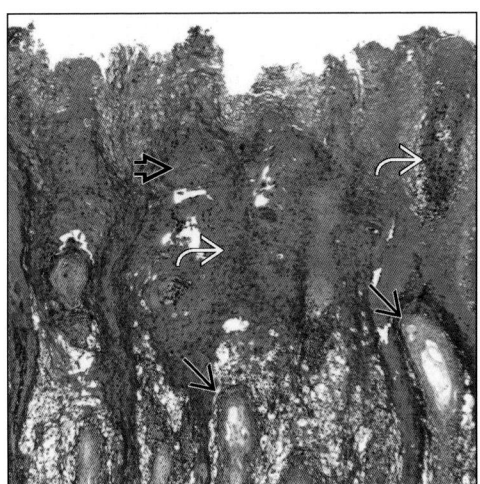 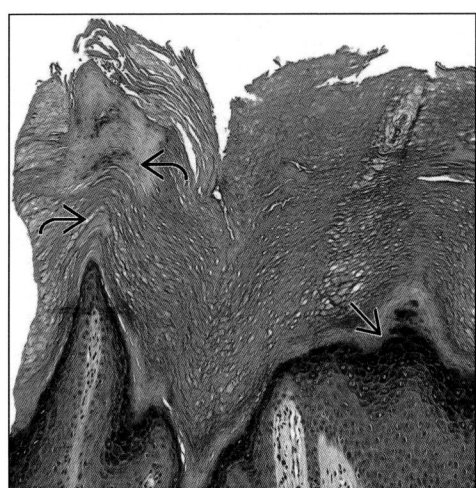

(Left) Warts often enter the differential diagnosis with papillomatous SKs but typically show more dense hyperkeratosis & parakeratosis. Palmoplantar wart (myrmecia) shows marked papillomatosis ➡ with thick overlying hyperkeratosis, parakeratosis ➡, & intracorneal hemorrhage ➡. (Right) Low magnification of the surface of a verruca vulgaris shows epidermal papillomatosis with hypergranulosis ➡ & overlying dense hyperkeratosis & tiers of parakeratosis ➡.

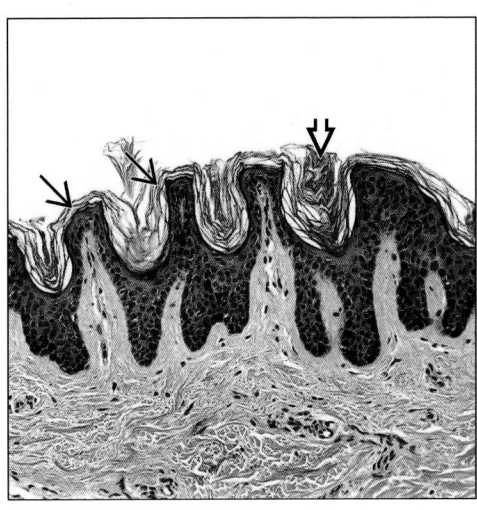 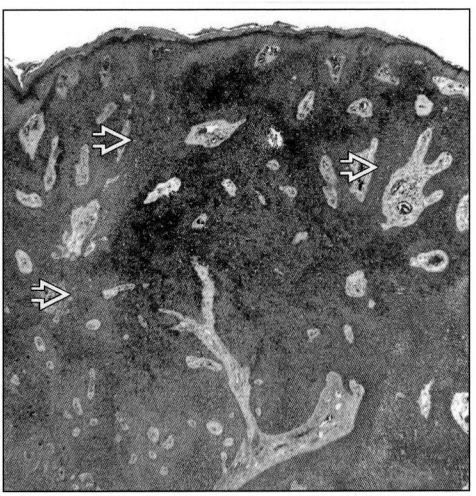

(Left) Epidermal nevus shows papillomatosis ➡, acanthosis, hyperkeratosis ➡, and minimal dermal perivascular lymphocytes. (Courtesy C. Cockerell, MD.) (Right) Pigmented poroma is a relatively common variant that can mimic a pigmented acanthotic SK in some cases. However, besides the heavy pigmentation, it shows features typical of poroma, being composed of basaloid to squamoid cells forming multiple thickened, anastomosing connections between tumor cords ➡.

PSEUDOEPITHELIOMATOUS HYPERPLASIA

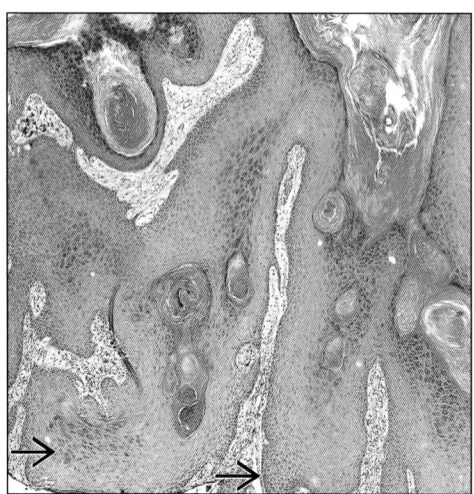

Pseudoepitheliomatous hyperplasia associated with a tattoo shows irregular downgrowths of the epidermis with bulbous rete ➡. Black tattoo pigment and inflammation are present in the dermis.

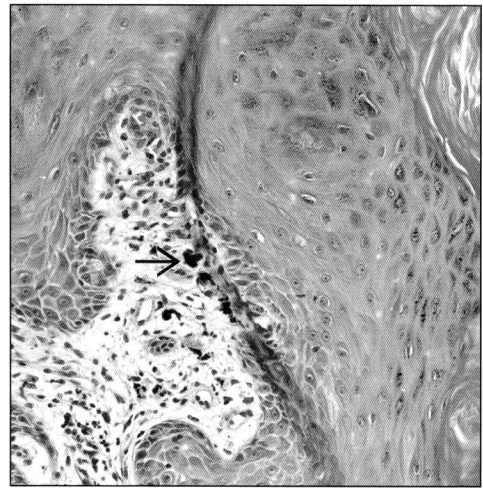

Medium-power view of pseudoepitheliomatous hyperplasia associated with a tattoo shows irregular downgrowths of epidermis without cytologic atypia. Dermal black tattoo pigment is present ➡.

TERMINOLOGY

Abbreviations
- Pseudoepitheliomatous hyperplasia (PEH)

Synonyms
- Pseudocarcinomatous hyperplasia

Definitions
- Florid proliferation of epidermis that mimics squamous cell carcinoma
- Reaction pattern that may be secondary to chronic irritation/trauma

ETIOLOGY/PATHOGENESIS

Associated or Underlying Conditions
- Tumors
  - e.g., granular cell tumor
- Inflammatory conditions
  - e.g., lupus erythematosus, lichen sclerosus
- Infections
  - Particularly deep fungal
  - Also consider syphilis, mycobacteria
- Tattoos

CLINICAL ISSUES

Presentation
- Variable, depending upon underlying condition

Prognosis
- Excellent, no malignant potential

MICROSCOPIC PATHOLOGY

Histologic Features
- Hyperplasia of epidermis

- Base of hyperplastic epidermis may show broad rete or jagged borders
- Varying depth (but never into subcutis)
- May seem to predominantly involve hair follicles and other adnexal structures
- Squamous eddies may be prominent
- Associated inflammation may be granulomatous
- Should prompt evaluation for underlying/associated process, including
  - Tumors
    - e.g., granular cell tumor, malignant melanoma, Spitz nevus, lymphoma
  - Infections
    - e.g., deep fungal, granuloma inguinale, syphilis, acid-fast bacilli
  - Inflammatory conditions
    - e.g., lupus erythematosus, lichen sclerosus
  - Tattoo
  - Prurigo nodularis/lichen simplex chronicus
    - May show areas of PEH

Cytologic Features
- Minimal keratinocyte atypia
- Cells are polygonal with central, round nuclei, small nucleoli, and intercellular bridges
- Individually necrotic cells rare

DIFFERENTIAL DIAGNOSIS

Squamous Cell Carcinoma (SCC)
- Well-differentiated SCC generally shows features not commonly seen in PEH, including
  - Infiltrative areas
  - Cytologic atypia, atypical mitoses
  - Squamous pearls

Keratoacanthoma
- Crateriform architecture with central keratin
- Keratinocytes with glassy pink cytoplasm

PSEUDOEPITHELIOMATOUS HYPERPLASIA

Key Facts

Terminology
- Pseudoepitheliomatous hyperplasia (PEH)
- Florid proliferation of epidermis that mimics squamous cell carcinoma

Etiology/Pathogenesis
- Tumors
- Inflammatory conditions
- Infections
- Tattoos

Microscopic Pathology
- Hyperplasia of epidermis
- Minimal keratinocyte atypia
- Varying depth (but never into subcutis)

Top Differential Diagnoses
- Squamous cell carcinoma (SCC)
- Keratoacanthoma
- Hypertrophic lupus erythematosus
- Hypertrophic lichen planus

- Elastic fiber trapping, dermal fibrosis, and eosinophilic/neutrophilic abscesses may be present
- Clinically should have history of rapid growth and should spontaneously resolve

Hypertrophic Lupus Erythematosus
- Adjacent features compatible with lupus should be present
  - Interface changes
  - Basement membrane thickening
  - Follicular plugging
  - Perivascular and periadnexal lymphocytic infiltrate

Hypertrophic Lichen Planus
- Hyperplasia of epidermis
- Lichenoid lymphocytic infiltrate concentrated at tips of elongated rete
- Clinically often on lower legs; pruritic

Pyodermatitis Vegetans
- Vegetating plaque with pustules
- May be associated with inflammatory bowel disease
- Florid epithelial hyperplasia with eosinophilic/neutrophilic abscesses
- Direct immunofluorescence negative
- Clinicopathologic correlation important

Pemphigus Vegetans
- Florid epithelial hyperplasia with eosinophilic abscesses
- Direct immunofluorescence positive for intercellular IgG &/or C3

Halogenoderma (Iododerma, Bromoderma)
- Florid hyperplasia of epidermis secondary to ingestion of halogens

DIAGNOSTIC CHECKLIST

Pathologic Interpretation Pearls
- Currently, evaluation of hematoxylin and eosin stained sections is gold standard
- Special stains for infectious organisms often performed
- Special immunohistochemical stains are not routinely performed

SELECTED REFERENCES
1. Kluger N et al: Pseudoepitheliomatous epidermal hyperplasia in tattoos: report of three cases. Am J Clin Dermatol. 9(5):337-40, 2008
2. Daldon PE et al: Hypertrophic lupus erythematosus: a clinicopathological study of 14 cases. J Cutan Pathol. 30(7):443-8, 2003
3. Lee ES et al: Pseudoepitheliomatous hyperplasia in lichen sclerosus of the vulva. Int J Gynecol Pathol. 22(1):57-62, 2003
4. Kamino H et al: Malignant melanoma with pseudocarcinomatous hyperplasia--an entity that can simulate squamous cell carcinoma. A light-microscopic and immunohistochemical study of four cases. Am J Dermatopathol. 12(5):446-51, 1990
5. Grunwald MH et al: Pseudocarcinomatous hyperplasia. Am J Dermatopathol. 10(2):95-103, 1988

IMAGE GALLERY

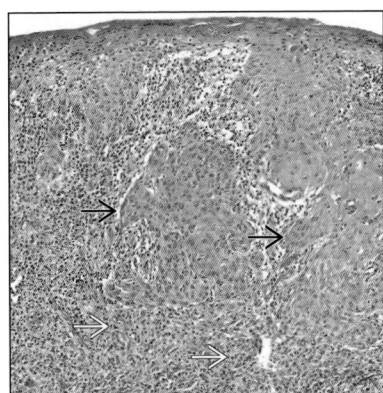 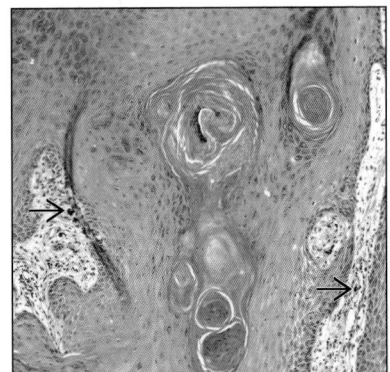 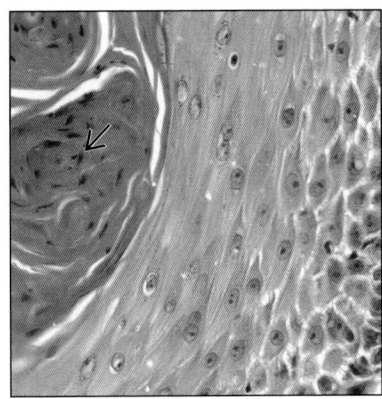

(Left) In this pseudoepitheliomatous hyperplasia ➔ above a primary cutaneous anaplastic large cell lymphoma, the epithelium is obscured by large lymphocytes ➔ and eosinophils. (Center) Pseudoepitheliomatous hyperplasia associated with a tattoo shows prominent epidermal hyperplasia above black tattoo pigment ➔. (Right) Cytologic atypia is absent in pseudoepitheliomatous hyperplasia. There is parakeratosis ➔, but a true squamous pearl is not evident.

WARTY DYSKERATOMA

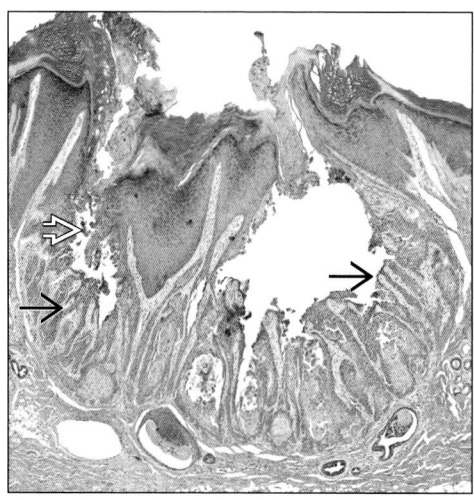

This is a low-power view of a warty dyskeratoma, a cup-shaped lesion. There is hyperkeratosis and parakeratosis above central acantholytic dyskeratosis ⇨ with villi at the base ⇨.

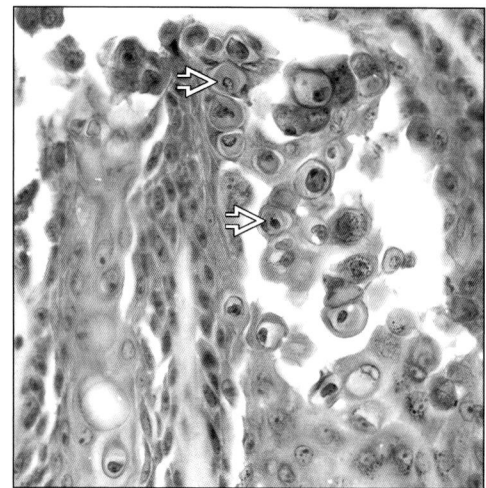

A high-power view shows the central acantholytic dyskeratosis in a warty dyskeratoma. There are corp ronds (central round to slightly oval shrunken nuclei with surrounding pink cytoplasm) ⇨.

TERMINOLOGY

Abbreviations
- Warty dyskeratoma (WD)

Definitions
- Cup-shaped epidermal proliferation
- Acantholysis is present
- Dyskeratosis (corp ronds and grains) is present

ETIOLOGY/PATHOGENESIS

Pathophysiology
- Germline mutations in *ATP2A2* not described (as are seen in Darier disease)
- Human papilloma virus infection has not been associated with WD

CLINICAL ISSUES

Epidemiology
- Age
  - Middle-aged to older patients

Site
- Often on head or neck
- May be in genital area
- Mucosal lesions uncommon but described

Presentation
- Solitary
- Very rarely multiple
- Umbilicated papule or nodule

Treatment
- Biopsy/excision generally curative

Prognosis
- Benign, no malignant potential

MICROSCOPIC PATHOLOGY

Histologic Features
- Cup-shaped lesion
- Occasionally cystic or nodular
- May be associated with hair follicles in some cases
- Hyperkeratosis and parakeratosis
- Suprabasilar acantholysis
- Corp ronds and grains
- Villi at base
- Mixed inflammatory infiltrate in dermis

Cytologic Features
- Corp ronds (dyskeratotic cells with round to slightly oval nucleus with eosinophilic cytoplasm)
- Grains (raisinoid nuclei with dense eosinophilic cytoplasm)
- Minimal to no cytologic atypia

DIFFERENTIAL DIAGNOSIS

Darier Disease
- Autosomal dominant genetic disorder
- Mutations in *ATP2A2* gene
- Multiple, hyperkeratotic, "greasy" papules
- Seborrheic (face, scalp, chest, upper back) distribution
- Histology similar to WD
  - Acantholysis and dyskeratosis beneath hyperkeratosis
  - Clinicopathologic correlation necessary

Grover Disease
- Multiple, slightly eroded papules
- May be pruritic
- Affects chest and upper back
- Middle-aged to older males
- Histology may be similar to WD

WARTY DYSKERATOMA

Key Facts

Clinical Issues
- Solitary (very rarely multiple)
- Umbilicated papule or nodule
- Often on head or neck

Microscopic Pathology
- Cup-shaped lesion
- Sometimes associated with hair follicles
- Hyperkeratosis and parakeratosis
- Suprabasilar acantholysis with villi at base

- Mixed inflammatory infiltrate in dermis
- Corp ronds (round to slightly oval nucleus with pink cytoplasm) are present
- Grains (raisinoid nuclei with pink cytoplasm) present
- Minimal to no cytologic atypia

Top Differential Diagnoses
- Darier disease
- Acantholytic dyskeratotic acanthoma
- Acantholytic squamous cell carcinoma

- o More commonly, acantholysis and dyskeratosis limited to a few rete, without prominent overlying hyperkeratosis
- Multiple patterns of acantholysis may be present
  - o Warty dyskeratoma-like
  - o Full-thickness acantholysis (Hailey-Hailey-like)
  - o Suprabasilar acantholysis (pemphigus vulgaris-like)
  - o Subcorneal acantholysis

Acantholytic Acanthoma
- Solitary lesion
- Often on trunk of middle-aged to older individuals
- Unlike WD, dyskeratosis is not present

Acantholytic Dyskeratotic Acanthoma
- Solitary lesion
- Often on trunk of middle-aged to older individuals
- Like WD, acantholysis and dyskeratosis present
- Unlike WD, overall architecture is flat
  - o Not cup-shaped
  - o Not associated with hair follicles

Acantholytic Actinic Keratosis
- Generally not cup-shaped
- Typically spares hair follicles
- Cytologic atypia present in basal layer with acantholysis
- Corp ronds and grains not prominent

Acantholytic Squamous Cell Carcinoma
- Endophytic lesion
- Infiltrative growth pattern

- Acantholysis present
- Corp ronds and grains not prominent
- Cytologic atypia and mitoses usually easily identified

Acantholytic Dermatosis of the Genital (Vulvocrural) Area
- Multiple papules and plaques in genital area
- Lesions with similar histology absent on other areas of body
- More common in women
- Histology may be WD-like or show acantholysis without dyskeratosis

DIAGNOSTIC CHECKLIST

Pathologic Interpretation Pearls
- Cup-shaped lesion with hyperkeratosis
- Suprabasilar acantholysis
- Corp ronds and grains
- Minimal to no cytologic atypia

SELECTED REFERENCES

1. Kaddu S et al: Warty dyskeratoma--"follicular dyskeratoma": analysis of clinicopathologic features of a distinctive follicular adnexal neoplasm. J Am Acad Dermatol. 47(3):423-8, 2002
2. Cooper PH: Acantholytic dermatosis localized to the vulvocrural area. J Cutan Pathol. 16(2):81-4, 1989
3. Brownstein MH: The benign acanthomas. J Cutan Pathol. 12(3-4):172-88, 1985

IMAGE GALLERY

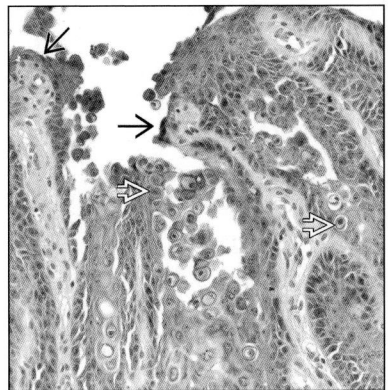
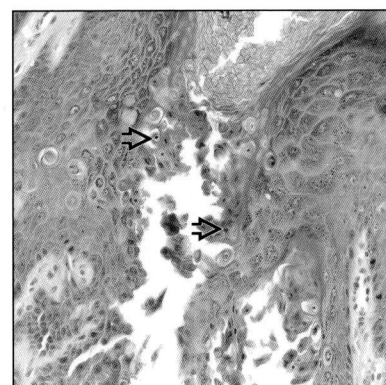
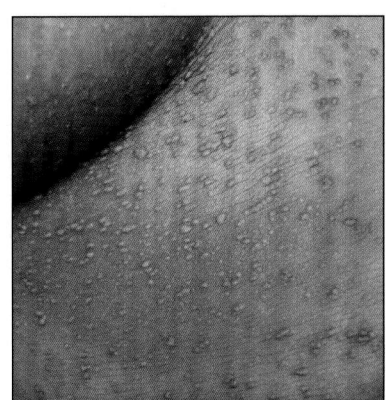

(Left) H&E shows villi (papillary dermis covered by a layer of epithelium) ➡ with central acantholytic dyskeratosis (corp ronds ▶). *(Center)* Higher magnification shows numerous grains ➡ below hyperkeratosis. *(Right)* Histopathologic findings of warty dyskeratoma and Darier disease can be identical; therefore, clinical findings are essential to distinguish these entities. Darier disease shows multiple papules (pictured). In contrast, warty dyskeratoma is a solitary lesion.

ACANTHOLYTIC AND ACANTHOLYTIC DYSKERATOTIC ACANTHOMA

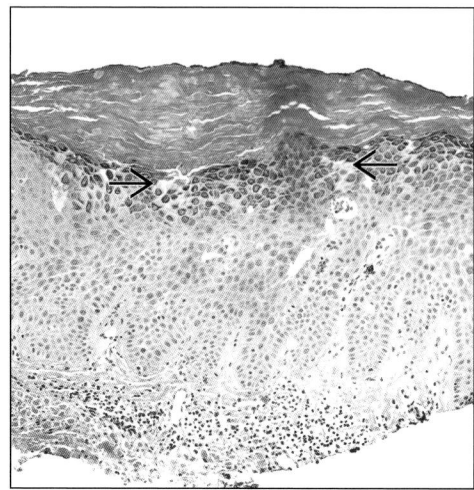

An acantholytic acanthoma is a solitary keratosis characterized by acantholysis (dyscohesion of keratinocytes) ➡, which is full thickness in this example. There is a lack of dyskeratosis (corp ronds and grains).

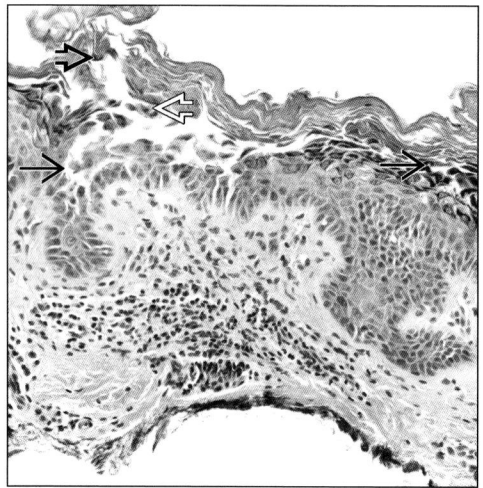

An acantholytic dyskeratotic acanthoma is a solitary keratosis with acantholysis ➡ and dyskeratosis (corp ronds ➡ and grains ➡). The overall architecture is flat and plaque-like.

TERMINOLOGY

Synonyms
- Some consider these 2 entities synonymous
- Criterion used to "split" these into 2 entities is presence or absence of dyskeratosis (corp ronds and grains)

Definitions
- Benign lesions with flat, plaque-like architecture and acantholysis
- **Acantholytic acanthoma**
  - Lacks dyskeratosis (corp ronds and grains)
- **Acantholytic dyskeratotic acanthoma**
  - Dyskeratosis (corp ronds and grains) present

CLINICAL ISSUES

Presentation
- Generally a solitary papule
- Often on trunk
- Often submitted as "rule out basal cell carcinoma"

Treatment
- Biopsy generally curative

Prognosis
- Benign, no malignant potential

MICROSCOPIC PATHOLOGY

Histologic Features
- Acantholytic and acantholytic dyskeratotic acanthoma
  - Flat, plaque-like architecture
- Acantholytic acanthoma
  - Acantholysis without dyskeratosis
  - Acantholysis may be suprabasilar or full thickness
- Acantholytic dyskeratotic acanthoma
  - Acantholysis with dyskeratosis (corp ronds and grains)
  - Acantholysis may be suprabasilar or subcorneal

Cytologic Features
- Acantholytic and acantholytic dyskeratotic acanthoma
  - Minimal to no cytologic atypia
  - Rounding up of keratinocytes (acantholysis)
- Acantholytic dyskeratotic acanthoma
  - Corp ronds (round to minimally oval nuclei with surrounding pink cytoplasm) present
  - Grains (raisinoid, shrunken nuclei with pink cytoplasm) present

DIFFERENTIAL DIAGNOSIS

Warty Dyskeratoma
- Often on head and neck
- Hyperkeratosis over cup-shaped lesion
- Sometimes associated with hair follicles
- Corp ronds and grains present

Acantholytic Actinic Keratosis
- Cytologic atypia present in basal layer with acantholysis
- Corp ronds and grains not prominent

Acantholytic Squamous Cell Carcinoma
- Endophytic and infiltrative growth pattern
- Acantholysis of atypical keratinocytes
- Corp ronds and grains not prominent
- Atypical mitoses present

Grover Disease
- Multiple slightly eroded papules
- Affects chest and upper back
- Affects middle-aged to older men
- Often is pruritic
- Acantholysis limited to a few rete
- Lacks prominent overlying hyperkeratosis

ACANTHOLYTIC AND ACANTHOLYTIC DYSKERATOTIC ACANTHOMA

Key Facts

Clinical Issues
- Generally a solitary papule
- Often on trunk
- Often submitted as "rule out basal cell carcinoma"

Microscopic Pathology
- Flat, plaque-like architecture
- Minimal to no cytologic atypia
- Acantholytic acanthoma
  - Acantholysis without dyskeratosis
- Acantholytic dyskeratotic acanthoma
  - Acantholysis with dyskeratosis (corp ronds and grains)

Top Differential Diagnoses
- Warty dyskeratoma
- Acantholytic actinic keratosis
- Grover disease
- Acantholytic dermatosis of genital area
- Hailey-Hailey disease

- Multiple patterns of acantholysis may be present
  - Darier-like (acantholysis and dyskeratosis)
  - Full-thickness acantholysis
  - Suprabasilar acantholysis
  - Subcorneal acantholysis

Acantholytic Dermatosis of Genital (Vulvocrural) Area
- Multiple papules and plaques in genital area
- Lesions with similar histology absent on other areas of body
- Histology can be identical to acantholytic acanthoma or acantholytic dyskeratotic acanthoma (clinical history key)

Hailey-Hailey Disease
- Eroded, macerated, erythematous plaques in intertriginous areas
- Histology shows full-thickness acantholysis
- Generally lacks dyskeratosis

Pemphigus Vulgaris and Foliaceus
- Immunobullous disorders with acantholysis
- Multiple flaccid blisters and erosions generally present
- Pemphigus vulgaris: Suprabasilar acantholysis, lacks dyskeratosis, involves adnexal structures
- Pemphigus foliaceus: Subcorneal acantholysis
- Direct immunofluorescence shows intercellular staining with IgG and C3

Darier Disease
- Autosomal dominant genetic disorder
- Multiple hyperkeratotic, "greasy" papules
- Seborrheic (face, scalp, chest, upper back) distribution
- Acantholysis and dyskeratosis beneath hyperkeratosis

DIAGNOSTIC CHECKLIST

Pathologic Interpretation Pearls
- Acantholytic and acantholytic dyskeratotic acanthoma
  - Flat, plaque-like architecture
  - Rounding up of keratinocytes (acantholysis)
  - Minimal to no cytologic atypia
- Acantholytic acanthoma
  - Acantholysis
    - Suprabasilar or full thickness
- Acantholytic dyskeratotic acanthoma
  - Acantholysis
    - Suprabasilar or subcorneal
  - Corp ronds (round to minimally oval nuclei with surrounding pink cytoplasm) present
  - Grains (raisinoid, shrunken nuclei with pink cytoplasm) present

SELECTED REFERENCES
1. Ko CJ et al: Acantholytic dyskeratotic acanthoma: a variant of a benign keratosis. J Cutan Pathol. 35(3):298-301, 2008
2. Omulecki A et al: Plaque form of warty dyskeratoma - acantholytic dyskeratotic acanthoma. J Cutan Pathol. 34(6):494-6, 2007
3. Cooper PH: Acantholytic dermatosis localized to the vulvocrural area. J Cutan Pathol. 16(2):81-4, 1989

IMAGE GALLERY

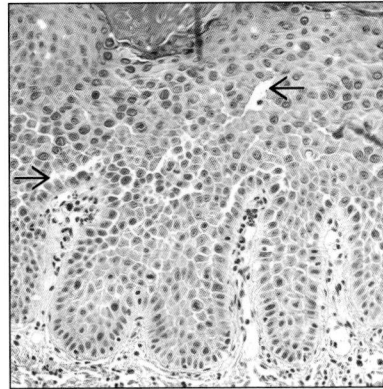 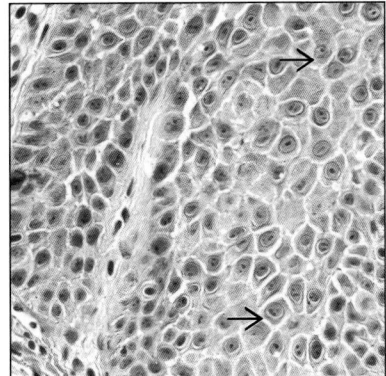 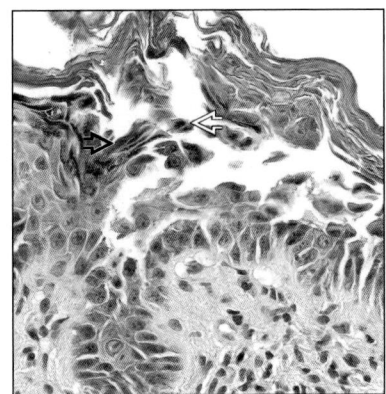

(Left) Intermediate-magnification view of an acantholytic acanthoma shows dyscohesion of keratinocytes (acantholysis) ➡. Dyskeratosis is absent. *(Center)* High-magnification view of an acantholytic acanthoma reveals acantholytic cells that lack cytologic atypia and have pink cytoplasm ➡ due to clumped tonofilaments. *(Right)* High-magnification view of an acantholytic dyskeratotic acanthoma with corp ronds ➡ and grains ➡ is shown. The lesion is flat and plaque-like.

VERRUCA VULGARIS (AND VARIANTS)

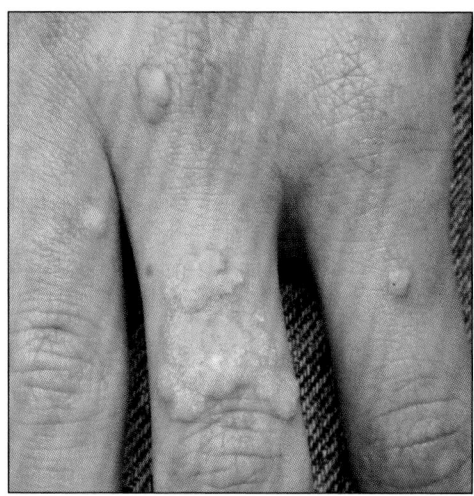

Clinical photograph shows multiple verrucae on the dorsal hand and fingers. (Courtesy J. Wu, MD.)

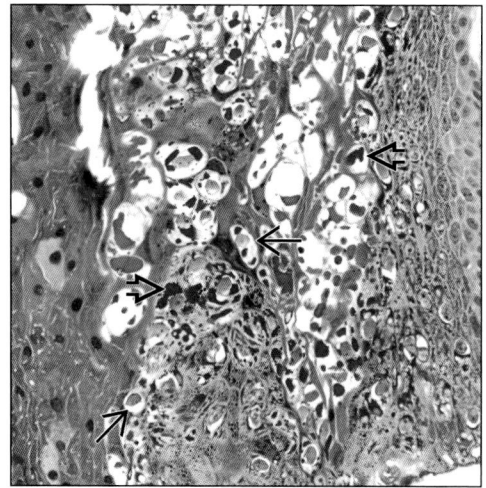

Palmoplantar warts (myrmecia) often show especially prominent koilocytes with perinuclear halos ➡ and large, dense keratohyaline inclusions ▷.

TERMINOLOGY

Abbreviations
- Verruca vulgaris (VV)

Synonyms
- Common warts
- **Variants**
  - Palmoplantar warts (myrmecia)
  - Flat warts (verruca plana)

Definitions
- HPV-related benign epidermal proliferation

ETIOLOGY/PATHOGENESIS

Infectious Agents
- Causal relationship established with numerous HPV types, including HPV 1, 2, 3, 4, 7, 10, 27, 29, 57
  - Most common types include 1, 2, 3, 4, 7, 10

CLINICAL ISSUES

Epidemiology
- Incidence
  - Very common lesions
- Age
  - Common in children and young adults but can occur at any age

Site
- Common sites include fingers and dorsal hands (verruca vulgaris), palms and soles (palmoplantar warts), face and dorsal hands (flat warts)

Presentation
- Small papular to plaque-like lesions

Natural History
- Grow rapidly, then stabilize

- Some lesions may regress

Treatment
- Surgical approaches
  - Complete excision is curative but not necessary in most cases
- Drugs
  - Topical therapy with podophyllin or other antiviral medications

Prognosis
- Excellent, unless immunosuppressed
  - Rare cases of cutaneous carcinoma are associated with various HPV types, especially in immunosuppressed patients

MACROSCOPIC FEATURES

General Features
- Often exophytic-appearing scaly (hyperkeratotic) lesion

Size
- May be small (several mm) papules to large plaques (several cm)

MICROSCOPIC PATHOLOGY

Histologic Features
- Exophytic and endophytic papillomatous epidermal proliferation
  - Epidermal acanthosis with hypergranulosis, dense overlying hyperkeratosis, and tiers of parakeratosis ("church spires")
    - Flat warts show acanthosis and hyperkeratosis, but they lack significant papillomatosis and parakeratosis
  - Intracorneal hemorrhage typically present

VERRUCA VULGARIS (AND VARIANTS)

Key Facts

Terminology
- Verruca vulgaris (VV)
- Common warts
- Palmoplantar warts (myrmecia)
- Flat warts (verruca plana)

Etiology/Pathogenesis
- Causal relationship with numerous HPV types

Clinical Issues
- Common sites include fingers and hands (verruca vulgaris), palms and soles (palmoplantar warts), face and dorsal hands (flat warts)

Microscopic Pathology
- Exophytic/endophytic papillomatous proliferation with hypergranulosis, dense overlying hyperkeratosis, and tiers of parakeratosis

- Intracorneal hemorrhage typically present
- Periphery often shows "pointing inward" of the basilar epidermis
- Superficial keratinocytes show perinuclear halos and prominent keratohyaline granules
  - Palmoplantar warts show especially prominent keratohyaline inclusions
- Lesions may be irritated and inflamed, often associated with reactive atypia

Top Differential Diagnoses
- Verrucous keratosis
- Seborrheic keratosis (SK)
- Lichen simplex chronicus (LSC)
- Hypertrophic lichen planus (LP)
- Verrucous carcinoma
- Epidermodysplasia verruciformis (EDV)

- Periphery of lesion shows pointing ("toeing") inward of the basilar epidermis
- Superficial keratinocytes may show perinuclear halos and prominent keratohyaline granules
  - Palmoplantar warts (myrmecia) show especially prominent keratohyaline inclusions, which appear basophilic
  - Palmoplantar warts may also show prominent intranuclear basophilic inclusions
- Keratinocytes may be mildly enlarged and atypical-appearing, but no high-grade cytologic atypia or pleomorphism is present
- Mitotic figures often present within basilar layer, especially in irritated/inflamed lesions, but are not present in upper levels of epidermis
- Lesions may be irritated and inflamed, often associated with reactive atypia
- Dermal papillae often show dilated capillaries

DIFFERENTIAL DIAGNOSIS

Verrucous Keratosis
- Epidermal proliferation with acanthosis and irregular papillomatosis; lacks diagnostic features of VV
- May represent a variant of hypertrophic seborrheic keratosis lacking more classic features
- Often used for partial, nondiagnostic biopsies, in which the lesion cannot be accurately classified due to incomplete examination

Seborrheic Keratosis (SK)
- Verrucous SK shows epidermal hyperplasia with papillomatous projections
- Intraepidermal pseudohorn cysts filled with keratin whorls
- Often pigmented, at least focally

Lichen Simplex Chronicus (LSC)
- Irregular epidermal hyperplasia with hypergranulosis and overlying hyperkeratosis
- Lacks tiers of parakeratosis and "toeing in" of peripheral epidermis

Hypertrophic Lichen Planus (LP)
- Shows irregular epidermal acanthosis, often with "sawtooth" pattern
- More endophytic than VV, which is endo-/exophytic
- Superficial dermis shows dense band-like chronic inflammatory infiltrate

Verrucous Carcinoma
- Papillomatous epidermal proliferation demonstrating prominent elongated, bulbous rete ridges extending deeply into dermis
- Lesion shows bland cytologic features, demonstrating large squamous keratinocytes with abundant dense eosinophilic cytoplasm

Epidermodysplasia Verruciformis (EDV)
- May be inherited (genodermatosis) or related to immunosuppression (i.e., AIDS)
- Typically associated with HPV types 3, 5, 10
- Histologic features are similar to verruca plana, but keratinocytes show basophilic cytoplasm and prominent keratohyaline granules

SELECTED REFERENCES

1. Joly P et al: Squamous cell carcinomas are associated with verrucokeratotic cutaneous lesions but not with common warts in organ-transplant patients. A case-control study. Transplantation. 89(10):1224-30, 2010
2. Barcelos AC et al: Comparative analysis of the expression of cytokeratins (1, 10, 14, 16, 4), involucrin, filaggrin and e-cadherin in plane warts and epidermodysplasia verruciformis plane wart-type lesions. J Cutan Pathol. 36(6):647-54, 2009
3. Dhar SB et al: Intralesional bleomycin in the treatment of cutaneous warts: a randomized clinical trial comparing it with cryotherapy. Indian J Dermatol Venereol Leprol. 75(3):262-7, 2009
4. Mammas I et al: High-risk human papilloma viruses (HPVs) were not detected in the benign skin lesions of a small number of children. Acta Paediatr. 97(12):1669-71, 2008
5. Nunes Mde G et al: Human papillomavirus detection and typification in cutaneous and mucosal lesions of HIV-seropositive patients. Int J STD AIDS. 19(9):611-6, 2008

Microscopic Features

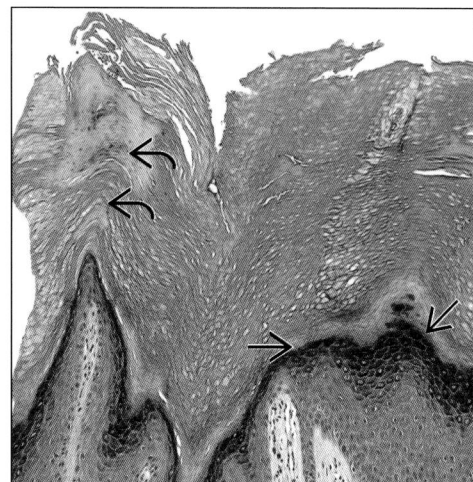

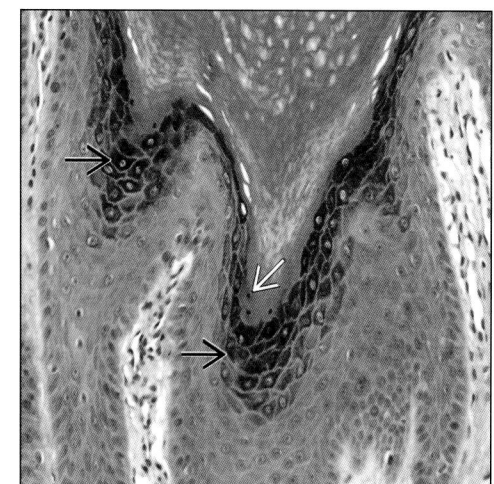

(Left) Low magnification of the surface of a VV shows epidermal papillomatosis with hypergranulosis ➡ and overlying dense hyperkeratosis and tiers of parakeratosis ➡. *(Right)* High magnification of a VV shows prominent granular layer ➡ with focal parakeratosis ➡.

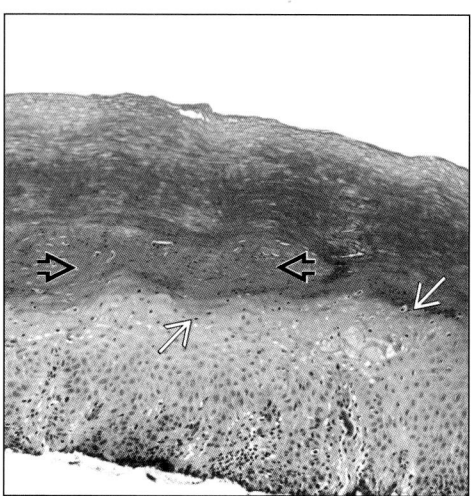

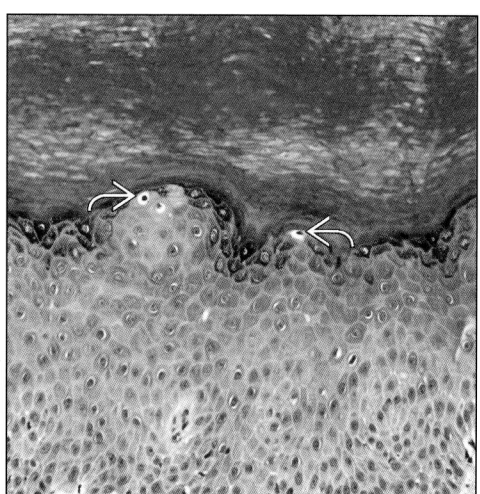

(Left) Low magnification of a flat wart demonstrates mild epidermal acanthosis and dense overlying hyperkeratosis and parakeratosis. This lesion was treated (with liquid nitrogen) prior to biopsy, and it shows prominent intracorneal hemorrhage ➡ and superficial necrosis ➡, consistent with treatment effects. *(Right)* High magnification of a flat wart shows hypergranulosis, dense hyperkeratosis, and scattered superficial koilocytic cells ➡ with perinuclear halos.

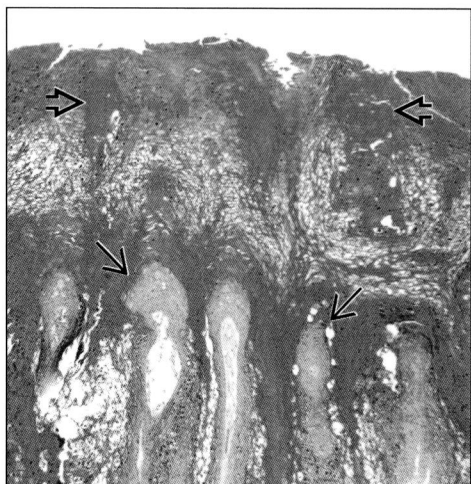

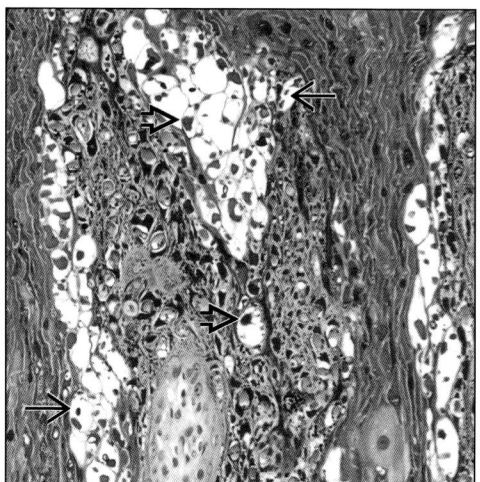

(Left) Scanning magnification of a palmoplantar wart (myrmecia) shows prominent papillomatosis ➡ with thick overlying hyperkeratosis and parakeratosis with areas of hemorrhage ➡. *(Right)* Palmoplantar wart at high magnification shows especially prominent koilocytes with perinuclear halos ➡ and large, dense keratohyaline inclusions ➡.

VERRUCA VULGARIS (AND VARIANTS)

Differential Diagnosis

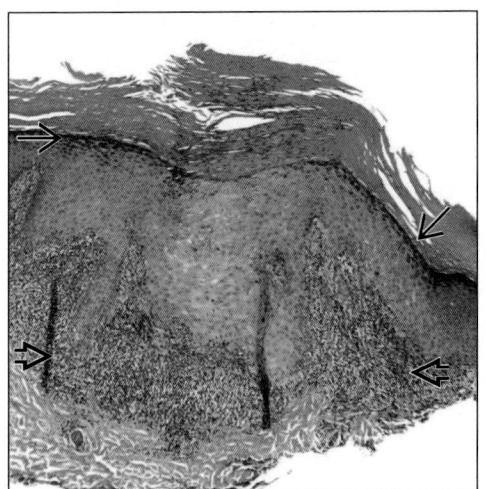

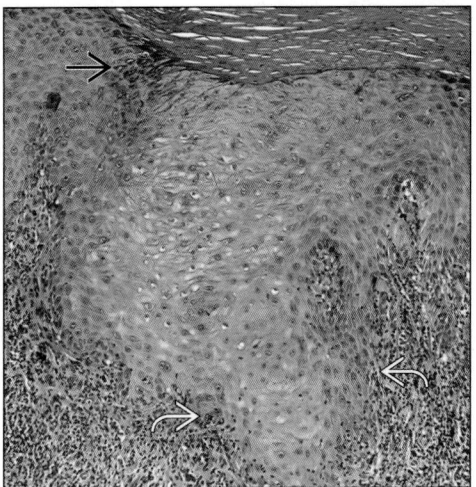

(Left) Hypertrophic lichen planus (LP) shows irregular epidermal acanthosis with an endophytic growth pattern and overlying hypergranulosis ➡ and hyperkeratosis. Note the band-like inflammatory infiltrate ➡ in the dermis, characteristic of LP. *(Right)* High magnification of hypertrophic LP shows epidermal acanthosis with hypergranulosis ➡. The superficial dermis shows a dense lymphoid infiltrate with scattered exocytosis into the basilar epithelium ➡.

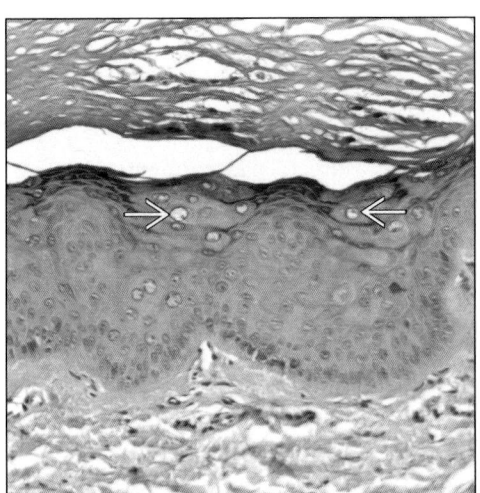

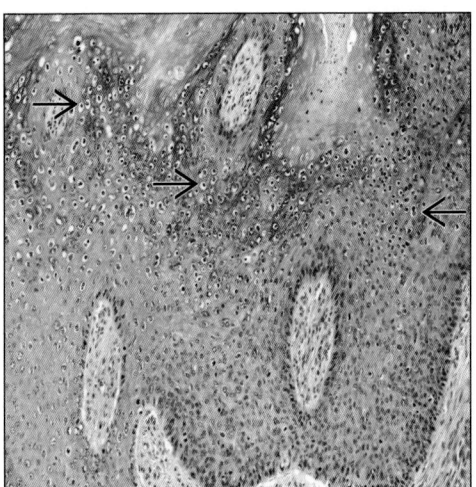

(Left) An example of epidermodysplasia verruciformis shows mild epidermal acanthosis and a proliferation of enlarged, bluish gray-staining keratinocytes with nuclear clearing ➡. *(Right)* A rare example of squamous cell carcinoma in situ (Bowen disease) arising in association with a VV is shown. Note the numerous superficial koilocytes ➡.

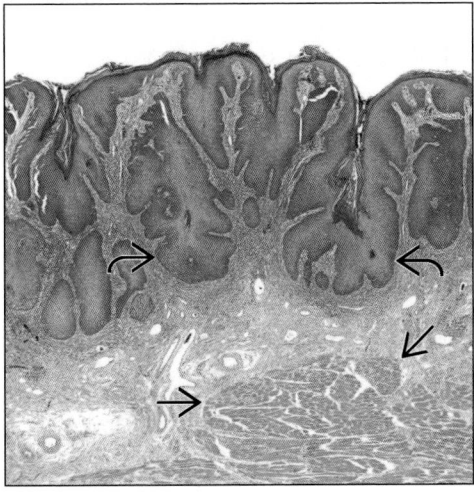

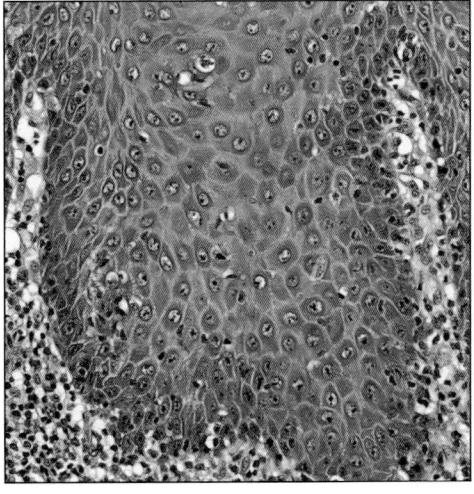

(Left) Verrucous carcinoma shows prominent endophytic downgrowths with bulbous rete ridges ➡ surrounded by chronic inflammation. Note the deep "pushing invasion" approaching bundles of skeletal muscle ➡. *(Right)* High magnification of a verrucous carcinoma shows the bland cytologic features of the squamous cells. The cells are enlarged and show abundant dense, eosinophilic cytoplasm, but there is minimal cytologic atypia.

CONDYLOMA ACUMINATUM (GENITAL WART)

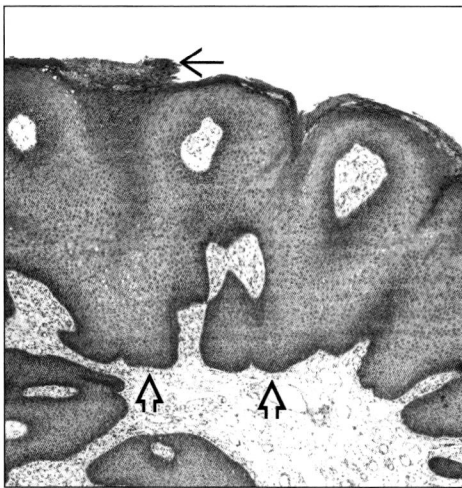

Condyloma acuminatum is characterized by marked acanthosis, slight (as in this example) to marked papillomatosis, and sharply demarcated bulbous base ➡. Note the focal parakeratosis ➡.

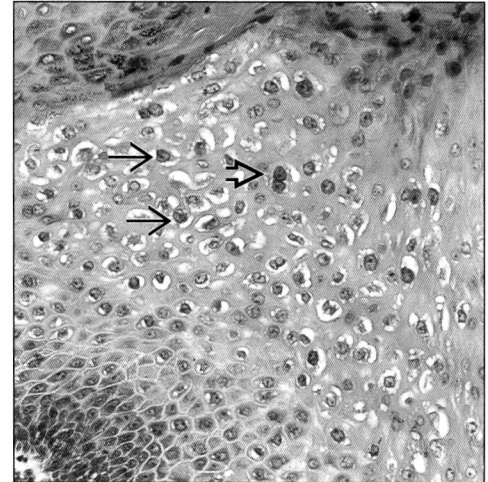

Koilocytes are characterized by clear perinuclear halos ➡ and wrinkled and hyperchromatic nuclei. Binucleation is common ➡. The cytoplasm is eosinophilic.

TERMINOLOGY

Synonyms
- Genital wart

Definitions
- Exophytic and verruciform nonmalignant epithelial lesions

ETIOLOGY/PATHOGENESIS

Infectious Agents
- Caused by human papillomavirus (HPV)
  - Low-risk serotypes 6 and 11 (90% of cases)
  - Other serotypes include 16, 18, 30-32, 42-44, 51-55
  - > 1 serotype may be found in a lesion

CLINICAL ISSUES

Epidemiology
- Incidence
  - Very common sexually transmitted disease
- Age
  - Most frequent in young adults (2nd and 3rd decades of life)
  - Uncommon in children
    - Such cases should raise suspicion of sexual abuse

Site
- Predilection for anogenital area
  - Males: Glans, prepuce, shaft
    - May extend to meatus
  - Females: Labia minora, interlabial sulcus, area around introitus
    - May extend into introitus
  - Both sexes: Perianal and more rarely oral cavity

Presentation
- Soft fleshy verruciform plaques
- Filiform lesions
- Lesion in coronal sulcus and vulva may be bulkier and macerated
- Some lesions may be almost flat and difficult to detect

Treatment
- For small tumors: Cryosurgery, electrofulguration, laser ablation, and topical treatments
- For medium-sized and large tumors: Surgical excision

Prognosis
- Malignant transformation is rare in condyloma acuminatum
- Patients with condyloma often have other sexually transmitted diseases

MACROSCOPIC FEATURES

General Features
- Size ranges from few mm to several cm

MICROSCOPIC PATHOLOGY

Histologic Features
- Arborescent acanthotic papillae with prominent fibrovascular cores
  - Some lesions may be flat
- Variable parakeratosis and orthokeratosis
- Koilocytosis
  - Best seen in upper portion of epithelium of papillae and upper portion of declivities
  - Koilocytes exhibit perinuclear vacuolization
  - Wrinkled and hyperchromatic nuclei
  - Frequent bi- and multinucleation
- Sharply defined base that is broad and flat
- Condylomata may show horn pseudocysts
- Old condylomata may show little to no koilocytosis
  - Old condylomata may look very similar to seborrheic keratoses

CONDYLOMA ACUMINATUM (GENITAL WART)

Key Facts

Etiology/Pathogenesis
- HPV-related lesion
- Low-risk HPV serotypes (6, 11) predominate

Macroscopic Features
- From flat to exophilic cauliflower-like lesions
- Measuring from a few mm to several cm

Microscopic Pathology
- Acanthosis with variable papillomatosis and prominent fibrovascular cores
- Broad and sharply defined lower border
- Conspicuous koilocytosis
  - Irregular wrinkled nuclei
  - Bi- and multinucleation
  - Perinuclear vacuolization

Top Differential Diagnoses
- Verrucous carcinoma
- Giant condyloma (Buschke-Löwenstein tumor)
- Warty carcinoma
- Papillary carcinoma, NOS
- Papillomatosis of glans corona (pearly penile papules)
- Bowenoid papulosis
- Squamous cell carcinoma in situ (SCCis)

  - Seborrheic keratosis-like lesions in genital areas are very often associated with HPV
- Condylomata treated with resin of podophyllin
  - May show pallor of upper epithelium
  - Nuclear enlargement
  - Increased numbers of mitotic figures (not atypical)
  - Scattered necrotic keratinocytes
  - Differential diagnosis includes carcinoma in situ and bowenoid papulosis
    - History of treatment is important
  - Changes disappear after a week

Cytologic Features
- Koilocytosis

DIFFERENTIAL DIAGNOSIS

Verrucous Carcinoma
- May be HPV-unrelated in some cases (no koilocytosis)
- Acanthotic papillae with thin fibrovascular cores
- Minimal cytologic atypia
- Broad and pushing tumor base

Giant Condyloma (Buschke-Löwenstein Tumor)
- Condyloma measuring > 5 cm in size
- More prominent endophytic pattern of growth
- May harbor foci of squamous cell carcinoma (SCC)
  - Malignant foci tend to be located in deep portions
  - Keratinizing SCC of usual type is most commonly associated subtype
  - Generous sampling of giant condylomata is recommended

Warty Carcinoma
- Affects older patients
- Associated with high-risk HPV
- Koilocytes frequently show pleomorphism and numerous mitoses
- Jagged and irregular tumor base
- Usually positive for p16 overexpression

Papillary Carcinoma, NOS
- HPV-unrelated (no koilocytosis)
- Complex papillae with irregular fibrovascular cores
- Cytologic atypia ranges from mild to moderate
- Jagged and irregular tumor base

Papillomatosis of Glans Corona (Pearly Penile Papules)
- Very common (about 1/3 of normal males)
- Uniform small lesions arranged in 2-3 rows on dorsal aspect of glans corona
- Histologically correspond to small fibroepithelial papillomas with no koilocytosis

Bowenoid Papulosis
- Condylomata after treatment with podophyllin may mimic bowenoid papulosis

Squamous Cell Carcinoma In Situ (SCCis)
- Condylomata after treatment with podophyllin may mimic SCCis
- Atypical mitosis should not be seen in treated condylomata
- History of treatment is important to make distinction

DIAGNOSTIC CHECKLIST

Pathologic Interpretation Pearls
- Condylomata treated with podophyllin may show degenerative changes including nuclear enlargement and metaphase arrest

SELECTED REFERENCES

1. Nordenvall C et al: Cancer risk among patients with condylomata acuminata. Int J Cancer. 119(4):888-93, 2006
2. Li J et al: "Seborrheic keratoses" that contain human papillomavirus are condylomata acuminata. Am J Dermatopathol. 16(4):398-405; discussion 406-8, 1994
3. Wade TR et al: The effects of resin of podophyllin on condyloma acuminatum. Am J Dermatopathol. 6(2):109-22, 1984

CONDYLOMA ACUMINATUM (GENITAL WART)

Microscopic Features

(Left) Condyloma acuminatum shows an exophytic papillomatous growth, regular and broad tumor base, and easily recognizable fibrovascular cores ➡. **(Right)** Condyloma acuminatum is characterized by papillomatosis with acanthotic epithelium and prominent fibrovascular cores ➡. Koilocytes ➡ are easily found.

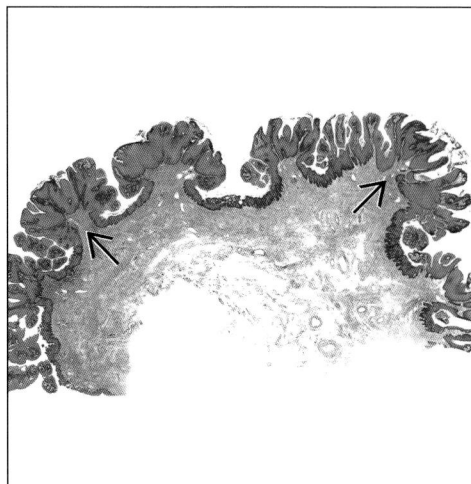
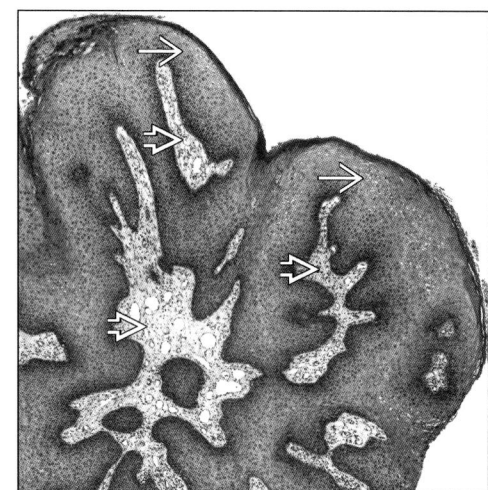

(Left) High magnification shows koilocytes ➡ with perinuclear vacuolization and wrinkled nuclei seen in the upper portions of the acanthotic papilla. There is also parakeratosis with large nuclei ➡. **(Right)** Koilocytosis may be less evident in older condylomata. Furthermore, such lesions may show horn pseudocysts, mimicking a seborrheic keratosis. However, most of these lesions are positive for HPV by in situ hybridization or immunohistochemistry.

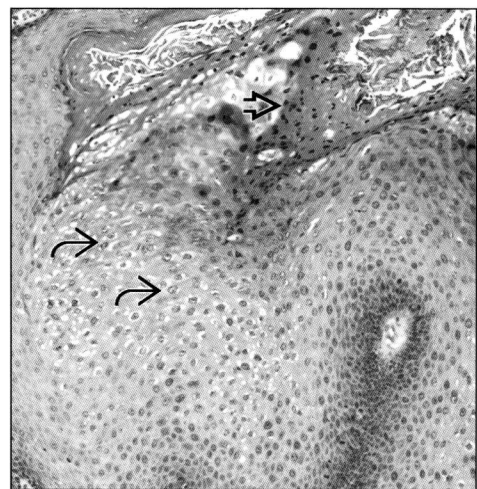
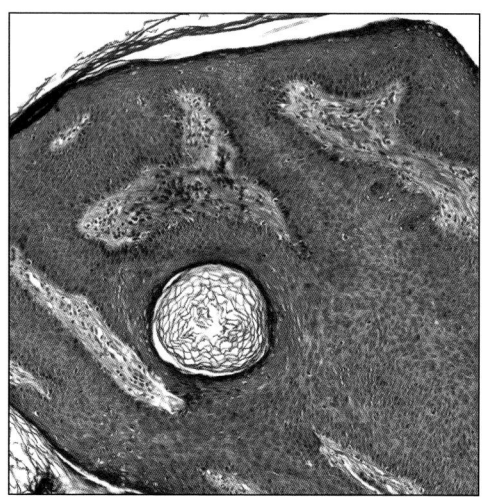

(Left) In situ hybridization shows strongly positive nuclear staining for low-risk HPV 6. **(Right)** HPV 6 is the most frequent genotype associated with condyloma acuminatum as supported by in situ hybridization in this case. Dark blue nuclear staining ➡ indicates a positive result.

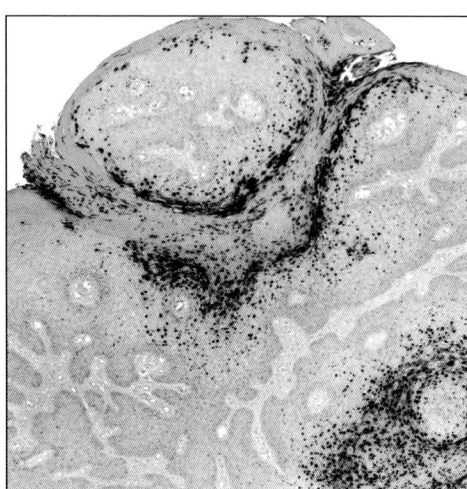
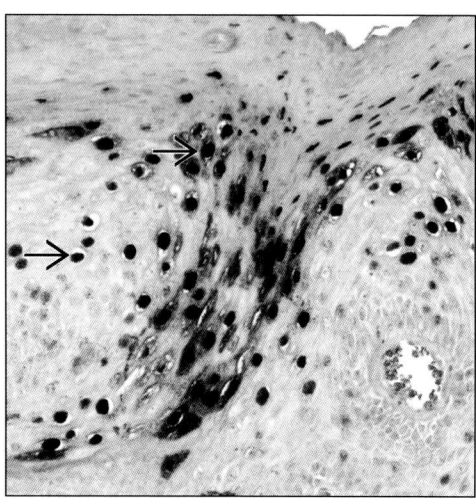

CONDYLOMA ACUMINATUM (GENITAL WART)

Giant Condyloma and Differential Diagnosis

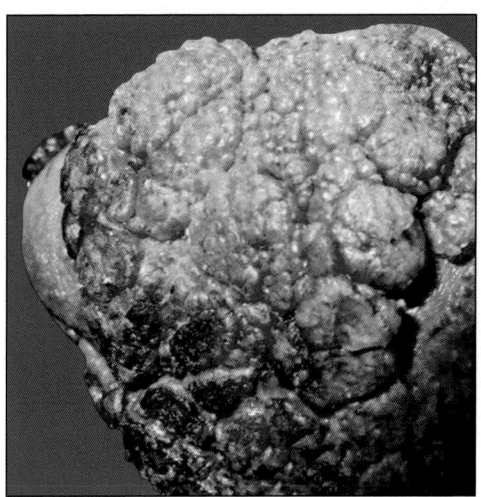

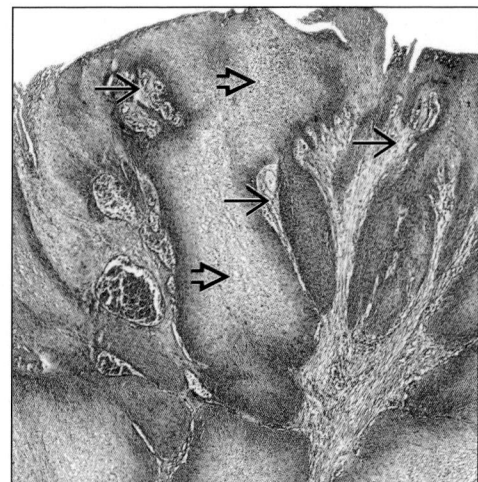

(Left) Giant condyloma affecting the distal penis is shown. Note the large exophytic tumoral growth with a "cobblestone" and cauliflower-like appearance. (Right) Giant condyloma is characterized by marked acanthosis and an endophytic pattern of growth with bulbous extension of the base, prominent fibrovascular cores ⊡, and clear areas ⊡, which correspond to koilocytosis at higher power.

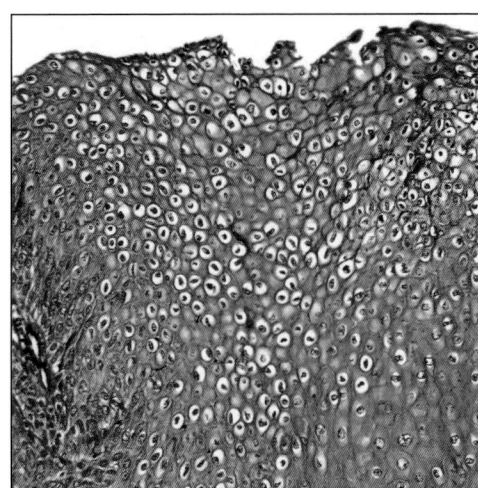

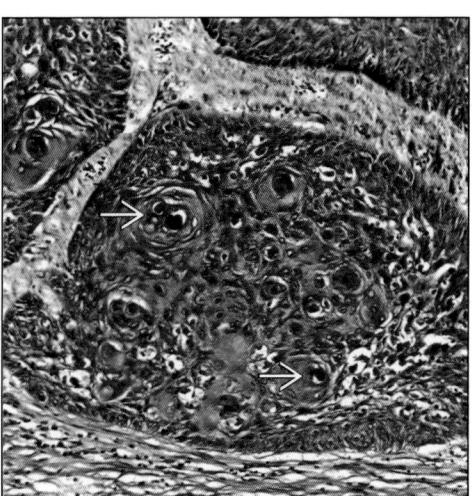

(Left) Hematoxylin & eosin shows giant condyloma with conspicuous koilocytosis. Note irregular hyperchromatic nuclei with perinuclear vacuolization. (Right) Giant condylomata may harbor foci of squamous cell carcinoma. Such carcinomatous foci usually correspond to keratinizing SCC of the usual type. Note foci of well-differentiated usual SCC with obvious keratinization ⊡.

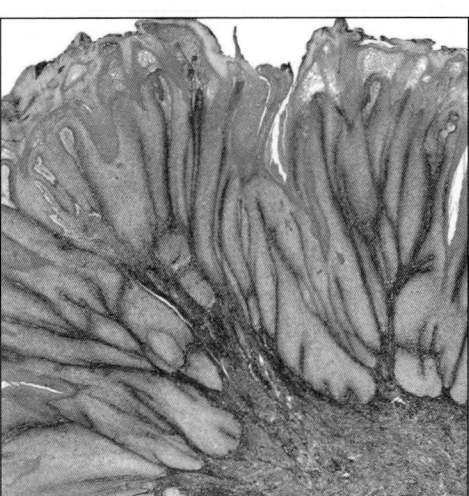

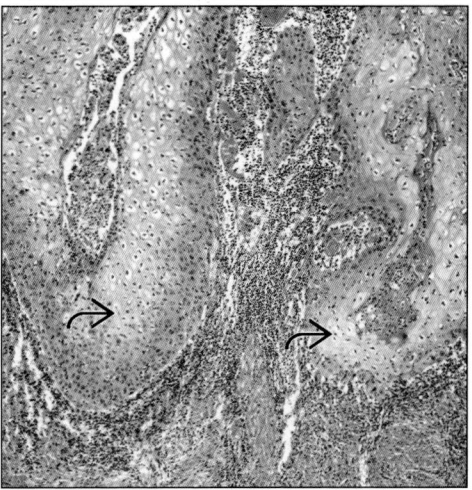

(Left) Verrucous carcinomas may appear similar to condylomata at low power due to the papillary surface and pushing base. However, verrucous carcinomas lack koilocytosis, & papillae tend to be more acanthotic with thin fibrovascular cores. (Right) Warty carcinomas are malignant tumors with a papillary surface; however, they exhibit nuclear pleomorphism and often have infiltrative deep borders. Koilocytosis is seen throughout the lesion including its deep portion ⊡.

PRURIGO NODULARIS

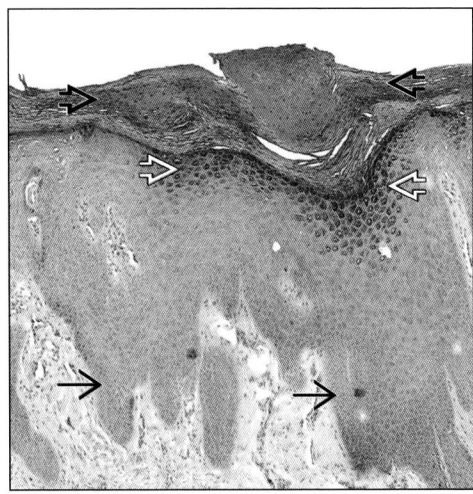

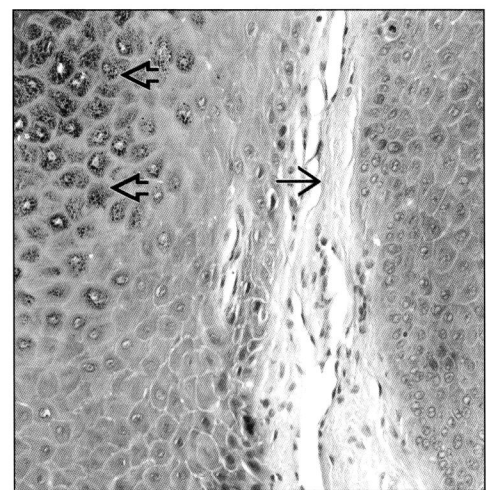

Low-power view of prurigo nodularis shows prominent hyperkeratosis ⊵, parakeratosis, and hypergranulosis ⊵ overlying irregular acanthosis ➔ with vertical streaking of collagen in the papillary dermis.

High magnification of prurigo nodularis shows hypergranulosis ⊵. There is vertical streaking of collagen bundles present in the papillary dermis ➔, a finding seen in both prurigo nodularis and lichen simplex chronicus.

TERMINOLOGY

Abbreviations
- Prurigo nodularis (PN)

Definitions
- Pruritic nodules
- Generally on extensor surfaces of extremities
- Secondary to chronic rubbing/scratching

ETIOLOGY/PATHOGENESIS

Pathophysiology
- Chronic rubbing/scratching induces discrete papules/ nodules
- True cause of pruritus leading to chronic rubbing/ scratching often unknown
- Papillary dermal nerves increased in number compared to normal skin
- Conditions sometimes present that cause pruritus include
  - Atopic dermatitis
  - Diabetes mellitus
  - Renal failure
  - Liver failure
  - Psychiatric disorders
  - Internal malignancy
  - HIV infection

CLINICAL ISSUES

Presentation
- Most commonly seen in middle-aged to elderly individuals
- Generally on extremities but sometimes on trunk or posterior scalp
- Discrete papules or nodules
  - Often slightly scaly
  - Sometimes hyperpigmented
  - May be crusted or show other signs of trauma

Laboratory Tests
- Depending on history, consider ordering
  - CBC
  - Liver function tests
  - Renal function tests

Treatment
- Prevent rubbing/scratching
  - Occlusion may be key
- Topical therapies to reduce pruritus may be helpful
  - Corticosteroids
  - Calcineurin inhibitors
  - Capsaicin
  - Menthol, pramoxine, other antipruritics
- Intralesional corticosteroids
- In some cases, UV light treatments or oral treatments (corticosteroids, antihistamines, anxiolytics, gabapentin, thalidomide) may be necessary

Prognosis
- Resolution with elimination of chronic rubbing/ scratching

MICROSCOPIC PATHOLOGY

Histologic Features
- Hyperkeratosis with stratum lucidum, focal parakeratosis
- Acanthosis and sometimes pseudoepitheliomatous hyperplasia
- Cup-shaped/exo-endophytic or more plaque-like with overlap with lichen simplex chronicus
- Vertical streaking of collagen in papillary dermis
- Perivascular lymphocytes, histiocytes, and sometimes neutrophils &/or eosinophils
- Thickened dermal nerve fibers sometimes present

PRURIGO NODULARIS

Key Facts

Etiology/Pathogenesis
- Chronic rubbing/scratching induces discrete papules/nodules

Clinical Issues
- Generally on extremities but sometimes on trunk or posterior scalp

Microscopic Pathology
- Hyperkeratosis, focal parakeratosis, hypergranulosis
- Acanthosis and sometimes pseudoepitheliomatous hyperplasia
- Vertical streaking of collagen in papillary dermis
- Minimal keratinocyte atypia

Top Differential Diagnoses
- Squamous cell carcinoma (SCC)
- Keratoacanthoma (KA)
- Lichen simplex chronicus (LSC)
- Deep fungal and atypical mycobacterial infection

Cytologic Features
- Minimal keratinocyte atypia
- Cells are polygonal with central round nuclei, small nucleoli, and intercellular bridges
- Individually necrotic cells rare

DIFFERENTIAL DIAGNOSIS

Squamous Cell Carcinoma (SCC)
- Infiltrative areas with cytologic atypia, atypical mitoses, squamous pearls
- May be difficult to exclude underlying SCC with certainty in superficial shave biopsy specimens

Keratoacanthoma (KA)
- Crateriform architecture with central keratin
- Keratinocytes with abundant glassy pink cytoplasm
- Elastic fiber trapping, dermal fibrosis, and eosinophilic/neutrophilic abscesses may be present
- Clinically, KA typically has history of rapid growth and spontaneously resolves

Lichen Simplex Chronicus (LSC)
- On histologic continuum with prurigo nodularis
- Clinically flat plaque rather than papule or nodule (clinical correlation necessary)

Deep Fungal Infection
- Histologic features of pseudoepitheliomatous hyperplasia
- Granulomatous inflammation and abscesses often present
- Special stains should highlight fungal organisms

Atypical Mycobacterial Infection
- Histologic features of pseudoepitheliomatous hyperplasia
- Special stains should highlight acid-fast bacteria
- Culture may be necessary

Pemphigoid Nodularis
- Clinically similar with pruritic papules and nodules
- Presence of bullous lesions a helpful clue
- Histologic findings similar to PN
- Direct immunofluorescence positive for linear IgG &/or C3 at dermoepidermal junction

SELECTED REFERENCES

1. Haas S et al: Low density of sympathetic nerve fibers relative to substance P-positive nerve fibers in lesional skin of chronic pruritus and prurigo nodularis. J Dermatol Sci. 58(3):193-7, 2010
2. Weigelt N et al: Prurigo nodularis: systematic analysis of 58 histological criteria in 136 patients. J Cutan Pathol. 37(5):578-86, 2010
3. Powell AM et al: Pemphigoid nodularis (non-bullous): a clinicopathological study of five cases. Br J Dermatol. 147(2):343-9, 2002
4. Tanaka M et al: Prurigo nodularis consists of two distinct forms: early-onset atopic and late-onset non-atopic. Dermatology. 190(4):269-76, 1995

IMAGE GALLERY

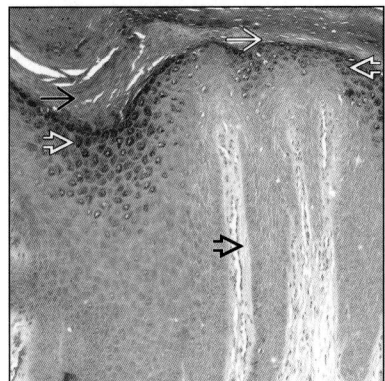 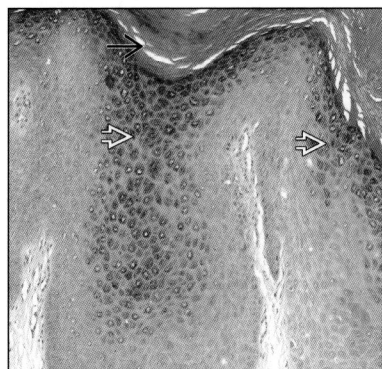 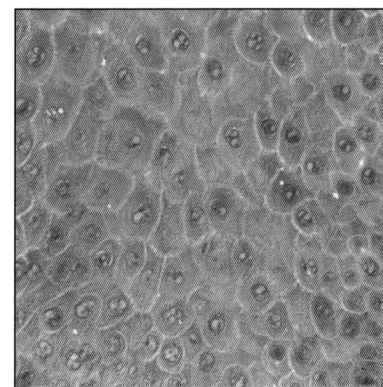

(Left) Prurigo nodularis shows hyperkeratosis ➡, a stratum lucidum ➡, hypergranulosis ➡, and vertical streaking of collagen bundles ➡ in the dermis. (Center) Prurigo nodularis shows hyperkeratosis ➡, hypergranulosis ➡, and acanthosis. Similar changes are seen in lichen simplex chronicus; clinicopathologic correlation separates these 2 entities, which lie on a spectrum. (Right) High magnification shows a lack of cytologic atypia in the keratinocytes.

LARGE CELL ACANTHOMA

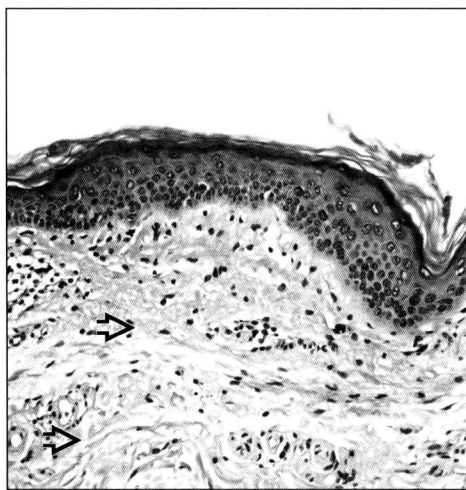

LCA shows an intraepidermal proliferation of enlarged keratinocytes in a disorganized pattern. There is no basilar budding or overlying parakeratosis typical of an actinic keratosis. Note prominent solar elastosis ⊵ in dermis.

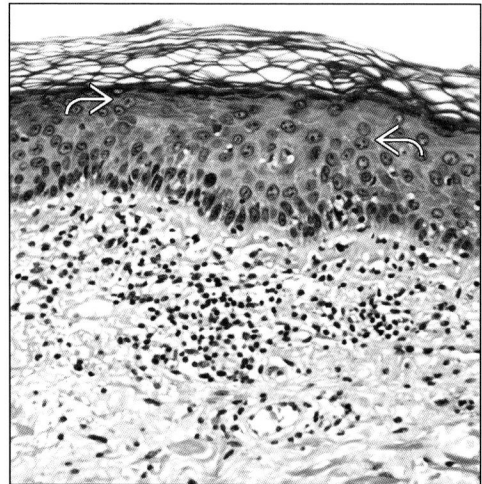

Higher power of LCA shows enlarged keratinocytes ➡ involving the mid to upper layers of epidermis with overlying basket-weave orthokeratosis. Dermis shows solar elastosis and mild chronic inflammatory infiltrate.

TERMINOLOGY

Abbreviations
- Large cell acanthoma (LCA)

Definitions
- Proliferation of enlarged and mildly atypical keratinocytes in sun-damaged skin without diagnostic features of actinic keratosis (AK)
  - Has been variously considered to be related to or a variant of solar lentigo, seborrheic keratosis (stucco keratosis), or AK

ETIOLOGY/PATHOGENESIS

Environmental Exposure
- Most cases associated with UV radiation (chronic solar damage)

Infectious Agents
- HPV types have been detected in some studies

CLINICAL ISSUES

Epidemiology
- Incidence
  - Uncommon lesions but may be underreported
- Age
  - Typically occur in older adults (mean age: 75 years)
- Gender
  - Approximately equal sex distribution or slight female predominance

Site
- Usually head and neck region or extremities

Presentation
- Hyperkeratotic patch, usually well-demarcated lesion

Natural History
- Most cases do not regress, but only rare cases are associated with squamous cell carcinoma in situ (Bowen disease)

Treatment
- Surgical approaches
  - Not necessary in most cases, given the benign behavior of majority of these lesions

Prognosis
- Excellent, very low malignant potential

MACROSCOPIC FEATURES

Size
- Small lesions, usually < 1 cm in greatest dimension

MICROSCOPIC PATHOLOGY

Histologic Features
- Epidermal acanthosis and intraepidermal proliferation of enlarged keratinocytes with proportionately enlarged nuclei
  - Cells show abundant eosinophilic cytoplasm and hyperchromatic-staining nuclei
- Overlying hypergranulosis and hyperkeratosis usually present
- Lesion is typically sharply demarcated from adjacent normal epidermis
- May show mild basilar pigmentation and elongated rete ridges in some cases, suggesting derivation from, or association with, solar lentigo
- Mitotic figures rare

Cytologic Features
- Enlarged, mildly atypical squamous keratinocytes with large nuclei and small to focally prominent nucleoli

LARGE CELL ACANTHOMA

Key Facts

Terminology
- Proliferation of enlarged and mildly atypical keratinocytes in sun-damaged skin without diagnostic features of actinic keratosis
- Variously considered to be related to solar lentigo, seborrheic keratosis, or actinic keratosis

Etiology/Pathogenesis
- Most cases associated with UV radiation
- HPV types have been detected in some studies

Clinical Issues
- Typically occur in older adults (mean age: 75 years)
- Usually head and neck region or extremities

Microscopic Pathology
- Epidermal acanthosis with proliferation of enlarged keratinocytes with proportionately enlarged nuclei
- Overlying hypergranulosis and hyperkeratosis usually present
- Mitotic figures rare

ANCILLARY TESTS

Immunohistochemistry
- Increased expression of nuclear proliferative markers including Ki-67 and PCNA

Cytogenetics
- Cells are mostly aneuploid

DIFFERENTIAL DIAGNOSIS

Actinic Keratosis (AK)
- Proliferation of atypical keratinocytes typically confined to basilar 1/3 of epidermis
- Overlying parakeratosis very common
- Basilar budding of atypical cells usually present
- Mitotic figures often easily identified (as opposed to rare in LCA)

Solar Lentigo (Lentigo Senilis)
- Elongated, hyperpigmented rete ridges
  - May also be seen in some case of LCA, suggesting association with, or derivation from, a solar lentigo
- Background of severe solar elastosis
- Lacks the degree of cellular and nuclear enlargement of LCA

Seborrheic Keratosis (SK)
- Classically shows prominent epidermal acanthosis with pseudohorn cysts
  - Degree of acanthosis is greater than that in LCA in most cases
  - Pseudohorn cysts lacking in LCA
- Stucco keratosis variant of SK shows milder acanthosis with papillomatosis and lacks pseudohorn cysts
- Lacks the degree of enlargement of lesional cells seen in LCA

SELECTED REFERENCES

1. Garrido-Ríos AA et al: Human papillomavirus detection in multiple large-cell acanthomas. J Eur Acad Dermatol Venereol. 23(4):454-5, 2009
2. Berger T et al: Multiple disseminated large-cell acanthomas of the skin associated with human papillomavirus type 6. J Am Acad Dermatol. 53(2):335-7, 2005
3. Mehregan DR et al: Large cell acanthoma. Int J Dermatol. 42(1):36-9, 2003
4. Argenyi ZB et al: Large-cell acanthoma of the skin. A study by image analysis cytometry and immunohistochemistry. Am J Dermatopathol. 16(2):140-4, 1994
5. Rabinowitz AD et al: Large-cell acanthoma. A distinctive keratosis. Am J Dermatopathol. 14(2):136-8; discussion 139, 1992
6. Sánchez Yus E et al: Large-cell acanthoma is a distinctive condition. Am J Dermatopathol. 14(2):140-7; discussion 148, 1992
7. Weinstock MA: Large-cell acanthoma. Am J Dermatopathol. 14(2):133-4; discussion 135, 1992
8. Rahbari H et al: Large cell acanthoma. One of the actinic keratoses. Arch Dermatol. 114(1):49-52, 1978

IMAGE GALLERY

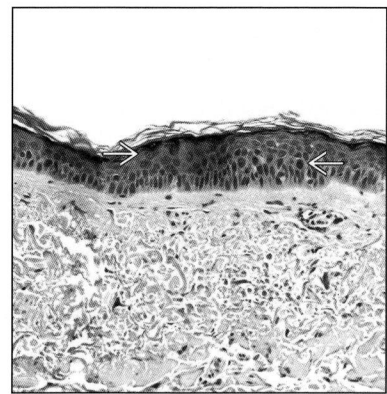 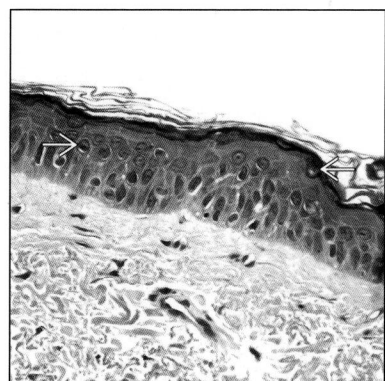 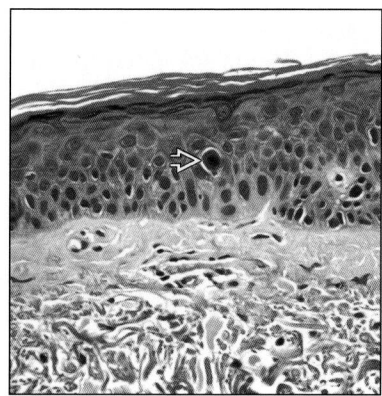

(Left) LCA shows an intraepidermal proliferation of enlarged, atypical-appearing keratinocytes ➡ with a disorganized pattern. (Center) Higher power of LCA shows intraepidermal proliferation of enlarged squamous cells in haphazard arrangement. The cells show nuclear enlargement, hyperchromasia, and focally prominent nucleoli ➡, but no mitotic figures. (Right) LCA shows a proliferation of enlarged, atypical-appearing keratinocytes, but no budding or overlying parakeratosis typical of actinic keratosis. Note presence of apoptotic figure ➡ in mid epidermis.

CLEAR CELL ACANTHOMA

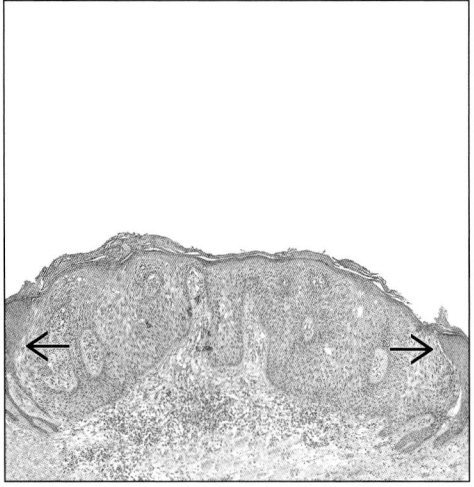

Clear cell acanthoma at low-power magnification shows clear/pale cells in an acanthotic epidermis. The lesion is sharply demarcated from the surrounding epidermis ➡.

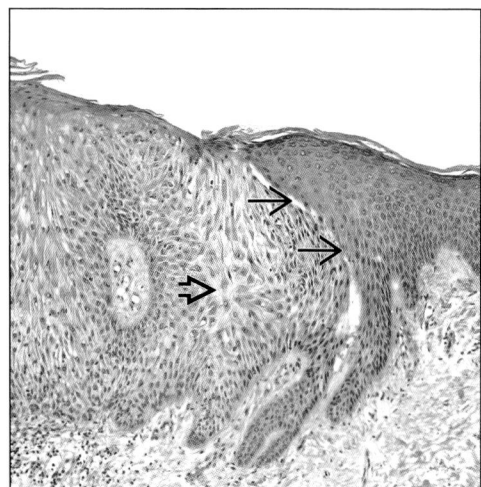

In this medium-power magnification of clear cell acanthoma, there are clear/pale cells ⧑ with overlying parakeratosis. The lesion is sharply demarcated from the adjacent normal epidermis ➡.

TERMINOLOGY

Abbreviations
- Clear cell acanthoma (CCA)

Synonyms
- Degos acanthoma, pale cell acanthoma

Definitions
- Benign epidermal tumor, generally on lower legs of women
- Epidermal acanthosis with pale or clear cells, often with overlying parakeratosis
- Pale or clear cells sharply demarcated from adjacent, normal epidermis

ETIOLOGY/PATHOGENESIS

Pathogenesis
- Some consider this a reactive proliferation of epidermis rather than a true neoplasm

CLINICAL ISSUES

Epidemiology
- Gender
  ○ More common in middle-aged women

Site
- Generally on lower legs

Presentation
- Solitary, pink-red, shiny papule or plaque
- White scale may be seen at periphery
- Rarely multiple lesions associated with ichthyosis

Treatment
- Biopsy/surgical removal is generally curative

Prognosis
- Benign, no malignant potential

MACROSCOPIC FEATURES

Dermatoscopy
- Characteristic dot-like vessels in linear arrangements

MICROSCOPIC PATHOLOGY

Histologic Features
- Epidermal acanthosis with a proliferation of pale or clear cells
- Often overlying parakeratosis, sometimes with neutrophils
- Pale or clear cells sharply demarcated from adjacent, normal epidermis
- Pale or clear cells stain bright pink/purple with periodic-acid Schiff (PAS), with diastase sensitivity

Cytologic Features
- Minimal to no cytologic atypia
- Keratinocytes have pale to clear cytoplasm

DIFFERENTIAL DIAGNOSIS

Psoriasis
- Varying clinical presentations
  ○ Commonly multiple plaques with silvery scale favoring elbows/knees/scalp/lower back
- Regular acanthosis with hypogranulosis
- Confluent parakeratosis with collections of neutrophils
- Unlike CCA
  ○ Not composed of pale or clear cells that are sharply demarcated from adjacent, normal epidermis
  ○ Has increased basilar and suprabasilar mitoses
  ○ Shows thinning of suprapapillary plates

CLEAR CELL ACANTHOMA

Key Facts

Clinical Issues
- Common in middle-aged women
- Generally on lower legs
- Solitary, pink-red, shiny papule or plaque

Microscopic Pathology
- Acanthosis of pale or clear cells
- Often overlying parakeratosis, sometimes with neutrophils

- Pale or clear cells (glycogen filled, PAS[+]) sharply demarcated from adjacent, normal epidermis
- Minimal to no cytologic atypia

Top Differential Diagnoses
- Psoriasis
- Psoriasiform keratosis
- Tricholemmoma
- Clear cell Bowen disease

---

    o Has dilated vessels in papillary dermis

Psoriasiform Keratosis
- Solitary papule
- Patient without history of psoriasis
- Hyperkeratosis and parakeratosis with neutrophils overlying acanthosis

Tricholemmoma
- 2 main clinical presentations
    - o Solitary papule on sun-damaged skin
    - o Multiple, slightly verrucous papules on central face associated with Cowden syndrome
- Hyperkeratosis and parakeratosis
- Sometimes papillomatous
- Hyperplastic epidermis composed of clear or pale cells with
    - o Peripheral palisaded basal layer
    - o Thickened basement membrane

Clear Cell Bowen Disease
- Confluent parakeratosis
- Regular or irregular acanthosis
- Atypical keratinocytes and atypical mitoses in full-thickness of epidermis
- Keratinocytes are clear or pale

Dermatophyte Infection
- Like CCA, may have confluent parakeratosis with neutrophils
- Unlike CCA, dermatophyte infection is characterized by

    o Epidermis not composed of pale/clear cells that are sharply demarcated from surrounding normal epidermis
    o Special stains (e.g., PAS) that highlight fungal hyphae in stratum corneum

Verruciform Xanthoma
- Like CCA, may have confluent parakeratosis with neutrophils
- Unlike CCA, verruciform xanthoma shows
    - o Often polypoid architecture
    - o Papillary dermis containing foamy cells

DIAGNOSTIC CHECKLIST

Pathologic Interpretation Pearls
- Acanthosis of pale or clear cells with overlying parakeratosis
- Pale or clear cells sharply demarcated from adjacent, normal epidermis
- Minimal to no cytologic atypia

SELECTED REFERENCES

1. Zalaudek I et al: How to diagnose nonpigmented skin tumors: a review of vascular structures seen with dermoscopy: part II. Nonmelanocytic skin tumors. J Am Acad Dermatol. 63(3):377-86; quiz 387-8, 2010
2. Zedek DC et al: Clear-cell acanthoma versus acanthosis: a psoriasiform reaction pattern lacking tricholemmal differentiation. Am J Dermatopathol. 29(4):378-84, 2007

IMAGE GALLERY

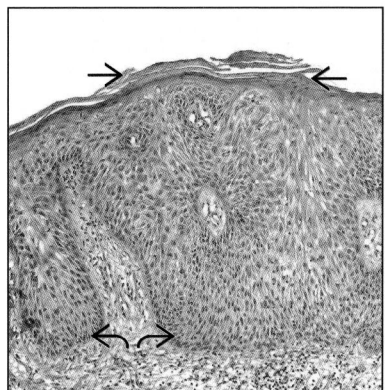 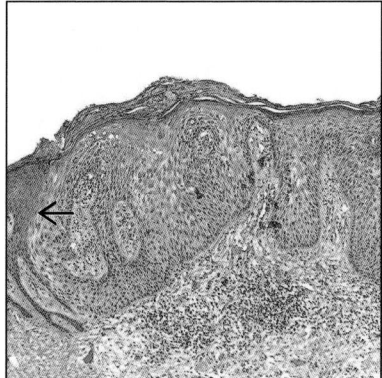 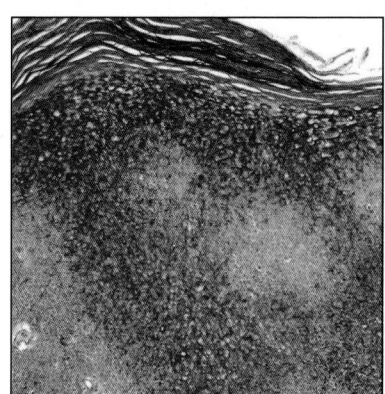

(Left) Clear cell acanthoma shows pale cells in a hyperplastic epidermis with confluent parakeratosis ➡ above regular acanthosis (the rete come down to the same level in the dermis ➡). (Center) CCA shows acanthosis, clear/pale cells, and overlying parakeratosis. The lesion is sharply demarcated from the adjacent, normal epidermis ➡. (Right) The lesional cells of CCA contain glycogen and are bright pink/purple with the periodic acid-Schiff (PAS) stain.

CLEAR CELL PAPULOSIS

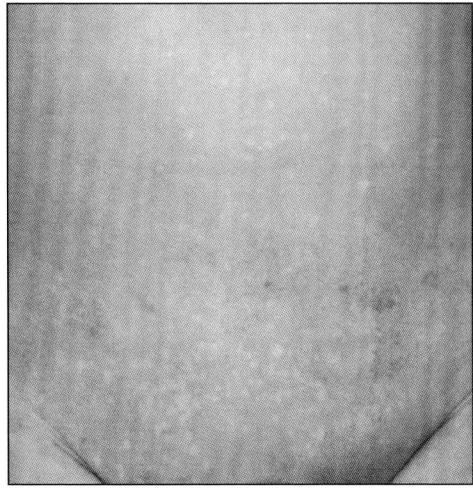

Symmetrically distributed hypopigmented macules and papules are seen on the abdomen and suprapubic region of a young child. (Courtesy R. Hui, MD.)

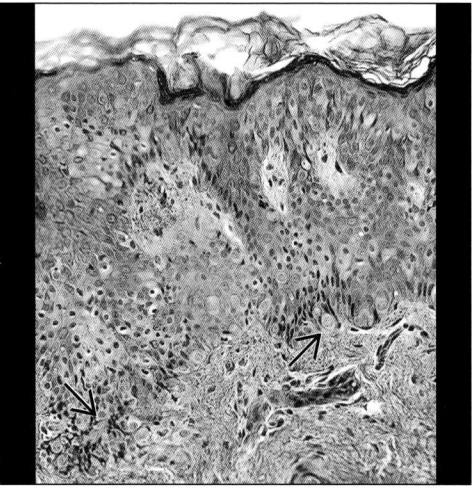

Clear/pale cells ⊡ are seen with abundant cytoplasm in the basal and suprabasal layers of a hyperkeratotic and acanthotic epidermis. (Courtesy R. Hui, MD.)

TERMINOLOGY

Definitions
- Rare disorder of multiple, hypopigmented to white, flat-topped papules and macules
- Generally on lower trunk
- Almost always in young children, often of Asian descent
- Histopathology characteristic, with clear/pale cells in basal layer of acanthotic epidermis

ETIOLOGY/PATHOGENESIS

Pathogenesis
- Clear cells may be normal component of epidermis along "milk lines," type of glandular epithelial cell
- Others postulate that clear cells are derived from eccrine secretory gland
  - Based on staining of clear cells with IKH-4, carcinoembryonic antigen, and CAM5.2
- Genetic component is postulated as siblings may be affected

CLINICAL ISSUES

Epidemiology
- Age
  - Young children, mean age = 1.7 years
  - Exceptional case report in an adult
- Gender
  - Slight female predominance
- Ethnicity
  - Often in patients of Asian descent

Site
- Generally on lower trunk/suprapubic area
- Also reported on chest, axillae, inguinal area, lower back/buttocks, and extremities

- Sometimes described as affecting trunk along "milk lines," which run from anterior axillae to upper medial thighs

Presentation
- Multiple, often symmetric, hypopigmented to white, flat-topped papules and macules
- 1-10 millimeters in diameter
- Number of skin lesions ranges from 2 to over 100; average of 10 to 20
- Asymptomatic

Natural History
- Lesions increase in number, become stable, and then regress with age

Treatment
- Treatment is not necessary as many patients develop spontaneous regression

Prognosis
- Benign condition
- No malignant potential

MICROSCOPIC PATHOLOGY

Histologic Features
- Clear to pale cells with abundant cytoplasm concentrated in basal layers of epidermis
- Cells single or in clusters
- Cells occasionally in suprabasal layers
- Epidermis acanthotic and hyperkeratotic
- Decreased basal layer melanin pigmentation
- Clear to pale cells stain with
  - Periodic acid-Schiff
  - Mucin stains (variable)
  - Cytokeratin stains (including CK7)
  - Carcinoembryonic antigen
  - Epithelial membrane antigen
  - Gross cystic disease fluid protein 15 (GCDFP-15)

CLEAR CELL PAPULOSIS

Key Facts

Terminology

- Rare disorder
- Multiple, hypopigmented to white, flat-topped papules and macules
- Generally on lower trunk/suprapubic area
- Almost always in young children
- More common in Asian populations

Microscopic Pathology

- Clear to pale cells with abundant cytoplasm

- Cells concentrated in basal layers of epidermis
- Cells single or in clusters
- Nuclear atypia and pleomorphism absent
- Cells positive with CK7

Top Differential Diagnoses

- Clear cells of Toker
- Pagetoid dyskeratosis
- Paget disease
- Extramammary Paget disease

- Clear to pale cells reportedly negative with HER2/neu

Cytologic Features

- Clear to pale cells with abundant cytoplasm
- Nuclei are round to oval and sometimes slightly indented
- Inconspicuous nucleoli
- Nuclear atypia and pleomorphism absent

DIFFERENTIAL DIAGNOSIS

Clear Cells of Toker

- Clinical history differs; incidental finding in nipple/areola, breast, and vulva
- Histologic findings similar to clear cell papulosis
  o Clear to pale cells with abundant cytoplasm in epidermis
- Unlike clear cell papulosis, clear/pale cells often scattered into upper portions of epidermis

Pagetoid Dyskeratosis

- Clinical history differs; incidental finding
- Clusters of pale cells in spinous layer

Paget Disease

- Clinical history differs; generally affects unilateral nipple/areola in older adults
- Clear to pale cells with abundant cytoplasm scattered at all levels in epidermis
- Nuclear atypia present

Extramammary Paget Disease

- Clinical history differs, with extramammary Paget disease presenting as erythematous patch or plaque, usually in groin/perineal area
- Clear to pale cells with abundant cytoplasm scattered at all levels in epidermis
- Nuclear atypia present

DIAGNOSTIC CHECKLIST

Pathologic Interpretation Pearls

- Clear to pale cells with abundant cytoplasm concentrated in basal layer of epidermis
- Clear cells single or in groups
- No nuclear atypia

SELECTED REFERENCES

1. Tseng FW et al: Long-term follow-up study of clear cell papulosis. J Am Acad Dermatol. 63(2):266-73, 2010
2. Yu Y et al: Clear cell papulosis: a connection of clear cells to toker cells or paget disease. Arch Dermatol. 145(9):1066-8, 2009
3. Farley-Loftus R et al: Clear cell papulosis. Dermatol Online J. 14(10):19, 2008
4. Kim YC et al: Clear cell papulosis: an immunohistochemical study to determine histogenesis. J Cutan Pathol. 29(1):11-4, 2002

IMAGE GALLERY

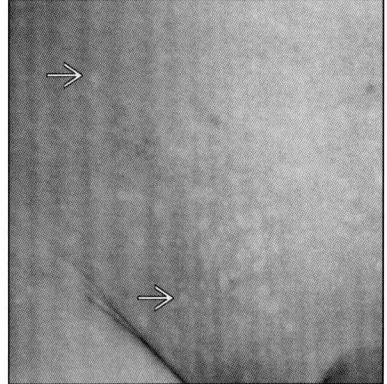
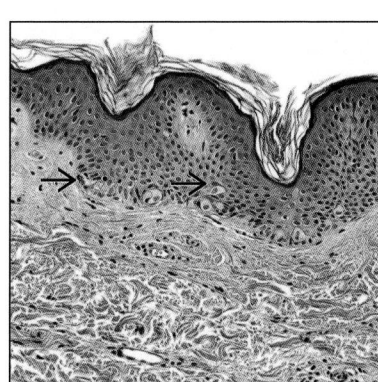
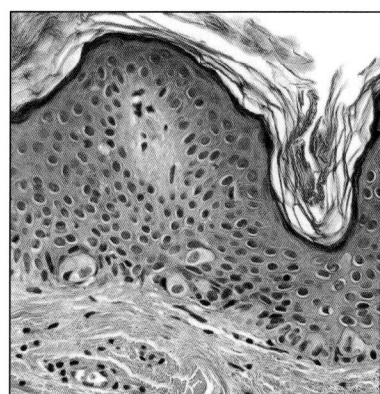

(Left) Hypopigmented macules and flat-topped papules ➡ are visible on the lower abdomen/suprapubic area. *(Courtesy R. Hui, MD.)* *(Center)* Clear cell papulosis shows scattered enlarged, clear-staining cells ➡ in the basal layer of the epidermis. *(Courtesy R. Hui, MD.)* *(Right)* High magnification shows clear cells with abundant cytoplasm in the basal layer of an acanthotic epidermis. *(Courtesy R. Hui, MD.)*

TOKER CELL HYPERPLASIA

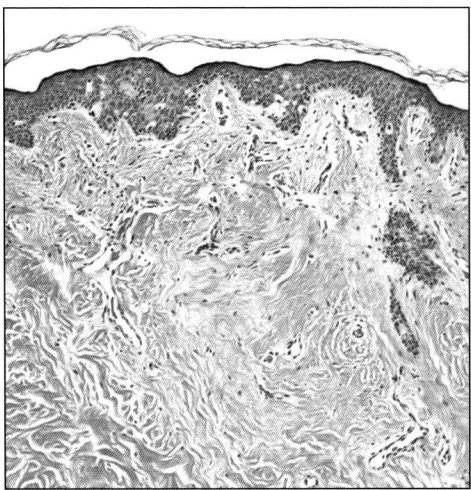

Toker cell hyperplasia is a rare histopathologic finding. Toker cells, a normal component of the nipple epithelium, are increased in number and may mimic Paget disease of the nipple.

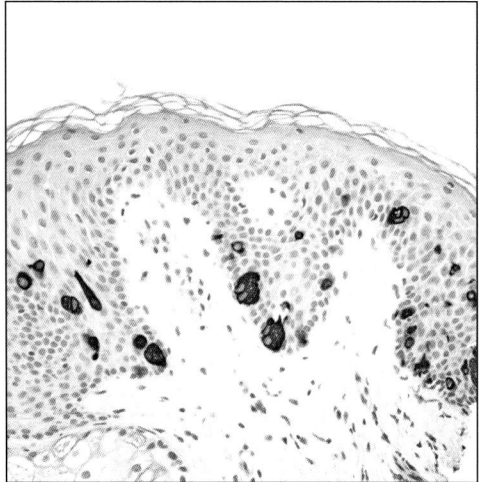

In Toker cell hyperplasia, Toker cells are evident by light microscopy, and they are also highlighted by CK7 staining. The bland cells are scattered in the basal and suprabasal layers.

TERMINOLOGY

Definitions
- Increase in number of Toker cells in epidermis
- Absence of underlying ductal carcinoma
- Mimics Paget disease of the nipple
- Awareness important to avoid overdiagnosis of Paget disease

CLINICAL ISSUES

Epidemiology
- Incidence
  - Toker cells present by light microscopy in ~ 10% of normal nipples
  - Toker cells also described in
    - Vulva
    - Accessory nipples
    - Along milk line of epidermis
    - Overlying nipple duct adenoma/florid papillomatosis of the nipple
  - Toker cell hyperplasia
    - Rare
    - Described in 2 cases out of 340 in Toker's original series
    - Increase in number of Toker cells, mimicking Paget disease of the nipple
    - Absence of underlying ductal carcinoma
    - Clinically normal nipple

Presentation
- Incidental finding
- Nipple normal grossly/clinically

Treatment
- Excision with clear margins has been recommended

Prognosis
- Hyperplasia that mimics Paget disease is rare; in reported cases, excision with negative margins seems to portend an excellent prognosis

MICROSCOPIC PATHOLOGY

Histologic Features
- Slightly enlarged cells in epidermis
- Cells without atypia or pleomorphism
- Cells concentrated in basal and suprabasal layers
- Often arranged in single units but occasionally clustered
- Mitoses should not be present in cells
- Inflammation absent
- Immunohistochemical findings
  - Positive with
    - CK7
    - EMA
    - CAM5.2
  - Negative with
    - CK20
    - GCDFP-15
    - 34bE12
    - S100
    - HER2

Cytologic Features
- Round to slightly oval nuclei
- Cytoplasm
  - Abundant
  - Slightly pale to clear
- No pleomorphism

DIFFERENTIAL DIAGNOSIS

Paget Disease of the Nipple
- Clinical history differs

TOKER CELL HYPERPLASIA

Key Facts

Terminology
- Increase in number of Toker cells in epidermis
- Absence of underlying ductal carcinoma
- Mimics Paget disease of the nipple

Clinical Issues
- Very rare
- Incidental finding
- Nipple normal clinically/grossly

Microscopic Pathology
- Round to slightly oval nuclei
- Abundant cytoplasm that is slightly pale to clear
- No pleomorphism
- CK7 positive

Top Differential Diagnoses
- Paget disease of the nipple
- Pagetoid dyskeratosis
- Clear cell papulosis

---

   o Generally affects unilateral nipple/areola in older adults
- Clear to pale cells with abundant cytoplasm scattered at all levels in epidermis
- Nuclear atypia present
   o Hyperchromatic nuclei
   o Prominent eosinophilic cytoplasm
- Variable mitotic activity

Extramammary Paget Disease
- Clinical history differs
   o Erythematous patch or plaque, usually in groin/perineal area
- Clear to pale cells with abundant cytoplasm scattered at all levels in epidermis
- Nuclear atypia present
- Variable mitotic activity

Pagetoid Dyskeratosis
- Clusters of somewhat pale or clear keratinocytes
   o Slightly shrunken nuclei
   o Perinuclear halo
- Possibly related to trauma
- Cells do not mark with CK7

Clear Cell Papulosis
- Clinical presentation differs
   o Child with multiple hypopigmented, white to flesh-colored papules on lower abdomen/groin area
- Scattered, benign-appearing cells in basal layer of acanthotic epidermis
- Cells stain with CK7

DIAGNOSTIC CHECKLIST

Pathologic Interpretation Pearls
- Slightly enlarged cells in basal and suprabasal epidermis
   o Without pleomorphism
   o Predominately single units
   o Occasionally clustered
   o CK7 positive
   o EMA positive
- Degree of hyperplasia mimics Paget disease, but cells are not atypical and mitoses are absent

SELECTED REFERENCES

1. Garijo MF et al: Pagetoid dyskeratosis of the nipple epidermis: an incidental finding mimicking Paget's disease of the nipple. APMIS. 116(2):139-46, 2008
2. Willman JH et al: Vulvar clear cells of Toker: precursors of extramammary Paget's disease. Am J Dermatopathol. 27(3):185-8, 2005
3. Willman JH et al: Clear cells of Toker in accessory nipples. J Cutan Pathol. 30(4):256-60, 2003
4. Lundquist K et al: Intraepidermal cytokeratin 7 expression is not restricted to Paget cells but is also seen in Toker cells and Merkel cells. Am J Surg Pathol. 23(2):212-9, 1999
5. Decaussin M et al: Paget's disease versus Toker cell hyperplasia in a supernumerary nipple. Virchows Arch. 432(3):289-91, 1998
6. Toker C: Clear cells of the nipple epidermis. Cancer. 25(3):601-10, 1970

IMAGE GALLERY

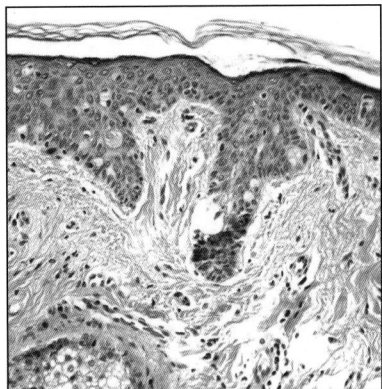 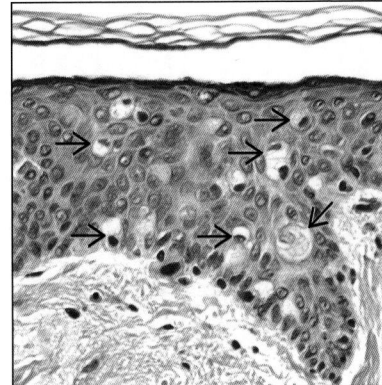 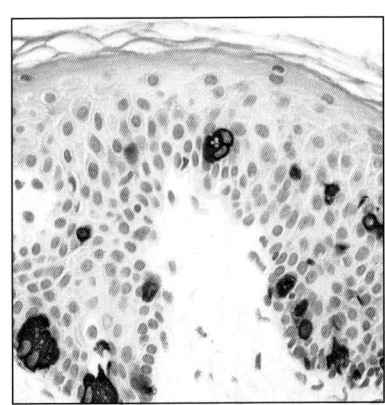

(Left) At this magnification, the scattered, hyperplastic Toker cells in the epidermis mimic Paget disease of the nipple. (Center) This is a high-magnification view of Toker cell hyperplasia. Toker cells ➔ have bland nuclei with expanded, somewhat clear cytoplasm. They are in the basal and suprabasal layers of the epidermis. (Right) Toker cells are CK7 positive. The cells lack atypia, are sometimes clustered, and are predominately in single units.

ACTINIC KERATOSIS

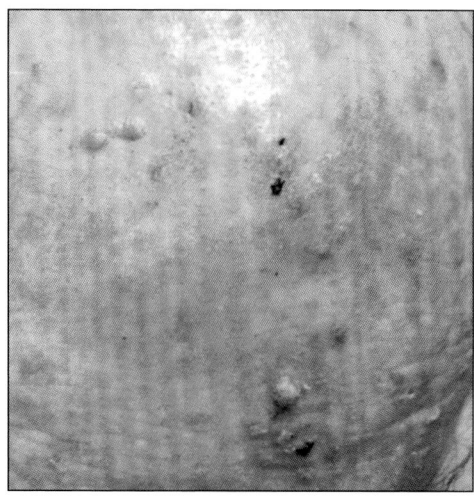

Clinical photograph of the scalp of an elderly patient shows multiple actinic keratoses with prominent crusting. (Courtesy J. Wu, MD.)

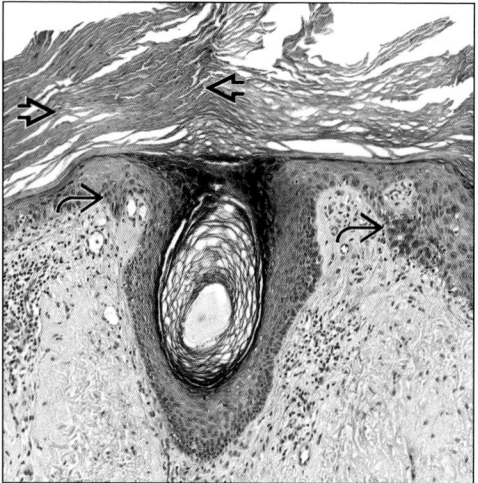

Low-magnification view of an actinic keratosis shows basilar keratinocytic budding and atypia ➡, with sparing of a central hair follicle. Prominent overlying parakeratosis ⇗ is typically present.

TERMINOLOGY

Abbreviations
- Actinic keratosis (AK)

Synonyms
- Solar keratosis
- Often considered a "precancer" or early squamous cell carcinoma in situ (SCCis)

Definitions
- Atypical intraepidermal proliferation of keratinocytes typically confined to basilar portion of epidermis, with very low risk for progression to invasive squamous cell carcinoma (SCC)

ETIOLOGY/PATHOGENESIS

Solar Damage
- Ultraviolet light (primarily UVB) induces mutations in DNA, which lead to abnormal proliferation of intraepidermal keratinocytes
- *P53* mutations are most common genetic alteration identified

CLINICAL ISSUES

Epidemiology
- Incidence
  - Very common lesions, estimated to affect up to 10-40% of adult Caucasians; higher incidence in areas with heavy sun exposure (i.e., Australia)
- Age
  - Older adults typically affected
- Gender
  - Males more common than females
- Ethnicity
  - Mostly occur in Caucasians; much less common in other races

Site
- Sun-exposed sites, especially face, head and neck, dorsal hands, and forearms

Presentation
- Scaly papules and plaques, often multiple

Natural History
- Minority of cases progress to invasive squamous cell carcinoma

Treatment
- Options, risks, complications
  - Controversial whether treatment is necessary in all cases, but most clinicians opt for treatment in order to avoid potential development of SCC
- Surgical approaches
  - Conservative excision of lesions is not necessary in most cases (unless there is clinical suspicion for invasive SCC), but is curative
- Drugs
  - Topical therapy with drugs such as 5-fluorouracil, diclofenac, or imiquimod may be used
  - Liquid nitrogen (cryotherapy) frequently used
  - Photodynamic therapy is also an emerging treatment that may be useful for extensive AKs

Prognosis
- Excellent in vast majority of cases, as only approximately 2-3% progress to invasive SCC
- Most invasive SCCs arising in AKs are low grade, but aggressive cases may also occur

MACROSCOPIC FEATURES

Size
- Usually small (< 1 cm) papules, but larger lesions may occur

ACTINIC KERATOSIS

Key Facts

Terminology
- Actinic keratosis (AK)
- Solar keratosis
- Atypical intraepidermal proliferation of keratinocytes typically confined to basilar portion of epidermis

Clinical Issues
- Older adults typically affected
- Mostly occur in Caucasians, much less common in other races
- Excellent in vast majority of cases, as only approximately 2-3% progress to invasive SCC

Microscopic Pathology
- Basilar budding of atypical cells
- Cells show nuclear enlargement, hyperchromasia, and prominent nucleoli

- Overlying parakeratosis present
- Lesional cells usually do not involve follicles (as opposed to Bowen disease)
- Histologic subtypes include hypertrophic, atrophic, pigmented, lichenoid, and bowenoid AK

Top Differential Diagnoses
- Squamous cell carcinoma (SCC)
- Bowen disease (SCC in situ)
- Basal cell carcinoma (BCC), superficial-multicentric and basosquamous types
- Melanoma in situ (lentigo maligna type)
- Discoid lupus erythematosus
- Lichen planus (LP) and lichen planus-like keratosis (benign lichenoid keratosis [BLK])

MICROSCOPIC PATHOLOGY

Histologic Features
- Intraepidermal proliferation of atypical keratinocytes, typically confined to basilar 1/3 of epithelium
  - Basilar budding of atypical cells
  - Cells show nuclear enlargement, hyperchromasia, and prominent nucleoli
  - Abundant eosinophilic-staining cytoplasm
  - Increased numbers of mitotic figures usually present
- Overlying parakeratosis present in vast majority of cases; hypogranulosis may also be present
- Lesional cells usually do not involve follicles (as opposed to Bowen disease) and adnexal ducts
  - Leads to alternating "red and blue" tiers of parakeratosis (overlying AK) and hyperorthokeratosis (overlying follicles and eccrine ducts)
- Histologic subtypes
  - **Hypertrophic AK**
    - Shows epidermal hyperplasia, often psoriasiform, with prominent overlying hyperkeratosis and parakeratosis
    - Dermal fibrosis and vertical collagen bundles often present, suggesting lichen simplex chronicus changes (due to chronic excoriation) superimposed on an AK
  - **Atrophic AK**
    - Shows thinning of epidermis and flattening of rete ridges, and may involve superficial portions of adnexal structures
    - Dense hyperkeratosis usually is present, parakeratosis is more focal than usual
  - **Acantholytic AK**
    - Shows dyscohesive atypical basilar cells and clefts between AK and overlying benign keratinocytes
    - Dyskeratotic cells often present
  - **Pigmented AK**
    - Shows basilar hyperpigmentation
    - Melanophages often present in dermis

  - May be confused with melanoma in situ in some cases
  - Immunohistochemistry for melanocytic markers and cytokeratins can be used to distinguish these lesions
  - **Lichenoid AK**
    - Has a dense, band-like inflammatory infiltrate present in superficial dermis
    - Shows mild basal-vacuolar alteration and scattered dyskeratotic keratinocytes
  - **Bowenoid AK**
    - Involves greater proportion of epidermis (up to 1/2 or 2/3 thickness)
    - Does not show full thickness involvement, which should be diagnosed as SCC in situ (Bowen disease)
  - **Proliferative AK (controversial variant)**
    - Closely related to hypertrophic AK, but nests and finger-like projections of atypical keratinocytes extend into upper dermis
    - Involvement of follicular epithelium frequently present
    - Many dermatopathologists would consider these lesions to be superficially invasive SCC

Cytologic Features
- Enlarged squamous cells with irregular, hyperchromatic-staining nuclei, enlarged nucleoli
- Abundant dense, eosinophilic-staining cytoplasm

ANCILLARY TESTS

Immunohistochemistry
- Not necessary except in very few special situations
  - **AK vs. superficial or basosquamous-type BCC**
    - BER-EP4 positive in BCC, negative in AK
    - Bcl-2 often strongly positive in BCC, weak or negative in AK
  - **Pigmented AK vs. melanoma in situ**
    - Cytokeratins (including pankeratin and high molecular weight cytokeratins) and melanocytic markers (S100, HMB-45, or tyrosinase)

- MART-1/Melan-A least useful in this situation, as it often shows staining of pigmented keratinocytes

DIFFERENTIAL DIAGNOSIS

Squamous Cell Carcinoma (SCC)
- Vast majority of cases of invasive SCC arise in associated AK (likely over 90%)
- Invasive cells extend through basement membrane into (at least) superficial dermis
- Cannot be excluded with certainty in cases where AK involves base of biopsy
  - Should be diagnosed as "at least an AK; underlying SCC cannot be excluded, given involvement of base of biopsy"

Bowen Disease (SCC In Situ)
- Involves full thickness of epidermis, with atypical cells extending into granular cell layer
- Usually spares basilar layer, producing so-called "eyeliner" sign
- Involves hair follicles and adnexal structures, as opposed to AK, which typically spares them

Basal Cell Carcinoma (BCC), Basosquamous and Superficial-Multicentric Types
- Proliferation of superficial basaloid cells with peripheral palisading
- May be difficult to distinguish in some cases of small, superficial shave biopsies, where lesional cells are transected at base of biopsy
  - Especially if ulceration and inflammation present (often associated with/induce squamoid features in BCC)
- Often see at least focal tumor-stromal retraction artifact and superficial surrounding mucinous stroma

Melanoma In Situ (Lentigo Maligna Type)
- May be difficult to separate from pigmented AK in some cases
- Cells are typically more spindle-shaped with angulated, hyperchromatic-staining nuclei; show lentiginous pattern ± nesting
- Lacks overlying parakeratosis (unless irritated)
- Immunohistochemistry for cytokeratins (including pankeratin and high molecular weight cytokeratins) and melanocytic markers (S100, HMB-45, or tyrosinase) allows distinction in most cases

Discoid Lupus Erythematosus
- Atrophic AK may occasionally be difficult to separate from lupus, as both show flattening of epidermis
- Reactive atypia may be present in basilar keratinocytes
- Interface changes with exocytosis of lymphocytes into basilar epidermis, basal vacuolization, and dyskeratotic cells should be present
- Additional findings may include follicular plugging, basement membrane thickening, and periadnexal inflammation

Lichen Planus (LP) and Lichen Planus-like Keratosis/Benign Lichenoid Keratosis (BLK)
- Lichenoid AK may mimic LP or BLK in some cases, especially at low magnification
- Basal vacuolization and dyskeratotic cells typical of LP and BLK, though also present in lichenoid AK
- Cytologic atypia and budding of keratinocytes are main diagnostic features for lichenoid AK

SELECTED REFERENCES

1. Fenske NA et al: Actinic keratoses: past, present and future. J Drugs Dermatol. 9(5 Suppl ODAC Conf Pt 1):s45-9, 2010
2. Cassarino DS et al: SIN, not KIN. J Cutan Pathol. 36(7):820, 2009
3. Puizina-Ivić N et al: An overview of Bcl-2 expression in histopathological variants of basal cell carcinoma, squamous cell carcinoma, actinic keratosis and seborrheic keratosis. Coll Antropol. 32 Suppl 2:61-5, 2008
4. Ferrándiz C: Update on actinic keratosis in clinical trial experience with imiquimod. Br J Dermatol. 157 Suppl 2:32-3, 2007
5. Roewert-Huber J et al: Pathology and pathobiology of actinic (solar) keratosis - an update. Br J Dermatol. 157 Suppl 2:18-20, 2007
6. Berman B et al: Mechanisms of action of new treatment modalities for actinic keratosis. J Drugs Dermatol. 5(2):167-73, 2006
7. Cassarino DS et al: Cutaneous squamous cell carcinoma: a comprehensive clinicopathologic classification. Part one. J Cutan Pathol. 33(3):191-206, 2006
8. Gold MH et al: Current treatments of actinic keratosis. J Drugs Dermatol. 5(2 Suppl):17-25, 2006
9. Cockerell CJ et al: New histopathological classification of actinic keratosis (incipient intraepidermal squamous cell carcinoma). J Drugs Dermatol. 4(4):462-7, 2005
10. Wheeland RG: The pitfalls of treating all actinic keratoses as squamous cell carcinomas. Semin Cutan Med Surg. 24(3):152-4, 2005
11. Anwar J et al: The development of actinic keratosis into invasive squamous cell carcinoma: evidence and evolving classification schemes. Clin Dermatol. 22(3):189-96, 2004
12. Epstein E: Quantifying actinic keratosis: assessing the evidence. Am J Clin Dermatol. 5(3):141-4, 2004
13. Oppel T et al: Actinic keratosis: the key event in the evolution from photoaged skin to squamous cell carcinoma. Therapy based on pathogenetic and clinical aspects. Skin Pharmacol Physiol. 17(2):67-76, 2004
14. Tran H et al: Summary of actinic keratosis studies with imiquimod 5% cream. Br J Dermatol. 149 Suppl 66:37-9, 2003
15. Ortonne JP: From actinic keratosis to squamous cell carcinoma. Br J Dermatol. 146 Suppl 61:20-3, 2002
16. Salasche SJ: Epidemiology of actinic keratoses and squamous cell carcinoma. J Am Acad Dermatol. 42(1 Pt 2):4-7, 2000
17. Tope WD et al: Ber-EP4-positive phenotype differentiates actinic keratosis from superficial basal cell carcinoma. Dermatol Surg. 26(5):415-8, 2000
18. Nakagawa K et al: bcl-2 expression in epidermal keratinocytic diseases. Cancer. 74(6):1720-4, 1994
19. Callen JP et al: Bowen's and non-Bowen's squamous intraepidermal neoplasia of the skin. Relationship to internal malignancy. Arch Dermatol. 116(4):422-6, 1980

ACTINIC KERATOSIS

Microscopic Features and Differential Diagnosis

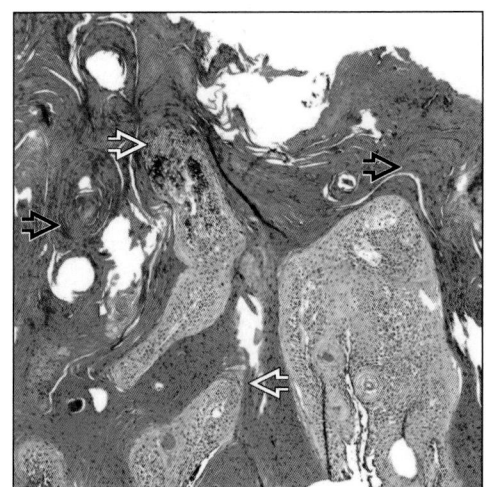

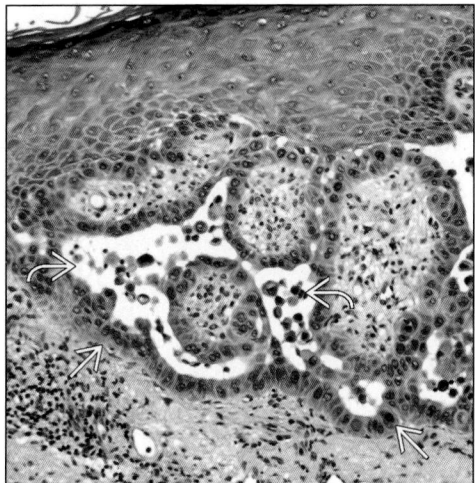

(Left) Scanning magnification view of a hypertropic actinic keratosis shows prominent hyperkeratosis and parakeratosis ⇗ overlying epidermal acanthosis with papillomatosis ➡. **(Right)** This is an example of an acantholytic AK demonstrating prominent suprabasilar acantholysis ➡ overlying atypical basilar keratinocytes ➡.

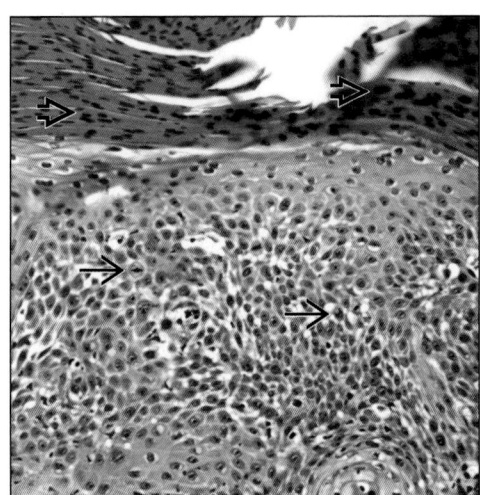

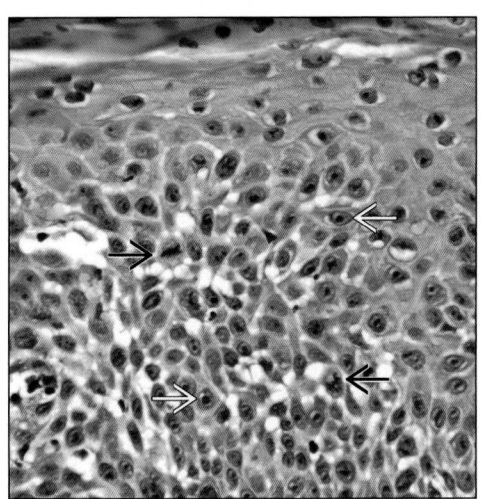

(Left) Bowenoid AK demonstrates prominent parakeratosis ⇗ overlying a proliferation of atypical keratinocytes involving the basilar 2/3 of the epidermis. Multiple suprabasilar mitotic figures are easily identified ➡. **(Right)** High magnification of a bowenoid AK shows markedly enlarged and atypical-appearing keratinocytes with hyperchromatic nuclei, prominent nucleoli ➡, and dense eosinophilic-staining cytoplasm. Mitotic figures ➡ are scattered throughout the lesion.

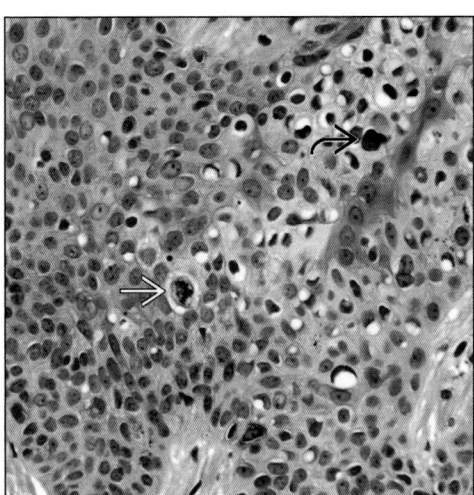

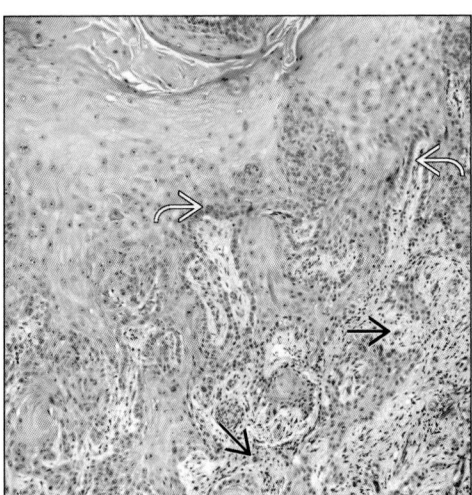

(Left) High magnification of SCC in situ (Bowen disease) shows atypical keratinocytes filling the entire epidermis. The cells show nuclear hyperchromasia, and mitotic figures ➡ and dyskeratotic cells ➡ are usually easily identified. **(Right)** Invasive well-differentiated SCC arising in an AK ➡ is shown. Irregular cords and islands with jagged edges, and a few single keratinocytes ➡, infiltrate an inflamed stroma.

ACTINIC CHEILITIS

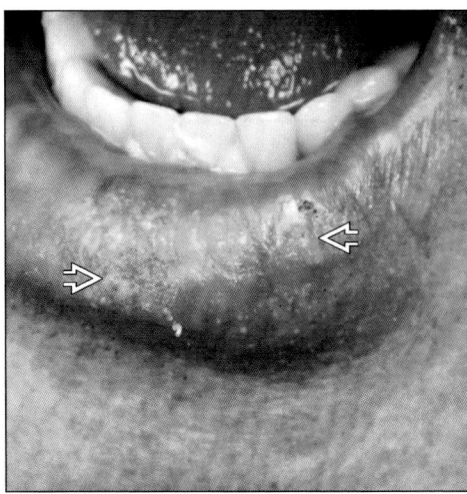

Clinical photograph shows actinic cheilitis diffusely involving the lower lip with associated crusting ➡. (Courtesy J. Wu, MD.)

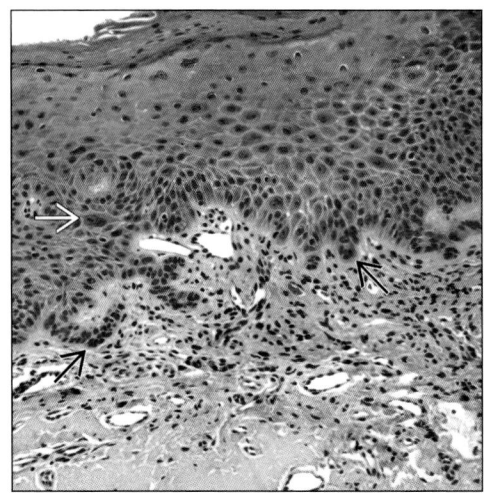

Histologic section of actinic cheilitis shows mucosal acanthosis with overlying parakeratosis. There is irregular budding ➡ and basilar atypia, with the cells showing enlarged, hyperchromatic-staining nuclei ➡.

TERMINOLOGY

Abbreviations
- Actinic cheilitis (AC)

Synonyms
- Actinic keratosis (AK) of lip
- Solar cheilosis
- Cheilosis exfoliativa

Definitions
- Proliferation of atypical keratinocytes involving basilar layers of mucosal epithelium
- Minority of cases may transform into squamous cell carcinoma in situ (SCCis) or invasive SCC

ETIOLOGY/PATHOGENESIS

Environmental Exposure
- Chronic sun exposure, especially UVB rays
- Smoking and chronic irritation are also risk factors

Infectious Agents
- Herpes virus infection and syphilis implicated in rare cases

CLINICAL ISSUES

Epidemiology
- Age
  - Occurs in older adults with longstanding sun damage
- Gender
  - Much more common in males than females
- Ethnicity
  - Most commonly occurs in Caucasians

Site
- Most often presents on lower lip in vermilion zone

Presentation
- Dry, whitish gray, scaly plaques with erythema
  - Recurrent crusting and healing may occur
- Erosions and ulcerations may be present
- Large areas of lip may be involved

Treatment
- Surgical approaches
  - Conservative excision may be performed to prevent development of SCC, but is not necessary in most cases
- Drugs
  - Similar to AKs, often treated with liquid nitrogen (cryotherapy), imiquimod, diclofenac, or 5-fluorouracil

Prognosis
- Excellent in most cases, low risk of developing SCCis and invasive SCC

MICROSCOPIC PATHOLOGY

Histologic Features
- Mucosa may be hyperplastic or atrophic
- Often show overlying parakeratosis alternating with orthokeratosis
- Basilar keratinocytic atypia with budding, similar to AK
  - May involve 1/2 to 2/3 of mucosal thickness (Bowenoid features) in some cases
- Increased mitotic activity typically present in basilar layers
- Submucosal tissue shows prominent solar elastosis, variable telangiectasia, and mild to moderately dense inflammatory infiltrate
  - Intense inflammatory infiltrate should raise the possibility of adjacent invasive SCC

ACTINIC CHEILITIS

Key Facts

Terminology

- Actinic cheilitis (AC)
- Actinic keratosis of lip

Etiology/Pathogenesis

- Chronic sun exposure, especially UVB rays

Clinical Issues

- Excellent in most cases, low risk of developing SCCis and invasive SCC

Microscopic Pathology

- Mucosa may be hyperplastic or atrophic
- Basilar keratinocytic atypia with budding
- Increased mitotic activity typically present in basilar layers

Top Differential Diagnoses

- Squamous cell carcinoma in situ (Bowen disease)
- Squamous cell carcinoma (SCC)
- Actinic cheilitis prurigo

Cytologic Features

- Cells show mild to moderate atypia, with nuclear enlargement, hyperchromasia, and enlarged nucleoli

DIFFERENTIAL DIAGNOSIS

Squamous Cell Carcinoma In Situ (Bowen Disease)

- Full thickness keratinocytic atypia (dysplasia), often with prominent suprabasilar mitoses and apoptotic figures
- May develop in some cases of actinic cheilitis

Squamous Cell Carcinoma (SCC)

- Invasive islands of atypical keratinocytes involving submucosal stroma
- Often associated with ulceration and dense inflammatory infiltrate
- May arise in preexisting actinic cheilitis
  - Prolonged ulceration should raise the possibility of development of SCC

Actinic Cheilitis Prurigo

- Most common in Native Americans, usually presents in summer months after sun exposure
- Epithelial spongiosis with superficial and deep perivascular lymphocytic infiltrate
- May show mucosal acanthosis and parakeratosis, but it lacks significant cytologic atypia

Contact Cheilitis

- Similar to contact dermatitis on cutaneous surfaces
- Spongiosis and intraepithelial lymphocytes present; eosinophils often present in stroma
- Lacks significant cytologic atypia of basilar keratinocytes

Plasma Cell Cheilitis

- Prominent plasmacytic infiltrate in submucosal stroma
- Lacks significant overlying epithelial atypia

SELECTED REFERENCES

1. Castiñeiras I et al: Actinic cheilitis: evolution to squamous cell carcinoma after carbon dioxide laser vaporization. A study of 43 cases. J Dermatolog Treat. 21(1):49-53, 2010
2. Cavalcante AS et al: Actinic cheilitis: clinical and histological features. J Oral Maxillofac Surg. 66(3):498-503, 2008
3. Rossi R et al: Photodynamic therapy: treatment of choice for actinic cheilitis? Dermatol Ther. 21(5):412-5, 2008
4. Ulrich C et al: Management of actinic cheilitis using diclofenac 3% gel: a report of six cases. Br J Dermatol. 156 Suppl 3:43-6, 2007
5. Picascia DD et al: Actinic cheilitis: a review of the etiology, differential diagnosis, and treatment. J Am Acad Dermatol. 17(2 Pt 1):255-64, 1987

IMAGE GALLERY

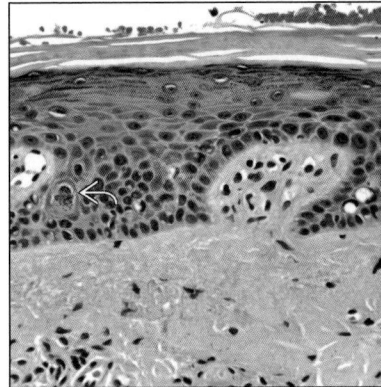 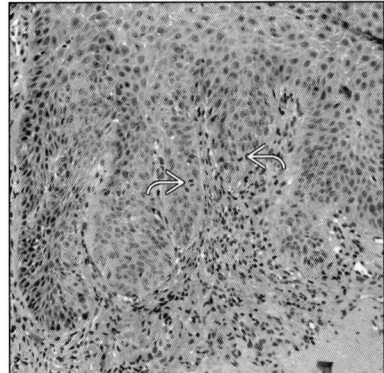 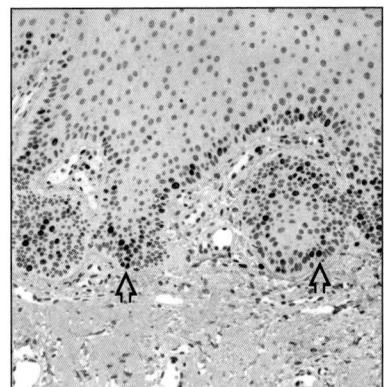

(Left) This example of AC shows mild basilar atypia, with enlarged, hyperchromatic-staining nuclei. Note the large, atypical mitotic figure ➡ just above the basilar layer. *(Center)* AC with prominent mucosal acanthosis and elongation of the rete ridges. Atypical keratinocytes involve the lower 1/3 of the epithelium, and scattered mitotic figures are easily identified ➡. *(Right)* Immunohistochemistry for Ki-67 shows increased proliferative activity with strong nuclear staining in numerous basilar keratinocytes ➡.

SQUAMOUS CELL CARCINOMA IN SITU (BOWEN DISEASE)

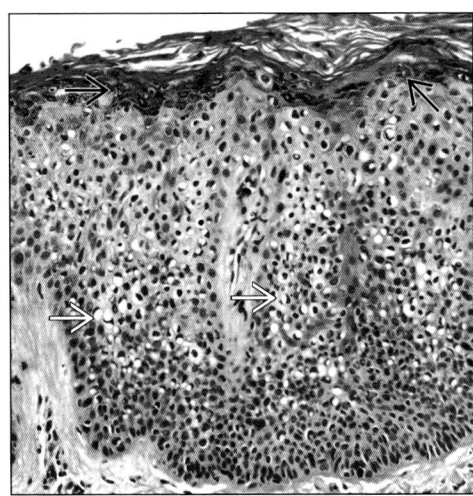

Bowen disease (SCCis) is characterized by a proliferation of atypical intraepidermal keratinocytes filling the entire epidermis, including the granular layer ➡. Many of the cells show cytoplasmic clearing ➡.

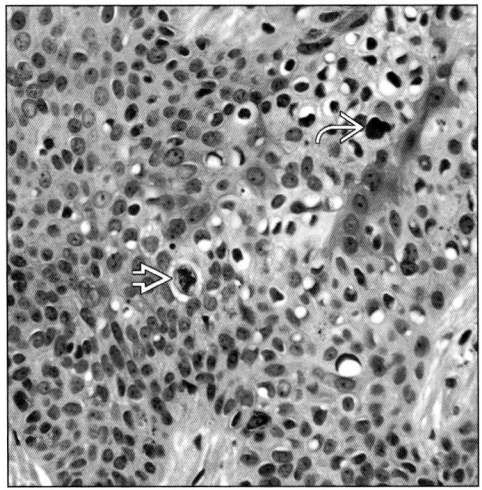

High magnification of Bowen disease shows prominent cytologic atypia, an atypical mitotic figure ➡ in the mid-epidermis, and apoptotic cells ➡.

TERMINOLOGY

Abbreviations
- Squamous cell carcinoma in situ (SCCis)

Synonyms
- Bowen disease
- Squamous intraepithelial neoplasia (SIN)

Definitions
- Full thickness intraepidermal atypia of squamous keratinocytes often with numerous mitotic figures and apoptotic cells

ETIOLOGY/PATHOGENESIS

Sun Exposure
- Chronic UV radiation strongly implicated in SCCis

Immunosuppression
- Increased risk of developing SCCis in immunosuppressed patients, especially organ transplant recipients

HPV Infection
- Some cases of SCCis are related to HPV infection, particularly in anogenital sites
  - SCCis also may arise in verrucae and condylomata

CLINICAL ISSUES

Site
- Most common on head and neck region, other sun-exposed sites

Presentation
- Scaly patch or plaque lesion
- Ulceration and hemorrhage may be present

Treatment
- Surgical approaches
  - Complete surgical excision is standard and definitive therapy
  - Mohs surgery often performed for facial lesions to minimize amount of tissue taken
  - Electrodessication and curettage (ED&C) may also be used
- Drugs
  - Topical therapy with immunomodulators, including imiquimod or 5-fluorouracil, may be used
    - Patients with extensive lesions or poor surgical candidates

Prognosis
- Excellent in most cases
- Small risk for invasive squamous cell carcinoma
  - Greater risk in patients with immunosuppression or numerous lesions

MACROSCOPIC FEATURES

General Features
- Broad, superficial lesion with epidermal thickening and overlying scale

MICROSCOPIC PATHOLOGY

Histologic Features
- Atypical intraepidermal proliferation of squamous cells extending into upper levels of the epidermis
  - Basilar keratinocytes are often spared, leading to so-called "eyeliner" sign
- Overlying parakeratosis often diffusely present, without skip areas over adnexal structures
- Follicular epithelial involvement is typically seen

SQUAMOUS CELL CARCINOMA IN SITU (BOWEN DISEASE)

Key Facts

Terminology

- Squamous cell carcinoma in situ (SCCis)
- Synonyms: Bowen disease, squamous intraepithelial neoplasia
- Full thickness intraepidermal atypia of squamous keratinocytes often with numerous mitotic figures and apoptotic cells

Etiology/Pathogenesis

- Chronic UV radiation strongly implicated in SCCis
- Some cases of SCCis are related to HPV infection, particularly in anogenital sites

Clinical Issues

- Small risk for invasive squamous cell carcinoma
- Most common on head and neck region, other sun-exposed sites

Microscopic Pathology

- Cells are usually markedly enlarged and atypical appearing, with nuclear hyperchromasia and enlarged nucleoli
- Basilar keratinocytes are often spared, leading to so-called "eyeliner" sign
- Overlying parakeratosis is usually diffusely present, without skip areas over adnexal structures
- Numerous intraepidermal mitotic figures and apoptotic figures typically present

Top Differential Diagnoses

- Actinic keratosis (AK)
- Invasive squamous cell carcinoma (SCC)
- Paget disease and other pagetoid in situ carcinomas

- Cells are usually markedly enlarged and atypical appearing, with nuclear hyperchromasia and enlarged nucleoli
- Numerous intraepidermal mitotic figures and apoptotic figures typically present

Cytologic Features

- Enlarged cells with dense eosinophilic-staining cytoplasm, enlarged hyperchromatic-staining nuclei, and prominent nucleoli

DIFFERENTIAL DIAGNOSIS

Actinic Keratosis (AK)

- Defined as atypical proliferation of basilar keratinocytes not involving the full epidermal thickness
  - However, bowenoid AK can be difficult and somewhat subjective to separate from SCCis, as it can involve 1/2 to 2/3 of the epidermal thickness
- Typically spares adnexal structures, while SCCis involves them
  - AKs often show parakeratosis (overlying the AK) alternating with orthokeratosis (overlying uninvolved adnexal structures), leading to an alternating "red and blue" pattern, as opposed to diffuse parakeratosis overlying SCCis

Invasive Squamous Cell Carcinoma (SCC)

- Shows infiltrative nests, cords, &/or single cells in the dermis
- May only be focally/superficially invasive in some cases, and can be easily overlooked on scanning magnification
- Superficial biopsies in which intraepidermal cells are transected at base of the biopsy cannot be definitively evaluated for invasion
  - Such cases should be signed out as "at least in situ," with a comment stating that underlying invasive carcinoma cannot be excluded with certainty

Paget Disease and Other Pagetoid In Situ Carcinomas

- In differential diagnosis with pagetoid Bowen disease
- Cells are epithelioid appearing and show abundant amphophilic to clear or foamy-appearing cytoplasm
- Gland formation may be seen in some Paget cases but is absent in most
- Immunohistochemistry typically shows strong positivity for CK7, CEA, EMA, and GCDFP-15; ER/PR positive in many cases, especially mammary Paget
  - Typically negative for CK20 and high molecular weight cytokeratins including CK5/6, CK903
- Other pagetoid carcinomas including pagetoid sebaceous carcinoma (EMA, CK7, and androgen R[+]) and Merkel cell carcinoma (CK20, synaptophysin, chromogranin[+]) may be in the differential

SELECTED REFERENCES

1. Cassarino DS et al: SIN, not KIN. J Cutan Pathol. 36(7):820, 2009
2. Nakanishi G et al: Human papillomavirus genome integration in multifocal vulvar Bowen's disease and squamous cell carcinoma. Clin Exp Dermatol. 34(8):e965-7, 2009
3. Neubert T et al: Bowen's disease - a review of newer treatment options. Ther Clin Risk Manag. 4(5):1085-95, 2008
4. Rosen T et al: Treatment of Bowen's disease with topical 5% imiquimod cream: retrospective study. Dermatol Surg. 33(4):427-31; discussion 431-2, 2007
5. Cassarino DS et al: Cutaneous squamous cell carcinoma: a comprehensive clinicopathologic classification--part two. J Cutan Pathol. 33(4):261-79, 2006
6. Hama N et al: Detection of mucosal human papilloma virus DNA in bowenoid papulosis, Bowen's disease and squamous cell carcinoma of the skin. J Dermatol. 33(5):331-7, 2006
7. Sun JD et al: Papillated Bowen disease, a distinct variant. Am J Dermatopathol. 28(5):395-8, 2006
8. Campbell C et al: p53 mutations are common and early events that precede tumor invasion in squamous cell neoplasia of the skin. J Invest Dermatol. 100(6):746-8, 1993

SQUAMOUS CELL CARCINOMA IN SITU (BOWEN DISEASE)

Microscopic Features

(Left) Low magnification of a SCCis shows epidermal acanthosis with expansion of the epidermis by atypical keratinocytes, many of which show pale to clear cytoplasmic staining ➡. Note the focal overlying parakeratosis ➡. *(Right)* Intermediate magnification of SCCis shows expansion of the epidermis by atypical keratinocytes. Numerous mitotic figures are easily identified ➡. Scattered intraepidermal pigmented cells and focal papillary dermal pigment incontinence are seen ➡.

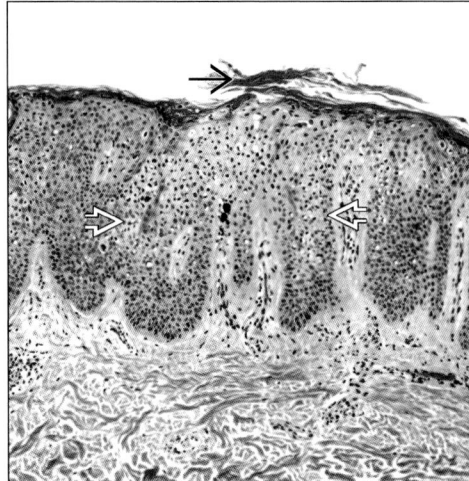
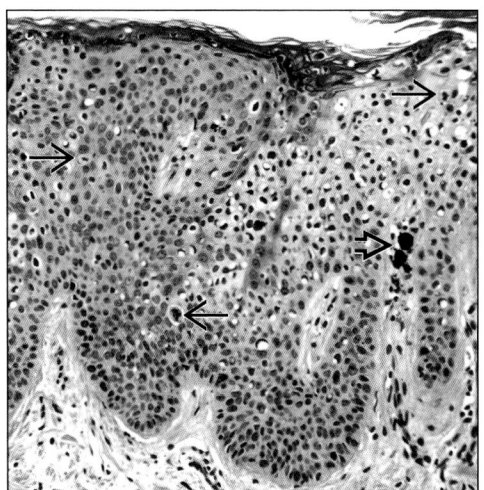

(Left) High magnification of a SCCis shows disordered proliferation of cells with prominent cytologic atypia, including nuclear hyperchromasia and enlarged nucleoli, as well as multiple mitotic figures ➡ in the mid- to upper epidermis. *(Right)* Pagetoid Bowen disease shows upward spread of clusters of atypical squamous cells ➡ with abundant clear cytoplasm extending into the granular layer with overlying parakeratosis. Note the preserved basilar layer ➡ of benign keratinocytes.

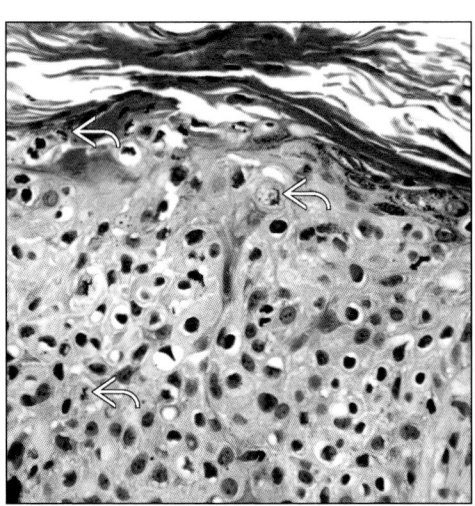
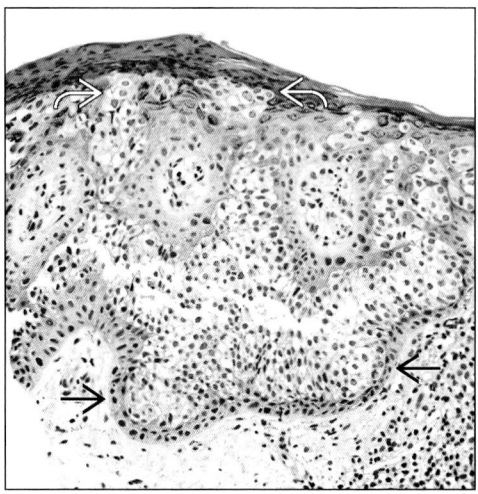

(Left) Verrucoid SCCis with hypergranulosis, mild papillomatosis, and superficial koilocytic-appearing cells, suggesting an HPV etiology. Note the scattered mitotic figures ➡ and enlarged, bizarre-appearing, hyperchromatic-staining nuclei ➡. *(Right)* This is a rare example of a SCCis arising in association with a longstanding verruca vulgaris. There is marked, full thickness atypia of the squamous cells, many of which show prominent perinuclear halos ➡, consistent with HPV effect.

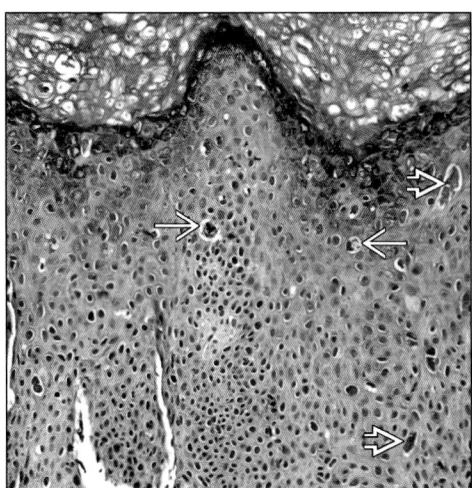
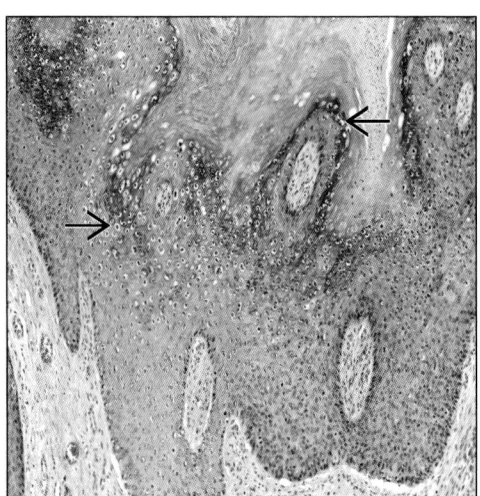

SQUAMOUS CELL CARCINOMA IN SITU (BOWEN DISEASE)

Differential Diagnosis

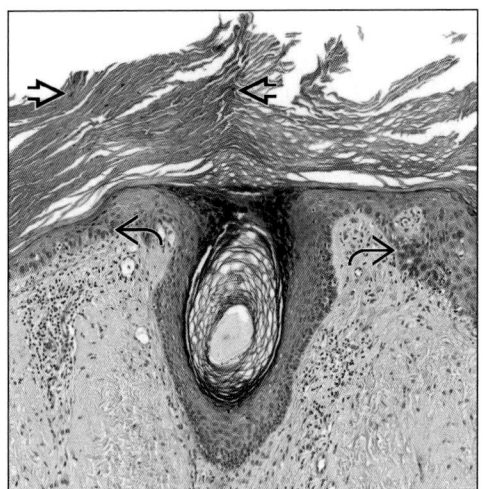

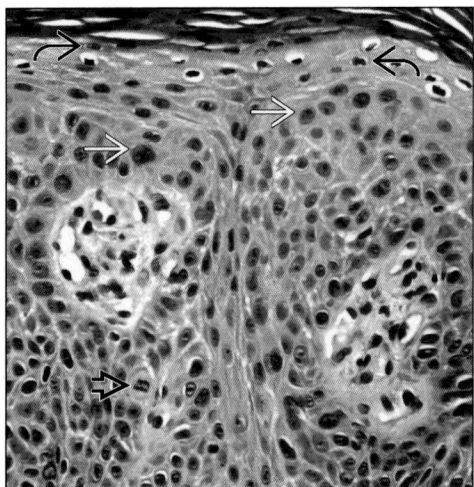

(Left) Actinic keratosis classically shows basilar keratinocytic atypia ⮕ surrounding, but sparing, a hair follicle (which are typically involved in Bowen disease). There is prominent overlying hyperkeratosis and parakeratosis ⮕. **(Right)** Bowenoid actinic keratosis shows atypical keratinocytes ⮕ involving the lower and mid-levels of the epidermis but sparing the upper levels, which show smaller, more bland-appearing keratinocytes ⮕. Basilar mitotic figures are identified ⮕.

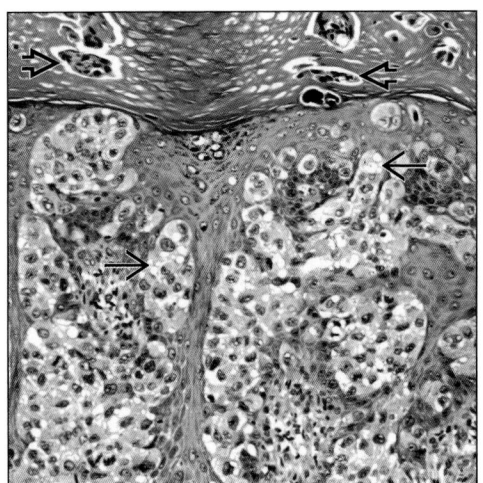

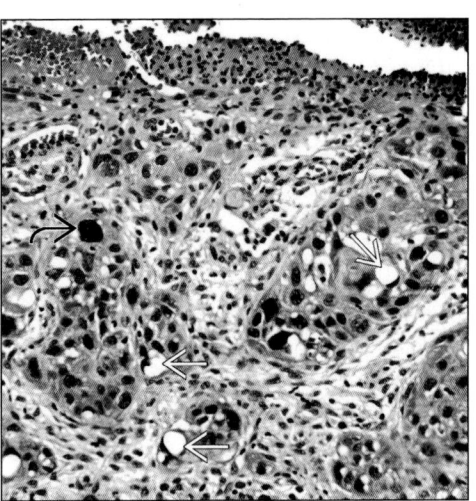

(Left) Extramammary Paget disease shows prominent intraepidermal nests of epithelioid cells with abundant eosinophilic to vacuolated ⮕ cytoplasm. Numerous pagetoid single cells and nests extend into the stratum corneum ⮕. **(Right)** Pagetoid sebaceous carcinoma is rare but often mimics clear cell SCCis and extramammary Paget disease. It is characterized by numerous atypical cells with nuclear hyperchromasia ⮕ and cytoplasmic vacuoles displacing and indenting the nuclei ⮕.

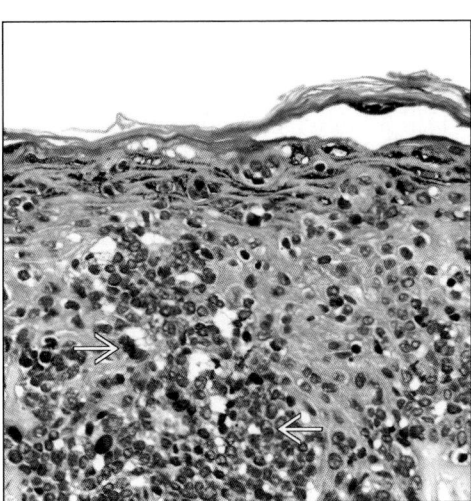

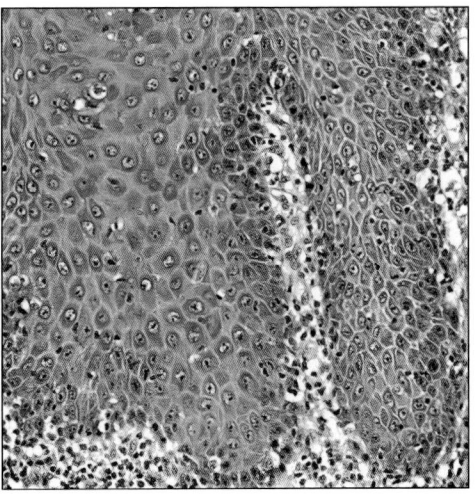

(Left) Pagetoid Merkel cell carcinoma shows a proliferation of atypical cells with hyperchromatic to vesicular nuclei with focal molding ⮕. Merkel cell carcinoma may show pagetoid spread in up to 15-20% of cases. IHC for CK20 and neuroendocrine markers confirms the diagnosis. **(Right)** Verrucous carcinoma shows expansion of the epidermis by enlarged squamous keratinocytes with minimal cytologic atypia. Cells typically show dense eosinophilic cytoplasm & vesicular chromatin.

BOWENOID PAPULOSIS

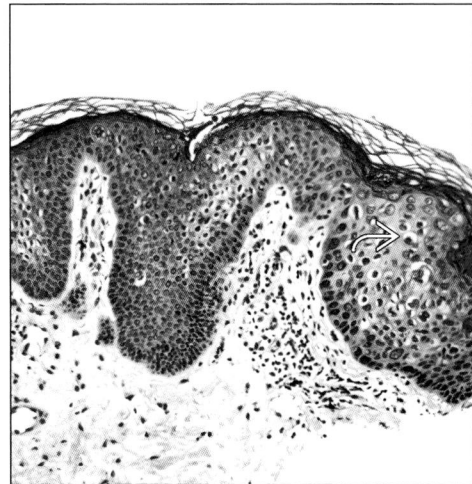

Patchy foci of full thickness keratinocytic atypia are usually seen in bowenoid papulosis. Atypical cells vary from small basaloid to larger and more pleomorphic with koilocytic-like changes ➡.

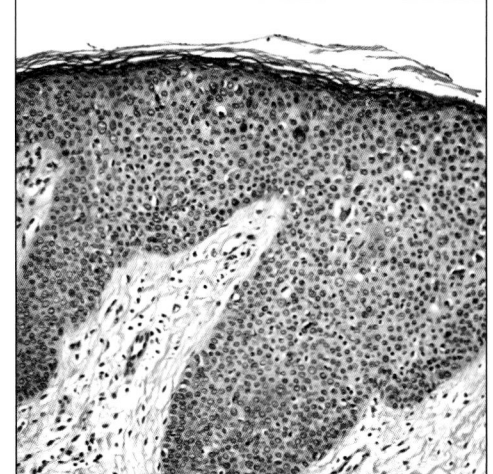

Bowenoid papulosis shows atypical keratinocytes throughout the full thickness of the epithelium. There are several mitoses and koilocytic change.

TERMINOLOGY

Abbreviations
- Bowenoid papulosis (BP)

Synonyms
- Multicentric pigmented Bowen disease

Definitions
- Multifocal HPV-related, papular, preneoplastic condition affecting anogenital region in sexually active young adults

ETIOLOGY/PATHOGENESIS

Etiology
- Related to high-risk types of HPV, especially type 16
- Other types of HPV (18, 31, 32, 33, 34, 35, 39, 42, 48, 51, 52, 53, and 54) have also been implicated
- Usually transmitted via sexual contact

Pathogenesis
- Oncogenic HPV elaborate proteins that interfere with normal cellular homeostasis

CLINICAL ISSUES

Epidemiology
- Incidence
  - Unknown and probably underestimated
  - Immunosuppression, including HIV infection, greatly increases risk for bowenoid papulosis
- Age
  - 20-40 years

Presentation
- Solitary or, more often, multiple soft papules and macules with flat surface
  - Surface may be verruciform
- Small (0.2-1 cm in diameter); red, brown, or flesh-colored
- In males
  - Affects skin of shaft, epithelium of glans, coronal sulcus, foreskin, or perianal area
- In females
  - Labia majora is most frequent site
  - Spread to other vulvar areas is common; perianal lesions may occur
  - Lesions tend to be bilateral and hyperpigmented
- Extraanogenital lesions are exceptional
- Usually asymptomatic
  - May be pruritic or painful
- Lesions in immunosuppressed patients tend to be more widespread

Treatment
- Usually may be treated with locally destructive modalities
  - Important to remember that BP may be multifocal and has malignant potential: Follow-up is advised

Prognosis
- Most BP lesions run benign course with spontaneous regression occurring within several months
- Some lesions (especially in older or immunocompromised patients) last longer or never regress at all
- Minority of lesions evolve to invasive squamous cell carcinoma (SCC)
- Females with BP and female partners of men with BP have increased risk of cervical intraepithelial neoplasia

MICROSCOPIC PATHOLOGY

Histologic Features
- Proliferation of atypical cells with high nuclear:cytoplasmic ratio (basaloid cells) that may be scattered throughout epidermis, often with preserved maturation

BOWENOID PAPULOSIS

Key Facts

Etiology/Pathogenesis
• Most often related to HPV 16

Clinical Issues
• Often multifocal
• Benign-looking papules
• Usually affecting skin of shaft in males
• Affecting labia majora in females
  ○ Lesions tend to be bilateral and hyperpigmented

Microscopic Pathology
• Proliferation of atypical basaloid and koilocytic cells as scattered single units or involving full thickness of epithelium
• Most cases are indistinguishable from SCCis

Top Differential Diagnoses
• Vulvar and penile intraepithelial neoplasia (VIN and PeIN)
• Treated condyloma

• Koilocytic-like changes are also seen in most cases
• Range of atypia from scattered atypical cells to low-grade dysplasia to full thickness atypia of the squamous epithelium
• Morphological features are indistinguishable from HPV-related vulvar and penile intraepithelial neoplasia (VIN and PeIN)
• Variable increased pigmentation of basal layer

Predominant Pattern/Injury Type
• Epithelial dysplasia

Predominant Cell/Compartment Type
• Epithelial, squamous

DIFFERENTIAL DIAGNOSIS

Squamous Cell Carcinoma In Situ (HPV-related VIN and PeIN)
• Despite clinically benign-looking appearance of BP, histopathologic findings reveal features that may be identical to those of SCCis
• Clinical correlation is crucial to make the distinction

Treated Flat Condyloma (after Podophyllin Application)
• Pallor of epithelium, nuclear enlargement, necrotic keratinocytes
• Increase in number of mitotic figures (metaphase arrest)

• Atypical mitoses should not be seen

DIAGNOSTIC CHECKLIST

Pathologic Interpretation Pearls
• Histologically, most cases are indistinguishable from SCCis
• Presence of only scattered atypical cells or more patchy pattern of full thickness squamous dysplasia may suggest BP
• Clinical correlation is crucial to make distinction

SELECTED REFERENCES

1. Liu H et al: Expression of p16 and hTERT protein is associated with the presence of high-risk human papillomavirus in Bowenoid papulosis. J Cutan Pathol. 33(8):551-8, 2006
2. Obalek S et al: Bowenoid papulosis of the male and female genitalia: risk of cervical neoplasia. J Am Acad Dermatol. 14(3):433-44, 1986
3. Wade TR et al: The effects of resin of podophyllin on condyloma acuminatum. Am J Dermatopathol. 6(2):109-22, 1984
4. Eisen RF et al: Spontaneous regression of bowenoid papulosis of the penis. Cutis. 32(3):269-72, 1983
5. Wade TR et al: Bowenoid papulosis. JAMA. 246(7):732-3, 1981
6. Wade TR et al: Bowenoid papulosis of the genitalia. Arch Dermatol. 115(3):306-8, 1979

IMAGE GALLERY

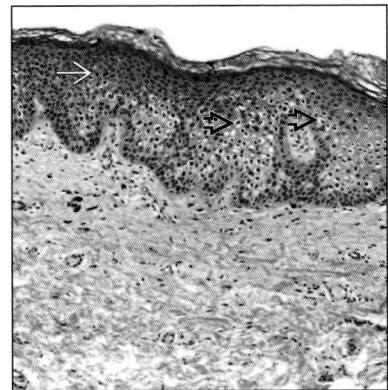 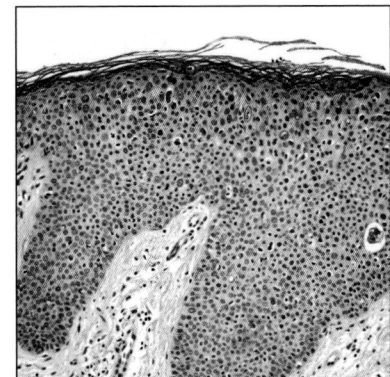 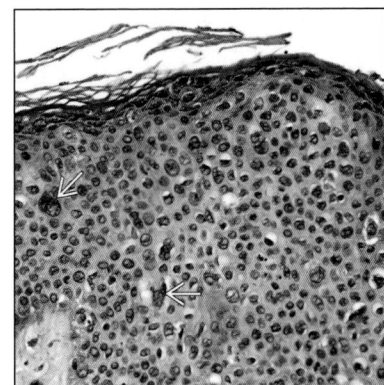

(Left) BP is seen with preserved maturation and scattered full thickness atypia. Dyskeratotic and apoptotic keratinocytes ➡ and koilocytic changes ⊳ are present. *(Center)* The changes in BP are indistinguishable from those seen in squamous carcinoma in situ (HPV-related VIN and PeIN). *(Right)* This higher power view shows basaloid and pleomorphic cells ➡ replacing the epidermis.

PENILE AND VULVAR INTRAEPITHELIAL NEOPLASIA

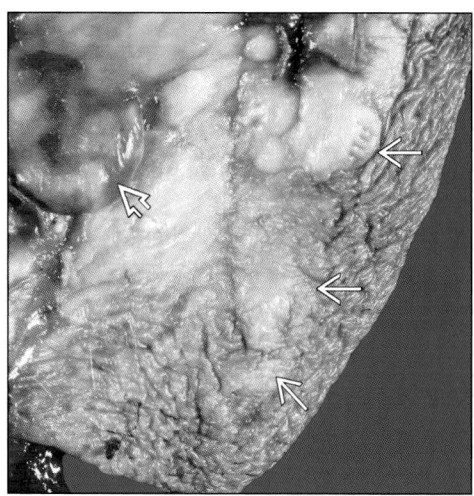

Vulvar intraepithelial neoplasia may appear as a raised, thickened white plaque ➡. This lesion is associated with an invasive component ➡ that is exophytic. (Courtesy T. Quinn, MD.)

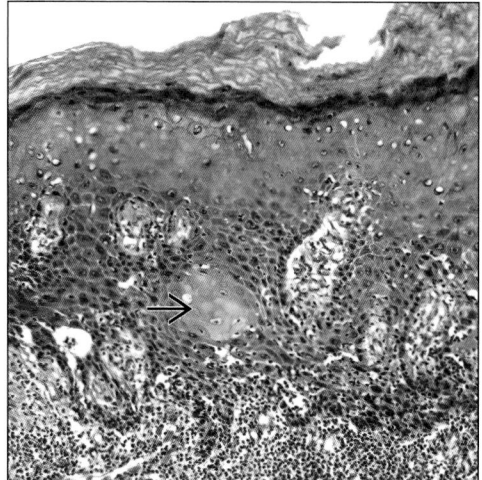

Enlarged keratinocytes with abundant eosinophilic cytoplasm throughout most of the epithelium are seen in differentiated PeIN/VIN. Characteristic keratin pearl formation is present ➡.

TERMINOLOGY

Abbreviations
- Penile intraepithelial neoplasia (PeIN)
- Vulvar intraepithelial neoplasia (VIN)

Synonyms
- Erythroplasia of Queyrat, Bowen disease, squamous cell carcinoma in situ (SCCis)

Definitions
- VIN and PeIN are considered intraepithelial (in situ) precursor lesions of invasive SCC

ETIOLOGY/PATHOGENESIS

Pathogenesis
- Bimodal pathway of tumor progression in vulvar and penile SCC (HPV-related and HPV-unrelated)
  - Basaloid, warty, and warty-basaloid (mixed) VIN and PeIN are HPV-related (especially HPV 16)
  - Differentiated (simplex) VIN and PeIN are HPV-unrelated
    - May be related to lichen sclerosus et atrophicus (LS&A)
    - May be associated with *P53* mutations

CLINICAL ISSUES

Epidemiology
- Incidence
  - Real incidence is unknown
  - 2/3 associated with invasive SCC
- Age
  - 5th and 6th decades
    - About 1/2 of patients with VIN are < 40 years old

Presentation
- Differentiated PeIN and VIN

  - Older patients
  - Usually arises in setting of chronic scarring, inflammatory dermatosis, especially lichen sclerosus et atrophicus (LS&A)
- Warty, basaloid, and mixed PeIN and VIN (a.k.a. VIN of usual type in vulvar pathology)
  - Younger patients
  - Patients may have history of condyloma

Treatment
- Surgery, locally destructive treatments

Prognosis
- Most studies are retrospective and real prognosis remains unknown

MACROSCOPIC FEATURES

General Features
- VIN and PeIN have heterogeneous gross appearance
- Solitary or multifocal
- Flat to slightly elevated hyperkeratotic or even condylomatous lesions
- Pearly white, moist, erythematous, dark brown/black macules, papules, or plaques

MICROSCOPIC PATHOLOGY

Histologic Features
- **Differentiated (simplex) PeIN and VIN**
  - Thickened epithelium
  - Elongated and anastomosing rete ridges
  - Atypical basal cells with hyperchromatic nuclei
  - Subtle abnormal maturation (enlarged keratinocytes with abundant eosinophilic cytoplasm)
  - Whorling and keratin pearl formation (usually in deep rete ridges)
  - Prominent intercellular bridges (spongiosis and sometimes acantholysis)

PENILE AND VULVAR INTRAEPITHELIAL NEOPLASIA

Key Facts

Terminology
- Most warty, basaloid, and mixed VIN and PeIN replace 2/3 to entire thickness of epithelium (VIN III and PeIN III) and represent carcinoma in situ
  - VIN/PeIN I-II is rare
- Differentiated VIN/PeIN is considered high-grade lesion

Microscopic Pathology
- Differentiated (simplex) PeIN and VIN (HPV-unrelated)
  - Elongated and anastomosing rete ridges
  - Atypical basal cells with hyperchromatic nuclei
  - Subtle abnormal maturation (large eosinophilic keratinocytes)
  - Whorling and keratin pearl formation
  - Usually associated with LS&A

- Preferential association with HPV-unrelated variants of invasive SCC (keratinizing SCC, verrucous carcinoma)
- Basaloid, warty, and mixed (warty-basaloid) PeIN and VIN (a.k.a. usual VIN) (HPV-related)
  - Basaloid VIN/PeIN: Basaloid cells replace most to full thickness of epithelium
  - Warty VIN/PeIN: Pleomorphic cells with koilocytic changes replace most to full thickness of epithelium
  - Warty-basaloid VIN/PeIN: Pleomorphic cells with koilocytic changes seen on upper epithelium and basaloid cells replace lower epithelium
  - Warty, basaloid, and mixed VIN/PeIN is usually seen adjacent to HPV-related variants of invasive SCC (basaloid and warty types)

  - Parakeratosis is frequent
  - Absence of koilocytosis
  - Usually associated with LS&A
- HPV-related PeIN and VIN (warty, basaloid, mixed warty-basaloid)
  - Most lesions are high-grade: PeIN III and VIN III (atypical cells replacing > 2/3 of squamous epithelium)
  - Atypical/dysplastic cells may extend down the epithelium of hair follicles
  - Low-grade PeIN/VIN I-II (atypical cells replacing < 2/3 of epithelium) is rare
- **Warty PeIN/VIN**
  - Undulating/spiky surface with atypical parakeratosis
  - Pleomorphic cells with koilocytic changes (multinucleation, irregular nuclear contours, perinuclear halos) replace epithelium
  - Mitoses tend to be numerous
- **Basaloid PeIN/VIN**
  - Epithelium replaced by monotonous population of small immature cells with high nuclear/cytoplasmic ratios
  - Apoptosis and mitotic figures are numerous
- **Mixed PeIN/VIN (warty-basaloid)**
  - Lower part of epithelium is replaced by small crowded cells with high nuclear/cytoplasmic ratios
  - Upper portion of epithelium shows features of warty PeIN/VIN
  - Surface often slightly undulated/papillary
  - Mitosis and apoptosis are prominent

Predominant Pattern/Injury Type
- Dysplasia

Predominant Cell/Compartment Type
- Epithelial, squamous

ANCILLARY TESTS

Immunohistochemistry
- p16 is typically positive

DIFFERENTIAL DIAGNOSIS

Squamous Hyperplasia/Lichen Simplex Chronicus
- Reactive condition may be confused with differentiated VIN/PeIN
- Basilar atypia and abnormal maturation are not seen

Condyloma
- Koilocytosis confined to upper epithelium
- Absence of nuclear pleomorphism
- Mitoses are scant and confined to lower epithelium
- Associated with low-risk HPV (usually 6 and 11)
- Usually p16 negative

Bowenoid Papulosis
- Indistinguishable from warty, basaloid, and mixed PeIN/VIN on histology alone
- Clinical correlation is essential for this diagnosis

DIAGNOSTIC CHECKLIST

Pathologic Interpretation Pearls
- Differentiated PeIN: At low power, atypia seems to be present only in lower levels of epidermis
  - At higher power, it is more clear that there is subtle but abnormal maturation in all levels of epithelium
- Warty, basaloid and mixed PeIN are HPV-related, and p16 may be useful morphologic surrogate

SELECTED REFERENCES
1. Chaux A et al: Distinctive association of p16INK4a overexpression with penile intraepithelial neoplasia depicting warty and/or basaloid features: a study of 141 cases evaluating a new nomenclature. Am J Surg Pathol. 34(3):385-92, 2010
2. Sideri M et al: Squamous vulvar intraepithelial neoplasia: 2004 modified terminology, ISSVD Vulvar Oncology Subcommittee. J Reprod Med. 50(11):807-10, 2005

Differentiated PeIN/VIN

(Left) Characteristic features of PeIN and VIN include elongated rete ridges and atypical basilar cells. Abnormal maturation, spongiosis, keratin pearl formation ➡, and parakeratosis are also appreciated. *(Right)* Atypia in the basilar/parabasal layer is easily recognized in differentiated VIN and PeIN. There are enlarged keratinocytes with plump vesicular nuclei and abundant eosinophilic cytoplasm, and parakeratosis is seen on the surface.

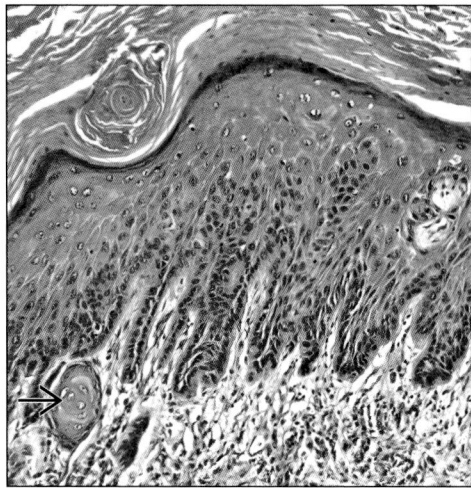
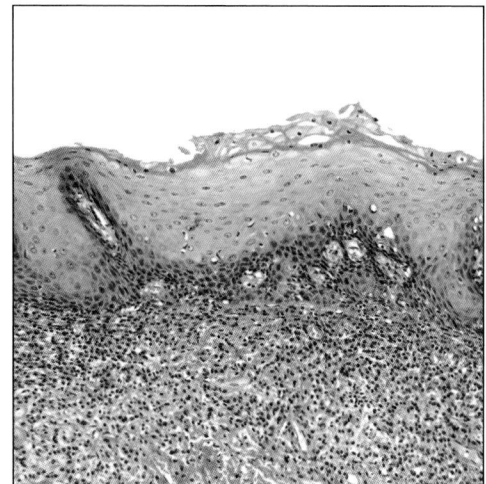

(Left) There is a markedly thickened epithelium with atypical basal and parabasal cells in this example of differentiated PeIN arising in a background of lichen sclerosus. *(Right)* Differentiated VIN/PeIN shows parakeratosis and atypical basilar cells. A few cells showing more frankly atypical nuclei ➡ are seen in this example. There is also a thickened basement membrane and hyalinization of the upper lamina propria corresponding to associated lichen sclerosus.

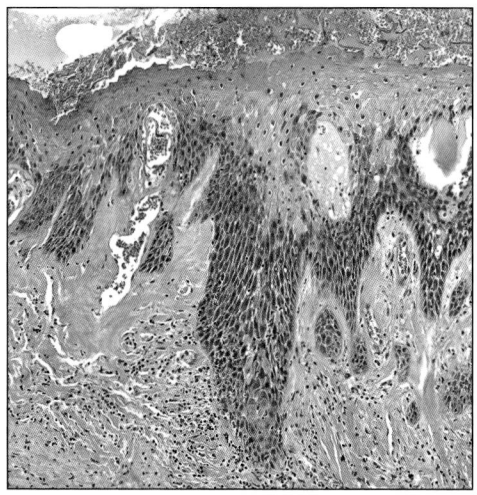
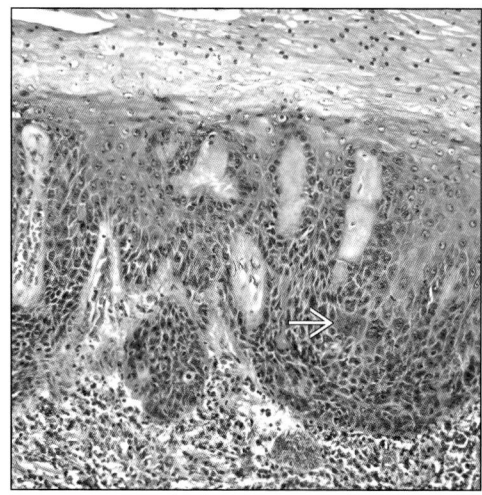

(Left) Differentiated PeIN and VIN ➡ are often seen adjacent to non-HPV-related variants of invasive keratinizing SCC ➡. Note the elongated rete ridges and basilar hyperchromasia of the precursor lesion. *(Right)* Differentiated PeIN ➡ is shown adjacent to an invasive SCC ➡. Note the elongation of the rete ridges and subtle abnormal maturation of the epithelium. Cytologic atypia is minimal.

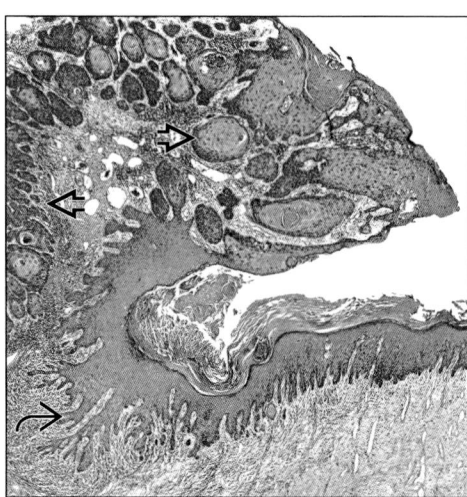
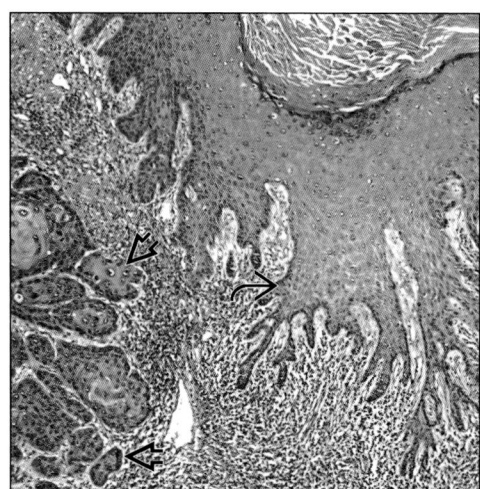

PENILE AND VULVAR INTRAEPITHELIAL NEOPLASIA

Warty, Basaloid, and Warty/Basaloid PeIN/VIN

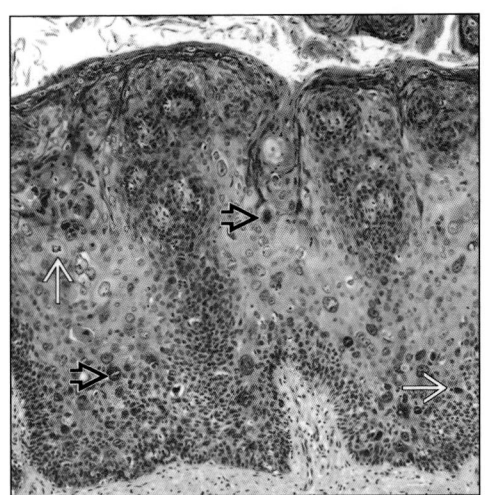

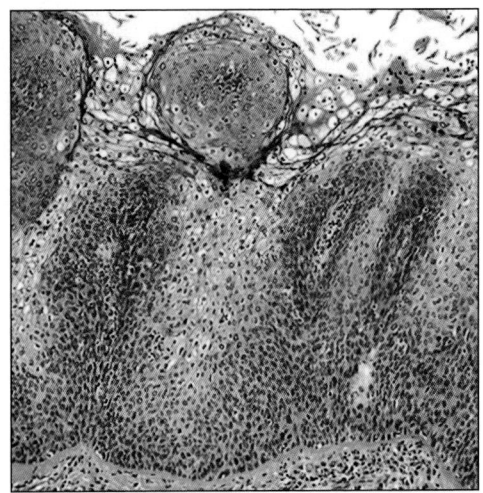

(Left) Warty PeIN and VIN show pleomorphic and hyperchromatic nuclei ⊡, bi- and multinucleation, and multiple mitoses ➡ throughout the epithelium. (Right) Note the full thickness replacement of the epithelium by atypical cells. The lower part of the epithelium is replaced by small basaloid cells, and the upper part is replaced by larger cells showing koilocytotic changes. These features characterize PeIN and VIN of warty-basaloid type.

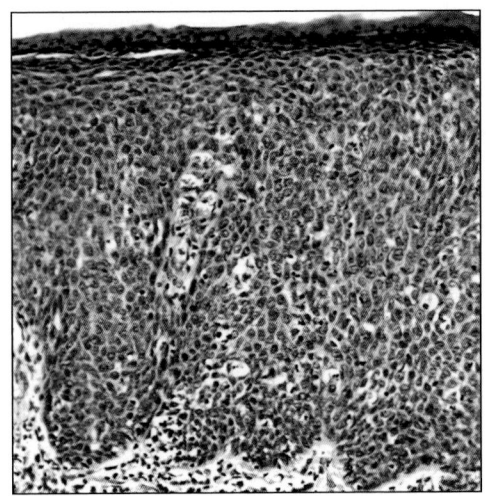

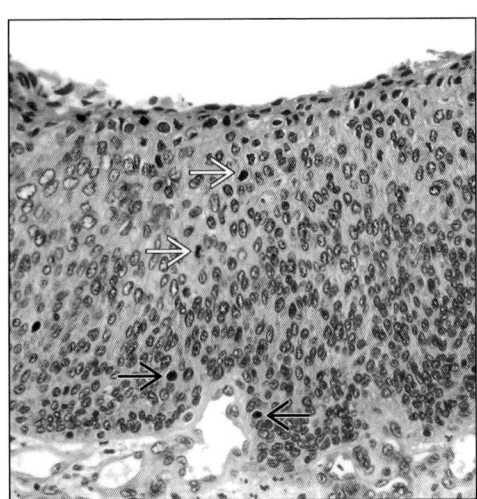

(Left) Proliferation of small round crowded cells with high nuclear/cytoplasmic ratios and hyperchromatic nuclei replacing the entire thickness of the epithelium is seen in the basaloid variant of VIN and PeIN. (Right) The epithelium is completely replaced by atypical cells with basaloid features. Numerous mitoses ➡ and apoptotic bodies ➡ are seen. The diagnosis of carcinoma in situ is easily achieved in high-grade basaloid PeIN and VIN.

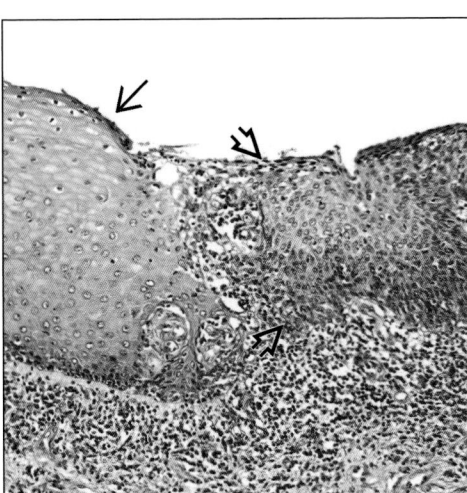

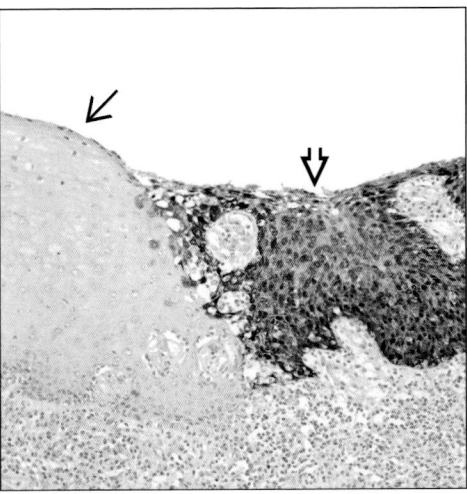

(Left) This picture illustrates a sharp demarcation between the atypical epithelium of basaloid PeIN ⊡ and adjacent hyperplastic squamous epithelium without atypia ➡. (Right) Immunohistochemistry with p16 (surrogate marker for oncogenic HPV) is strongly positive in the area of basaloid PeIN ⊡. The adjacent hyperplastic epithelium is negative ➡.

EPIDERMODYSPLASIA VERRUCIFORMIS

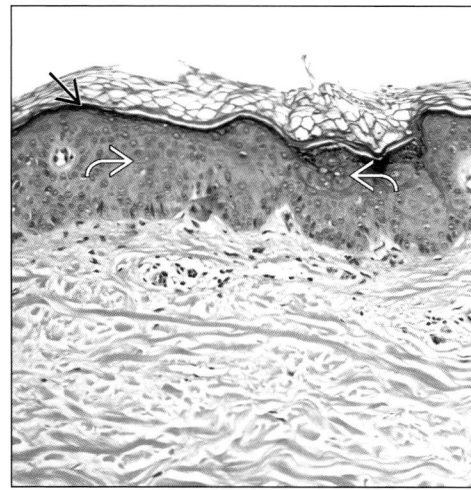

EDV is characterized by irregular epidermal acanthosis associated with an intraepidermal proliferation of enlarged, bluish-gray staining keratinocytes ➔. Note the overlying hypergranulosis ➔.

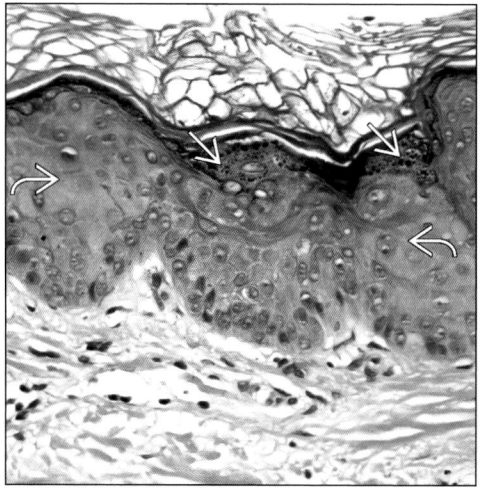

Higher magnification of EDV shows a proliferation of enlarged, bluish-gray staining keratinocytes ➔ with prominent keratohyaline granules ➔.

TERMINOLOGY

Abbreviations
- Epidermodysplasia verruciformis (EDV)

Definitions
- HPV-related intraepidermal proliferation of enlarged, often bluish-gray staining keratinocytes

ETIOLOGY/PATHOGENESIS

Environmental Exposure
- HPV infection is established as etiologic agent
- Subtypes implicated include HPV 3, 5, 8, 9, 10, 12

Genetic Condition
- Majority of cases are familial (genodermatosis)
- Inherited mutations in *EVER1/TMC6* or *EVER2/TMC8* lead to susceptibility to infections with HPV
  - Increased risk for development of in situ and invasive squamous cell carcinoma (SCC)

CLINICAL ISSUES

Presentation
- Scaly papules or plaques

Treatment
- Options, risks, complications
  - As most cases are benign, aggressive treatment not usually indicated
  - Radiotherapy reported to increase risk for malignant transformation and should be avoided
- Surgical approaches
  - Excision may be considered in patients considered at higher risk for SCC
- Drugs
  - Topical antivirals (similar to those used for verruca vulgaris) may be used

  - Liquid nitrogen (cryotherapy) is usually effective

Prognosis
- Risk for malignant transformation increased in genetic forms
- Up to 25-50% of patients may eventually develop in situ or invasive SCC

MICROSCOPIC PATHOLOGY

Histologic Features
- Epidermal acanthosis with expansion of the epidermis by enlarged, mildly atypical-appearing cells
- Cells typically show abundant bluish-gray staining cytoplasm
- Nuclei can be hyperchromatic or cleared out with small nucleoli
  - Perinuclear halos usually prominent
- Mitotic figures are rare
- High-grade atypia usually not present
  - If full thickness frank atypia present, should be diagnosed as SCCis (Bowen disease), which can arise in EDV

Cytologic Features
- Enlarged squamous cells with abundant bluish-gray cytoplasm
- Nuclear clearing may be seen in some of the cells

Predominant Pattern/Injury Type
- Epithelial proliferation of atypical enlarged squamous cells

DIFFERENTIAL DIAGNOSIS

Verruca Plana
- Clinically shows overlapping features with EDV

EPIDERMODYSPLASIA VERRUCIFORMIS

Key Facts

Terminology
- Epidermodysplasia verruciformis (EDV)
- HPV-related intraepidermal proliferation of enlarged, often bluish-gray staining keratinocytes

Etiology/Pathogenesis
- Subtypes implicated include HPV 3, 5, 8, 9, 10, 12
- Majority of cases are familial (genodermatosis)
  - Increased risk for development of in situ and invasive SCC

Microscopic Pathology
- Epidermal acanthosis with proliferation of enlarged cells with abundant bluish-gray staining cytoplasm
- Perinuclear halos usually prominent

Top Differential Diagnoses
- Verruca plana
- Actinic keratosis (AK)
- Bowen disease/squamous cell carcinoma in situ
- EDV acanthoma

- Histologically shows epidermal acanthosis with hypergranulosis and overlying orthokeratosis or hyperkeratosis
- Superficial koilocytic cells with nuclear hyperchromasia and prominent perinuclear halos
- Lacks prominent bluish-gray staining cells of EDV

Actinic Keratosis (AK)
- Basilar keratinocytes show nuclear enlargement and atypia
- Basilar budding and overlying parakeratosis usually present
- Mitotic figures usually easily identified
- No bluish-gray staining cells as in EDV

Bowen Disease/Squamous Cell Carcinoma In Situ (SCCis)
- Full thickness epidermal atypia with enlarged squamous cells
- Numerous mitotic figures usually present
- No bluish-gray staining cells as in EDV

EDV Acanthoma
- Rarely, histologic changes typical of EDV can be seen as a single lesion
- May be the only finding or may be associated with another benign lesion, including nevus, seborrheic keratosis, or acantholytic acanthoma
- If the patient has only 1 lesion, it may be referred to as "EDV acanthoma"

DIAGNOSTIC CHECKLIST

Pathologic Interpretation Pearls
- Intraepidermal proliferation of enlarged, often bluish-gray staining keratinocytes with perinuclear halos

SELECTED REFERENCES

1. Kim T et al: Development of aggressive squamous cell carcinoma in epidermodysplasia verruciformis associated with human papillomavirus type 22b. Dermatology. 220(4):326-8, 2010
2. Dell'Oste V et al: High beta-HPV DNA loads and strong seroreactivity are present in epidermodysplasia verruciformis. J Invest Dermatol. 129(4):1026-34, 2009
3. Rogers HD et al: Acquired epidermodysplasia verruciformis. J Am Acad Dermatol. 60(2):315-20, 2009
4. Mitsuishi T et al: Epidermodysplasia verruciformis with keratoacanthoma, Bowen's disease and squamous cell carcinoma: isolation of high-risk types of HPV 5 and unknown type of human papillomavirus. J Eur Acad Dermatol Venereol. 22(9):1126-7, 2008
5. Ko CJ et al: Changes of epidermodysplasia verruciformis in benign skin lesions: the EV acanthoma. J Cutan Pathol. 34(1):44-8, 2007
6. Cassarino DS et al: Cutaneous squamous cell carcinoma: a comprehensive clinicopathologic classification. Part one. J Cutan Pathol. 33(3):191-206, 2006
7. Orth G: Genetics of epidermodysplasia verruciformis: Insights into host defense against papillomaviruses. Semin Immunol. 18(6):362-74, 2006

IMAGE GALLERY

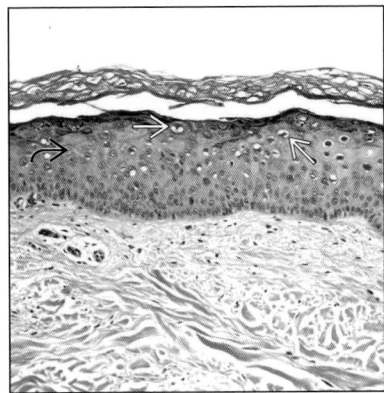 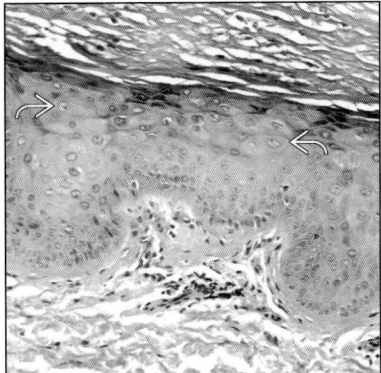 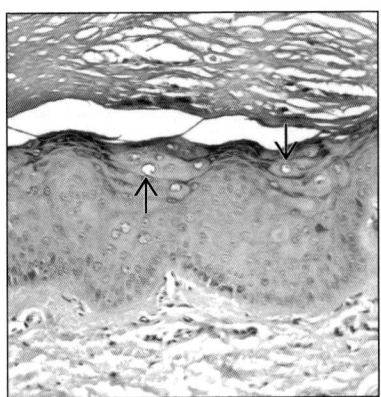

(Left) EDV shows epidermal acanthosis and a proliferation of enlarged keratinocytes ➔ involving the upper levels of the epidermis. Note the perinuclear halos in many of the keratinocytes ➔. *(Center)* Higher magnification of EDV shows a proliferation of enlarged bluish-gray keratinocytes ➔ involving the mid to upper layers of the epidermis. There is dense overlying hyperkeratosis and parakeratosis. *(Right)* Some of the cells show prominent nuclear clearing ➔.

VERRUCOUS CARCINOMA (AND VARIANTS)

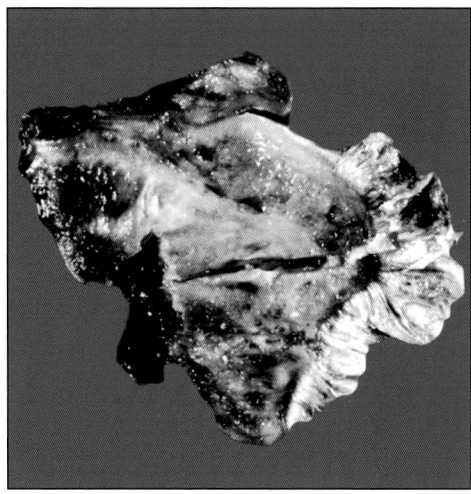

Cut section of a partial penectomy specimen shows a verruciform tumor with sharp bulbous base confined to the lamina propria. Note the papillomatous and spiky surface.

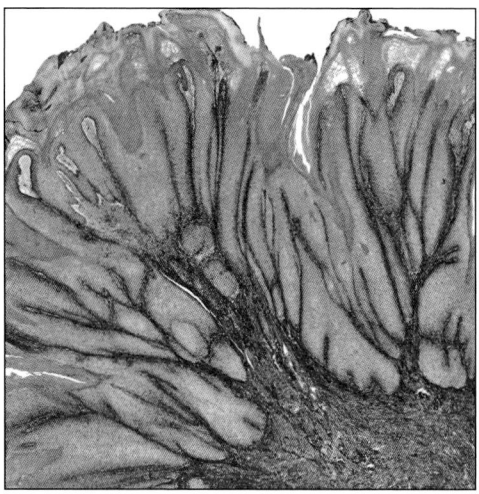

Low-power view of a verrucous carcinoma illustrates the thick acanthotic papillae, thin fibrovascular cores, and the classic piling up of keratin between papillae.

TERMINOLOGY

Abbreviations
- Verrucous carcinoma (VC), squamous cell carcinoma (SCC)

Synonyms
- Buschke-Loewenstein tumor
- Ackerman tumor (oral florid papillomatosis)

Definitions
- Very well-differentiated verruciform SCC with bulbous deep borders and lack of koilocytosis

ETIOLOGY/PATHOGENESIS

Unknown Pathogenesis
- Cutaneous (particularly plantar) lesions may be associated with HPV and arise within preexisting warts
- Cutaneous lesions may be related to scarring and chronic inflammation
- Oral VC (Ackerman tumor) may be related to tobacco chewing
- Anogenital cases may be associated with phimosis and lichen sclerosus
- Anogenital VC are associated with HPV6 in some cases

CLINICAL ISSUES

Epidemiology
- Incidence
  - Rare
- Age
  - 6th-7th decade

Site
- Originally described by Lauren Ackerman in the oral cavity

- May also affect anogenital area and skin (sole of the foot, finger, nail bed, scalp, wrist, buttocks, etc.)

Presentation
- Exophytic white-gray neoplasm
- Unicentric tumors are more frequent than multicentric ones

Treatment
- Surgical

Prognosis
- Pure VCs have excellent prognosis
  - Tumors may recur but almost never metastasize
- Hybrid/mixed VCs have worse prognosis than pure VC
- Sporadic reports of sarcomatoid/anaplastic transformation after radiation therapy

MACROSCOPIC FEATURES

General Features
- Exophytic white-gray neoplasms with papillary, sometimes spiky surface
- Cut sections reveal broad base between tumor and stroma
- Tumors may invade deep dermis and deeper structures
- Irregular jagged borders or foci of necrosis are not features of pure verrucous carcinoma

Size
- 1-3 cm in diameter

MICROSCOPIC PATHOLOGY

Histologic Features
- Extremely well-differentiated squamous neoplasm
- Thick acanthotic papillae with slender fibrovascular cores
- Papillae are separated by prominent keratin craters
- Orthokeratosis with presence of granular layer

VERRUCOUS CARCINOMA (AND VARIANTS)

Key Facts

Clinical Issues
- Unicentric tumors are more frequent but multicentric ones may occur
- Some cases may be associated with viral warts (plantar lesions)
- VC may arise in the setting of longstanding lichen sclerosus (genital tumors)

Macroscopic Features
- Exophytic papillary tumor
- Broad and pushing base
- Deep burrowing pattern is hallmark of carcinoma cuniculatum (VC variant)

Microscopic Pathology
- Acanthotic papillae
- Slender fibrovascular cores
- Prominent (orange) keratin craters between papillae
- Lack of koilocytosis
- Extremely well differentiated
- Epithelium of papillae and keratin predominate over fibrovascular core
- Pushing, club-shaped base
- Higher grade areas &/or infiltrative borders are not features of pure VC and raise possibility of hybrid (mixed) VC

Top Differential Diagnoses
- Carcinoma cuniculatum (VC variant)
- Mixed/hybrid VC with foci of SCC of usual type
- Condyloma acuminatum/giant condyloma
- Warty (condylomatous) carcinoma
- Papillary carcinoma (SCC variant)

- Parakeratosis may be occasional
- Absence of koilocytosis
- Pushing, club-shaped deep borders
- Adjacent epithelium often shows verrucous squamous hyperplasia &/or differentiated vulvar or penile intraepithelial neoplasia (differentiated VIN or PeIN)
- Some cases associated with background of lichen sclerosus (genital)

Predominant Pattern/Injury Type
- Papillary

Predominant Cell/Compartment Type
- Epithelial, squamous

DIFFERENTIAL DIAGNOSIS

Carcinoma Cuniculatum
- Overlapping features with VC, but with characteristic burrowing pattern
- Bulk of the tumor has classical features of VC
- Focal higher grade areas and jagged borders

Mixed (Hybrid) Verrucous Carcinoma
- VC admixed with foci of SCC of usual type
- Tumors showing classical areas of VC associated with other foci that are less differentiated and more infiltrative

Giant Condyloma
- More rounded, arborescent papillae
- Koilocytosis on surface

Warty Carcinoma
- Vulvar or penile locations
- Higher histological grade
- Prominent koilocytosis throughout neoplasm
- Usually infiltrative deep borders

Papillary Carcinoma (SCC Variant)
- Well to moderately differentiated SCC
- Infiltrative borders

DIAGNOSTIC CHECKLIST

Pathologic Interpretation Pearls
- Acanthotic papillae with thin fibrovascular cores
- Piling up of keratin (usually orange in color) between papillae (keratin craters) is characteristic
- Epithelium and keratin predominate over fibrovascular cores
- Club-shaped pushing base
- In a partial biopsy, recommended diagnosis is "well-differentiated squamous cell carcinoma, with verrucous features"
  - Acknowledges possibility of unsampled moderately or poorly differentiated invasive conventional carcinoma in definitive excision
  - VCs with foci of moderately or poorly differentiated SCC are considered hybrid/mixed VC
- Carcinoma cuniculatum is a variant of VC (usually a hybrid VC) with classical burrowing pattern of growth

SELECTED REFERENCES

1. Arduino PG et al: Verrucous oral carcinoma: clinical findings and treatment outcomes in 74 patients in Northwest Italy. Minerva Stomatol. 57(7-8):335-9, 339-41, 2008
2. Velazquez EF et al: Penile squamous cell carcinoma: anatomic, pathologic and viral studies in Paraguay (1993-2007). Anal Quant Cytol Histol. 29(4):185-98, 2007
3. Kato N et al: Penile hybrid verrucous-squamous carcinoma associated with a superficial inguinal lymph node metastasis. Am J Dermatopathol. 22(4):339-43, 2000
4. McKee PH et al: Carcinoma (epithelioma) cuniculatum: a clinico-pathological study of nineteen cases and review of the literature. Histopathology. 5(4):425-36, 1981
5. Wilkinson JD et al: A case of carcinoma cuniculatum with coexistant viral plantar wart. Clin Exp Dermatol. 6(6):619-23, 1981

Microscopic Features

(Left) Verrucous carcinoma shows prominent, deeply endophytic downgrowths with bulbous rete ridges ➔ surrounded by chronic inflammation. Note the deep "pushing invasion" approaching bundles of skeletal muscle ➔. *(Right)* Abundant keratin-filled craters are usually seen in VC. In a superficial biopsy specimen in which the entire lesion cannot be examined, the diagnosis of VC can be challenging. Clinical correlation and recommendation for additional sampling may be necessary.

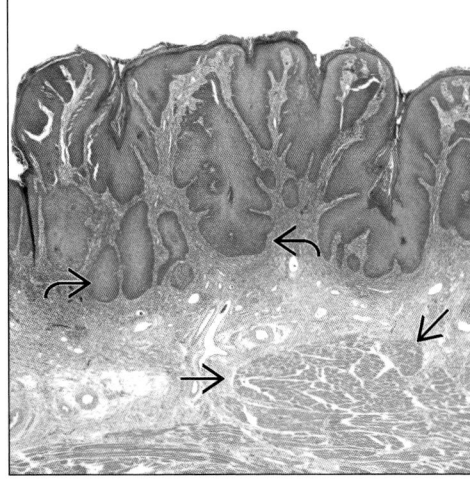
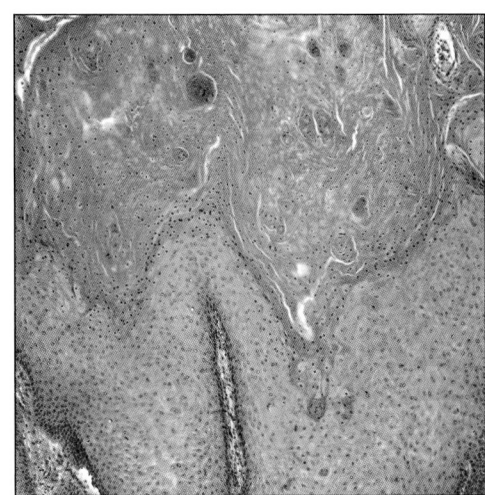

(Left) Abundant orange keratin ➔ and bulbous bases are typical of VC. The acanthotic epithelium and abundant keratin are much more prominent than the thin fibrovascular cores. *(Right)* Pure VC is extremely well differentiated, including its deep portion. The bulbous ➔ base is a key differentiating feature from pseudoepitheliomatous hyperplasia, which has narrow elongated rete ridges. The absence of koilocytosis helps to distinguish it from condyloma acuminatum.

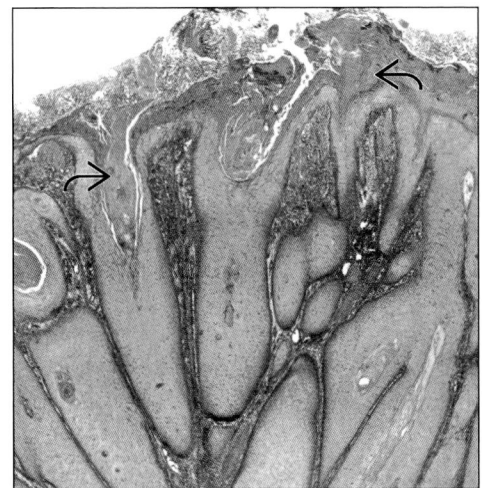
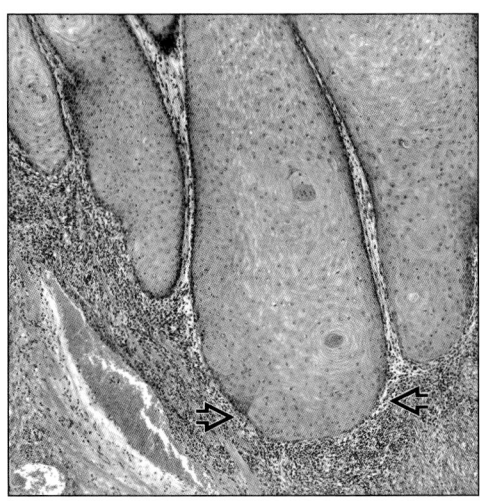

(Left) High magnification of VC shows a very well-differentiated squamous tumor with craters containing abundant (orange-staining) keratin material ➔ with parakeratosis. *(Right)* High magnification of VC shows enlarged, bland-appearing squamous cells with abundant, dense eosinophilic to amphophilic-staining cytoplasm ➔, and nuclei with vesicular chromatin and small to mildly enlarged nucleoli ➔.

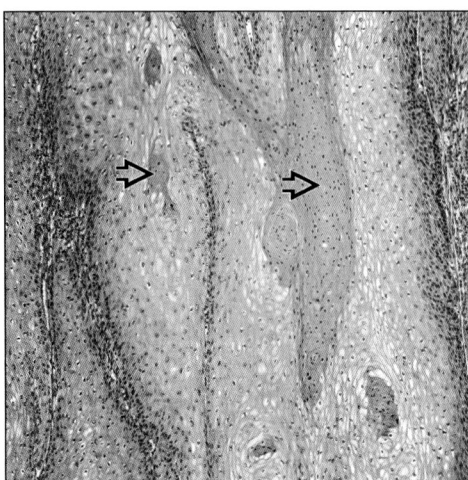
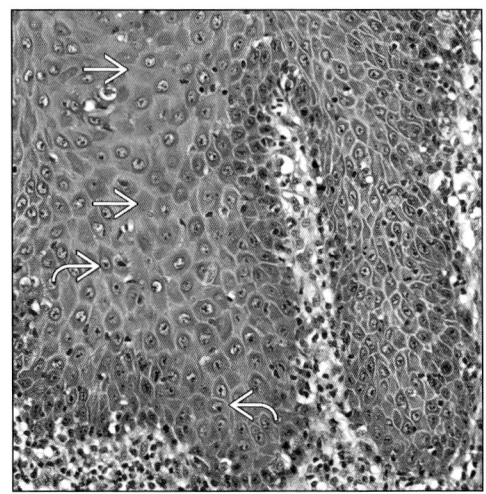

VERRUCOUS CARCINOMA (AND VARIANTS)

Differential Diagnosis

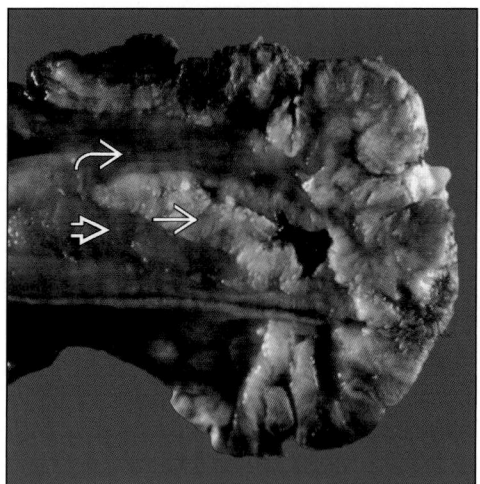

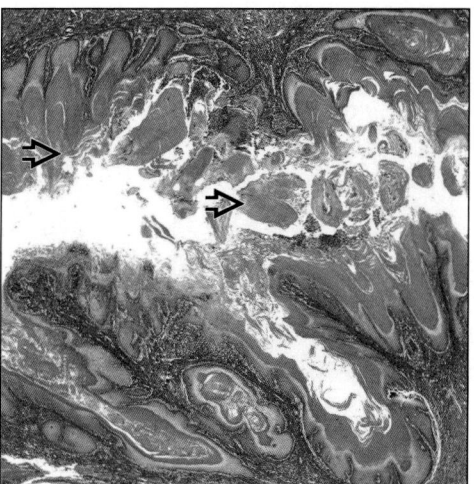

(Left) Cut section of a penectomy specimen with a carcinoma cuniculatum shows the "burrowing pattern," which is the hallmark of this tumor. A deep penetrating "burrow" ➡ is seen growing along the tunica albuginea ➔ and invading the corpus cavernosum ▶. *(Right)* H&E shows microscopic features of a carcinoma cuniculatum. Most authors consider this tumor to be a variant of VC with hybrid foci. Note the tumoral burrows containing abundant keratin ▷.

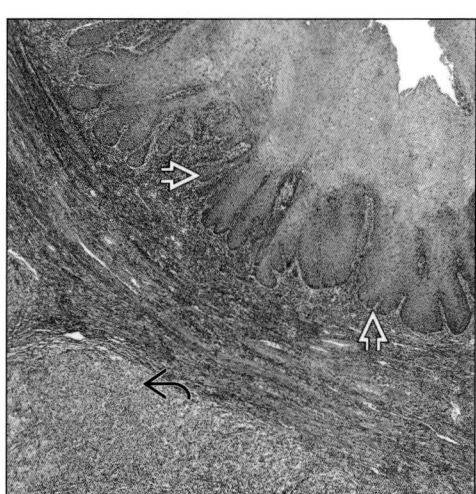

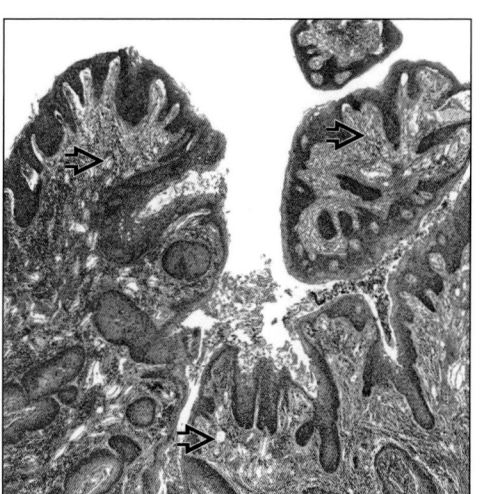

(Left) Hybrid (mixed) VC shows areas of classic VC ➡ associated with less differentiated areas ➔. These tumors have worse prognosis than pure VC. *(Right)* Papillary carcinoma, NOS, shows arborescent papillae. Fibrovascular cores ▷ are more prominent than in VC. Papillary carcinoma is less well differentiated than VC and shows infiltrative deep borders. It is distinguished from warty carcinoma by the lack of koilocytic changes.

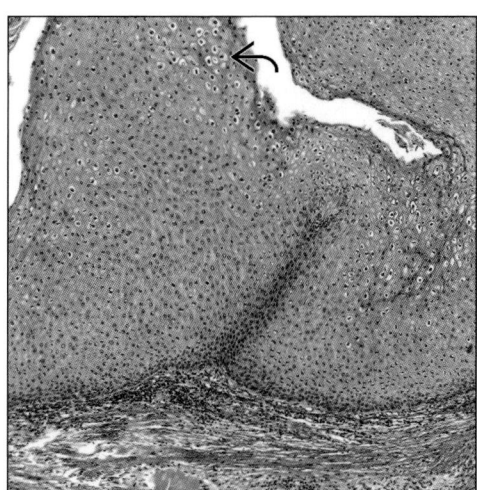

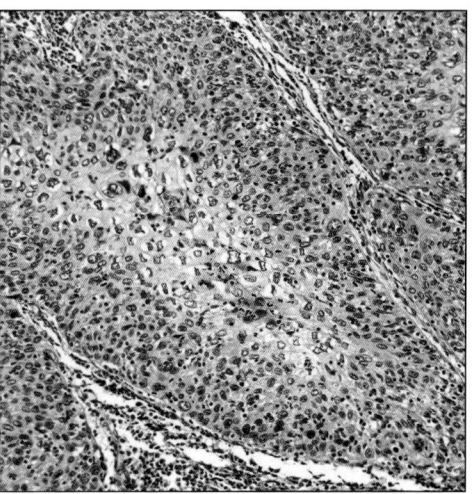

(Left) In this case of condyloma acuminatum, the lesion has some features reminiscent of verrucous carcinoma. However, there is prominent koilocytosis on the surface ➔. *(Right)* Warty carcinoma shows atypical koilocytic changes throughout the tumor. In addition to frankly malignant cytologic features, the bases of warty carcinomas tend to be more infiltrative and jagged appearing.

SQUAMOUS CELL CARCINOMA (AND VARIANTS)

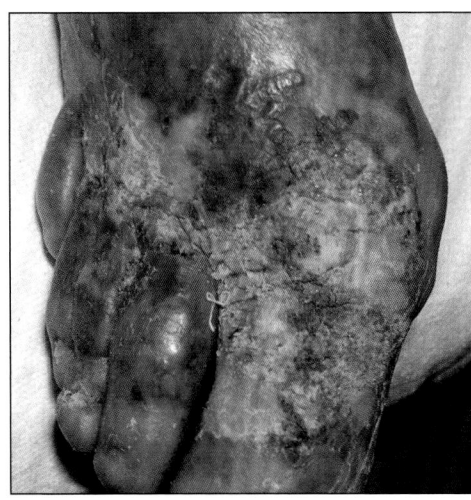

Clinical photograph shows an extensive SCC arising on the distal foot in a patient with a history of previous burn injury. (Courtesy S. Yashar, MD.)

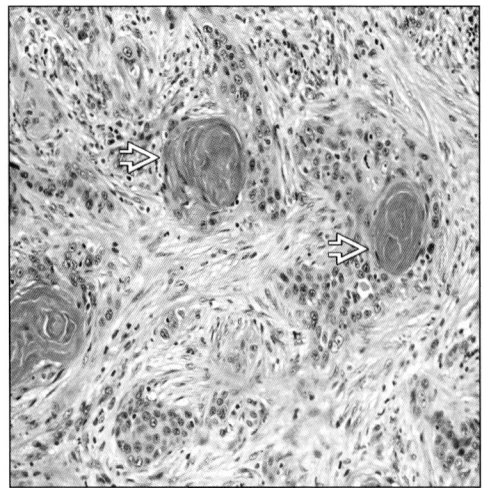

Moderately differentiated invasive SCC shows prominent keratin pearls ⊳ and a sclerotic stroma with scattered inflammatory cells.

TERMINOLOGY

Abbreviations
- Squamous cell carcinoma (SCC)

Synonyms
- Epidermoid carcinoma
- Sarcomatoid carcinoma/spindle cell carcinoma/carcinosarcoma/metaplastic carcinoma
- Acantholytic/adenoid/pseudoglandular SCC
- Verrucous carcinoma (well-differentiated variant)
- Keratoacanthoma (KA) (well-differentiated variant, regresses spontaneously)

Definitions
- Malignant tumor of squamous keratinocytes

ETIOLOGY/PATHOGENESIS

Environmental Exposure
- Most cases are related to UV radiation
- Some cases are likely related to chronic inflammation (i.e., SCC arising in burns, lupus, lichen planus)
- Previous radiation therapy is implicated in some cases, usually associated with more aggressive SCC
- Chronic wounds and burn scars also can be associated with high-risk SCC
- HPV is associated with some cases
  - Especially verrucous carcinoma (low grade) and SCC in immunosuppressed patients (high grade)

CLINICAL ISSUES

Epidemiology
- Age
  - Usually in the elderly, especially solar-related lesions
  - However, can present in a wide age range (34-95 years)
    - Rare cases in children (should prompt genetic studies)
- Gender
  - Slightly more common in males, overall

Presentation
- Slow-growing papular, nodular, or plaque lesion
- Often arises in sun-damaged skin (head and neck tumors)
  - Vast majority of cases associated with preexisting actinic keratosis (AK)
- May be ulcerated or bleeding
- Ear canal and middle ear tumors may present with pain, hearing loss, and discharge

Treatment
- Surgical approaches
  - Complete surgical excision is optimal and definitive therapy
    - Mohs surgery has been shown to be highly effective for most tumors
- Drugs
  - If patients are not surgical candidates, topical chemotherapeutics or immunomodulators may be used
- Radiation
  - May be used for very advanced cases where surgical therapy is not curative

Prognosis
- Usually excellent in most cases
- Worse prognosis with poorly differentiated, deeply invasive, or rare aggressive subtypes
- Site of tumor important for prognosis
  - Lip and ear tumors more aggressive, regardless of degree of differentiation

SQUAMOUS CELL CARCINOMA (AND VARIANTS)

Key Facts

Terminology
- Squamous cell carcinoma (SCC)
  - Malignant epithelial tumor of squamous keratinocytes

Etiology/Pathogenesis
- Most cases are related to UV radiation
- Previous radiation therapy implicated in some cases, usually associated with more aggressive SCC

Clinical Issues
- Often arises in sun-damaged skin of elderly patients (usually head and neck)
  - Vast majority of cases associated with preexisting actinic keratosis (AK)
- Complete surgical excision is optimal and definitive therapy

- Prognosis usually good in superficial and well-differentiated cases
- Worse prognosis with poorly differentiated, deeply invasive, or aggressive subtypes

Microscopic Pathology
- Proliferation of invasive atypical keratinocytes, often with areas of keratinization (keratin pearls) and squamous eddies
- Cells are present in nests, sheets, and cords
- Cytologically, cells show abundant eosinophilic cytoplasm, and large nucleus with vesicular chromatin and prominent nucleoli
- Degree of differentiation is variable, ranging from well- to moderately to poorly differentiated
- Multiple variants of differing malignant potential described

MACROSCOPIC FEATURES

General Features
- Papular to nodular or plaque-like lesion; can be exophytic
  - May be ulcerated or hemorrhagic

Size
- Variable; can be small or large lesions

MICROSCOPIC PATHOLOGY

Histologic Features
- Proliferation of invasive atypical keratinocytes
  - Cells are present in nests, sheets, and infiltrative cords
  - Often show areas of keratinization (keratin pearls) and squamous eddies
  - Attachments to overlying epidermis in most cases
  - Associated AK is very common; less likely, may be associated with SCC in situ (Bowen disease)
  - Cytologically, cells show abundant eosinophilic cytoplasm and large nucleus with vesicular chromatin and prominent nucleoli
  - Intercellular bridges (desmosomes) should be present on high-power examination
  - Presence of dyskeratotic cells (apoptotic keratinocytes) is reliable sign of squamous differentiation
  - If no definite squamous differentiation is present, immunohistochemistry should be used to confirm diagnosis
- Degree of differentiation is variable, ranging from well- to moderately to poorly differentiated
  - Amount of keratinization typically decreases and cytologic atypia increases with higher grades
  - Mitotic figures are usually numerous, and atypical forms are found especially in moderately to poorly differentiated cases
- Multiple variants of differing malignant potential described

  - Low-risk variants include well-differentiated SCC arising in AK, keratoacanthoma, verrucous carcinoma, and tricholemmal (variant of clear cell) carcinoma
  - Intermediate-risk variants include acantholytic (adenoid/pseudoglandular) and lymphoepithelioma-like carcinoma of the skin (LELCS)
  - High-risk variants include spindle cell/sarcomatoid, basaloid, adenosquamous, and desmoplastic
    - Also, radiation, burn scar, and immunosuppression-related SCCs
  - Rare variants of uncertain malignant potential include clear cell SCC, signet ring cell SCC, follicular SCC, papillary SCC, pigmented SCC, and SCC arising from adnexal ducts or cysts

Predominant Pattern/Injury Type
- Epithelioid/squamoid

Predominant Cell/Compartment Type
- Squamous cell

ANCILLARY TESTS

Immunohistochemistry
- Immunohistochemistry is not necessary in well-/moderately differentiated cases but may be needed in poorly differentiated and spindle cell cases
- Cytokeratins are most important markers, especially high molecular weight cytokeratins (HMWCKs)
  - HMWCKs are most sensitive markers for poorly differentiated and spindle cell/sarcomatoid SCC
    - Pankeratin can be lost in poorly differentiated and spindle cell cases
  - p63 is also a very sensitive marker and can be used in addition to HMWCK to confirm diagnosis
- Vimentin may be positive in spindle cell/sarcomatoid cases
- Negative staining for other markers, including
  - S100, MART-1/Melan-A, and HMB-45 (melanoma)
  - CD10, CD68, and CD99 (AFX)
  - Actin-sm and desmin (leiomyosarcoma)

SQUAMOUS CELL CARCINOMA (AND VARIANTS)

○ BER-EP4, androgen receptor (AR), and D2-40 (BCC and sebaceous carcinoma)

DIFFERENTIAL DIAGNOSIS

Basal Cell Carcinoma (BCC)
- Cells are typically smaller, more hyperchromatic, and show peripheral palisading, mucinous stroma, and retraction artifact
- Cytokeratins do not distinguish BCC from SCC, but BER-EP4 and AR are almost always positive in BCC, negative in SCC

Atypical Fibroxanthoma (AFX)
- Usually a large, nodular lesion in heavily sun-damaged (typically head and neck) skin
- Immunohistochemistry is essential in excluding poorly differentiated SCC
  ○ SCC is typically positive for HMWCKs and p63; AFX is negative for these markers and often CD10(+) and CD99(+)

Poorly Differentiated Carcinoma (Including Metastatic)
- Clinical history and imaging studies are paramount, as immunohistochemistry may not be able to distinguish some cases from primary SCC
- Adenocarcinomas may show varying degree of ductal/glandular differentiation
  ○ If present, ductal spaces can be highlighted with markers such as EMA and CEA

Pseudoepitheliomatous Hyperplasia
- Can mimic SCC, especially SCC in situ, but does not show infiltrative features or high-grade cytologic atypia
- Mitotic figures can be numerous but should be in basilar keratinocytes and nonatypical

Keratoacanthoma (KA)
- Essentially a well-differentiated variant of SCC that spontaneously regresses in most cases
- Typically composed of large, crateriform (cup-like) lesion filled with abundant keratin debris
- Cells are enlarged, with abundant glassy-appearing/hyalinized cytoplasm
- Most cases regress, but giant KA and subungual KA can be aggressive; some may metastasize in immunosuppressed patients

DIAGNOSTIC CHECKLIST

Clinically Relevant Pathologic Features
- Degree of differentiation
- Depth of invasion
  ○ Deeply invasive tumors have much higher rates of recurrence and metastasis
- Perineural invasion
  ○ Tumors with perineural invasion have high rates of local recurrence and increased risk of metastasis

- Location of tumor important (i.e., lip, mucosal lesions more aggressive)

Pathologic Interpretation Pearls
- Invasive proliferation of epithelioid cells, with areas of keratinization (keratin pearls) and squamous eddies
  ○ Intercellular bridges (desmosomes) and dyskeratotic cells confirm squamous differentiation in poorly differentiated cases
- Adjacent or overlying AK often present in external ear cases

SELECTED REFERENCES

1. Yang A et al: Primary cutaneous myxoid spindle cell squamous cell carcinoma: a clinicopathologic study and review of the literature. J Cutan Pathol. 37(4):465-74, 2010
2. Bridges MN et al: Cutaneous squamous cell carcinoma of the external auditory canal. Dermatol Online J. 15(2):13, 2009
3. McGuire JF et al: Nonmelanoma skin cancer of the head and neck I: histopathology and clinical behavior. Am J Otolaryngol. 30(2):121-33, 2009
4. Garcia-Zuazaga J et al: Cutaneous squamous cell carcinoma. Adv Dermatol. 24:33-57, 2008
5. Ulrich C et al: Skin cancer in organ transplant recipients--where do we stand today? Am J Transplant. 8(11):2192-8, 2008
6. Yang HM et al: Immunohistochemical expression of D2-40 in benign and malignant sebaceous tumors and comparison to basal and squamous cell carcinomas. Am J Dermatopathol. 30(6):549-54, 2008
7. Renzi C et al: Sentinel lymph node biopsy for high risk cutaneous squamous cell carcinoma: case series and review of the literature. Eur J Surg Oncol. 33(3):364-9, 2007
8. Weinberg AS et al: Metastatic cutaneous squamous cell carcinoma: an update. Dermatol Surg. 33(8):885-99, 2007
9. Cassarino DS et al: Cutaneous squamous cell carcinoma: a comprehensive clinicopathologic classification--part one. J Cutan Pathol. 33(3):191-206, 2006
10. Cassarino DS et al: Cutaneous squamous cell carcinoma: a comprehensive clinicopathologic classification--part two. J Cutan Pathol. 33(4):261-79, 2006
11. Veness MJ et al: High-risk cutaneous squamous cell carcinoma of the head and neck: results from 266 treated patients with metastatic lymph node disease. Cancer. 106(11):2389-96, 2006
12. Leibovitch I et al: Cutaneous squamous cell carcinoma treated with Mohs micrographic surgery in Australia I. Experience over 10 years. J Am Acad Dermatol. 53(2):253-60, 2005
13. Lindelöf B et al: Cutaneous squamous cell carcinoma in organ transplant recipients: a study of the Swedish cohort with regard to tumor site. Arch Dermatol. 141(4):447-51, 2005
14. Baker NJ et al: Surgical management of cutaneous squamous cell carcinoma of the head and neck. Br J Oral Maxillofac Surg. 39(2):87-90, 2001
15. Weinstock MA: Epidemiologic investigation of nonmelanoma skin cancer mortality: the Rhode Island Follow-Back Study. J Invest Dermatol. 102(6):6S-9S, 1994
16. Rowe DE et al: Prognostic factors for local recurrence, metastasis, and survival rates in squamous cell carcinoma of the skin, ear, and lip. Implications for treatment modality selection. J Am Acad Dermatol. 26(6):976-90, 1992

SQUAMOUS CELL CARCINOMA (AND VARIANTS)

Microscopic Features

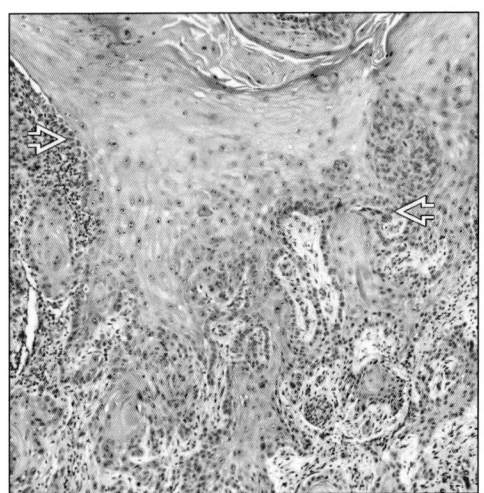
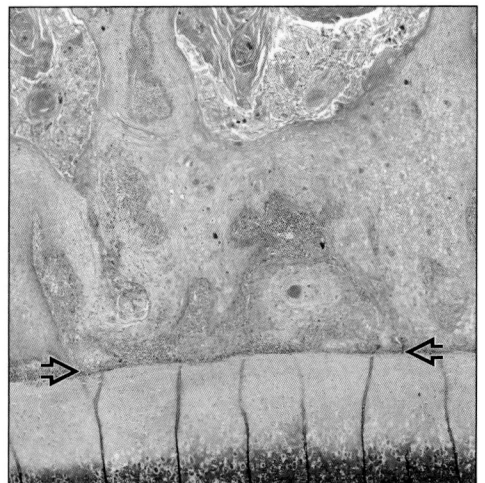

(Left) Invasive, well-differentiated SCC is seen arising in association with an actinic keratosis ⮩. *(Right)* Invasive, well-differentiated squamous cell carcinoma of the ear invading up to ⮩ (but not into) the auricular cartilage is shown.

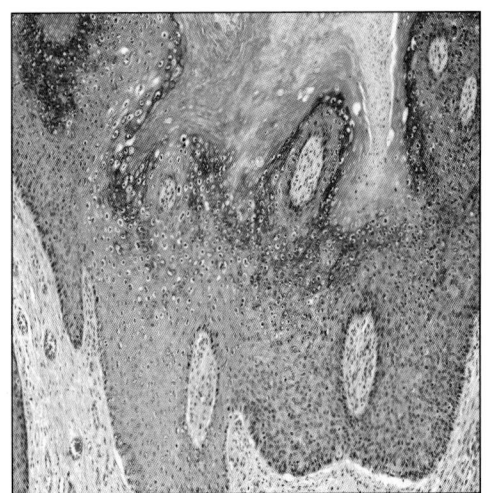
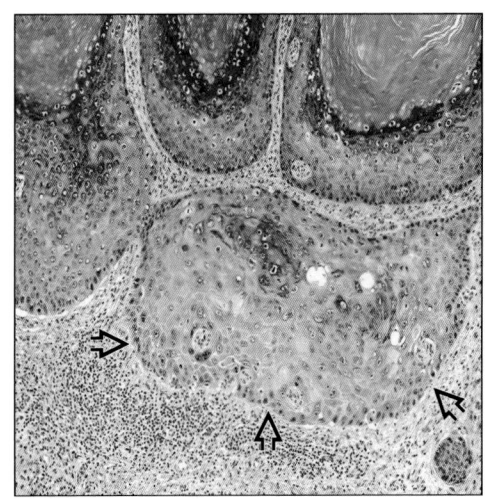

(Left) SCC in situ (Bowen disease) is seen arising in a longstanding large verruca vulgaris. *(Right)* Higher power view of the base of the lesion shows tangentially sectioned SCC in situ with smooth borders ⮩ and lack of an infiltrative growth pattern. There is an associated inflammatory cell infiltrate.

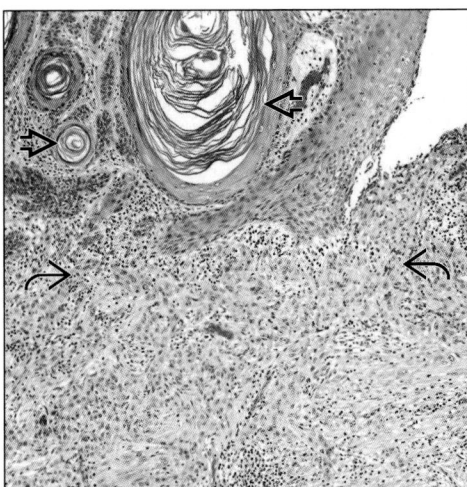
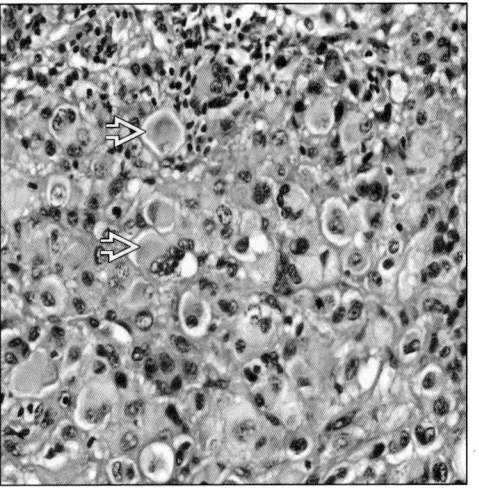

(Left) A rare invasive SCC arising in association with a seborrheic keratosis shows sheets of moderately to poorly differentiated infiltrating squamous cells ⮩, with an overlying seborrheic keratosis with pseudohorn cysts present ⮩. *(Right)* High-grade invasive SCC shows a sheet-like proliferation of atypical and pleomorphic epithelioid and multinucleated cells with hyperchromatic nuclei, prominent nucleoli, and abundant glassy-appearing eosinophilic cytoplasm ⮩.

Variant Microscopic Features

(Left) Acantholytic (adenoid) type of invasive squamous cell carcinoma shows scattered cystic spaces containing dyscohesive squamous cells ➡. This variant of SCC may mimic an adenocarcinoma ("pseudoglandular SCC") or even an angiosarcoma ("pseudovascular SCC"). *(Right)* High-power view of acantholytic SCC shows large epithelioid cells with dense eosinophilic cytoplasm and scattered dyskeratotic (apoptotic) cells ➡. There is an associated heavy inflammatory cell infiltrate.

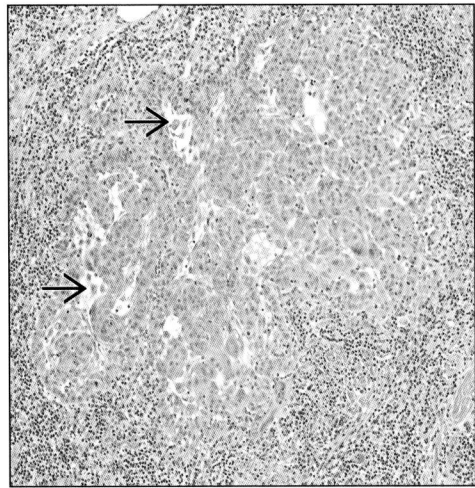
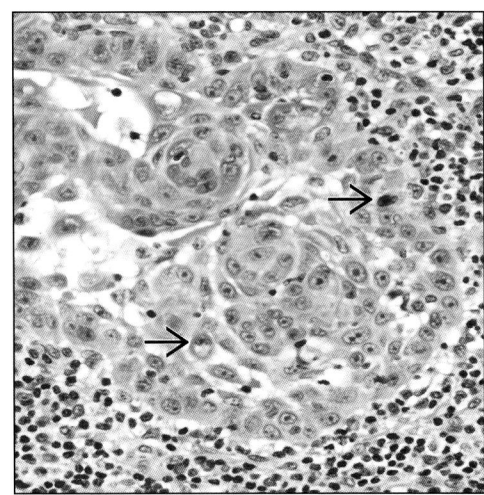

(Left) Poorly differentiated invasive SCC shows signet ring cell-like features and areas of myxoid stroma ➡ (myxoid SCC). *(Right)* Higher power view of poorly differentiated myxoid SCC shows epithelioid to signet ring-like eosinophilic-staining cells with focal extracellular mucin ➡.

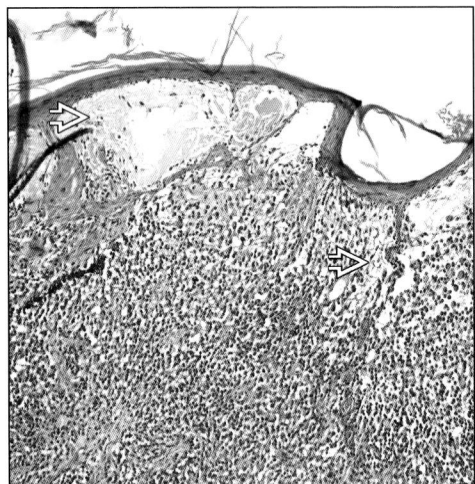
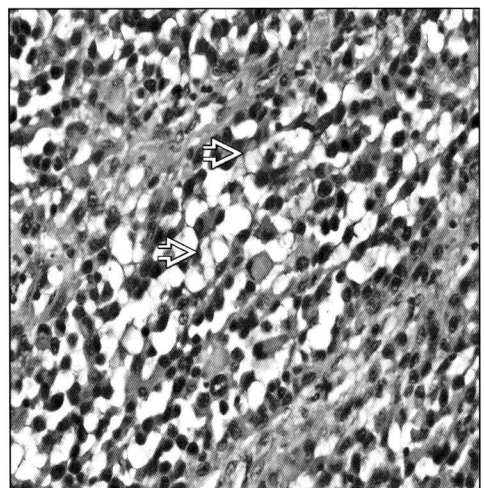

(Left) Poorly differentiated infiltrating SCC ➡ associated with a sclerotic (desmoplastic) stroma is shown. This is a high malignant potential variant of SCC. *(Right)* Heavily inflamed invasive SCC with moderately differentiated tumor islands ➡ composed of basaloid to squamoid cells is surrounded by a sea of inflammatory cells, features suggestive of the lymphoepithelioma-like carcinoma of the skin (LELCS) variant.

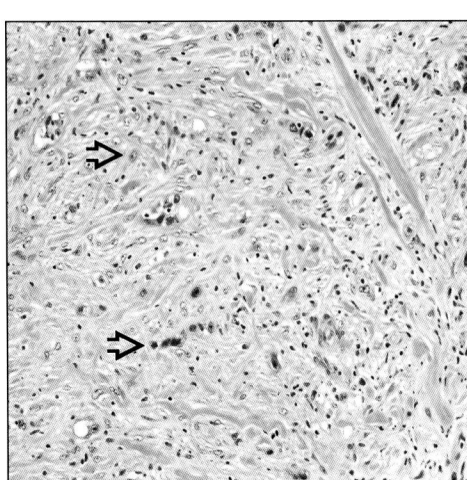
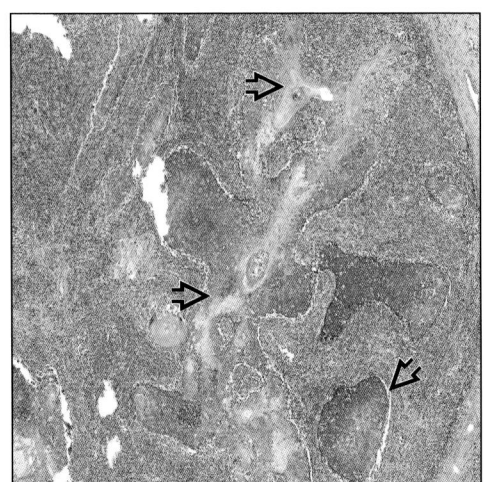

SQUAMOUS CELL CARCINOMA (AND VARIANTS)

Immunohistochemical Features

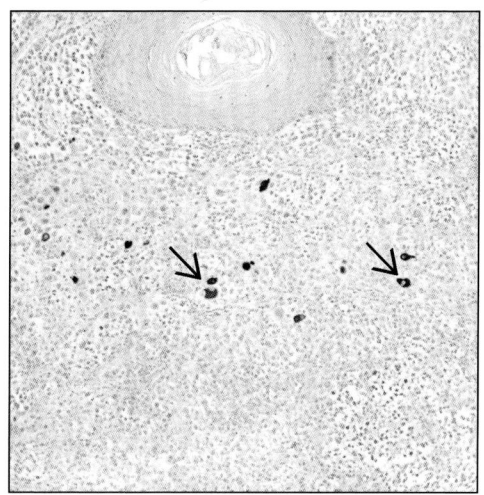

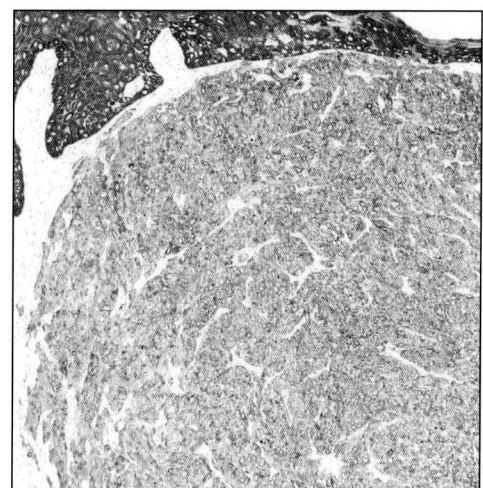

(Left) CK-PAN immunohistochemistry (IHC) shows only focal staining of a few scattered single cells ➡ in a case of poorly differentiated SCC. CK-PAN is much less sensitive than HMWCKs and p63 in identifying poorly differentiated and sarcomatoid SCC cases. **(Right)** CK903 (HMWCK) immunohistochemistry shows strong staining of an invasive, poorly invasive SCC (with strong internal control staining of the overlying epidermis).

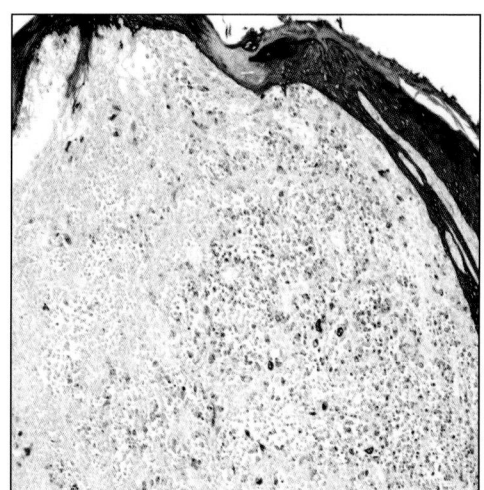

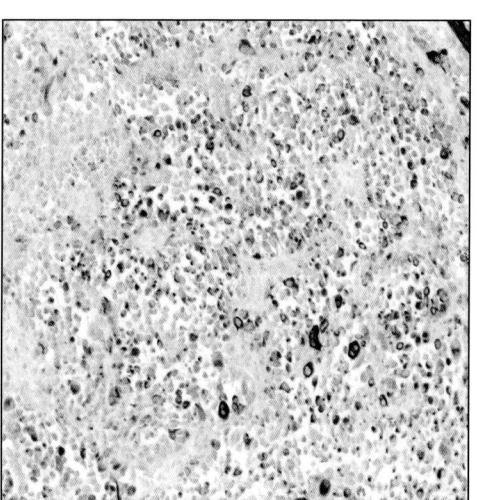

(Left) CK5/6 (HMWCK) IHC shows strong staining of the epidermis and scattered single cells in a poorly differentiated SCC. **(Right)** Higher power view of CK5/6 shows moderate to strong cytoplasmic staining of many of the tumor cells.

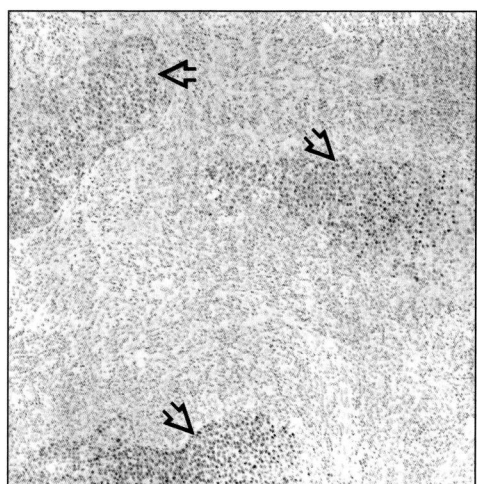

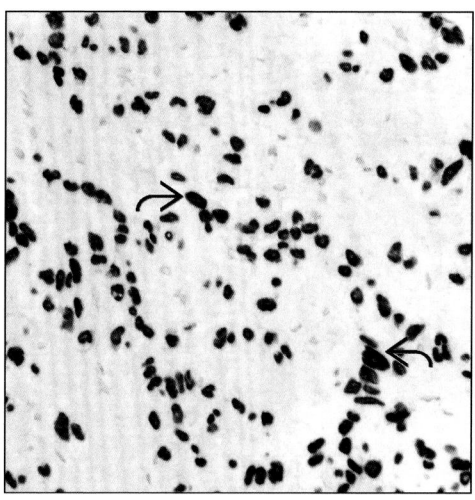

(Left) IHC stain for p63 in an LELCS shows strong and diffuse nuclear staining in islands of epithelial tumor cells ➡. **(Right)** High-power view of p63 immunohistochemistry shows strong and diffuse nuclear staining of large, irregularly shaped nuclei ➡ in a poorly differentiated infiltrating SCC.

KERATOACANTHOMA

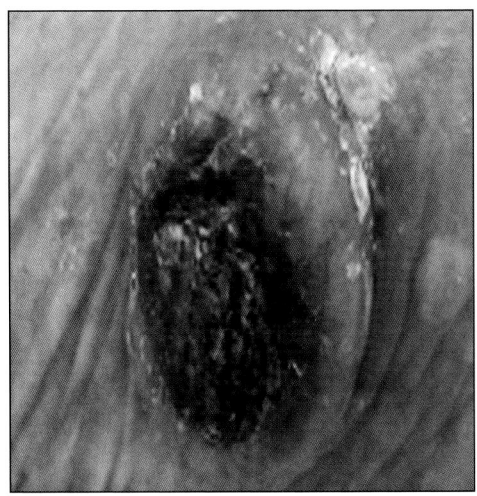

Clinical photograph shows a tumor with raised borders and a central, crateriform keratin-filled defect, consistent with a keratoacanthoma. (Courtesy S. Yashar, MD.)

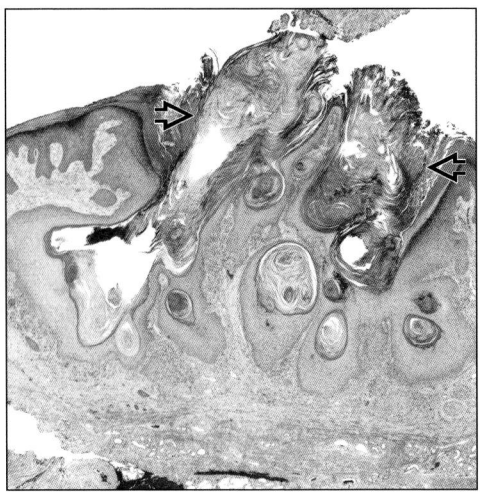

Scanning magnification of a keratoacanthoma shows an endophytic-appearing atypical squamous proliferation with prominent, central keratin-filled cavities ➤.

TERMINOLOGY

Abbreviations
- Keratoacanthoma (KA)

Synonyms
- Crateriform ulcer
- Self-healing squamous cell carcinoma

Definitions
- Very well-differentiated form of cutaneous squamous cell carcinoma (SCC), which often spontaneously regresses

ETIOLOGY/PATHOGENESIS

Environmental Exposure
- Similar to other forms of SCC, typically related to chronic solar (UV) damage
  - Vast majority of lesions occur in sun-damaged skin of older adults
  - Regression is thought to be due to immune-mediated destruction of the squamous cells

CLINICAL ISSUES

Epidemiology
- Incidence
  - Relatively common, may represent up to 25% of cases of cutaneous SCC
- Age
  - Older adults, mean age is mid 60s
- Gender
  - More common in males
- Ethnicity
  - Most common in Caucasians

Site
- Head and neck most common, followed by arms, legs

Presentation
- Rapidly growing nodular lesion
  - Often dome-shaped with central keratinous plug
  - May reach large size, up to 10 cm (giant keratoacanthoma)

Treatment
- Options, risks, complications
  - Surgical excision is mainstay of treatment although observation may be acceptable in many cases
- Surgical approaches
  - Complete excision is curative but likely not necessary in most cases due to spontaneous regression
  - Patients with giant KAs, subungual KAs, and immunosuppressed patients should have complete excision, as lesions may not regress in these patients

Prognosis
- Excellent; vast majority of cases spontaneously regress
- Rare case reports of metastatic KA, but most of these are in giant or subungual KAs or immunosuppressed patients

MACROSCOPIC FEATURES

General Features
- Typically large, scaly lesions with central keratinous crater

MICROSCOPIC PATHOLOGY

Histologic Features
- Scanning magnification shows a large, nodular, well-differentiated squamous tumor
- Lesion typically appears symmetric with central keratin-filled crater present
- Cells may show infiltrative features at periphery of tumor

KERATOACANTHOMA

Key Facts

Terminology
- Keratoacanthoma (KA)
- Very well-differentiated SCC variant

Etiology/Pathogenesis
- Similar to other forms of SCC, typically related to chronic solar (UV) damage

Clinical Issues
- Often dome-shaped with central keratinous plug
- May reach large size, up to 10 cm (giant KA)
- Excellent prognosis; vast majority of cases spontaneously regress
- Head and neck most common, followed by arms, legs

Microscopic Pathology
- Scanning magnification shows a large, nodular, well-differentiated tumor

- Typically appears symmetric with central keratin-filled crater present
- Large squamous cells with abundant dense eosinophilic-staining cytoplasm and enlarged, hyperchromatic to vesicular-appearing nuclei with prominent nucleoli
- Prominent inflammatory infiltrate, usually with abundant eosinophils and neutrophils
- Regressing lesions often show epidermal atrophy and bland cytologic features

Top Differential Diagnoses
- Conventional well-differentiated SCC
- Squamous cell carcinoma in situ (SCCis) (Bowen disease)
- Verrucous carcinoma

- o Perineural and even lymphovascular invasion have been reported in rare cases but do not seem to correlate with increased metastatic potential
- Cells are enlarged, with large nuclei and abundant dense eosinophilic-staining cytoplasm
  - o Dyskeratotic cells and mitotic figures usually present, especially in growing lesions
- Prominent inflammatory infiltrate, usually with abundant eosinophils and neutrophils
- Regressing lesions often show epidermal atrophy and bland cytologic features
  - o Dermal fibrosis and chronic inflammation typically present

Cytologic Features
- Enlarged squamous cells with abundant dense eosinophilic-staining cytoplasm and enlarged, hyperchromatic to vesicular-appearing nuclei with prominent nucleoli

DIFFERENTIAL DIAGNOSIS

Conventional Squamous Cell Carcinoma
- Well-differentiated SCC may occasionally mimic or arise in KA
- Lacks a central keratin-filled crater
- More atypia, mitoses, and infiltrative features
- If lesion appears to be a KA but is only partially sampled, possibility of SCC cannot be excluded
  - o Complete conservative excision should be recommended in these cases

Squamous Cell Carcinoma In Situ (SCCis) (Bowen Disease)
- Not often difficult to distinguish from KA except in some superficial/partial shave biopsies in which the lesion cannot be completely visualized
- Lacks the central crateriform area of KA
- Typically shows prominent cytologic atypia with numerous mitotic figures present throughout the full thickness of epidermis

Verrucous Carcinoma
- Shows prominent endophytic and exophytic architecture with deep, bulbous rete ridges
- Lacks central crater of KA
- Cells are large and bland appearing and show similar cytologic features to KA with abundant dense/glassy eosinophilic cytoplasm

DIAGNOSTIC CHECKLIST

Pathologic Interpretation Pearls
- Symmetric-appearing atypical squamous proliferation with central keratin-filled crater
- Cells are enlarged with large nuclei and abundant dense eosinophilic-staining cytoplasm

SELECTED REFERENCES

1. Ko CJ: Keratoacanthoma: facts and controversies. Clin Dermatol. 28(3):254-61, 2010
2. Weedon DD et al: Squamous cell carcinoma arising in keratoacanthoma: a neglected phenomenon in the elderly. Am J Dermatopathol. 32(5):423-6, 2010
3. Smith KJ et al: Eruptive keratoacanthoma-type squamous cell carcinomas in patients taking sorafenib for the treatment of solid tumors. Dermatol Surg. 35(11):1766-70, 2009
4. Connolly M et al: Immunohistochemical staining for the differentiation of subungual keratoacanthoma from subungual squamous cell carcinoma. Clin Exp Dermatol. 33(5):625-8, 2008
5. Magalhães RF et al: Diagnosis and follow-up of keratoacanthoma-like lesions: clinical-histologic study of 43 cases. J Cutan Med Surg. 12(4):163-73, 2008
6. Cassarino DS et al: Cutaneous squamous cell carcinoma: a comprehensive clinicopathologic classification--part two. J Cutan Pathol. 33(4):261-79, 2006
7. Clausen OP et al: Are keratoacanthomas variants of squamous cell carcinomas? A comparison of chromosomal aberrations by comparative genomic hybridization. J Invest Dermatol. 126(10):2308-15, 2006
8. Monroe WM: Keratoacanthoma: a frequent but rarely recognized skin lesion confused with squamous carcinoma. South Med J. 50(7):852-4, 1957

KERATOACANTHOMA

Microscopic Features

(Left) *Scanning power examination of a relatively small KA shows a symmetric-appearing atypical squamous proliferation with a dilated, central keratin-filled crater ➡ and dense overlying parakeratosis ➡. **(Right)** High magnification shows enlarged keratinocytes with abundant, glassy amphophilic- ➡ to eosinophilic-staining cytoplasm. Note the numerous dyskeratotic cells ➡ in the foci of keratinization.*

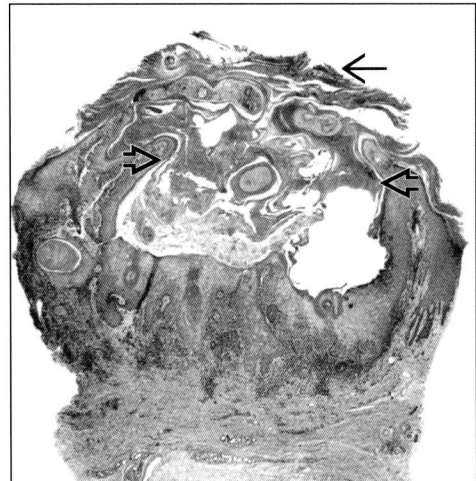
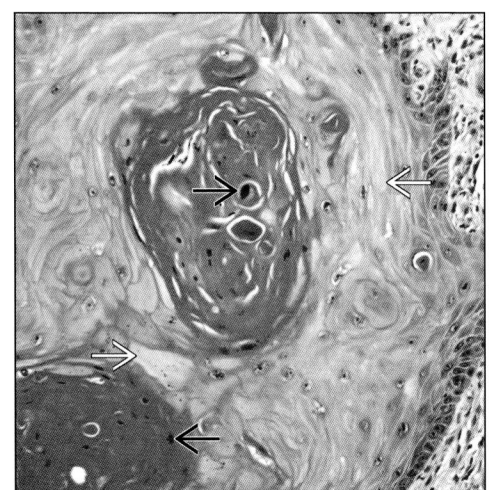

(Left) *High magnification of an area with significant cytologic atypia is characterized by enlarged squamous cells with hyperchromatic nuclei and prominent nucleoli ➡. Note the inflamed surrounding stroma ➡. **(Right)** Acute inflammation is common in KAs, and intraepithelial microabscesses ➡ filled with eosinophils and neutrophils are often seen.*

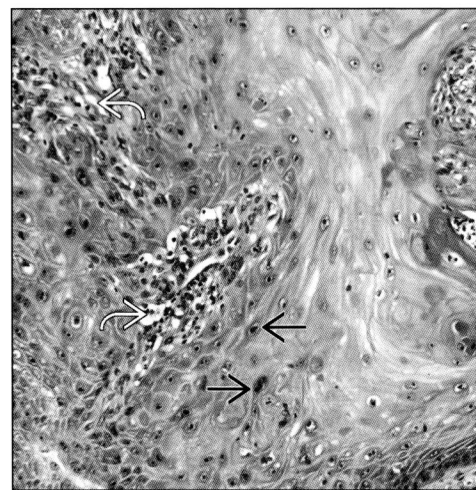
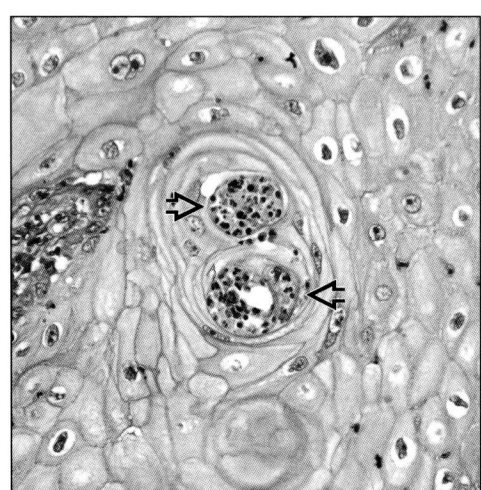

(Left) *Low magnification of another example of a KA shows an endophytic-appearing, multilobulated ➡ atypical squamous proliferation lined by a squamous epithelium with prominent, central keratin-filled cavities ➡. **(Right)** Higher magnification of this KA shows enlarged, relatively bland-appearing squamous cells with abundant pale- to eosinophilic-staining cytoplasm. Note the scattered dyskeratotic keratinocytes ➡.*

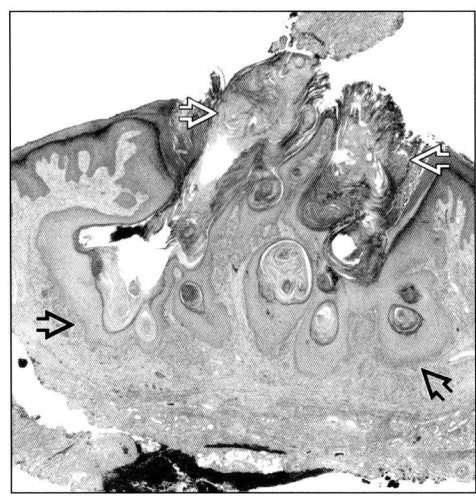
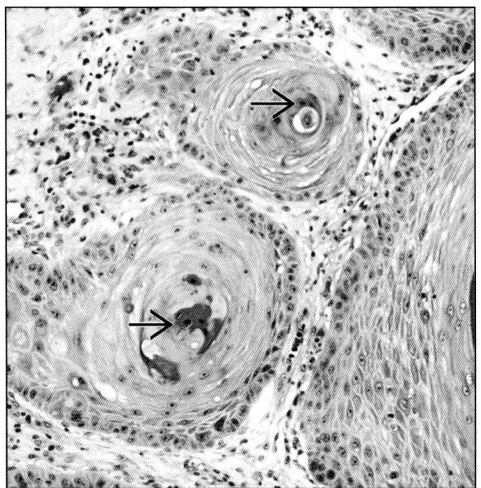

KERATOACANTHOMA

Differential Diagnosis

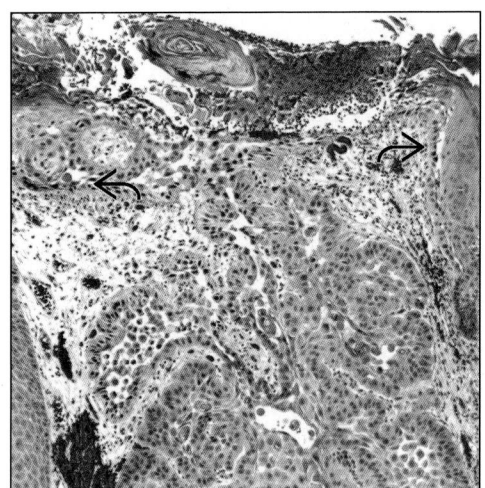

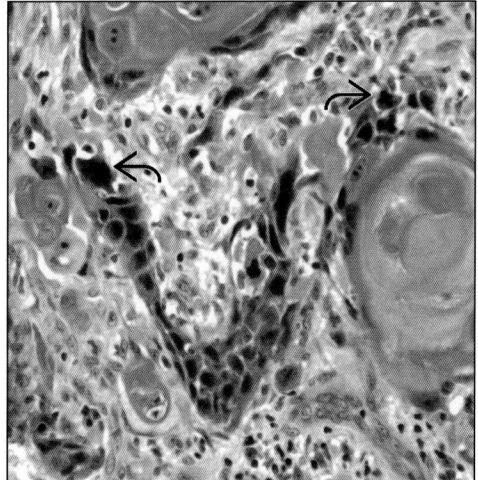

(Left) KA should be distinguished from cases of conventional SCC, which can be more aggressive. This is an example of an invasive SCC with acantholytic features arising in association with an AK ➡. *(Right)* High magnification of an infiltrating, moderately differentiated SCC shows prominent nuclear atypia, pleomorphism, and scattered atypical mitotic figures ➡. This degree of atypia should not be seen in KA.

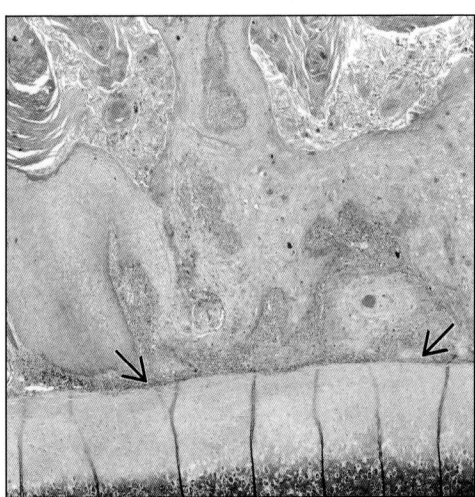

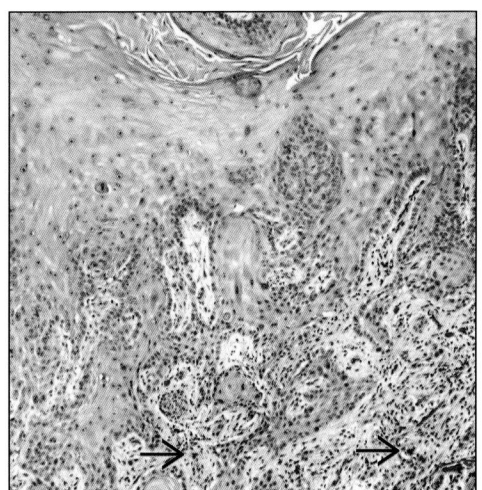

(Left) This is an example of a well-differentiated SCC with large, glassy-appearing tumor cells mimicking a KA. This case arose on the ear and invaded deeply to abut the cartilage ➡. *(Right)* This is another example of a well-differentiated SCC with some features mimicking a KA, including enlarged squamous cells with abundant glassy-appearing eosinophilic cytoplasm. However, this tumor lacks a central keratin-filled crater and shows infiltrating single atypical cells in the dermis ➡.

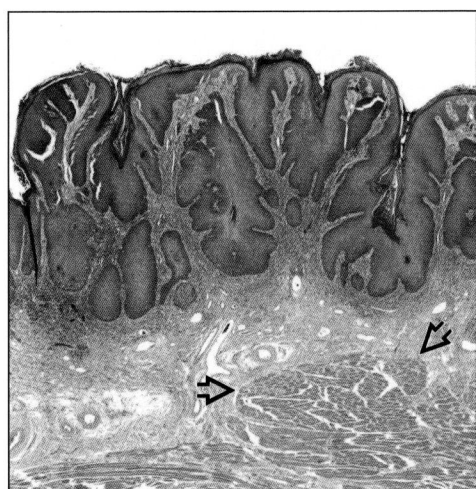

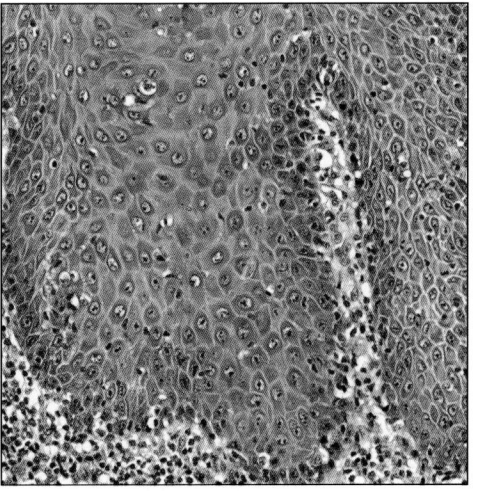

(Left) Verrucous carcinoma (VC) shows exophytic and endophytic growth patterns with deep "pushing" invasion. Note underlying skeletal muscle bundles ➡, indicating deep extent of invasion. *(Right)* High-power examination of VC shows enlarged keratinocytes with dense eosinophilic cytoplasm and nuclei with vesicular chromatin and focally enlarged nucleoli. While the cytologic features can be similar to KA, the architectural features are very different in these tumors.

LYMPHOEPITHELIOMA-LIKE CARCINOMA OF THE SKIN

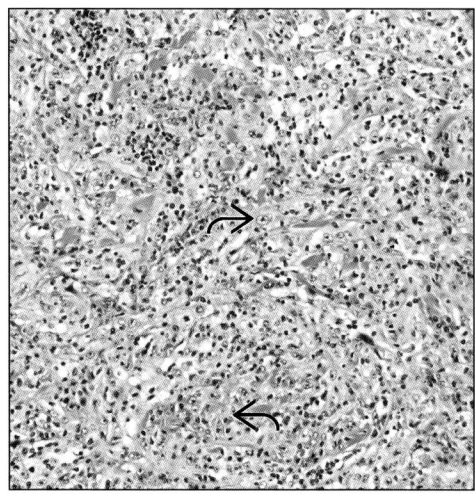

LELCS is characterized by a prominent lymphohistiocytic infiltrate obscuring a background of large, undifferentiated epithelioid-appearing cells ⤳.

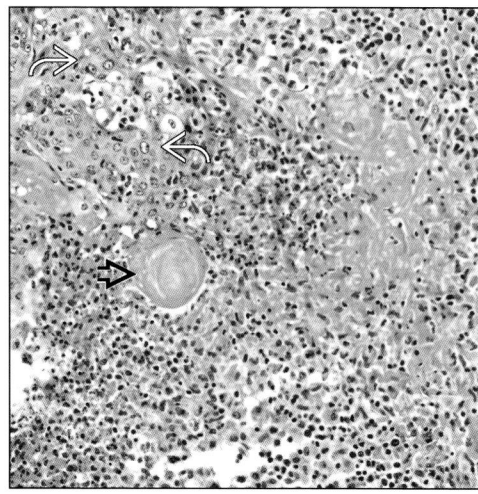

High-magnification examination of a LELCS shows areas of squamous differentiation ⇨ and prominent keratinization ⇥.

TERMINOLOGY

Abbreviations
- Lymphoepithelioma-like carcinoma of the skin (LELCS)

Definitions
- Poorly differentiated carcinoma, most likely variant of squamous cell carcinoma (SCC), with prominent inflammatory infiltrate mimicking lymphoepithelioma-like carcinoma of the nasopharynx

ETIOLOGY/PATHOGENESIS

Unknown
- No proven relationship with Epstein-Barr virus (EBV) (unlike nasopharyngeal lymphoepitheliomas)

CLINICAL ISSUES

Epidemiology
- Incidence
  - Extremely rare variant of SCC; less than 50 cases reported to date
- Age
  - Typically occurs in elderly patients
- Gender
  - Males > females

Site
- Most common in head and neck region

Presentation
- Nodular erythematous lesion

Treatment
- Surgical approaches

  - Complete excision is definitive treatment, similar to invasive SCC

Prognosis
- Low risk of metastasis, but several cases of metastatic disease have been reported
- Currently classified as a variant of SCC with intermediate malignant potential

MICROSCOPIC PATHOLOGY

Histologic Features
- Dermal infiltrate of predominantly lymphoid cells associated with enlarged, atypical epithelioid cells
- Epithelioid cells may form small nests or clusters
  - Tumor cells may be difficult to discern due to heavy lymphoid infiltrate
  - On high-magnification examination, epithelioid cells show enlarged nuclei with vesicular chromatin and prominent nucleoli
- Focal overlying SCC in situ may be identified
- Rare cases may represent a poorly differentiated adnexal carcinoma

ANCILLARY TESTS

Immunohistochemistry
- Epithelioid cells are positive for cytokeratins, especially high molecular weight cytokeratins (CK5/6, CK903) and p63
- EMA also positive in most cases
- Lymphoid markers, especially T-cell markers, will highlight the dense background lymphoid infiltrate

DIFFERENTIAL DIAGNOSIS

Lymphoma
- Atypical lymphocytes lacking epithelial component

LYMPHOEPITHELIOMA-LIKE CARCINOMA OF THE SKIN

Key Facts

Terminology

- Lymphoepithelioma-like carcinoma of the skin (LELCS)
- Poorly differentiated carcinoma, most likely variant of SCC, with prominent inflammatory infiltrate

Etiology/Pathogenesis

- No relationship with EBV (unlike nasopharyngeal lymphoepitheliomas)

Clinical Issues

- Extremely rare variant of SCC; less than 50 cases reported to date

Microscopic Pathology

- Dense dermal infiltrate of predominantly lymphoid cells associated with scattered large epithelioid cells
- Epithelioid cells may form nests or clusters, although they may be difficult to discern due to heavy lymphoid infiltrate
- Epithelioid cells typically show enlarged nuclei with vesicular chromatin and prominent nucleoli
- Cytokeratins and EMA will highlight epithelial cells
- Lymphoid markers show mixed lymphocytic population

- Positive for B- or T-cell markers; negative for cytokeratins and EMA

Poorly Differentiated Inflamed Carcinoma

- Look for areas of well-differentiated carcinoma or overlying carcinoma in situ
- Typically lacks the zonation pattern of LELCS
- Immunohistochemistry will be similar to LELCS
- If metastatic tumor, p63 and CK5/6 are typically negative; additional organ-specific markers, such as TTF-1, CDX-2, or PSA, may be positive

Regressing Melanoma with Heavy Inflammation

- May be difficult to recognize if only a few residual melanocytes are present
- Overlying melanoma in situ often present
- Immunohistochemistry should show positivity for melanocytic markers including S100, Melan-A, HMB-45

DIAGNOSTIC CHECKLIST

Clinically Relevant Pathologic Features

- Size of tumor and depth of invasion likely correlate with prognosis

Pathologic Interpretation Pearls

- Dense dermal infiltrate of predominantly lymphoid cells associated with scattered large atypical epithelioid cells

SELECTED REFERENCES

1. López V et al: Lymphoepitelioma-like carcinoma of the skin: report of three cases. J Cutan Pathol. 38(1):54-8, 2011
2. Welch PQ et al: Lymphoepithelioma-like carcinoma of head and neck skin: a systematic analysis of 11 cases and review of literature. Oral Surg Oral Med Oral Pathol Oral Radiol Endod. 111(1):78-86, 2011
3. Kazakov DV et al: Absence of Epstein-Barr virus, human papillomavirus, and simian virus 40 in patients of central european origin with lymphoepithelioma-like carcinoma of the skin. Am J Dermatopathol. 29(4):365-9, 2007
4. Cassarino DS et al: Cutaneous squamous cell carcinoma: a comprehensive clinicopathologic classification--part two. J Cutan Pathol. 33(4):261-79, 2006
5. Wick MR et al: Lymphoepithelioma-like carcinoma of the skin with adnexal differentiation. J Cutan Pathol. 18(2):93-102, 1991
6. Swanson SA et al: Lymphoepithelioma-like carcinoma of the skin. Mod Pathol. 1(5):359-65, 1988

IMAGE GALLERY

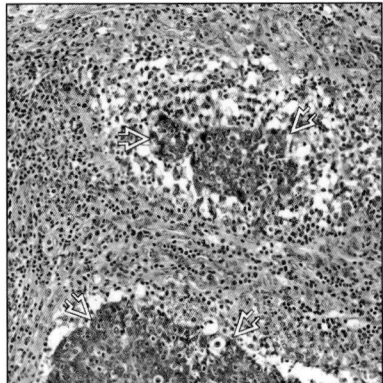 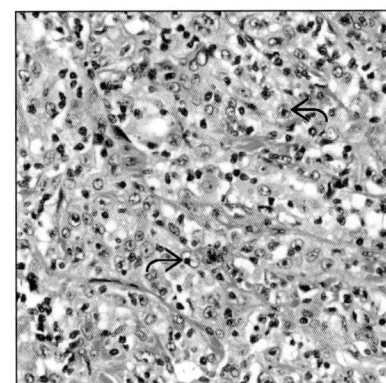 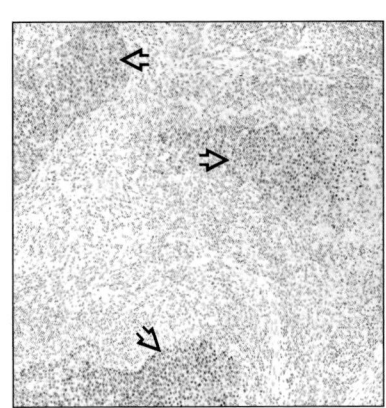

(Left) Another example of LELCS shows islands of more basaloid-appearing epithelial cells ⧩ surrounded by a dense inflammatory infiltrate. *(Center)* High magnification of a LELCS shows enlarged, atypical epithelioid cells with vesicular chromatin and prominent nucleoli ⧩. *(Right)* Immunohistochemistry for p63 shows diffuse nuclear staining ⧩ of the epithelial cells, which are in islands surrounded by inflammatory cells.

BASAL CELL CARCINOMA

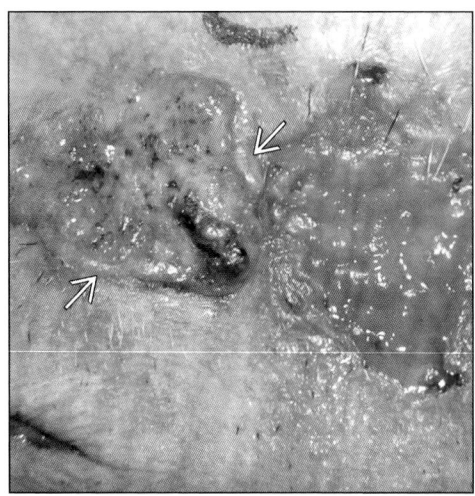

Clinical photograph of a large facial BCC shows areas of ulceration and granulation-like tissue surrounded by a raised border ➡. (Courtesy S. Yashar, MD.)

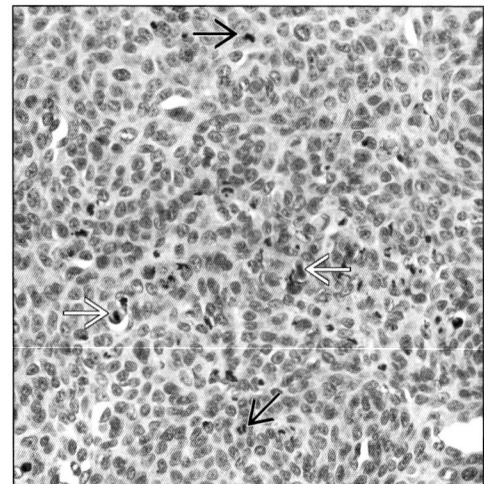

High magnification of a nodular BCC shows a sheet-like proliferation of atypical basaloid cells with high N:C ratios and numerous apoptotic ➡ and mitotic figures ➡.

TERMINOLOGY

Abbreviations
- Basal cell carcinoma (BCC)

Synonyms
- Basal cell epithelioma (BCE)
- Trichoblastic carcinoma (not well accepted and should be discouraged)

Definitions
- Low-grade malignancy of basaloid-appearing keratinocytes

ETIOLOGY/PATHOGENESIS

Multifactorial
- Related to sun exposure (vast majority of cases)
  - Some cases may also be associated with radiation, immunosuppression (organ transplantation), burn scars
    - These cases tend to be more aggressive
- May actually be derived from follicular stem cells (hence, "trichoblastic carcinoma")

Genetics
- Rare cases are associated with genetic syndromes including nevoid basal cell carcinoma (Gorlin) syndrome, xeroderma pigmentosum, basex syndrome, Rombo syndrome, and McKusick syndrome
  - Genes implicated include *PTCH1* (Gorlin syndrome), *P53, SOX9, BMI1, BAX, RMRP*

CLINICAL ISSUES

Epidemiology
- Incidence
  - Extremely common: Most common cancer in humans when skin cancers are included
    - Accounts for 70% of primary cutaneous malignancies
- Age
  - Typically older adults; few cases in young adults
    - If in a child, should consider a genetic syndrome
- Gender
  - Slightly greater incidence in males
- Ethnicity
  - Caucasian/light-skinned individuals
  - Rare in darker skin types

Site
- Most common in head and neck region (up to 80% of cases)
  - About 15% occur on trunk and shoulders
  - Very rare cases involve lips, breast, axillae, groin, inguinal region, and genitalia

Presentation
- Typically papular, plaque-like, or nodular lesion
  - Often present as a pearly, translucent papule with telangiectasia
  - Larger lesions often ulcerated with bleeding &/or overlying crusting
  - Minority of cases are pigmented, more often in Asians and Africans

Treatment
- Surgical approaches
  - Complete excision or electrodessication and curettage (ED&C)
  - Mohs micrographic surgery often used in facial cases

Prognosis
- Usually excellent, cured by local excision
- More aggressive subtypes, including micronodular, infiltrative, desmoplastic, and basosquamous, have higher rate of recurrence and increased risk of metastasis
  - Overall risk of metastasis estimated at 0.05%

BASAL CELL CARCINOMA

Key Facts

Terminology
- Low-grade malignancy of basal keratinocytes

Etiology/Pathogenesis
- Related to sun exposure, radiation, immunosuppression
- May be derived from follicular stem cells

Clinical Issues
- Very common: Most common cancer in humans
- Prognosis usually excellent, most cases cured by excision
- More aggressive subtypes, including infiltrative, micronodular, desmoplastic, and basosquamous, have higher rate of recurrence and low risk of metastasis
- Treated by complete excision or electrodessication and curettage

Microscopic Pathology
- Proliferation of nodules, nests, and cords of small basaloid cells with peripheral palisading, stromal retraction artifact, and mucinous material
- Numerous mitotic and apoptotic figures typically present
- Cells show enlarged hyperchromatic nuclei with inconspicuous nucleoli and scant amounts of eosinophilic cytoplasm

Top Differential Diagnoses
- Squamous cell carcinoma
- Actinic keratosis (on superficial shave biopsy)
- Follicular neoplasms (trichoepithelioma and trichoblastoma)
- Merkel cell carcinoma

MACROSCOPIC FEATURES

Size
- Variable, small (few mm) to large (several cm)

MICROSCOPIC PATHOLOGY

Histologic Features
- Tumor is composed of nodules, nests, &/or infiltrative cords
  - Overlying ulceration and serum crusting often present in large tumors
- Proliferation of small basaloid cells with peripheral palisading
- Stromal retraction artifact
  - Between tumor cells and stroma
- Mucinous material may be present
- Numerous mitotic and apoptotic figures present
- Cells show enlarged hyperchromatic nuclei with inconspicuous or small nucleoli and scant eosinophilic cytoplasm

Variants
- **Superficial-multicentric**: Superficial nests attached to epidermis separated by areas of uninvolved epidermis
- **Nodular**: Large, rounded predominantly dermal-based nests with prominent peripheral palisading
- **Micronodular**: Predominantly dermal-based infiltrative proliferation of small nests
- **Infiltrative**: Small cords and nests, often deeply invasive
- **Desmoplastic/sclerosing/morpheaform**: Infiltrative strands and nests associated with dense sclerotic stroma
- **Infundibulocystic**: Mature folliculocystic spaces containing keratinous material
- **Basosquamous/metatypical**: Prominent areas of squamous differentiation (may mimic squamous cell carcinoma [SCC]), less peripheral palisading present

- **Fibroepithelioma of Pinkus**: Numerous small, anastomosing cords of basaloid cells attached to the epidermis
- Rare variants include adenoid, clear cell, signet ring cell, plasmacytoid/myoepithelial, and BCC with neuroendocrine differentiation

ANCILLARY TESTS

Immunohistochemistry
- Not necessary in most cases except when unusual features present
- Basal cell carcinoma vs. trichoepithelioma and trichoblastoma
  - BCC shows greater staining for Bcl-2, p53, and Ki-67
- BCC vs. SCC
  - BCC is positive for BER-EP4; SCC is almost always negative
  - CK-PAN, HMWCKs, and p63 are not useful as they are positive in both tumors

DIFFERENTIAL DIAGNOSIS

Squamous Cell Carcinoma (SCC)
- Most cases are easily separated; however, basosquamous type of BCC shows prominent squamous differentiation
  - Usually, areas of more typical BCC are present, especially at periphery of tumor
  - Overlying actinic keratosis or Bowen disease often seen in association with SCC
  - BER-EP4 strongly positive in BCC, almost always negative in SCC
- Superficial shave biopsies of ulcerated/inflamed cases may be very difficult or impossible to accurately separate

Actinic Keratosis (AK)
- Can be difficult to distinguish on very superficial shave biopsies

- o AK typically shows basilar budding of atypical squamous cells and overlying parakeratosis
- o No mucinous stroma, peripheral palisading, or tumor-stromal retraction artifact should be seen
- o Numerous apoptotic and mitotic figures favor BCC

Follicular Neoplasms (Trichoepithelioma and Trichoblastoma)

- Dermal-based basaloid adnexal neoplasms, may be large and nodular (trichoblastoma)
  - o Usually symmetric and well circumscribed at scanning magnification
- Typically lack the degree of cytologic atypia, mitoses, and apoptotic figures of BCC
- May show peripheral palisading, but mucinous stroma and tumor-stromal retraction artifact typically lacking in benign follicular neoplasms

Merkel Cell Carcinoma

- Nodular to sheet-like proliferation of highly atypical basaloid cells
  - o Mucinous stroma and tumor-stromal retraction artifact only rarely identified
  - o Peripheral palisading usually absent or only focally present
- Nuclei typically show speckled ("salt and pepper") chromatin pattern or nuclear clearing
- Perinuclear dot-like staining with CK20, pancytokeratin, and CAM5.2
- Positive immunoreactivity with neuroendocrine markers

Sebaceous Carcinoma

- Can show prominent areas of basaloid differentiation
- Focal atypical clear/multivacuolated cells with nuclear indentations should be present
- Lacks peripheral palisading, mucinous stroma, or stromal retraction artifact
- Immunohistochemistry may be useful
  - o Androgen receptor (+), but also frequently positive in BCC
  - o CAM5.2 and CK7(+/-); typically negative in BCC
  - o EMA often positive in clear cells, although it is often lost in poorly differentiated cases
  - o Strong BER-EP4 and Bcl-2 favor BCC, but they are positive in some sebaceous carcinomas

DIAGNOSTIC CHECKLIST

Clinically Relevant Pathologic Features

- Aggressive subtypes (micronodular, infiltrative, sclerosing/morpheaform, and basosquamous)
- Deep subcutaneous invasion
- Perineural invasion

Pathologic Interpretation Pearls

- Proliferation of nodules, nests, and cords of small basaloid cells with peripheral palisading, stromal retraction artifact, and mucinous material

SELECTED REFERENCES

1. Begnini A et al: PTCH1 gene haplotype association with basal cell carcinoma after transplantation. Br J Dermatol. 163(2):364-70, 2010
2. Plaza JA et al: Value of p63 and podoplanin (D2-40) immunoreactivity in the distinction between primary cutaneous tumors and adenocarcinomas metastatic to the skin: a clinicopathologic and immunohistochemical study of 79 cases. J Cutan Pathol. 37(4):403-10, 2010
3. Garcia C et al: Basosquamous carcinoma. J Am Acad Dermatol. 60(1):137-43, 2009
4. Krokowski M et al: Basal cell carcinoma with neuroendocrine differentiation arising in a scar: A case report. Dermatol Online J. 15(10):4, 2009
5. Mosterd K et al: Destructive basal cell carcinoma in a patient with basal cell nevus syndrome and an interstitial deletion of chromosome 9q22. Dermatol Surg. 35(12):2051-3, 2009
6. Cohen PR et al: Basal cell carcinoma with mixed histology: a possible pathogenesis for recurrent skin cancer. Dermatol Surg. 32(4):542-51, 2006
7. Farley RL et al: Aggressive basal cell carcinoma with invasion of the parotid gland, facial nerve, and temporal bone. Dermatol Surg. 32(2):307-15; discussion 315, 2006
8. Tschen JP et al: Pleomorphic basal cell carcinoma: case reports and review. South Med J. 99(3):296-302, 2006
9. Wadhera A et al: Metastatic basal cell carcinoma: a case report and literature review. How accurate is our incidence data? Dermatol Online J. 12(5):7, 2006
10. Ackerman AB et al: Fibroepithelial tumor of pinkus is trichoblastic (Basal-cell) carcinoma. Am J Dermatopathol. 27(2):155-9, 2005
11. Ting PT et al: Metastatic basal cell carcinoma: report of two cases and literature review. J Cutan Med Surg. 9(1):10-5, 2005
12. Bogdanov-Berezovsky A et al: Risk factors for incomplete excision of basal cell carcinomas. Acta Derm Venereol. 84(1):44-7, 2004
13. Colvett KT et al: Atypical presentation of metastatic basal cell carcinoma. South Med J. 97(3):305-7, 2004
14. Saldanha G et al: Basal cell carcinoma: a dermatopathological and molecular biological update. Br J Dermatol. 148(2):195-202, 2003
15. Kim YC et al: Signet ring cell basal cell carcinoma: a basal cell carcinoma with myoepithelial differentiation. Am J Dermatopathol. 23(6):525-9, 2001
16. Meehan SA et al: Basal cell carcinoma with tumor epithelial and stromal giant cells: a variant of pleomorphic basal cell carcinoma. Am J Dermatopathol. 21(5):473-8, 1999
17. Jones MS et al: The immunohistochemical characteristics of the basosquamous cell carcinoma. Dermatol Surg. 23(3):181-4, 1997
18. Lobo CJ et al: Basal cell carcinoma of the external auditory canal and Gorlin-Goltz syndrome: a case report. J Laryngol Otol. 111(9):850-1, 1997
19. Kazantseva IA et al: Immunohistochemical study of primary and recurrent basal cell and metatypical carcinomas of the skin. Am J Dermatopathol. 18(1):35-42, 1996
20. Sina B et al: Fibroepithelioma of Pinkus: eccrine duct spread of basal cell carcinoma. Am J Dermatopathol. 17(6):634-6, 1995
21. Suster S et al: Myoepithelial differentiation in basal cell carcinoma. Am J Dermatopathol. 13(4):350-7, 1991
22. Pinkus H: Epithelial and fibroepithelial tumors. Arch Dermatol. 91:24-37, 1965

BASAL CELL CARCINOMA

Microscopic Features

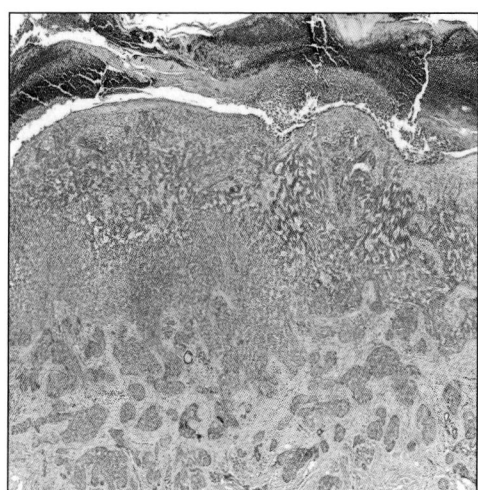
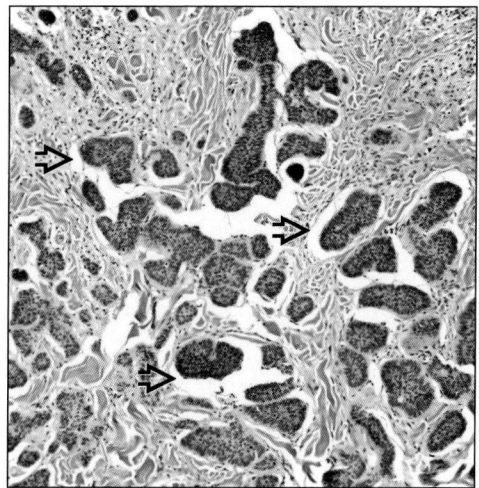

(Left) Low magnification shows a large nodular- and micronodular-type BCC with diffuse overlying ulceration and dense serum crusting. *(Right)* Histologic section of a micronodular-type BCC shows a proliferation of small nests of basaloid cells with a prominent retraction artifact ⇨ in a somewhat sclerotic-appearing stroma.

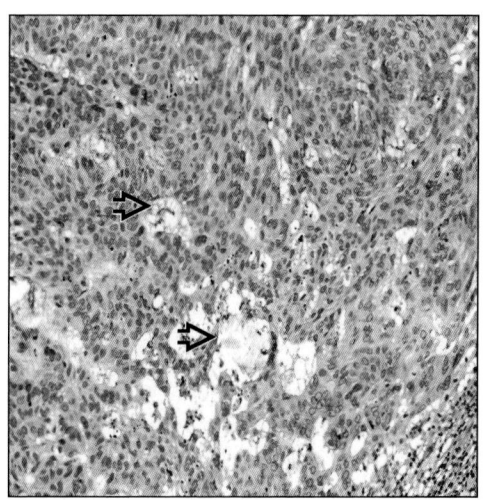
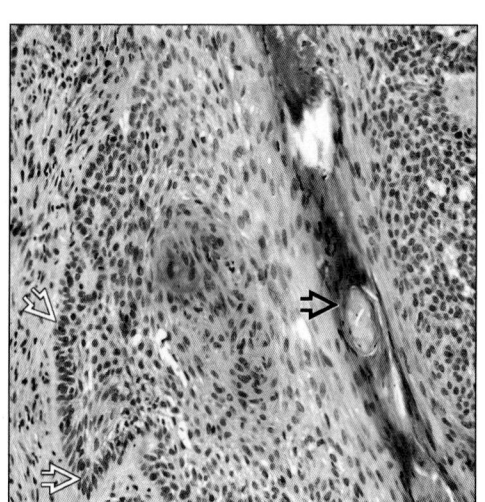

(Left) Basosquamous-type BCC shows a proliferation of large, squamoid-appearing cells with abundant eosinophilic cytoplasm and focal mucin collections ⇨. *(Right)* Another example of basosquamous-type BCC shows traditional areas of BCC with peripheral palisading ⇨ surrounding collections of larger, squamoid-appearing cells associated with follicular differentiation and focal keratinization ⇨.

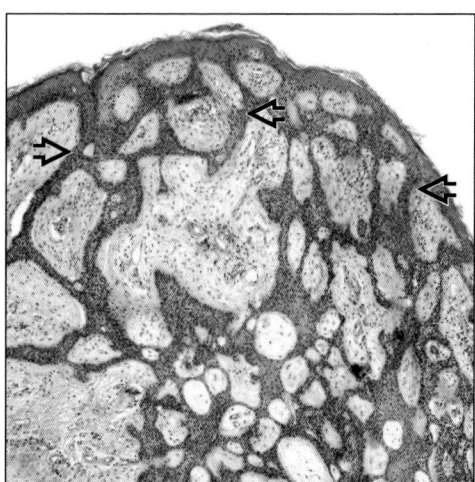
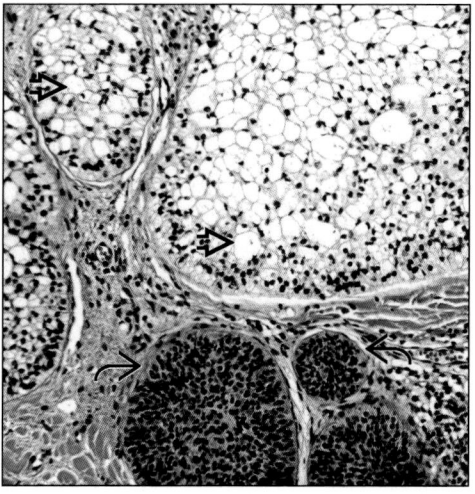

(Left) Scanning magnification of a fibroepithelioma of Pinkus-type BCC is characterized by numerous small anastomosing cords of basaloid cells with multiple epidermal connections ⇨. *(Right)* Clear cell BCC is composed of large cells with abundant clear cytoplasm ⇨, and can mimic clear cell squamous cell carcinoma or sebaceous carcinoma in some cases. However, areas of more conventional-appearing BCC are often present, as are seen in the lower portion of this photomicrograph ⇨.

Microscopic and Immunohistochemical Features

(Left) Low-power view of a large pigmented nodular BCC shows prominent pigmentation ➡ throughout the nodule. *(Right)* High magnification of a nodular BCC shows a rare markedly enlarged, pleomorphic tumor cell with a macronucleolus ⊵.

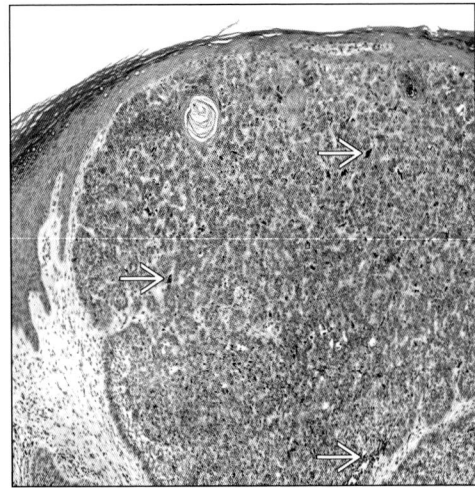 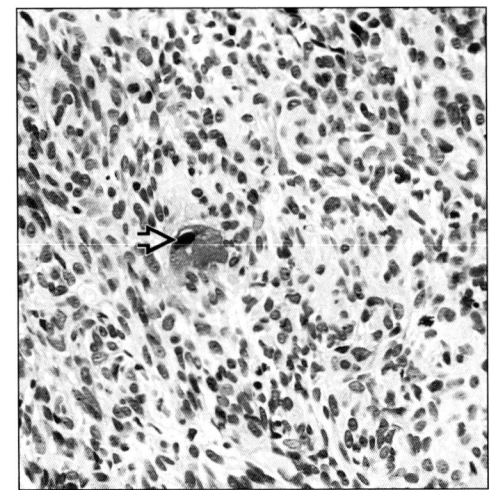

(Left) Morpheaform (desmoplastic/sclerosing) BCC shows cords of atypical basaloid cells infiltrating a dense, desmoplastic stroma. *(Right)* High-power magnification of a plasmacytoid BCC shows dense eosinophilic cytoplasmic inclusions ⊵ and displaced nuclei. These cases have been shown to exhibit myoepithelial differentiation.

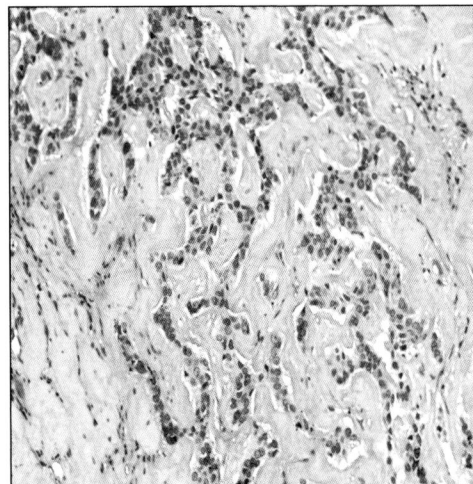 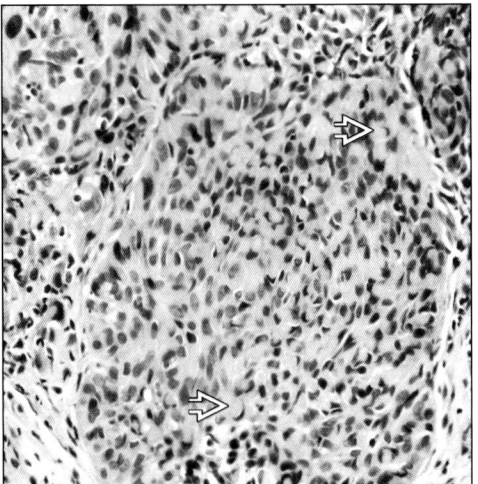

(Left) BER-EP4/CD326 immunohistochemistry of a plasmacytoid BCC shows moderate to strong membranous staining of many of the tumor cells. *(Right)* Bcl-2 immunohistochemistry in a micronodular BCC shows moderate to strong cytoplasmic staining of the tumor cells.

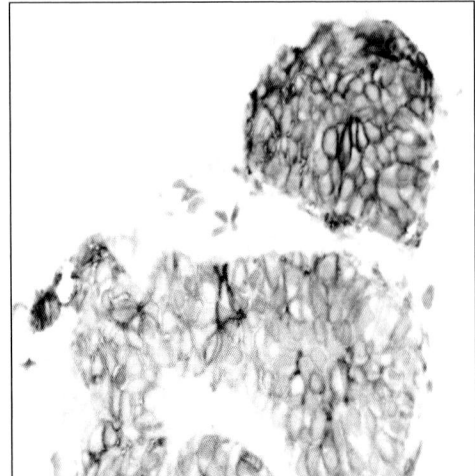 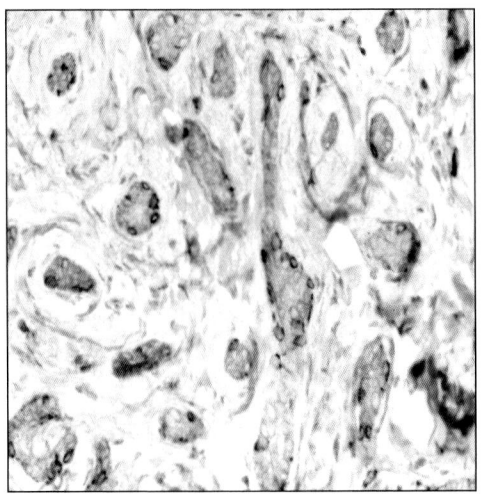

BASAL CELL CARCINOMA

Differential Diagnosis

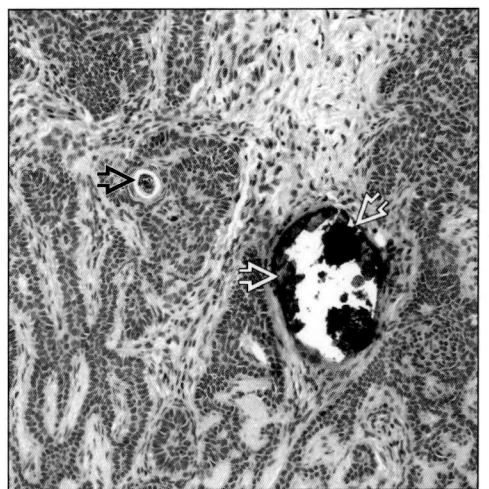

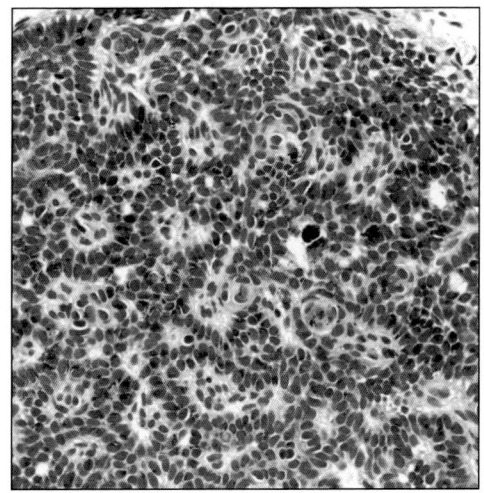

(Left) Histologic section of a trichoblastoma shows a bland-appearing basaloid tumor in a fibromyxoid stroma lacking tumor-stromal retraction artifact (as in BCC). There is focal pigmentation ➔ and an area of calcification ➔, findings typical of this neoplasm. (Right) High magnification shows a trichoblastoma with diffuse pigmentation. The lesion is composed of bland-appearing basaloid cells in anastomosing ribbons. Note the bland cytology and lack of mitotic or apoptotic figures.

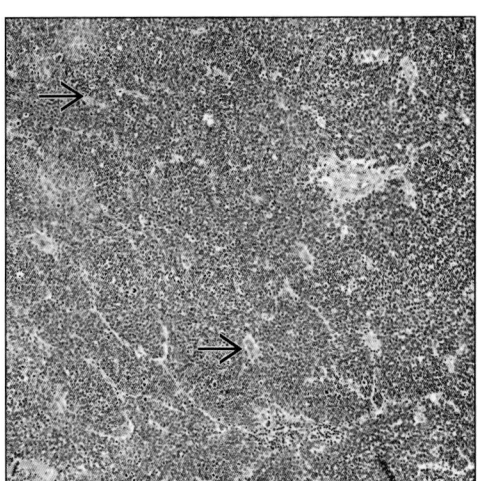

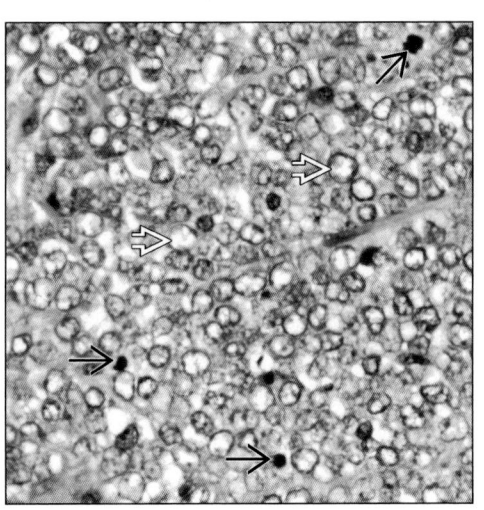

(Left) Merkel cell carcinoma is typically composed of broad cords and sheet-like collections of highly atypical basaloid cells. There is scant stroma ➔ intervening between the neoplastic cells, and no tumor-stromal retraction, peripheral palisading, or mucinous material is present. (Right) Nuclear clearing ➔ is often seen in Merkel cell carcinoma, a feature not seen in basal cell carcinoma. Note the numerous apoptotic and mitotic figures ➔.

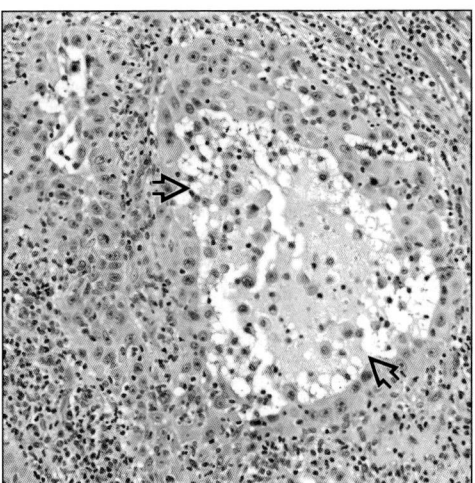

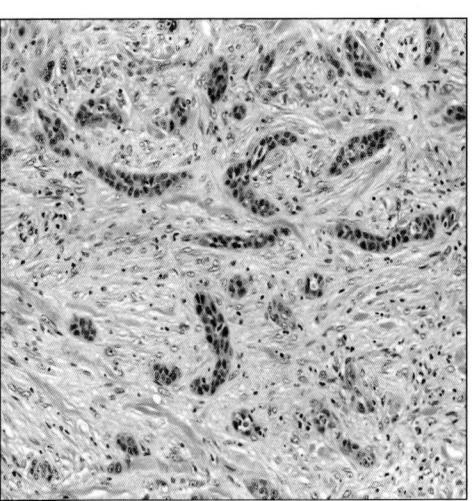

(Left) Squamous cell carcinoma can rarely show mucin production ➔, as in this example of acantholytic SCC, but it is typically found within the center of a tumor island, not in the stroma (as in BCC). (Right) Infiltrative SCC with cord-like structures associated with a desmoplastic stroma can mimic desmoplastic/morpheaform BCC or, less likely, microcystic adnexal carcinoma (MAC).

EXTRAMAMMARY PAGET DISEASE

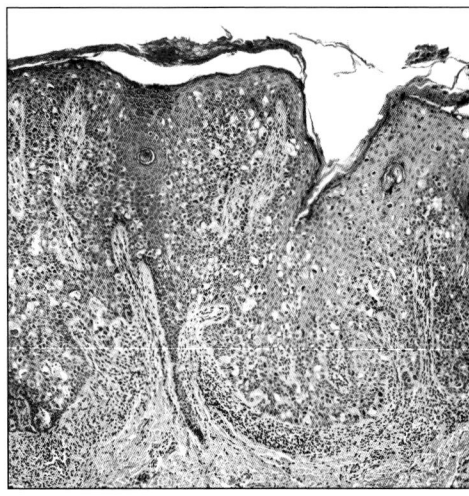

Large pale-staining neoplastic cells extensively infiltrate all levels of a hyperplastic epidermis in EMPD. There is a chronic inflammatory infiltrate in the upper dermis.

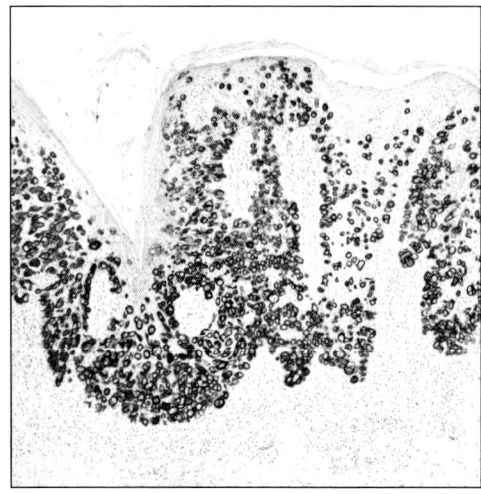

Cytokeratin 7 immunohistochemical stain strongly highlights the neoplastic cells throughout the epidermis. The use of CK7 may also assist in defining the margins of the disease.

TERMINOLOGY

Abbreviations
- Extramammary Paget disease (EMPD)

Definitions
- Adenocarcinoma involving epidermis and commonly extending to epithelium of eccrine glands &/or hair follicles (adenocarcinoma in situ)
- May involve dermis in minority of cases

ETIOLOGY/PATHOGENESIS

Pathogenesis
- Uncertain in most cases
- Cases limited to epidermis are postulated to originate from intraepidermal portion of sweat glands or from intraepidermal stem cells
- Heterogeneous condition; can be classified as primary (cutaneous origin) and secondary (extracutaneous origin)
  - Rarely, primary EMPD is associated with underlying sweat gland adenocarcinoma (usually apocrine)
  - Secondary EMPD may represent extension from urethral, bladder, anal/rectal, prostatic, or endocervical carcinoma
    - Incidence of association with internal carcinoma is about 15%
    - Especially true in perianal EMPD, which is associated with rectal carcinoma in 1/3 of cases

CLINICAL ISSUES

Epidemiology
- Age
  - 6th-8th decade
- Gender
  - Female predominance

Site
- Skin regions rich in apocrine glands
  - Most common sites are vulva and perianal region
  - Other sites include scrotum, perineum, penis, axilla, umbilicus
  - Exceptional sites include eyelid (accompanying carcinoma of Moll gland), external auditory meatus (associated with ceruminous carcinoma), face, scalp, chest, abdomen, and extremities

Presentation
- Circinate or annular moist erythematous scaly patches or plaques
- Gray-white eczematous patches are also common
- Hypopigmented macules, ulceration, crusting, or palpable tumor may be present
- Pruritus is frequent
- Bleeding, oozing, tenderness, or burning sensation can occur
- EMPD may mimic eczema
- Lesions may be multifocal

Treatment
- Complete surgical excision is treatment of choice for primary EMPD
- Treatment in secondary lesions will depend on associated carcinoma

Prognosis
- Primary EMPD confined to epidermis and epithelium of adnexal structures (in situ carcinoma) has good prognosis when completely excised
- Patients require long-term follow-up because of multifocal nature of condition and high recurrence rate
- Dermal invasion is associated with worse prognosis
- Prognosis in secondary Paget disease is related to underlying carcinoma and is usually poor

EXTRAMAMMARY PAGET DISEASE

Key Facts

Terminology
- Extramammary Paget disease (EMPD)

Clinical Issues
- Erythematous patches or plaques with sharply defined borders
- May clinically mimic chronic eczema

Microscopic Pathology
- Round large pale cells in all levels of epidermis arranged as single units or confluent aggregates
- Round vesicular nuclei with prominent nucleoli
- Abundant clear cytoplasm
- Absence of intercellular bridges
- Paget cells often extend to adnexal structures
- Flattened basal keratinocytes

Ancillary Tests
- Paget cells positive for mucin
- Primary EMPD positive for CK7 and negative for CK20
- Secondary EMPD has more variable immunohistochemical profile
  - Secondary EMPD associated with urothelial carcinoma positive for CK7 and CK20
  - Secondary EMPD associated with anal/rectal carcinoma positive for CK20 and negative for CK7

Top Differential Diagnoses
- Squamous cell carcinoma in situ
- Melanoma in situ
- Clear cell papulosis
- Benign mucinous metaplasia of penis

MACROSCOPIC FEATURES

General Features
- Erythematous patches or plaques with sharply defined borders

Sections to Be Submitted
- Important to carefully evaluate margins because neoplastic cells may extend beyond clinical borders

Size
- A few millimeters to several centimeters
- Focal or multicentric

MICROSCOPIC PATHOLOGY

Histologic Features
- Intraepithelial proliferation of large round atypical cells (Paget cells)
- Epithelium varied from hyperplastic to atrophic
- Epithelium may be eroded or ulcerated
- Cytoplasm of neoplastic cells is abundant and pale or vacuolated
- Melanin pigment may be present within cytoplasm of Paget cells
- Intercellular bridges not appreciated between Paget cells on light microscopy
- Nuclei are large and vesicular
- Nucleoli prominent
- Mitoses may be numerous
- Early lesions show only scattered single Paget cells in epidermis
- As lesions evolve, Paget cells are more numerous and are arranged as single cells and confluent aggregates
- Paget cells compress squamous cells
- Flattened basal keratinocytes lying between neoplastic cells and underlying dermis are observed
- Neoplastic cells often extend to epithelium of adnexal structures
- Neoplastic cells may form true intraepidermal glandular lumina
- Dermal mixed cell infiltrate is usually present
- Dermal involvement by tumoral cells may occur

Predominant Pattern/Injury Type
- Adenocarcinoma

Predominant Cell/Compartment Type
- Paget cells

ANCILLARY TESTS

Histochemistry
- Mucicarmine
  - Reactivity: Positive
  - Staining pattern
    - Cytoplasmic

Immunohistochemistry
- Primary EMPD is positive for CEA, low molecular weight cytokeratins (especially CK7 and CAM5.2), EMA/MUC1, and GCDFP-15
- Primary EMPD is negative for CK20
- Primary and secondary EMPD are negative for melanocytic markers such as S100, MART-1/Melan-A, tyrosinase, and HMB-45
- Immunohistochemical expression profile of secondary EMPD is related to associated carcinoma
  - Secondary EMPD associated with urothelial carcinoma
    - Usually expresses both CK7 and CK20
    - Also expresses uroplakin-3
    - Negative for CEA
  - EMPD secondary to anal/rectal carcinomas
    - Expresses CK20 and CEA
    - CDX-2 expression would be another indicator of associated anal/rectal malignancy
    - CK7 usually negative
    - GCDFP-15 negative

EXTRAMAMMARY PAGET DISEASE

DIFFERENTIAL DIAGNOSIS

Squamous Cell Carcinoma In Situ with Pagetoid Pattern
- Dense eosinophilic-staining cytoplasm and presence of intercellular bridges between neoplastic cells
- Positive for HMWCKs (34βE12 and CK5/6) and p63
- Negative for mucicarmine and PAS-D
- Negative for CEA, GCDFP-15, ER/PR
- Negative for CK20, and usually weak/negative for CK7

Melanoma In Situ
- Melanoma cells are present in all levels of epidermis, including basal layer
- No flattened basal cells are seen between melanoma cells and dermis
- Presence of melanin pigment in neoplastic cells does not necessarily indicate melanoma, as some Paget cells can be pigmented
- Melanoma invades dermis much more frequently than does Paget disease
- Immunohistochemical expression of melanocytic markers such as S100, MART-1/Melan-A, and HMB-45

Clear Cell Papulosis
- Young children (more often Asian or Hispanic)
- Small macules or papules affecting the lower part of the trunk, face
- Predominantly milk line location
- Clear cells with pagetoid features in lower part of epidermis
- PAN-CK (AE1/AE3) and CEA positive

Benign Mucinous Metaplasia of Penis
- Elderly patients
- Prepuce or glans
- Benign mucin-containing cells in squamous epithelium
- Usually associated with chronic inflammatory conditions

Pagetoid Dyskeratosis
- Reactive process
- Intertriginous and genital area
- Lesional cells are keratinocytes showing early keratinization

Pagetoid Reticulosis
- Rare variant of cutaneous T-cell lymphoma
- Exclusive epidermal infiltration by medium- to large-sized T cells with abundant pale cytoplasm
- T cells are CD45 (LCA) and CD3 positive
- T cells may be either CD4 or CD8 positive or double negative
- T-cell gene rearrangement can be demonstrated

Merkel Cell Carcinoma
- Rare cases may have prominent epidermotropic component
- Small round blue cells with scant cytoplasm
- No true glandular formation
- Characteristic dot-like pattern with CK20 and PAN-CK (AE1/AE3)

- In a minority of cases, may express CK7
- Positive expression of neuroendocrine markers such as chromogranin and synaptophysin

DIAGNOSTIC CHECKLIST

Clinically Relevant Pathologic Features
- Tissue distribution
  ○ Important to distinguish in situ lesions, in which Paget cells are confined within epidermis and epithelium of adnexal structures, from tumors showing dermal invasion
  ○ Important to recognize EMPD associated with underlying sweat gland carcinoma
  ○ Important to rule out an associated internal carcinoma

Pathologic Interpretation Pearls
- Large round cells with abundant pale cytoplasm in all levels of epidermis (Paget cells)
- Sometimes true glandular formation by these neoplastic cells in epidermis
- Flattened basal keratinocytes lying between Paget cells and underlying basement membrane
- Presence of melanin does not rule out Paget disease

SELECTED REFERENCES

1. Wang Z et al: Penile and scrotal Paget's disease: 130 Chinese patients with long-term follow-up. BJU Int. 102(4):485-8, 2008
2. Liegl B et al: Mammary and extramammary Paget's disease: an immunohistochemical study of 83 cases. Histopathology. 50(4):439-47, 2007
3. De Nisi MC et al: Usefulness of CDX2 in the diagnosis of extramammary Paget disease associated with malignancies of intestinal type. Br J Dermatol. 153(3):677-9, 2005
4. Brown HM et al: Uroplakin-III to distinguish primary vulvar Paget disease from Paget disease secondary to urothelial carcinoma. Hum Pathol. 33(5):545-8, 2002
5. van Randenborgh H et al: Extramammary Paget's disease of penis and scrotum. J Urol. 168(6):2540-1, 2002
6. Kuan SF et al: Differential expression of mucin genes in mammary and extramammary Paget's disease. Am J Surg Pathol. 25(12):1469-77, 2001
7. Ohnishi T et al: The use of cytokeratins 7 and 20 in the diagnosis of primary and secondary extramammary Paget's disease. Br J Dermatol. 142(2):243-7, 2000
8. Parker LP et al: Paget's disease of the vulva: pathology, pattern of involvement, and prognosis. Gynecol Oncol. 77(1):183-9, 2000
9. Val-Bernal JF et al: Benign mucinous metaplasia of the penis. A lesion resembling extramammary Paget's disease. J Cutan Pathol. 27(2):76-9, 2000
10. Val-Bernal JF et al: Pagetoid dyskeratosis of the prepuce. An incidental histologic finding resembling extramammary Paget's disease. J Cutan Pathol. 27(8):387-91, 2000
11. Lee JY: Clear cell papulosis: a unique disorder in early childhood characterized by white macules in milk-line distribution. Pediatr Dermatol. 15(4):328-9, 1998
12. Goldblum JR et al: Vulvar Paget's disease: a clinicopathologic and immunohistochemical study of 19 cases. Am J Surg Pathol. 21(10):1178-87, 1997

EXTRAMAMMARY PAGET DISEASE

Microscopic and Immunohistochemical Features

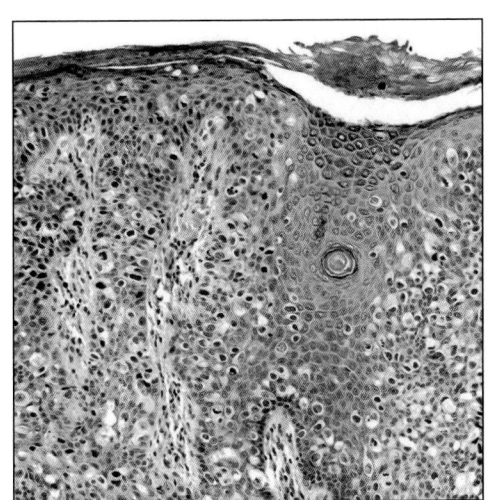

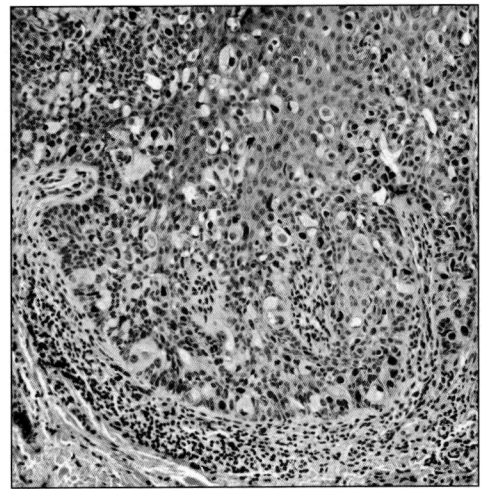

(Left) Numerous pagetoid cells are present in all levels of the epidermis in this case of extramammary Paget disease. The epidermis is hyperplastic with overlying foci of parakeratosis. (Right) Paget cells are large, round to oval, and show ample pale cytoplasm.

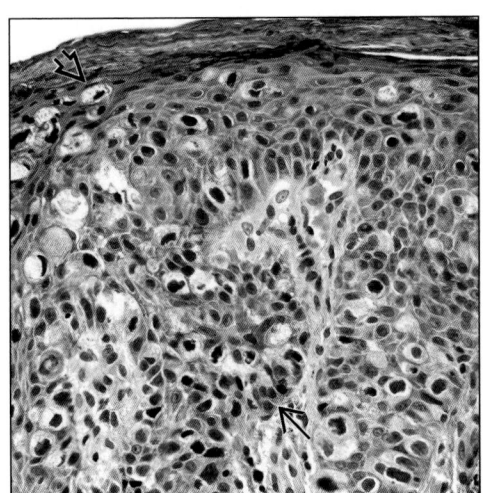

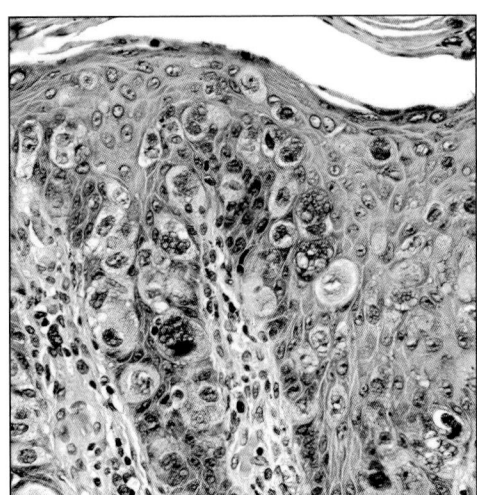

(Left) Numerous Paget cells ⮥ arranged as single units are seen in all levels of the epidermis, including the cornified layer. Note the flattened basal keratinocytes ➡. (Right) A mucicarmine stain shows reddish pink staining of the cytoplasm in most cases of EMPD.

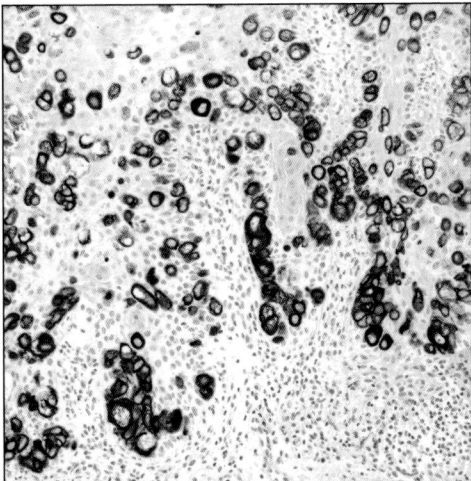

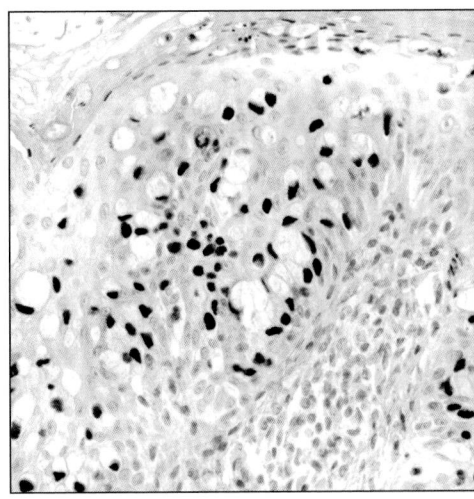

(Left) Strong CK20 expression by the neoplastic cells is seen in this case of EMPD secondary to underlying rectal/anal carcinoma. (Right) CDX-2 expression by the Paget cells would be another strong indicator of an associated synchronous or metachronous anal/rectal malignancy in cases of EMPD.

SQUAMOMELANOCYTIC TUMOR

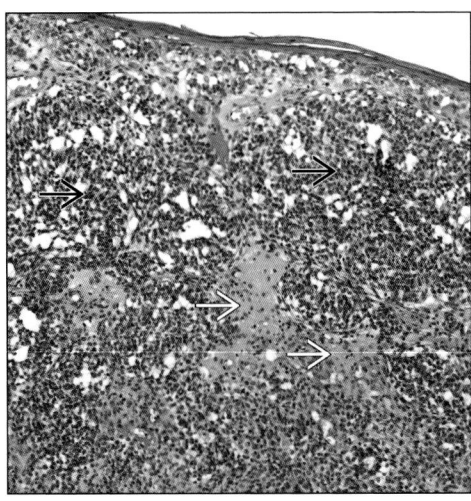

Squamomelanocytic tumor is a dermal-based tumor composed of 2 populations of cells: Epithelioid melanocytic cells ⇒ and larger squamoid cells ➡. (Courtesy P. Amerio, MD, PhD.)

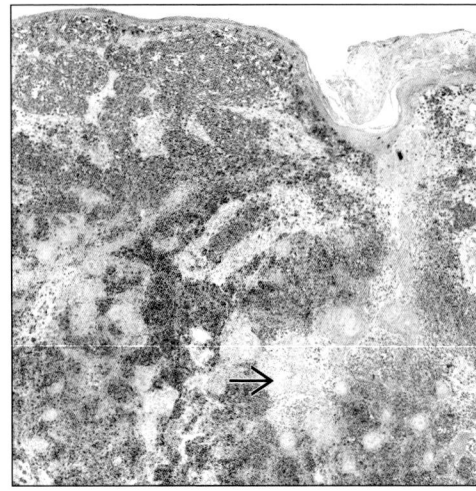

Squamomelanocytic tumor shows distinctive staining of the epithelioid cells with S100. The squamoid cells are negative ⇒ with S100. (Courtesy P. Amerio, MD, PhD.)

TERMINOLOGY

Definitions
- Admixed histopathologic features of both squamoid cells and cells that stain with melanocytic markers
  - 2 cell types generally within < 1 mm of each other
- Original descriptions were of dermal-based tumors

CLINICAL ISSUES

Presentation
- Very rare tumor
  - < 10 cases reported in the literature
- Generally elderly patients
- Predilection for head and neck
- Nondescript papule or nodule
  - Blue-black to red or flesh colored

Treatment
- Excision

Prognosis
- Unclear as so few cases have been reported
- Nodal micrometastasis reported in 1 case

MICROSCOPIC PATHOLOGY

Histologic Features
- Intermingled cell populations in dermal nodules
  - Atypical epithelioid cells
    - Pink cytoplasm, hyperchromatic nuclei, atypical mitoses
    - Keratin pearls may be evident
    - Cytokeratin positive
    - 1 case describes focal ductal differentiation
  - Melanocytes
    - Dermal-based cases
    - Melanocytes not obvious on histologic sections; dendritic cells highlighted with S100 staining; or

- Atypical epithelioid cells in nests
- In 1 published case, arranged as irregular nests and as single cells (with pagetoid scatter); cells with scant cytoplasm and pleomorphic nuclei
  - In some published cases of dermal-based tumors, 3rd population of cells reported
    - Difficult to appreciate on H&E sections
    - Do not mark with melanocytic or epithelial immunohistochemical stains
- 1 published case had intermingled cells mostly within epidermis
- Changes of lentigo maligna may overlie dermal-based tumors

Cytologic Features
- Squamoid cells
  - Nuclei often hyperchromatic
  - Pink cytoplasm
  - Keratin pearls may be present
  - Mitoses
- Melanocytic population
  - May be spindled with clear cytoplasm with fine melanin pigment
  - May be difficult to appreciate; highlighted by melanocytic immunohistochemical stains in dermal-based nodules
  - In 1 published case, atypical melanocytes in nests in epidermis
    - Hyperchromatic nuclei, scant cytoplasm, nucleoli prominent

ANCILLARY TESTS

Immunohistochemistry
- Squamoid cells
  - Stain with cytokeratins
- Melanocytic population
  - Stains with S100 and other melanocytic markers

SQUAMOMELANOCYTIC TUMOR

Key Facts

Terminology
- Admixed histopathologic features of both squamous cell carcinoma and malignant melanoma
- Original descriptions were of dermal-based tumors

Clinical Issues
- Very rare tumor
- Often elderly patients
- Predilection for head and neck
- Unclear prognosis as so few cases reported

Microscopic Pathology
- Intermingled populations of cells in dermal nodules
- Squamoid population
- Melanocytic population

Top Differential Diagnoses
- Squamous cell carcinoma with colonization of melanocytes
- Pseudoepitheliomatous hyperplasia associated with malignant melanoma

DIFFERENTIAL DIAGNOSIS

Squamous Cell Carcinoma with Colonization by Melanocytes
- Predominantly composed of atypical squamous cells, with scattered melanocytes
  - Melanocytes
    - Of low density
    - Single, not nested
    - Dendritic-shaped
    - Nuclei not atypical

Pseudoepitheliomatous Hyperplasia Associated with Malignant Melanoma
- Keratinocytes in hyperplastic areas not atypical and connect to epidermal surface
- Mitoses not prominent
- Dyskeratosis absent

Melanocytic Matrixoma
- Dermal nodule of cells
  - Dendritic melanocytes intermingled with epithelial cells
  - Epithelial cells are small, basaloid (matrical), similar to pilomatrixoma
  - Shadow cells also present

Atypical Solid-Cystic Hidradenoma
- Lacks population of spindled cells with clear cytoplasm and fine melanin pigment

DIAGNOSTIC CHECKLIST

Pathologic Interpretation Pearls
- Generally dermal nodule of atypical cells
  - Origin of cells may be difficult to determine
  - Some keratin pearls may be evident
  - Immunohistochemistry shows
    - Intermingled cytokeratin-positive epithelioid cells, dendritic cells positive with melanocytic markers, and usually a 3rd cell type that is negative with both epithelial and melanocytic stains
- 1 case report of "in situ" intermingled atypical keratinocytes and melanocytes

SELECTED REFERENCES

1. Amerio P et al: Metastasizing dermal squamomelanocytic tumour. J Eur Acad Dermatol Venereol. 25(4):489-91, 2011
2. Leonard N et al: Squamomelanocytic tumor: an unusual and distinctive entity of uncertain biological potential. Am J Dermatopathol. 31(5):495-8, 2009
3. Miteva M et al: A rare case of a cutaneous squamomelanocytic tumor: revisiting the histogenesis of combined neoplasms. Am J Dermatopathol. 31(6):599-603, 2009
4. Rongioletti F et al: Squamomelanocytic tumor: a new case of a unique biphenotypic neoplasm of uncertain biological potential. J Cutan Pathol. 36(4):477-81, 2009
5. Pool SE et al: Dermal squamo-melanocytic tumor: a unique biphenotypic neoplasm of uncertain biological potential. Hum Pathol. 30(5):525-9, 1999

IMAGE GALLERY

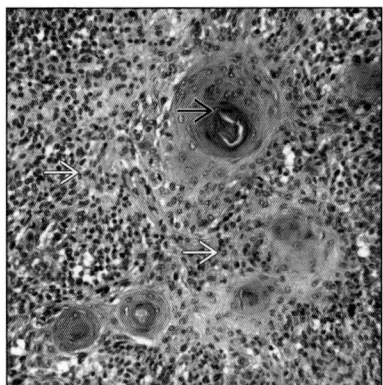 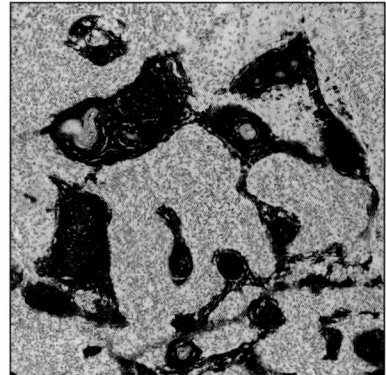 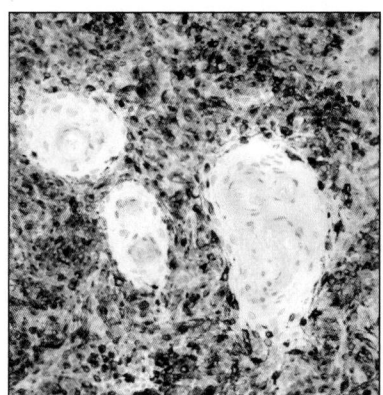

(Left) Squamomelanocytic tumor shows cells with pink cytoplasm in islands, forming keratin pearls ➡, surrounded by cells ➡ with less distinctive cytoplasm. (Courtesy P. Amerio, MD PhD.) *(Center)* Cytokeratin AE1/AE3 highlights the islands of cells forming keratin. (Courtesy P. Amerio, MD, PhD.) *(Right)* Melan-A staining is positive in cells surrounding the negative islands of squamoid cells forming keratin. (Courtesy P. Amerio, MD, PhD.)

PROTOCOL FOR SPECIMENS OF SQUAMOUS CELL CARCINOMA OF THE SKIN

Squamous Cell Carcinoma of the Skin

Biopsy, Excision, Reexcision, Lymphadenectomy

Procedure

____ Biopsy, punch

____ Biopsy, shave

____ Biopsy, other (specify): _____

____ Excision, ellipse

____ Excision, wide

____ Excision, other (specify): _____

____ Reexcision, ellipse

____ Reexcision, wide

____ Reexcision, other (specify): _____

____ Lymphadenectomy, sentinel node(s)

____ Lymphadenectomy, regional nodes (specify): _____

____ Other (specify): _____

____ Not specified

Tumor Site

Specify, if known: _____

____ Not specified

Tumor Size

Greatest dimension: _____ cm

*Additional dimensions: _____ x _____ cm

____ Cannot be determined

Histologic Type (select all that apply)

____ Squamous cell carcinoma (SCC)

*____ Acantholytic SCC

*____ Spindle cell (sarcomatoid) SCC

*____ Verrucous SCC

*____ Pseudovascular SCC

*____ Adenosquamous carcinoma

*____ Squamous cell carcinoma, type not otherwise specified

*____ Other (specify): _____

Histologic Grade

____ GX: Cannot be assessed

____ G1: Well differentiated

____ G2: Moderately differentiated

____ G3: Poorly differentiated

____ G4: Undifferentiated

Maximum Tumor Thickness

____ Not applicable

Thickness: _____ mm

Thickness: At least _____ mm

Margins (select all that apply)

Peripheral margins

____ Cannot be assessed

____ Uninvolved by invasive carcinoma

*Distance of invasive carcinoma from closest peripheral margin: _____ mm

*Specify location(s), if possible: _____

____ Involved by invasive carcinoma

Specify location(s), if possible: _____

____ Uninvolved by carcinoma in situ

PROTOCOL FOR SPECIMENS OF SQUAMOUS CELL CARCINOMA OF THE SKIN

    *Distance of carcinoma in situ from closest peripheral margin: _____ mm

    *Specify location(s), if possible: _____

____ Involved by carcinoma in situ

    Specify location(s), if possible: _____

Deep margin

____ Cannot be assessed

____ Uninvolved by invasive carcinoma

    *Distance of invasive carcinoma from margin: _____ mm

    *Specify location(s), if possible: _____

____ Involved by invasive carcinoma

    Specify location(s), if possible: _____

Lymph-Vascular Invasion

____ Not identified

____ Present

____ Indeterminate

Perineural Invasion

____ Not identified

____ Present

____ Indeterminate

Lymph Nodes

____ No nodes submitted or found

Number of lymph nodes examined

Specify: _____

____ Number cannot be determined (explain): _____

Number of lymph nodes involved by metastatic carcinoma

Specify: _____

____ Number cannot be determined (explain): _____

*Extranodal extension

*____ Present

*____ Not identified

Pathologic Staging (pTNM)

TNM descriptors (required only if applicable) (select all that apply)

____ m (multiple)

____ r (recurrent)

____ y (post treatment)

Primary tumor (pT)

____ pTX: Primary tumor cannot be assessed

____ pT0: No evidence of primary tumor

____ pTis: Carcinoma in situ

____ pT1: Tumor ≤ 2 cm in greatest dimension with < 2 high-risk features

____ pT2: Tumor > 2 cm in greatest dimension ± 1 additional high-risk feature, or any size with ≥ 2 high-risk features

____ pT3: Tumor with invasion of maxilla, mandible, orbit, or temporal bone

____ pT4: Tumor with direct or perineural invasion of skull base or axial skeleton

Regional lymph nodes (pN)

____ pNX: Regional lymph nodes cannot be assessed

____ pN0: No regional lymph node metastasis

____ pN1: Metastasis in a single ipsilateral lymph node ≤ 3 cm in greatest dimension

____ pN2: Metastasis in a single ipsilateral lymph node, > 3 cm but ≤ 6 cm in greatest dimension, or multiple ipsilateral lymph nodes, none > 6 cm in greatest dimension, or in bilateral or contralateral lymph nodes, none > 6 cm in greatest dimension

    ____ pN2a: Metastasis in a single ipsilateral lymph node, > 3 cm but ≤ 6 cm in greatest dimension

    ____ pN2b: Metastasis in multiple ipsilateral lymph nodes, none > 6 cm in greatest dimension

    ____ pN2c: Metastasis in bilateral or contralateral lymph nodes, none > 6 cm in greatest dimension

____ pN3: Metastasis in a lymph node, > 6 cm in greatest dimension

PROTOCOL FOR SPECIMENS OF SQUAMOUS CELL CARCINOMA OF THE SKIN

Distant metastasis (pM)

____ Not applicable

____ pM1: Distant metastasis

*Specify site(s), if known: _____

*Additional Pathologic Findings

*Specify: _____

*Adapted with permission from College of American Pathologists, "Protocol for the Examination of Specimens from Patients with Squamous Cell Carcinoma of the Skin." Web posting date: February 2011, www.cap.org. Protocol applies to invasive squamous cell carcinomas of the skin. Squamous cell carcinomas of the eyelid, vulva, and penis are not included. Note: Use of checklist is optional for tumors < 2 cm. *Data elements with asterisks are not required. These elements may be clinically important but are not yet validated or regularly used in patient management.*

PROTOCOL FOR SPECIMENS OF SQUAMOUS CELL CARCINOMA OF THE SKIN

Staging of Cutaneous Squamous Cell Carcinoma

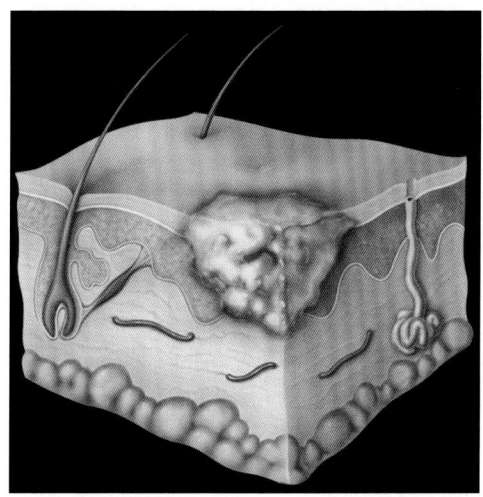
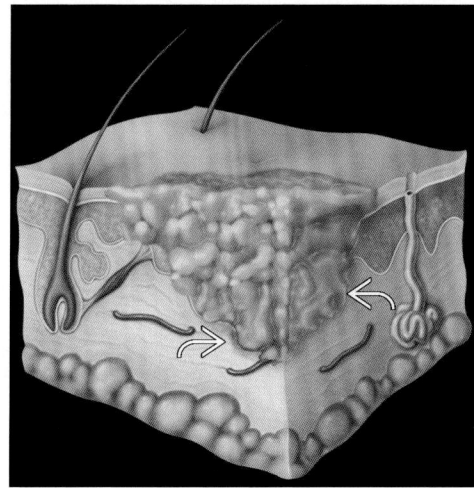

(Left) Squamous carcinoma in situ (Bowen disease) shows growth limited to the epidermis (Tis). *(Right)* Invasive squamous cell carcinoma (SCC) shows superficial invasion into the dermis ➡. This is a tumor ≤ 2 cm in greatest dimension with < 2 high-risk features (T1).

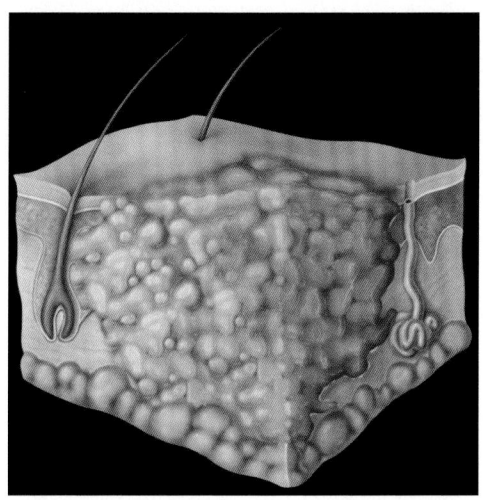
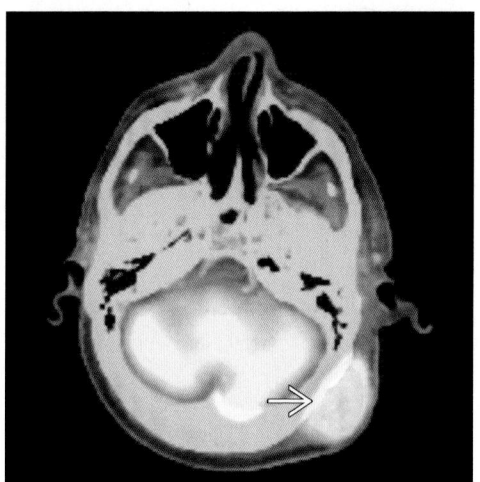

(Left) A tumor > 2 cm in greatest dimension ± 1 additional high-risk feature, or any size with ≥ 2 high-risk features is staged as T2. *(Right)* Axial fused PET/CT scan shows an increase in size and metabolic activity of a left scalp mass ➡; excision confirmed an invasive SCC of greater than 2cm in greatest dimension (T2).

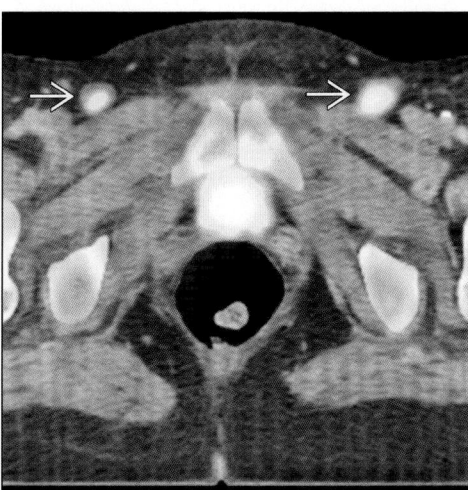
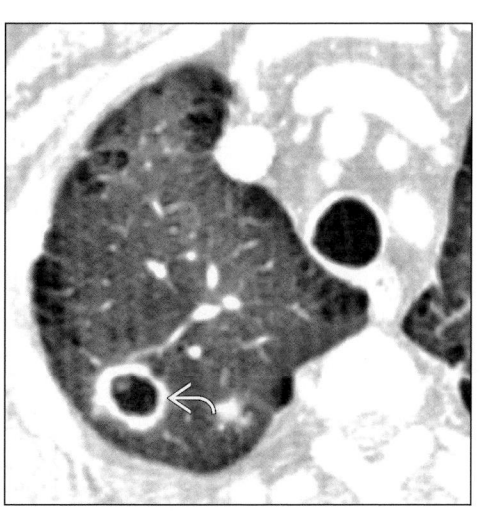

(Left) Axial fused PET/CT shows bilateral intense inguinal FDG activity ➡, compatible with metastatic nodes (N2c). This is a patient with a known primary anal squamous cell carcinoma. *(Right)* Axial HRCT of a patient with metastatic squamous cell carcinoma shows 2 right upper lobe metastases (M1), 1 of which exhibits cavitation ➡. Note the thick nodular cavity wall, typical of malignancy.

Tumors and Tumor-like Conditions of the Hair Follicle

NEVUS SEBACEUS AND FOLLICULAR HAMARTOMAS

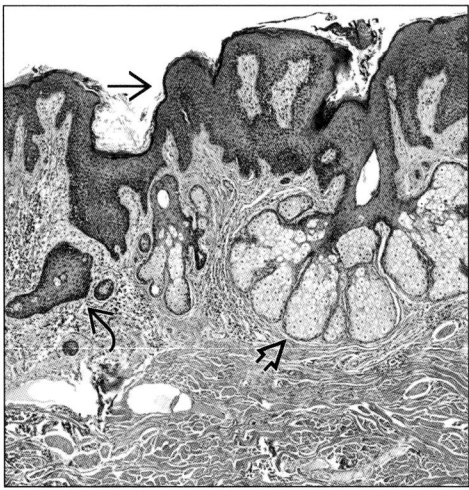

Nevus sebaceus has an acanthotic epidermis, often with a papillomatous surface ➡. The follicles have a disorganized appearance ➡, and there are often associated large sebaceous glands ➡.

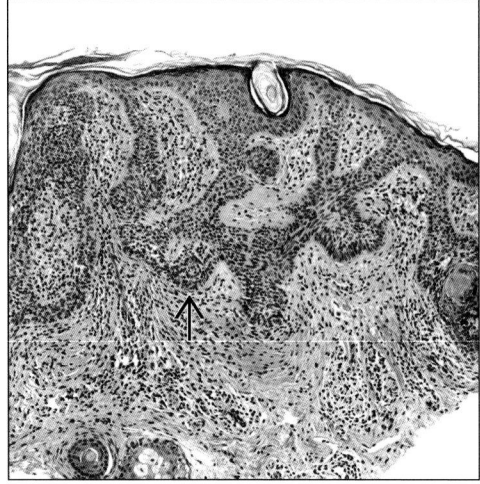

Basaloid follicular hamartoma is characterized by multifocal islands of basaloid epithelium ➡ resembling primitive follicles that are surrounded by a fibroblastic stroma.

TERMINOLOGY

Synonyms
- Nevus sebaceus: Organoid nevus, Jadassohn nevus

Definitions
- Nevus sebaceus
  - Hamartoma with abnormalities of epidermis, follicles, sebaceous glands, and apocrine glands
- Basaloid follicular hamartoma (main type of follicular hamartoma)
  - Hamartoma that consists of proliferation of basaloid epithelium resembling primitive follicles

ETIOLOGY/PATHOGENESIS

Developmental Anomaly
- Nevus sebaceus
  - Deletion of *PTCH* gene may play a role
- Basaloid follicular hamartoma
  - Possible role for Sonic Hedgehog signaling pathway

CLINICAL ISSUES

Presentation
- Nevus sebaceus
  - Usually presents in infancy, often at birth
  - Usually involves scalp
  - Less commonly on face
  - Presents as yellowish flat to warty plaque
  - Often enlarges during puberty
- Follicular hamartomas
  - Solitary
    - Elderly patients
    - Face most common site
    - Flesh-colored papule
    - May clinically mimic basal cell carcinoma (BCC)
  - Localized

- Presents in 3rd-4th decade
- Presents on head as erythematous to hyperpigmented plaque
  - Linear nevoid
    - Large surface area with linear pattern
    - May follow dermatome
    - Pale brown plaque with follicular papules
  - Generalized
    - Infiltrative plaques on face
    - Associated with alopecia totalis and autoimmune disease: Lupus erythematosus and myasthenia gravis
  - Inherited
    - Autosomal dominant
    - Presents in adulthood with numerous flesh-colored or hyperpigmented papules on head and neck, trunk, and anogenital areas
    - May be associated with alopecia &/or cystic fibrosis

Treatment
- Surgical approaches
  - Excision

Prognosis
- Benign
  - Nevus sebaceus
    - Rarely, BCC can arise in association with nevus sebaceus

MICROSCOPIC PATHOLOGY

Histologic Features
- **Nevus sebaceus**
  - Abnormalities of epidermis
    - Frequently acanthotic with papillomatosis
  - Abnormalities of follicles
    - Follicles are disorganized with primitive germ-like areas
    - Reduction in number of mature follicles

Key Facts

Clinical Issues
- Nevus sebaceus
  - Usually presents on scalp in infancy, often at birth
  - Presents as yellowish flat to warty plaque
  - Often enlarges during puberty
- Basaloid follicular hamartoma
  - Usually presents in adults

Microscopic Pathology
- Nevus sebaceus
  - Abnormalities of epidermis, follicles, and sebaceous glands: Follicles are disorganized with primitive germs; sebaceous hyperplasia
  - Abnormalities of apocrine glands
  - Associated tumors arising within nevus sebaceus: Trichoblastoma (most common), syringocystadenoma papilliferum, BCC (rare)
- Basaloid follicular hamartoma
  - Multifocal islands of basaloid epithelium: No retraction artifact; mitotic activity absent to rare

Top Differential Diagnoses
- DDx of nevus sebaceus
  - Epidermal nevus: Lacks abnormalities of follicles and sweat glands
  - Sebaceous adenoma: Lacks epidermal acanthosis and follicular structures
  - Sebaceous hyperplasia: Mature follicles
- DDx of basaloid follicular hamartoma
  - BCC: More cytologic atypia and mitotic activity, retraction spaces, inflammatory stroma

---

- Abnormalities of sebaceous glands
  - Sebaceous glands disorganized and abnormally high in dermis
  - May communicate with epidermal surface
  - May not be associated with a follicle
  - Sebaceous glands may not be prominent in tumors from young children
- Abnormalities of sweat glands
  - Dilated apocrine glands in deep dermis
  - Apocrine glands appear during/after puberty
- Associated other tumors arising within nevus sebaceus
  - Trichoblastoma (most common), syringocystadenoma papilliferum (next most common), and rarely, BCC
- **Basaloid follicular hamartoma**
  - Multiple islands of basaloid epithelium affecting most or all pilosebaceous units
    - Islands arranged as anastomosing cords of basaloid epithelium
    - May have squamoid areas and focal horn cyst formation
    - Epithelium weakly positive for Bcl-2
  - Islands surrounded by loose fibroblastic stroma
    - Stroma positive for CD34
  - Absence of mature follicular elements (i.e., sebaceous glands)
  - No retraction artifact
  - Mitotic activity absent to rare
  - No atypia

DIFFERENTIAL DIAGNOSIS

DDx of Nevus Sebaceus
- Epidermal nevus
  - Lacks abnormalities of follicles and sebaceous glands
- Sebaceous adenoma
  - Usually has more prominent germinative layer of immature sebocytes
  - Lacks epidermal acanthosis and papillomatosis and primitive follicular structures

- Sebaceous hyperplasia
  - Enlarged sebaceous glands associated with mature hair follicles

DDx of Basaloid Follicular Hamartoma
- BCC
  - Retraction artifact (often) and more cytologic atypia and mitotic activity with inflammatory mucinous stroma
  - Immunohistochemistry
    - Epithelium strongly positive for Bcl-2; stroma negative for CD34
  - Trichoepithelioma
    - Areas of basaloid follicular hamartoma can be indistinguishable from trichoepithelioma
    - Not multifocal like basaloid follicular hamartoma

DIAGNOSTIC CHECKLIST

Pathologic Interpretation Pearls
- Nevus sebaceus: Abnormalities of epidermis, follicles, and sweat glands; features dependent on patient age
- Basaloid follicular hamartoma: Lacks retraction spaces, lacks mitotic activity, stroma fibroblastic

SELECTED REFERENCES

1. Mills O et al: Basaloid follicular hamartoma. Arch Pathol Lab Med. 134(8):1215-9, 2010
2. Walsh N et al: Basaloid follicular hamartoma: solitary and multiple types. J Am Acad Dermatol. 29(1):125-9, 1993
3. Alessi E et al: Nevus sebaceus is associated with unusual neoplasms. An atlas. Am J Dermatopathol. 10(2):116-27, 1988
4. Alessi E et al: Nevus sebaceus. A clinicopathologic study of its evolution. Am J Dermatopathol. 8(1):27-31, 1986
5. Jones EW et al: Naevus sebaceus. A report of 140 cases with special regard to the development of secondary malignant tumours. Br J Dermatol. 82(2):99-117, 1970

Nevus Sebaceus

(Left) This nevus sebaceus demonstrates a papillomatous acanthotic epidermis ➡ overlying disorganized follicles with prominent sebaceous glands ⊳. (Right) In this nevus sebaceus from a young child, there are disorganized, immature follicles ➡, but sebaceous glands are not prominent.

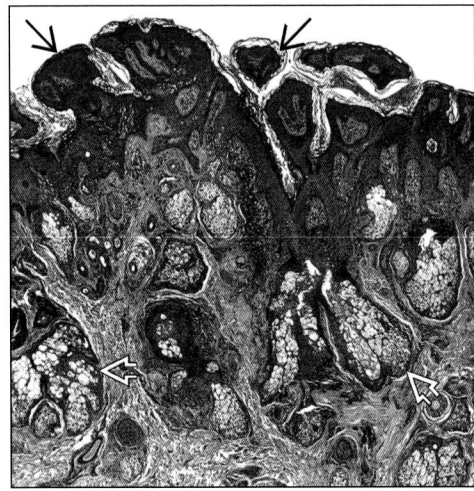
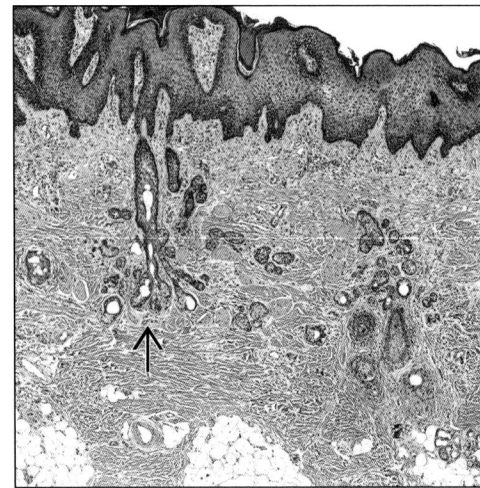

(Left) In this nevus sebaceus, there is prominent papillomatosis ➡, but the enlarged sebaceous glands ⊳ lack conspicuous attachment to the epidermis. (Right) This abnormal sebaceous gland directly communicates with the epidermal surface ➡ and lacks a well-formed associated follicle.

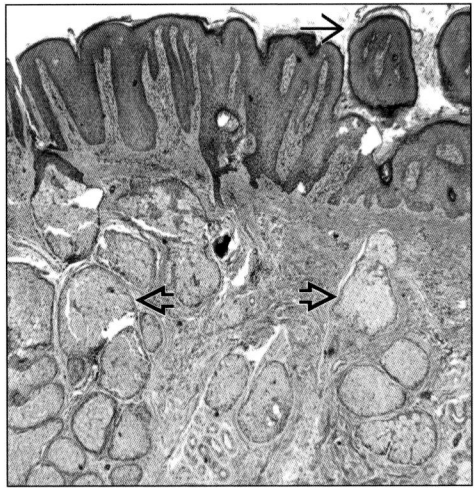
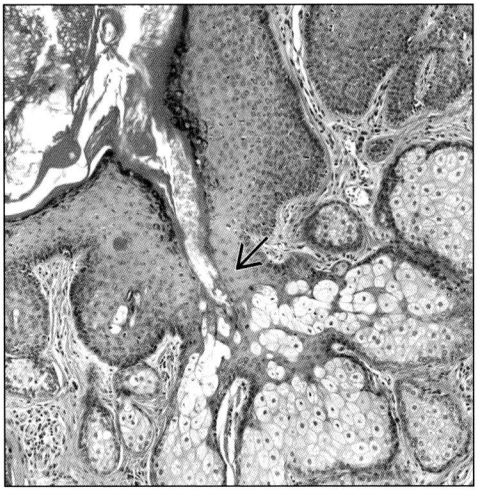

(Left) In addition to the primitive follicles and enlarged sebaceous glands ⊳, there are ectatic apocrine glands ➡. (Right) High-power image of apocrine glands from nevus sebaceus demonstrates characteristic decapitation secretion ➡.

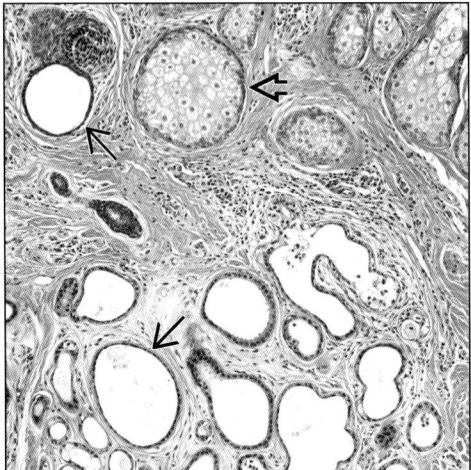
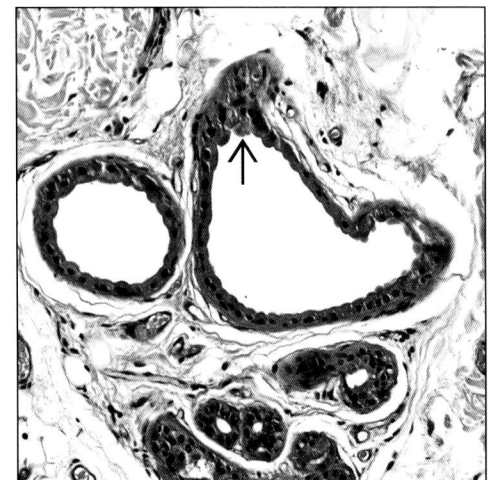

NEVUS SEBACEUS AND FOLLICULAR HAMARTOMAS

Nevus Sebaceus and Basaloid Follicular Hamartoma

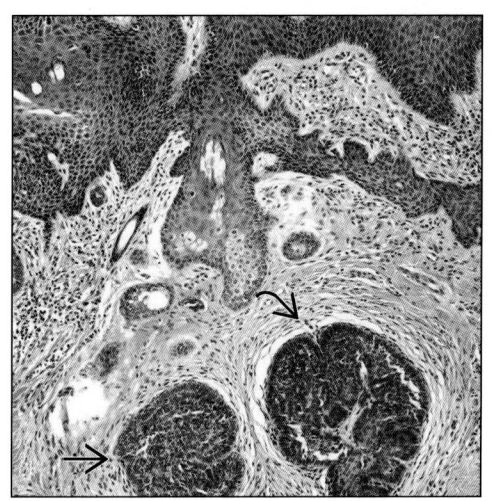

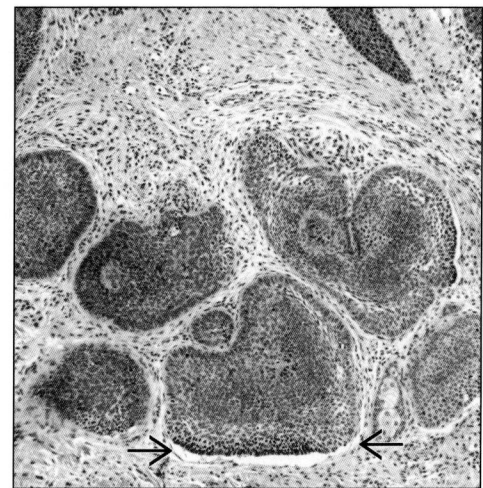

(Left) Beneath the nevus sebaceus in the upper part of the image, there is a focal area of trichoblastoma ➡ formation. Although there are retraction spaces, there is a thin rim of stroma still surrounding the nodule of trichoblastoma ➡. *(Right)* In this nevus sebaceus, there is an associated nodular basal cell carcinoma with prominent peripheral palisading and tumor-stroma retraction spaces ➡. High magnification showed multiple mitoses and apoptotic bodies.

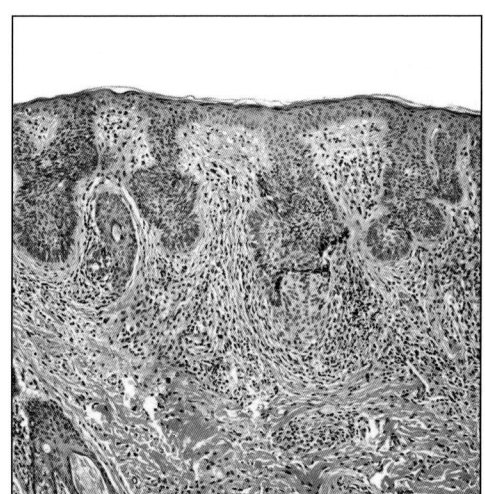

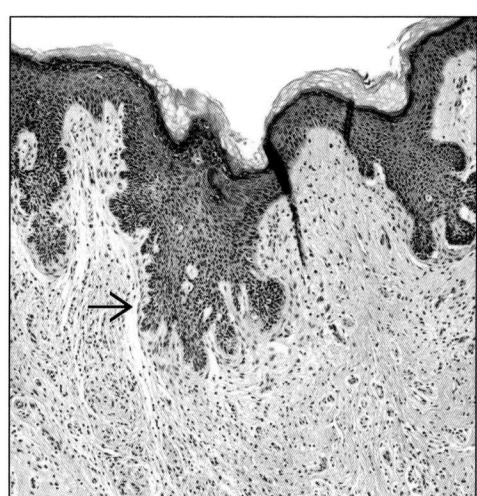

(Left) Basaloid follicular hamartoma is characterized by a proliferation of basaloid epithelium recapitulating primitive follicles. *(Right)* In this early basaloid follicular hamartoma, the primitive follicular structures ➡ are not well developed.

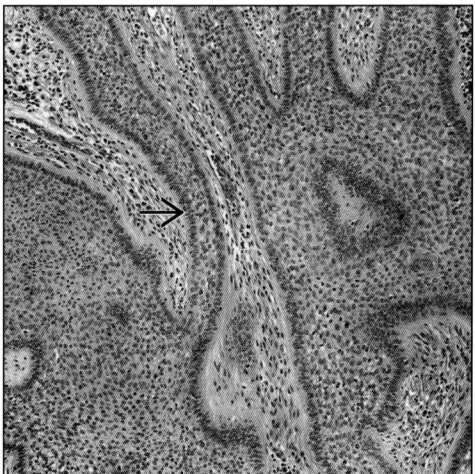

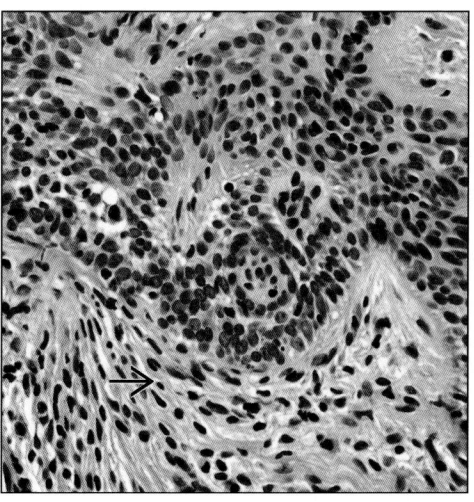

(Left) This higher power image from a basaloid follicular hamartoma demonstrates anastomosing cords of basaloid epithelium with peripheral palisading ➡. However, there is a conspicuous absence of atypia and mitotic activity. *(Right)* The epithelium of basaloid follicular hamartoma is surrounded by a fibroblastic stroma ➡. Note the absence of retraction spaces between the stroma and epithelium and the lack of mitotic activity.

TRICHOFOLLICULOMA

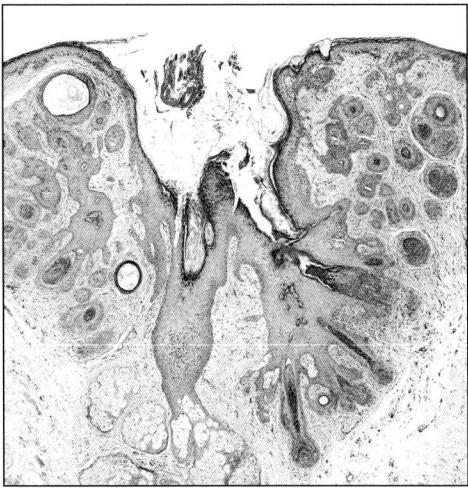

Trichofolliculoma is an invaginated cystic tumor lined by keratinizing squamous epithelium that communicates with the overlying epidermis. The central cystic space is usually filled with keratinous debris.

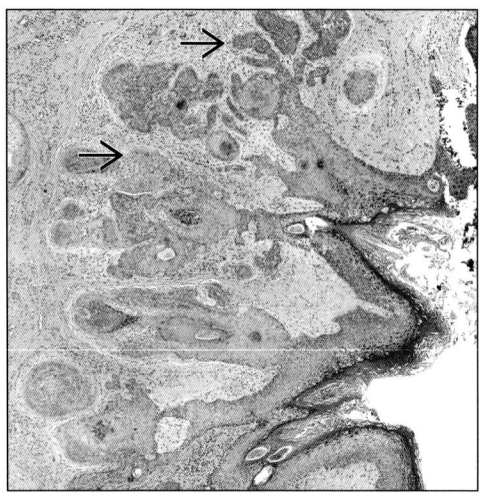

Radiating around the central cystic space are numerous primitive follicles that connect with the central cystic space. The follicles often have secondary branching ➡.

TERMINOLOGY

Definitions
- Hamartoma with prominent follicular differentiation

ETIOLOGY/PATHOGENESIS

Unknown
- Majority of cases are sporadic
- Likely represents a hamartoma rather than a true tumor

CLINICAL ISSUES

Epidemiology
- Incidence
  - Rare
- Age
  - Usually presents in adults
- Gender
  - Males and females equally affected

Presentation
- Dome-shaped papule with central dilated pore
  - Tuft of white hairs often emerges from the opening
- Face is most common location, especially around the nose
- Occasionally on scalp or neck or other locations

Treatment
- Surgical approaches
  - Simple excision is curative, but usually not necessary due to benign behavior

Prognosis
- Benign; no malignant potential

MICROSCOPIC PATHOLOGY

Histologic Features
- Cystic tumor that communicates to overlying epidermis
  - Cystic space filled with keratinous debris and hair shafts
  - Lined by squamous epithelium with thin granular layer
- Numerous small, primitive follicles radiate around periphery of the tumor and communicate with central cystic space
  - Follicles demonstrate some architectural complexity with secondary budding
  - May have small attached sebaceous glands
- Follicles surrounded by perifollicular stromal sheath
- Focal granulomatous inflammation secondary to rupture may be present

Cytologic Features
- Bland adnexal cells with small nuclei and basophilic- to eosinophilic-staining cytoplasm

Sebaceous Trichofolliculoma (Variant)
- Same architecture as conventional trichofolliculoma
  - Connects to epidermis
  - Central cystic space lined by squamous epithelium
  - Follicles radiating around periphery
- Primary difference is presence of numerous mature sebaceous lobules

DIFFERENTIAL DIAGNOSIS

Folliculosebaceous Cystic Hamartoma
- May also represent a later stage/regressing variant of trichofolliculoma, but is typically a dermal-based tumor
- Prominent sebaceous glands

TRICHOFOLLICULOMA

Key Facts

Clinical Issues
- Usually presents on the face
- Benign hamartomatous lesion
- Face is most common location

Microscopic Pathology
- Cystic tumor that communicates to overlying epidermis
- Cystic space filled with keratinous debris and hair shafts

- Numerous small, primitive follicles radiate around periphery of the tumor and communicate with central cystic space
- May have small attached sebaceous glands
- Follicles surrounded by perifollicular stromal sheath

Top Differential Diagnoses
- Folliculosebaceous cystic hamartoma
- Dilated pore of Winer
- Trichoepithelioma

- Much more than rare sebaceous glands seen in conventional trichofolliculoma
- Prominent collagenous stroma surrounding tumor lobules with fibroblastic proliferation
- Tumor lobules often have distinct clefts

Dilated Pore of Winer
- Cystically dilated follicle that communicates with overlying epidermis
- Irregular epithelial budding radiating out from cyst
- Lacks numerous primitive true follicular structures of trichofolliculoma

Trichoepithelioma
- Lobules and nests of basaloid epithelium with peripheral palisading
- Small keratocysts present; often associated with rupture and granulomatous inflammation
- Lacks central cystic space lined by keratinizing squamous epithelium

Dermoid Cyst
- Usually presents in infants and young children, often on the midline face
- Cystic lesion lined by bland squamous epithelium with follicular structures and sebaceous glands
  - Up to 25% of cases also have eccrine &/or apocrine glands
- Lacks communication with overlying epidermis

DIAGNOSTIC CHECKLIST

Pathologic Interpretation Pearls
- Cystic follicular structure lined by mature squamous epithelium
- Communication with surface epidermis
- Numerous primitive follicular structures radiating from cystic lumen

SELECTED REFERENCES

1. Wu YH: Folliculosebaceous cystic hamartoma or trichofolliculoma? A spectrum of hamartomatous changes inducted by perifollicular stroma in the follicular epithelium. J Cutan Pathol. 35(9):843-8, 2008
2. Kurokawa I et al: Trichofolliculoma: case report with immunohistochemical study of cytokeratins. Br J Dermatol. 148(3):597-8, 2003
3. Peterdy GA et al: Trichofolliculoma of the vulva associated with vulvar intraepithelial neoplasia: report of three cases and review of the literature. Int J Gynecol Pathol. 21(3):224-30, 2002
4. Kimura T et al: Folliculosebaceous cystic hamartoma. A distinctive malformation of the skin. Am J Dermatopathol. 13(3):213-20, 1991
5. Steffen C et al: Trichofolliculoma of the upper eyelid. Cutis. 30(3):343-5, 1982
6. Plewig G: Sebaceous trichofolliculoma. J Cutan Pathol. 7(6):394-403, 1980
7. Macmillan A et al: Trichofolliculoma. Br J Dermatol. 85(5):491-2, 1971
8. Gore HC Jr: Trichofolliculoma. Arch Dermatol. 89:385-6, 1964

IMAGE GALLERY

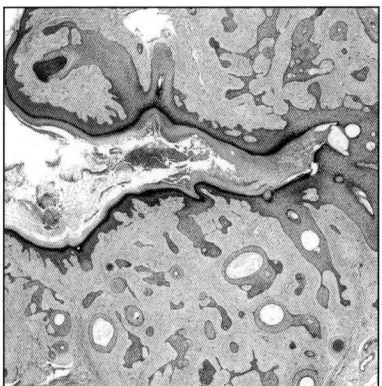 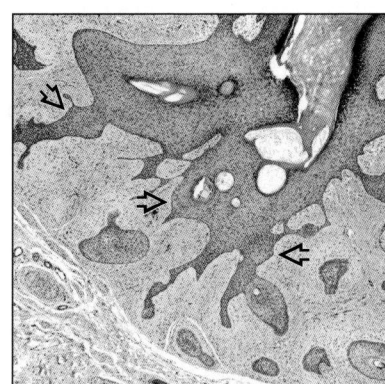 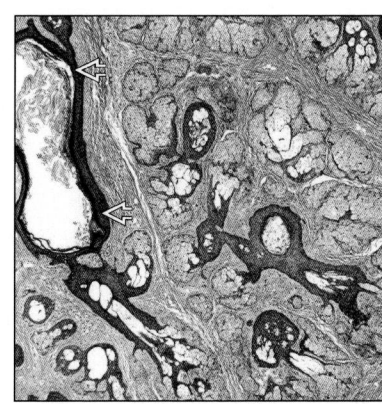

(Left) Trichofolliculoma is characterized by an invaginated cystic lesion lined by mature, keratinizing squamous epithelium that communicates with the overlying epidermis. (Center) Small, branching follicles ➦ radiate out from, and communicate with, the central cystic space. (Right) Folliculosebaceous cystic hamartoma is likely a mature variant of trichofolliculoma with very prominent sebaceous glands surrounding follicular structures. Note the dilated follicular lumen at the edge ➮.

TRICHOADENOMA

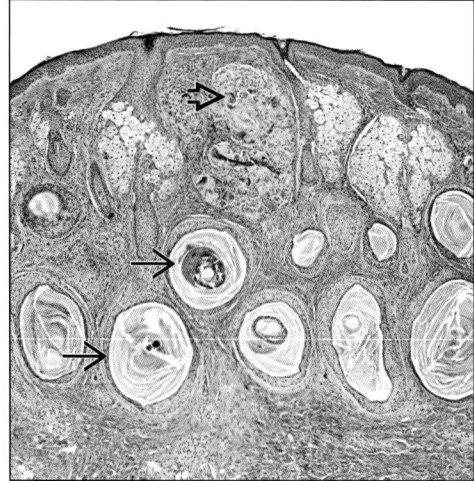

Low-magnification view of a trichoadenoma shows a dome-shaped lesion based in the dermis. Note numerous mature horn cysts ➡. There is focal granulomatous inflammation surrounding the keratin debris ⟴.

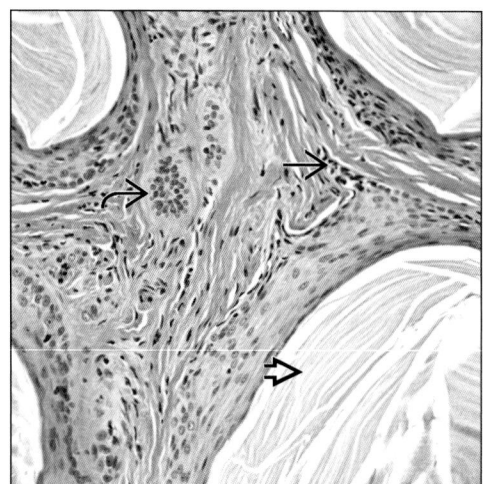

High magnification view of a trichoadenoma highlights the sclerotic stroma and the loose keratin debris within the horn cysts ⟴. There are basaloid buds off of horn cysts ➡ and in the stroma ⬈.

TERMINOLOGY

Synonyms
- Trichoadenoma of Nikolowski

Definitions
- Benign follicular tumor
- Predominance of mature folliculocystic structures in dermis
- Epithelial tubules and cords interspersed
- Sclerotic stroma

CLINICAL ISSUES

Site
- Often on the face
- Sometimes on buttock or other sites

Presentation
- Solitary papule

Prognosis
- Benign lesions
- No malignant potential

MICROSCOPIC PATHOLOGY

Histologic Features
- Multiple cystic structures in dermis, showing epidermal-type keratinization and the following features
  - Granular layer
  - Flaky central keratin (may see keratin granulomas)
  - Cytokeratin-10 positivity, suggesting infundibular differentiation
- Occasional cysts may show tricholemmal differentiation with
  - Absent granular layer
  - Abrupt keratinization into dense, pink keratin

- Interspersed among cystic structures are basaloid tubules and cords
- Cytokeratin-20 positive cells are present in cysts and tubules/cords
- Sclerotic stroma
- Well-circumscribed
- Not infiltrative

Cytologic Features
- No cytologic atypia

DIFFERENTIAL DIAGNOSIS

Trichoepithelioma
- Basaloid islands, some in grape-like arrangements, with occasional horn cysts
- Papillary mesenchymal bodies present
- Sclerotic stroma

Trichoepithelioma, Desmoplastic
- Occasional horn cysts (but not predominating as in trichoadenoma)
- Basaloid tubules and cords
- Often show calcifications and occasional foreign body giant cell reaction surrounding ruptured cysts
- Sclerotic stroma
- Limited to upper dermis
- Not infiltrative

Trichofolliculoma
- Central, dominant hair follicle
- Secondary, smaller hair follicles radiating away from central follicle

Panfolliculoma
- May show numerous dermal cystic structures with loose keratin and granular layer
- Also has other islands that show differentiation toward other parts of hair follicle
  - Bulbar

TRICHOADENOMA

Key Facts

Terminology
- Benign follicular tumor

Clinical Issues
- Often on the face
- Solitary papule

Microscopic Pathology
- Multiple mature cystic structures in dermis, showing epidermal-type keratinization

- Cysts have granular layer and flaky central keratin
- Interspersed among cystic structures are basaloid tubules and cords
- Sclerotic stroma
- Well circumscribed and not infiltrative

Top Differential Diagnoses
- Trichoepithelioma
- Trichofolliculoma
- Microcystic adnexal carcinoma

- May show matrical cells
  - Isthmic
    - May show clear cells or trichohyalin granules

Microcystic Adnexal Carcinoma (MAC)
- Sometimes has scattered cystic structures in superficial dermis
- Cords, tubules, and small clusters of cells with ductal differentiation infiltrate deep into dermis/subcutaneous tissues
- Cytologic atypia may be minimal
- Often perineural invasion present

Syringoma
- Lacks component of cysts with loose keratin
- Small cords and "tadpoles" of cells, with ductal differentiation (eosinophilic cuticle)
- Clear cells often present in islands

Nevus Comedonicus
- Multiple cysts in upper dermis with granular cell layer and loose keratin
- Lacks basaloid tubules/cords
- Clinically typically a linear lesion, often present from birth

Favre-Racouchot Disease
- Multiple milia (small cysts with granular layer and loose keratin) in background of solar elastosis
- Lacks basaloid tubules/cords
- Clinically numerous open comedones on heavily sun-damaged skin, especially malar area

Seborrheic Keratosis, Reticulated Type
- Plate-like proliferation off base of epidermis (not based in dermis)
- Reticulated strands, may be basaloid, but all interconnecting
- Horn cysts may be interspersed within reticulated strands

DIAGNOSTIC CHECKLIST

Pathologic Interpretation Pearls
- Predominance of cystic islands with rare basaloid tubules/cords in sclerotic stroma
- Well circumscribed and limited to dermis

SELECTED REFERENCES

1. Shimanovich I et al: Trichoadenoma of Nikolowski is a distinct neoplasm within the spectrum of follicular tumors. J Am Acad Dermatol. 62(2):277-83, 2010
2. Kurokawa I et al: Trichoadenoma: cytokeratin expression suggesting differentiation towards the follicular infundibulum and follicular bulge regions. Br J Dermatol. 153(5):1084-6, 2005
3. Yamaguchi J et al: A case of trichoadenoma arising in the buttock. J Dermatol. 19(8):503-6, 1992
4. Goldstein DJ et al: Microcystic adnexal carcinoma: a distinct clinicopathologic entity. Cancer. 50(3):566-72, 1982

IMAGE GALLERY

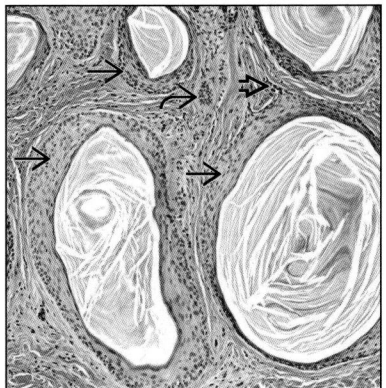 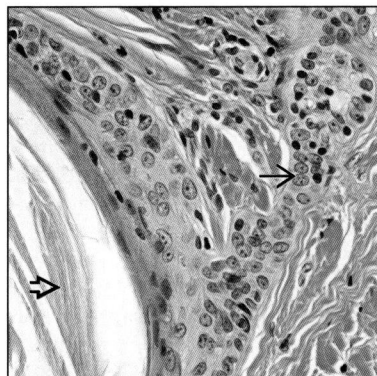 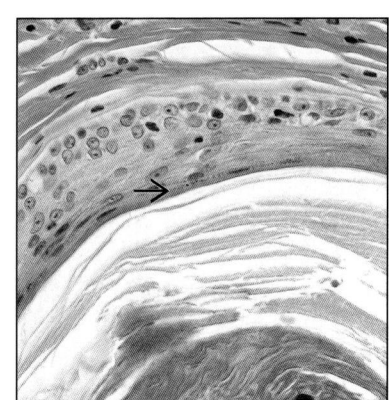

(Left) In this medium-power view of a trichoadenoma, there are numerous horn cysts ➡ embedded in a sclerotic stroma. There are basaloid buds in the stroma ➡ and emanating off the borders of the horn cysts ➡. *(Center)* In this high-power view of a trichoadenoma, flaky keratin ➡ is seen within a horn cyst, at the border of which there is a basaloid tubule ➡. The stroma is sclerotic. *(Right)* The horn cysts have abundant loose, flaky keratin debris and a granular layer ➡.

TRICHOEPITHELIOMA

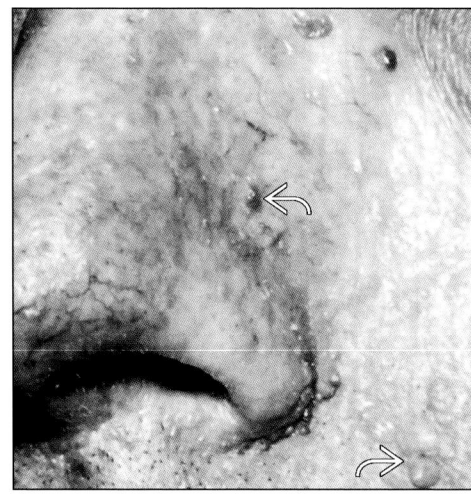

Multiple trichoepitheliomas (epithelioma adenoides cysticum) are scattered over the central face and nasolabial area presenting as flesh-colored, 1-4 mm papules. (Courtesy B. Hall, MD.)

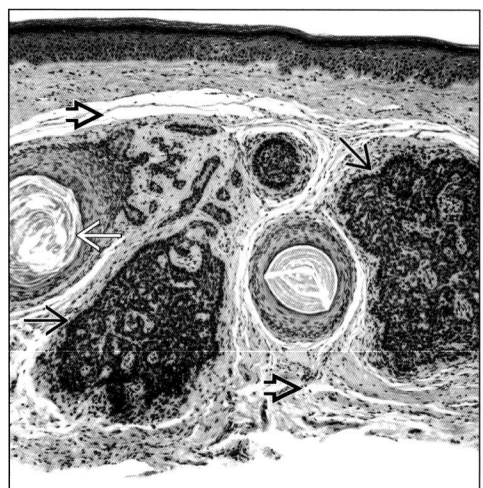

Scanning magnification of trichoepithelioma shows islands of basaloid cells with prominent horn cysts and clefts between collagen bundles, rather than tumor-stromal retraction artifact as in BCC.

TERMINOLOGY

Abbreviations
- Trichoepithelioma (TE)

Synonyms
- Superficial trichoblastoma

Definitions
- Basaloid follicular proliferation with mixture of primitive follicular structures and mature infundibulocystic keratinizing areas

ETIOLOGY/PATHOGENESIS

Genetic
- Some cases are inherited as part of a genetic syndrome, including Brooke-Spiegler syndrome, familial trichoepitheliomas, or Rombo syndrome
- Autosomal dominant inheritance
- Present as multiple lesions, often with cylindromas and spiradenomas (Brooke-Spiegler syndrome)

CLINICAL ISSUES

Epidemiology
- Incidence
  - Relatively common tumors
- Age
  - Usually present in adults
    - Genetic forms present in adolescence
- Gender
  - Slight male predominance

Site
- Most commonly occur on the face, but may involve other head and neck sites

Presentation
- Solitary or multiple papules
  - Sporadic cases are typically solitary
  - Inherited cases are usually multiple
  - Usually small (< 5 mm), especially the sporadic cases
  - Large or "giant" trichoepitheliomas are better referred to as trichoblastoma

Treatment
- Options, risks, complications
  - Surgical excision is curative
  - Should be recommended in partial biopsies in order to exclude basal cell carcinoma (BCC)

Prognosis
- Excellent; very low recurrence or malignant potential
- However, rare cases have been associated with (or progressed to) BCC

MACROSCOPIC FEATURES

General Features
- Small, superficial dermal-based lesion

MICROSCOPIC PATHOLOGY

Histologic Features
- Multiple lobules and nests of basaloid cells, typically confined to superficial dermis
- Areas of infundibulocystic differentiation (keratinizing cysts) are present
- Tumor is associated with fibrotic and cellular stroma
  - Stromal-stromal cleft artifact may be present, but no tumor-stromal clefts (as are seen in BCC)
  - Mucin is almost always absent in the stroma
- Papillary mesenchymal bodies
  - Characterized by invagination of fibroblastic stroma into basaloid nest
  - Represent abortive attempts at follicular induction

TRICHOEPITHELIOMA

Key Facts

Terminology

- Trichoepithelioma (TE)
- Synonyms: Superficial trichoblastoma
- Basaloid follicular proliferation with a mixture of primitive follicular structures and mature infundibulocystic keratinizing areas

Etiology/Pathogenesis

- Some cases are inherited as part of a genetic syndrome, including Brooke-Spiegler syndrome, familial trichoepitheliomas, or Rombo syndrome

Clinical Issues

- Most commonly occur on the face, but may involve other head and neck sites
- Excellent, very low recurrence or malignant potential

Microscopic Pathology

- Multiple lobules and nests of basaloid cells, typically confined to superficial dermis
- Scattered areas of infundibulocystic differentiation (keratinizing cysts) are typically present
- Tumor is associated with fibrotic and cellular stroma
- Papillary mesenchymal bodies classically are present
- Calcifications and granulomatous inflammation (reaction to ruptured cysts) are often present

Top Differential Diagnoses

- Basal cell carcinoma (BCC)
- Microcystic adnexal carcinoma (MAC)
- Trichoblastoma
- Trichoadenoma
- Sebaceoma

- Calcifications and granulomatous inflammation (reaction to ruptured cysts) are often present

Cytologic Features

- Basaloid cells with small, hyperchromatic nuclei, inconspicuous nucleoli, and eosinophilic cytoplasm

Subtype

- **Desmoplastic trichoepithelioma (dTE)**
  o More common in women
  o Firm or indurated papule/nodule
  o Shows superficial folliculocystic structures and calcifications
  o Deeper infiltrative-appearing cords and small islands in densely fibrotic stroma

DIFFERENTIAL DIAGNOSIS

Basal Cell Carcinoma (BCC)

- BCC usually shows multiple attachments to overlying epidermis (focal or absent in TE)
- BCC also shows the following features, which are not typically seen in TE
  o Prominent peripheral palisading
  o Mucinous stroma
  o Tumor-stroma retraction artifact (stromal-stromal retraction seen in TE)
  o Numerous mitotic and apoptotic figures
- Immunohistochemistry may be useful in some cases (especially small, partial biopsies)
  o Bcl-2, p53, and Ki-67 all elevated in BCC (low to negative in TE)
  o CK20 highlights Merkel cells in TE (absent in BCC)

Microcystic Adnexal Carcinoma (MAC)

- Can be difficult, if not impossible, to distinguish from dTE in superficial biopsies
- Need to see the base of lesion to evaluate for perineural invasion and deep invasion

Trichoblastoma (TB)

- Larger, more nodular tumor that often extends into deep dermis/superficial subcutis
- Histologic features of TB overlap with those of TE, which some dermatopathologists regard as "superficial trichoblastoma"
  o However, infundibulocystic differentiation more common in TE
  o Calcifications and granulomatous inflammation also more typical of TE

Trichoadenoma

- Mature follicular lesion composed of numerous infundibular cysts
- Squamoid cells line cysts, rather than basaloid cells of TE

Sebaceoma

- Superficial dermal adnexal neoplasm composed of lobules and nests of predominantly basaloid cells
- Scattered mature sebaceous cells with multivacuolated cytoplasm

SELECTED REFERENCES

1. Kazakov DV et al: Brooke-Spiegler syndrome: report of a case with a novel mutation in the CYLD gene and different types of somatic mutations in benign and malignant tumors. J Cutan Pathol. 37(8):886-90, 2010
2. Mamelak AJ et al: Desmoplastic trichoepithelioma. J Am Acad Dermatol. 62(1):102-6, 2010
3. Lum CA et al: Proliferative characterization of basal-cell carcinoma and trichoepithelioma in small biopsy specimens. J Cutan Pathol. 31(8):550-4, 2004
4. Shaffelburg M et al: Treatment of multiple trichoepithelioma with electrosurgery. Dermatol Surg. 24(10):1154-6, 1998
5. Sawchuk WS et al: CO2 laser treatment of trichoepithelioma with focused and defocused beam. J Dermatol Surg Oncol. 10(11):905-7, 1984
6. Andrews GC: Trichoepithelioma. Arch Dermatol Syph. 55(5):726, 1947

TRICHOEPITHELIOMA

Microscopic Features

(Left) Scanning magnification of trichoepithelioma shows irregular islands of bland basaloid cells ⧉ with prominent horn cysts ➡ and clefts between collagen bundles ⧉, rather than the tumor-stromal retraction artifact seen in BCC. (Right) Trichoepithelioma often shows variably sized nests of more primitive basaloid cells ➡ alternating with areas of more mature-appearing squamous cells ➡ lining follicular cysts. (Courtesy A. Bowen, MD.)

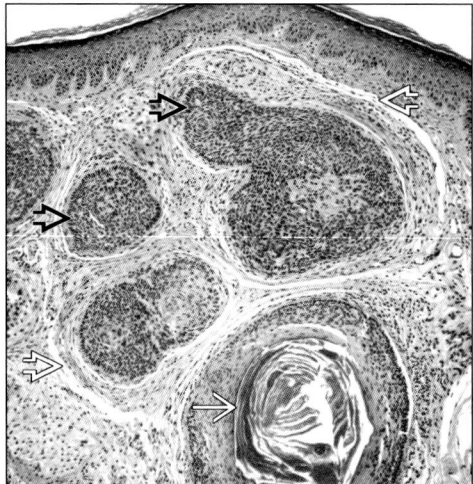
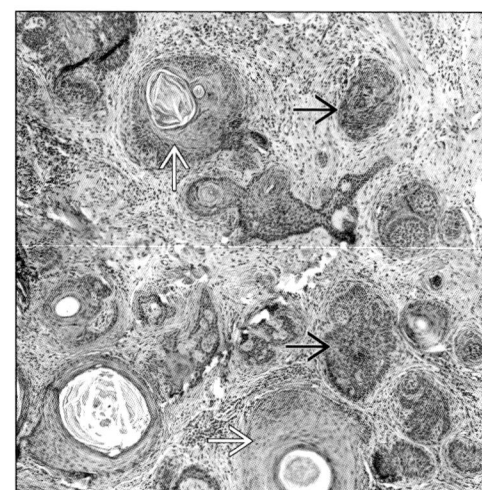

(Left) Higher magnification of trichoepithelioma shows basaloid nests with areas of peripheral palisading ➡. Focal intratumoral collections of mucin ➡ can be seen in some cases, but no stromal mucin is present. (Right) High-power view of a trichoepithelioma demonstrates characteristic papillary mesenchymal bodies ⧉ invaginating into the basaloid cells. (Courtesy A. Bowen, MD.)

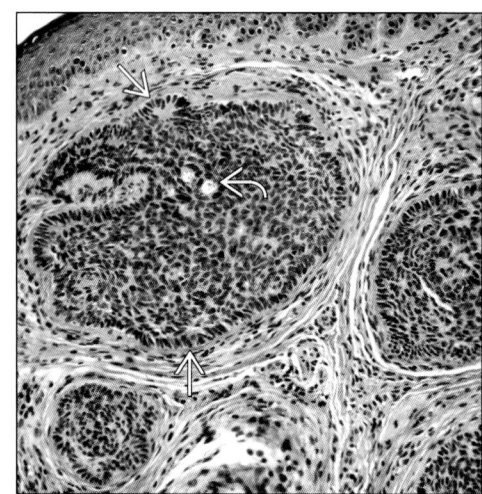
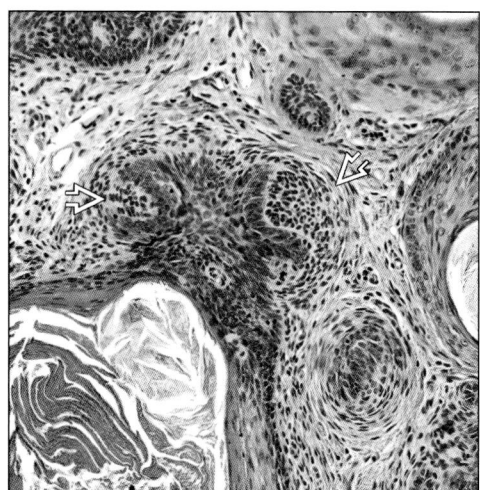

(Left) Desmoplastic trichoepithelioma can mimic a morpheaform BCC in some cases. However, the prominent horn cysts ➡ and calcifications ⧉ are more consistent with a trichoepithelioma. (Courtesy G. Fraga, MD.) (Right) A deeper area of dTE shows multiple infiltrative-appearing cords of cells ➡ mimicking a desmoplastic BCC. (Courtesy G. Fraga, MD.)

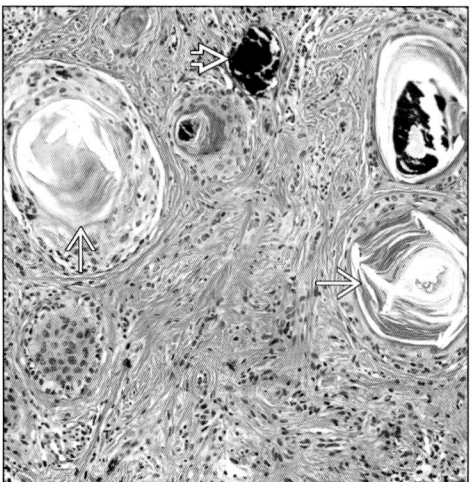
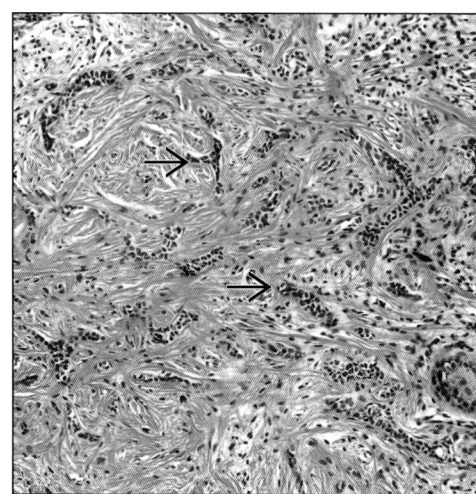

TRICHOEPITHELIOMA

Differential Diagnosis and Immunohistochemistry

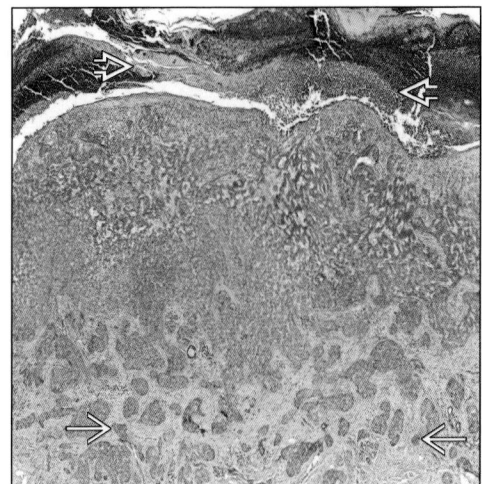
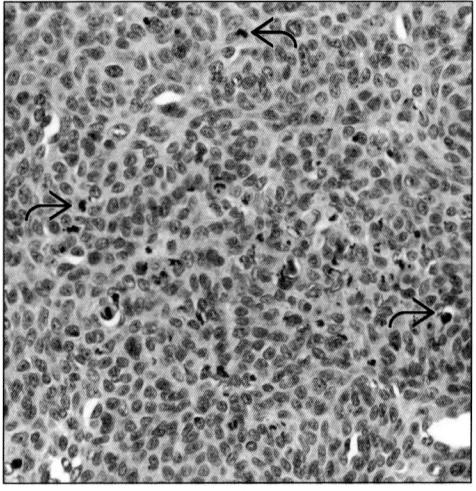

(Left) BCC is the main differential diagnostic consideration and should be excluded. BCC typically shows multiple attachments to the epidermis, and there is often overlying ulceration with thick serum crusting ➤ and impetiginization. This BCC is composed of superficial nodular areas progressing to deeper, more infiltrative micronodular areas ➤. (Right) High magnification of a BCC shows numerous mitotic and apoptotic figures ➚, which should be absent or rare in TE.

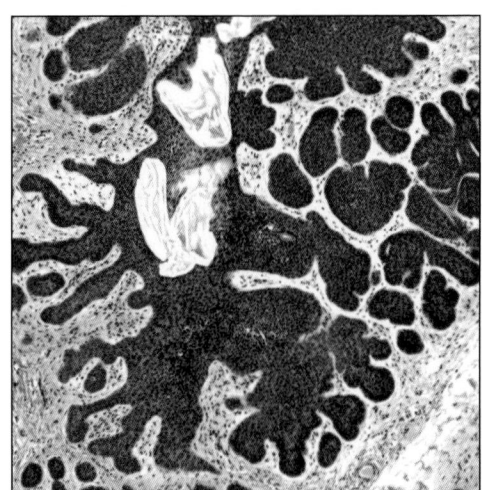
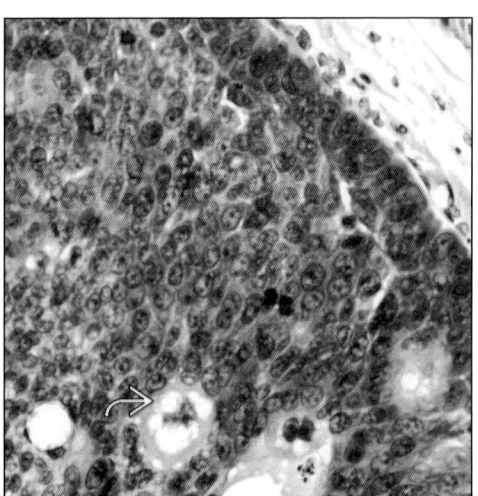

(Left) Trichoblastoma (TB) is closely related to TE, and some pathologists consider TE a "superficial trichoblastoma." While the histologic findings are similar, TB is typically a larger and deeper nodular lesion, which may even extend into the subcutaneous tissue. (Right) Sebaceoma is a basaloid sebaceous neoplasm that may occasionally enter the differential diagnosis. However, on high-power examination, multivacuolated sebocytes ➤ with nuclear indentations should be present.

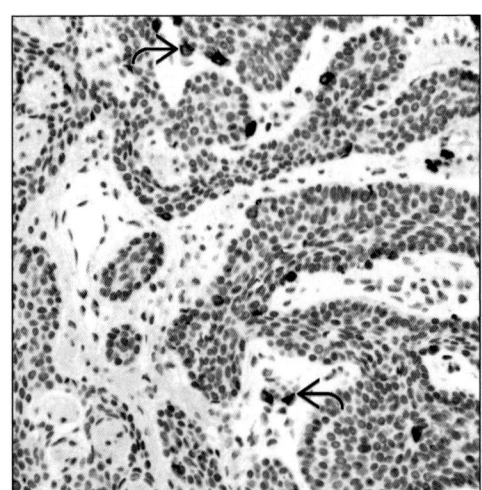
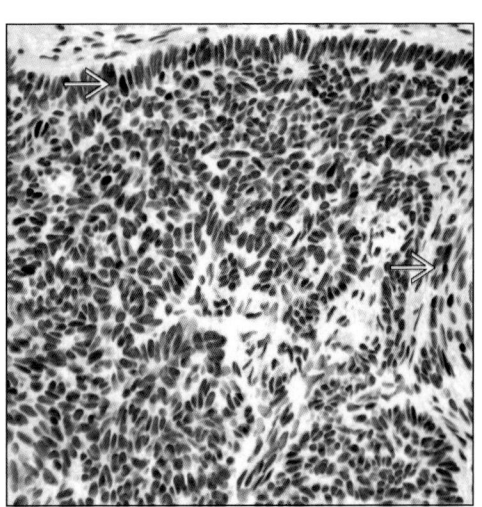

(Left) CK20 strongly highlights significant numbers of Merkel cells in a trichoepithelioma ➚. These cells are almost always present in benign follicular neoplasms and absent in BCC. (Right) Other markers that are useful in the differential diagnosis of TE vs. BCC include p53 and Ki-67, both of which are typically low in TE and significantly elevated in BCC. This is an example of p53 staining in a TE and shows only a few scattered positive nuclei ➤, mostly at the periphery of the tumor.

TRICHOBLASTOMA

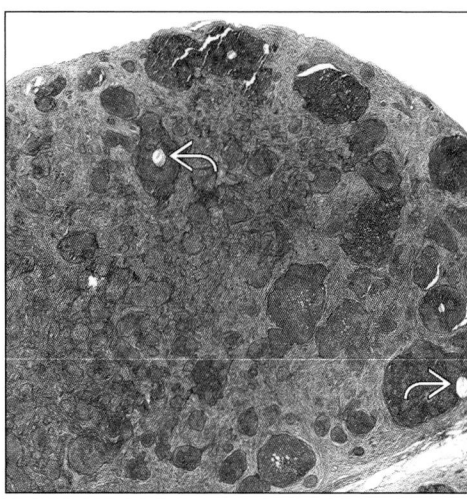

Scanning magnification of a trichoblastoma shows a nodular basaloid proliferation associated with a fibrotic stroma. Note the presence of scattered folliculocystic structures ➥.

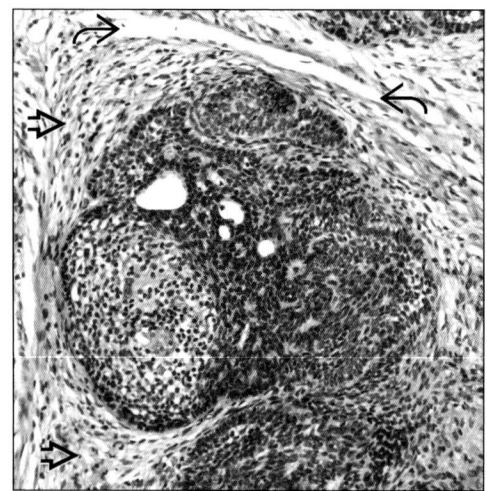

High magnification of a trichoblastoma shows a lobular basaloid proliferation associated with a cellular, fibrotic stroma ⊟. *Note the prominent stromal-stromal retraction artifact* ⊟.

TERMINOLOGY

Abbreviations
- Trichoblastoma (TB)

Synonyms
- Giant trichoepithelioma (TE)
- Trichogerminoma
- Rippled pattern trichomatricoma
- Trichoblastic fibroma
- Cutaneous lymphadenoma

Definitions
- Benign dermal-based adnexal tumor showing primitive follicular differentiation

CLINICAL ISSUES

Epidemiology
- Incidence
  - Uncommon tumors
- Age
  - Usually occur in adults

Site
- Head and neck area, especially the scalp

Presentation
- Dermal nodule/mass lesion
  - Usually single but may rarely be multiple
- Usually asymptomatic

Treatment
- Surgical approaches
  - Complete excision is curative
  - Should be recommended in cases of partial biopsy in order to exclude basal cell carcinoma (BCC)

Prognosis
- Excellent in most cases

- Rare recurrences and association with, or progression to, malignancy (BCC)

MACROSCOPIC FEATURES

General Features
- Nodular lesion involving the deep dermis and subcutis

Size
- Large, typically > 1 cm in diameter

MICROSCOPIC PATHOLOGY

Histologic Features
- Large, basaloid-appearing deep dermal-based nodule
  - Usually symmetric and shows well-circumscribed borders
  - Composed of irregular lobules and nests of basaloid cells
  - No epidermal connections
  - May extend into superficial subcutis
- Associated fibrotic stroma with increased numbers of fibroblasts
  - Stromal amyloid may be present
  - Calcifications and granulomatous inflammation occasionally seen but less common than in TE
- Papillary mesenchymal bodies classically present, similar to TE
  - Invagination of fibroblastic stroma into primitive follicular structures
  - Represents abortive follicular induction

Subtypes
- **Trichogerminoma**
  - Tightly packed lobules of primitive basaloid cells with minimal stroma
- **Rippled pattern trichomatricoma**
  - Palisading ribbons of basaloid cells; may resemble Verocay bodies

TRICHOBLASTOMA

Key Facts

Terminology
- Trichoblastoma (TB)
- Synonym: Giant trichoepithelioma
- Benign adnexal tumor showing primitive follicular differentiation

Clinical Issues
- Head and neck area, especially the scalp
- Rare recurrences and association with, or progression to, malignancy (BCC)

Macroscopic Features
- Nodular lesion involving the deep dermis and subcutis
- Large, typically > 1 cm in diameter

Microscopic Pathology
- Large, basaloid-appearing deep dermal-based nodule

- Composed of irregular lobules and nests of basaloid cells
- No epidermal connections
- Associated fibrotic stroma with increased numbers of fibroblasts
- Papillary mesenchymal bodies classically present, similar to TE
- Subtypes include trichogerminoma, rippled pattern trichomatricoma, trichoblastic fibroma, and cutaneous lymphadenoma

Top Differential Diagnoses
- Basal cell carcinoma (BCC)
- Trichoepithelioma (TE)
- Sebaceoma
- Cylindroma
- Spiradenoma

- **Trichoblastic fibroma**
  - Less epithelial structures, more prominent stroma, which may appear desmoplastic
- **Cutaneous lymphadenoma**
  - Rare variant with a prominent lymphocytic infiltrate and clear cell features

DIFFERENTIAL DIAGNOSIS

Basal Cell Carcinoma
- BCC usually shows multiple attachments to the overlying epidermis (focal or absent in TB)
- BCC also shows the following features (which are not seen in TB)
  - Prominent peripheral palisading
  - Mucinous stroma
  - Tumor-stromal retraction artifact (stromal-stromal retraction seen in TB)
  - Numerous mitotic and apoptotic figures
- Immunohistochemistry may be useful in some cases (particularly small, partial biopsies)
  - Bcl-2, p53, and Ki-67 all elevated in BCC (should be low in TB)
  - CK20 highlights Merkel cells in TB (absent in BCC)

Trichoepithelioma
- Small, papular lesion clinically
- Overlapping histologic features, but TE is smaller, more superficial than TB
- Usually shows more prominent folliculocysts, calcifications, and granulomatous inflammation

Sebaceoma
- More superficial, epidermal- or follicular-based adnexal neoplasm
- Composed of lobules and nests of predominantly basaloid cells with minor population of clear cells
- May show rippled pattern with nuclear palisading, similar to rippled pattern trichomatricoma
- Scattered mature sebaceous cells with multivacuolated cytoplasm

Cylindroma
- Dermal-based neoplasm composed of basaloid cells with ductal differentiation
- Irregular, "jigsaw puzzle" pattern of variably shaped lobules and nests
  - Surrounded by hyalinized basement membrane, and nests contain hyalinized globules
- Focal ductal lumina present (may be highlighted by EMA &/or CEA)

Spiradenoma
- Dermal-based nodular basaloid neoplasm with ductal differentiation
- Biphasic cellular population of smaller, darker cells and larger, pale cells
- Numerous lymphocytes typically sprinkled throughout the tumor
- Ductal structures usually numerous

SELECTED REFERENCES

1. Córdoba A et al: Bcl-2 and CD10 expression in the differential diagnosis of trichoblastoma, basal cell carcinoma, and basal cell carcinoma with follicular differentiation. Int J Dermatol. 48(7):713-7, 2009
2. Rofagha R et al: Trichoblastic carcinoma: a report of two cases of a deeply infiltrative trichoblastic neoplasm. Dermatol Surg. 27(7):663-6, 2001
3. Graham BS et al: Rippled-pattern sebaceous trichoblastoma. J Cutan Pathol. 27(9):455-9, 2000
4. Jaqueti G et al: Trichoblastoma is the most common neoplasm developed in nevus sebaceus of Jadassohn: a clinicopathologic study of a series of 155 cases. Am J Dermatopathol. 22(2):108-18, 2000
5. Diaz-Cascajo C et al: Cutaneous lymphadenoma. A peculiar variant of nodular trichoblastoma. Am J Dermatopathol. 18(2):186-91, 1996
6. Requena L et al: Trichogenic trichoblastoma. An unusual neoplasm of hair germ. Am J Dermatopathol. 12(2):175-81, 1990
7. Hashimoto K et al: Rippled-pattern trichomatricoma. Histological, immunohistochemical and ultrastructural studies of an immature hair matrix tumor. J Cutan Pathol. 16(1):19-30, 1989

Microscopic Features

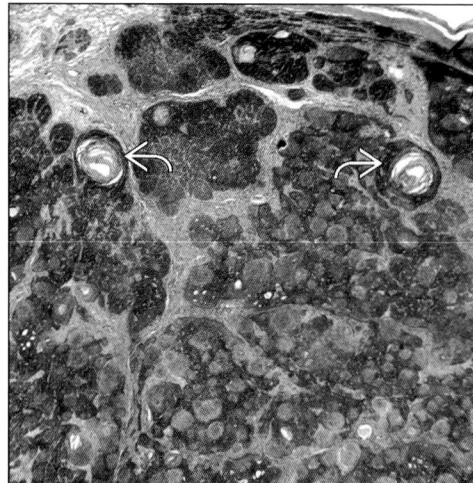
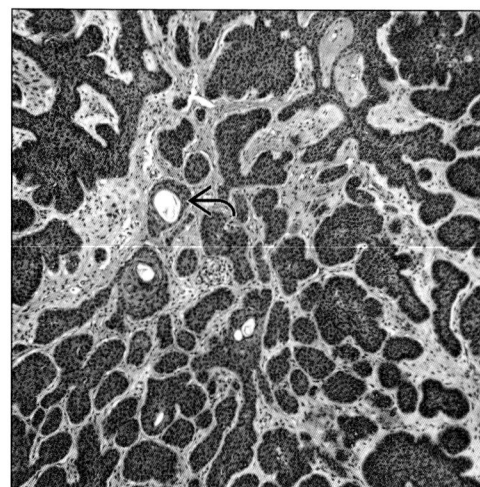

(Left) Scanning magnification of a trichoblastoma shows a multinodular basaloid proliferation associated with a fibrotic stroma. Note the scattered folliculocystic structures ➡. *(Right)* This example of trichoblastoma shows a proliferation of smaller nests and cords of basaloid cells associated with a fibrotic stroma with scattered lymphocytes. Note the small mature folliculocystic structures ➔.

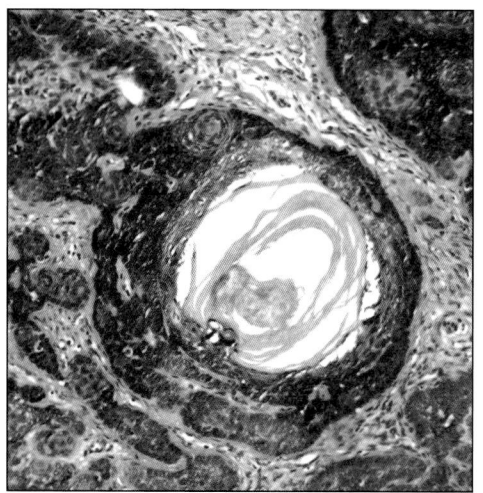
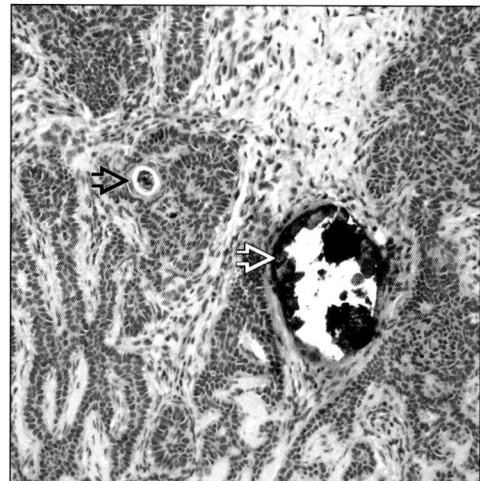

(Left) Well-differentiated keratinizing folliculocystic structures are often present in trichoblastoma, although they are less common than in trichoepithelioma. *(Right)* Areas of calcification ➡ are often seen in trichoblastoma and represent calcified folliculocystic structures. Focal pigmented material is also present ➔.

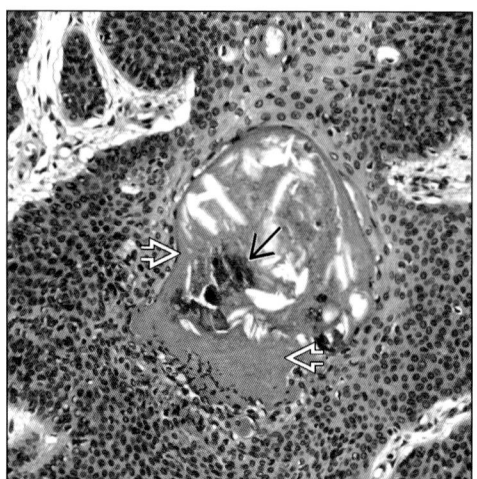
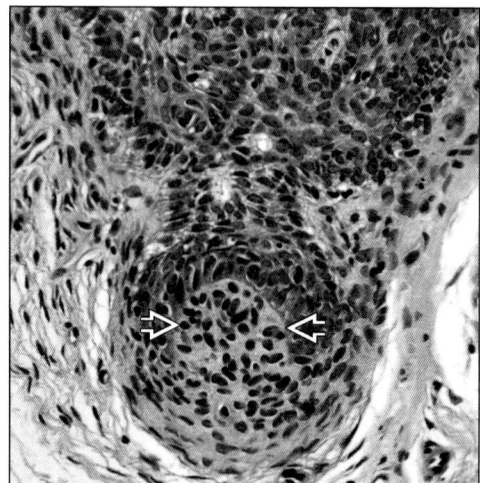

(Left) High magnification of a folliculocystic structure shows pilar-type keratinization with a central lumen containing dense keratin ➡ and a few calcifications ➔. *(Right)* High magnification of a papillary mesenchymal body shows invagination of cellular fibroblastic stroma ➡ into a peripheral bulb-like area of the tumor.

TRICHOBLASTOMA

Variant Microscopic Features

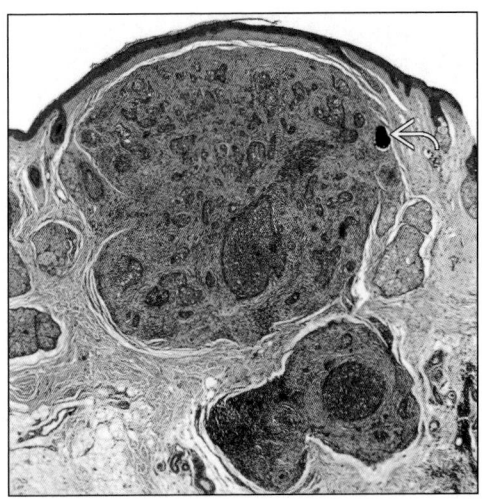

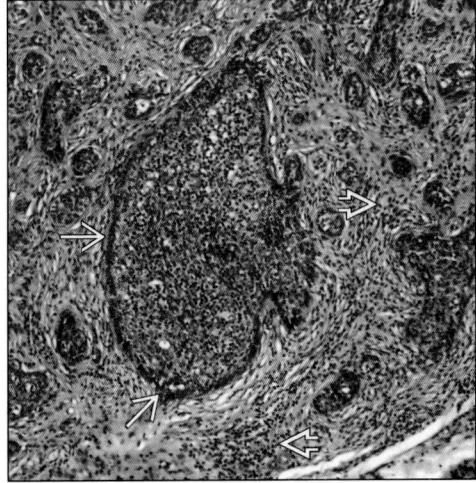

(Left) Low magnification of a cutaneous lymphadenoma shows a multinodular tumor in the dermis associated with a prominent fibrotic stroma and focal microcalcifications ➡. (Right) Intermediate-power view of cutaneous lymphadenoma shows small lobules and nests of basaloid cells with peripheral palisading ➡. Note the associated cellular fibrotic stroma with chronic inflammation ➡.

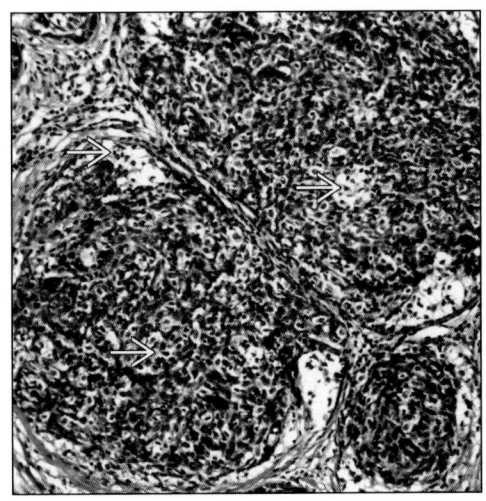

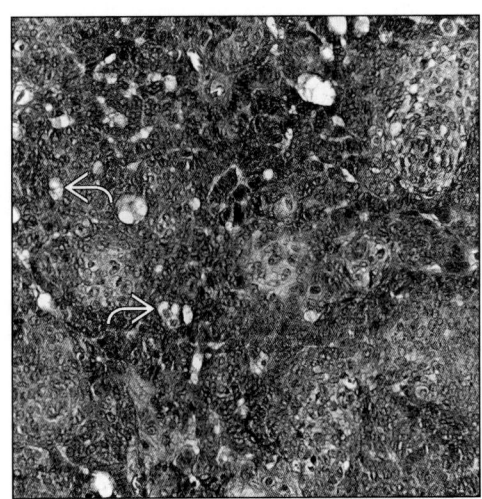

(Left) High magnification of another example of cutaneous lymphadenoma shows lobular collections of basaloid cells infiltrated by numerous small lymphocytes ➡. (Right) Trichoblastoma can show sebaceous differentiation in some cases. Scattered clear cells with multivacuolated cytoplasm are identified ➡.

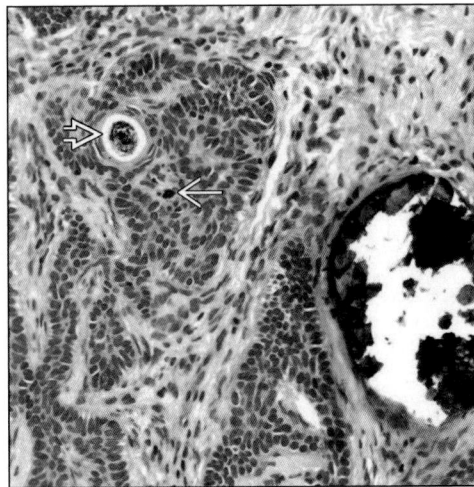

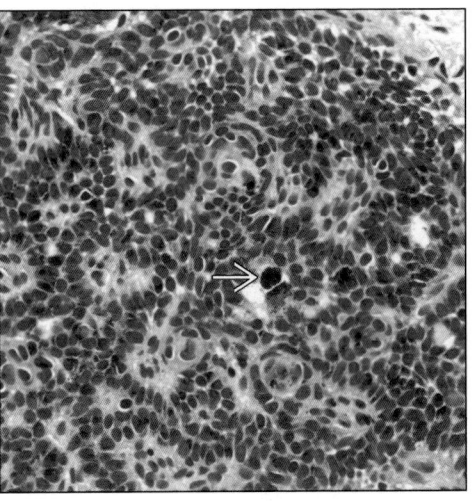

(Left) Pigmented trichoblastoma is a relatively common type that shows occasional cystic spaces ➡ and a few cells ➡ with melanin pigmentation. Note the adjacent microcalcification. (Right) High magnification of another pigmented trichoblastoma shows a bland, cellular proliferation of monomorphous basaloid cells with numerous melanin pigment deposits, including several large globules ➡.

Nonmelanocytic Tumors of the Skin: Tumors and Tumor-like Conditions of the Hair Follicle

Differential Diagnosis

(Left) Trichoepithelioma *(TE) is a closely related tumor and may even be considered a superficial variant of TB. However, TE is usually smaller and often shows more prominent well-differentiated folliculocystic structures* ⊡ *than does TB.* ***(Right)*** *This is another trichoepithelioma showing a mixture of superficial basaloid nests and mature infundibulocystic structures containing abundant keratin debris* ⊡. *These cystic structures often rupture and elicit a granulomatous infiltrate* ⊡.

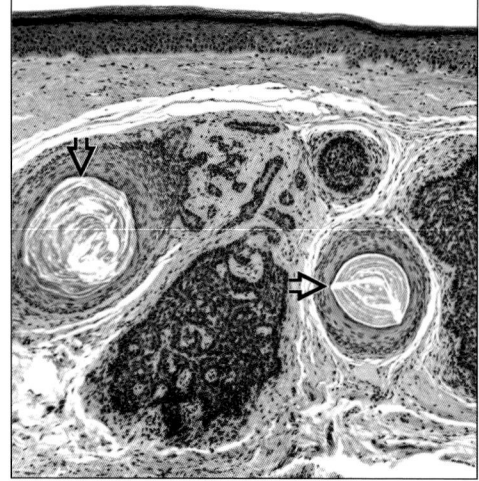
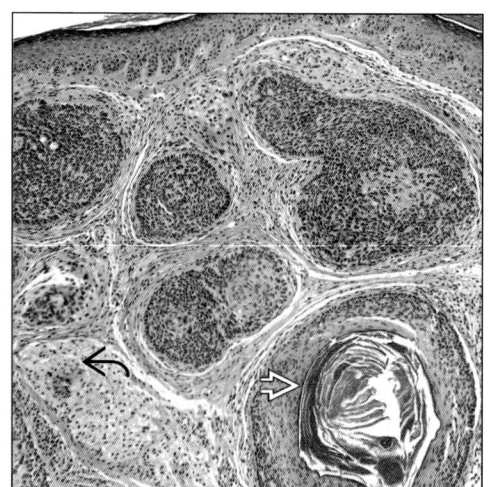

(Left) Sebaceoma is a basaloid adnexal neoplasm that can present as a nodular, dermal-based tumor, mimicking TB. However, on high-power examination, multiple well-differentiated sebocytes with multivacuolated clear cytoplasm ⊡ are identified. ***(Right)*** *Cylindroma is another nodular, dermal-based basaloid neoplasm. However, cylindroma is composed of irregularly shaped nests of cells surrounded by hyalinized basement membrane* ⊡, *and ductal structures are easily identified* ⊡.

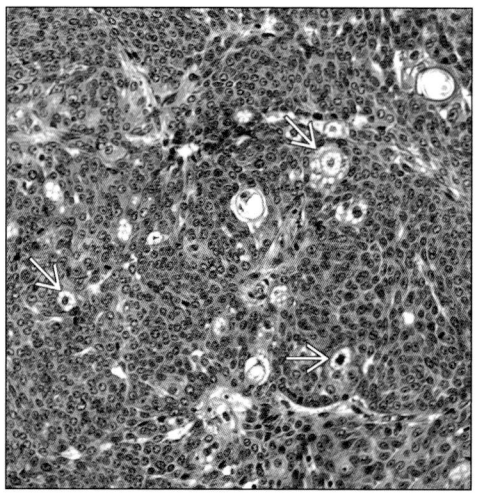
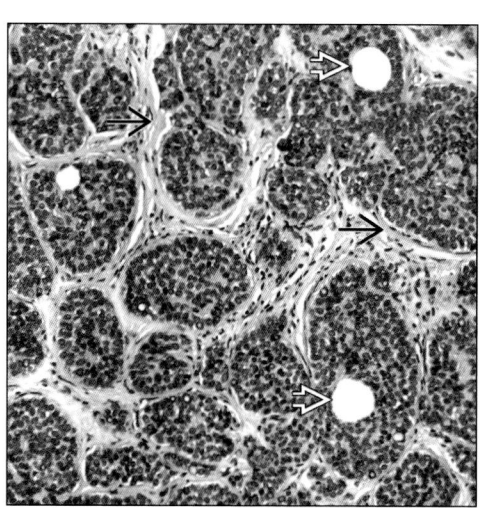

(Left) Hidradenoma typically presents as a nodular, dermal-based adnexal tumor, which may simulate TB at low power. However, hidradenoma typically shows clear cells and areas of ductal differentiation but lacks any evidence of follicular differentiation. The stroma also shows more of a hyalinized appearance ⊡. ***(Right)*** *Higher magnification of a hidradenoma shows areas with prominent clear cells* ⊡, *which would be unusual in TB. Focal ductal lumina can also be identified* ⊡.

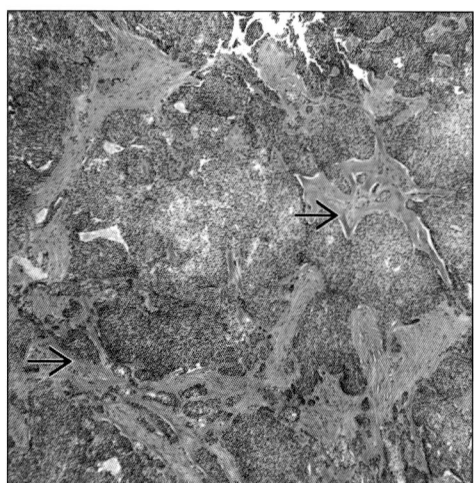
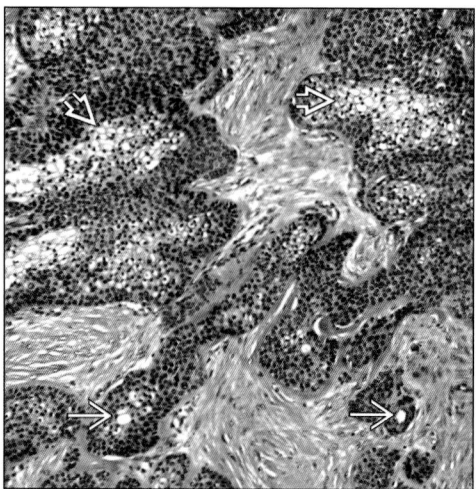

Differential Diagnosis and Ancillary Techniques

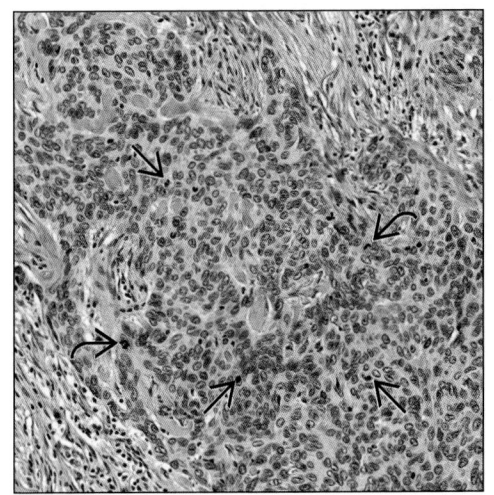

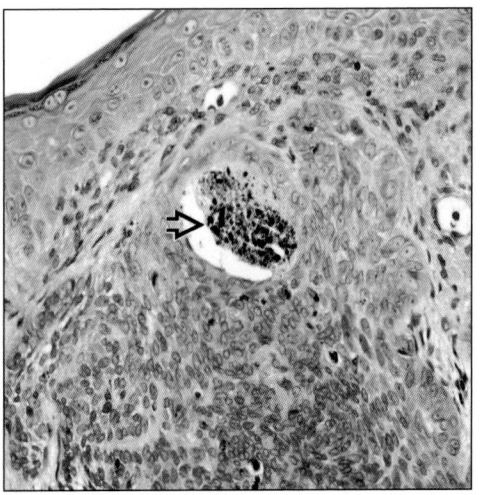

(Left) Basal cell carcinoma (BCC) may occasionally be difficult to distinguish from TB, especially if classic features, such as mucinous stroma and tumor-stromal retraction artifact, are absent. However, on high-power examination, mitotic ⊐ and apoptotic ⊐ figures are abundant, as opposed to rare in TB. (Right) High magnification of a pigmented BCC shows a nodular collection of enlarged, atypical basaloid cells closely approaching the epidermis. Note the pigmented material in a cystic space ⊳.

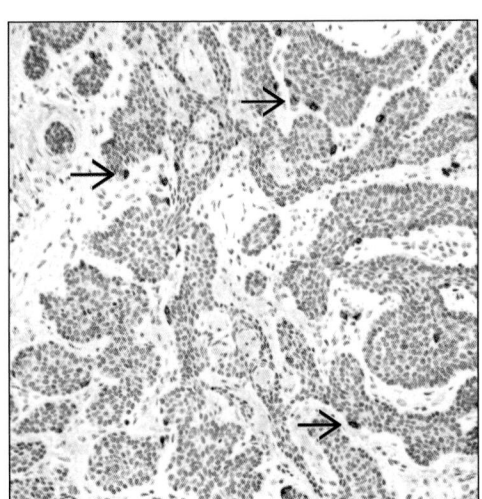

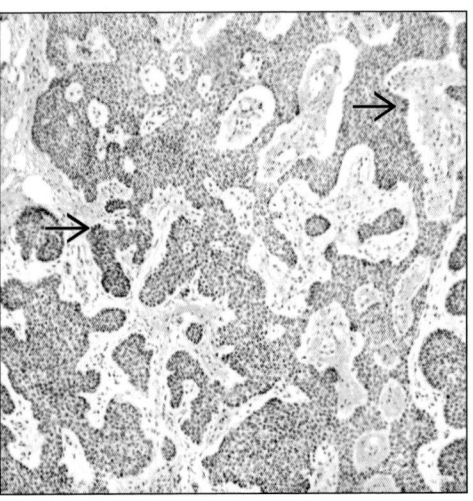

(Left) Cytokeratin 20 (CK20) highlights Merkel cells ⊐ in TB, which are often quite numerous. Merkel cells are almost always completely absent in BCC, making this a useful marker in their distinction. (Right) p53 protein immunohistochemistry usually shows only focal staining (< 10% of cells staining) in trichoblastoma, usually within scattered peripheral cells ⊐. BCC usually shows much greater labeling with this marker (> 30-40% of cells).

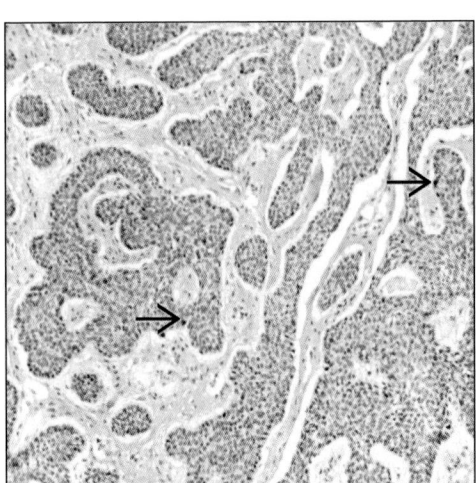

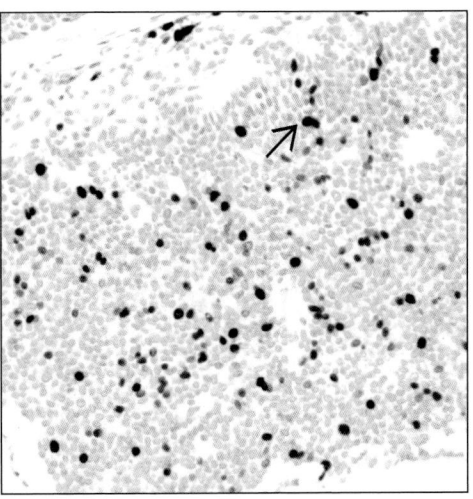

(Left) Ki-67 highlights a low nuclear proliferative rate in TB (typically < 5% of cells staining ⊐), as opposed to a much higher rate of staining in most cases of BCC (> 15-20% of cells). (Right) Ki-67 stains many more nuclei in this example of BCC, including scattered enlarged, irregular-appearing nuclei ⊐.

PANFOLLICULOMA

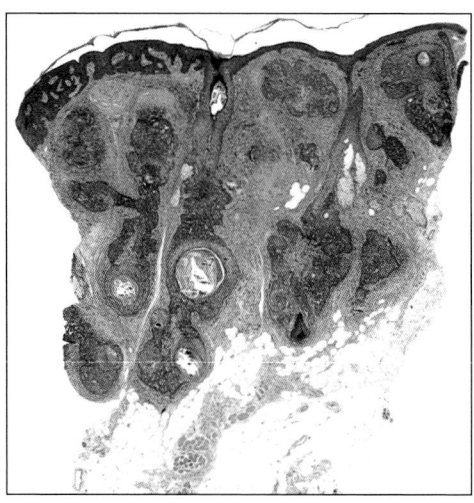

Panfolliculoma is characterized by a dermal-based adnexal proliferation recapitulating all levels of the hair follicle.

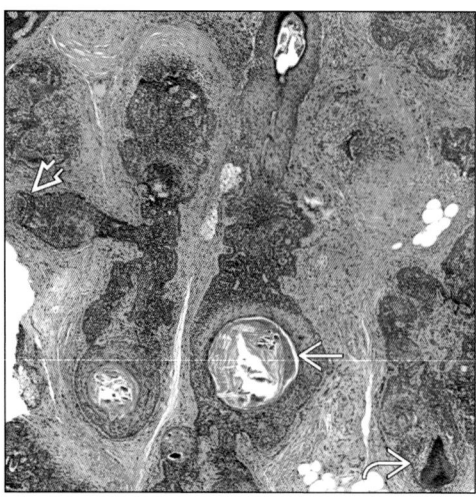

Panfolliculoma shows cystic areas lined by stratified squamous epithelium with a granular layer ➡, basaloid epithelium with papillary mesenchymal bodies ➡, and inner and outer root sheath ➡.

TERMINOLOGY

Definitions
- Benign tumor with differentiation that represents all segments of the hair follicle

CLINICAL ISSUES

Epidemiology
- Incidence
  - Very rare
- Age
  - Adults
- Gender
  - Men and women affected equally

Site
- Usually involving face or scalp but may occur elsewhere

Presentation
- Mass lesion
  - Slowly growing

Treatment
- Surgical approaches
  - Simple excision is usually curative

Prognosis
- Benign
  - Rare recurrence
  - No malignant transformation

MACROSCOPIC FEATURES

General Features
- Nodular, dermal-based tumor

Size
- Generally < 3 cm

MICROSCOPIC PATHOLOGY

Histologic Features
- Well-circumscribed, noninfiltrative, typically dermal-based lesion
- Closely set solid and partially cystic structures with follicular differentiation
- Follicular differentiation represents all components of follicular epithelium
  - Cystic areas resembling infundibulum
    - With stratified squamous epithelium showing a granular layer and basket-weave stratum corneum
  - Areas resembling internal and external root sheath, with the latter showing clear cell features
  - Areas with matrical epithelium
  - Areas resembling hair bulb with papillary mesenchymal body formation
- Rare intraepidermal cases also described

Cytologic Features
- Small, bland, basaloid, squamoid, and clear cells lacking nuclear irregularities and enlarged nucleoli
- Mitotic figures absent

DIFFERENTIAL DIAGNOSIS

Trichoblastoma
- May have similar low-power appearance
- More primitive follicular neoplasm that typically lacks more advanced follicular differentiation
  - Fewer keratin-filled cysts
  - No external root sheath differentiation with clear cell features
  - Lacks matrical epithelium

Trichoepithelioma
- May have similar low-power appearance, but is usually smaller and more superficial
- Lacks more advanced follicular differentiation

PANFOLLICULOMA

Key Facts

Microscopic Pathology

- Closely set solid and partially cystic structures with follicular differentiation
- Well circumscribed
- Follicular differentiation represents all areas of follicular unit
  - Cystic areas resembling infundibulum with stratified squamous epithelium with granular layer and basket-weave stratum corneum
  - Areas resembling internal and external root sheath
  - Areas with matrical epithelium
  - Areas resembling hair bulb

Top Differential Diagnoses

- Trichoblastoma
  - Lacks more advanced follicular differentiation
- Trichoepithelioma
  - Also lacks more advanced follicular differentiation

- No external root sheath differentiation with clear cell features
- Lacks matrical epithelium
- Often shows calcifications and ruptured cysts with associated granulomatous inflammation

Trichofolliculoma

- Multiple secondary follicles connecting to large, central, cystically dilated follicular structure
  - Panfolliculoma lacks central dilated follicular structure
- Often has sebaceous glands, which are not seen in panfolliculoma
  - Numerous sebaceous glands present in folliculocystic sebaceous hamartoma, which may be considered a trichofolliculoma variant

Pilomatrixoma

- Typically occurs in children or young adults
- Consists of basaloid matrical epithelium and shadow (or "ghost") cells
- Cystic spaces often present
- Lacks more advanced follicular differentiation
  - No keratin-filled cysts
  - No root sheath differentiation
- Often shows rupture with calcifications and associated granulomatous inflammation

DIAGNOSTIC CHECKLIST

Pathologic Interpretation Pearls

- Closely packed basaloid tumor nodules
- Key feature: All aspects of follicular differentiation present
  - Cystic areas resembling infundibulum
  - Areas with external and internal root sheath differentiation
  - Areas with matrical differentiation
  - Hair bulb formation with papillary mesenchymal bodies

SELECTED REFERENCES

1. Harris A et al: Epidermal panfolliculoma: A report of 2 cases. Am J Dermatopathol. 33(1):e7-10, 2011
2. Tellechea O et al: Trichogerminoma. Am J Dermatopathol. 31(5):480-3, 2009
3. Hoang MP et al: Cystic panfolliculoma. Arch Pathol Lab Med. 130(3):389-92, 2006
4. Ackerman AB et al: Panfolliculoma. In Neoplasms with Follicular Differentiation. London: Lea & Febiger: 461-76, 1993

IMAGE GALLERY

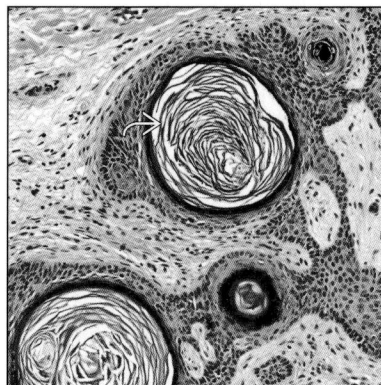 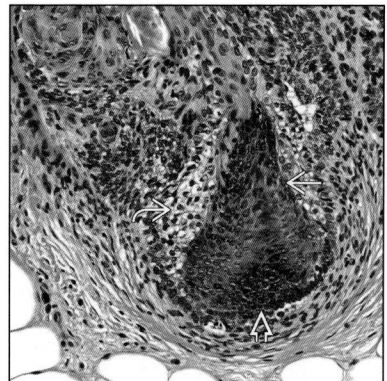 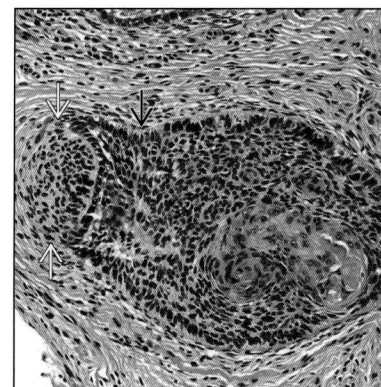

(Left) The cystic areas are lined by stratified squamous epithelium with a granular layer and filled with abundant laminated keratin ➔, consistent with infundibular differentiation. *(Center)* There is advanced follicular differentiation with external ➔ and internal ➔ root sheath formation, as well as matrical ➔ epithelium. *(Right)* This area of panfolliculoma shows immature basaloid cells ➔ as well as papillary mesenchymal body ➔ formation.

TUMOR OF THE FOLLICULAR INFUNDIBULUM

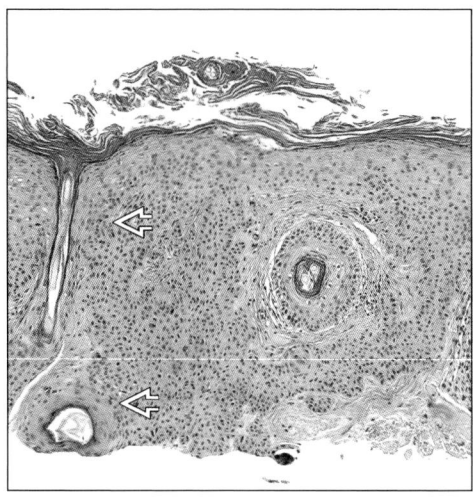

Tumor of the follicular infundibulum (TFI) is characterized by a superficial, plate-like distribution parallel to the epidermis. Note the multiple connections to an adjacent follicular structure ➡.

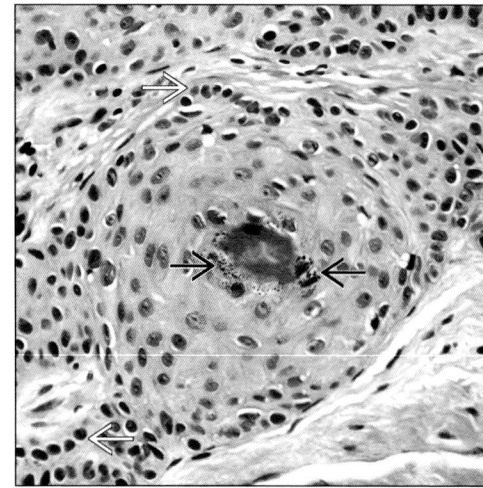

High magnification of TFI shows a central area of infundibular-type keratinization surrounded by bland squamous cells showing focal cytoplasmic granules ➡. Note the focal areas of peripheral palisading ➡.

TERMINOLOGY

Abbreviations
- Tumor of the follicular infundibulum (TFI)

Synonyms
- Basal cell hamartoma with follicular differentiation
- Mehregan tumor of follicular infundibulum

Definitions
- Benign proliferation of mature adnexal keratinocytes showing a superficial plate-like formation with multiple epidermal attachments

ETIOLOGY/PATHOGENESIS

Unknown
- Most cases are sporadic
- Some cases may be associated with nevus sebaceous (organoid nevus)

Genetic Syndrome
- May represent a manifestation of Cowden syndrome
  - Typically multiple lesions, often present with tricholemmomas

CLINICAL ISSUES

Epidemiology
- Incidence
  - Uncommon lesions
- Age
  - Usually presents in elderly adults
- Gender
  - More common in women

Site
- Typically presents on face and in head and neck region
- May also occur on upper chest

Presentation
- Small, slow-growing papule
  - Smooth or slightly keratotic appearing
  - Rarely may present as multiple lesions ("eruptive infundibulomas")

Natural History
- Stable lesions that do not regress

Treatment
- Options, risks, complications
  - Surgical excision is curative but not necessary due to benign nature of this lesion

Prognosis
- Excellent; little recurrence potential and no malignant potential

MICROSCOPIC PATHOLOGY

Histologic Features
- Superficial, plate-like proliferation parallel to epidermis
- Multiple anastomosing connections between lesion and epidermis
- Tumor is composed of mildly enlarged, bland-appearing squamous keratinocytes
  - Cells typically show abundant pale to clear-staining cytoplasm
  - Peripheral cells are more basaloid and show palisading
- Small follicular structures blend into deeper portions of lesion, but do not emerge from surface
  - Other evidence of follicular differentiation may include small follicular bulbs, papillary mesenchymal bodies, and occasional hair shafts
- Rarely, ductal structures may be present
- Stroma shows abundant elastic fibers

TUMOR OF THE FOLLICULAR INFUNDIBULUM

Key Facts

Terminology

- Tumor of the follicular infundibulum (TFI)
- Basal cell hamartoma with follicular differentiation
- Bland, superficial, plate-like adnexal proliferation with multiple epidermal attachments

Etiology/Pathogenesis

- May be sporadic (most cases) or part of Cowden syndrome (multiple, often with tricholemmomas)

Microscopic Pathology

- Multiple connections between lesion and epidermis
- Cells show abundant pale to clear-staining cytoplasm
- Peripheral cells often show palisading

Top Differential Diagnoses

- Basal cell carcinoma
- Inverted follicular keratosis
- Tricholemmoma

DIFFERENTIAL DIAGNOSIS

Basal Cell Carcinoma (BCC)

- TFI may mimic superficial BCC, as both show peripheral palisading; however
  - Cells are pale to clear staining in TFI
  - TFI lacks significant cytologic atypia, mitoses, and apoptotic bodies
- BCC typically lacks plate-like distribution of TFI
- Some dermatopathologists have claimed that TFI is an unusual variant of BCC, but this is not well accepted

Inverted Follicular Keratosis

- Acanthotic, endophytic proliferation of mature squamous keratinocytes
- Squamous eddies and scattered pseudohorn cysts present
- Typically considered a variant of irritated seborrheic keratosis

Tricholemmoma

- Lobular proliferation of mature squamoid cells with pale to clear-staining cytoplasm
- Multiple broad connections to epidermis and follicles present
- Lacks plate-like architecture of TFI

Pilar Sheath Acanthoma

- Central dell-like depression
- Composed of thickened epithelium with enlarged, pale-staining keratinocytes
- Lacks superficial, plate-like architecture of TFI

Dilated Pore of Winer

- Central dilated keratin-filled space
- Enlarged comedone-like follicular structure with acanthotic squamous lining
- Lacks superficial, plate-like architecture of TFI

SELECTED REFERENCES

1. Abbas O et al: Tumor of the follicular infundibulum: an epidermal reaction pattern? Am J Dermatopathol. 31(7):626-33, 2009
2. MacGregor JL et al: Basal cell and squamous cell carcinoma occurring within a field of multiple tumors of the follicular infundibulum. Dermatol Surg. 34(11):1567-70, 2008
3. Mahalingam M et al: Tumor of the follicular infundibulum with sebaceous differentiation. J Cutan Pathol. 28(6):314-7, 2001
4. Kolenik SA 3rd et al: Multiple tumors of the follicular infundibulum. Int J Dermatol. 35(4):282-4, 1996
5. Cribier B et al: Tumor of the follicular infundibulum: a clinicopathologic study. J Am Acad Dermatol. 33(6):979-84, 1995
6. Horn TD et al: Multiple tumors of follicular infundibulum with sweat duct differentiation. J Cutan Pathol. 22(3):281-7, 1995
7. Mehregan AH et al: A tumor of follicular infundibulum. Report of a case. Arch Dermatol. 83:924-7, 1961

IMAGE GALLERY

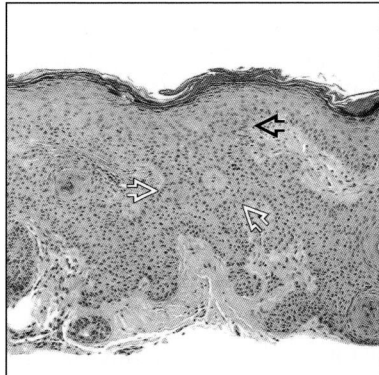 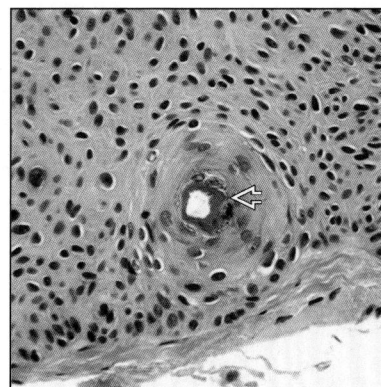 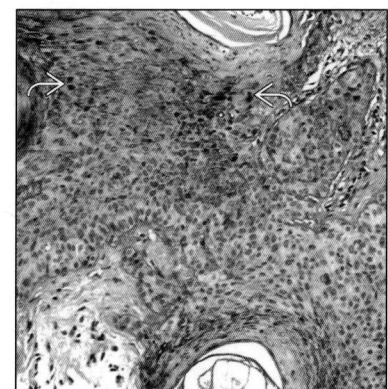

(Left) Low magnification of TFI shows a superficial, plate-like distribution parallel to the epidermis. Note the multiple anastomosing connections both between the tumor cords ⊳ and with the overlying epidermis ⊳. *(Center)* High magnification of TFI shows an area of infundibular-type keratinization ⊳ surrounded by relatively bland squamous cells with mild nuclear hyperchromasia. *(Right)* A PAS stain (without digestion) highlights focally prominent cytoplasmic glycogen collections ⊳.

DILATED PORE OF WINER

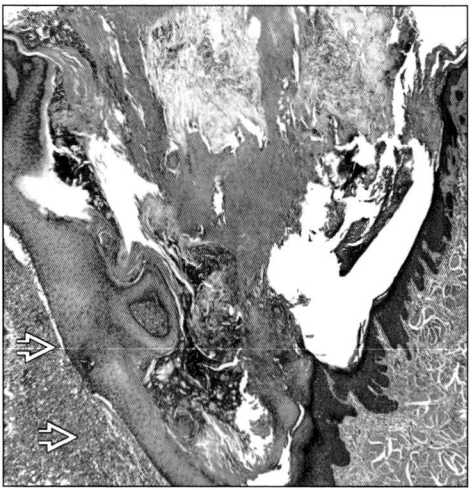 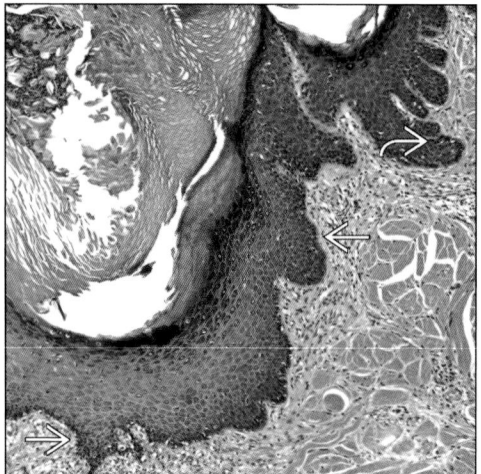

Dilated pore of Winer (DPW) at low-power examination shows a follicular structure with a dilated opening filled with keratin debris. This lesion shows focal rupture and associated inflammation ➡.

Intermediate magnification of a DPW shows the acanthotic squamous lining epithelium with focal finger-like projections ➡ and mild basilar hyperpigmentation ➡.

TERMINOLOGY

Abbreviations
- Dilated pore of Winer (DPW)

Definitions
- Enlarged follicular structure with acanthotic squamous lining and central keratin-filled space

ETIOLOGY/PATHOGENESIS

Unknown
- May be related to preceding inflammatory cystic acne in some cases
- Solar damage also implicated as most cases occur in elderly

CLINICAL ISSUES

Epidemiology
- Incidence
  - Uncommon lesions
- Age
  - Usually elderly patients

Site
- Head and neck region most common
  - May also occur on the trunk

Presentation
- Comedone-like lesion
  - May be solitary or multiple

Treatment
- Options, risks, complications
  - Surgery not necessary, but conservative excision or ablation is curative

Prognosis
- Excellent, completely benign (likely nonneoplastic) lesion

MACROSCOPIC FEATURES

General Features
- Markedly dilated comedone-like lesion

Size
- Variable; may be up to 2 cm

MICROSCOPIC PATHOLOGY

Histologic Features
- Enlarged, dilated follicular structure
- May extend into deep dermis
- Often filled with abundant keratin debris
  - Infundibular-type keratinization with a granular layer
- Squamous epithelial lining shows acanthosis and finger-like projections into surrounding dermis
  - No infiltrative features present
  - No significant cytologic atypia or mitotic activity present
- Small sebaceous glands and vellus hair follicles may be attached to base of lesion
- Follicular epithelium may show prominent pigmentation in some cases

Cytologic Features
- Bland squamous keratinocytes

DIFFERENTIAL DIAGNOSIS

Pilar Sheath Acanthoma
- Infundibular structure lined by acanthotic epithelium

DILATED PORE OF WINER

Key Facts

Terminology

- Dilated pore of Winer (DPW)
- Enlarged follicular structure with acanthotic squamous lining and central keratin-filled space

Etiology/Pathogenesis

- May be related to preceding inflammatory cystic acne in some cases
- Solar damage also implicated as most cases occur in elderly

Clinical Issues

- Head and neck region most common
- Excellent, completely benign (likely nonneoplastic) lesion

Microscopic Pathology

- Enlarged, dilated follicular structure
- Infundibular-type keratinization with a granular layer
- Squamous epithelial lining shows acanthosis and finger-like projections into surrounding dermis

---

- o Less dilated and more acanthotic appearing than dilated pore of Winer
- o Fewer finger-like projections than dilated pore of Winer
- Cells show abundant pale- to clear-staining (glycogen-containing, PAS[+], diastase-sensitive) cytoplasm

Comedone

- Enlarged, dilated follicular structure, similar to dilated pore of Winer
- Filled with abundant keratin debris, acute inflammatory cells, and numerous bacterial organisms
- Clinical presentation different from dilated pore of Winer
  - o Much more likely to present in adolescents and young adults

Hair Cortex Comedo

- Very rare lesion that is closely related to dilated pore of Winer
- Dilated follicular structure showing central keratinous plug with cornification (similar to cortex of hair shaft)
- Epithelium may show melanin pigmentation
- Stroma may show surrounding granulomatous inflammation

Regressing Keratoacanthoma

- Usually shows irregularly dilated crateriform area
- Epithelium appears more atrophic
- Often lacks significant cytologic atypia or mitotic activity

- Associated with dermal fibrosis and chronic inflammation

DIAGNOSTIC CHECKLIST

Pathologic Interpretation Pearls

- Enlarged, dilated follicular structure filled with keratinous debris
- Squamous epithelial lining shows acanthosis and finger-like projections into surrounding dermis

SELECTED REFERENCES

1. Moreira A et al: Dermoscopy of a dilated pore of Winer. Eur J Dermatol. 20(2):229, 2010
2. Walsh SN et al: Hair cortex comedo: a series of 34 cases. Am J Dermatopathol. 32(8):749-54, 2010
3. Jakobiec FA et al: Winer's dilated pore of the eyelid. Ophthal Plast Reconstr Surg. 25(5):411-3, 2009
4. Carlson-Sweet KL et al: Trichoid basal cell carcinoma found in a dilated pore on the nose. Dermatol Surg. 26(9):874-6, 2000
5. Resnik KS et al: Dilated pore nevus. A histologic variant of nevus comedonicus. Am J Dermatopathol. 15(2):169-71, 1993
6. Hausmann G et al: [The Winer dilated pore.] Med Cutan Ibero Lat Am. 17(1):45-7, 1989
7. Winer LH: The dilated pore, a tricho-epithelioma. J Invest Dermatol. 23(3):181-8, 1954

IMAGE GALLERY

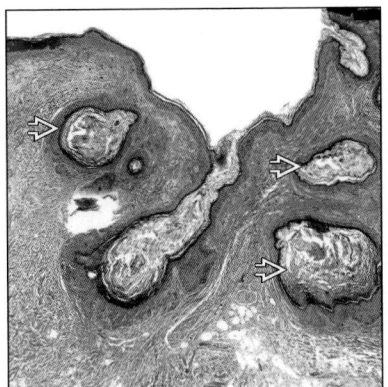 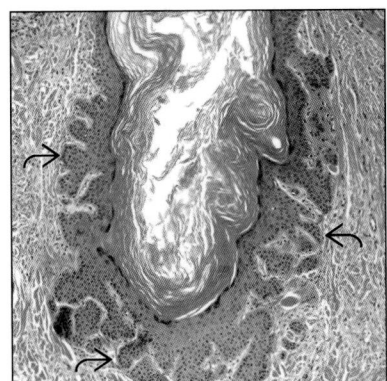 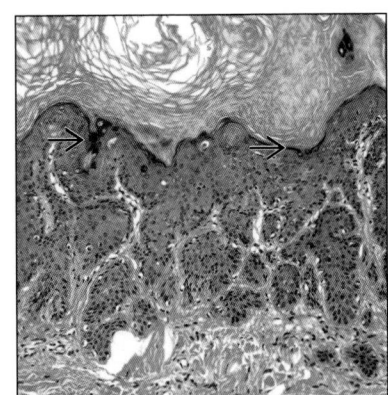

(Left) Dilated pore of Winer (DPW) at low-power examination shows a follicular structure with a patulous opening and several tangentially sectioned, surrounding follicular lumina ➡. *(Center)* A tangentially sectioned area shows a central keratin-filled follicular structure with multiple irregular, radiating finger-like projections ➡. *(Right)* Higher magnification of the finger-like projections surrounding a follicular lumen shows bland squamous epithelial cells forming a granular layer ➡.

PILAR SHEATH ACANTHOMA

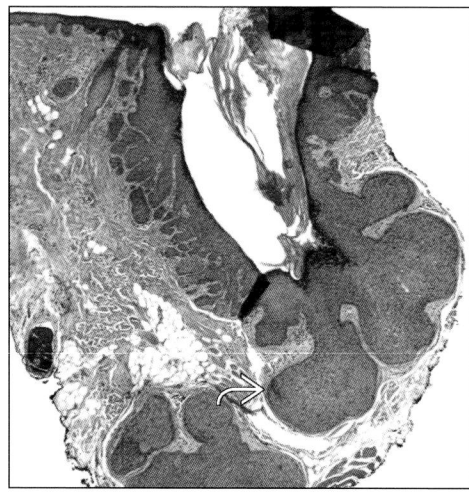

Scanning magnification of a pilar sheath acanthoma shows a dilated follicular structure lined by a thickened squamous epithelium with endophytic, lobulated areas ➡.

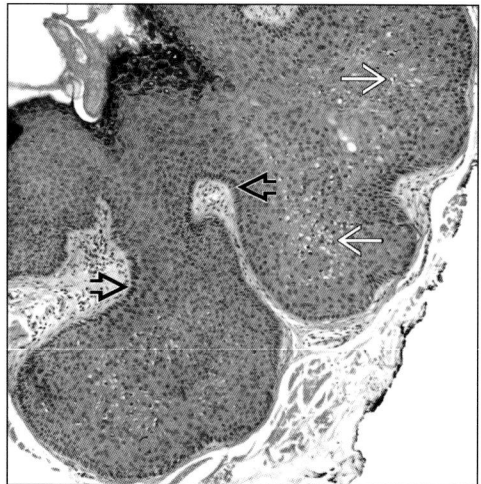

Higher magnification of the lobular areas shows acanthotic squamous epithelium with peripheral palisading ⊳ and scattered clear-staining cells ➡.

TERMINOLOGY

Abbreviations
- Pilar sheath acanthoma (PSA)

Definitions
- Mature adnexal proliferation composed of thickened epithelium with enlarged pale-staining keratinocytes

ETIOLOGY/PATHOGENESIS

Unknown
- No known causes/associations

CLINICAL ISSUES

Epidemiology
- Incidence
  - Rare lesions
- Age
  - Usually occur in middle-aged to older adults
- Gender
  - Males and females equally affected

Site
- Most often occur on upper lip

Presentation
- Keratotic papular lesion with central pore-like area

Natural History
- Slow-growing, stable lesion
  - Often present for years

Treatment
- Options, risks, complications
  - Complete surgical excision is curative but not necessary in most cases due to benign nature

Prognosis
- Excellent, benign behavior; no evidence of malignant transformation

MACROSCOPIC FEATURES

General Features
- Superficial keratotic papule

Size
- Generally small, < 1 cm

MICROSCOPIC PATHOLOGY

Histologic Features
- Endophytic, lobular proliferation of enlarged, mature squamous cells with prominent acanthosis
  - Lobules typically surround a central dilated follicular structure
  - Granular layer and foci of infundibular-type keratinization are present
  - Abortive follicles may be present
  - Peripheral palisading and thickened basement membrane may be seen (similar to tricholemmoma)
- Cells show abundant pale eosinophilic to clear-staining cytoplasm and small nuclei
  - Clear cells contain glycogen, which can be demonstrated by PAS (without diastase digestion)
- Lesion is usually superficial, well circumscribed, and noninfiltrative
  - Rare cases may extend deeply into subcutis
- Mitotic figures absent to rare, limited to basilar layer

Cytologic Features
- Bland-appearing squamoid cells with uniform nuclei, small nucleoli, and abundant pale- to clear-staining cytoplasm

PILAR SHEATH ACANTHOMA

Key Facts

Terminology
- Pilar sheath acanthoma (PSA)
- Mature adnexal proliferation composed of thickened epithelium with enlarged pale-staining keratinocytes

Clinical Issues
- Usually in middle-aged to older adults
- Most often occur on upper lip
- Slow-growing, stable lesion
- Keratotic papule with central pore-like area

Microscopic Pathology
- Endophytic, lobular proliferation of enlarged, mature squamous cells with prominent acanthosis
- Usually superficial, well circumscribed, and noninfiltrative
- Lobules typically surround a follicular structure
- Foci of infundibular-type keratinization
- Cells show abundant pale eosinophilic to clear-staining cytoplasm and small nuclei

Predominant Cell/Compartment Type
- Adnexal cell showing outer root sheath differentiation

DIFFERENTIAL DIAGNOSIS

Dilated Pore of Winer (DPW)
- Larger, more dilated follicular opening (comedone-like) than pilar sheath acanthoma
  - Filled with abundant keratin debris
- Does not show degree of acanthosis and clear cell features typical of pilar sheath acanthoma
- Small sebaceous glands and vellus hairs may attach to the base (absent in PSA)

Trichofolliculoma
- Central dilated follicular structure with multiple small, immature radiating follicles
  - Central follicle opens to epidermal surface
- Fibrotic and cellular stroma (which is lacking in PSA)
- Sebaceous glands may be prominent in some cases (sebaceous trichofolliculoma or folliculosebaceous cystic hamartoma)

Inverted Follicular Keratosis (IFK)
- Typically considered a variant of irritated seborrheic keratosis
- Endophytic-appearing lesion composed of mature squamous keratinocytes
- Often shows numerous keratinizing pseudohorn cysts and squamous eddies

- Usually lacks pale to clear cells seen in pilar sheath acanthoma

Tumor of the Follicular Infundibulum (TFI)
- Proliferation of mature adnexal keratinocytes showing a superficial plate-like formation with multiple epidermal attachments
- Cells show abundant pale- to clear-staining cytoplasm similar to pilar sheath acanthoma, but architectural features are different
- Peripheral palisading of tumor cells typically present

DIAGNOSTIC CHECKLIST

Pathologic Interpretation Pearls
- Endophytic proliferation of thickened epithelium with enlarged pale-staining keratinocytes

SELECTED REFERENCES

1. Choi YS et al: Pilar sheath acanthoma--report of a case with review of the literature. Yonsei Med J. 30(4):392-5, 1989
2. Lee JY et al: Pilar sheath acanthoma. Arch Dermatol. 123(5):569-70, 1987
3. Dudley K et al: Nevus comedonicus in association with widespread, well-differentiated follicular tumors. J Am Acad Dermatol. 15(5 Pt 2):1123-7, 1986
4. Bhawan J: Pilar sheath acanthoma. A new benign follicular tumor. J Cutan Pathol. 6(5):438-40, 1979
5. Mehregan AH et al: Pilar sheath acanthoma. Arch Dermatol. 114(10):1495-7, 1978

IMAGE GALLERY

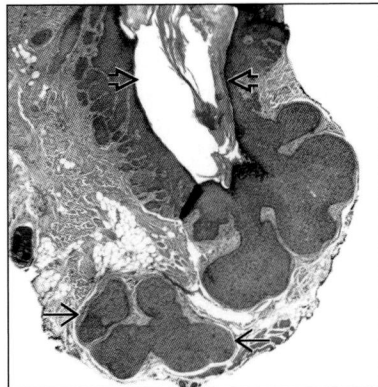 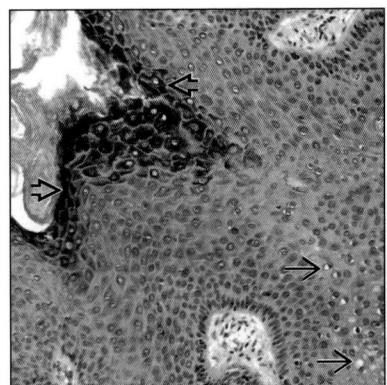 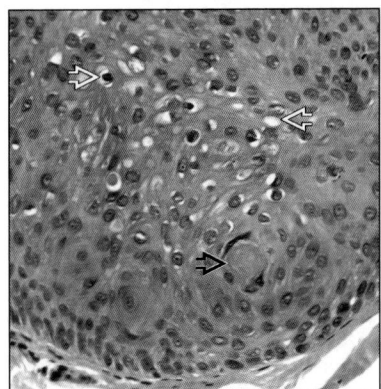

(Left) Low magnification of a PSA shows a central dilated follicular lumen ⊵ lined by a thickened epithelium with endophytic lobulated areas, some of which extend into the deeper dermis ➡. *(Center)* High magnification of the epithelium shows a prominent granular layer ⊵ (consistent with infundibular keratinization). The cells are mildly enlarged and squamoid appearing, with scattered pale/clear cells ➡. *(Right)* Foci of keratinization with squamous pearls ⊵ may be seen surrounded by bland squamoid to clear ⊳ cells.

INVERTED FOLLICULAR KERATOSIS

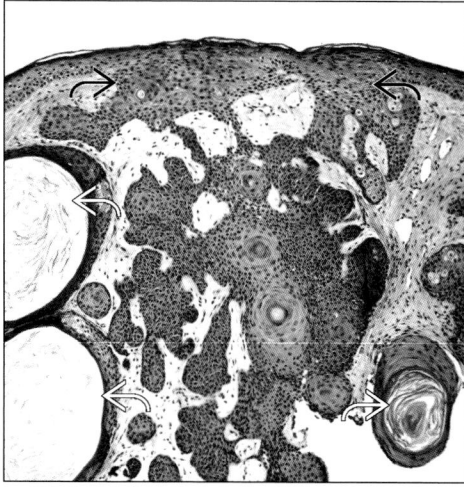

Inverted follicular keratosis (IFK) is a well-circumscribed, endophytic epithelial proliferation. This tumor shows multiple connections to the epidermis ➔, and multiple folliculocystic structures (similar to milia) are present ➔.

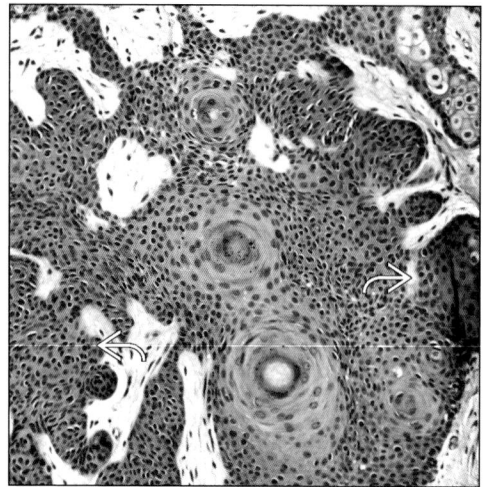

High magnification of the center of this lesion shows bland squamoid cells surrounding small follicular lumina and smaller, peripheral, more basaloid-appearing cells ➔.

TERMINOLOGY

Abbreviations
- Inverted follicular keratosis (IFK)

Synonyms
- Irritated seborrheic keratosis variant

Definitions
- Benign tumor of follicular infundibulum considered by many to be identical to irritated seborrheic keratosis

ETIOLOGY/PATHOGENESIS

Etiology
- Lesions arise from follicular infundibula, which explains the downward proliferation of these lesions
- IFK is considered to be identical to seborrheic keratosis derived from follicular infundibulum instead of surface epidermis
- Epithelium of follicular infundibulum has the same histology and keratinization as surface epidermis

CLINICAL ISSUES

Epidemiology
- Incidence
  - Relatively common
- Age
  - Older adults
- Gender
  - More common in men

Site
- 90% on head and neck
  - Upper cutaneous lip and cheeks are most commonly affected

Presentation
- Usually present as asymptomatic, solitary, dome-shaped or filiform, skin-colored papule

Treatment
- Not necessary
- Usually a biopsy for diagnosis removes the entire lesion

Prognosis
- Excellent: Benign lesion

MICROSCOPIC PATHOLOGY

Histologic Features
- Usually endophytic papillomatous proliferation of epithelium
  - Exophytic and exo-endophytic growth pattern can be seen
  - Composed predominately of squamous cells
  - Numerous squamous eddies are present and are characteristic feature
    - Squamous eddies are concentric layers of squamous cells with keratin at their centers
    - Presence of many squamous eddies is due to irritation of these lesions
  - Basaloid cells are often present at periphery of lesion
    - Mitotic figures often present in basaloid cells
- Overlying hyperkeratosis and parakeratosis
  - Prominent keratin-filled invagination
  - Cutaneous horn can be present

Cytologic Features
- Predominately squamous cells with basaloid cells at periphery of lesion
- No significant cytologic atypia or pleomorphism

INVERTED FOLLICULAR KERATOSIS

Key Facts

Terminology
- Inverted follicular keratosis (IFK)
- Benign tumor of follicular infundibulum

Clinical Issues
- Common benign tumor found mostly in men
- 90% on head and neck

Microscopic Pathology
- Hyperkeratosis and parakeratosis

- Endophytic papillomatous proliferation of epithelium
- Numerous squamous eddies are typically present and are characteristic feature
- Mitotic figures present in basaloid cells
- No significant cytologic atypia or pleomorphism

Top Differential Diagnoses
- Irritated seborrheic keratosis
- Well-differentiated squamous cell carcinoma

DIFFERENTIAL DIAGNOSIS

Irritated Seborrheic Keratosis (ISK)
- Many consider IFK to be the same as ISK except it is derived from the follicular infundibulum
- Clinical
  - IFK often on upper cutaneous lip or cheek
  - ISK shows variable location
- Histology
  - ISK often has horizontal growth pattern, while IFK has endophytic growth pattern
  - Bcl-2 positive dendritic cells present in increased numbers in suprabasilar areas of IFKs compared to ISKs

Well-Differentiated Squamous Cell Carcinoma (In Situ or Invasive)
- If squamous eddies are present, usually not as many as in IFKs
- Cytologic atypia with pleomorphic cells present
- Dyskeratotic cells and multiple mitotic figures usually present
- Bcl-2 positive dendritic cells present in increased numbers in suprabasilar areas of IFK compared to squamous cell carcinomas

Tumor of the Follicular Infundibulum
- Benign proliferation of enlarged pale to clear-staining squamous keratinocytes
- Often shows a plate-like pattern parallel to epidermis
- Peripheral palisading of basaloid cells typically present

DIAGNOSTIC CHECKLIST

Clinically Relevant Pathologic Features
- Age distribution

Pathologic Interpretation Pearls
- Benign, endophytic, epithelial proliferation with numerous squamous eddies is characteristic of IFK

SELECTED REFERENCES

1. Noiles K et al: Are all seborrheic keratoses benign? Review of the typical lesion and its variants. J Cutan Med Surg. 12(5):203-10, 2008
2. Ko CJ et al: Bcl-2-positive epidermal dendritic cells in inverted follicular keratoses but not squamous cell carcinomas or seborrheic keratoses. J Cutan Pathol. 33(7):498-501, 2006
3. Roth LM et al: Inverted follicular keratosis of the vulvar skin: a lesion that can be confused with squamous cell carcinoma. Int J Gynecol Pathol. 19(4):369-73, 2000
4. Mehregan AH: Inverted follicular keratosis is a distinct follicular tumor. Am J Dermatopathol. 5(5):467-70, 1983
5. Morales A et al: Seborrheic verruca and intraepidermal basal cell epithelioma of Jadassohn. Arch Dermatol. 91(4):342-4, 1965

IMAGE GALLERY

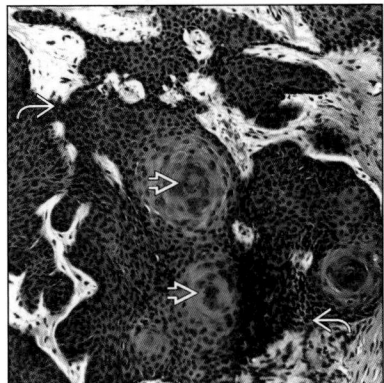 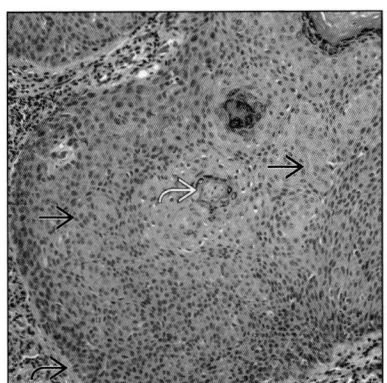 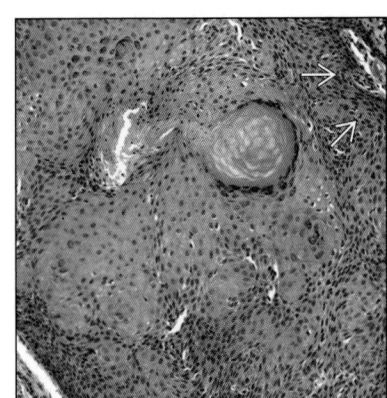

(Left) Squamous eddies with central keratinization ⊃ are shown. The proliferation is composed of keratinizing squamous cells and basaloid cells ⊃ at the periphery of the lesion. *(Center)* Numerous whorls of squamous cells ⊃ are a characteristic feature of IFK. This lesion is composed mostly of squamous cells with focal keratinization ⊃. Basaloid cells are seen at the periphery ⊃. *(Right)* The cells are cytologically bland, but several mitotic figures ⊃ may be seen in many cases, especially toward the periphery of the lesion.

TRICHOLEMMOMA

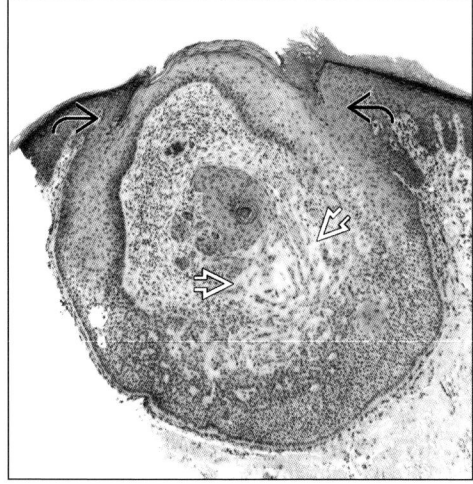

Scanning magnification of a small tricholemmoma shows a symmetric, well-circumscribed, lobular neoplasm with epidermal attachments ➔. Centrally, the lesion shows desmoplastic TL features ➔.

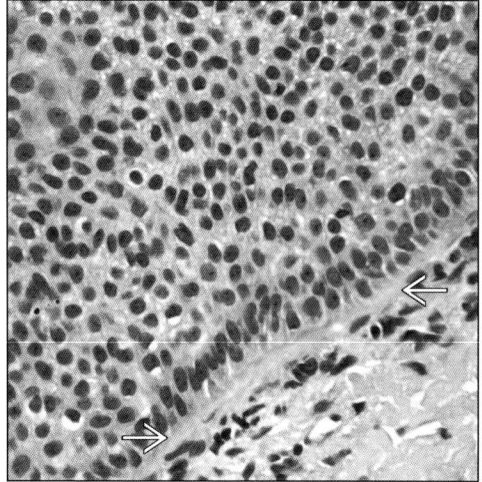

High magnification of a TL shows bland-appearing small cells with pale to clear-staining cytoplasm and small nucleoli. There is a thickened peripheral basement membrane ➔.

TERMINOLOGY

Abbreviations
- Tricholemmoma (TL)
- Desmoplastic tricholemmoma (dTL)

Synonyms
- Trichilemmoma

Definitions
- Benign clear cell adnexal proliferation with external root sheath differentiation

ETIOLOGY/PATHOGENESIS

Unknown in Most Cases
- Some have considered TL to be related to HPV infection ("tricholemmal verrucae")
  - Not generally accepted, and most PCR studies for HPV have been negative

Genetic
- Some cases are associated with Cowden syndrome (PTEN hamartoma syndrome)
  - Characterized by multiple tricholemmomas, hamartomas, and visceral tumors including breast and thyroid carcinomas
  - Mutation of *PTEN*, a tumor suppressor gene, on 10q23.31

CLINICAL ISSUES

Epidemiology
- Incidence
  - Relatively common tumors
- Age
  - Usually adults, although Cowden syndrome patients present earlier

Site
- Most occur on face, especially nose and upper lip

Presentation
- Small papular lesion
  - Usually flesh-colored
  - Often clinically mimics basal cell carcinoma or verruca

Treatment
- Surgical approaches
  - Usually not necessary, as these are benign tumors
  - Complete conservative excision is curative

Prognosis
- Excellent, no malignant potential
- Cowden syndrome patients have high risk of internal malignancies

MICROSCOPIC PATHOLOGY

Histologic Features
- Lobular proliferation of mature squamoid cells with pale- to clear-staining cytoplasm
- Peripheral palisading of basaloid cells
  - Cells are surrounded by thickened, glassy-appearing basement membrane
- Squamous eddies and small foci of tricholemmal (pilar)-type keratinization often present
- Multiple broad connections to epidermis and follicles
  - Early lesions often surround a follicle, consistent with follicular derivation

Predominant Cell/Compartment Type
- Adnexal keratinocyte with external root sheath differentiation

Subtype
- **Desmoplastic tricholemmoma (dTL)**
  - Variant with prominent desmoplastic stroma

TRICHOLEMMOMA

Key Facts

Terminology
- Tricholemmoma (TL)
  - Benign clear cell adnexal proliferation with external root sheath differentiation
- Subtype: Desmoplastic tricholemmoma (dTL)

Etiology/Pathogenesis
- Some cases are associated with Cowden syndrome (PTEN hamartoma syndrome)
  - Characterized by multiple tricholemmomas, hamartomas, and visceral tumors including breast and thyroid carcinomas
  - Mutation of *PTEN* gene on 10q23.31

Microscopic Pathology
- Lobular proliferation of mature squamoid cells with pale- to clear-staining cytoplasm

- Peripheral palisading of basaloid cells
- Cells are surrounded by thickened, glassy-appearing basement membrane
- Multiple broad connections to epidermis and follicles
- Desmoplastic tricholemmoma
  - Variant with prominent desmoplastic stroma
  - Typically in center of tumor, surrounded by conventional-appearing TL

Top Differential Diagnoses
- Tumor of follicular infundibulum (TFI)
- Clear cell acanthoma
- Tricholemmal carcinoma
- Clear cell squamous cell carcinoma in situ (clear cell Bowen disease)
- Basal cell carcinoma (BCC)

- Typically in center of tumor
- Can mimic invasive carcinoma
  - However, infiltrative areas are usually surrounded by conventional-appearing tricholemmoma

DIFFERENTIAL DIAGNOSIS

Tumor of Follicular Infundibulum (TFI)
- Superficial, plate-like growth pattern parallel to epidermis
- Peripheral palisading and clear cells present, but
  - TFI is more plate-like, less lobular than TL
  - TFI shows multiple anastomosing connections between tumor cells and with epidermis
  - Hair follicles merge with undersurface of TFI, not TL

Clear Cell Acanthoma
- Psoriasiform epidermal acanthosis
- Epidermal cells show prominent clear cell changes, similar to TL, but
  - Clear cell acanthoma shows overlying hypogranulosis and parakeratosis
  - Lacks lobular configuration and thickened peripheral basement membrane
  - Sharp demarcation from adjacent normal epidermis

Tricholemmal Carcinoma
- Shows lobular proliferation of clear cells with peripheral palisading
- However, tricholemmal carcinoma also shows
  - Significant cytologic atypia, mitotic activity, infiltrative features, and may show necrosis
  - Typically lacks symmetry and circumscription of TL
  - Desmoplastic areas at periphery, not in center of tumor (unlike dTL)

Clear Cell Squamous Cell Carcinoma In Situ (Clear Cell Bowen Disease)
- Atypical intraepidermal proliferation of clear-staining keratinocytes
  - Prominent nuclear atypia with hyperchromasia and large nucleoli

- Multiple mitotic figures, including atypical forms, typically present
- Lacks lobular architecture and peripheral thickened basement membrane of TL

Basal Cell Carcinoma (BCC)
- Can occasionally show prominent clear cell features
- Peripheral palisading seen in both BCC and TL, however
  - Prominent mitoses, apoptoses, and infiltrative feature characteristic of BCC
  - Tumor-stromal retraction artifact and mucinous stroma typical of BCC

SELECTED REFERENCES

1. Dalton SR et al: Squamous cell carcinoma with clear cells: how often is there evidence of tricholemmal differentiation? Am J Dermatopathol. 30(4):333-9, 2008
2. Cabral ES et al: Desmoplastic tricholemmoma of the eyelid misdiagnosed as sebaceous carcinoma: a potential diagnostic pitfall. J Cutan Pathol. 34 Suppl 1:22-5, 2007
3. Schweiger E et al: A case of desmoplastic trichilemmoma of the lip treated with Mohs surgery. Dermatol Surg. 30(7):1062-4, 2004
4. Trojan J et al: Activation of a cryptic splice site of PTEN and loss of heterozygosity in benign skin lesions in Cowden disease. J Invest Dermatol. 117(6):1650-3, 2001
5. Nelen MR et al: Novel PTEN mutations in patients with Cowden disease: absence of clear genotype-phenotype correlations. Eur J Hum Genet. 7(3):267-73, 1999
6. Hanssen AM et al: Cowden syndrome. J Med Genet. 32(2):117-9, 1995
7. Headington JT: Tricholemmoma. To be or not to be? Am J Dermatopathol. 2(3):225-6, 1980

TRICHOLEMMOMA

Clinical and Microscopic Features

(Left) Multiple tricholemmomas ⊞ on the nose of a patient with Cowden syndrome are shown. (Courtesy D. Kaplan, MD.) *(Right)* Traumatized TL at low-power magnification shows epidermal erosion with dense serum crusting and impetiginization overlying a symmetric, well-circumscribed, lobular neoplasm with epidermal attachments.

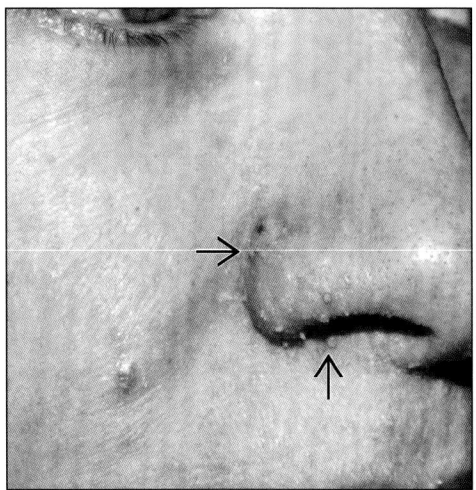
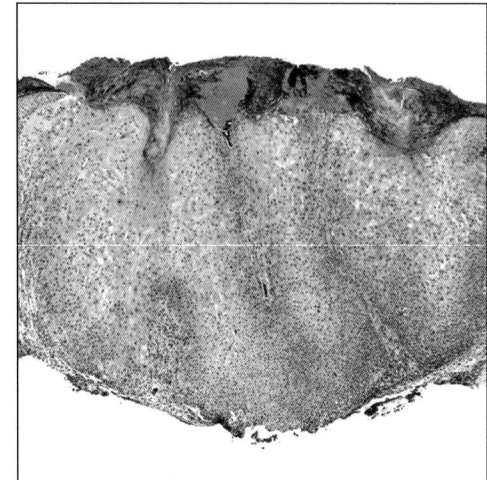

(Left) Desmoplastic TL shows focal areas of infiltrative-appearing cells ⊞ associated with a prominent hyalinized stroma in the center of a large, more conventional tumor. *(Right)* Intermediate magnification of a desmoplastic TL shows a central area of tumor cords set in a hyalinized stroma ⊞, surrounded by areas of more typical-appearing TL ⊞.

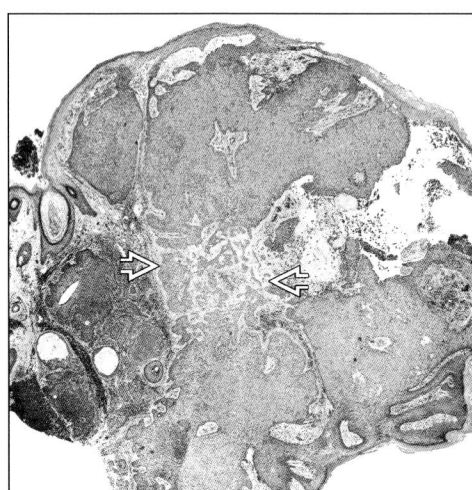
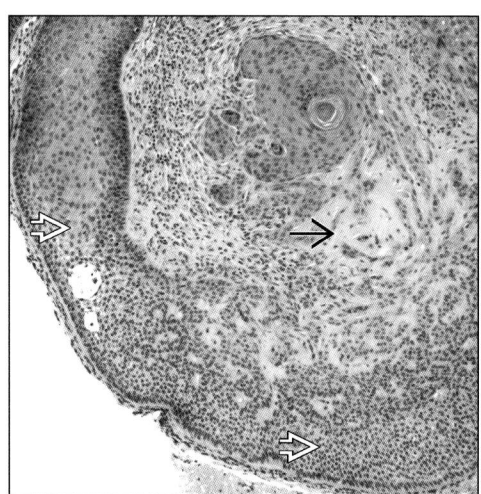

(Left) High magnification of desmoplastic TL shows areas of infiltrative-appearing cords and nests of eosinophilic-staining cells associated with a prominent hyalinized stroma ⊞. This variant may be mistaken for an infiltrative carcinoma. *(Right)* Periodic acid-Schiff (PAS) stain without diastase digestion is usually strongly positive in TL, due to cytoplasmic glycogenation.

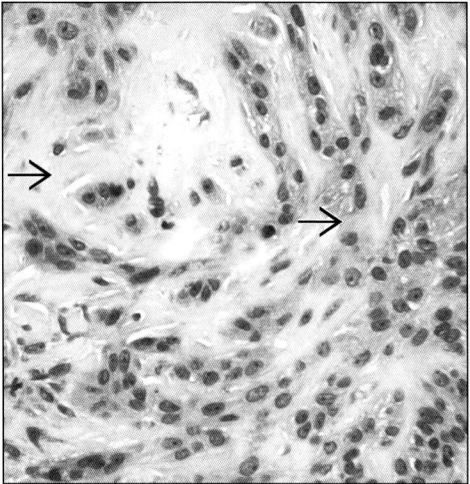
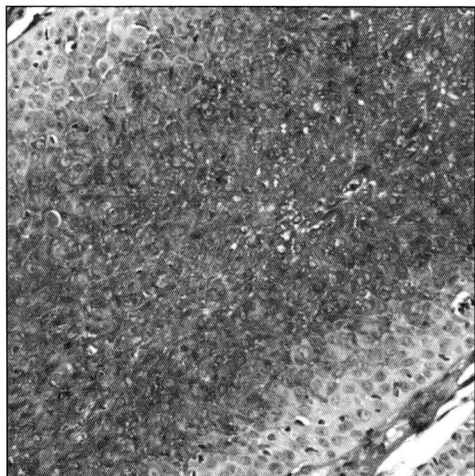

Differential Diagnosis

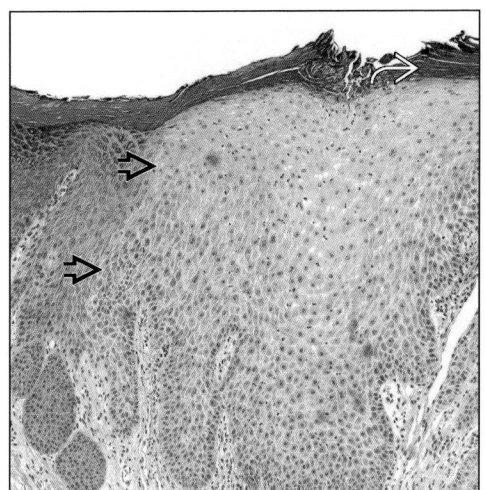

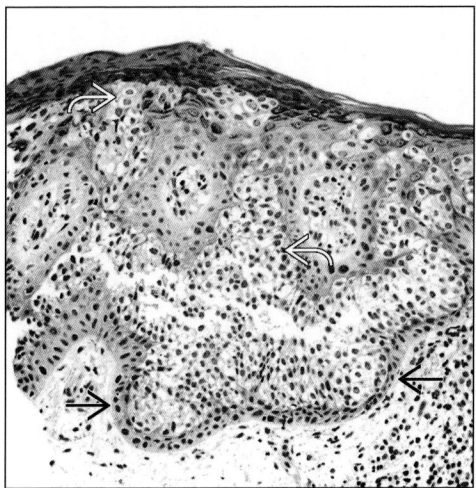

(Left) Clear cell acanthoma shows psoriasiform acanthosis, parakeratosis ⊿, and a proliferation of bland-appearing pale eosinophilic to clear-staining keratinocytes. Note the sharp demarcation from the adjacent epidermis ⊅. (Right) Clear cell pagetoid SCC in situ (Bowen disease) shows an intraepidermal proliferation of atypical squamous cells ➔ with abundant clear-staining cytoplasm extending into the granular layer. Note the preserved basilar layer ⊅ of benign keratinocytes.

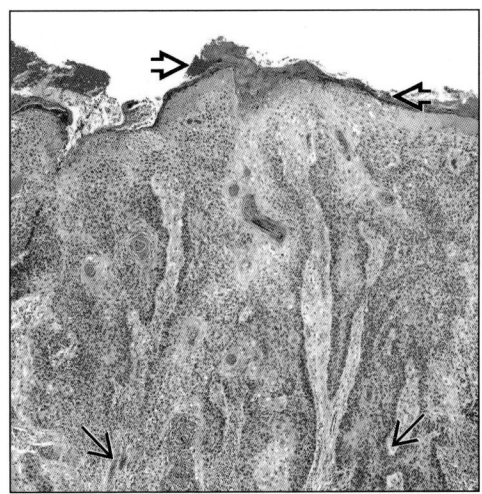

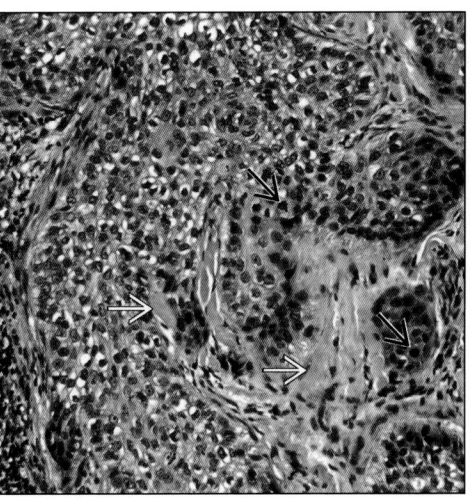

(Left) Tricholemmal carcinoma is typically a larger tumor than TL and shows deep, irregular downgrowths ➔ of atypical basaloid to clear-staining cells. There is overlying epidermal erosion and serum crusting ⊅. (Right) High magnification of a tricholemmal carcinoma shows cytologic atypia, mitotic figures ➔, and a hyalinized-appearing desmoplastic stroma ➔.

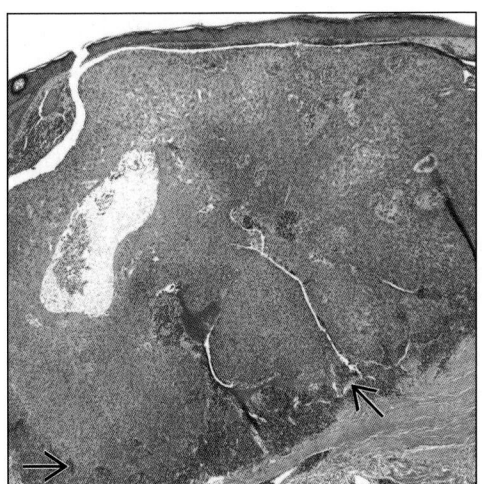

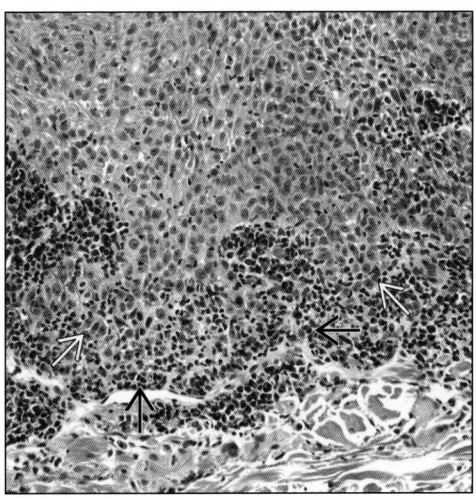

(Left) Another tricholemmal carcinoma shows a large, multilobulated, eosinophilic to clear cell neoplasm with irregular jagged borders ➔ and relatively dense surrounding chronic inflammation. (Right) Peripheral edge of a tricholemmal carcinoma shows jagged borders ➔, as opposed to the smooth, rounded borders and thickened basement membrane typical of TL. The lesion is associated with an inflammatory infiltrate including lymphocytes and numerous eosinophils ➔.

TRICHOLEMMAL CARCINOMA

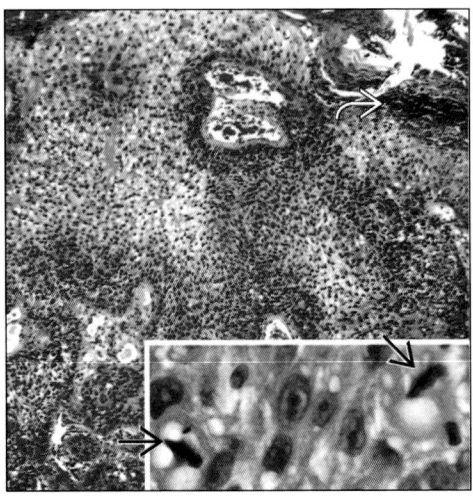

TLC is a clear cell neoplasm that may show multiple attachments to the epidermis and overlying ulceration and crusting ⤵. Inset shows atypical cells with prominent nucleoli and multiple mitotic figures ➔.

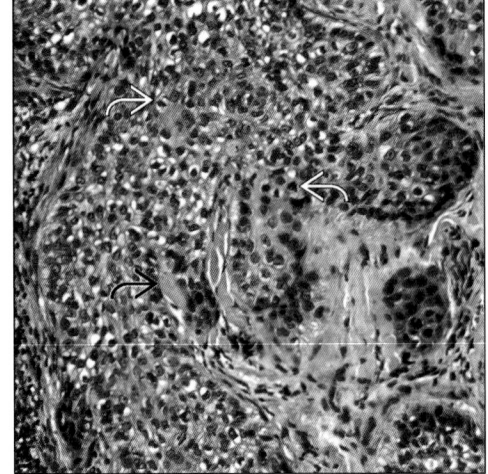

High magnification of another case of TLC shows a proliferation of pale to clear cells with cytologic atypia, mitotic figures ⤵, and a focally thickened basement membrane ➔.

TERMINOLOGY

Abbreviations
- Tricholemmal carcinoma (TLC)

Synonyms
- Trichilemmal carcinoma
- Malignant tricholemmoma

Definitions
- Low-grade malignant tumor of clear-staining squamous cells with tricholemmal/outer root sheath differentiation
- Has been classified as a low malignant potential variant of squamous cell carcinoma (SCC)

ETIOLOGY/PATHOGENESIS

Environmental Exposure
- Most cases likely due to ultraviolet light exposure
- Rare cases reportedly associated with radiation or immunosuppression

CLINICAL ISSUES

Epidemiology
- Incidence
  - Tumors rare but may be underreported due to classification as clear cell SCC or other tumors
- Age
  - Occurs in elderly patients
- Gender
  - No definite gender predilection

Site
- Most often presents in head and neck region

Presentation
- Papule or nodule with overlying crusting &/or ulceration

Treatment
- Surgical approaches
  - Complete excision should be performed and is curative

Prognosis
- Excellent, local recurrence potential but no confirmed metastatic cases
  - Reported metastatic cases likely represent malignant proliferating tricholemmal/pilar tumors, not TLC

MACROSCOPIC FEATURES

Size
- Generally small, less than 2-3 cm

MICROSCOPIC PATHOLOGY

Histologic Features
- Lobulated to nodular tumor with dermal invasion
  - Composed of a proliferation of large clear cells with cytologic atypia
    - Cells show nuclear hyperchromasia with prominent nucleoli and abundant clear-staining cytoplasm
    - Some cells may show prominent keratohyaline granules
  - Lobules may show connections to the epidermis &/or hair follicles
  - Areas of tricholemmal (pilar)-type keratinization without intervening granular layer
  - Peripheral palisading and thickened basement membrane often seen
  - Mitotic figures usually abundant; necrosis may be present

TRICHOLEMMAL CARCINOMA

Key Facts

Terminology
- Tricholemmal carcinoma (TLC)
- Low-grade malignant tumor of clear-staining squamous cells with tricholemmal differentiation

Clinical Issues
- Occurs in sun-damaged skin of the elderly
- Excellent, local recurrence potential but no confirmed metastatic cases

Microscopic Pathology
- Lobulated to nodular, predominantly dermal-based tumor
- Typically composed of a proliferation of large clear cells with cytologic atypia
- Areas of tricholemmal (pilar)-type keratinization without intervening granular layer
- Peripheral palisading and thickened basement membrane often seen

Cytologic Features
- Large cells with nuclear hyperchromasia, prominent nucleoli, and abundant clear-staining cytoplasm

DIFFERENTIAL DIAGNOSIS

Tricholemmoma
- Usually smaller and more superficial than TLC
- Symmetric, well-circumscribed lobular proliferation
- Lacks significant cytologic atypia and mitotic activity

Clear Cell Squamous Cell Carcinoma (SCC)
- TLC may be considered a low-grade variant of clear cell SCC
- Therefore, distinction from clear cell SCC may be subjective in some cases
  - However, conventional clear cell SCC does not show tricholemmal differentiation, peripheral palisading, or thickened basement membrane
- Some cases of clear cell SCC are higher grade, and may behave aggressively, with metastatic disease
  - No well-documented cases of metastatic TLC reported

Clear Cell Basal Cell Carcinoma (BCC)
- Most cases show areas of conventional BCC with atypical basaloid cells in nodules, cords, or islands
- Presence of peripheral palisading seen in both TLC and BCC, but
  - Other features such as mucinous stroma and retraction artifact are lacking in TLC
  - Lobular architecture and thickened basement membrane are lacking in BCC

Sebaceous Carcinoma
- Composed of nodules &/or lobules of atypical clear cells, often with attachments to the epidermis &/or hair follicles
- Cells typically show abundant multivacuolated cytoplasm with nuclear indentations, unlike the uniformly clear-staining cytoplasm of TLC
- Lacks areas of tricholemmal keratinization and thickened basement membrane
- IHC shows positivity for EMA, androgen receptor, CAM5.2, and usually for CK7

SELECTED REFERENCES

1. Cassarino DS et al: Cutaneous squamous cell carcinoma: a comprehensive clinicopathologic classification. Part one. J Cutan Pathol. 33(3):191-206, 2006
2. Wong TY et al: Tricholemmal carcinoma. A clinicopathologic study of 13 cases. Am J Dermatopathol. 16(5):463-73, 1994
3. Boscaino A et al: Tricholemmal carcinoma: a study of seven cases. J Cutan Pathol. 19(2):94-9, 1992
4. Swanson PE et al: Tricholemmal carcinoma: clinicopathologic study of 10 cases. J Cutan Pathol. 19(2):100-9, 1992

IMAGE GALLERY

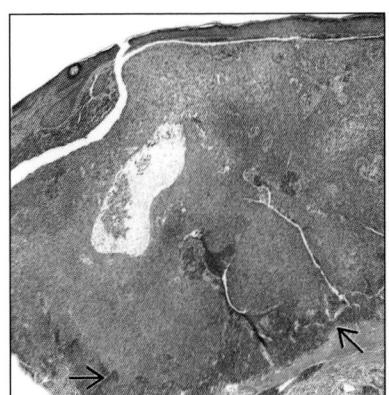 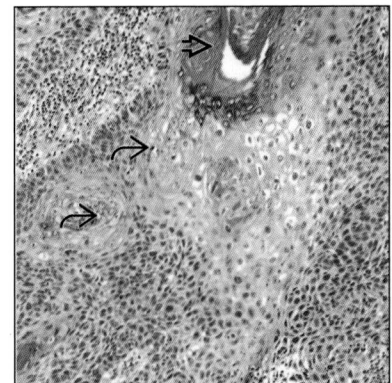 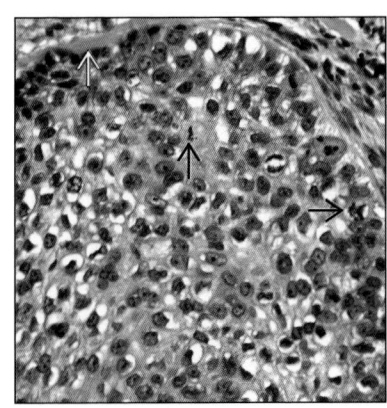

(Left) Scanning magnification of a TLC shows a large, multilobulated eosinophilic to clear cell neoplasm with irregular borders ➡ and relatively dense surrounding chronic inflammation. *(Center)* TLC often shows attachments to follicular structures ➡. The tumor cells show prominent enlargement and clear-staining cytoplasm with focal keratohyaline granules ➡. *(Right)* High magnification of a TLC shows prominent atypia, mitotic figures ➡, and a thickened basement membrane ➡.

PILOMATRIXOMA AND PILOMATRICAL CARCINOMA

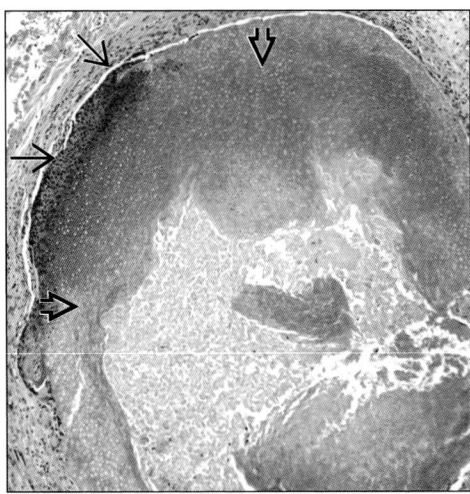

Low magnification of a pilomatrixoma shows a nodular-cystic dermal-based lesion with a thin, partial rim of peripheral basaloid cells ➡ surrounding central collections of eosinophilic and shadow cells ⇒.

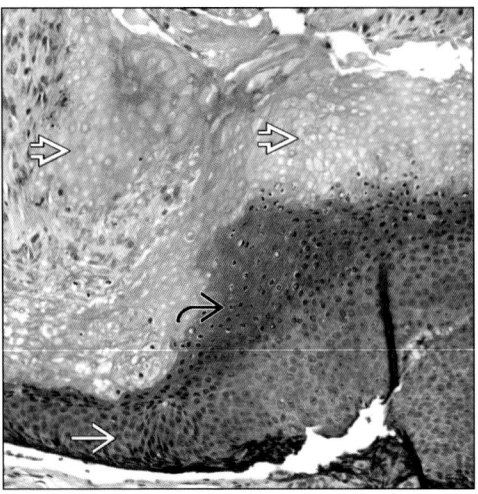

Higher magnification shows the 2 cell types of PMX: Basaloid ⇒ and shadow cells ⇒. In this case, transitional cells ↗ with pyknotic nuclei (prior to becoming shadow cells) are also seen.

TERMINOLOGY

Abbreviations
- Pilomatrixoma (PMX)

Synonyms
- Pilomatrixoma
  - Pilomatricoma
  - Calcifying epithelioma of Malherbe
  - Trichomatricoma
- Pilomatrical carcinoma
  - Matrical carcinoma
  - Malignant pilomatrixoma
  - Pilomatrix carcinoma

Definitions
- Pilomatrixoma
  - Benign dermal &/or subcutaneous tumor
  - Derived from matrical portion of hair follicle
- Pilomatrical carcinoma
  - Malignant counterpart of pilomatrixoma

ETIOLOGY/PATHOGENESIS

Differentiation
- Derived from matrix of hair follicle
- Mutation in the *CTNNB1* gene seen in both pilomatrixoma and pilomatrical carcinomas
  - *CTNNB1* gene encodes β-catenin

Genetics
- Rare cases are associated with myotonic dystrophy and Rubinstein-Taybi syndrome
  - Usually multiple pilomatrixomas present
- Cysts of Gardner syndrome can show pilomatricoma-like changes

CLINICAL ISSUES

Epidemiology
- Incidence
  - Pilomatrixoma
    - Relatively common
  - Pilomatrical carcinoma
    - Very rare
- Age
  - Pilomatrixoma
    - Young children (1st and 2nd decade)
    - Rare in adults
  - Pilomatrical carcinoma
    - Elderly
- Gender
  - Pilomatrixoma
    - No gender predilection
  - Pilomatrical carcinoma
    - Male predominance (M:F = 5:1)

Site
- Pilomatrixoma and pilomatrical carcinoma
  - Head and neck and upper limbs

Presentation
- Pilomatrixoma
  - Solitary, rarely multiple
  - Rubbery or hard
  - May be faceted, which lifts surface of skin
    - "Tent" sign is the appearance of skin when lifted by underlying pilomatrixoma
  - Rarely can perforate or rapidly enlarge
    - Rapid enlargement could be due to hematoma within tumor
- Pilomatrical carcinoma
  - Solitary
  - Usually occurs de novo
    - Rarely arises in preexisting pilomatrixoma (usually large, longstanding tumor)
  - Recurrence after excision is common

PILOMATRIXOMA AND PILOMATRICAL CARCINOMA

Key Facts

Terminology
- Calcifying epithelioma of Malherbe

Etiology/Pathogenesis
- Derived from matrix of hair follicle

Clinical Issues
- Pilomatrixoma
  - Relatively common, rubbery to hard solitary tumor mostly seen in young children
  - Head and neck and upper limbs
- Pilomatrical carcinoma
  - Very rare, solitary tumor of the elderly
  - Male predominance (M:F = 5:1)

Macroscopic Features
- On gross sectioning, PMX often shows chalky material due to calcifications

Microscopic Pathology
- Pilomatrixoma
  - Well-circumscribed, dermal to subcutaneous tumor with mixture of basaloid and shadow cells
  - Lesion often surrounded by fibrous connective tissue capsule
  - Dystrophic calcification is frequently seen
  - Foreign-body giant cell reaction surrounding tumor is common
- Pilomatrical carcinoma
  - Ulcerated, asymmetrical, dermal to subcutaneous nodule
  - Poorly circumscribed, cellular, and infiltrative tumor
  - Numerous mitoses and tumor necrosis often present

Treatment
- Surgical approaches
  - Pilomatrixoma
    - Simple excision is curative
  - Pilomatrical carcinoma
    - Wide local excision
    - Radiation &/or chemotherapy for recurrence and nodal metastasis

Prognosis
- Pilomatrixoma
  - Excellent
  - Very rare malignant transformation to pilomatrical carcinoma
- Pilomatrical carcinoma
  - Local recurrence is common if not widely excised
  - Metastasis is rare

MACROSCOPIC FEATURES

General Features
- Pilomatrixoma
  - On gross sectioning, chalky material due to calcification often found

Size
- Pilomatrixoma
  - 0.5-3 cm
- Pilomatrical carcinoma
  - 0.6-10 cm

MICROSCOPIC PATHOLOGY

Histologic Features
- Pilomatrixoma
  - Well-circumscribed, dermal to subcutaneous nodule
  - 2 cell types: Basaloid cells and shadow cells
    - Basaloid cells with variable thickness make up periphery of lesion
    - Basaloid cells are small, homogeneous, and monotonous
    - Basaloid cells have scant cytoplasm and indistinct cellular borders
    - Basaloid cells merge gradually or abruptly with keratinizing eosinophilic cells called shadow cells
    - Shadow cells have abundant pink cytoplasm and open space at their center where the nucleus used to be
    - Newer lesions usually have significant basaloid cells
    - Established lesions have predominately shadow cells
  - Lesion often surrounded by fibrous connective tissue capsule
  - Newer lesions might be cystic
  - Dystrophic calcification is commonly seen
    - Calcium deposits are seen in about 75% of tumors (can be highlighted with von Kossa stain)
    - They are present as fine granules within cytoplasm of shadow cells or as large deposits replacing shadow cells
  - Ossification is occasionally present
    - Seen in 15-20% of cases
    - Present in stroma near shadow cells
    - Older lesions have more calcification and ossification
  - Foreign-body giant cell reaction surrounding tumor is common
  - Melanin might be present
    - Melanin is often within shadow cells or melanophages of stroma
    - Melanocytic matricoma is a variant of pilomatrixoma with prominent dendritic melanocytes
  - Extramedullary hematopoiesis
    - Focal areas can rarely be present
- Pilomatrical carcinoma
  - Often connected to epidermis
  - Ulcerated, asymmetrical, dermal to subcutaneous nodule
  - Poorly circumscribed, cellular, and infiltrative
  - Focal areas of en masse necrosis
  - Basophilic cells

3

37

- Pleomorphic with prominent nucleoli
- Numerous mitoses
○ Foci of shadow cells are helpful in diagnosis
○ Rare vascular/lymphatic invasion
○ Melanocytes and melanin pigment within some tumors
  - Probably the malignant counterpart of melanocytic matricoma

Cytologic Features
- Pilomatrixoma
  ○ Basaloid cells
    - Deeply basophilic nuclei
    - Scant cytoplasm
    - Indistinct cell borders
    - Mitoses easily identified
  ○ Shadow cells
    - Central unstained areas where nuclei used to reside
    - Abundant eosinophilic cytoplasm
    - Distinct cell borders
- Pilomatrical carcinoma
  ○ Basaloid cells
    - Pleomorphic with prominent nucleoli
    - Numerous mitoses
  ○ Shadow cells
    - Same features as in PMX

ANCILLARY TESTS

Immunohistochemistry
- Hair matrix and precortex keratins are positive in pilomatrical carcinomas, as in PMX
  ○ hHa5 and hHa1
- β-catenin is positive, as in PMX
- Keratins 5, 14, and 17 often positive in pilomatrical carcinomas, but negative in PMX

DIFFERENTIAL DIAGNOSIS

DDx of Pilomatrixoma
- Basal cell carcinoma
  ○ Lacks shadow cells
  ○ Often has mucinous stroma
  ○ Often shows connections with overlying epidermis
  ○ Less likely to have calcifications and ossifications, although they may be present in some cases
  ○ Does not commonly have granulomatous inflammation, typically seen in PMX due to reaction to keratin
- Neuroendocrine (Merkel cell) carcinoma
  ○ Lacks shadow cells
  ○ Tumor often shows foci of trabecular pattern that might be limited to periphery of lesion
  ○ Cells are often small, uniform, hyperchromatic-staining and have vesicular nuclei with small nucleoli
  ○ Cytokeratin 20 stains tumoral cells in paranuclear dot-like pattern
- Proliferating tricholemmal cyst

○ On low power: Large symmetrical and well-circumscribed tumor, which may show cystic areas
○ Cells are squamoid with large eosinophilic cytoplasm, unlike basaloid small cells seen in PMX
○ Lacks shadow cells
- Melanocytic matricoma
  ○ Prominent pigment
  ○ Dendritic melanocytes present
  ○ Some consider this tumor to be a variant of PMX with dendritic melanocytes and melanin pigment

DDx of Pilomatrical Carcinoma
- Basal cell carcinoma with matrical differentiation
  ○ Very rare and difficult to differentiate from pilomatrical carcinoma
  ○ Considered to be basal cell carcinoma derived from hair follicle epithelium
    - Shadow cells present
    - β-catenin can be positive in both tumors and is not helpful in differentiating them
- Squamous cell carcinoma
  ○ Cells show more abundant and eosinophilic cytoplasm
  ○ Keratinization more common
  ○ Lacks shadow cells

DIAGNOSTIC CHECKLIST

Pathologic Interpretation Pearls
- Pilomatrixomas are well-circumscribed dermal tumors with peripheral basaloid cells that merge into shadow cells and often show calcification
- Pilomatrical carcinomas are very rare and, in the absence of shadow cells, can be difficult to diagnose

SELECTED REFERENCES
1. Nishioka M et al: Pilomatrix carcinoma arising from pilomatricoma after 10-year senescent period: Immunohistochemical analysis. J Dermatol. 37(8):735-9, 2010
2. Yadia S et al: Pilomatrix carcinoma of the thoracic spine: case report and review of the literature. J Spinal Cord Med. 33(3):272-7, 2010
3. Autelitano L et al: Pilomatrix carcinoma with visceral metastases: case report and review of the literature. J Plast Reconstr Aesthet Surg. 62(12):e574-7, 2009
4. Del Sordo R et al: Basal cell carcinoma with matrical differentiation: expression of beta-catenin [corrected] and osteopontin. Am J Dermatopathol. 2007 Oct;29(5):470-4. Erratum in: Am J Dermatopathol. 30(3):317, 2008
5. Lawrence C: Skin excision and osteophyte removal is not required in the surgical treatment of digital myxoid cysts. Arch Dermatol. 141(12):1560-4, 2005
6. Kim SH et al: Basal cell carcinoma with matrical differentiation. Yonsei Med J. 44(3):523-5, 2003
7. Haferkamp B et al: [Pilomatrix carcinoma in an unusual location. Case report and review of the literature.] Hautarzt. 50(5):355-9, 1999

PILOMATRIXOMA AND PILOMATRICAL CARCINOMA

Microscopic Features

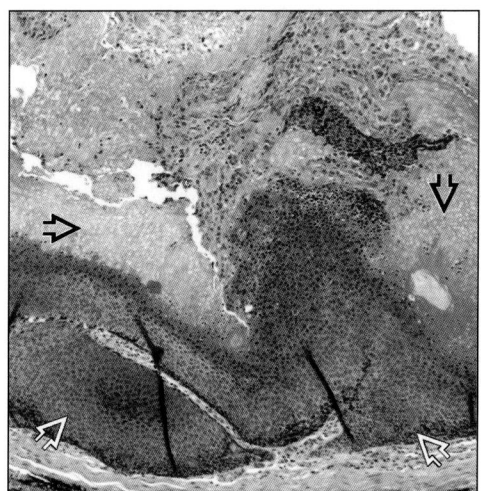

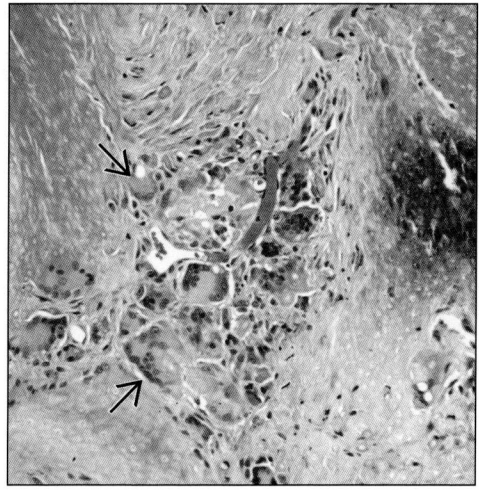

(Left) Basaloid cells with variable thickness make up the periphery of the lesion ➡, and they merge gradually or abruptly with keratinizing eosinophilic cells called shadow cells ➡. *(Right)* Foreign-body giant cell reaction ➡ to keratin often surrounds ruptured areas in pilomatrixomas.

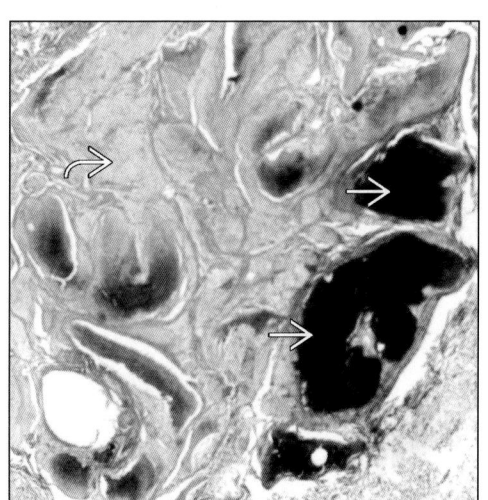

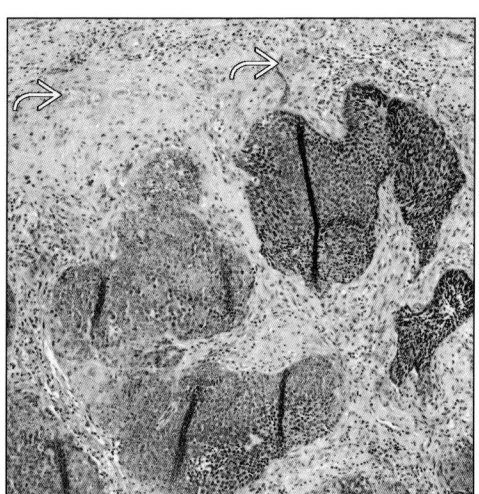

(Left) In older, or so-called "burned out" lesions, there are minimal to no basaloid cells, and the tumor is often composed only of shadow cells ➡ and large deposits of calcium ➡. *(Right)* Pilomatrical carcinomas typically show poor circumscription and an infiltrative pattern. The tumor is often composed predominately of basaloid cells, although larger, more squamoid-appearing cells can also be present ➡.

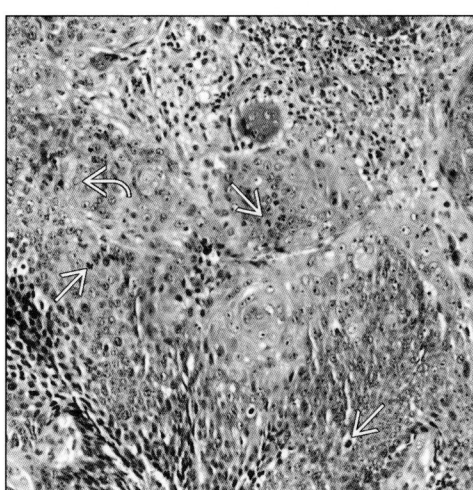

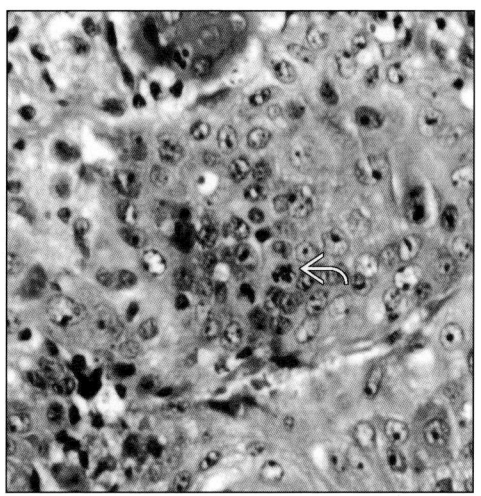

(Left) The basaloid cells, as in PMX, show foci of monotonous cells with scant cytoplasm and indistinct cellular borders ➡. However, in pilomatrical carcinoma, the cells are markedly atypical and pleomorphic appearing, and multiple mitotic figures are easily identified ➡. *(Right)* High magnification of pilomatrical carcinoma shows pleomorphic cells with prominent nucleoli and an atypical mitotic figure ➡. In the absence of shadow cells, it can be difficult to make this diagnosis.

FIBROFOLLICULOMA AND TRICHODISCOMA

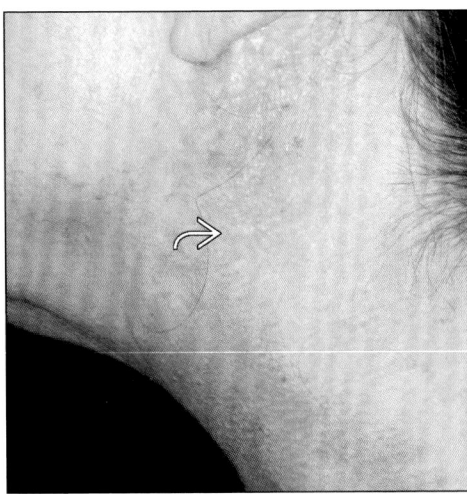

Clinical examination of a patient with Birt-Hogg-Dubé syndrome shows numerous small, flesh-colored papules on the lateral cheek and neck ➡. (Courtesy J. Wu, MD.)

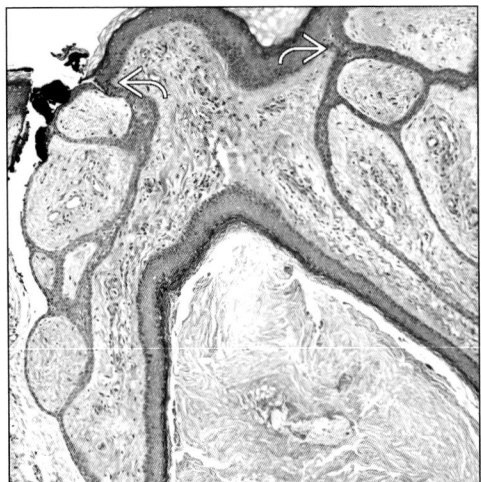

Fibrofolliculoma shows a central dilated (cystic) follicular structure with keratin debris. There are multiple thin, radiating epithelial strands attached to the overlying epidermis ➡.

TERMINOLOGY

Abbreviations
- Fibrofolliculoma (FF)
- Trichodiscoma (TD)

Synonyms
- Mantleoma (likely fibrofolliculoma variant with sebaceous differentiation)

Definitions
- Closely related hamartomatous proliferations with follicular and mesenchymal differentiation
- Trichodiscoma likely represents a late stage in evolution of fibrofolliculoma showing stromal predominance

ETIOLOGY/PATHOGENESIS

Genetic Syndrome
- Multiple lesions are strongly correlated with Birt-Hogg-Dubé syndrome (BHD)
  - Due to mutations in folliculin (*FLCN*) gene
    - Tumor suppressor gene that interacts with TGF-beta signaling pathway
  - High risk of internal malignancies, especially renal cell carcinoma
    - Often low-grade chromophobe or mixed chromophobe/oncocytoma type
  - Also predisposed to pulmonary cysts and pneumothoraces

CLINICAL ISSUES

Epidemiology
- Incidence
  - Very rare lesions
- Age

  - Usually present in young adults, especially in Birt-Hogg-Dubé syndrome
- Gender
  - More common in men

Site
- Facial area most common but also may involve other head and neck sites, trunk, and arms

Presentation
- Small, asymptomatic papule(s) on face
  - Usually multiple (even hundreds), especially in BHD
- Typically small, smooth dome-shaped lesions

Treatment
- Options, risks, complications
  - Excision is curative but not necessary in most cases given the benign nature of these lesions
  - Work-up for underlying disease (including renal cell carcinoma) is indicated for patients suspected of having syndromic form

Prognosis
- Skin lesions are completely benign
- Patients with BHD syndrome have high incidence of internal organ involvement, which may be fatal

MICROSCOPIC PATHOLOGY

Histologic Features
- **Fibrofolliculoma**
  - Bland epithelial proliferation composed of thin, anastomosing cords
    - Numerous attachments to follicular structures and epidermis present
    - Cells are small, bland-appearing basaloid to squamoid cells
  - Typically a central, dilated follicular structure is present

FIBROFOLLICULOMA AND TRICHODISCOMA

Key Facts

Terminology
- Closely related hamartomas with follicular and mesenchymal differentiation

Etiology/Pathogenesis
- Multiple lesions are strongly correlated with Birt-Hogg-Dubé syndrome
  - High risk of renal cell carcinoma
  - Also, pulmonary cysts and pneumothoraces

Clinical Issues
- Small papule(s) on face

Microscopic Pathology
- FF shows proliferation of thin, anastomosing epithelial cords
- Numerous attachments to follicular structures and epidermis
- Typically find a central, dilated follicular structure
- **TD** is a stromal-predominant lesion

- Fibromyxoid stroma, similar to trichodiscoma, with decreased or lost elastic fibers
- **Trichodiscoma**
  - Stromal-predominant lesion
  - Consists of a proliferation of small, bland-appearing fibroblastic cells within a loose, fibromyxoid stroma
    - Elastic fibers markedly reduced or absent
  - Peripheral follicular structure and epithelial strands usually present
    - May need to examine multiple deeper level sections to identify

DIFFERENTIAL DIAGNOSIS

Tumor of the Follicular Infundibulum
- Superficial, plate-like proliferation of bland pale to clear squamoid cells
- Anastomosing strands of epithelium present, but they are usually thicker than those in fibrofolliculoma
- Multiple follicles merge with undersurface of tumor
- Lacks fibromyxoid stroma of fibrofolliculoma and trichodiscoma

Inverted Follicular Keratosis
- Endophytic epithelial proliferation with numerous squamous eddies
  - Cells are larger and more squamoid appearing than those in fibrofolliculoma
- Typically shows multiple pseudohorn cysts, supporting theory that these are variants of irritated seborrheic keratoses

- Lacks fibromyxoid stroma of fibrofolliculoma and trichodiscoma

Basal Cell Carcinoma, Infundibulocystic Type
- BCC shows areas of peripheral palisading and tumor-stromal retraction artifact
- Tumor cells are larger and more atypical, with hyperchromatic nuclei and multiple mitotic and apoptotic figures
- Mucinous stroma usually prominent (less fibromyxoid than that in fibrofolliculoma and trichodiscoma)

SELECTED REFERENCES

1. Menko FH et al: Birt-Hogg-Dubé syndrome: diagnosis and management. Lancet Oncol. 10(12):1199-206, 2009
2. Toro JR et al: BHD mutations, clinical and molecular genetic investigations of Birt-Hogg-Dubé syndrome: a new series of 50 families and a review of published reports. J Med Genet. 45(6):321-31, 2008
3. Toro JR: Birt-Hogg-Dubé syndrome. GeneReviews [Internet]. 1-12, 2006
4. Schmidt LS: Birt-Hogg-Dubé syndrome, a genodermatosis that increases risk for renal carcinoma. Curr Mol Med. 4(8):877-85, 2004
5. Ubogy-Rainey Z et al: Fibrofolliculomas, trichodiscomas, and acrochordons: the Birt-Hogg-Dubé syndrome. J Am Acad Dermatol. 16(2 Pt 2):452-7, 1987
6. Birt AR et al: Hereditary multiple fibrofolliculomas with trichodiscomas and acrochordons. Arch Dermatol. 113(12):1674-7, 1977

IMAGE GALLERY

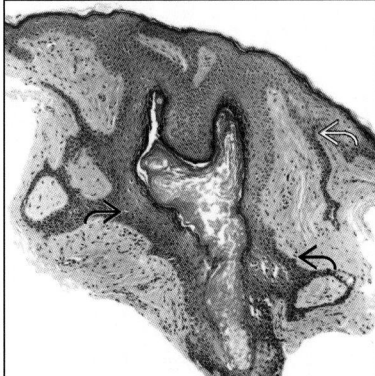 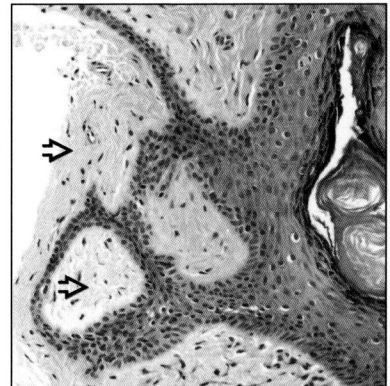 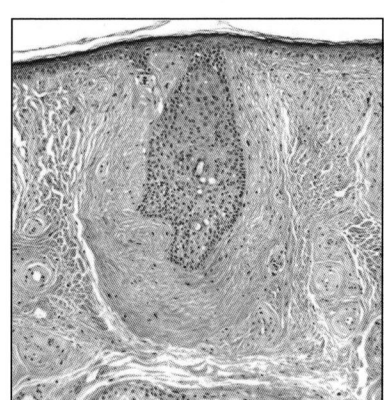

(Left) Fibrofolliculoma shows a central follicular structure with a dilated lumen and thin, radiating epithelial strands attached to both the follicle ⮕ and the epidermis ⮕. *(Center)* High magnification shows the radiating epithelial strands consisting of small, bland squamous cells embedded in a fibromyxoid stroma ⮕. *(Right)* Trichodiscoma is composed mostly of fibromyxoid stroma, but will often demonstrate a follicular structure if multiple deeper level sections are examined.

Tumors and Tumor-like Conditions with Sebaceous Differentiation

SEBACEOUS HYPERPLASIA

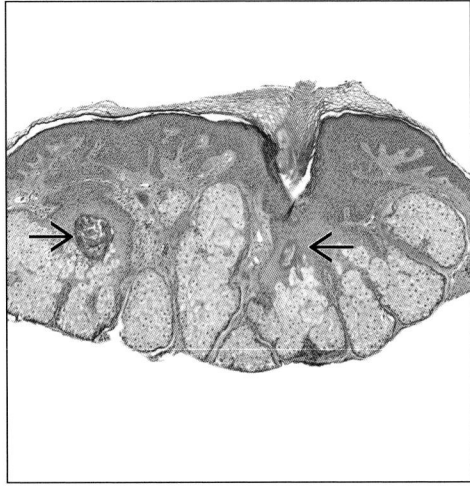

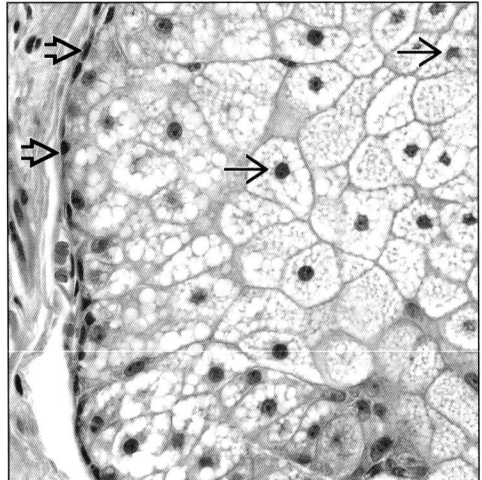

H&E shows low-magnification view of sebaceous hyperplasia. There are normal-appearing lobules of sebocytes surrounding invaginations of epidermis that resemble the infundibulum of hair follicles ➡.

High-magnification view of the edge of a lobule of sebocytes shows that central sebocytes ➡ with round to scalloped nuclei and bubbly cytoplasm are rimmed by a compressed layer of small, basaloid cells ➡.

TERMINOLOGY

Definitions
- Benign
- Hyperplasia (overgrowth) of sebaceous glands
- Plump lobules of sebaceous glands arranged around central follicles

CLINICAL ISSUES

Site
- Commonly on face
- Rarely on the trunk or other sites

Presentation
- Yellow to flesh-colored to slightly pink papule
- Often there is central dell
- Telangiectasias may be present
- Often biopsied to rule out basal cell carcinoma

Laboratory Tests
- Generally not performed
- Some have suggested that sebaceous hyperplasia on sites other than face is sufficiently rare
  - Recommend evaluation for Muir-Torre syndrome
    - Clinical history and examination
    - Immunohistochemical testing for mismatch repair proteins (e.g., MSH-2, MLH-1)
    - Microsatellite instability testing
    - Mutation analysis

Treatment
- Not necessary
- Biopsy (shave removal) may be curative

Prognosis
- Benign
- No malignant potential

MACROSCOPIC FEATURES

Dermoscopic Findings
- "Crown-like," thin, red vessels
- Vessels surround white to yellow globules

MICROSCOPIC PATHOLOGY

Histologic Features
- Lobules of sebocytes
  - Arranged around infundibulum of central hair follicle
  - Rarely connect to epidermal surface
- Basaloid cells
  - 1 layer of basaloid cells compressed at periphery of sebocytes
  - Layers of basaloid cells not increased in number

Cytologic Features
- No cytologic atypia
- Sebocytes
  - Round to scalloped central nucleus
  - Bubbly cytoplasm

DIFFERENTIAL DIAGNOSIS

Sebaceous Adenoma
- May have a similar low-power architecture to sebaceous hyperplasia
  - Sebocytes in lobules in clusters or around follicle
- Several layers of basaloid cells bordering sebocytes

Nevus Sebaceus
- Lobules of sebocytes directly connecting to epidermal surface
- Germinative (basaloid) cell layers not increased
- Abortive/vellus follicles may be present
- Apocrine glands may be present in deep dermis

SEBACEOUS HYPERPLASIA

Key Facts

Clinical Issues
- Commonly on face
- Yellow to flesh-colored to slightly pink papule
- Often there is central dell
- Often biopsied to rule out basal cell carcinoma

Microscopic Pathology
- Lobules of sebocytes arranged around infundibulum of central hair follicle

- 1 layer of basaloid cells compressed at periphery of sebocytes
- No cytologic atypia

Top Differential Diagnoses
- Sebaceous adenoma
- Ectopic sebaceous glands in other sites (e.g., nipple)
- Phymatous rosacea
- Sebaceous trichofolliculoma
- Folliculosebaceous (cystic) hamartoma

Ectopic Sebaceous Glands in Other Sites
- Montgomery tubercle
  - Sebaceous glands on nipple
  - Lobules of sebocytes directly connecting to epithelial surface
- Fordyce spot
  - Sebaceous glands on mucosa
  - Lobules of sebocytes directly connecting to epithelial surface

Phymatous Rosacea
- Prominent sebaceous glands, edema, and fibrosis on different sites
  - Rhinophyma (nose)
  - Otophyma (ear)
  - Gnatophyma (chin)
  - Metophyma (forehead)
  - Blepharophyma (eyelid)
- Clinical history is key

Sebaceous Trichofolliculoma
- Central main follicle
- Surrounding secondary hair follicles
- Sebaceous glands seen connecting to hair follicles

Folliculosebaceous (Cystic) Hamartoma
- Central dilated infundibulum
  - May be so dilated as to be cystic
  - Surrounding sebaceous glands and hair follicles
- Fibrocytic stroma

Sebaceous Induction
- Sebaceous glands connecting to epidermal surface
- May be seen above dermatofibroma

Juxtaclavicular Beaded Lines
- Hypertrophy of hair follicles and associated sebaceous glands on neck/upper trunk
- Clinical history is key

DIAGNOSTIC CHECKLIST

Pathologic Interpretation Pearls
- Normal sebocytes in lobules
- Single layer of compressed basaloid cells
- Lobules of sebocytes surround infundibulum of hair follicle
- No atypia

SELECTED REFERENCES

1. Gupta M et al: Otophyma: a rare and frequently misdiagnosed entity. Am J Otolaryngol. 31(3):199-201, 2010
2. Zalaudek I et al: How to diagnose nonpigmented skin tumors: a review of vascular structures seen with dermoscopy: part II. Nonmelanocytic skin tumors. J Am Acad Dermatol. 63(3):377-86; quiz 387-8, 2010
3. Eisen DB et al: Sebaceous lesions and their associated syndromes: part I. J Am Acad Dermatol. 61(4):549-60; quiz 561-2, 2009

IMAGE GALLERY

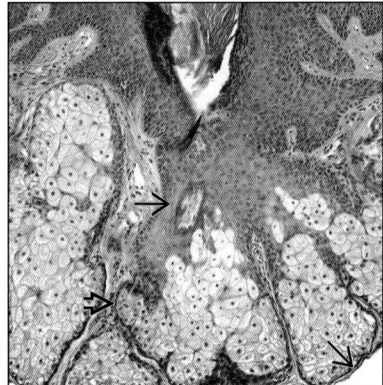 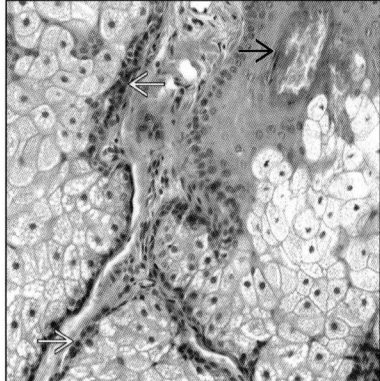 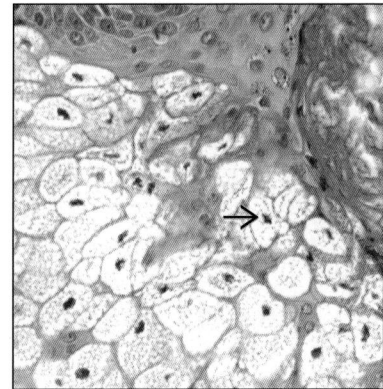

(Left) Lobules of sebocytes surround an invagination of epidermis ➡ that resembles the infundibulum of a hair follicle. The lobules of sebocytes are rimmed by a compressed layer of small basaloid cells ➡. *(Center)* High magnification shows lobules of sebocytes that are rimmed by compressed basaloid cells ➡, surrounding an infundibulum-like structure ➡. *(Right)* High-power view of sebocytes shows bubbly cytoplasm and a central round or scalloped ➡ nucleus.

SEBACEOMA (SEBACEOUS EPITHELIOMA)

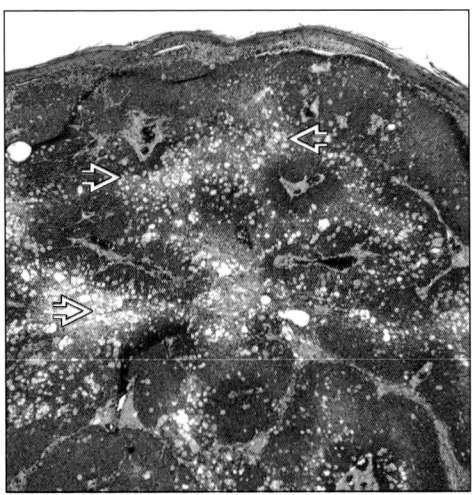

Low magnification of a sebaceoma shows a dermal-based basaloid to clear cell neoplasm with peripheral basaloid cells surrounding central collections of clear cells ⮞ and sebaceous secretions.

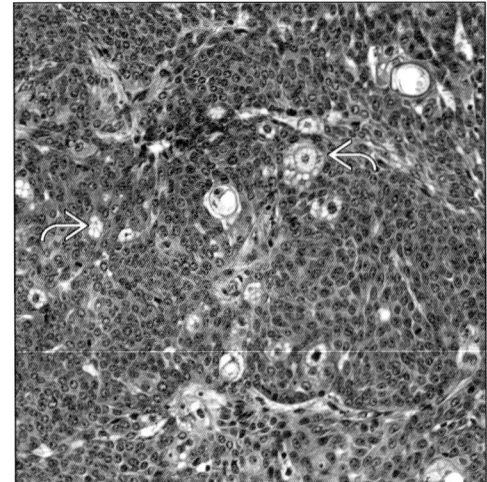

High magnification of a sebaceoma shows a predominantly basaloid population of cells surrounding several large clear cells ⮞ with abundant, multivacuolated cytoplasm.

TERMINOLOGY

Synonyms
- Sebaceous epithelioma (older term, should be discouraged)

Definitions
- Benign proliferation of mature sebaceous cells associated with a predominant basaloid cell population

ETIOLOGY/PATHOGENESIS

Unknown in Most Cases
- Some cases are part of Muir-Torre syndrome (MTS)
  - Autosomal dominant disease due to mutations in mismatch repair genes *MLH1*, *MSH2*, *MSH6*
  - Patients present with multiple sebaceous tumors including sebaceous adenomas, sebaceomas, and sebaceous carcinomas
  - Also associated with internal malignancies including gastrointestinal carcinomas (most common), genitourinary, breast, and ovarian tumors
- Rare cases arise in nevus sebaceous of Jadassohn

CLINICAL ISSUES

Epidemiology
- Incidence
  - Rare tumors
- Age
  - Typically occur in adults

Site
- Often occur on face, but may also present on trunk

Presentation
- Slow-growing papular to nodular lesion

- Usually single, but may be multiple, especially in MTS
- Flesh-colored to yellowish

Treatment
- Surgical approaches
  - Complete conservative excision is curative

Prognosis
- Excellent; very low malignant potential
  - Possible transformation to sebaceous carcinoma in longstanding lesions

MACROSCOPIC FEATURES

Size
- Usually measure between 0.5-3 cm in diameter

MICROSCOPIC PATHOLOGY

Histologic Features
- Nodular, dermal-based adnexal tumor
  - Usually located in mid to upper dermis
  - Well-circumscribed, noninfiltrative appearing
  - May show association with hair follicle in some cases
  - Epidermal attachments in rare cases
  - Cysts and (sebaceous) ductal structures often present
  - Rare apocrine differentiation has been reported
- Composed mostly of immature-appearing basaloid cells
  - Basaloid cells may show mild cytologic atypia and increased mitotic figures
  - Atypical mitoses should be absent
- Minority of tumor consists of clear cells with multivacuolated cytoplasm, consistent with mature sebaceous cells
  - Show nuclear hyperchromasia with indentations, typical of sebocytes

SEBACEOMA (SEBACEOUS EPITHELIOMA)

Key Facts

Terminology
- Sebaceous epithelioma is older term (discouraged)
- Benign proliferation of mature sebaceous cells with predominant basaloid cell population

Etiology/Pathogenesis
- Some cases are part of Muir-Torre syndrome
  - Autosomal dominant disease due to mutations in mismatch repair genes *MLH1*, *MSH2*, *MSH6*
- Multiple sebaceous tumors including sebaceous adenomas > carcinomas and sebaceomas

Clinical Issues
- Rare tumors; typically occur in adults
- Most common on the face
- Usually single but may be multiple, especially in MTS patients

Microscopic Pathology
- Nodular, dermal-based adnexal tumor
- Well-circumscribed, noninfiltrative appearing
- Composed mostly of basaloid cells
- Minor population of clear cells with multivacuolated cytoplasm, consistent with mature sebaceous cells
  - Show nuclear hyperchromasia with indentations
- Basaloid cells may show mild cytologic atypia and increased mitotic figures
- Sebaceous cells do not show significant atypia or mitotic activity

Top Differential Diagnoses
- Basal cell carcinoma with sebaceous differentiation, sebaceous carcinoma, sebaceous adenoma, trichoblastoma with sebaceous differentiation

---

- Sebaceous cells do not show significant atypia or mitotic activity
- Rarely, overlying changes similar to verruca vulgaris or seborrheic keratosis may be seen
- **Rippled pattern sebaceoma**: Rare variant showing palisading of basaloid nuclei
  - Similar to rippled pattern trichoblastoma but lacks evidence of follicular differentiation

ANCILLARY TESTS

Immunohistochemistry
- EMA usually positive in clear cells; BER-EP4 negative (+ in BCC)
- Low p53, Ki-67 (higher in sebaceous carcinoma)

DIFFERENTIAL DIAGNOSIS

Basal Cell Carcinoma (BCC) with Sebaceous Differentiation
- Basal cells show greater atypia and peripheral palisading
- Mucinous stroma and retraction artifact often present (lacking in sebaceoma)
- Some cases have previously been reported as "sebaceous epithelioma"; therefore, this term is confusing and should not be used

Sebaceous Carcinoma
- Sebaceous cells show greater cytologic atypia and pleomorphism
- Mitotic figures usually numerous and often atypical
- Basaloid sebaceous carcinoma can be very difficult to separate from sebaceoma in some cases, especially in small, partial biopsies
  - If findings are not definitive in partial biopsy, complete excision should be recommended to allow for definitive diagnosis

Sebaceous Adenoma
- Mature sebaceous cells predominate over basaloid cells

- Basaloid cells confined to peripheral layers of sebaceous lobules
- Frequent attachment to hair follicles and epidermis

Trichoblastoma with Sebaceous Differentiation
- Typically larger, deeper dermal nodular lesions
- Sebaceous differentiation, when present, is very focal
- Areas of follicular differentiation, including papillary mesenchymal bodies and infundibulocystic structures with keratin debris
- May show rippled pattern in rare cases, similar to rippled pattern sebaceoma

Superficial Epithelioma with Sebaceous Differentiation
- Very rare, solitary lesion that presents on face in older adults
- Superficial, plate-like proliferation with multiple attachments to the epidermis (similar to tumor of the follicular infundibulum)
  - Composed mostly of basaloid to squamoid cells with scattered clusters of mature sebocytes

SELECTED REFERENCES

1. Yang HM et al: Immunohistochemical expression of D2-40 in benign and malignant sebaceous tumors and comparison to basal and squamous cell carcinomas. Am J Dermatopathol. 30(6):549-54, 2008
2. Fan YS et al: Characteristic Ber-EP4 and EMA expression in sebaceoma is immunohistochemically distinct from basal cell carcinoma. Histopathology. 51(1):80-6, 2007
3. Lazar AJ et al: Sebaceous neoplasia and Torre-Muir syndrome. Curr Diagn Pathol. 13(4):301-319, 2007
4. Cabral ES et al: Distinction of benign sebaceous proliferations from sebaceous carcinomas by immunohistochemistry. Am J Dermatopathol. 28(6):465-71, 2006
5. Misago N et al: Basal cell carcinoma with sebaceous differentiation. Am J Dermatopathol. 26(4):298-303, 2004
6. Troy JL et al: Sebaceoma. A distinctive benign neoplasm of adnexal epithelium differentiating toward sebaceous cells. Am J Dermatopathol. 6(1):7-13, 1984

SEBACEOMA (SEBACEOUS EPITHELIOMA)

Microscopic and Immunohistochemical Features

(Left) Low magnification of a sebaceoma shows a dermal-based basaloid to clear cell neoplasm with peripheral basaloid cells surrounding clear cells ➔, sebaceous secretions, and a focal cystic space ⇨. *(Right)* Intermediate magnification of a cystic area of sebaceoma shows a proliferation of predominantly basaloid ⇨ and focal clear cells ➔ surrounding the cystic space.

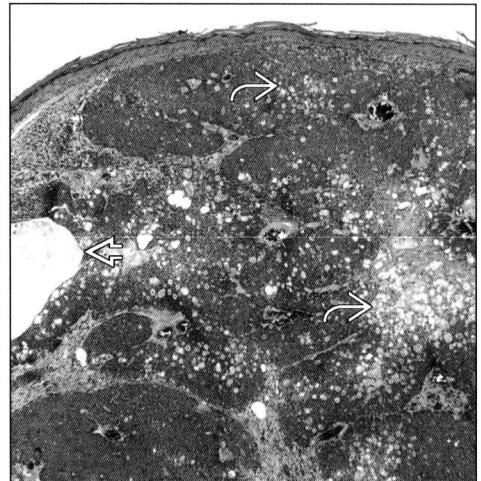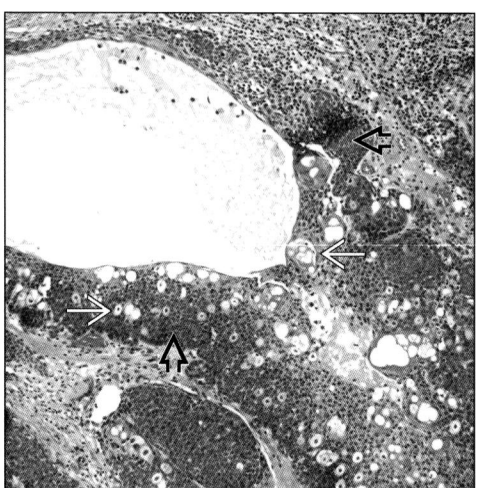

(Left) Higher magnification of sebaceoma showing a superficial, well-circumscribed lobule of predominantly basaloid cells with a smaller population of bland-appearing, mature sebaceous cells ⇨. *(Right)* High magnification of a sebaceoma shows a population of scattered bland-appearing, multivacuolated clear cells demonstrating nuclear hyperchromasia and nuclear indentations ➔, which are due to cytoplasmic lipids.

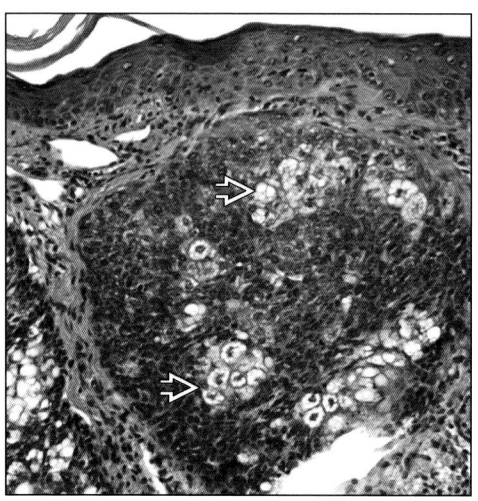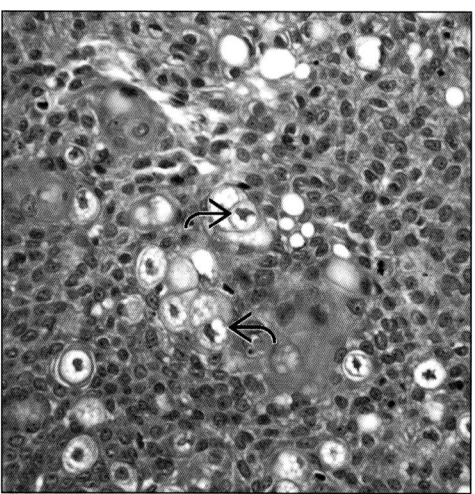

(Left) Podoplanin (D2-40) is often moderately to strongly positive in sebaceoma (especially in the basaloid cells ⇨), but usually weak to absent in sebaceous carcinoma. *(Right)* Ki-67 immunohistochemistry highlights many of the peripheral basaloid cells ➔, but note its complete absence of staining in the large clear cells ⇨ (which are also positive in sebaceous carcinoma). Both Ki-67 and p53 are typically low in sebaceomas, but elevated in sebaceous carcinomas.

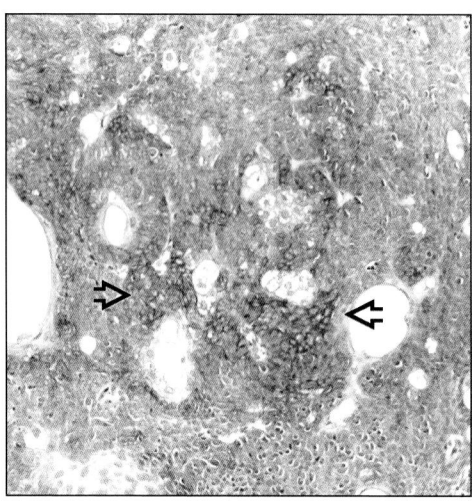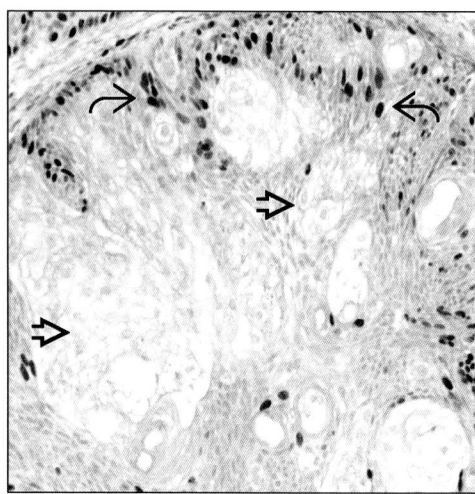

SEBACEOMA (SEBACEOUS EPITHELIOMA)

Differential Diagnosis

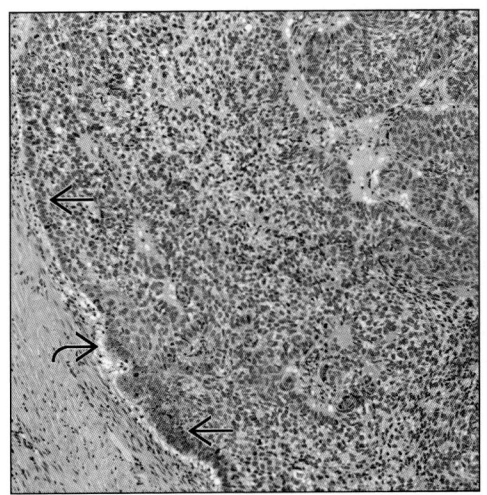
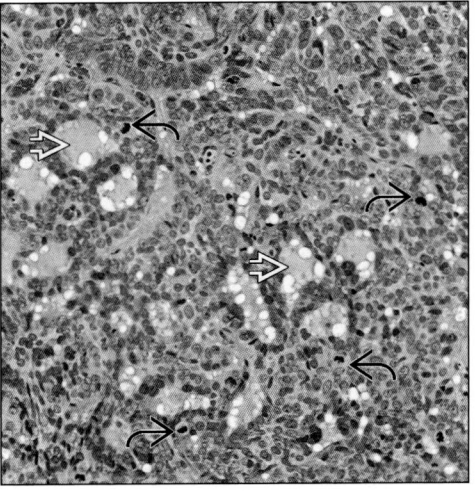

(Left) Basal cell carcinoma (BCC) with clear cell features. This is a nodular and adenoid-type BCC with areas of clear cell change. Note the peripheral palisading ⇨ and tumor-stromal retraction artifact ⇨ with mucinous material in the retraction space, findings lacking in sebaceoma. (Right) Higher magnification of BCC with adenoid features shows prominent pools of mucin ⇨ within the tumor. Numerous mitotic figures ⇨ are easily found.

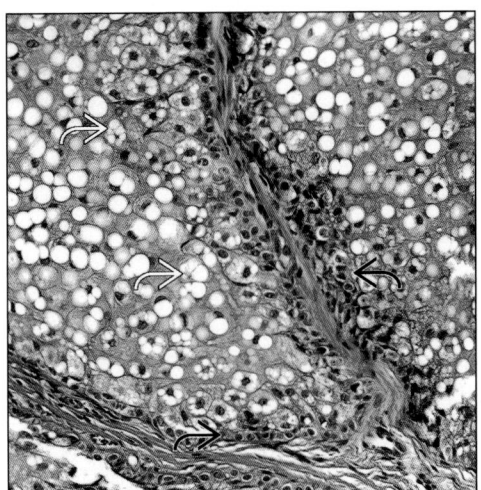
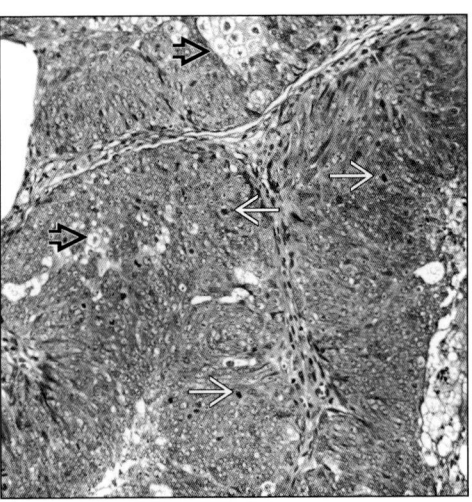

(Left) Sebaceous adenoma is a benign sebaceous tumor characterized by a predominant population of enlarged bland, clear-staining multivacuolated sebocytes ⇨, with only a minor component of peripheral, small basaloid cells ⇨. (Right) Basaloid sebaceous carcinoma shows prominent nuclear crowding and hyperchromasia with increased mitotic figures ⇨ in the basaloid population. Scattered well-differentiated sebaceous cells ⇨ are present.

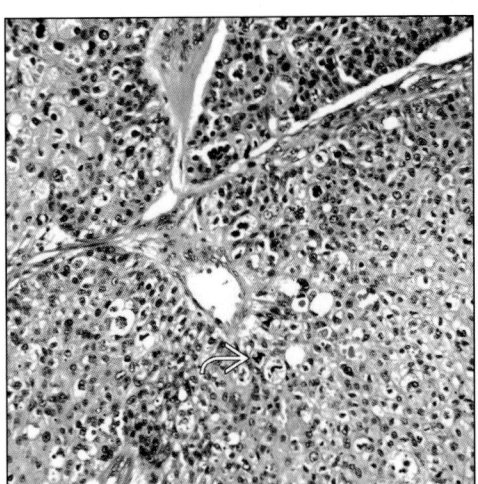
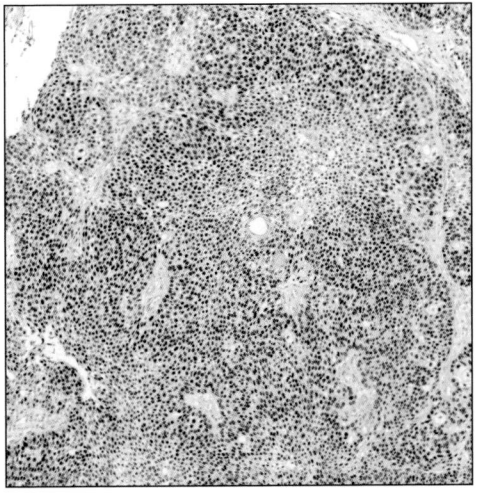

(Left) High-grade sebaceous carcinoma shows larger basaloid to squamoid and clear cells with prominent nuclear atypia with hyperchromasia, enlarged nucleoli, and multiple mitotic figures ⇨. (Right) p53 immunohistochemistry shows very strong, diffuse nuclear staining in a sebaceous carcinoma. Sebaceoma typically shows low p53 staining and a low nuclear proliferative rate by Ki-67 (< 20% of cells staining).

SEBACEOUS ADENOMA

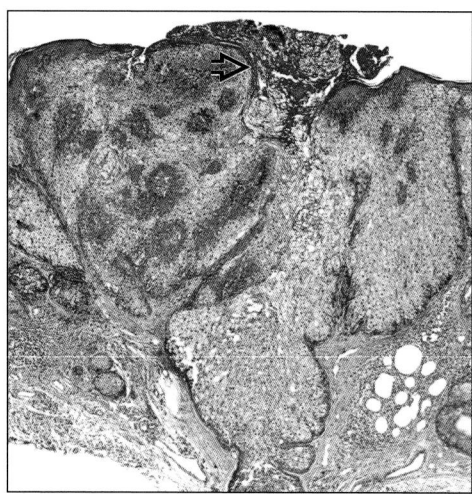

In this low magnification of a large sebaceous adenoma, the tumor is a well-circumscribed, multilobular proliferation with multiple attachments to the epidermis and superficial holocrine necrosis ⊳.

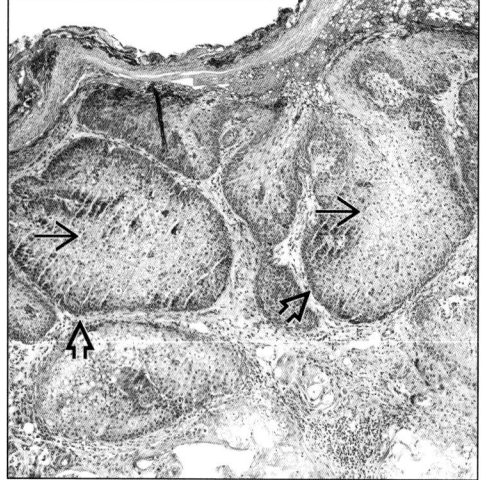

Higher magnification of the lobules shows central sebocytes ⊳ and peripheral basaloid cells ⊳. The basaloid cells form more than 1 layer at the periphery of lobules.

TERMINOLOGY

Definitions
- Benign tumor
- More than 50% of the tumor is composed of sebocytes
- More than 1 layer of basaloid/germinative cells at periphery of sebocyte-filled lobules

CLINICAL ISSUES

Site
- Often on the head and neck, but any site possible

Presentation
- Yellow, tan, to pink papule

Treatment
- Reexcision not necessary

Prognosis
- Benign tumor
- No malignant potential

Associated Syndromes
- Even 1 sebaceous adenoma can be associated with Muir-Torre syndrome
  - Muir-Torre syndrome
    - Defined as the association of sebaceous tumors (sebaceous adenoma, sebaceoma, sebaceous carcinoma) or multiple keratoacanthomas with internal malignancy
    - May be autosomal dominant; thus, syndrome has implications for screening of family members
    - Proportion of Muir-Torre cases are a subset of Lynch (hereditary nonpolyposis colon cancer) syndrome
    - At a minimum, patients should have age-appropriate screening for internal malignancy

- If desired, immunohistochemistry (MSH2, MLH1, possibly MLH6) &/or microsatellite instability testing can be performed on tumor tissue
- Loss of immunohistochemical staining with MSH2, MLH1 (or possibly MLH6), &/or presence of microsatellite instability are supportive of hereditary germline mutation

MICROSCOPIC PATHOLOGY

Histologic Features
- Lobular downgrowth from the epidermis
- Predominance (> 50%) of mature sebocytes
- Basaloid/germinative cells at periphery of lobules form more than 1 layer
  - Generally cytokeratin 7 positive
- Sebocytes arranged centrally, basaloid/germinative cells peripherally
- Cytologic atypia not prominent

Cytologic Features
- Sebocytes
  - Central, scalloped/crenulated nuclei
  - Bubbly, multivacuolated cytoplasm
  - Positive with EMA or androgen receptor
- Basaloid/germinative cells
  - Round nuclei with small nucleoli
  - Minimal cytoplasm

DIFFERENTIAL DIAGNOSIS

Sebaceoma
- Composed of > 50% germinative/basaloid cells
- < 50% sebocytes
- Sebocytes and germinative/basaloid cells often arranged haphazardly
- May or may not connect to epidermis

SEBACEOUS ADENOMA

Key Facts

Clinical Issues
- Often on the head and neck, but any site possible
- Yellow, tan, to pink papule
- Even 1 sebaceous adenoma can be associated with Muir-Torre syndrome, which is the association of sebaceous tumors or multiple keratoacanthomas with internal malignancy

Microscopic Pathology
- Lobular downgrowth from epidermis

- Predominance (> 50%) of sebocytes
  - Located centrally within lobules
- Basaloid/germinative cells at periphery of lobules
- Cytologic atypia not prominent

Top Differential Diagnoses
- Sebaceoma
- Sebaceous hyperplasia
- Clear cell basal cell carcinoma
- Tricholemmoma

Sebaceous Hyperplasia
- Superficial sebaceous lobules surrounding dilated follicle/pore
- Lobules increased in number, but normal in size
- 1 layer of germinative/basaloid cells at periphery of sebocytes

Clear Cell Basal Cell Carcinoma
- Clear cells in variably sized islands
- Clear cells characterized by
  - Lack of scalloped nuclei
  - Cytoplasm not truly bubbly
- Some islands show peripheral palisading
- Positive with BER-EP4

Tricholemmoma
- Lobular downgrowth from epidermis
- Cells are pale/clear
- Clear cells lack scalloped nuclei and cytoplasm not truly bubbly
- Peripheral palisading with thickened basement membrane at periphery of lobules
- Surface may be papillated/verrucous

Nevus Sebaceus
- Lobular downgrowth of sebaceous glands from epidermis
- Absence of mature hair follicles
- Basaloid proliferations (i.e., trichoblastoma) may be present
- Apocrine glands may be present in deep dermis

Sebaceous Carcinoma
- Often larger, infiltrative tumors
- Basaloid/germinative cells generally predominate
- Often prominent cytologic atypia
- Numerous mitoses

DIAGNOSTIC CHECKLIST

Pathologic Interpretation Pearls
- Lobular downgrowth from the epidermis
- Predominance (> 50%) of sebocytes
  - Located centrally within lobules
- Basaloid/germinative cells at periphery of lobules form more than 1 layer
- Cytologic atypia not prominent

SELECTED REFERENCES

1. Ko CJ: Muir-Torre syndrome: Facts and controversies. Clin Dermatol. 28(3):324-9, 2010
2. Shalin SC et al: Sebaceous neoplasia and the Muir-Torre syndrome: important connections with clinical implications. Histopathology. 56(1):133-47, 2010
3. Eisen DB et al: Sebaceous lesions and their associated syndromes: part I. J Am Acad Dermatol. 61(4):549-60; quiz 561-2, 2009
4. Cabral ES et al: Distinction of benign sebaceous proliferations from sebaceous carcinomas by immunohistochemistry. Am J Dermatopathol. 28(6):465-71, 2006

IMAGE GALLERY

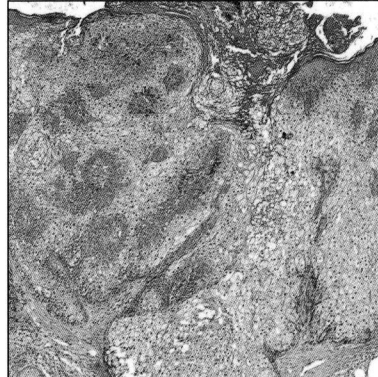 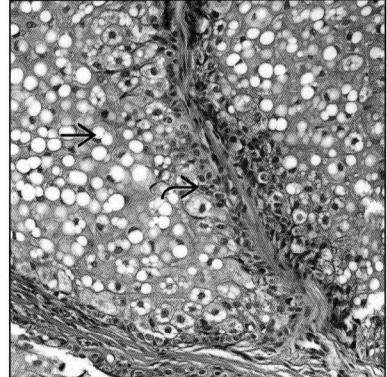 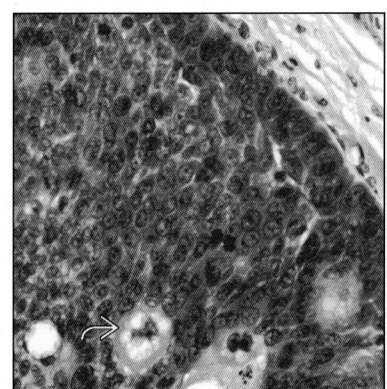

(Left) Low-power view of a sebaceous adenoma shows lobules of sebocytes with peripheral basaloid cells, descending from the surface of the epidermis. *(Center)* Sebocytes have central, scalloped/crenulated nuclei with bubbly cytoplasm ➡. Basaloid/germinative cells rim the sebocytes ➡. *(Right)* The differential diagnosis includes sebaceoma. Sebaceoma shows numerous crowded basaloid cells surrounding a few large clear cells with abundant, multivacuolated cytoplasm ➡.

SEBACEOUS CARCINOMA

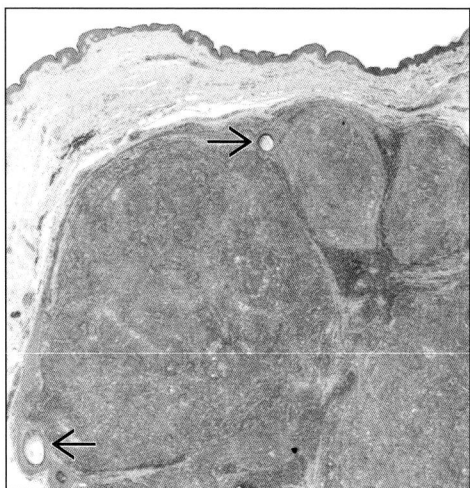

Scanning magnification of a sebaceous carcinoma shows a very large, nodular tumor in the dermis. Note the lack of epidermal attachments; however, there are focal entrapped follicular structures ➡.

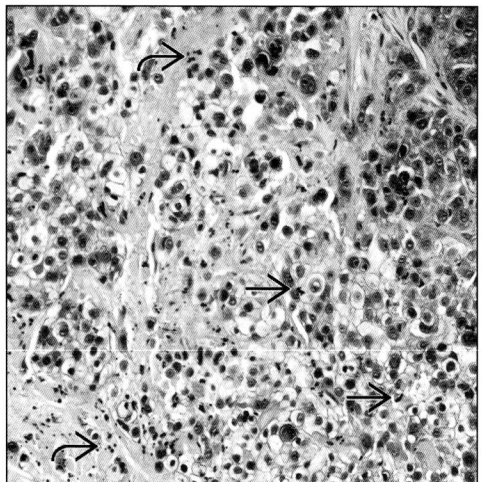

Higher power examination of a sebaceous carcinoma shows a proliferation of markedly atypical clear cells with numerous mitotic figures ➡ and abundant apoptotic cellular debris ➡.

TERMINOLOGY

Synonyms
- Sebaceous adenocarcinoma

Definitions
- Malignant adnexal tumor of sebaceous cells
- Often lacks clear cell features in poorly differentiated cases and may show basaloid or squamoid features, leading to high incidence of misdiagnosis

ETIOLOGY/PATHOGENESIS

Unknown in Most Cases
- Some cases likely due to solar (UV) damage, as most occur on sun-damaged skin of elderly

Genetic
- Strong association with Muir-Torre syndrome (MTS) in patients who have multiple sebaceous tumors &/or multiple keratoacanthomas and internal organ malignancies
  - Genes implicated include *MLH1, MSH2, MSH6*
    - Encode mismatch repair proteins
    - Mutations lead to microsatellite instability (MSI)
    - MSI assays and immunohistochemistry can be used to screen for Muir-Torre syndrome

CLINICAL ISSUES

Epidemiology
- Incidence
  - Uncommon tumors, but one of the more common types of adnexal carcinoma
- Age
  - Most occur in elderly patients
- Gender
  - Females have slightly higher incidence

Site
- Eyelids are by far the most common site (~ 75% of cases)
- Remainder of cases occur in other head and neck sites, followed by trunk, extremities

Presentation
- Nodular, firm, yellow-tan lesions
- Often ulcerated

Treatment
- Surgical approaches
  - Complete excision is necessary to ensure local removal
  - Mohs excision is reported to be effective in most cases
  - Sentinel lymph node biopsy may be useful for staging purposes

Prognosis
- Aggressive tumors with high incidence of metastasis (> 30% of cases) and generally poor prognosis unless discovered early

MACROSCOPIC FEATURES

General Features
- Dermal-based firm, nodular lesion

Size
- Usually 1-4 cm

MICROSCOPIC PATHOLOGY

Histologic Features
- Dermal-based infiltrative, nodular to sheet-like tumor
- Often with focal follicular &/or epidermal connections
  - Pagetoid involvement of epidermis may be seen in up to 30% of cases

SEBACEOUS CARCINOMA

Key Facts

Terminology
- Adnexal carcinoma that often lacks clear cell features in poorly differentiated cases

Etiology/Pathogenesis
- Strong association with MTS if patients have multiple sebaceous tumors

Clinical Issues
- Eyelids are the most common site (~ 75% of cases)
- Mohs excision is effective in most cases
- Aggressive tumors with high incidence of metastasis (> 30%) and generally poor prognosis unless discovered early

Microscopic Pathology
- Dermal-based infiltrative, nodular to sheet-like tumor
- Often focal follicular &/or epidermal connections
- Well-differentiated tumors show clear cell changes
- Moderately and poorly differentiated tumors show few to rare clear cells
- Often show basaloid or squamoid features
- Mitotic figures are usually abundant
- Areas of comedonecrosis are common

Ancillary Tests
- EMA(+) in well-differentiated cases, but often lost in poorly differentiated tumors
- AR(+) in most cases, including poorly differentiated

Top Differential Diagnoses
- Clear cell squamous cell carcinoma (SCC)
- Clear cell basal cell carcinoma (BCC)
- Other primary cutaneous adnexal carcinomas
- Metastatic carcinoma to the skin

- Tumor consists of variably differentiated epithelioid cells
  - Clear cells often present but vary greatly in number
  - Well-differentiated tumors show prominent clear cell changes
    - Cells contain abundant cytoplasmic lipid, often producing multiple vacuoles and nuclear indentation
    - Nuclei are enlarged and vesicular or hyperchromatic-staining, with prominent nucleoli
  - Moderately and poorly differentiated tumors show few to rare clear cells
    - May be composed predominantly of basaloid or squamoid cells
    - Show prominent cytologic atypia and pleomorphism
    - Mitotic figures, including atypical forms, are usually abundant
  - Areas of necrosis, with comedonecrosis pattern, are common
  - Lymphovascular invasion present in significant percentage of cases

Cytologic Features
- Enlarged, epithelioid cells with abundant cytoplasm and hyperchromatic or vesicular nuclei with enlarged nucleoli
  - Clear cells usually show cytoplasmic vacuoles and nuclear indentation
  - However, cells can also be basaloid (common) or squamoid (rare)

ANCILLARY TESTS

Histochemistry
- Sudan black B and oil red O (need frozen tissue)
  - Reactivity: Positive
  - Staining pattern
    - Cytoplasmic staining
- Periodic acid-Schiff
  - Reactivity: Usually negative (indicating lack of glycogen)

Immunohistochemistry
- EMA is positive in most well-differentiated cases, but is often negative in poorly differentiated tumors
  - EMA is negative in BCC, but often shows at least focal staining in SCC
  - EMA often highlights ductal structures in other adnexal carcinomas (i.e., porocarcinoma and hidradenocarcinoma), but not in sebaceous carcinoma
- Androgen receptor (AR) is positive (nuclear staining) in most cases, including poorly differentiated carcinomas
  - SCC and most other primary cutaneous carcinomas are negative for AR
  - However, AR is often positive in BCC (> 60% of cases) and some metastatic carcinomas to the skin
- HMWCKs (i.e., CK5/6 and CK903/34βE12) and p63 are typically strongly and diffusely positive
  - Help to exclude metastatic tumors (most of which are negative for both of these markers) but do not distinguish from other primary cutaneous tumors
- D2-40 (podoplanin) is positive in a subset of cases, especially in more basaloid sebaceous carcinomas
  - Can also highlight areas of lymphovascular invasion
- Other markers that may be positive include CAM5.2, BER-EP4, CK7 (~ 50% of cases), and CD10 (~ 50%)
- Negative for CEA-M, CK20, GCDFP-15, RCA/PRNA, TTF-1, S100
- Muir-Torre patients show loss of staining for MLH1, MSH2, &/or MSH6

Molecular Genetics
- Muir-Torre syndrome in patients with multiple sebaceous tumors and internal organ carcinomas
  - Genes include MLH1, MSH2, MSH6
  - Mutations lead to loss of mismatch repair capabilities
  - Can be identified directly through PCR for specific mutations or indirectly through MSI studies
    - MSI studies are less sensitive than PCR and immunohistochemistry

SEBACEOUS CARCINOMA

DIFFERENTIAL DIAGNOSIS

Squamous Cell Carcinoma (SCC)

- SCC with clear cell features can be difficult to distinguish from sebaceous carcinoma in some cases
- Often associated with overlying actinic keratosis or SCC in situ (Bowen disease)
- Clear cells in SCC are due to either degenerative changes or glycogen accumulation
  ○ Lack cytoplasmic lipid and nuclear indentations
  ○ PAS (without diastase) is positive in cases with cytoplasmic glycogen (negative in sebaceous carcinoma)
- Areas of squamous eddies and keratinization typically present (only rarely seen in sebaceous carcinoma)
- Sebaceous carcinoma is usually diffusely positive for EMA (weak/focal in SCC) and AR (negative in SCC)

Basal Cell Carcinoma (BCC)

- Most cases are not difficult to distinguish from sebaceous carcinoma
- However, some cases of sebaceous carcinoma are predominantly composed of basaloid cells
  ○ Usually, at least focal clear cells with sebaceous features are present
  ○ Lack peripheral palisading, mucinous stroma, and tumor-stromal retraction artifact of BCC
- Some cases of BCC are predominantly clear cell, **but**
  ○ Typically show at least focal areas of more conventional BCC with peripheral palisading and mucinous stroma
- Sebaceous carcinoma is usually diffusely positive for EMA (negative in BCC) and AR (often focally positive in BCC)

Other Primary Cutaneous Adnexal Carcinomas

- Porocarcinoma and hidradenocarcinoma with clear cell features may enter the differential diagnosis in some cases
- Porocarcinoma shows multiple epidermal attachments, whereas hidradenocarcinoma is dermal-based tumor typically lacking epidermal connections
- Both tumors show at least focal ductal differentiation (rare in sebaceous carcinoma)
  ○ May be highlighted by EMA and CEA
- Sebaceous carcinoma is usually diffusely positive for EMA and AR

Metastatic Carcinomas to the Skin

- Metastatic carcinomas with clear cell features should be considered in the differential, especially if no epidermal or follicular connections are identified
- Metastatic clear cell renal cell carcinoma (RCC) is the most likely consideration
  ○ Prominent capillary-type vasculature typically present (lacking in sebaceous carcinoma)
  ○ Cells are typically relatively low-grade appearing
  ○ Show uniform cytoplasmic clearing rather than multivacuolization of sebaceous carcinoma
  ○ IHC: Positive for RCA/PRNA, pax-8, CD10 (positive in ~ 50% of sebaceous carcinomas); EMA is positive in both RCC and sebaceous carcinoma

DIAGNOSTIC CHECKLIST

Pathologic Interpretation Pearls

- Well-differentiated cells contain abundant cytoplasmic lipid, often producing multiple vacuoles and nuclear indentation
- Poorly differentiated cells often lack vacuoles and may appear basaloid or squamoid

SELECTED REFERENCES

1. Dasgupta T et al: A retrospective review of 1349 cases of sebaceous carcinoma. Cancer. 115(1):158-65, 2009
2. Buitrago W et al: Sebaceous carcinoma: the great masquerader: emgerging concepts in diagnosis and treatment. Dermatol Ther. 21(6):459-66, 2008
3. Yang HM et al: Immunohistochemical expression of D2-40 in benign and malignant sebaceous tumors and comparison to basal and squamous cell carcinomas. Am J Dermatopathol. 30(6):549-54, 2008
4. Cabral ES et al: Desmoplastic tricholemmoma of the eyelid misdiagnosed as sebaceous carcinoma: a potential diagnostic pitfall. J Cutan Pathol. 34 Suppl 1:22-5, 2007
5. Ho VH et al: Sentinel lymph node biopsy for sebaceous cell carcinoma and melanoma of the ocular adnexa. Arch Otolaryngol Head Neck Surg. 133(8):820-6, 2007
6. Cabral ES et al: Distinction of benign sebaceous proliferations from sebaceous carcinomas by immunohistochemistry. Am J Dermatopathol. 28(6):465-71, 2006
7. Curry ML et al: Muir-Torre syndrome: role of the dermatopathologist in diagnosis. Am J Dermatopathol. 26(3):217-21, 2004
8. Nelson BR et al: Sebaceous carcinoma. J Am Acad Dermatol. 33(1):1-15; quiz 16-8, 1995
9. Cohen PR et al: Association of sebaceous gland tumors and internal malignancy: the Muir-Torre syndrome. Am J Med. 90(5):606-13, 1991
10. Nakamura S et al: Sebaceous carcinoma--with special reference to histopathologic differential diagnosis. J Dermatol. 15(1):55-9, 1988
11. Burgdorf WH et al: Muir-Torre syndrome. Histologic spectrum of sebaceous proliferations. Am J Dermatopathol. 8(3):202-8, 1986
12. Ratz JL et al: Sebaceous carcinoma of the eyelid treated with Mohs' surgery. J Am Acad Dermatol. 14(4):668-73, 1986
13. Wolfe JT 3rd et al: Sebaceous carcinoma of the eyelid. Errors in clinical and pathologic diagnosis. Am J Surg Pathol. 8(8):597-606, 1984
14. Russell WG et al: Sebaceous carcinoma of meibomian gland origin. The diagnostic importance of pagetoid spread of neoplastic cells. Am J Clin Pathol. 73(4):504-11, 1980

SEBACEOUS CARCINOMA

Microscopic Features

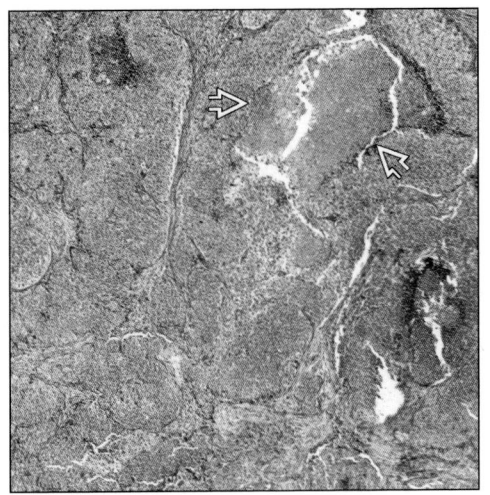 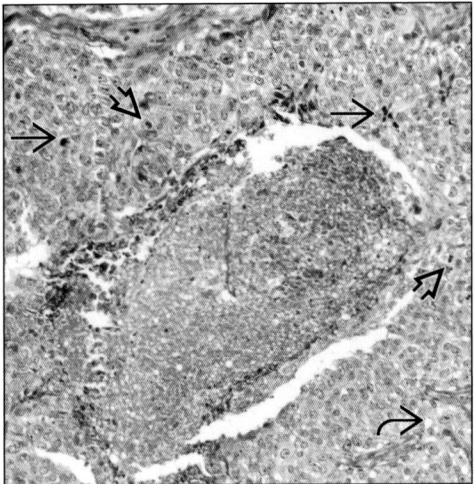

(Left) Scanning magnification view shows an atypical cellular, nodular basaloid-appearing proliferation with large areas of comedonecrosis ➡. *(Right)* High magnification of an area of comedonecrosis is surrounded by atypical clear to basaloid cells with apoptotic bodies ➡ and mitoses ➡. Some of the cells show clear cytoplasmic vacuoles ➡.

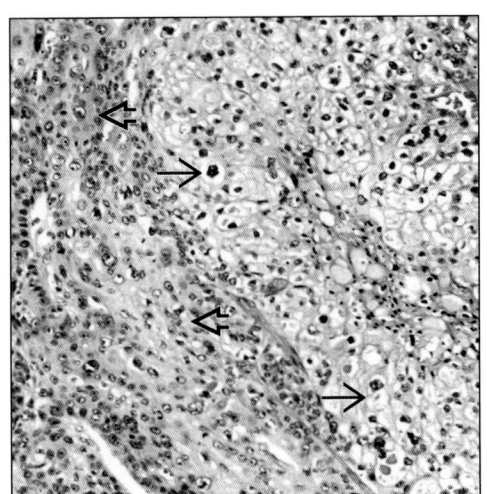 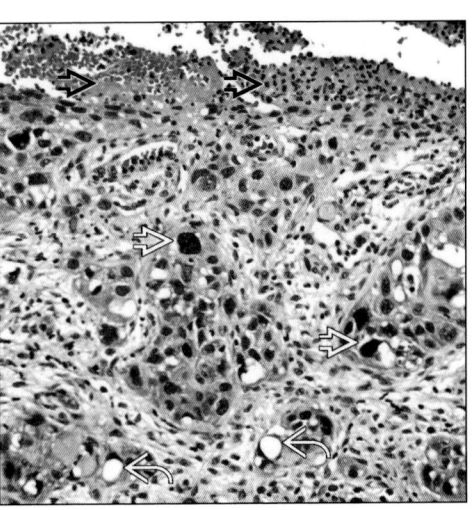

(Left) Sebaceous carcinoma shows areas of squamous differentiation ➡ adjacent to more typical areas with clear cell differentiation ➡. *(Right)* Invasive poorly differentiated sebaceous carcinoma with squamoid features shows markedly enlarged, atypical, and pleomorphic-appearing cells ➡. Note the overlying epidermal ulceration with serum crusting and neutrophils ➡. Scattered cells show nuclear indentations by cytoplasmic vacuoles ➡.

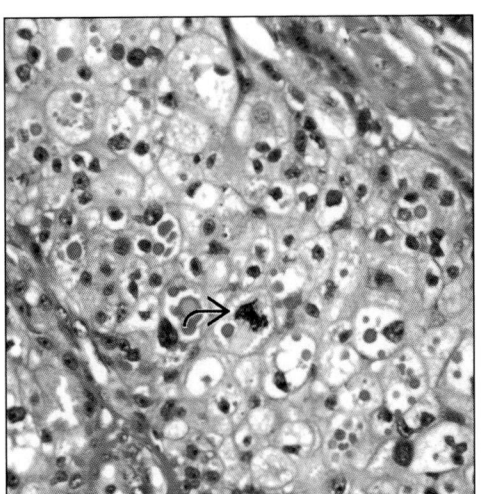 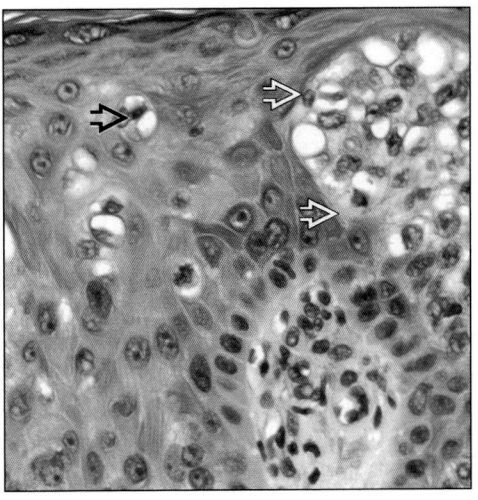

(Left) High magnification shows a sebaceous carcinoma with abundant red blood cells, some of which appear to be within the cytoplasm of the atypical clear cells. However, the abundant vascularity of renal cell carcinoma is lacking. Note the central atypical mitotic figure ➡. *(Right)* High magnification shows nests ➡ and atypical single pagetoid clear cells ➡ in the epidermis. Pagetoid involvement may be present in a minority of cases, and it may rarely be entirely in situ.

Ancillary Techniques

(Left) High magnification shows a sebaceous carcinoma composed of atypical clear to basaloid cells with mitoses ➡. Many of the cells show multiple small to large clear cytoplasmic vacuoles ➡. *(Right)* Strong immunohistochemical staining for EMA, which is often positive in well- and moderately differentiated tumors and highlights the cytoplasmic membrane and intracytoplasmic vacuoles ➤.

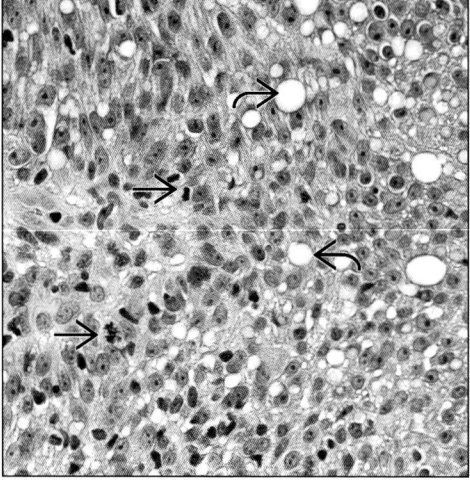 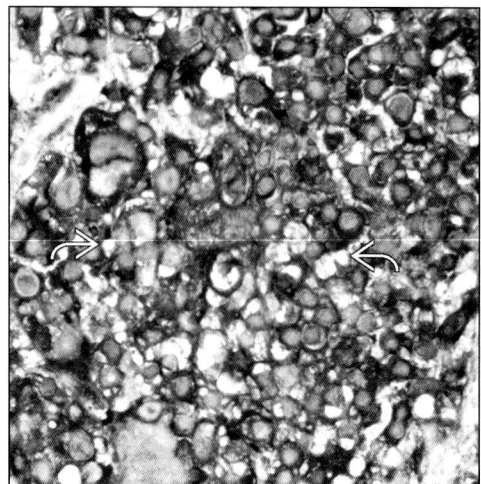

(Left) CK7 may be positive, but only in approximately 50% of cases. It often shows patchy, moderate to strong cytoplasmic staining, as in this case. *(Right)* Androgen receptor (AR) immunohistochemistry is positive in most cases and shows moderate, diffuse nuclear staining in the majority of the tumor cells.

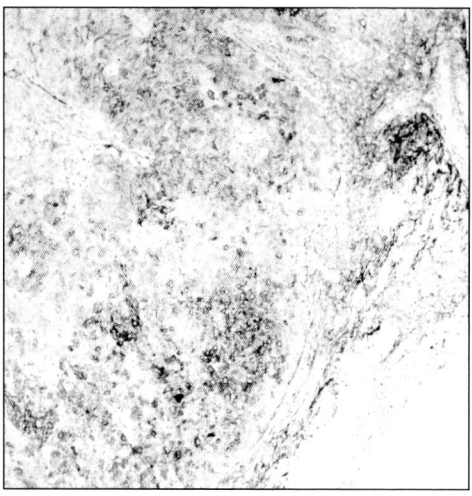 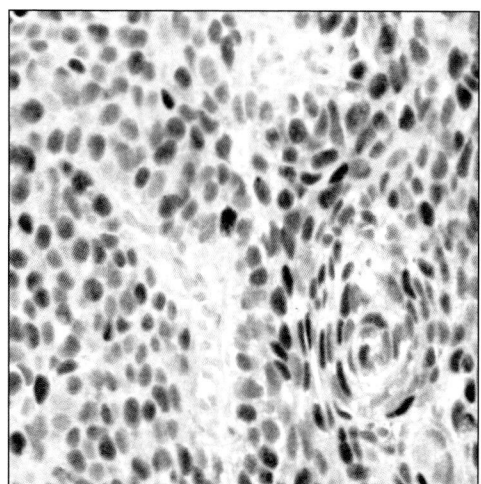

(Left) D2-40 (podoplanin) is positive in some cases of sebaceous carcinoma, especially basaloid variants. This case shows strong cytoplasmic staining of many of the basaloid and spindled cells ➤ without significant staining of the well-differentiated clear cells ➤. *(Right)* Diffuse nuclear staining for p53 is seen in this example of sebaceous carcinoma. p53 and Ki-67 are usually elevated in sebaceous carcinomas, and Bcl-2 is lost, compared with sebaceous adenomas and sebaceomas.

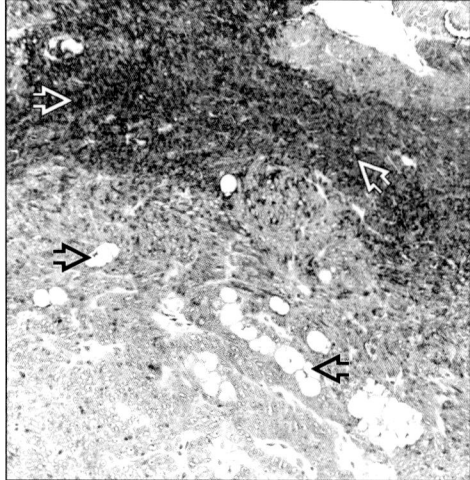 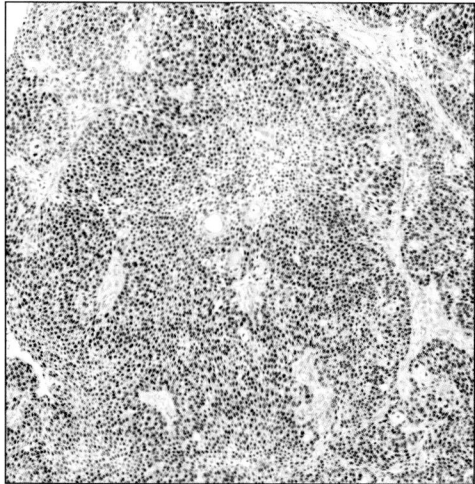

4

SEBACEOUS CARCINOMA

Differential Diagnosis

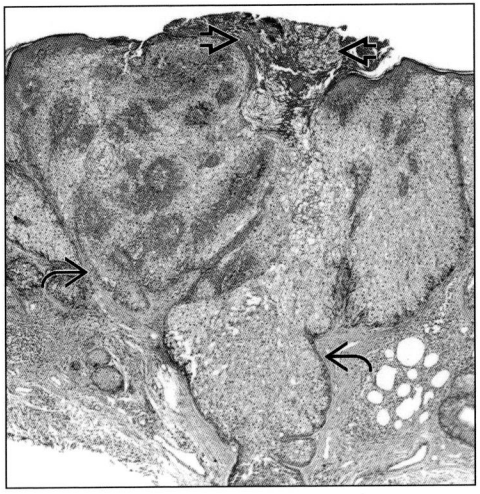

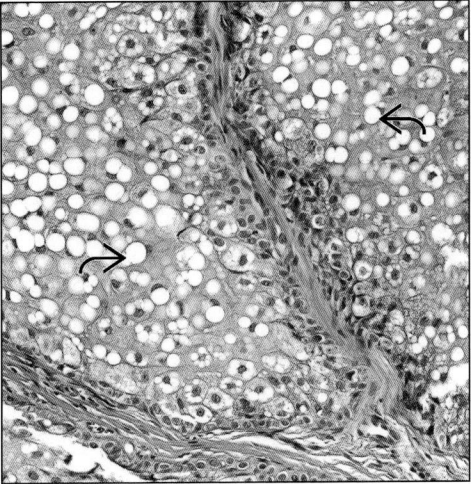

(Left) Low magnification shows a large sebaceous adenoma. The tumor is a well-circumscribed fusing lobular proliferation with superficial holocrine necrosis ⊃ (recapitulating normal sebaceous glands), composed of bland clear cells surrounded by a thin layer of basaloid cells ⊅. (Right) High magnification of a sebaceous adenoma shows the bland cytologic appearance of the mature sebocytes and surrounding basaloid cells. Note the prominent intracytoplasmic lipid vacuoles ⊅.

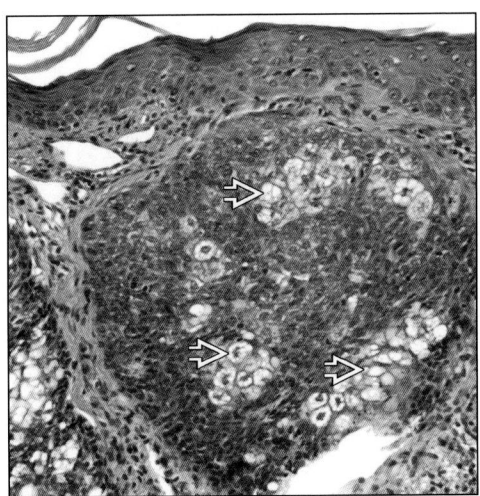

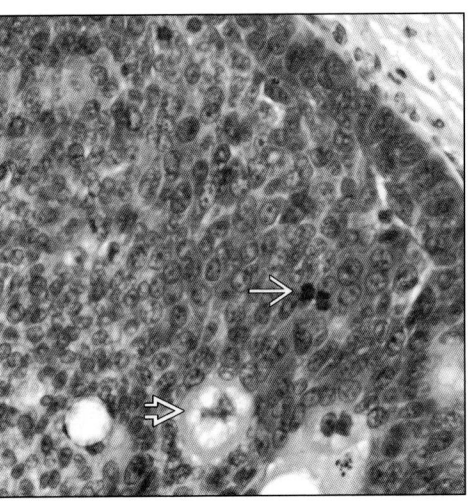

(Left) Sebaceoma shows well-circumscribed lobules of predominantly basaloid cells with a smaller population of bland-appearing mature sebaceous cells ⊃. (Right) High magnification of an atypical sebaceoma shows a predominantly basaloid population of enlarged, moderately atypical cells with nuclear hyperchromasia surrounding several large clear cells ⊃ with abundant, multivacuolated cytoplasm. Several mitotic figures are seen ⊃, but these can be quite numerous in some sebaceomas.

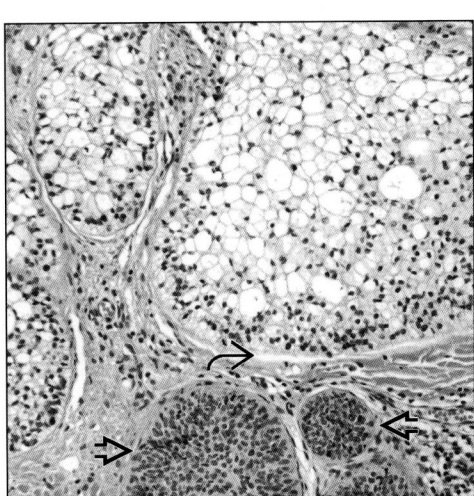

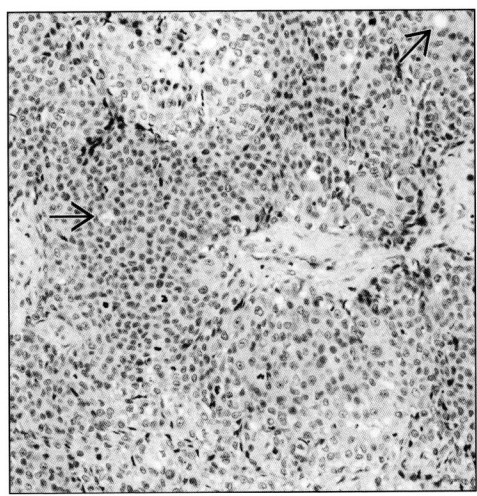

(Left) Clear cell BCC shows uniform cytoplasmic clearing without the vacuoles and nuclear indentations seen in sebaceous carcinoma. Note the focal retraction artifact ⊅ and adjacent areas of conventional-type BCC ⊃. (Right) Hidradenocarcinoma is another malignant adnexal tumor that often shows clear cell features. However, the cells lack cytoplasmic vacuoles and nuclear indentations. In addition, a few ductal structures are often seen ⊅, which are rare in sebaceous carcinoma.

Neoplasms and Proliferations of Eccrine and Apocrine Sweat Glands

APOCRINE TUBULAR ADENOMA

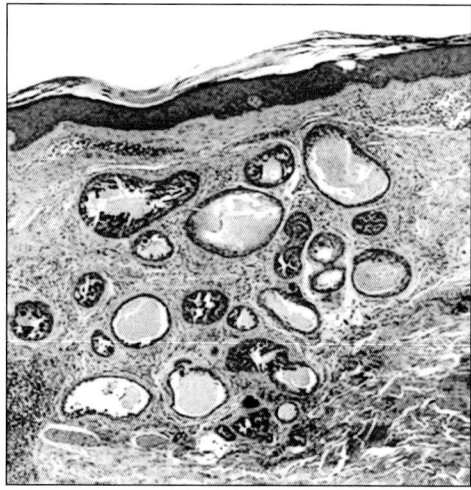

Apocrine tubular adenoma is usually a well-circumscribed intradermal nodule composed of variably sized and shaped tubules. Some tubular structures are cystically dilated.

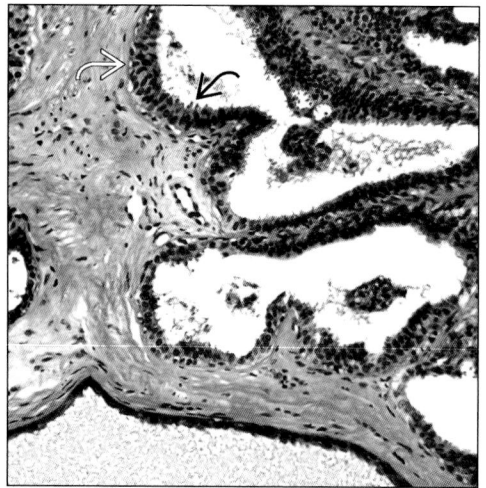

The tubules are lined by at least 2 layers of cells. The outer layer is composed of small myoepithelial cells ⊋, and the luminal layer is composed of columnar apocrine cells ⊐ with apical snouts.

TERMINOLOGY

Synonyms
- Apocrine adenoma, tubulopapillary hidradenoma, papillary tubular adenoma

Definitions
- Rare benign adnexal neoplasm with apocrine differentiation

CLINICAL ISSUES

Epidemiology
- Incidence
  ○ Rare tumor
- Age
  ○ Wide age distribution (range: 18-78 years)
- Gender
  ○ Female predominance (2:1)

Presentation
- Scalp nodule
  ○ Other locations include face, axilla, anogenital area, extremities
- < 2 cm in diameter

Treatment
- Complete excision is curative

Prognosis
- Excellent

MACROSCOPIC FEATURES

General Features
- Well-circumscribed intradermal nodule

Size
- < 2 cm in diameter
  ○ Larger lesions are exceptional

MICROSCOPIC PATHOLOGY

Histologic Features
- Intradermal nodule
  ○ Well-circumscribed
    ▪ Infiltrative borders should not be seen in apocrine tubular adenoma
  ○ Subcutaneous tissue may rarely be involved
  ○ Rarely tumor communicates with epidermis through ducts or infundibula of hair follicles
- Variable-sized tubules
  ○ Double or multilayered
  ○ Some cystically dilated
  ○ Some with papillary projections
    ▪ Usually without fibrovascular cores
- Peripheral (outer) layer
  ○ Flattened to cuboidal myoepithelial cells
- Luminal (inner) layer
  ○ Lined by columnar cells with apocrine differentiation
  ○ Eosinophilic cytoplasm
  ○ Often showing decapitation secretion
  ○ Regular round to oval nuclei
  ○ Nuclear pleomorphism absent to minimal
  ○ Mitoses are very rare
- Eosinophilic proteinaceous material may be seen in the lumen
- Connective tissue stroma
  ○ Scattered blood vessels and few inflammatory cells
- May arise in a background of nevus sebaceous
  ○ Sometimes associated with syringocystadenoma papilliferum

Cytologic Features
- Apocrine cells with decapitation secretion (apical snouts and secretions)

APOCRINE TUBULAR ADENOMA

Key Facts

Clinical Issues
- Scalp
- Nodule measuring < 2 cm

Microscopic Pathology
- Intradermal tumor
- Sometimes arises in association with nevus sebaceous and syringocystadenoma papilliferum
- Tubules of different size and shape
- Some cystically dilated

- Papillary projections devoid of fibrovascular cores
- Outer layer composed of myoepithelial cells
- Inner layer composed of apocrine cells

Top Differential Diagnoses
- Syringocystadenoma papilliferum
- Papillary eccrine adenoma
- Apocrine hamartoma
- Apocrine carcinoma

ANCILLARY TESTS

Immunohistochemistry
- Luminal cells are positive for
  - EMA and CEA (surface expression)
  - HMFG-1 and GCDFP-15
- Myoepithelial cells are positive for
  - S100 and SMA

DIFFERENTIAL DIAGNOSIS

Syringocystadenoma Papilliferum
- Connects to epidermis
- Papillae with true fibrovascular cores
- Dense plasma cell-rich inflammatory infiltrate
- Some apocrine tubular adenomas arise in association with syringocystadenoma papilliferum
  - Especially when arising in background of nevus sebaceous

Papillary Eccrine Adenoma
- Lacks true apocrine differentiation
- Lacks surface decapitation
- Rare tumors may have mixed features of eccrine and apocrine tubular adenomas
  - Distinction may be impossible in such cases

Apocrine Hamartoma (Apocrine Nevus)
- Often affect the axilla
- May affect chest, neck, inguinal area

- Excess of normal-appearing apocrine glands
  - Usually located in reticular dermis

Apocrine Carcinoma
- Infiltrative tumor
- Nuclear pleomorphism
- Numerous mitoses usually present

DIAGNOSTIC CHECKLIST

Pathologic Interpretation Pearls
- 2 or more cell layers with outer layer composed of myoepithelial cells
- Luminal cells show decapitation secretion
- Infiltrative pattern is not a feature of apocrine tubular adenoma
  - Should raise suspicion for apocrine carcinoma

SELECTED REFERENCES

1. Mitsuishi T et al: Tubular apocrine adenoma of the nose. Eur J Dermatol. 21(1):132, 2011
2. Tellechea O et al: Tubular apocrine adenoma with eccrine and apocrine immunophenotypes or papillary tubular adenoma? Am J Dermatopathol. 17(5):499-505, 1995
3. Fox SB et al: Tubular apocrine adenoma and papillary eccrine adenoma. Entities or unity? Am J Dermatopathol. 14(2):149-54, 1992
4. Toribio J et al: Tubular apocrine adenoma. J Cutan Pathol. 14(2):114-7, 1987
5. Rabens SF et al: Apocrine gland organic hamartoma (apocrine nevus). Arch Dermatol. 112(4):520-2, 1976

IMAGE GALLERY

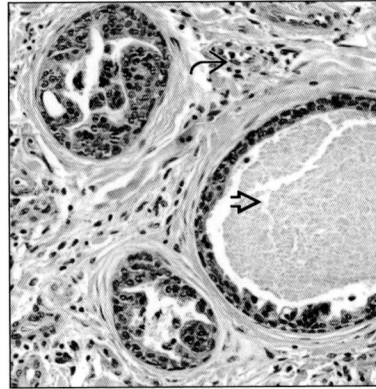 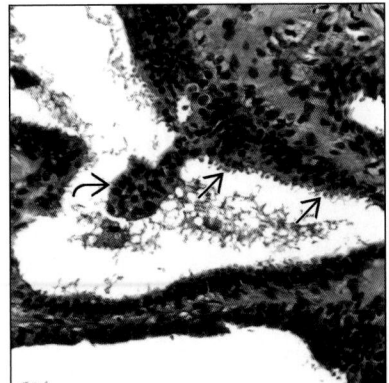 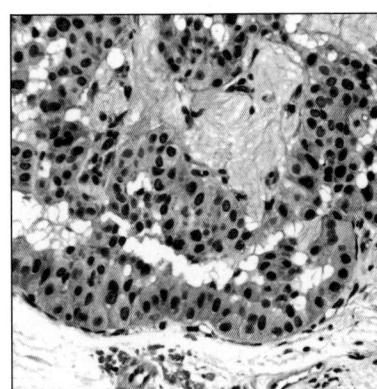

(Left) The tubules may contain eosinophilic secretion and debris ➡. The tubular structures are separated by a connective tissue stroma with few blood vessels ➡ and scant chronic inflammation. *(Center)* Papillary projections ➡ are common and usually devoid of fibrovascular cores. Note the decapitation secretions on the surface of the apocrine cells ➡. *(Right)* High magnification shows cells with relatively uniform round to oval nuclei and low mitotic activity.

SYRINGOCYSTADENOMA PAPILLIFERUM

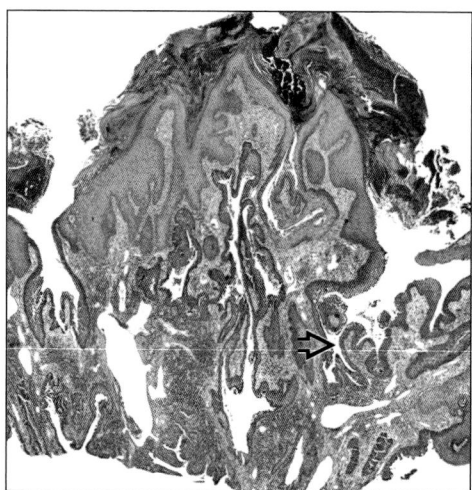

Syringocystadenoma papilliferum has an endo/exophytic growth pattern with invaginations into the underlying dermis that have a papillary architecture ⊳.

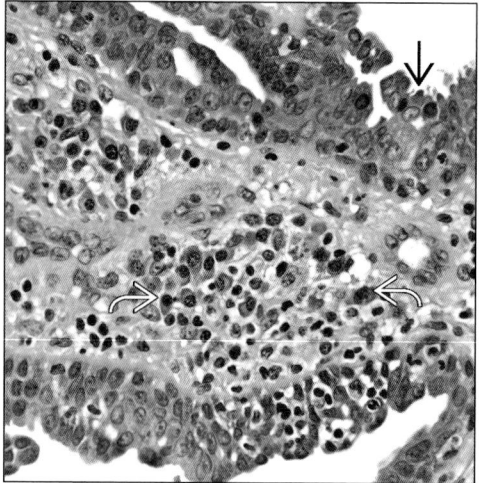

The glandular epithelium in this case shows evidence of apocrine differentiation ⊳, with focal apical snouts and secretions. The stroma contains numerous plasma cells ⊳.

TERMINOLOGY

Abbreviations
- Syringocystadenoma papilliferum (SCP)

Definitions
- Benign adnexal tumor with endophytic/exophytic growth pattern

ETIOLOGY/PATHOGENESIS

Cytogenetics
- Subset of tumors have loss of heterozygosity for *PTCH* &/or *P16*, suggesting a role for loss of these tumor suppressor genes in some cases

CLINICAL ISSUES

Epidemiology
- Age
  - Approximately 1/2 present at birth or childhood

Presentation
- Scalp most common location, followed by face
- Presents as solitary gray to dark brown papillomatous lesion
- Rarely multiple
- Often associated with nevus sebaceus (present in 5-19% of cases of nevus sebaceus)
  - Typically in scalp lesions
- May rarely be associated with other neoplasms (e.g., tricholemmoma, apocrine hidrocystoma)

Treatment
- Surgical approaches
  - Simple excision is curative

Prognosis
- Benign

- Rare cases may have a basal cell carcinoma develop within the syringocystadenoma papilliferum
- Rare cases may transform to syringocystadenocarcinoma papilliferum

MICROSCOPIC PATHOLOGY

Histologic Features
- Endo-/exophytic tumors
- Invaginations that communicate with epidermal surface
  - Superficial aspects often lined by squamous epithelium that transitions to glandular epithelium
- Invaginations have papillary architecture
  - Papillary structures lined by glandular epithelium with a double layer
    - Basal layer is flattened to cuboidal (myoepithelial cells)
    - Luminal layer usually columnar
    - Goblet cells occasionally present
    - Papillae may communicate with duct-like structures in deeper aspects
- Characteristic stroma
  - Fibrovascular connective tissue within papillae
  - Numerous plasma cells admixed with some lymphocytes

ANCILLARY TESTS

Immunohistochemistry
- Glandular epithelium positive for AE1/AE3, CAM5.2, EMA, and CEA
  - Epithelium variably positive for GCDFP-15, consistent with apocrine differentiation
- Basal layer positive for SMA, CK5/6, and p63, consistent with myoepithelial differentiation

SYRINGOCYSTADENOMA PAPILLIFERUM

Key Facts

Clinical Issues
- Approximately 1/2 present at birth or childhood
- Scalp most common location, followed by face
- Often associated with nevus sebaceus (present in 5-19% of cases of nevus sebaceus)
- Benign tumors, but
  - Rarely, basal cell carcinoma may develop within syringocystadenoma papilliferum
  - Rare cases may transform to syringocystadenocarcinoma papilliferum

Microscopic Pathology
- Endophytic/exophytic adnexal tumors
  - Invaginations that communicate with epidermal surface
  - Invaginations have papillary architecture

- Papillary structures lined by glandular epithelium with a double layer
  - Papillae communicate with duct-like structures in deeper aspects
  - Basal layer is flattened to cuboidal
  - Luminal layer usually columnar
- Characteristic stroma
  - Fibrovascular connective tissue within papillae
  - Numerous plasma cells admixed with some lymphocytes

Top Differential Diagnoses
- Hidradenoma papilliferum
- Tubular apocrine adenoma
- Syringocystadenocarcinoma papilliferum/malignant syringocystadenoma

DIFFERENTIAL DIAGNOSIS

Hidradenoma Papilliferum
- Usually presents on vulva or perineum of women
- More delicate papillary architecture
- Usually does not communicate with surface epithelium
- Lacks plasma cell-rich stroma

Tubular Apocrine Adenoma
- Closely related tumors; both components may be found in same lesion
- Dermal component of SCP appears similar to tubular apocrine adenoma, however
  - Overlying epidermal attachments lacking
  - Plasma cells not as common as in SCP

Syringocystadenocarcinoma Papilliferum/ Malignant Syringocystadenoma
- Very rare tumors
- Adult patients
- May present with history of rapid growth in longstanding lesion
- Recognizable precursor syringocystadenoma papilliferum usually present
  - Malignant transformation characterized by increased nuclear atypia, multilayering of glandular epithelium, and increased mitotic activity
    - May be in situ or invasive
    - In situ tumors have silhouette of syringocystadenoma papilliferum
    - Invasive tumors have invasive adenocarcinoma component
    - May have a squamous cell carcinoma component

DIAGNOSTIC CHECKLIST

Pathologic Interpretation Pearls
- Usually presents on scalp of children
- Low-power examination demonstrates invaginations into underlying dermis

- Communicates with overlying epidermis
  - Superficial aspects may have squamous epithelium where underlying tumor communicates with surface
- Papillary architecture
- Papillae lined by glandular epithelium with double layer
- Numerous plasma cells in stroma

SELECTED REFERENCES

1. Kazakov DV et al: Morphologic diversity of syringocystadenocarcinoma papilliferum based on a clinicopathologic study of 6 cases and review of the literature. Am J Dermatopathol. 32(4):340-7, 2010
2. Leeborg N et al: Diagnostic pitfalls in syringocystadenocarcinoma papilliferum: case report and review of the literature. Arch Pathol Lab Med. 134(8):1205-9, 2010
3. Karg E et al: Congenital syringocystadenoma papilliferum. Pediatr Dermatol. 25(1):132-3, 2008
4. Nakai K et al: Sebaceoma, trichoblastoma and syringocystadenoma papilliferum arising within a nevus sebaceous. J Dermatol. 35(6):365-7, 2008
5. Laxmisha C et al: Linear syringocystadenoma papilliferum of the scalp. J Eur Acad Dermatol Venereol. 21(2):275-6, 2007
6. Rammeh-Rommani S et al: Syringocystadenoma papilliferum: report of 8 cases. Pathologica. 98(3):178-80, 2006
7. Arai Y et al: A case of syringocystadenocarcinoma papilliferum in situ occurring partially in syringocystadenoma papilliferum. J Dermatol. 30(2):146-50, 2003
8. Böni R et al: Syringocystadenoma papilliferum: a study of potential tumor suppressor genes. Am J Dermatopathol. 23(2):87-9, 2001
9. Cribier B et al: Tumors arising in nevus sebaceus: A study of 596 cases. J Am Acad Dermatol. 42(2 Pt 1):263-8, 2000
10. Bondi R et al: Syringocystadenocarcinoma papilliferum. Histopathology. 28(5):475-7, 1996
11. Mammino JJ et al: Syringocystadenoma papilliferum. Int J Dermatol. 30(11):763-6, 1991
12. Niizuma K: Syringocystadenoma papilliferum: light and electron microscopic studies. Acta Derm Venereol. 56(5):327-36, 1976

SYRINGOCYSTADENOMA PAPILLIFERUM

Microscopic Features

(Left) Syringocystadenoma papilliferum often has a partially exophytic, as well as endophytic growth pattern. The superficial aspects have squamous epithelium ⮕, and the deeper aspects have glandular epithelium ⮕. *(Right)* The tumor is characterized by invaginations with a papillary architecture that extend into the dermis.

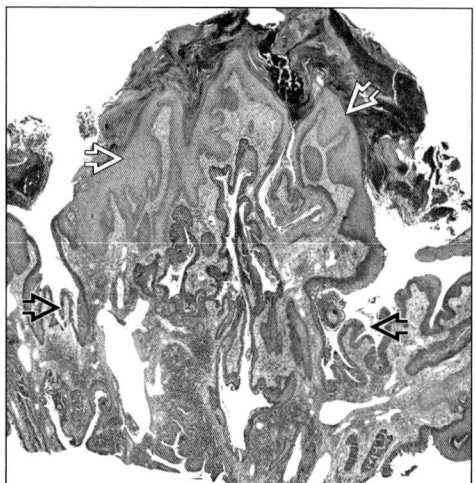
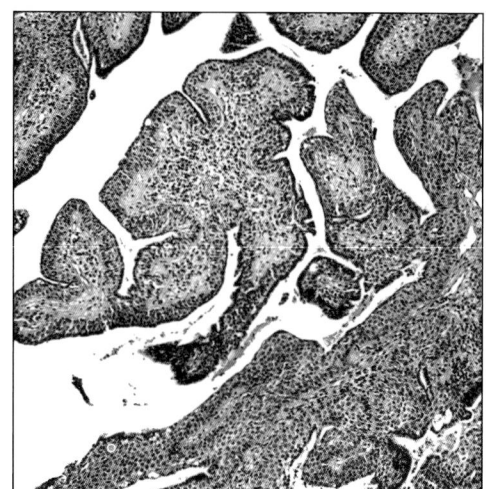

(Left) The epithelium lining the papillae demonstrates a transition from squamous to glandular epithelium ⮕. The stroma contains numerous plasma cells ⮕. *(Right)* The stroma of syringocystadenoma papilliferum characteristically has numerous plasma cells ⮕. The epithelium in this case has focal goblet cells ⮕.

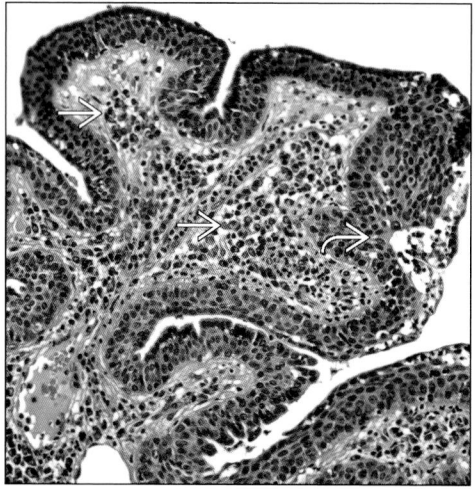
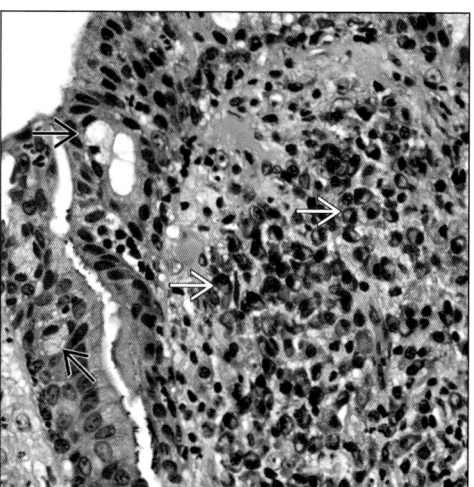

(Left) This example of SCP has a predominantly endophytic growth pattern extending below the level of the adjacent epidermis. Note the overlying serum crusting ⮕, likely due to excoriation/trauma. *(Right)* The papillae are typically lined by squamous epithelium superficially that transitions to glandular epithelium.

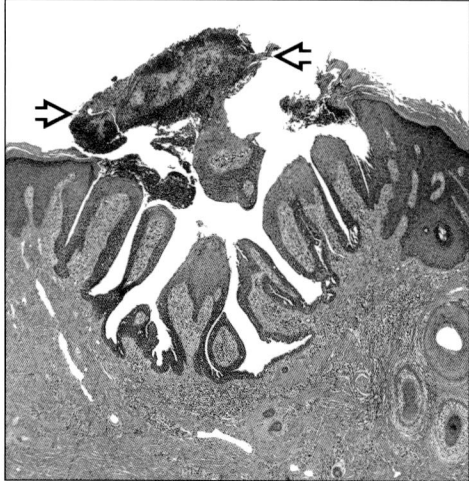
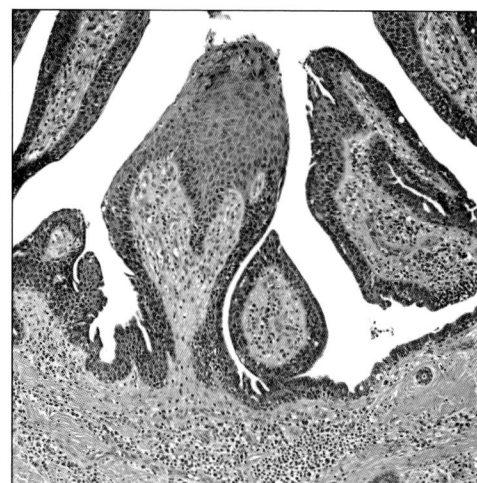

Syringocystadenocarcinoma Papilliferum

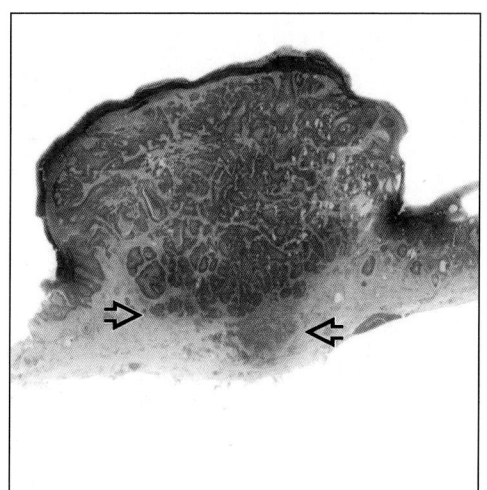
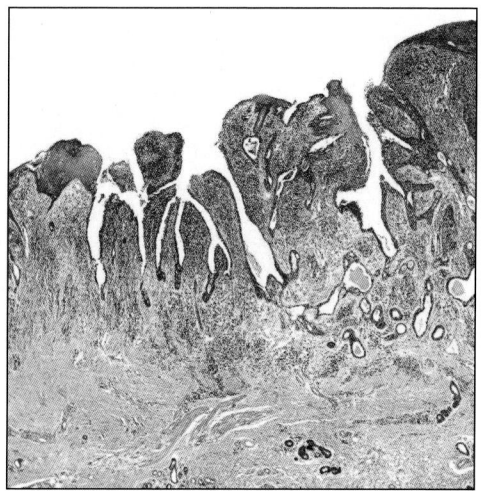

(Left) Scanning image of a syringocystadenocarcinoma papilliferum shows a large, endophytic-appearing tumor with deep invasion into the dermis ⇒. *(Right)* The periphery of the syringocystadenocarcinoma papilliferum has remnants of the precursor syringocystadenoma papilliferum.

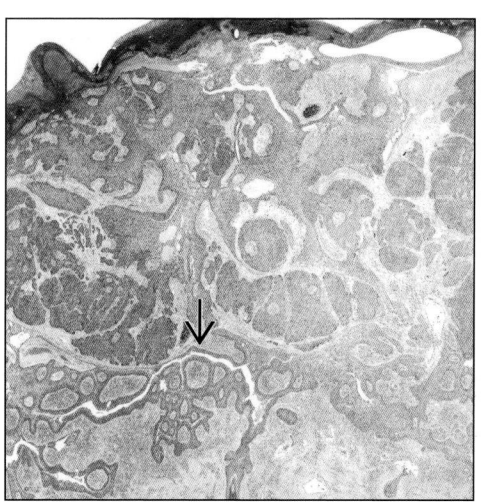
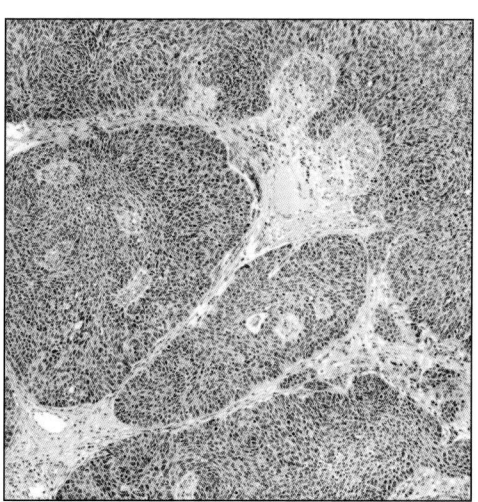

(Left) This syringocystadenocarcinoma papilliferum demonstrates central areas of squamous cell carcinoma that transitions to an in situ adenocarcinoma component with a papillary architecture in the deeper aspects of the tumor ⇒. *(Right)* In central areas of this syringocystadenocarcinoma papilliferum, there was squamous differentiation.

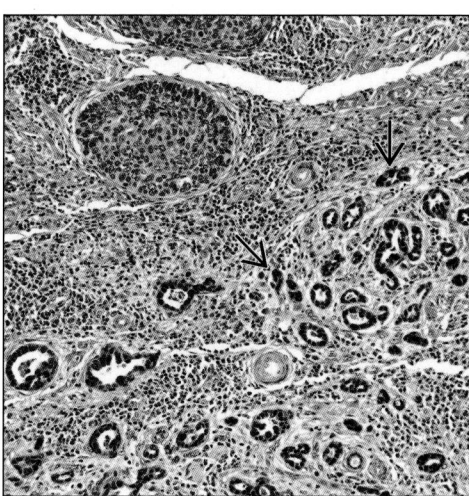
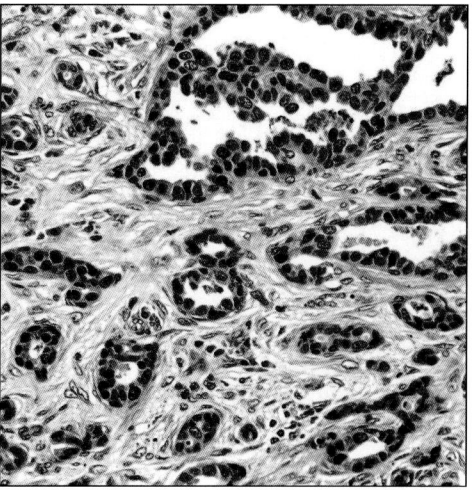

(Left) The invasive adenocarcinoma component of syringocystadenocarcinoma papilliferum ⇒ often loses the papillary architecture. *(Right)* Invasive adenocarcinoma component of syringocystadenocarcinoma papilliferum is characterized by irregular glands lined by atypical cells with hyperchromatic nuclei. The invasive tumor has an irregular growth pattern and is surrounded by a desmoplastic stroma.

HIDRADENOMA PAPILLIFERUM

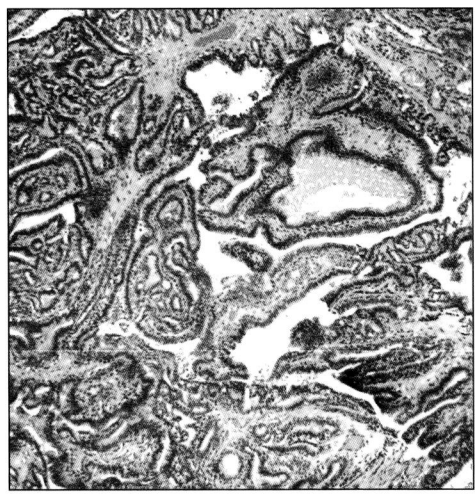

Hidradenoma papilliferum at low magnification shows a proliferation of papillary, cystic, and glandular areas with a complex, arborizing architecture. The tumors are dermal-based and well circumscribed.

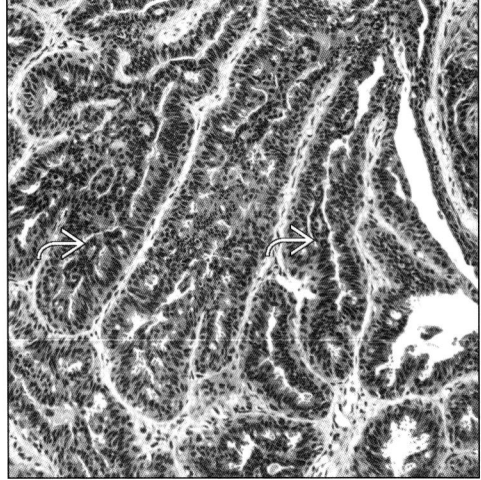

Higher magnification of a hidradenoma papilliferum shows the elongated, arborizing papillary structures ➡ lined by 2-3 cell layers of bland columnar luminal cells and underlying myoepithelial cells.

TERMINOLOGY

Abbreviations
- Hidradenoma papilliferum (HP)

Synonyms
- Papillary hidradenoma

Definitions
- Small, well-circumscribed, dermal-based adenoma with apocrine differentiation

CLINICAL ISSUES

Epidemiology
- Incidence
  - Rare
- Age
  - Adult
- Gender
  - Almost always women
- Ethnicity
  - No race predilection

Site
- Vulva or perianal region
  - Rarely other sites (and termed ectopic HP)

Treatment
- Conservative surgical excision

Prognosis
- Generally excellent
- Extremely rare malignant transformation to hidradenocarcinoma papilliferum or aggressive adenosquamous carcinoma

MACROSCOPIC FEATURES

General Features
- Solid or, rarely, cystic skin-colored papule

Sections to Be Submitted
- Representative sections

Size
- Small, less than 1 cm in most cases

MICROSCOPIC PATHOLOGY

Histologic Features
- Dermal-based, well-circumscribed tumor
  - Surrounded by fibrous capsule
- No connection to epidermis
- Maze-like glandular spaces
- Tubular and cystic structures
- Papillary folds
  - Often project into cystic spaces
- Inner layer of columnar apocrine secretory cells
  - Often with "decapitation" secretion
- Outer layer of cuboidal myoepithelial cells
- Cuboidal cells with eosinophilic cytoplasm and small nuclei present in 1/3 of cases
  - Resemble apocrine metaplasia seen in breast tissue
- Variable degree of mitotic index
  - High mitotic rate does not necessarily indicate malignancy (need to see cytologic atypia, pleomorphism, &/or infiltrative features)
- Minimal inflammation

Cytologic Features
- Benign apocrine secretory and myoepithelial cells

HIDRADENOMA PAPILLIFERUM

Key Facts

Terminology
- Well-circumscribed adenoma with apocrine differentiation

Clinical Issues
- Rare, benign tumor
- Vulvar or perianal area, predominately in women

Microscopic Pathology
- Well-circumscribed, dermal-based tumor

- No connections to the epidermis
- Maze-like glandular spaces and papillary foldings
- Apocrine differentiation is usually seen

Top Differential Diagnoses
- Tubular apocrine adenoma
- Syringocystadenoma papilliferum
- Nipple adenoma
- Papillary eccrine adenoma
- Hidradenoma

DIFFERENTIAL DIAGNOSIS

Tubular Apocrine Adenoma
- Simpler lesions composed predominantly of tubular structures
  - No maze-like glandular spaces
- No characteristic location

Syringocystadenoma Papilliferum (SCP)
- Location is on head and neck
- Similar histologic features, indicating that these are likely closely related tumors; however
  - Epidermal connections are seen in SCP but not HP
  - Characteristic prominent plasma cell infiltrate present in SCP, rare in HP

Nipple Adenoma (Erosive Adenomatosis of the Nipple, Florid Papillomatosis)
- Location is on the nipple
- Histology is similar to SCP and hidradenoma papilliferum

Papillary Eccrine Adenoma
- Rare tumors composed of small tubular structures with no decapitation secretion
  - Eccrine differentiation

Hidradenoma
- Nodular dermal-based tumor lacking epidermal connections

- More cellular; nodular to sheet-like collections of pale to clear-staining cells
  - Squamoid cells may also be present
- Lacks the intricate, maze-like features of hidradenoma papilliferum

DIAGNOSTIC CHECKLIST

Pathologic Interpretation Pearls
- Small, dermal-based apocrine adenoma with maze-like appearance

SELECTED REFERENCES

1. Duhan N et al: Hidradenoma papilliferum of the vulva: case report and review of literature. Arch Gynecol Obstet. 284(4):1015-7, 2011
2. Vazmitel M et al: Hidradenoma papilliferum with a ductal carcinoma in situ component: case report and review of the literature. Am J Dermatopathol. 30(4):392-4, 2008
3. Virgili A et al: Vulvar hidradenoma papilliferum. A review of 10.5 years' experience. J Reprod Med. 45(8):616-8, 2000
4. Vang R et al: Ectopic hidradenoma papilliferum: a case report and review of the literature. J Am Acad Dermatol. 41(1):115-8, 1999

IMAGE GALLERY

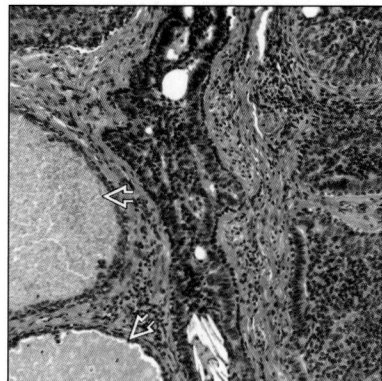 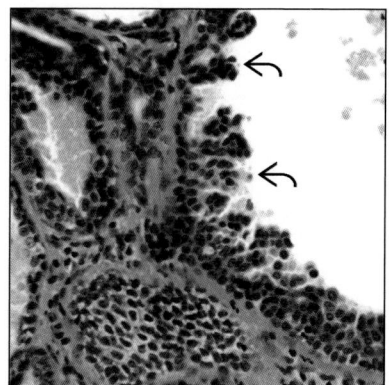 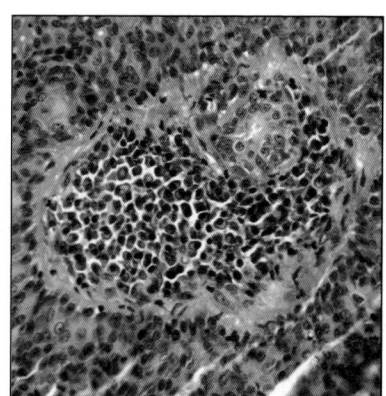

(Left) Hidradenoma papilliferum is typically composed mostly of cellular trabecular areas but may also show cystic areas ➡. *(Center)* H&E shows high magnification of a cystic area with evidence of apocrine differentiation. The surface-lining cells show apical snouts and secretions ➡. Note the lack of cytologic atypia or pleomorphism. *(Right)* Cross-section of a papillary area shows numerous stromal plasma cells, similar to syringocystadenoma papilliferum (which are likely closely related tumors).

HIDRADENOMA

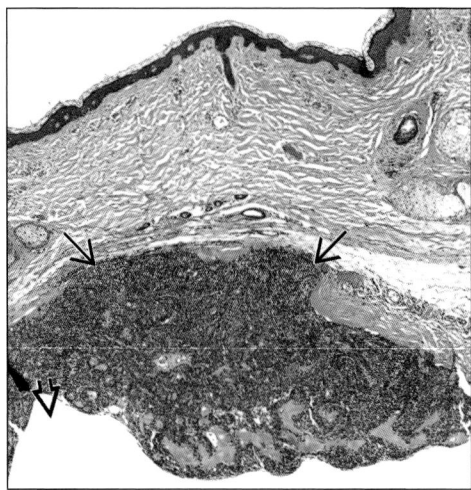

Low-magnification view of a hidradenoma shows a dermal-based, nodular-appearing solid ➡ to cystic ⇗ tumor.

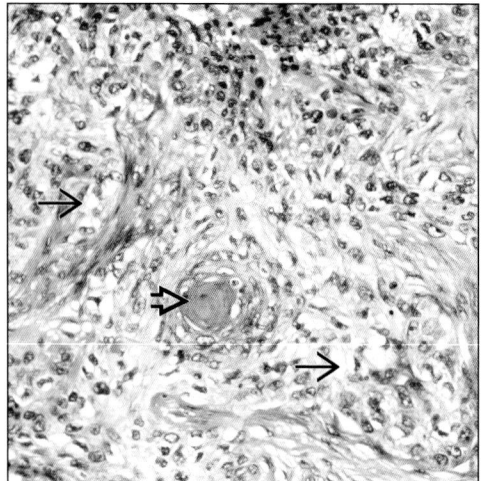

High-power view shows a hidradenoma. Variable proportions of cell types are seen in any given tumor. In this field, clear cells ➡ and squamoid cells forming focal keratin pearls ⇗ are present.

TERMINOLOGY

Synonyms
- Clear cell hidradenoma, nodular hidradenoma, solid-cystic hidradenoma, cystic hidradenoma, eccrine acrospiroma, eccrine sweat gland adenoma, clear cell myoepithelioma, poroid hidradenoma, apocrine hidradenoma

Definitions
- Benign tumor showing apocrine or eccrine differentiation

CLINICAL ISSUES

Presentation
- Solitary dermal nodule

Treatment
- Excision is generally curative

Prognosis
- Benign
- Low malignant potential; may rarely transform to hidradenocarcinoma

MICROSCOPIC PATHOLOGY

Histologic Features
- Well-circumscribed dermal-based tumor
  - Classically does not connect to epidermis and is deep-seated
- May be primarily composed of solid areas, or cystic areas, or both
- Solid areas composed of varying proportion of clear cells, poroid cells, squamoid cells, and rarely mucinous cells
- Ducts with eosinophilic cuticles present in solid areas

- Cystic areas lined by cuboidal cells, sometimes with evidence of decapitation secretion
- Stroma between solid islands &/or cystic areas is prominently hyalinized appearing
- Prominent cytologic atypia not present
- Mitoses can be present, but usually not numerous
- Necrosis usually absent
- Generally does not show infiltrative pattern

Cytologic Features
- Variable cell composition
  - Clear cells
    - Clear cytoplasm
    - Nuclei oval to round with small nucleoli
    - Contain glycogen and are PAS positive (diastase-sensitive)
  - Squamoid cells
    - Resemble keratinocytes with eosinophilic cytoplasm and well-demarcated cytoplasmic borders
  - Poroid cells
    - Basaloid cells with little cytoplasm
    - Nuclei have blue outlines and single nucleoli or occasionally multiple small nucleoli

DIFFERENTIAL DIAGNOSIS

Metastatic Renal Cell Carcinoma
- Composed of clear cells arranged in variably sized islands
- Vascular pattern may be prominent
- Often extravasated erythrocytes numerous
- Generally does not show cystic areas
- More commonly CD10 and EMA positive
- Positive with renal cell carcinoma antigen (RCA)

Hidradenocarcinoma
- Cellular, atypical nodular dermal-based tumor
- Shows greater cytologic atypia and mitotic figures and often has infiltrative features

HIDRADENOMA

Key Facts

Clinical Issues
- Solitary dermal nodule

Microscopic Pathology
- May be primarily composed of solid areas, cystic areas, or both
- Classically does not connect to epidermis and is deep-seated
- Solid areas composed of varying proportion of
  - Clear cells
  - Poroid cells
  - Squamoid cells
  - Rarely mucinous cells
- Ducts with eosinophilic cuticles present in solid areas
- Cystic areas lined by cuboidal cells, sometimes with evidence of decapitation secretion

- Stroma between solid islands &/or cystic areas is prominently hyalinized
- Well circumscribed
- Necrosis usually absent
- Prominent cytologic atypia not present
- Mitoses not numerous

Top Differential Diagnoses
- Metastatic renal cell carcinoma
- Other clear cell tumors
  - Basal cell carcinoma
  - Squamous cell carcinoma
- Other adnexal tumors
  - Lymphadenoma
  - Sebaceous adenoma
  - Cystadenoma

Clear Cell Basal Cell Carcinoma
- Composed of clear cells arranged in variably sized islands
- Some islands may have peripheral palisading
- Some foci of conventional basal cell carcinoma may be present
- Generally does not show cystic areas
- Positive with BER-EP4 and androgen receptor (AR)

Clear Cell Squamous Cell Carcinoma
- Composed of clear cells arranged in variably sized islands
- Some foci of conventional squamous cell carcinoma may be present
- Absence of ductal differentiation
- Generally does not show cystic areas

Squamous Cell Carcinoma
- When a hidradenoma has few clear cells and mostly squamoid cells, squamous cell carcinoma enters the differential
- Keratin pearls often present
- Epidermal connection often more prominent
- Ductal/glandular differentiation generally absent
- Hyalinized stroma usually absent
- May be infiltrative

Lymphadenoma
- Jagged islands composed of clear cells with peripheral palisading
- Variably dense infiltrate of lymphocytes may obscure islands

Sebaceous Adenoma
- Lobular downgrowth from epidermal surface (not deep-seated in dermis)
- Lobules composed of sebocytes with scalloped/crenulated nuclei and bubbly cytoplasm with peripheral rim of 2 or more layers of basaloid cells

Sebaceoma
- When a hidradenoma has few clear cells and mostly basaloid cells, sebaceoma may enter the differential

- Sebaceoma has scattered bubbly cells with scalloped nuclei
- AR and adipophilin positive

Papillary Hidrocystoma (Cystadenoma)
- If a hidradenoma is primarily cystic, cystadenoma enters the differential
- Cystadenoma resembles traditional hidrocystoma, except there is increased cellularity and papillations

DIAGNOSTIC CHECKLIST

Pathologic Interpretation Pearls
- May be primarily composed of solid areas, cystic areas, or both
- Classically does not connect to epidermis and is deep-seated
- Solid areas composed of varying proportion of clear cells, poroid cells, squamoid cells, and rarely mucinous cells
- Ducts with eosinophilic cuticles present in solid areas
- Cystic areas lined by cuboidal cells, sometimes with evidence of decapitation secretion
- Hyalinized stroma
- Well-circumscribed
- Prominent cytologic atypia not present
- Mitoses not numerous

SELECTED REFERENCES

1. Battistella M et al: From hidroacanthoma simplex to poroid hidradenoma: clinicopathologic and immunohistochemic study of poroid neoplasms and reappraisal of their histogenesis. Am J Dermatopathol. 32(5):459-68, 2010
2. Plaza JA et al: Value of p63 and podoplanin (D2-40) immunoreactivity in the distinction between primary cutaneous tumors and adenocarcinomas metastatic to the skin: a clinicopathologic and immunohistochemical study of 79 cases. J Cutan Pathol. 37(4):403-10, 2010
3. Yavel R et al: Hidradenomas and a hidradenocarcinoma of the scalp managed using Mohs micrographic surgery and a multidisciplinary approach: case reports and review of the literature. Dermatol Surg. 35(2):273-81, 2009

Microscopic Features

(Left) This hidradenoma shows both solid ⇒ and cystic areas ⇒. The lesion extends to the tissue margins, so circumscription cannot be assessed. Necrosis is not evident, and there are no infiltrative features. *(Right)* Hidradenomas can be variably cystic and solid. In this view, a cystic area is seen in the upper right corner ⇒. Most of the tumor in this field, however, is composed of solid islands with mostly clear cells ⇒.

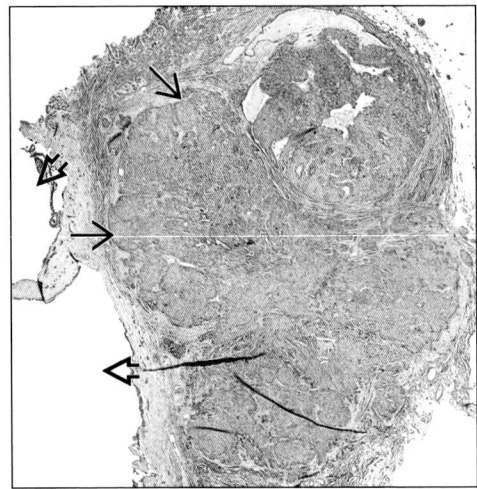
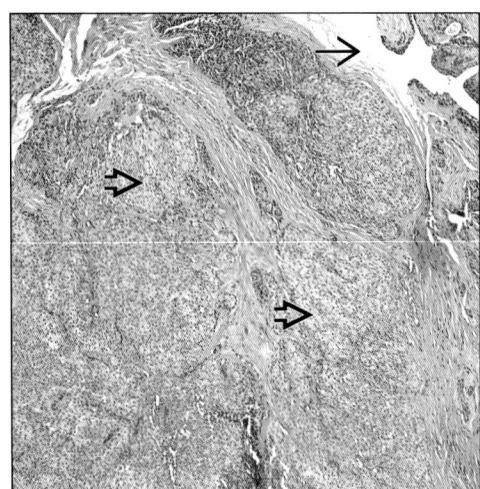

(Left) The cells lining cystic/ glandular areas ⇒ may show decapitation secretion. The solid area ⇒ contains cells that are basaloid without prominent cytologic atypia. Occasional clear cells ⇒ are also present. *(Right)* Hidradenoma often has a prominent hyalinized stroma ⇒. Islands are composed of clear cells and poroid cells with some evidence of ductal ⇒ and glandular ⇒ differentiation.

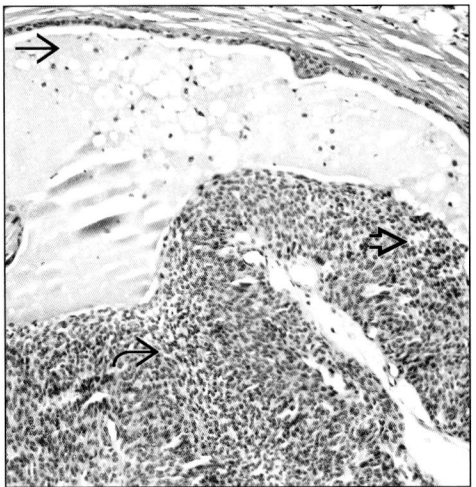
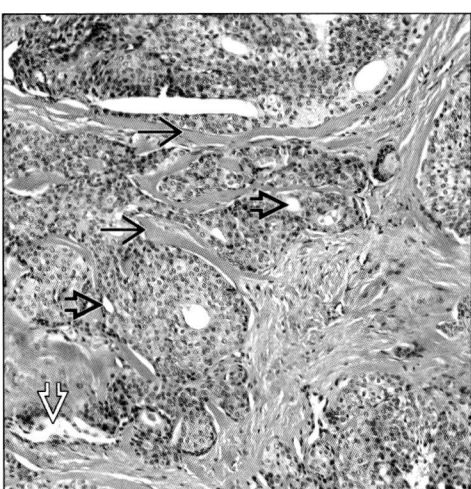

(Left) This area of a hidradenoma shows an admixture of clear ⇒ and poroid cells ⇒. There is minimal cytologic atypia. Mitoses are not prominent, and necrosis is absent. *(Right)* This area of hidradenoma shows an admixture of clear cells ⇒ and basaloid/poroid cells ⇒. Basaloid/poroid cells have minimal cytoplasm that is eosinophilic to basophilic-staining and round/oval nuclei. Mitoses and cytologic atypia are not present.

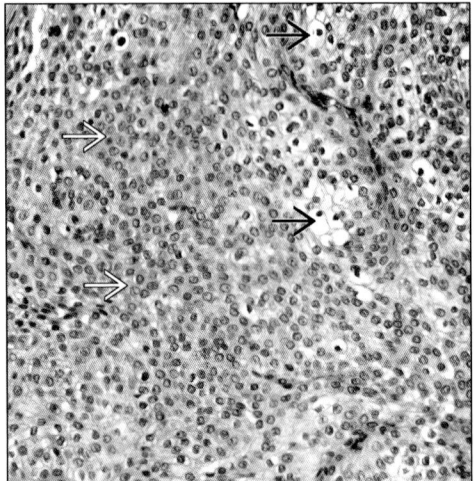
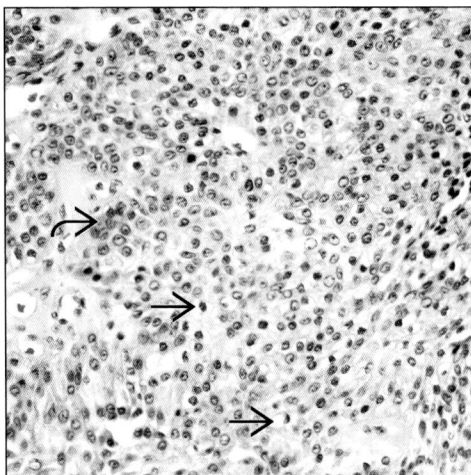

HIDRADENOMA

Variant Microscopic Features and Differential Diagnosis

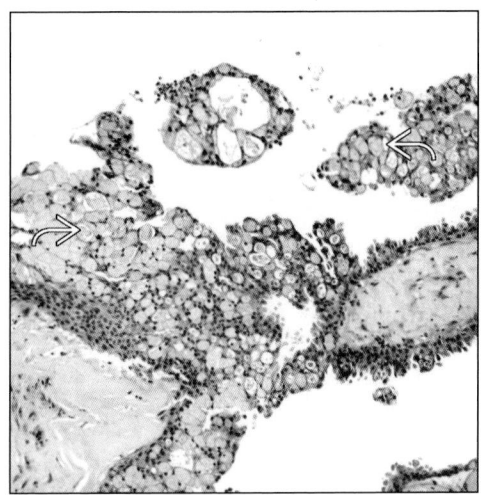 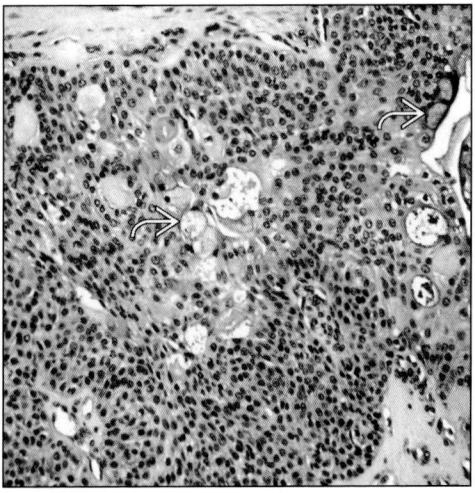

(Left) Mucinous differentiation can be seen in a minority of cases of hidradenoma (and more rarely in hidradenocarcinoma). In this area, numerous goblet-like cells ⇗ containing abundant cytoplasmic mucin are seen lining cystic spaces. (Right) High magnification of a more solid area of a mucinous hidradenoma shows scattered goblet-like cells ⇗ with prominent cytoplasmic mucin.

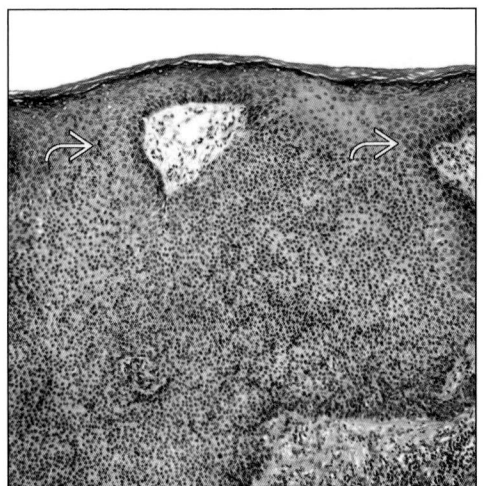 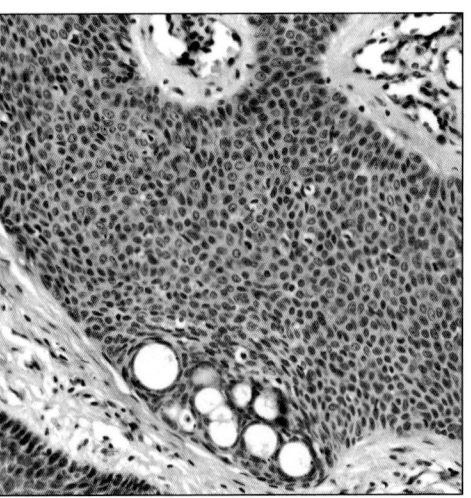

(Left) Low magnification of a poroma shows basaloid to squamoid cells with thickened, anastomosing connections between the tumor cells and the overlying epidermis ⇗. Although closely related tumors, hidradenomas are typically deeper-seated, dermal-based tumors lacking epidermal connections. (Right) Poromas are composed of poroid cells with oval to round nuclei, small nucleoli, and indistinct cytoplasmic borders. Clear cell features are less common than in hidradenoma.

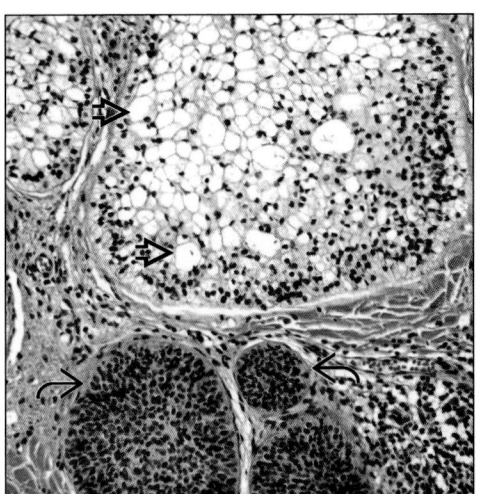 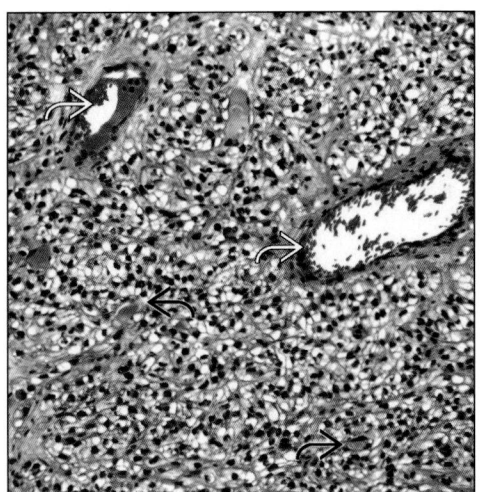

(Left) Clear cell BCC is composed of large cells with abundant clear cytoplasm ⇗ and can mimic clear cell hidradenoma in some cases. However, areas of more conventional BCC are often present as are seen in the lower corner of this field ⇗. (Right) Metastatic clear cell renal cell carcinoma to the skin can present as a dermal nodule, mimicking clear cell hidradenoma. However, RCC shows numerous small ⇗ to medium-sized blood vessels ⇗, which are much sparser in hidradenoma.

HIDRADENOCARCINOMA

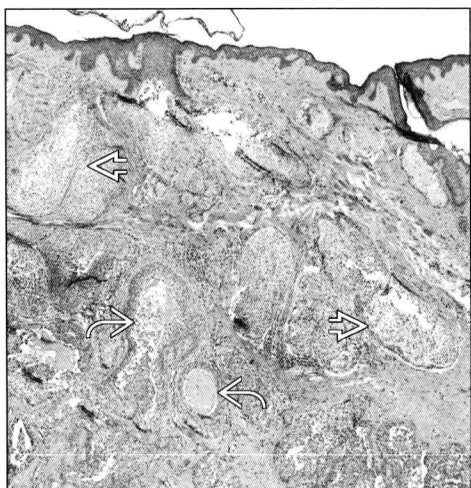

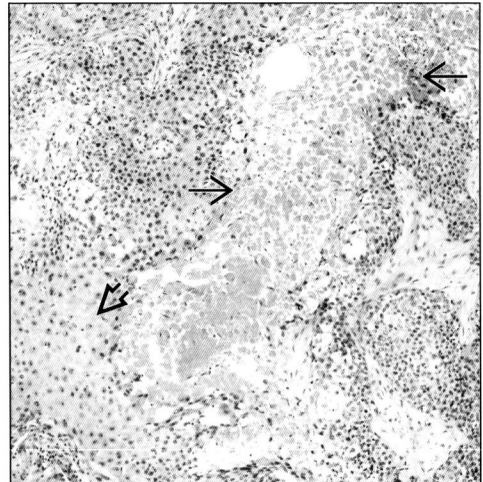

Low magnification of a hidradenocarcinoma shows a dermal-based, atypical, multilobular neoplasm with clear cell features ⊇ and cystic spaces ⊅ containing mucinous material and cellular debris.

Areas of squamous differentiation ⊇ and prominent tumoral cell necrosis ⊅ are present in this example of hidradenocarcinoma. Squamous differentiation is much less common than in porocarcinoma.

TERMINOLOGY

Synonyms
- Malignant acrospiroma, malignant hidradenoma

Definitions
- Malignant adnexal tumor arising from, or showing areas similar to, a hidradenoma

CLINICAL ISSUES

Site
- Most frequently in head and neck region

Presentation
- Nodule or mass

Treatment
- Surgical approaches
  - Wide, local excision of tumor
  - Mohs micrographic surgery may be best option to ensure clear margins
- Drugs
  - For metastatic hidradenocarcinoma, if surgery is not an option
    - Various chemotherapeutic regimens reported
    - Case reports of sunitinib and capecitabine treatment
- Radiation
  - Variable response

Prognosis
- Excision is sometimes curative
- Course can be aggressive
  - Local recurrences
  - Metastatic disease
    - Lymph nodes, distant skin, internal organs

MICROSCOPIC PATHOLOGY

Histologic Features
- Epithelial islands with interspersed glands/ducts
- Architecture may be predominantly solid islands; sometimes cystic areas present
  - Cells composing the islands are variable
    - Clear, poroid, less commonly squamoid, rarely mucinous
- Hyalinized stroma
- Infiltrative growth pattern; not well-circumscribed
- Deep extension
- Necrosis may be evident
- Nuclear pleomorphism may be present
- Mitoses often present
  - May be > 4 per 10 high-power fields
- Perineural or vascular invasion may be identified
- Area of tumor compatible with benign hidradenoma may be seen

Cytologic Features
- May show high-grade cytologic atypia
- Some cases may be composed of relatively bland cells without prominent cytologic atypia
- Mitoses may be few or many
- Varying proportions of clear, poroid, and squamoid cells
  - Poroid cells have dark blue nuclear outline with finely granular nucleoplasm

ANCILLARY TESTS

Immunohistochemistry
- Positive with p63, cytokeratin 5/6, consistent with a primary cutaneous tumor
- Carcino-embryonic antigen (CEA) and EMA highlight glandular/ductal foci
- p53 positive, and Ki-67 generally shows a high proliferative index

HIDRADENOCARCINOMA

Key Facts

Terminology
- Malignant acrospiroma, malignant hidradenoma
- Malignant adnexal tumor arising from, or showing areas similar to, a hidradenoma

Clinical Issues
- Most frequently occurs on head and neck region
- Presents as nodule or mass lesion
- Excision is sometimes curative
- Mohs micrographic surgery may be best option to ensure clear margins
- Course can be aggressive, with local recurrences and metastases

Microscopic Pathology
- Epithelial islands with interspersed glands/ducts
- Cells composing islands are variable

- ○ Clear, poroid, squamoid (less common), rarely mucinous
- Hyalinized stroma (similar to hidradenoma)
- Infiltrative growth pattern (not well-circumscribed, unlike hidradenoma)
- Deep extension
- Perineural or vascular invasion may be present
- Ki-67 generally shows a high proliferative index

Top Differential Diagnoses
- Hidradenoma
- Metastatic renal cell carcinoma
- Clear cell squamous cell carcinoma
- Clear cell basal cell carcinoma
- Sebaceous carcinoma
- Porocarcinoma

- Generally negative with Her2/neu

DIFFERENTIAL DIAGNOSIS

Hidradenoma
- Nodular, well-circumscribed, dermal-based tumor
- Composed of varying proportion of clear cells, poroid cells, squamoid cells (less common than in porocarcinomas), and rarely mucinous cells
- Lacks high-grade atypia, necrosis, infiltrative features, and atypical mitoses

Metastatic Renal Cell Carcinoma
- Clear cells in variably sized islands
- No true ductal differentiation present
- Prominence of small, capillary-type vessels and extravasated erythrocytes
- Hyalinized stroma absent
- More commonly positive with EMA (cytoplasmic, not ductal) and CD10

Clear Cell Squamous Cell Carcinoma
- Clear cells in variably sized nests and islands
- Dyskeratotic cells and areas of keratinization often present
- Poroid cells absent
- No true ductal differentiation present

Clear Cell Basal Cell Carcinoma
- Clear cells in variably sized islands
  - ○ Some islands show peripheral palisading
- Poroid cells absent
- Ductal differentiation absent to minimal
- Positive with BER-EP4

Sebaceous Carcinoma
- Invasive basaloid to squamoid tumor with interspersed clear cells with bubbly cytoplasm
- Ducts with pink cuticles may be present but are rare
- EMA (cytoplasmic staining), adipophilin, and AR staining are typically positive

Porocarcinoma
- Invasive poroid neoplasm with anastomosing cords of tumor cells
- Typically shows multiple epidermal attachments (absent in hidradenocarcinoma)
- More frequent squamous differentiation and fewer clear cell features compared to hidradenocarcinoma

DIAGNOSTIC CHECKLIST

Pathologic Interpretation Pearls
- Epithelial islands with interspersed glands/ducts
- Cells composing islands are variable
  - ○ Clear, poroid, squamoid, rarely mucinous
- Hyalinized-appearing stroma
- Infiltrative growth pattern
  - ○ Not well circumscribed (unlike hidradenoma)
- Deep extension; necrosis
- Mitoses usually, but not always, prominent

SELECTED REFERENCES

1. Cohen M et al: Apocrine hidradenocarcinoma of the scalp: a classification conundrum. Head Neck Pathol. 3(1):42-6, 2009
2. Nazarian RM et al: Atypical and malignant hidradenomas: a histological and immunohistochemical study. Mod Pathol. 22(4):600-10, 2009
3. Wahl CE et al: Apocrine hidradenocarcinoma showing Paget's disease and mucinous metaplasia. J Cutan Pathol. 36(5):582-5, 2009
4. Yavel R et al: Hidradenomas and a hidradenocarcinoma of the scalp managed using Mohs micrographic surgery and a multidisciplinary approach: case reports and review of the literature. Dermatol Surg. 35(2):273-81, 2009
5. Ko CJ et al: Hidradenocarcinoma: a histological and immunohistochemical study. J Cutan Pathol. 33(11):726-30, 2006
6. Hernández-Pérez E et al: Nodular hidradenoma and hidradenocarcinoma. A 10-year review. J Am Acad Dermatol. 12(1 Pt 1):15-20, 1985

HIDRADENOCARCINOMA

Microscopic Features

(Left) Scanning magnification of a hidradenocarcinoma from the axilla shows normal apocrine glands ⇨ at the top of the photo. The tumor is deep-seated, has cystic areas containing necrotic cellular debris ⇗, and is composed of basaloid and clear cells. **(Right)** Nodular hidradenocarcinoma at low magnification demonstrates a large tumor with sheets of cells showing prominent cytologic atypia, pleomorphism, and focal ductal lumina ⇨.

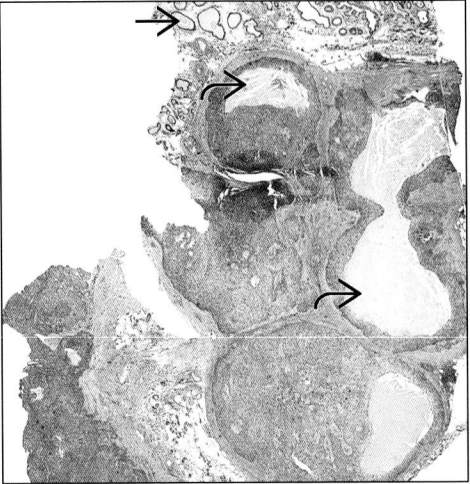 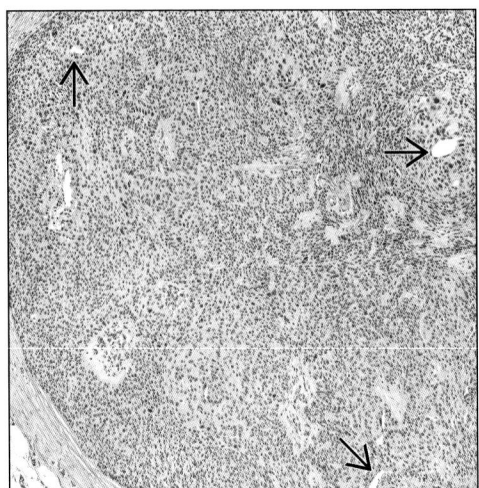

(Left) Higher power view of a hidradenocarcinoma shows infiltrative islands ⇨ of cytologically atypical cells in a densely hyalinized stroma. There is focal perineural invasion ⇗. Larger tumor islands are both solid and cystic ⇲. **(Right)** Hidradenocarcinoma with an infiltrative, cord-like proliferation of basaloid to clear-staining cells also shows a focal cystic area containing mucinous material ⇲.

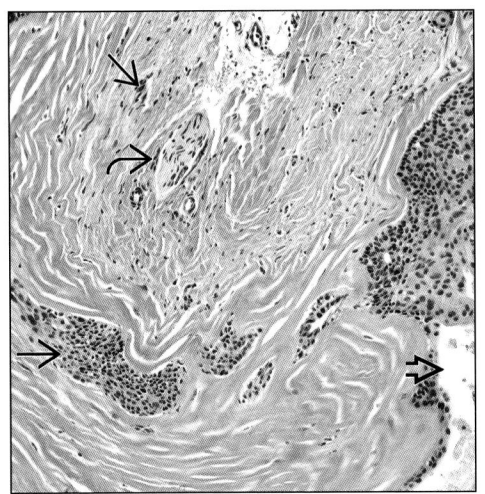 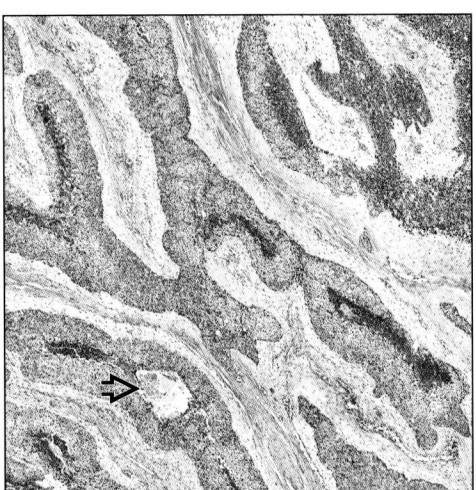

(Left) High magnification of an area of hidradenocarcinoma with predominantly clear cell features and focal ductal differentiation ⇲ demonstrates mitotic figures ⇨, areas of apoptotic cells ⇢, and necrotic cellular debris ⇗. **(Right)** Infiltrative islands of a hidradenocarcinoma show clear to squamoid cells with atypia, demonstrating enlarged nuclei and prominent nucleoli. There is an atypical mitosis ⇨ in the center of the field.

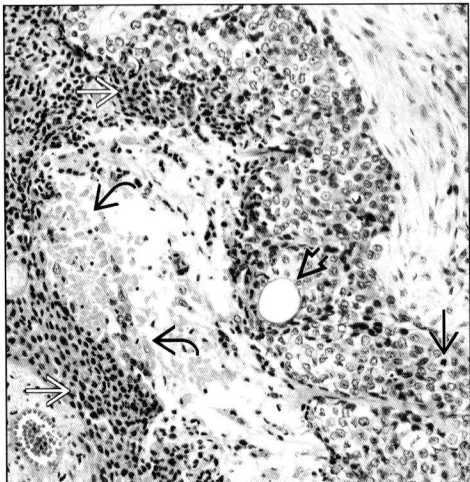 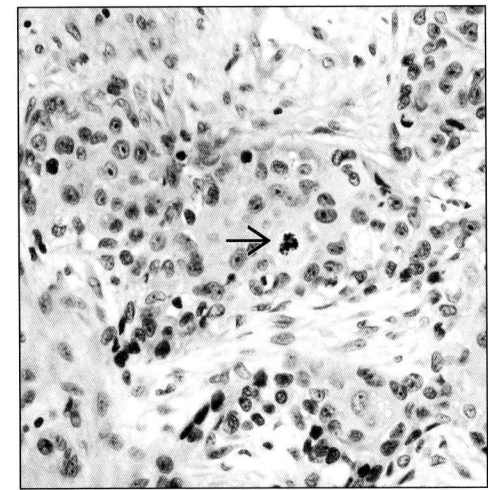

HIDRADENOCARCINOMA

Ancillary Techniques and Differential Diagnosis

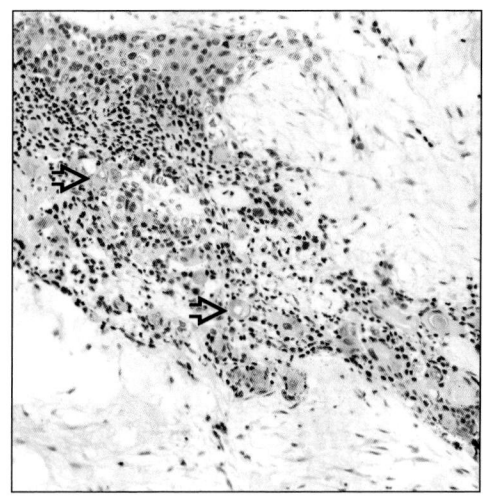

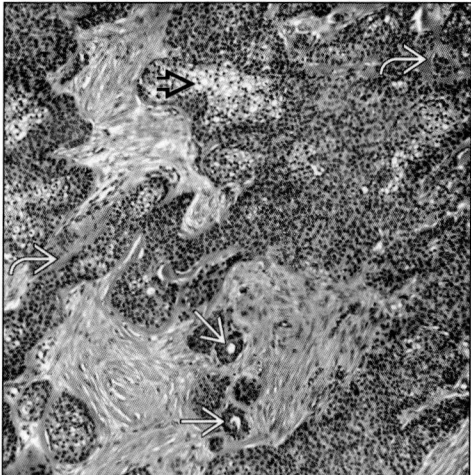

(Left) CEA-M weakly highlights numerous small ductal lumina ⊃ and their contents in this example of an infiltrative hidradenocarcinoma. (Right) Low magnification of a hidradenoma shows hyalinized stroma �“, which can suggest an infiltrative tumor, but is common in hidradenomas. The tumor cells are basaloid to focally clear ⊃. There is focal ductal differentiation ➙.

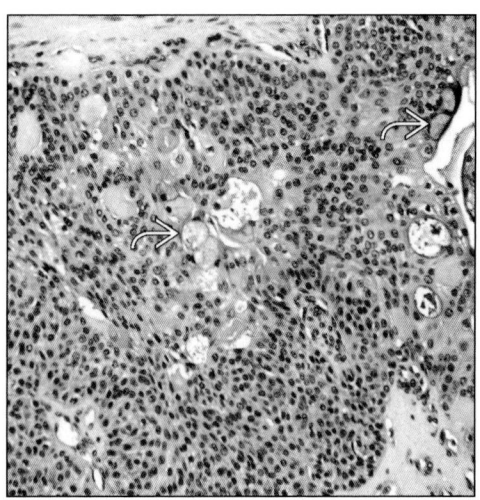

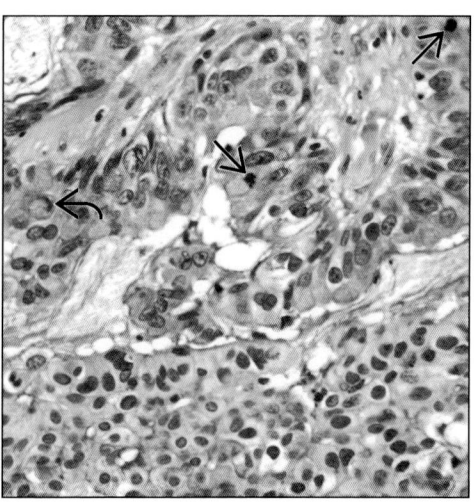

(Left) Mucinous differentiation can be seen in a minority of cases of hidradenoma (and very rarely in hidradenocarcinoma). In this area, numerous goblet-like cells ➙ containing abundant cytoplasmic mucin are seen lining cystic spaces. (Right) Rare mucinous hidradenocarcinoma shows a proliferation of markedly enlarged and atypical-appearing, eosinophilic-staining cells with focal cytoplasmic mucin ➙. Several mitotic figures ➙ are present in this field.

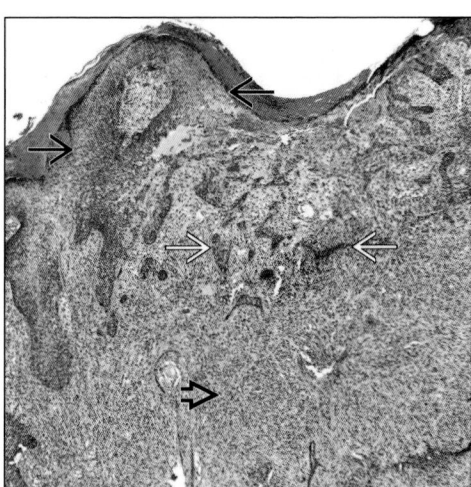

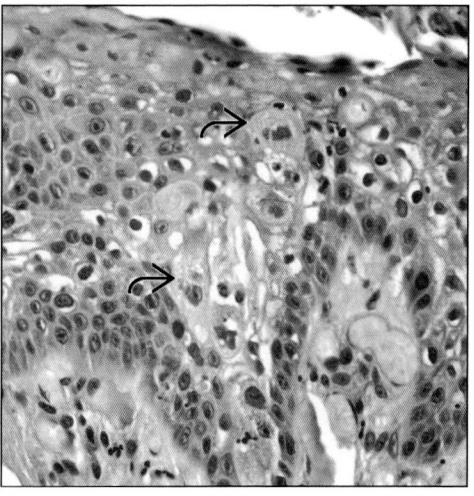

(Left) Porocarcinoma with an in situ component ➙ and ulceration overlies an invasive tumor with epithelial islands ➙ and poorly differentiated spindle cells ⊃. Hidradenocarcinomas only very rarely show epidermal involvement. (Right) Pagetoid spread in a mucinous hidradenocarcinoma shows intraepidermal spread of enlarged, atypical-appearing cells with abundant mucinous-appearing cytoplasm ➙. This is a very rare finding that has been reported in only a few cases.

POROMA AND DERMAL DUCT TUMOR

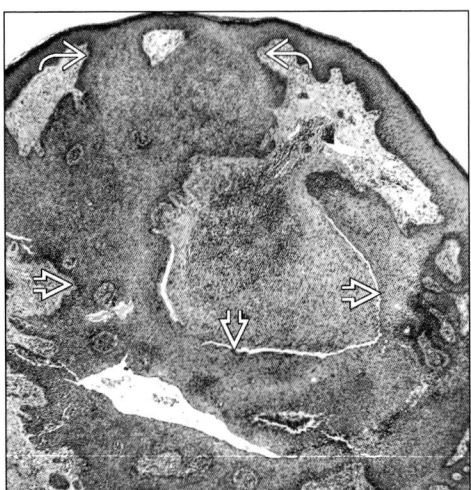

Low magnification of a poroma shows a basaloid to squamoid tumor with multiple thickened, anastomosing connections between the tumor cords ⇒ and to the overlying epidermis ⇒.

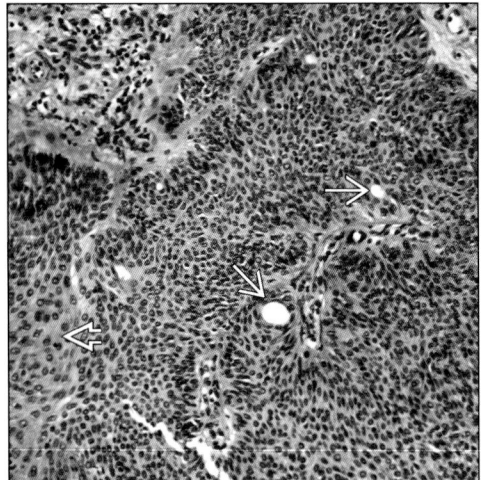

Higher magnification of a poroma shows a proliferation of small basaloid to focally squamoid ⇒ cells forming thick, anastomosing cords. Note the scattered small ductal lumina ⇒.

TERMINOLOGY

Synonyms
- Apocrine poroma
- Eccrine poroma
- Hidroacanthoma simplex (intraepidermal poroma, syringoacanthoma)
- Acrospiroma (older term, includes both poroma and hidradenoma)

Definitions
- Benign adnexal proliferation with anastomosing cords of tumor cells exhibiting ductal differentiation
- Typically has multiple epidermal attachments, except for dermal duct tumor

ETIOLOGY/PATHOGENESIS

Unknown
- Rare cases associated with radiation therapy and pregnancy
  - May rarely be multiple ("poromatosis")
- Formerly considered eccrine, but many cases likely of apocrine differentiation
  - May see sebaceous &/or follicular differentiation in apocrine cases

CLINICAL ISSUES

Epidemiology
- Incidence
  - Relatively common tumors
- Age
  - Usually occur in middle-aged adults
- Gender
  - Equal incidence in males and females

Site
- Most common on the extremities, especially the palmar and plantar surfaces
  - May also occur on the trunk, head and neck

Presentation
- Solitary pink to reddish papular or nodular lesion
  - Some cases may be very vascular and bleed easily
  - Minority of cases are pigmented

Natural History
- Stable lesions; do not usually regress

Treatment
- Surgical approaches
  - Complete conservative excision is curative
    - Typically recommended to prevent recurrence and rare transformation to porocarcinoma

Prognosis
- Excellent; most cases do not show aggressive behavior

MACROSCOPIC FEATURES

General Features
- Superficial, firm papule or nodule

Size
- Generally < 1 cm but may be larger

MICROSCOPIC PATHOLOGY

Histologic Features
- Symmetric, well-circumscribed tumor with multiple epidermal attachments
  - Intraepidermal component is typically sharply demarcated from adjacent normal epidermis
- Broad, anastomosing columns and thickened cords of tumor cells
- Ductal lumina typically numerous

Key Facts

Terminology
- Eccrine poroma
- Apocrine poroma
- Hidroacanthoma simplex (intraepidermal poroma, syringoacanthoma)
- Acrospiroma (older term, includes poroma and hidradenoma)
- Benign adnexal proliferation with anastomosing cords of cells and ductal differentiation

Clinical Issues
- Relatively common tumors
- Usually occur in middle-aged adults
- Most common on the extremities, especially the palmar and plantar surfaces
- Solitary pink to reddish papular or nodular lesion
- Excellent prognosis in most cases

Microscopic Pathology
- Symmetric, well-circumscribed tumor with multiple epidermal attachments (except in dermal duct tumor)
- Broad, anastomosing columns and thickened cords of tumor cells
- Ductal lumina typically well-formed, numerous
- Cells may be basaloid, squamoid, clear, or pigmented
- Mitotic figures may be present, and can be numerous in traumatized lesions

Top Differential Diagnoses
- Hidradenoma
- Irritated/clonal seborrheic keratosis (SK)
- Basal cell carcinoma (BCC)
- Squamous cell carcinoma (SCC)
- Porocarcinoma (malignant poroma)

○ A few small cystic structures may also be present
- Composed of basaloid to squamoid-appearing cells
  ○ Most cells are small, cuboidal-shaped and have bland nuclei with uniform chromatin
  ○ Cells may also be clear (clear cell poroma) or pigmented (pigmented poroma)
    ▪ Clear cells contain glycogen, which is confirmed by PAS without diastase
- Mitotic figures may be present and can be numerous in traumatized lesions
  ○ But are usually localized to basilar layers and are not atypical

Subtypes
- **Dermal duct tumor (DDT)**
  ○ Similar-appearing tumor in the dermis
  ○ Ductal structures usually numerous
  ○ Epidermal attachments often found if multiple deeper level sections examined
- **Hidroacanthoma simplex (intraepidermal poroma)**
  ○ Intraepidermal proliferation of nests of monotonous basaloid cells
    ▪ Appears similar to clonal seborrheic keratosis, but cells are smaller and show ductal differentiation
  ○ Likely represents example of so-called "intraepidermal epithelioma of Borst-Jadassohn"

DIFFERENTIAL DIAGNOSIS

Hidradenoma
- Closely related tumors (grouped together under "acrospiroma"), **but**
  ○ Typically deep dermal-based nodule
  ○ Lacks epidermal connections
  ○ More commonly shows clear cell features

Irritated/Clonal Seborrheic Keratosis (SK)
- Irritated SK may occasionally mimic poroma (and hidroacanthoma simplex); **however**
  ○ SK shows follicular differentiation with keratinizing pseudohorn cysts, no ductal differentiation
  ○ Cells are typically larger than those in poroma

Basal Cell Carcinoma (BCC)
- Not difficult to separate from poroma except in small superficial biopsies
  ○ Areas of peripheral palisading, mucinous stroma, and tumor-stromal retraction artifact present
  ○ Cells more atypical, and mitotic and apoptotic figures usually abundant

Squamous Cell Carcinoma (SCC)
- Usually not difficult to separate from poroma except in small biopsies
  ○ Poromas show squamoid features in many cases
  ○ SCC lacks evidence of ductal differentiation
  ○ Greater cytologic atypia, dyskeratotic cells in SCC

Porocarcinoma (Malignant Poroma)
- Malignant poroid tumor; can be in situ or invasive
- Often arise in longstanding poroma
- Increased cytologic atypia, pleomorphism, and mitotic figures (including atypical forms)

SELECTED REFERENCES

1. Battistella M et al: From hidroacanthoma simplex to poroid hidradenoma: clinicopathologic and immunohistochemic study of poroid neoplasms and reappraisal of their histogenesis. Am J Dermatopathol. 32(5):459-68, 2010
2. Mitsuishi T et al: Pigmented poroid neoplasm mimicking nodular melanoma. J Dermatol. 37(6):542-4, 2010
3. Ansai S et al: Assessment of cellular proliferation of eccrine acrospiromas and eccrine sweat gland carcinomas by AgNOR counting and immunohistochemical demonstration of proliferating cell nuclear antigen (PCNA) and Ki-67. Clin Exp Dermatol. 20(1):27-34, 1995
4. Galadari E et al: Malignant transformation of eccrine tumors. J Cutan Pathol. 14(1):15-22, 1987
5. Kitamura K et al: Hidroacanthoma simplex with invasive growth. Cutis. 32(1):83-4, 86-8, 1983
6. Pylyser K et al: The histology of eccrine poromas: a study of 14 cases. Dermatologica. 167(5):243-9, 1983
7. Goldman P et al: Eccrine poroma; tumors exhibiting features of the epidermal sweat duct unit. AMA Arch Derm. 74(5):511-21, 1956

POROMA AND DERMAL DUCT TUMOR

Variant Microscopic Features

(Left) Traumatized poroma shows overlying erosion, dense serum crusting ⇒, and impetiginization ⇒. Reactive atypia may be seen in cases with recent irritation/trauma. *(Right)* Higher magnification of a traumatized poroma shows mild nuclear enlargement and hyperchromasia ⇒, as well as a few (nonatypical) mitotic figures ⇒, consistent with reactive changes due to irritation/trauma.

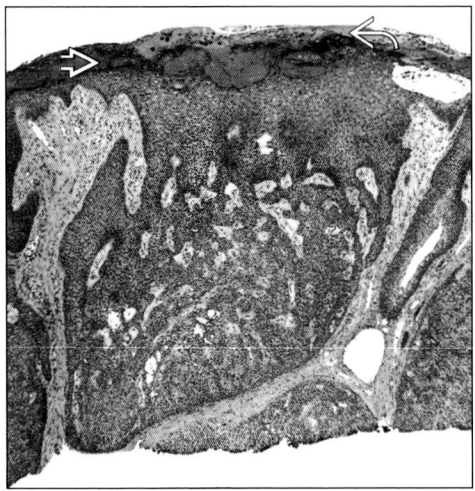
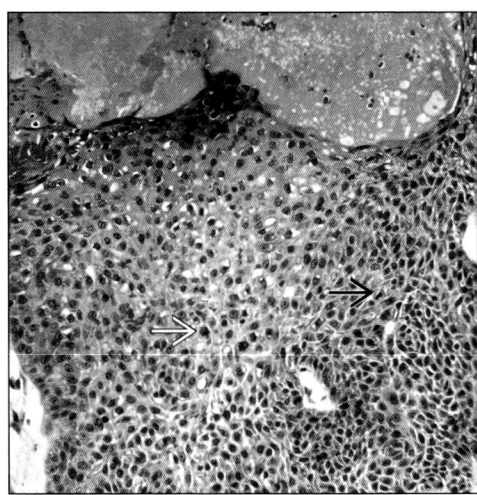

(Left) Scanning magnification of a poroma with clear cell features shows a basaloid to clear cell ⇒ neoplasm with multiple anastomosing connections between thickened cords of tumor cells and to epidermis ⇒. *(Right)* Higher magnification of a clear cell area of poroma shows a proliferation of small cells with abundant pale to clear-staining cytoplasm ⇒ and small nuclei lacking atypia.

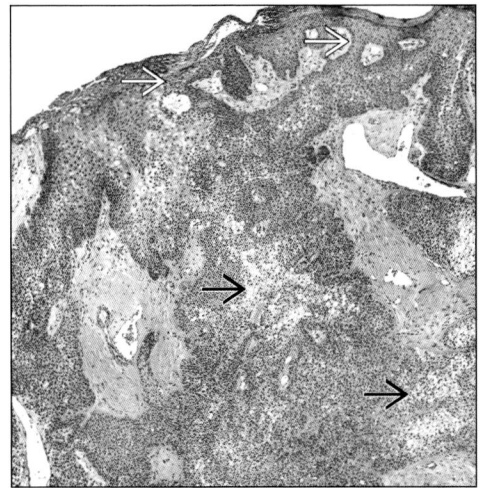
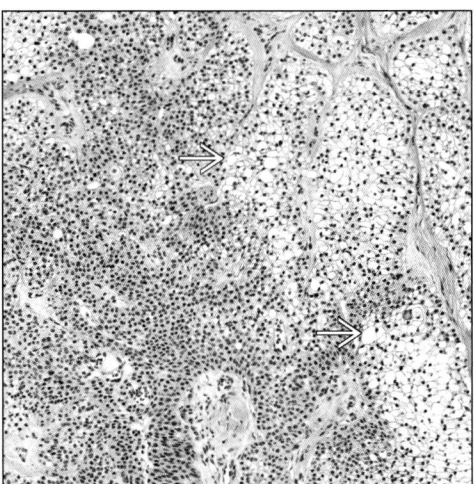

(Left) Pigmented poroma is not an uncommon variant. Although many of the cells are darkly pigmented ⇒, it otherwise shows features typical of poroma, being composed of basaloid to squamoid cells forming multiple thickened, anastomosing connections between the tumor cords ⇒. *(Right)* High magnification of a pigmented poroma shows a bland-appearing population of small basaloid to squamoid cells with prominent cytoplasmic pigmentation. Colonizing melanocytes ⇒ are present.

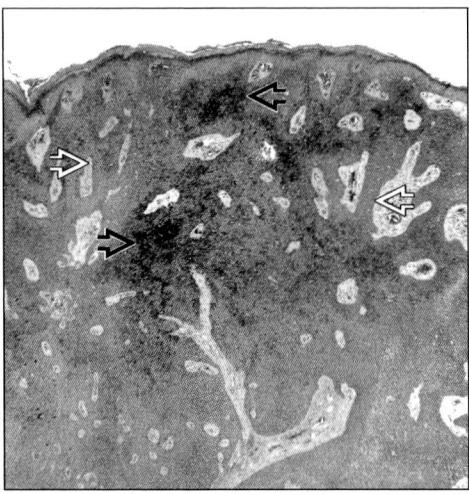
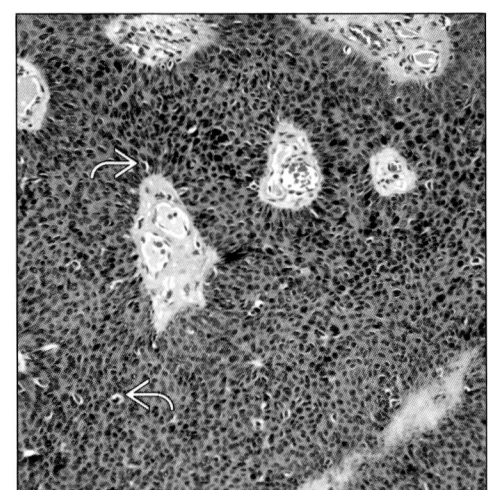

Differential Diagnosis and Ancillary Techniques

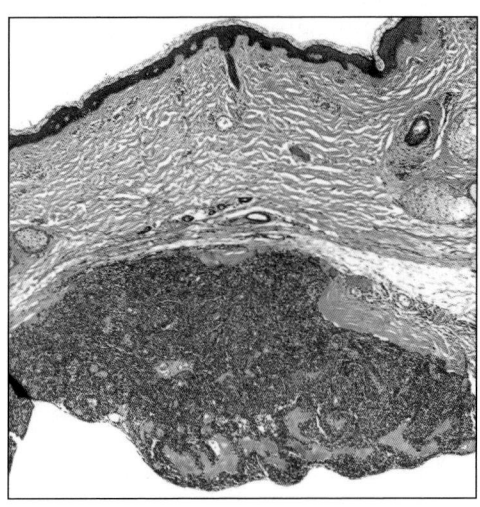

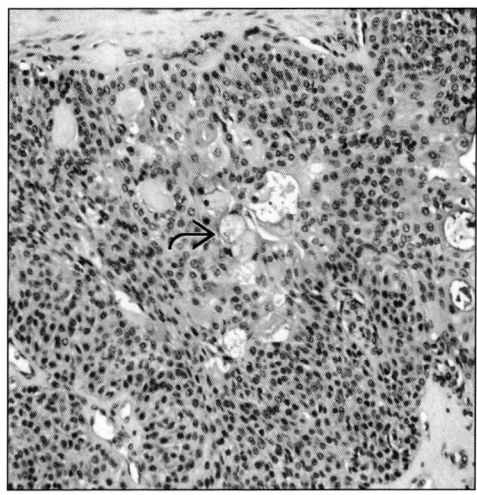

(Left) Nodular-cystic hidradenoma is a closely related tumor (and may be grouped together under the term "acrospiroma"), but it is typically situated deeper in the dermis, often shows clear cell features, and lacks connections to the epidermis. *(Right)* High magnification shows mucinous metaplasia with goblet cells ⮞ in a hidradenoma. This is not an uncommon finding in hidradenomas, but is extremely rare in poromas.

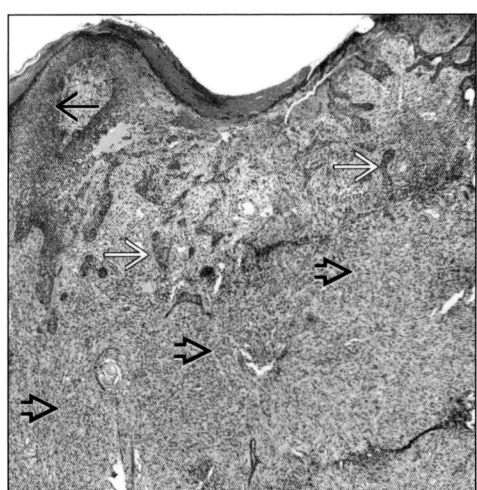

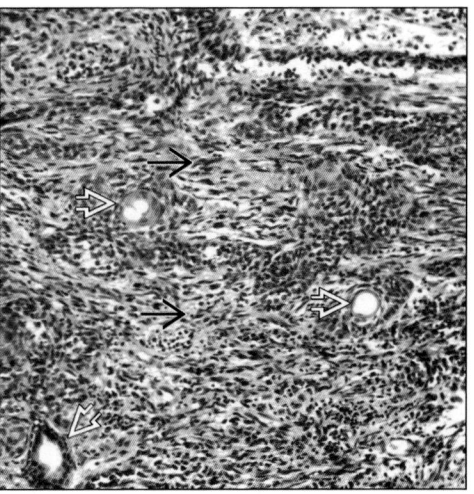

(Left) Scanning magnification of sarcomatoid porocarcinoma shows an in situ component ⮞ with areas of ulceration that is overlying an invasive tumor composed of epithelial islands ⮞ surrounded by poorly differentiated spindle cells ⮞. *(Right)* Invasive porocarcinoma with sarcomatoid features. Note the scattered well-differentiated ductal structures ⮞ that are surrounded by infiltrative atypical spindle cells ⮞.

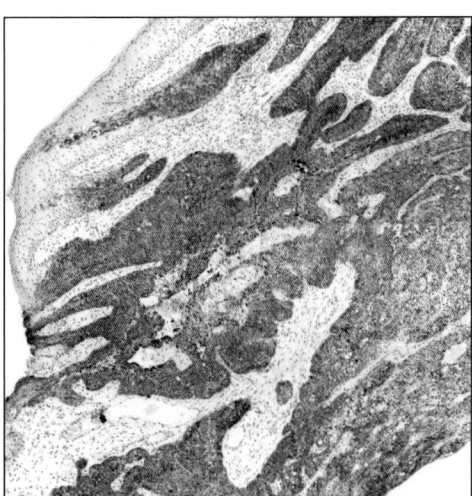

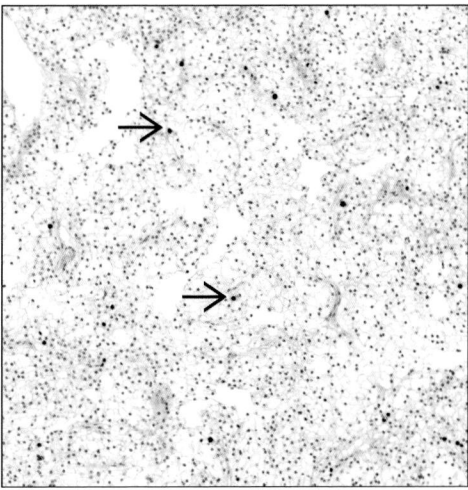

(Left) High molecular weight cytokeratins including CK5/6 and CK903/34βE12 are typically strongly and diffusely positive in poroma and porocarcinoma, similar to most adnexal tumors. *(Right)* Ki-67 highlights scattered nuclei ⮞ in a poroma, consistent with a low nuclear proliferative rate (< 5% in most cases).

POROCARCINOMA

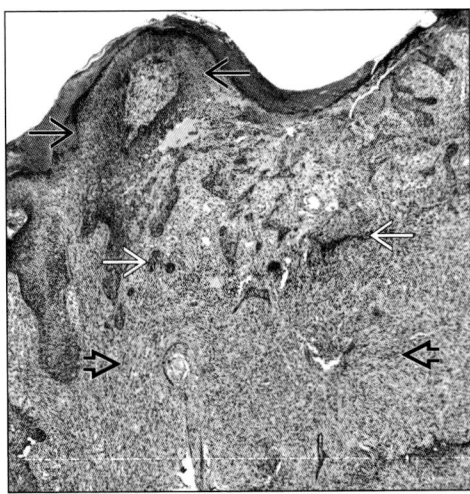

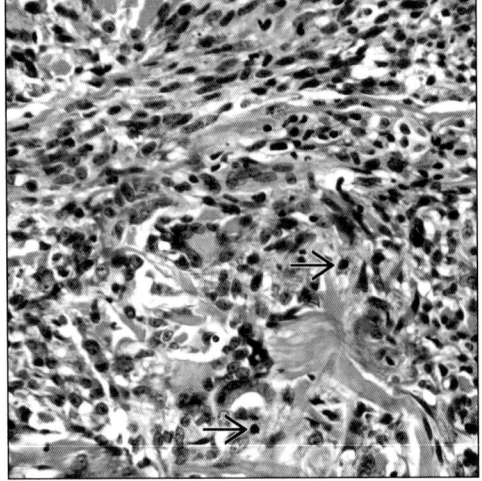

Scanning magnification of porocarcinoma shows an situ component ⇨ overlying an invasive tumor composed of epithelial islands ⇨ surrounded by poorly differentiated spinell cells ⇱.

High magnification of an invasive sarcomatoid porocarcinoma shows atypical infiltrative spindle cells with hyperchromatic nuclei and scattered mitotic figures ⇨.

TERMINOLOGY

Synonyms
- Malignant poroma

Definitions
- Malignant adnexal tumor with ductal differentiation that may arise in a poroma

ETIOLOGY/PATHOGENESIS

Unknown
- May arise from malignant transformation of longstanding poroma
- Rare cases have been reported in nevus sebaceous

CLINICAL ISSUES

Epidemiology
- Incidence
  ○ Rare tumors; approximately 200 cases reported
- Age
  ○ Usually occur in elderly patients

Site
- Predilection for extremities
  ○ Acral surfaces most common

Presentation
- Plaque or polypoid tumor

Treatment
- Surgical approaches
  ○ Complete surgical excision is recommended to ensure complete removal
    ▪ Mohs surgery reported to be effective
  ○ Some investigators recommend performing sentinel lymph node biopsy for staging purposes

Prognosis
- Significant rate of metastasis (up to 40-50% reported, usually to lymph nodes)

MACROSCOPIC FEATURES

Size
- Typically large tumors, several centimeters

MICROSCOPIC PATHOLOGY

Histologic Features
- Epidermal-based atypical adnexal tumor with anastomosing cords of tumor cells
  ○ Most cases are invasive, but some show only intraepidermal growth (porocarcinoma in situ)
- Ductal structures are typically found and are often numerous in well-differentiated cases
- Cells are usually basaloid, but may show clear cell or squamoid features
- Rare sarcomatoid variants have been reported, with an invasive spindle cell component
- Mitotic figures usually numerous and may be atypical

Cytologic Features
- Cells show cytologic atypia, with enlarged, hyperchromatic-staining nuclei and prominent nucleoli

ANCILLARY TESTS

Immunohistochemistry
- Immunohistochemistry usually not necessary, but can be useful to confirm diagnosis
  ○ Ductal/glandular lumina usually positive for EMA and CEA-M
    ▪ Squamous cell carcinoma and basal cell carcinoma lack luminal staining

POROCARCINOMA

Key Facts

Etiology/Pathogenesis

• May arise from malignant transformation of longstanding poroma

Clinical Issues

• Rare tumors; approximately 200 cases reported
• Usually occur in elderly patients
• Acral surfaces most common
• Significant rate of metastasis (up to 50%)

Microscopic Pathology

• Epidermal-based atypical adnexal tumor with anastomosing cords of tumor cells
• Most cases are invasive, but some may be in situ (porocarcinoma in situ)
• Cells are usually basaloid but may show clear cell, squamoid, or spindle cell features
• Mitotic figures are usually numerous and may be atypical

---

    o Tumor cells are usually diffusely positive for pancytokeratins, high molecular weight cytokeratins (i.e., CK5/6), and p63
       ■ Metastatic tumors to the skin are typically negative for CK5/6 and p63

DIFFERENTIAL DIAGNOSIS

Poroma

• May be difficult to distinguish from porocarcinoma on superficial shave biopsy
    o Particularly if tumor is traumatized &/or inflamed and shows reactive changes
• Epidermal-based neoplasm with multiple anastomosing cords of tumor cells
• Lacks dermal invasion, significant cytologic atypia, and necrosis
• Mitoses often present, but not numerous or atypical

Hidradenoma and Hidradenocarcinoma

• Dermal-based tumors without prominent anastomosing connections (unlike poroma and porocarcinoma)
• Usually nodular, well-circumscribed tumors, although hidradenocarcinomas are usually infiltrative
• Clear cell change more common, and squamoid features less common, than in poroid neoplasms

Squamous Cell Carcinoma (SCC)

• Invasive epithelial tumor composed of large squamoid cells with abundant eosinophilic cytoplasm

• Squamoid variant of porocarcinoma may be difficult to distinguish from SCC, **but**
    o SCC lacks ductal structures (can be highlighted with EMA and CEA)
    o Porocarcinoma shows more anastomosing tumor cords

Basal Cell Carcinoma (BCC)

• Most cases easily distinguishable
• BCC shows peripheral palisading, mucinous stroma, and tumor-stroma retraction artifact
• Porocarcinoma shows more anastomosing cords and at least focal ductal structures

SELECTED REFERENCES

1. Mahomed F et al: The squamous variant of eccrine porocarcinoma: a clinicopathological study of 21 cases. J Clin Pathol. 61(3):361-5, 2008
2. Kolde G et al: Metastasizing eccrine porocarcinoma. Report of two cases with fatal outcome. Pathol Res Pract. 187(4):477-81, 1991
3. Tarkhan II et al: Metastasizing eccrine porocarcinoma developing in a sebaceous nevus of Jadassohn. Report of a case. Arch Dermatol. 121(3):413-5, 1985
4. Mehregan AH et al: Eccrine adenocarcinoma. A clinicopathologic study of 35 cases. Arch Dermatol. 119(2):104-14, 1983
5. Gschnait F et al: Eccrine porocarcinoma. J Cutan Pathol. 7(6):349-53, 1980
6. Bardach H: Hidroacanthoma simplex with in situ porocarcinoma. A case suggesting malignant transformation. J Cutan Pathol. 5(5):236-48, 1978

IMAGE GALLERY

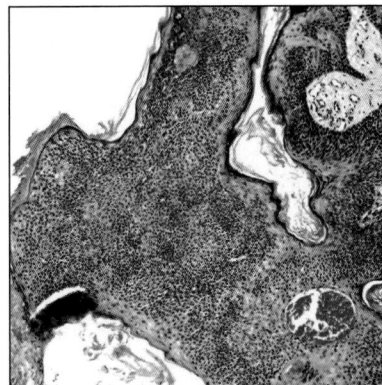 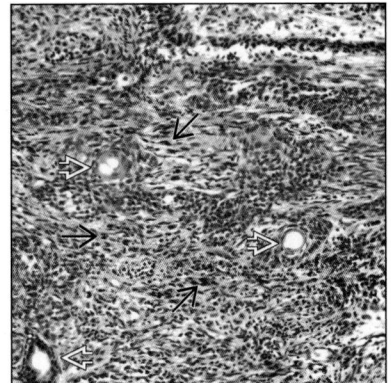 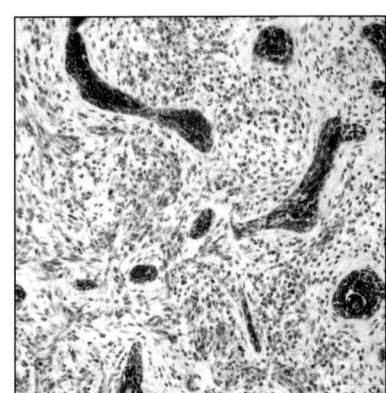

(Left) Scanning magnification of the superficial portion of a porocarcinoma shows a relatively bland-appearing area consistent with a preexisting poroma. *(Center)* Invasive porocarcinoma with sarcomatoid features. Note the scattered well-differentiated ductal structures ⬄, which are surrounded by infiltrative atypical spindle cells ➡. *(Right)* High molecular weight cytokeratin (HMWCK) diffusely highlights both the epithelial structures and infiltrative spindle cells in this case of sarcomatoid porocarcinoma.

CYLINDROMA

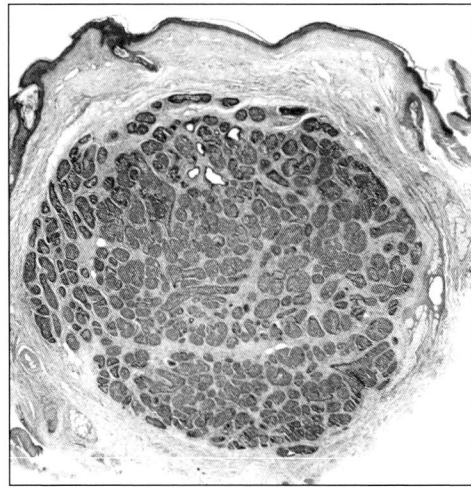

Cylindroma is typically a dermal-based, well-circumscribed, but unencapsulated tumor without connections to the overlying dermis.

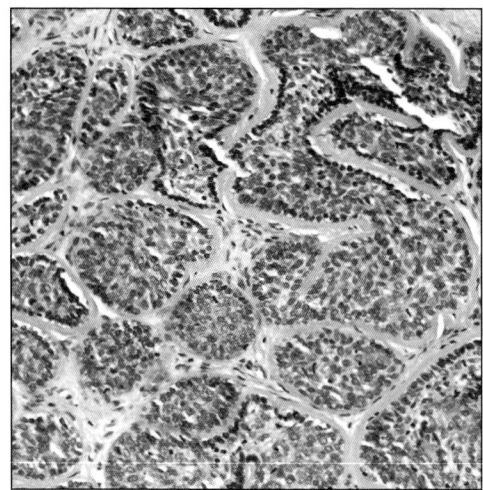

The tumor is composed of irregular lobules, surrounded by dense hyalinized membranous material, which appear to fit together in a pattern reminiscent of a jigsaw puzzle.

TERMINOLOGY

Synonyms
- Dermal cylindroma
- Turban tumor (clinical term for multiple tumors on head)

Definitions
- Benign dermal-based adnexal tumor with distinctive, "jigsaw puzzle" pattern
- May show evidence of apocrine differentiation rather than eccrine differentiation in most cases

ETIOLOGY/PATHOGENESIS

Loss of Heterozygosity of Tumor Suppressor Gene CYLD
- Mutation of *CYLD* found in both sporadic and familial cases

Sporadic or Familial
- Familial cases associated with Brooke-Spiegler syndrome
  - Also known as familial cylindromatosis or turban tumor syndrome
  - Autosomal dominant
  - Predilection for women
  - Multiple eccrine spiradenomas and trichoepitheliomas often present as well

CLINICAL ISSUES

Epidemiology
- Incidence
  - Common adnexal tumor of sweat glands
- Age
  - Usually early adulthood
- Gender
  - Marked female predominance (F:M = 9:1)

Site
- 90% present on head and neck
- 60% present on scalp

Presentation
- Dermal mass

Treatment
- Surgical approaches
  - Complete excision is curative

Prognosis
- Benign; may recur if incompletely excised
- Rare transformation to malignant cylindroma (cylindrocarcinoma), usually in large, longstanding tumors

MICROSCOPIC PATHOLOGY

Histologic Features
- Usually located in upper dermis
- No attachment to epidermis
- Circumscribed but not encapsulated
- Composed of multiple nodules/lobules of basaloid cells
- Tumor lobules have complex pattern where tumor lobules appear to fit together in an irregular, "jigsaw puzzle" pattern
- Tumor lobules surrounded by dense eosinophilic basement membrane material
- Tumor lobules have 2 cell types
  - Outer, small basaloid cells with small hyperchromatic nuclei
  - Inner cells have larger oval nuclei with vesicular chromatin
  - Tumor cells positive for CK6, CK7, CK19, and EMA

CYLINDROMA

Key Facts

Etiology/Pathogenesis
- Familial cases associated with Brooke-Spiegler syndrome

Clinical Issues
- Marked female predominance (F:M = 9:1)
- 90% present on head and neck

Microscopic Pathology
- Dermal-based tumor, circumscribed but not encapsulated
- Composed of multiple nodules/lobules of basaloid cells
- Tumor lobules have complex pattern where they appear to fit together in a "jigsaw puzzle" pattern
- Tumor lobules surrounded by dense eosinophilic basement membrane material

- Lobules have 2 cell types: Small basaloid cells and larger pale cells
- Focal ductal lumen formation
- Globules of hyaline basement membrane material often present in interior of tumor nodules

Top Differential Diagnoses
- Spiradenoma
  - Can have areas indistinguishable from cylindroma
  - Usually encapsulated
  - Tumor stroma has prominent vasculature
- Malignant cylindroma/cylindrocarcinoma
- Trichoblastoma
  - Tumor lobule surrounded by fibroblastic stroma; not thick basement membrane
- Basal cell carcinoma
  - Peripheral palisading with tumor-stroma retraction

- Basaloid cells may be positive for SMA, calponin, and S100, consistent with myoepithelial differentiation
- Focal ductal lumen formation
  - Lumina positive for CEA and EMA
- Globules of hyaline basement membrane material often present in interior of tumor nodules
  - PAS positive, diastase resistant
- Mitotic figures rare

DIFFERENTIAL DIAGNOSIS

Spiradenoma
- Encapsulated tumor composed of nodules of small basophilic tumor cells
- 2 cell types
  - Outer, small basaloid cells with hyperchromatic nuclei
  - Inner cells have larger oval nuclei with vesicular chromatin
- Significant histologic overlap with cylindroma
  - Tumor nodules can have thickened basement membrane
  - Tumor nodules can have globules of hyaline material
  - Can have areas indistinguishable from cylindroma
  - Essentially same immunophenotype as cylindroma
- Ductal lumen formation (usually more frequent than cylindroma)
- Tumor stroma has prominent vasculature and often hemorrhage

Malignant Cylindroma/Cylindrocarcinoma
- Rare tumor
- Precursor cylindroma should be present
  - Can arise in large, longstanding cylindromas (i.e., turban tumors) or cylindromas that have been irradiated
- Infiltrative growth with loss of jigsaw pattern
- Loss of thickened basement membrane and biphasic cell population of cylindroma
- Overt cytologic atypia

- Frequent mitotic figures, including atypical forms

Trichoblastoma
- Dermal-based basaloid tumor, which is circumscribed but not encapsulated
- Lobules of basaloid epithelium with peripheral palisading surrounded by condensed fibroblastic stroma
- No thickened hyalinized basement membranes
- Papillary mesenchymal bodies

Basal Cell Carcinoma
- Attachments to epidermis often present
- Peripheral palisading with tumor-stroma retraction
- Lacks jigsaw pattern and duct formation
- Lacks thickened basement membrane
- Mitotic and apoptotic figures often present

SELECTED REFERENCES

1. Kazakov DV et al: Morphologic diversity of malignant neoplasms arising in preexisting spiradenoma, cylindroma, and spiradenocylindroma based on the study of 24 cases, sporadic or occurring in the setting of Brooke-Spiegler syndrome. Am J Surg Pathol. 33(5):705-19, 2009
2. Scheinfeld N et al: Identification of a recurrent mutation in the CYLD gene in Brooke-Spiegler syndrome. Clin Exp Dermatol. 28(5):539-41, 2003
3. van der Putte SC: The pathogenesis of familial multiple cylindromas, trichoepitheliomas, milia, and spiradenomas. Am J Dermatopathol. 17(3):271-80, 1995
4. Eckert F et al: Myoepithelial differentiation in benign sweat gland tumors. Demonstrated by a monoclonal antibody to alpha-smooth muscle actin. J Cutan Pathol. 19(4):294-301, 1992
5. Lotem M et al: Multiple dermal cylindroma undergoing a malignant transformation. Int J Dermatol. 31(9):642-4, 1992
6. Rubin MG et al: Generalized cutaneous cylindromatosis. Cutis. 33(6):568-9, 1984
7. Goette DK et al: Cylindroma and eccrine spiradenoma coexistent in the same lesion. Arch Dermatol. 118(4):274-4, 1982
8. Crain RC et al: Dermal cylindroma (dermal eccrine cylindroma). Am J Clin Pathol. 35:504-15, 1961

Microscopic Features

(Left) This low-power image of cylindroma demonstrates the "jigsaw puzzle" arrangement of the tumor lobules filling the dermis. *(Right)* The tumor lobules are surrounded by a dense, eosinophilic basement membrane ⮕ and show intratumoral hyalinized globules ⮕.

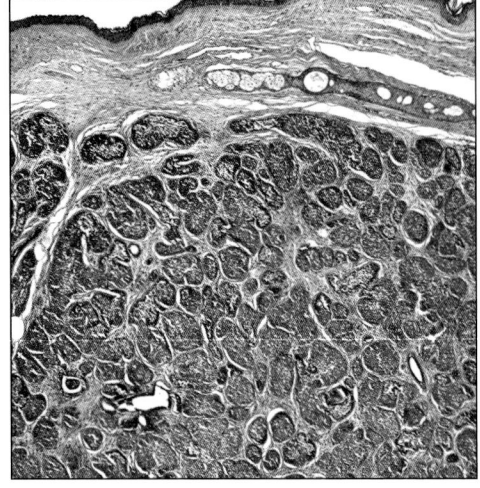 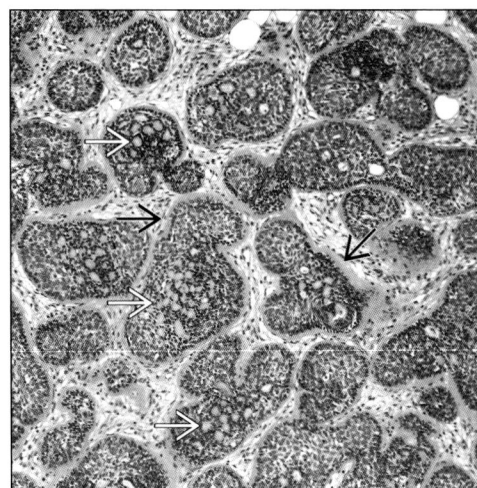

(Left) Duct lumen ⮕ formation is present. The presence of true lumina can aid in the distinction of cylindroma from basal cell carcinoma. Lumen formation is often a focal finding. *(Right)* This higher power image demonstrates how the tumor lobules fit together in an irregular, "jigsaw-puzzle" pattern. Note the prominent basement membranes surrounding the tumor lobules that are characteristic of cylindroma.

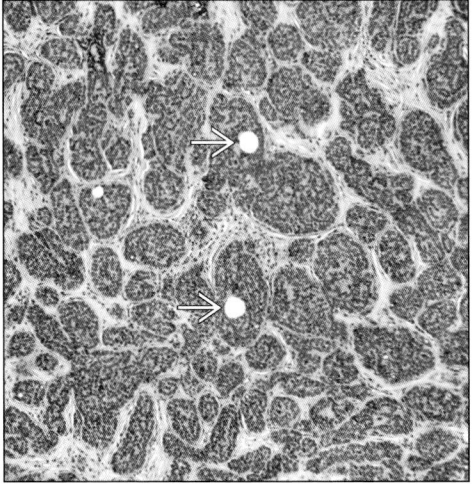 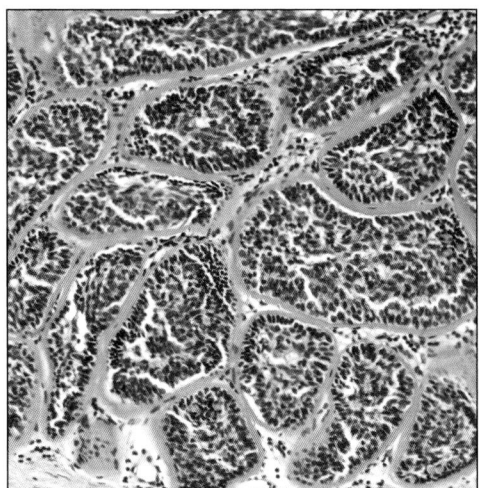

(Left) High magnification reveals that the individual tumor lobules are composed of small, relatively bland-appearing basaloid cells with hyperchromatic cells ⮕, typically at the periphery of the tumor lobule, and larger pale cells with more vesicular nuclei ⮕ in the central portion of the tumor lobule. *(Right)* PAS stain with diastase digestion shows strong, purplish staining of the hyalinized membranes ⮕ surrounding the tumor nests and lobules.

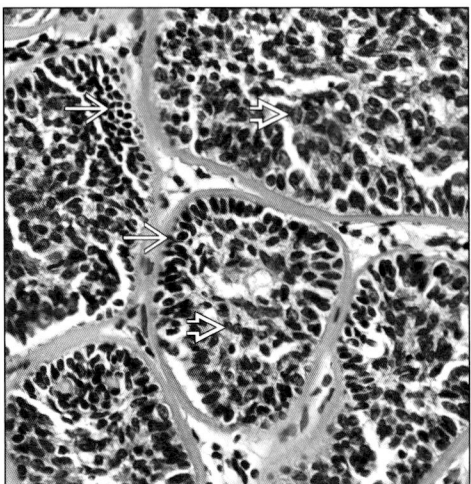 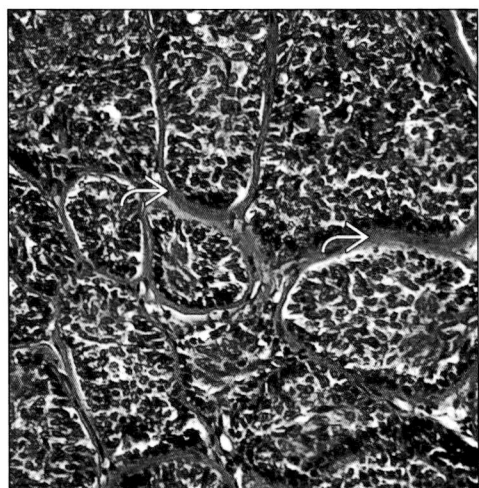

Differential Diagnosis

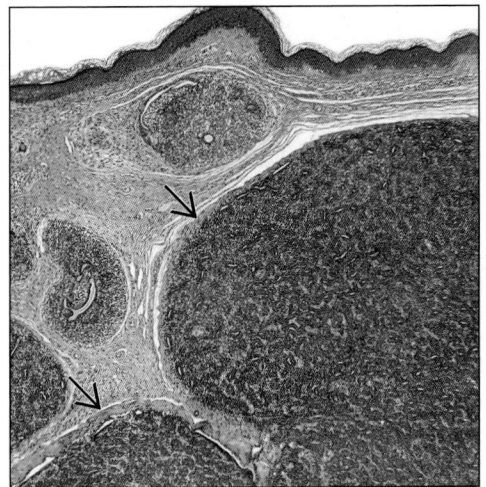

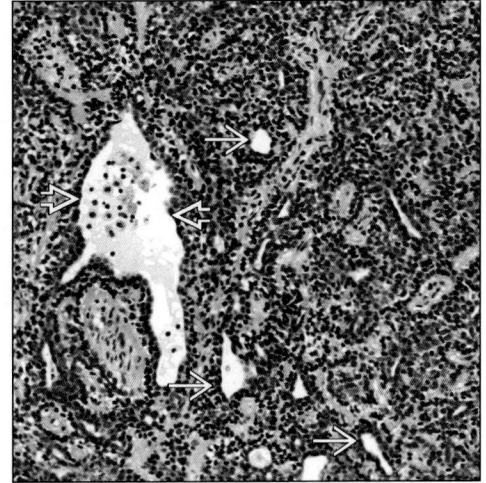

(Left) *Spiradenoma has overlapping features with cylindroma but is characterized by multiple cellular basophilic lobules in the dermis, often with a surrounding fibrous capsule* ⇢*, which is lacking in cylindroma. (Right) Higher magnification of spiradenoma shows a proliferation of small blue cells and lymphocytes surrounding a dilated glandular lumen* ⇥ *and multiple small ductal lumina* ⇥*, which are more numerous than in cylindromas.*

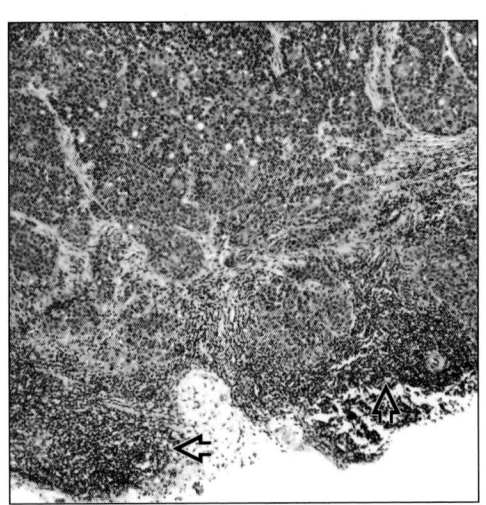

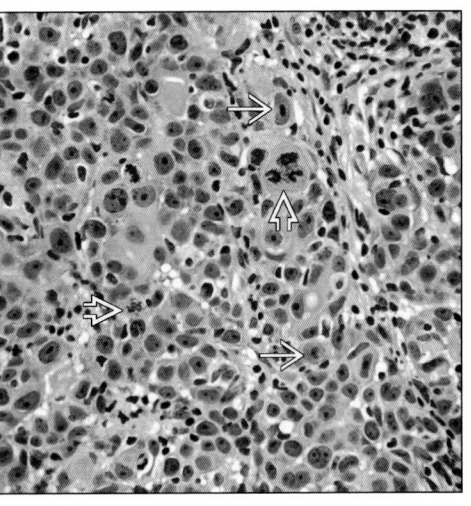

(Left) *Cylindrocarcinoma is a malignant tumor, which can arise in a large, longstanding cylindroma, and is characterized by infiltrative islands of atypical adnexal cells. Note the relatively dense surrounding lymphoid infiltrate* ⇒*. (Right) High magnification of cylindrocarcinoma shows enlarged, atypical cells with prominent nucleoli* ⇥ *and multiple mitotic figures* ⇥*.*

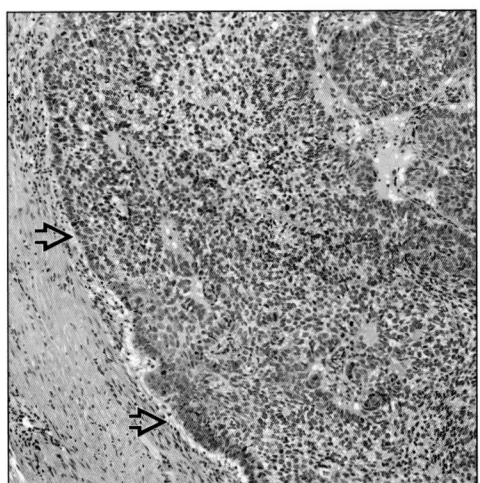

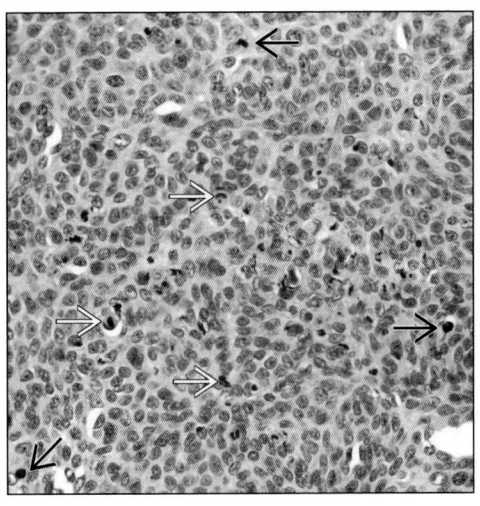

(Left) *Histologic section of a nodular-type basal cell carcinoma shows a proliferation of atypical basaloid cells with peripheral palisading and prominent retraction artifact* ⇒*, findings that are lacking in cylindromas. (Right) High magnification of a nodular basal cell carcinoma shows a sheet-like proliferation of atypical basaloid cells with high nuclear to cytoplasmic ratios and numerous apoptotic* ⇥ *and mitotic figures* ⇥*.*

SPIRADENOMA

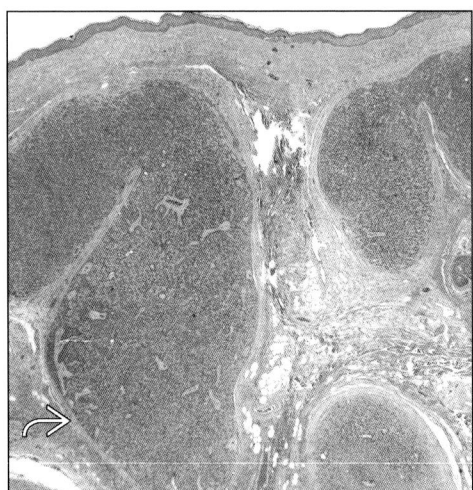

Spiradenoma is characterized by circumscribed basophilic tumor nodules or lobules in the dermis. The tumor lobules often have at least a partial fibrous capsule ➜.

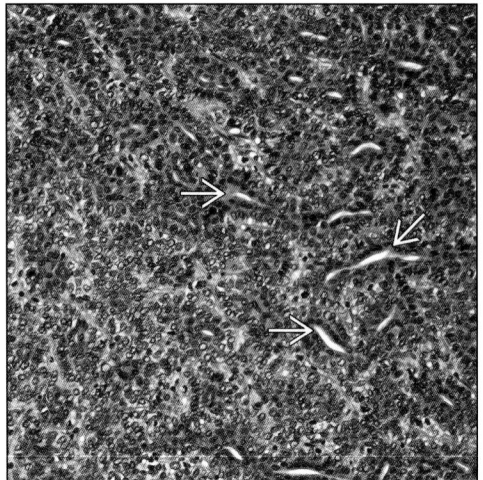

The tumor is composed of a biphasic population of smaller basaloid cells and larger pale cells. Duct lumen formation ➜ is present and may be focal or relatively prominent, as in this case.

TERMINOLOGY

Synonyms
• "Eccrine" spiradenoma

Definitions
• Benign adnexal tumor composed of nodules of basaloid cells with ductal differentiation
• May show evidence of apocrine differentiation rather than eccrine differentiation

ETIOLOGY/PATHOGENESIS

Genetic Syndrome
• Familial cases associated with Brooke-Spiegler syndrome
  ○ Also known as familial cylindromatosis or turban tumor syndrome
  ○ Autosomal dominant
  ○ Multiple cylindromas, but can also have spiradenomas and trichoepitheliomas

CLINICAL ISSUES

Epidemiology
• Age
  ○ Most common in young adults, but can present at any age

Site
• Upper 1/2 of body most commonly involved
  ○ > 75% present on ventral surface

Presentation
• Dermal mass/nodular lesion
  ○ Often tender or painful
  ○ May have bluish color
  ○ Usually solitary, but may be multiple

  ▪ Multiple lesions may be part of Brooke-Spiegler syndrome, and associated with multiple cylindromas and trichoepitheliomas

Treatment
• Surgical approaches
  ○ Complete surgical excision is curative

Prognosis
• Benign, but local recurrence may occur
• Very rare malignant transformation

MACROSCOPIC FEATURES

General Features
• Dermal-based, bluish nodule

Size
• Typically small, < 1-2 cm

MICROSCOPIC PATHOLOGY

Histologic Features
• Basophilic tumor nodules in dermis
• Tumor lobules may be partially encapsulated
• Biphasic appearance with 2 cell types
  ○ Small cells with scant cytoplasm and small hyperchromatic nuclei
  ○ Small cells are typically at periphery of tumor lobules
  ○ Larger cells with eosinophilic cytoplasm and oval, vesicular nuclei ± a distinct nucleolus
  ○ Larger cells are typically in the centers of tumor lobules
• Focal duct lumen formation
  ○ Lumina can be highlighted by immunohistochemical stains for EMA and CEA
• Tumor lobules sometimes surrounded by thickened basement membrane, similar to cylindroma

SPIRADENOMA

Key Facts

Clinical Issues
- Upper 1/2 of body most commonly involved
- Dermal mass/nodule, < 2 cm in size
- Often tender or painful lesion

Microscopic Pathology
- Basophilic tumor lobules/nodules in dermis
- Tumor may be partially encapsulated
- Biphasic appearance with 2 cell types
  - Small cells with scant cytoplasm and small hyperchromatic nuclei; typically at periphery of tumor lobules
  - Larger cells with eosinophilic cytoplasm and oval, vesicular nuclei; typically in centers of tumor lobules
- Focal to diffuse duct lumen formation

- Tumor lobules associated with vascularized stroma, hemorrhage may be present

Top Differential Diagnoses
- Cylindroma
  - Significant overlap with spiradenoma, and may have combined tumors
  - Lobules in cylindroma are typically smaller and have a "jigsaw puzzle" pattern
- Spiradenocarcinoma (malignant spiradenoma)
  - Associated with precursor spiradenoma, usually with abrupt transition
- Merkel cell carcinoma
  - More cytologic atypia and high mitotic rate
- Basal cell carcinoma
  - Peripheral palisading with tumor-stroma retraction
- Lymphoid infiltrate (pseudolymphoma)

- Tumor lobules associated with vascularized stroma, hemorrhage sometimes present
- Mitotic activity absent to rare

ANCILLARY TESTS

Immunohistochemistry
- Tumor cells positive for cytokeratins 7, 8, and 18 (CAM5.2), CK5/6, and p63; EMA and CEA highlight ducts
- Some immunoreactivity for SMA, calponin, and S100, consistent with myoepithelial differentiation

DIFFERENTIAL DIAGNOSIS

Cylindroma
- Significant overlap with spiradenoma, and may have combined tumors or areas that are indistinguishable
  - Combined tumors more common in Brooke-Spiegler patients
- Tumor lobules in cylindroma are typically smaller and have a distinct "jigsaw puzzle" pattern
- Lobules typically unencapsulated, but surrounded by dense hyalinized membranes

Spiradenocarcinoma (Malignant Spiradenoma)
- Associated with precursor spiradenoma, usually with abrupt transition to malignant component
- Infiltrative, not circumscribed
- Prominent atypia and numerous mitotic figures
- Variable tumor necrosis

Merkel Cell Carcinoma
- Lacks biphasic pattern of 2 cell types
- No ductal differentiation
- More cytologic atypia and high mitotic rate
- Positive for CK20 and neuroendocrine markers

Basal Cell Carcinoma (BCC)
- Attachments to epidermis often present

- Peripheral palisading with tumor-stroma retraction
- Lacks evidence of ductal differentiation
- Mitotic and apoptotic figures often present

Lymphoid Infiltrate (Pseudolymphoma)
- In small biopsies, duct lumen formation may be difficult to appreciate
- Immunostains for cytokeratins and CD45 can distinguish

DIAGNOSTIC CHECKLIST

Pathologic Interpretation Pearls
- Basophilic tumor nodules in dermis
- Biphasic population of small and larger cells
- Tumor lobules, especially larger ones, often encapsulated
- Vascular stroma

SELECTED REFERENCES

1. Tanese K et al: Malignant eccrine spiradenoma: case report and review of the literature, including 15 Japanese cases. Clin Exp Dermatol. 35(1):51-5, 2010
2. Bumgardner AC et al: Trichoepitheliomas and eccrine spiradenomas with spiradenoma/cylindroma overlap. Int J Dermatol. 44(5):415-7, 2005
3. Gupta S et al: Multiple eccrine spiradenomas in zosteriform distribution in a child. Pediatr Dermatol. 17(5):384-6, 2000
4. Wright S et al: Multiple familial eccrine spiradenoma with cylindroma. Acta Derm Venereol. 70(1):79-82, 1990
5. Cooper PH et al: Malignant transformation of eccrine spiradenoma. Arch Dermatol. 121(11):1445-8, 1985
6. Mambo NC: Eccrine spiradenoma: clinical and pathologic study of 49 tumors. J Cutan Pathol. 10(5):312-20, 1983
7. Goette DK et al: Cylindroma and eccrine spiradenoma coexistent in the same lesion. Arch Dermatol. 118(4):274-4, 1982
8. Evans HL et al: Carcinoma arising in eccrine spiradenoma. Cancer. 43(5):1881-4, 1979
9. Kersting DW et al: Eccrine spiradenoma. AMA Arch Derm. 73(3):199-227, 1956

SPIRADENOMA

Microscopic Features

(Left) Low magnification of a spiradenoma shows a dermal-based tumor characterized by irregularly shaped nodules and smaller lobules ➤ in the dermis. *(Right)* Spiradenoma is characterized by circumscribed, cellular basophilic nodules or lobules in the dermis. The tumor lobules often have a surrounding fibrous capsule ➡.

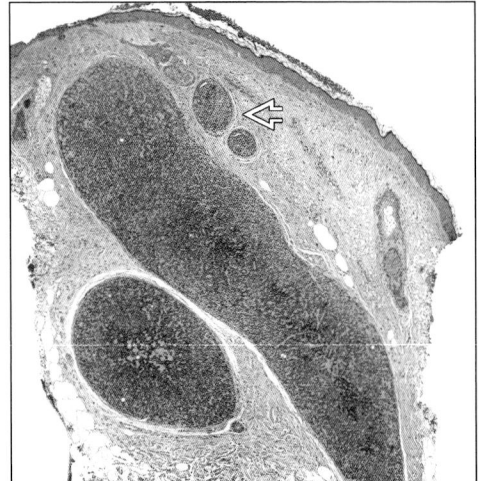
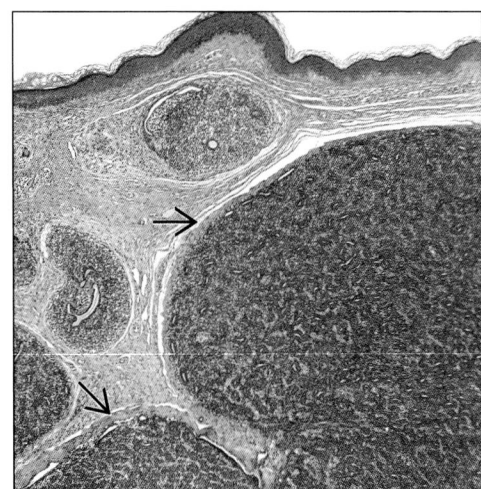

(Left) The stroma in this case is edematous and highlights the associated capillary vasculature ➡. *(Right)* The tumor is composed of 2 cell types: Small cells with scant cytoplasm and hyperchromatic nuclei, and larger cells with oval vesicular nuclei ➡. Scattered lymphocytes are also present throughout the tumor ➤.

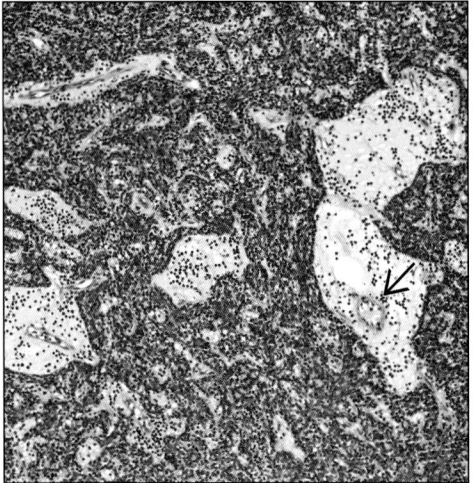
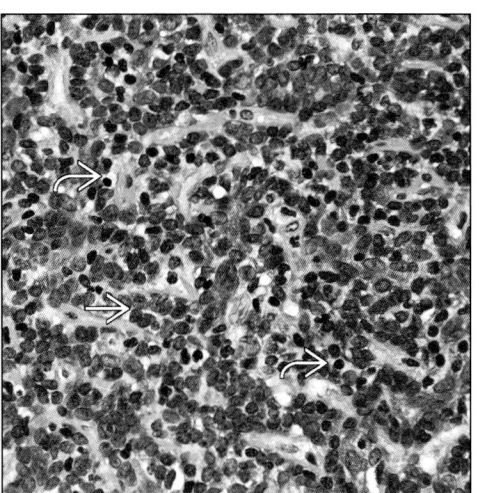

(Left) High magnification of a spiradenoma with a very prominent, hyalinized stroma. Note the focal duct formation surrounded by cells with vesicular nuclei ➡. *(Right)* This case has overlapping features of spiradenoma and cylindroma. The tumor lobules on the left ➡ have a jigsaw-like pattern reminiscent of cylindroma, while the right side demonstrates circumscribed nodules ➤ more typical of spiradenoma.

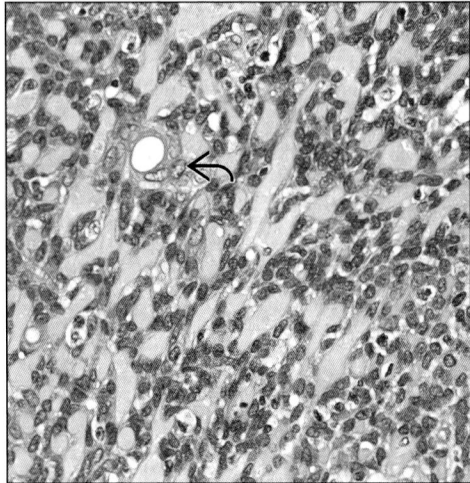
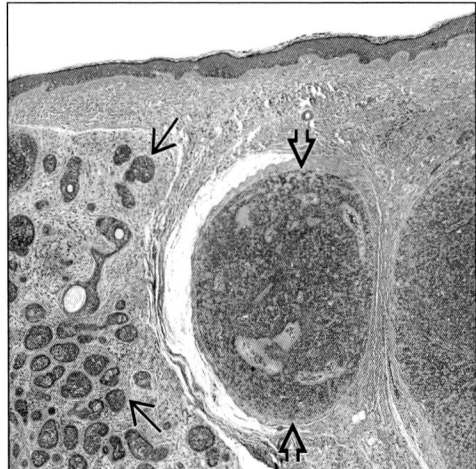

Differential Diagnosis

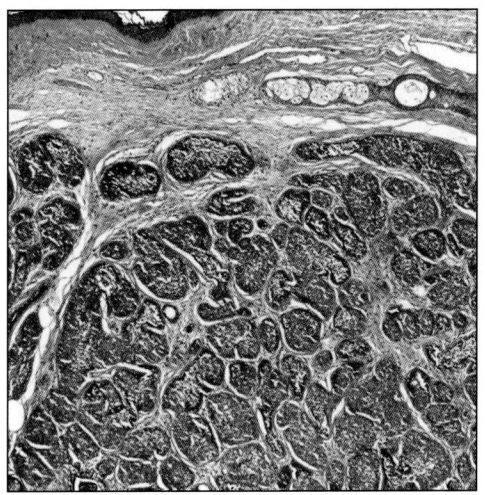
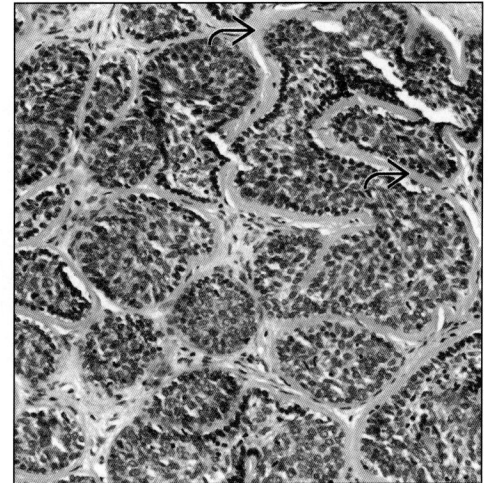

(Left) Cylindromas are closely related tumors, but typically demonstrate the characteristic jigsaw puzzle-like arrangement of the tumor lobules (which are usually smaller than those in spiradenoma) filling the dermis. (Right) Higher magnification of cylindroma shows a proliferation composed of irregular lobules of small, bland basaloid cells, which are surrounded by dense hyalinized membranous material ➡.

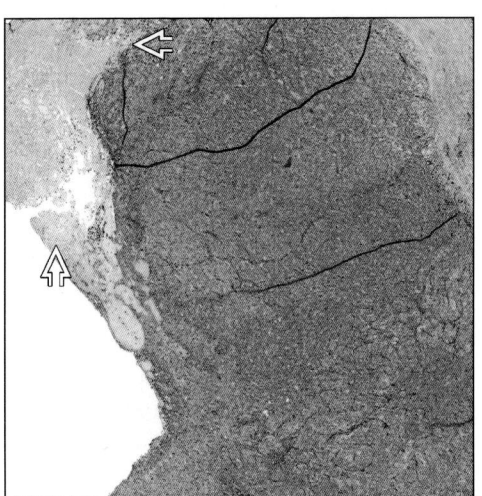
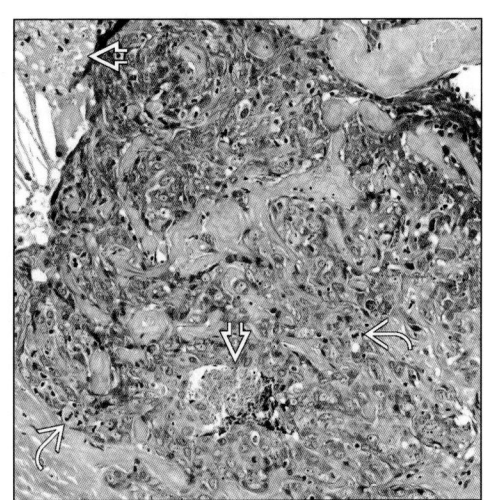

(Left) Spiradenocarcinoma is a very rare adnexal carcinoma which may arise in large, longstanding spiradenomas. This is a very cellular tumor composed of nodular to sheet-like collections of basaloid cells with a large area of tumor necrosis ➡. (Right) Spiradenocarcinoma at high-power magnification shows infiltrative nests and cords of markedly enlarged and atypical-appearing cells. Note the presence of mitoses ➡ and tumor necrosis ➡.

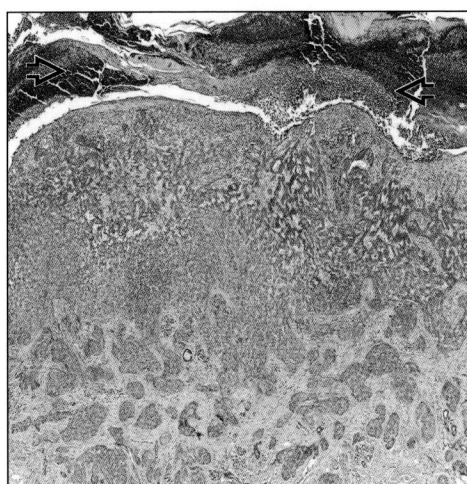
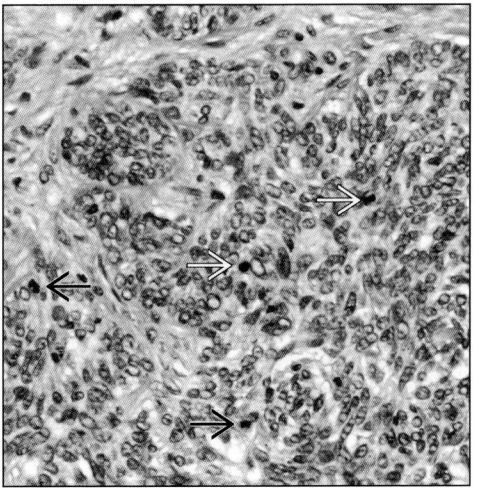

(Left) Histologic section of a nodular- and micronodular-type BCC shows a proliferation of atypical basaloid cells with epidermal attachments and overlying ulceration and dense serum crusting ➡, findings which are lacking in spiradenomas and spiradenocarcinomas. (Right) High magnification of BCC shows a proliferation of atypical basaloid cells with high N:C ratios and numerous apoptotic ➡ and mitotic figures ➡.

ADENOID CYSTIC CARCINOMA

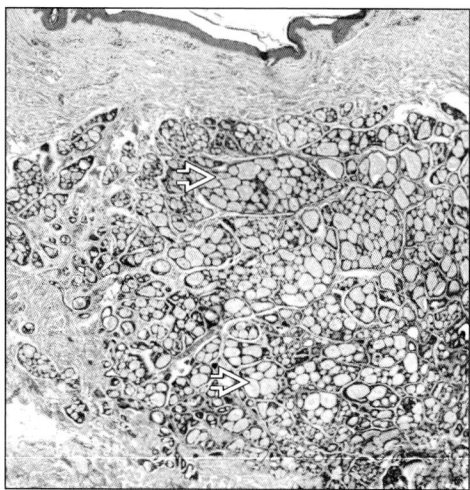

Adenoid cystic carcinoma at low magnification shows a dermal-based basaloid neoplasm with numerous cribriform spaces ⮊ containing basophilic mucin and showing a prominent Swiss cheese-like pattern.

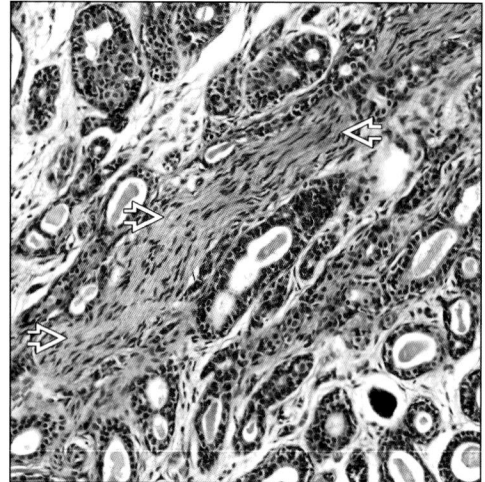

Adenoid cystic carcinoma frequently shows perineural invasion, which accounts for its high local recurrence rate. Here, a large central nerve ⮊ is surrounded by multiple tumor cords and ducts.

TERMINOLOGY

Abbreviations
- Adenoid cystic carcinoma (ACC)

Synonyms
- Primary cutaneous adenoid cystic carcinoma

Definitions
- Rare adnexal tumor showing prominent cribriform pattern and perineural invasion

ETIOLOGY/PATHOGENESIS

Unknown
- May be related to chronic sun damage in some cases

CLINICAL ISSUES

Epidemiology
- Incidence
  - Rare tumors
- Age
  - Typically occur in adults

Presentation
- Dermal mass
  - Slow-growing, skin-colored nodule

Treatment
- Surgical approaches
  - Complete and wider excision is necessary to prevent recurrence given high incidence of perineural invasion
  - Mohs surgery may be effective to minimize recurrence

Prognosis
- Up to 70% of cases have been reported to recur (due to perineural invasion)
- Only a few cases have metastasized, usually to lymph nodes and lungs

MACROSCOPIC FEATURES

Size
- Usually a few centimeters, can be up to 8 cm

MICROSCOPIC PATHOLOGY

Histologic Features
- Poorly circumscribed dermal-based tumor
- Composed of lobules, islands, and cords of basaloid cells with numerous cystic and ductular spaces
  - Typically shows prominent cribriform pattern, similar to that seen in adenoid cystic carcinoma of the salivary glands and breast
  - Spaces are filled with mucinous material that stains with mucicarmine, Alcian blue, and colloidal iron
  - Cells are typically small, relatively monomorphic-appearing, and cuboidal-shaped
  - Mitotic figures are usually not prominent
- Perineural invasion is very common
  - Multiple sections should be examined if it is not initially identified

Cytologic Features
- Nuclei are typically hyperchromatic-staining with small nucleoli

ANCILLARY TESTS

Immunohistochemistry
- ACC stains positive with EMA, CEA-M, and cytokeratins, including low and high molecular weight keratins

ADENOID CYSTIC CARCINOMA

Key Facts

Terminology

- Adenoid cystic carcinoma (ACC)
- Rare adnexal tumor showing prominent cribriform pattern and perineural invasion

Clinical Issues

- Up to 70% of cases reported to recur (due to perineural invasion)
- Only a few cases have metastasized, usually to lymph nodes and lungs

Microscopic Pathology

- Composed of lobules, islands, and cords of basaloid cells
  - Numerous cystic and ductular spaces with prominent cribriform pattern
- Cells are typically small, relatively monomorphic-appearing, and cuboidal-shaped
- By immunohistochemistry, ACC stains positive with EMA, CEA-M, cytokeratins, p63, S100, and actin

- S100, p63, GFAP, and muscle markers including SMA, MSA, and calponin often stain peripheral cells, consistent with myoepithelial cells

DIFFERENTIAL DIAGNOSIS

Basal Cell Carcinoma (BCC)

- Can show adenoid cystic carcinoma-like features (adenoid-type BCC)
- Should have areas of peripheral palisading, tumor-stromal retraction, and mucinous stroma

Metastatic Adenoid Cystic Carcinoma

- Shows essentially identical histologic features
- Very rarely metastatic, but must be excluded based on clinical history and imaging studies

Other Primary Cutaneous Adnexal Tumors

- Cylindroma
  - Composed of irregularly shaped nests and islands of basaloid cells surrounded by dense basement membranes
  - Does not show the prominent degree of cystic/ductal spaces seen in ACC
- Spiradenoma
  - Large nodules composed of biphasic population of small, hyperchromatic-staining basaloid cells and larger clear cells
  - Often associated with dilated vascular spaces and numerous lymphocytes scattered throughout tumor
- Both tumors lack perineural invasion

SELECTED REFERENCES

1. Dores GM et al: Primary cutaneous adenoid cystic carcinoma in the United States: incidence, survival, and associated cancers, 1976 to 2005. J Am Acad Dermatol. 63(1):71-8, 2010
2. Singh A et al: Primary cutaneous adenoid cystic carcinoma with distant metastasis: a case report and brief literature review. Indian J Dermatol Venereol Leprol. 76(2):176-9, 2010
3. Xu YG et al: Cutaneous adenoid cystic carcinoma with perineural invasion treated by mohs micrographic surgery-a case report with literature review. J Oncol. 2010:469049, 2010
4. Doganay L et al: Primary cutaneous adenoid cystic carcinoma with lung and lymph node metastases. J Eur Acad Dermatol Venereol. 18(3):383-5, 2004
5. Matsumura T et al: Adenoid cystic carcinoma of the skin-- an immunohistochemical and ultrastructural study. J Dermatol. 20(3):164-70, 1993
6. Bergman R et al: A comparative immunohistochemical study of adenoid cystic carcinoma of the skin and salivary glands. Am J Dermatopathol. 13(2):162-8, 1991
7. Wick MR et al: Primary adenoid cystic carcinoma of the skin. A clinical, histological, and immunocytochemical comparison with adenoid cystic carcinoma of salivary glands and adenoid basal cell carcinoma. Am J Dermatopathol. 8(1):2-13, 1986
8. Cooper PH et al: Primary cutaneous adenoid cystic carcinoma. Arch Dermatol. 120(6):774-7, 1984

IMAGE GALLERY

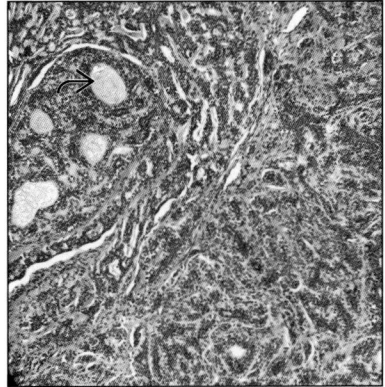 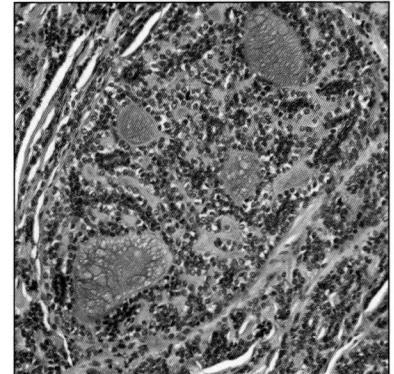 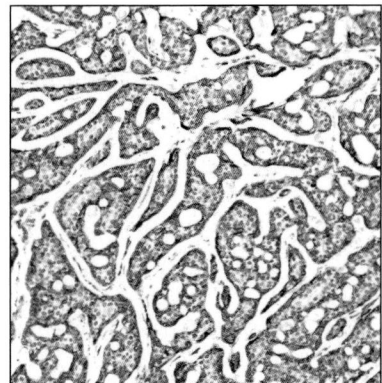

(Left) Adenoid cystic carcinoma is characterized by a proliferation of ductal structures that often show well-formed lumina containing basophilic mucinous material ➡. *(Center)* Higher magnification of ACC shows relatively bland basaloid cells surrounding the ductal lumina containing blue mucinous material. *(Right)* Adenoid cystic carcinoma typically demonstrates expression of myoepithelial markers including SMA (shown here), MSA, calponin, cytokeratins, S100, and GFAP.

PRIMARY CUTANEOUS MUCINOUS CARCINOMA

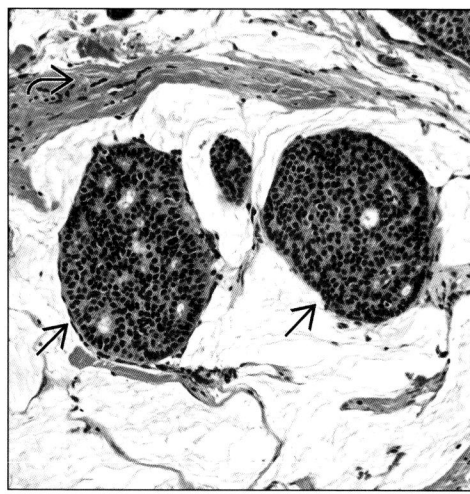

Medium-power view of primary cutaneous mucinous carcinoma shows islands of epithelial cells ➡ in pools of mucin. Fibrous septa ➡, which characteristically divide the tumor into compartments, are present.

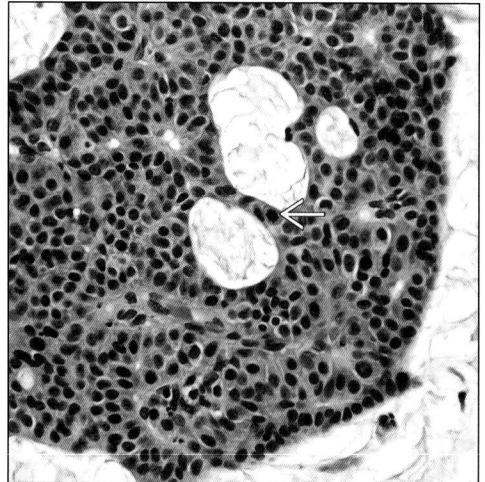

Higher magnification shows uniform cells with hyperchromatic nuclei and eosinophilic cytoplasm. An occasional mitotic figure is identified ➡, but necrosis and marked cytologic atypia are not present.

TERMINOLOGY

Abbreviations
- Primary cutaneous mucinous carcinoma (PCMC)

Synonyms
- Mucinous carcinoma, mucinous eccrine carcinoma, mucinous eccrine adenocarcinoma

Definitions
- Malignant cutaneous tumor with classic histology of epithelial islands "floating" in pools of mucin

CLINICAL ISSUES

Epidemiology
- Gender
  - Men affected more often than women

Presentation
- Very rare tumor
- Occurs in adults and elderly
- Commonly on face, with higher incidence on eyelids
- Slow-growing, asymptomatic, solitary, reddish papule, ulcer, or cyst

Treatment
- Surgical approaches
  - Wide local excision, ± dissection of regional lymph nodes
  - Mohs micrographic surgery
  - Antiestrogen drugs have been tried for patients with estrogen receptor (ER) positive tumors
  - Chemotherapy and radiation have not been helpful in recurrent tumors

Prognosis
- Up to 36% local recurrence and up to 15% metastasis to regional lymph nodes or distant metastasis

MACROSCOPIC FEATURES

Size
- 0.5-7 cm; rare larger lesions

MICROSCOPIC PATHOLOGY

Histologic Features
- Highly distinct low-power histologic appearance
  - Composed of epithelial cells in nests and cords present in large pools of mucin
- Well-circumscribed, dermal-based tumor with occasional extension into subcutaneous tissues
- Occasional overlying ulceration
- Strands of fibrous tissue divide tumor into different compartments
- Epithelial component
  - Usually denser at tumor periphery
  - Nests and cords of epithelial cells with ductal and tubular spaces
  - Glandular or tubular spaces have mucin
  - Cribriform pattern can be seen
- Mucinous component
  - Strongly positive with PAS, mucicarmine, and colloidal iron
  - Resistant to diastase and hyaluronidase, sensitive to digestion with sialidase
  - Positive with Alcian blue (AB) at pH 2.5, negative with AB at pH 1.0 and 0.4, confirming mucin to be epithelial mucin/sialomucin

Cytologic Features
- Small cuboidal cells
  - Uniform in size and shape with minimal atypia
  - Some have vacuolated cytoplasm, and rare signet ring cells are found
  - Electron microscopy shows peripheral dark cells (may be myoepithelial cells) and inner pale cells

PRIMARY CUTANEOUS MUCINOUS CARCINOMA

Key Facts

Terminology
- Malignant tumor with characteristic histology of epithelial islands "floating" in pools of mucin

Clinical Issues
- Very rare tumor, commonly on eyelids
- Slow-growing, asymptomatic, solitary, reddish papule, ulcer, or cyst
- Up to 36% local recurrence and up to 15% metastasis to regional lymph nodes or distant metastasis

Microscopic Pathology
- Well-circumscribed, dermal-based tumor with occasional extension to subcutaneous or deeper tissue
- Strands of fibrous tissue divide tumor into different compartments

- Within compartments, epithelial cells in nests and cords appear to float in large pools of mucin

Ancillary Tests
- CK5/6 and p63 are typically positive and favor cutaneous primary
- CK7 is typically positive, CK20 negative
- ER, PR, and GCDFP-15 are often positive but not useful in excluding metastatic breast carcinoma

Top Differential Diagnoses
- Metastatic mucinous carcinoma (MMC)
  - Mucinous breast carcinoma
  - Mucinous colonic carcinoma
- Other primary cutaneous tumors with mucin
  - Basal cell carcinoma
  - Adenoid cystic carcinoma

ANCILLARY TESTS

Immunohistochemistry
- CK5/6 and p63 are typically positive
  - p63 can only show very focal staining in some cases
  - May indicate presence of myoepithelial cells/differentiation
- CK7 is typically positive, CK20 negative
- ER, PR, and GCDFP-15 are often positive, but are not useful in excluding metastatic breast carcinoma

DIFFERENTIAL DIAGNOSIS

Metastatic Mucinous Carcinoma (MMC)
- **Metastasis from breast and colon are most likely**
- Lesions on breast, chest wall, axillae suggest metastasis from breast
- Exclusion of metastatic visceral carcinoma by histology alone is essentially impossible
- Definitive diagnosis of PCMC should be made only after thorough work-up for visceral carcinoma is found to be negative
- Histologic features that can help distinguish PCMC from MMC
  - Tumor cells in MMC infiltrate surrounding collagen bundles
  - Characteristic "dirty necrosis" is often present in metastatic lesions (especially from colon)
  - Epithelial tumor cells in MMC show higher degree of atypia
  - In situ component is commonly seen in PCMC
  - Presence of myoepithelial cells can help in identifying PCMC
- Immunohistochemical stains might be of some help in distinguishing PCMC from MMC
  - CK5/6 and p63 staining favor primary over metastatic MCC
  - CK20 and CDX-2 staining favor metastasis from colon/gastrointestinal tract
  - Breast carcinoma is much more difficult to separate from PCMC

  - CK7 staining is seen in both PCMC and metastatic mucinous breast carcinoma
  - Staining with GCDFP-15 and ER/PR are also not helpful (typically positive in both breast carcinoma and PCMC)

Other Primary Cutaneous Tumors with Prominent Mucin
- Basal cell carcinoma
  - Shows focal stromal mucin, but not nearly as prominent as that in PCMC
  - Tumor-stromal retraction artifact, peripheral palisading, and numerous mitoses and apoptoses typically present
- Adenoid cystic carcinoma
  - Prominent cribriform appearance
  - Mucin present in ductal lumina, but not prominent in stroma (as in PCMC)

DIAGNOSTIC CHECKLIST

Pathologic Interpretation Pearls
- Characteristic low-power finding of abundant mucin with islands of epithelial cells

SELECTED REFERENCES

1. Levy G et al: Immunohistochemical techniques to compare primary vs. metastatic mucinous carcinoma of the skin. J Cutan Pathol. 37(4):411-5, 2010
2. Kazakov DV et al: Mucinous carcinoma of the skin, primary, and secondary: a clinicopathologic study of 63 cases with emphasis on the morphologic spectrum of primary cutaneous forms: homologies with mucinous lesions in the breast. Am J Surg Pathol. 29(6):764-82, 2005
3. Qureshi HS et al: Primary cutaneous mucinous carcinoma: presence of myoepithelial cells as a clue to the cutaneous origin. Am J Dermatopathol. 26(5):353-8, 2004
4. Ohnishi T et al: Immunohistochemical analysis of cytokeratin and human milk fat globulin expression in mucinous carcinoma of the skin. J Cutan Pathol. 29(1):38-43, 2002

PRIMARY CUTANEOUS MUCINOUS CARCINOMA

Microscopic Features and Differential Diagnosis

(Left) Low-power view of primary cutaneous mucinous carcinoma (PCMC) shows islands of epithelial cells ➡ floating in pools of mucin ⮊. Fibrous septa ➔ are present between areas of epithelial islands. *(Right)* More cellular areas are typically present at the periphery of the tumor and are composed of nodular collections of basophilic tumor cells surrounding multiple ductal lumina ⮞.

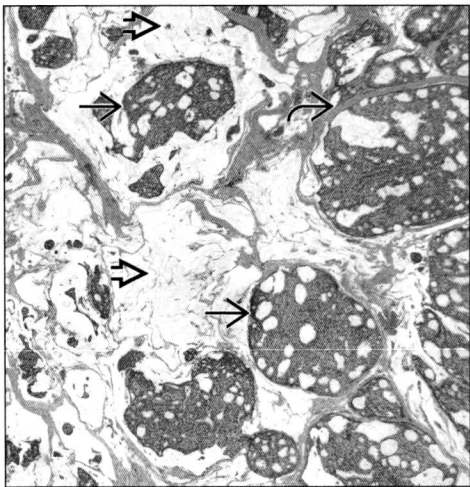
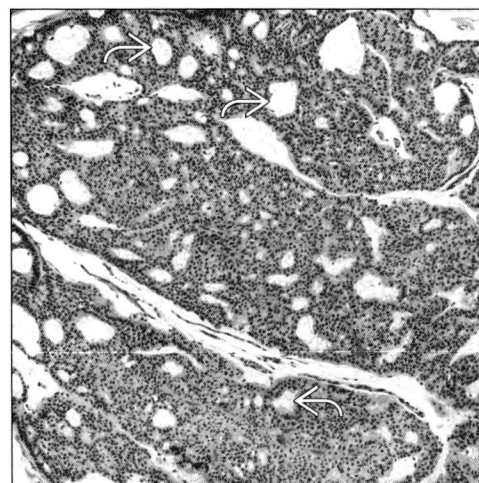

(Left) Intermediate magnification of PCMC shows cribriforming ductal structures ➔ containing mucin. *(Right)* Higher magnification shows the relatively bland, monomorphous appearance of the tumor cells. Rare mitotic figures ⮞ can sometimes be seen.

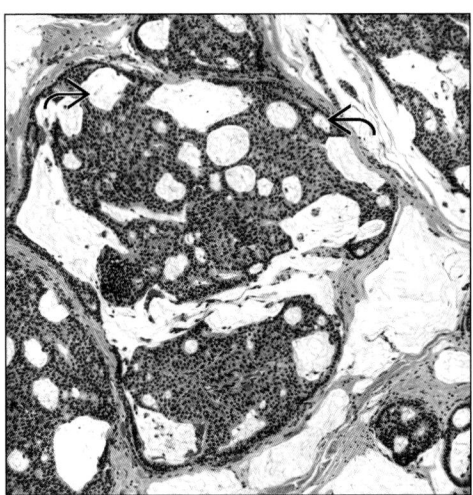
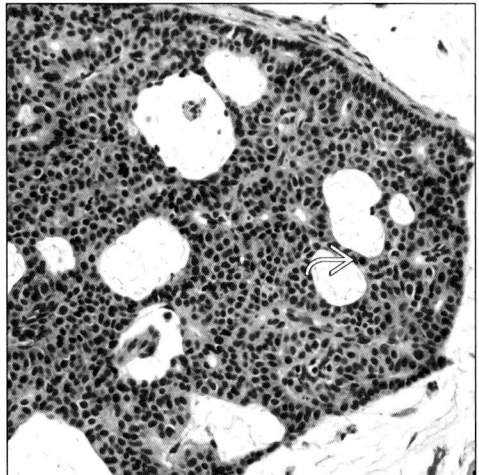

(Left) Metastatic mucinous carcinoma of the colon or appendix can appear histologically identical to primary cutaneous mucinous carcinoma, and can only be excluded by immunohistochemistry for markers such as CK20 and CDX-2. *(Right)* Adenoid cystic carcinoma of the skin shows a prominent cribriforming pattern and bluish mucinous material within ductal lumina ⮞ but not in the stroma (unlike PCMC).

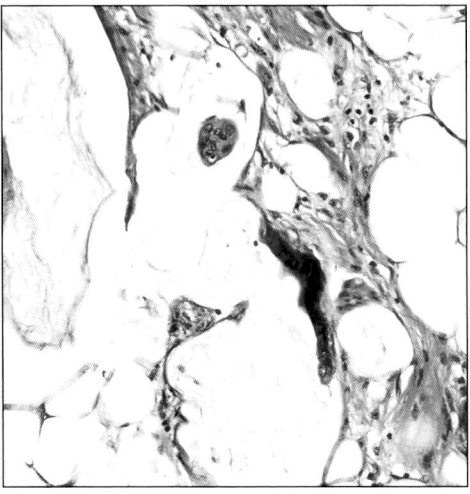
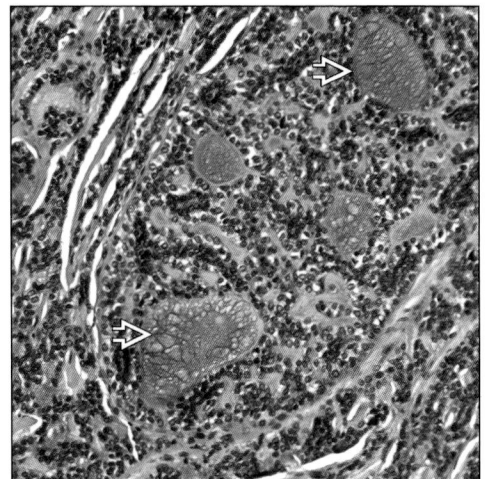

Ancillary Techniques and Differential Diagnosis

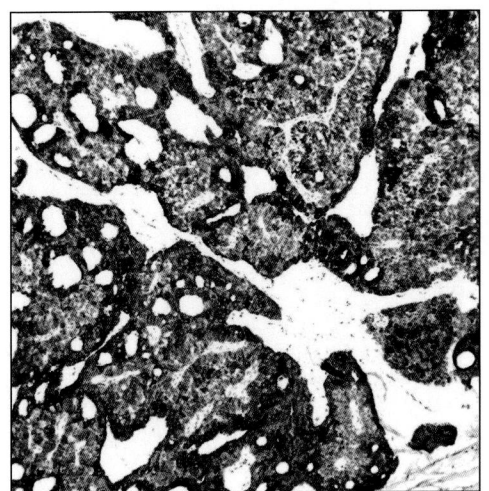

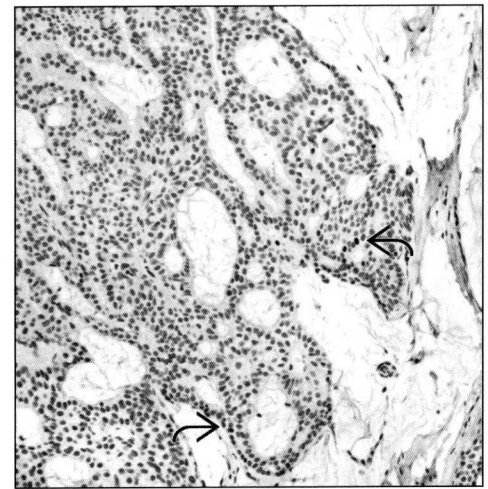

(Left) CK5/6 shows strong staining of many of the cells, especially around the periphery of the tumor, possibly indicating myoepithelial cells. This finding can help distinguish PCMC from metastatic mucinous carcinoma, which is typically negative for this marker. (Right) p63 shows only very focal nuclear staining ⊃ in a few cells in some cases of primary cutaneous mucinous carcinoma.

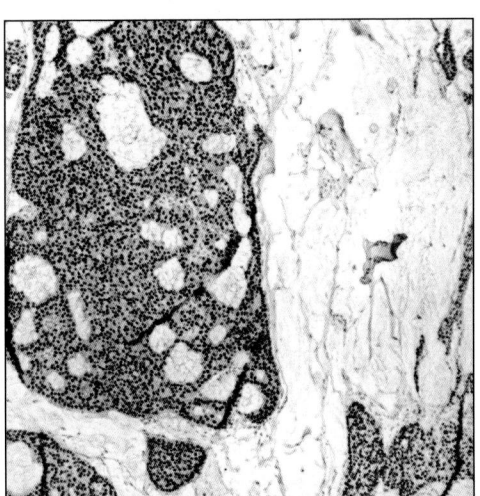

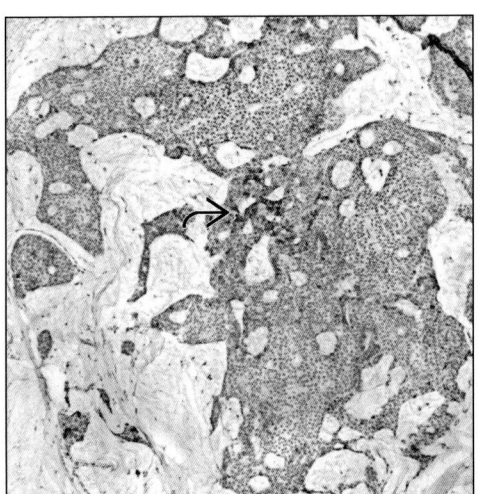

(Left) Estrogen receptor (ER) shows strong and diffuse nuclear staining in almost 100% of the tumor cells. This is a useful finding in excluding a metastatic mucinous colonic carcinoma, but it is not useful in excluding a metastatic breast carcinoma. (Right) GCDFP-15 shows patchy peripheral positive staining in a subset of the tumor cells ⊃, a finding that is also typical of PCMC, but not helpful in excluding a metastatic mucinous breast carcinoma.

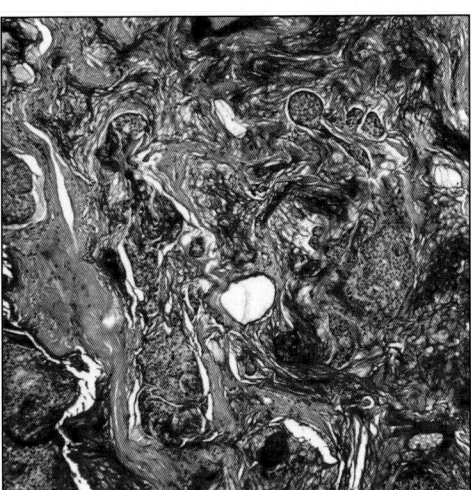

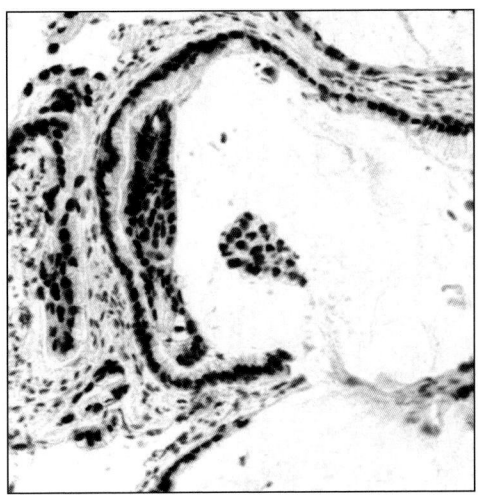

(Left) PAS staining with diastase shows strong and diffuse purplish/reddish staining of the pools of mucin in PCMC. (Right) CDX-2 in a metastatic mucinous pancreatic carcinoma to the skin shows strong and diffuse nuclear staining. This marker is not expressed in PCMC, and is strong evidence for a metastatic tumor of gastrointestinal origin.

APOCRINE CARCINOMA (APOCRINE ADENOCARCINOMA)

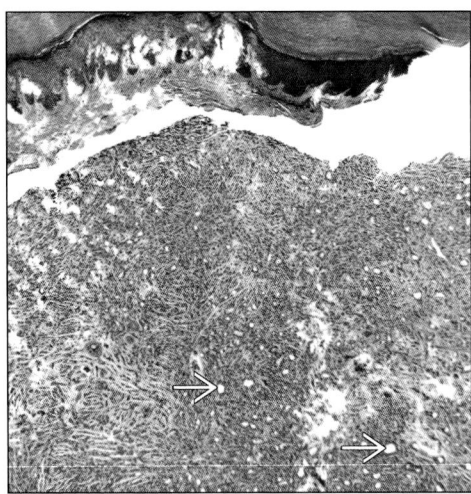

Low magnification of apocrine carcinoma shows a dermal mass composed of crowded, tubular, branching, thin cords and islands, many of which contain lumina ➡.

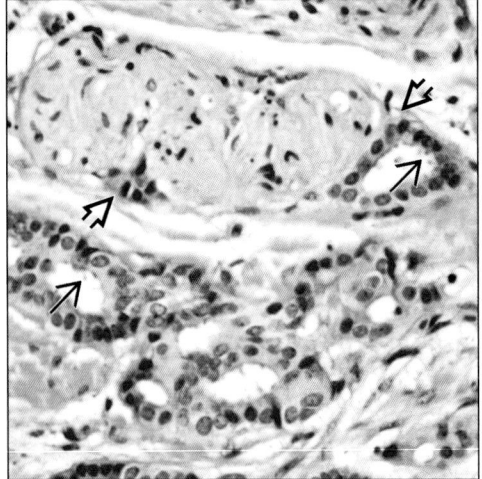

High-magnification view of apocrine carcinoma with perineural invasion ⇗ shows glands lined by cuboidal cells surrounding a nerve. Focal snouts and secretions of cytoplasm ➩ are present within the lumina.

TERMINOLOGY

Synonyms
- Cribriform apocrine carcinoma

Definitions
- Malignant tumor with apocrine differentiation

CLINICAL ISSUES

Site
- Axilla most common site, but other sites described

Presentation
- Dermal nodule
- Often asymptomatic
- No history of breast carcinoma

Treatment
- Wide local excision
- Role of chemotherapy or radiotherapy unclear

Prognosis
- Variable: Indolent or aggressive course
- Local recurrence common
- Metastases to lymph nodes or other internal organs in 25% or more of cases

MICROSCOPIC PATHOLOGY

Histologic Features
- Dermal tumor composed of islands, cords, and ductal/glandular structures
- May extend into subcutaneous tissue
- Surface may be ulcerated
- Pagetoid spread may be present
- Variable architecture of islands
  - Tubular
  - Papillary
  - Solid
  - Complex
- Islands generally interconnecting
- May have cribriform pattern in areas
- Glandular areas lined by cells showing decapitation secretion
- Cells often atypical and pleomorphic appearing
- Mitoses often present
- Infiltrative growth pattern
- Variable necrosis
- Vascular invasion may be present

Cytologic Features
- Eosinophilic, granular cytoplasm
- Hyperchromatic nuclei

ANCILLARY TESTS

Immunohistochemistry
- Generally positive with GCDFP-15
- Often positive with estrogen receptor and androgen receptor
- Negative or only patchy staining with mammaglobin

DIFFERENTIAL DIAGNOSIS

Metastatic Breast Carcinoma
- History of primary breast carcinoma
- May be indistinguishable histologically and immunohistochemically from apocrine carcinoma
  - ER, PR, and GCDFP-15 are all typically positive in both tumors
  - However, strong diffuse staining of majority of cells with mammaglobin supports breast carcinoma

Primary Cutaneous Adenoid Cystic Carcinoma
- Cribriform pattern within islands
- Islands relatively uniform in size/shape

APOCRINE CARCINOMA (APOCRINE ADENOCARCINOMA)

Key Facts

Clinical Issues
- Axilla most common site, but other sites described
- No history of breast carcinoma
- Indolent or aggressive course

Microscopic Pathology
- Dermal/subcutaneous tumor
- Tubular, papillary, cord-like, solid, or complex interconnecting glandular patterns
- May have cribriform pattern to islands

- Cells often hyperchromatic/pleomorphic
- Glandular areas lined by cells showing decapitation secretion
- Infiltrative growth pattern

Top Differential Diagnoses
- Metastatic breast carcinoma
- Primary cutaneous adenoid cystic carcinoma
- Tubular apocrine adenoma
- Hidradenocarcinoma

- Islands not interconnected
- Deeply infiltrative, almost always with perineural invasion

Tubular Apocrine Adenoma
- Well-circumscribed, noninfiltrative
- Tubular islands with evidence of decapitation secretion
- Islands not crowded together
- Cytologic atypia not prominent
- Often a myoepithelial cell layer present around islands

Hidradenocarcinoma
- Larger solid and cystic nodules, infiltrative
- Admixture of cell types
  - Clear, squamoid, poroid, mucinous
- Hyalinized stroma

Microcystic Adnexal Carcinoma
- Horn cysts often present superficially
- Mid-dermal islands may be solid or tubular
- Deeply infiltrative tubular cords with perineural invasion
- Cytologic atypia often not prominent

Papillary Eccrine Adenoma
- Well-circumscribed
- Not infiltrative
- Islands with papillations
- Islands not crowded together
- Cytologic atypia not prominent
- Often a myoepithelial cell layer present around islands

DIAGNOSTIC CHECKLIST

Clinically Relevant Pathologic Features
- No history of breast carcinoma

Pathologic Interpretation Pearls
- Dermal/subcutaneous tumor with variable architecture
  - Tubular, papillary, cord-like, solid, cribriform, or complex interconnecting glandular patterns
- Cells often hyperchromatic and pleomorphic appearing
- Infiltrative growth pattern

SELECTED REFERENCES

1. Fernandez-Flores A: Podoplanin immunostaining in cutaneous apocrine carcinoma and in cutaneous metastasis from the breast. Appl Immunohistochem Mol Morphol. 18(6):573-4, 2010
2. Maury G et al: [Unusual axillary apocrine carcinoma of the skin: histological diagnostic difficulties.] Ann Dermatol Venereol. 137(8-9):555-9, 2010
3. Rütten A et al: Primary cutaneous cribriform apocrine carcinoma: a clinicopathologic and immunohistochemical study of 26 cases of an under-recognized cutaneous adnexal neoplasm. J Am Acad Dermatol. 61(4):644-51, 2009
4. Robson A et al: Primary cutaneous apocrine carcinoma: a clinico-pathologic analysis of 24 cases. Am J Surg Pathol. 32(5):682-90, 2008

IMAGE GALLERY

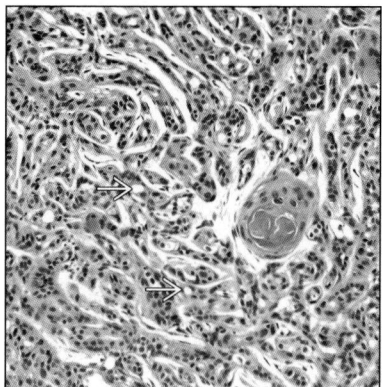 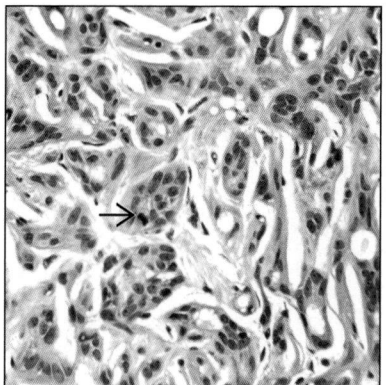 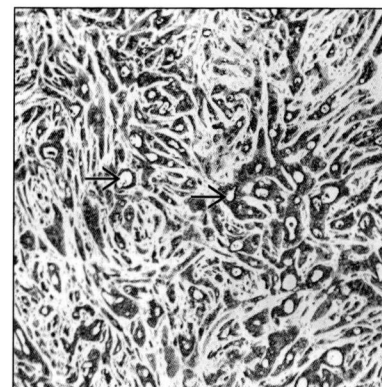

(Left) This apocrine carcinoma shows densely packed islands of cells with lumina ➡ within many of the islands. Nuclear hyperchromasia and pleomorphism are evident. *(Center)* In this view of apocrine carcinoma, nuclear pleomorphism and a mitosis ➡ can be seen. A myoepithelial cell layer is not evident around many of the islands. *(Right)* Apocrine carcinoma stains diffusely with GCDFP-15. The islands are crowded together, and lumina ➡ can be seen in many of the islands.

ECCRINE HAMARTOMAS

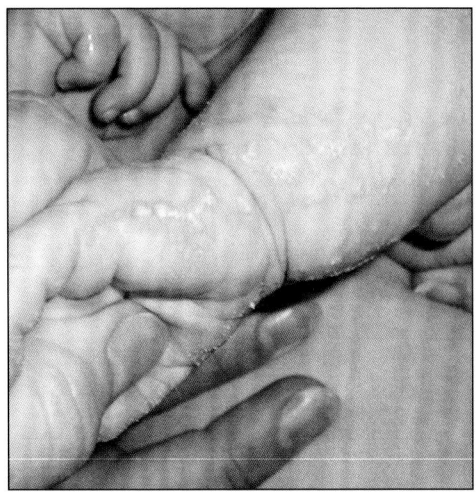

This is a porokeratotic eccrine ostial and dermal duct nevus with light pink, hyperkeratotic streaks following Blaschko lines. There are focal spines. (Courtesy J. McNiff, MD and R. Antaya, MD.)

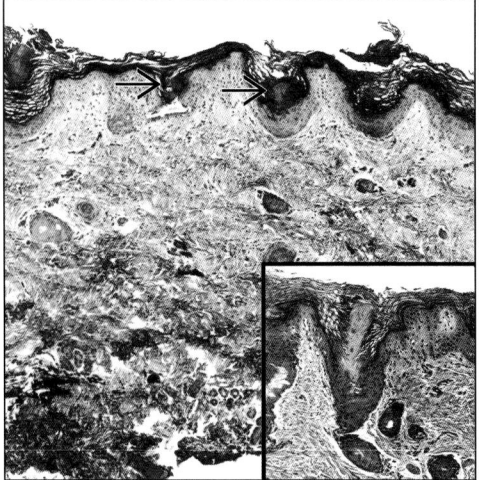

Biopsy of porokeratotic eccrine ostial and dermal duct nevus shows tiers of parakeratosis (cornoid lamellae) ➜ overlying acrosyringeal ostia. The inset is another example. (Courtesy J. McNiff, MD.)

TERMINOLOGY

Synonyms
- Eccrine angiomatous hamartoma
  - Sweating angiomatous hamartoma
  - Sudoriparous angioma
  - Functioning sudoriparous angiomatous hamartoma
- Porokeratotic eccrine ostial and dermal duct nevus
  - Porokeratotic eccrine duct and hair follicle nevus
  - Porokeratotic adnexal ostial nevus

Definitions
- Lesions, often congenital, with prominent component of eccrine glands

CLINICAL ISSUES

Presentation
- **Eccrine angiomatous hamartoma**
  - Congenital or develops in childhood; may present in adulthood
  - Occasionally familial
  - Symptoms/signs
    - May be asymptomatic
    - Tends to grow slowly over time
    - May be hyperhidrotic or painful
    - Hypertrichosis may be evident
  - Macule or plaque (0.3-11 cm), generally solitary
    - Occasionally papular or nodular
    - Rarely surface is verrucous or hyperkeratotic
    - Variable color: Red, blue, yellow, purple, or brown
    - Overlying telangiectasias may be present
  - Commonly on palms/soles or extremities, but other sites described
- **Eccrine nevus**
  - Rarely congenital; develops in childhood or adulthood
  - Solitary or multiple (may follow Blaschko lines)
  - Nondescript macule/patch; may display hyperhidrosis
- **Coccygeal polypoid eccrine nevus**
  - Often congenital
  - Skin tag-like papule over the coccygeal area
  - Generally asymptomatic
- **Porokeratotic eccrine ostial and dermal duct nevus**
  - Often congenital
  - May be solitary and localized to palms/soles and adjacent limb
  - May be generalized, following Blaschko lines
    - Rarely associated with systemic abnormalities (e.g., deafness)
  - Tend to be asymptomatic
  - Rarely spontaneously involute
  - Rarely may develop malignancy

Treatment
- Excision is not necessary for eccrine hamartomas
- Conservative excision may be performed if symptomatic (e.g., hyperhidrotic)

Prognosis
- Eccrine hamartomas are benign

MICROSCOPIC PATHOLOGY

Histologic Features
- **Eccrine angiomatous hamartoma**
  - Epidermis
    - May be normal
    - Or may display hyperkeratosis, acanthosis, &/or papillomatosis
  - Dermal eccrine glands appear normal (occasionally enlarged) but may be increased in numbers
  - Adipose tissue, hair follicles, &/or mucin may be increased
  - Endothelial cell-lined, thin-walled vascular spaces intimately admixed with eccrine glands

ECCRINE HAMARTOMAS

Key Facts

Microscopic Pathology
- Eccrine angiomatous hamartoma
  - Eccrine glands normal (occasionally enlarged) or increased in number
  - Endothelial cell-lined, thin-walled vascular spaces intimately admixed with eccrine glands
  - Differential diagnosis includes eccrine nevus
- Coccygeal polypoid eccrine nevus
  - Polypoid shape

- Increased number of eccrine glands
- Differential diagnosis includes skin tag
- Porokeratotic eccrine ostial and dermal duct nevus
  - Cornoid lamellae (tiers of parakeratosis over diminished granular layer) above acrosyringeal ducts &/or hair follicles
  - Differential diagnosis includes porokeratosis
- Eccrine nevus
  - Increased number or size of eccrine glands
  - No increase in vessels; not polypoid

- Papillary and upper reticular dermis may show increased vessels, sometimes resembling an angioma (i.e., verrucous hemangioma or angiokeratoma-like)
- Immunohistochemistry
  - Eccrine glands stain as normal (positive with S100, CEA, EMA)
  - Vascular structures stain with CD34 and other vascular markers
- Eccrine nevus
  - Increased number or size of eccrine glands
  - Mucin may be increased (if so, termed "mucinous eccrine nevus")
  - No increase in vessels; not polypoid
- Coccygeal polypoid eccrine nevus
  - Polypoid shape
  - Dermis contains increased number of eccrine glands
  - No increase in vessels or nerves
- Porokeratotic eccrine ostial and dermal duct nevus
  - Cornoid lamellae (tiers of parakeratosis over diminished granular layer) overlying acrosyringeal ducts &/or hair follicles

DIFFERENTIAL DIAGNOSIS

DDx of Eccrine Angiomatous Hamartoma
- Eccrine nevus
  - Shows enlargement of eccrine glands
  - Lacks increase in vessels

DDx of Eccrine Nevus
- Normal eccrine glands

- In eccrine nevus, eccrine glands are often enlarged

DDx of Coccygeal Polypoid Eccrine Nevus
- Skin tag/acrochordon or soft fibroma
  - Polypoid shape
  - No increase in eccrine glands in dermis

DDx of Porokeratotic Eccrine Ostial and Dermal Duct Nevus
- Porokeratosis
  - Cornoid lamellae are not centered over acrosyringeal ducts
- Inflammatory linear verrucous epidermal nevus
  - Hyperkeratosis alternating with orthokeratosis, acanthotic epidermis
  - True cornoid lamellae absent

SELECTED REFERENCES

1. Masferrer E et al: Porokeratotic eccrine ostial and dermal duct naevus: report of 10 cases. J Eur Acad Dermatol Venereol. 24(7):847-51, 2010
2. Chen J et al: Mucinous eccrine nevus: a case report and literature review. Am J Dermatopathol. 31(4):387-90, 2009
3. García-Arpa M et al: Multiple and familial eccrine angiomatous hamartoma. Acta Derm Venereol. 85(4):355-7, 2005
4. Cebreiro C et al: Eccrine angiomatous hamartoma: report of seven cases. Clin Exp Dermatol. 23(6):267-70, 1998

IMAGE GALLERY

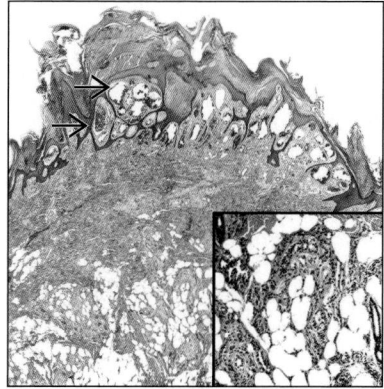 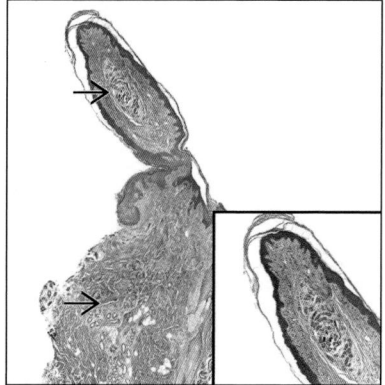 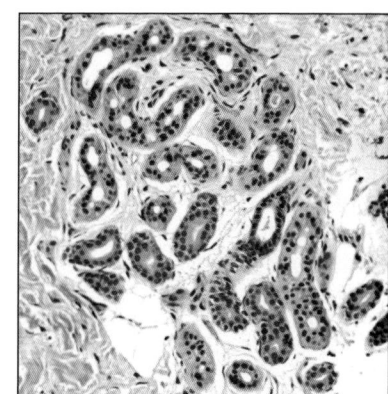

(Left) In eccrine angiomatous hamartoma, the epidermis is often normal; this example has an overlying verrucous hemangioma ➡. Dermal eccrine glands are intimately admixed with fat and vessels. (Courtesy A. Galan, MD.) *(Center)* In this coccygeal polypoid eccrine nevus, there are increased numbers of eccrine glands ➡ in the dermis. *(Right)* Mucinous eccrine nevus shows increased numbers of normal-appearing eccrine glands/ducts in a mucinous stroma.

PAPILLARY ECCRINE ADENOMA

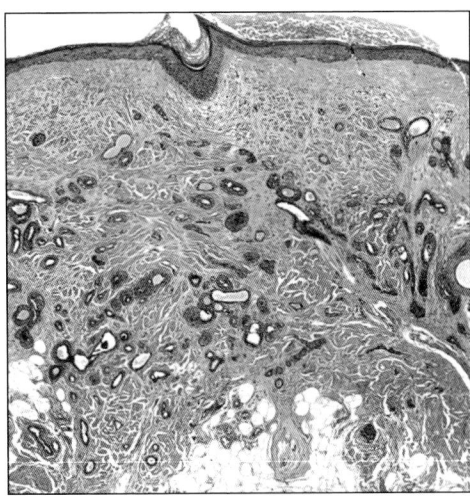

Low-power examination shows a dermal adnexal tumor with variably sized ductal and glandular spaces associated with a fibrous stroma.

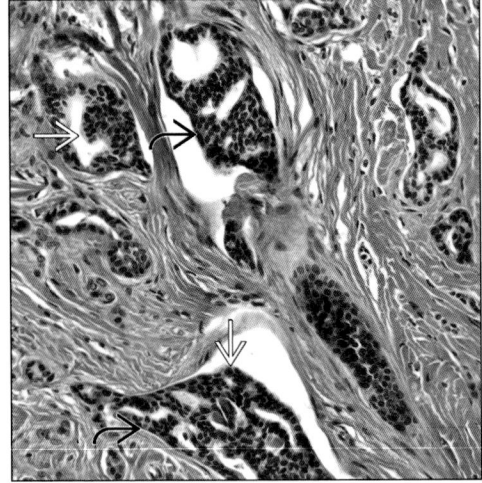

On high magnification, the glands show low-cuboidal eccrine cells ⤳ and areas with cribriforming and papillary projection of variable complexity ⮞. (Courtesy J. McNiff, MD.)

TERMINOLOGY

Abbreviations
- Papillary eccrine adenoma (PEA)

Synonyms
- Tubulopapillary hidradenoma with eccrine differentiation

Definitions
- Rare benign adnexal tumor with evidence of eccrine derivation/differentiation
  - In the past, many cases with apocrine features were included in this category
  - However, most authorities now separate PEAs from tubular apocrine adenomas

CLINICAL ISSUES

Epidemiology
- Incidence
  - Rare
- Gender
  - Women
- Ethnicity
  - More common in Africans/African-Americans

Site
- Distal extremity
  - Other sites include the trunk and head and neck

Presentation
- Firm or hard nodule
- Asymptomatic
  - Occasionally tender
- Slowly growing

Treatment
- Surgical approaches
  - Treatment is not usually necessary

- If treatment is desired, simple excision is best
- Mohs micrographic surgery
  - May be done in cases where possibility of aggressive digital papillary adenocarcinoma cannot be ruled out due to superficial nature of biopsy

Prognosis
- Excellent
- Can recur if partially removed

MICROSCOPIC PATHOLOGY

Histologic Features
- Circumscribed, symmetric-appearing dermal tumor
- Rare connections to epidermis
- Dilated ductal and glandular structures of various sizes
- Microcysts from dilated ducts may be present
- Inner layer often forms 1 or multiple papillae of variable complexity
- Ducts are lined by ≥ 2 layers of cuboidal cells
- Some lumina contain eosinophilic amorphous material
- Rare keratin-filled cysts
- Lesion embedded in dense fibrous stroma
- Stroma often forms bands around ducts
- Foci of loosely arranged spindled cells and hyalinized collagen present in stroma
- Rare histologic features
  - Focal squamous differentiation
  - Clear cell change
  - Epidermal connections of ducts
  - Follicular and sebaceous differentiation
  - Proliferation of nerves within stroma
  - Human papillomavirus-like epidermal changes
- Term "tubulopapillary hidradenoma" is used for lesions with both eccrine and apocrine differentiation

Cytologic Features
- Cuboidal to columnar cells

PAPILLARY ECCRINE ADENOMA

Key Facts

Terminology

- Rare benign adnexal tumor with eccrine differentiation
- Most authorities separate PEAs from tubular apocrine adenomas

Clinical Issues

- Presentation: Firm or hard nodules
- Site: Distal extremity
- Prognosis: Excellent

Microscopic Pathology

- Circumscribed, symmetrical dermal tumor with rare connections to epidermis
- Dilated glandular structures of various sizes
- Ducts lined by ≥ 2 layers of cuboidal cells

Top Differential Diagnoses

- Tubular apocrine adenoma
- Aggressive digital papillary adenocarcinoma
- Metastatic adenocarcinoma

ANCILLARY TESTS

Immunohistochemistry

- Epithelial cells often show S100 protein, carcinoembryonic antigen (CEA), and epithelial membrane antigen (EMA) reactivity

DIFFERENTIAL DIAGNOSIS

Tubular Apocrine Adenoma

- Similar histology as PEA, but with evidence of apocrine glandular differentiation
- Shows decapitation secretion
- Some consider PEA and tubular apocrine adenoma to be synonymous, but most separate these entities

Aggressive Digital Papillary Adenocarcinoma

- Predominately in young adult males
- Larger nodular tumor with ductal structures
- More cellular and shows infiltrative features
- Cytologic atypia and increased mitoses usually present
- High recurrence rate

Metastatic Adenocarcinoma

- Usually large, nodular, and infiltrative tumor
- Cytologic atypia and mitoses usually prominent

DIAGNOSTIC CHECKLIST

Pathologic Interpretation Pearls

- Dermal-based adnexal tumor with variably dilated eccrine ducts
- Projection of papillae into lumen of ducts

SELECTED REFERENCES

1. Kazakov DV et al: Tubular adenoma of the skin with follicular and sebaceous differentiation: A report of two cases. Am J Dermatopathol. 28(2):142-6, 2006
2. Hsu PJ et al: Mixed tubulopapillary hidradenoma and syringocystadenoma papilliferum occurring as a verrucous tumor. J Cutan Pathol. 30(3):206-10, 2003
3. Mizuoka H et al: Papillary eccrine adenoma: immunohistochemical study and literature review. J Cutan Pathol. 25(1):59-64, 1998
4. Hattori N et al: Papillary tubular adenoma with marked tubular vacuolization. J Dermatol. 24(12):777-80, 1997
5. Ishiko A et al: Is tubular apocrine adenoma a distinct clinical entity? Am J Dermatopathol. 15(5):482-7, 1993
6. Falck VG et al: Papillary eccrine adenoma. A tubulopapillary hidradenoma with eccrine differentiation. Am J Dermatopathol. 8(1):64-72, 1986
7. Rulon DB et al: Papillary eccrine adenoma. Arch Dermatol. 113(5):596-8, 1977

IMAGE GALLERY

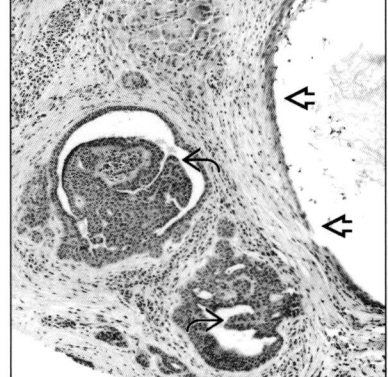 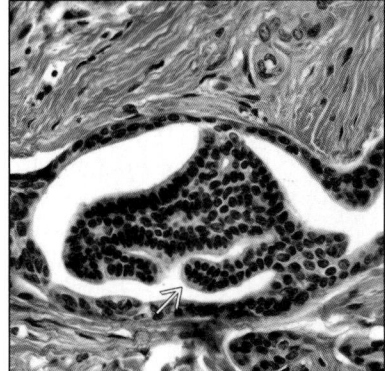 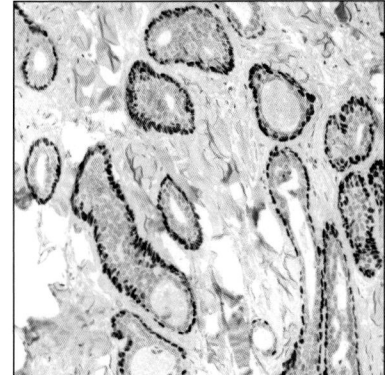

(Left) Complex papillary projections arising from the inner cells and extending into the lumen are seen ➡. A dilated duct forming a microcyst ➡ is also present. *(Center)* High magnification shows uniform, small cuboidal cells lining the glands and forming papillary projections ➡. *(Courtesy J. McNiff, MD.)* *(Right)* p63 immunohistochemistry shows strong staining of the peripheral myoepithelial cell layer, consistent with a benign tumor. *(Courtesy J. McNiff, MD.)*

SYRINGOMA

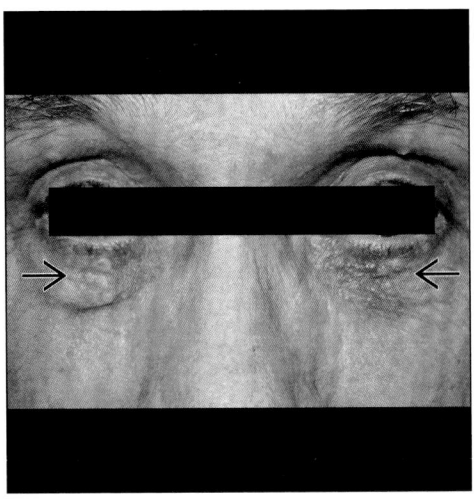

Multiple, small, skin-colored to white papules on the eyelids ➡ are the classic presentation of a syringoma.

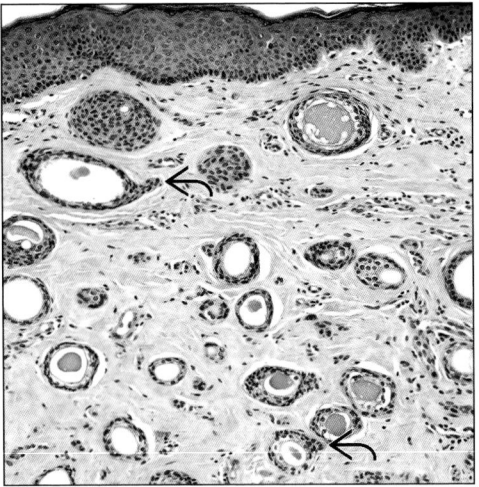

In the superficial dermis, a proliferation of ductal structures embedded in fibrotic stroma is seen. Some of the ducts have comma-like tails ➡.

TERMINOLOGY

Definitions
- Benign eccrine ductal proliferation in superficial dermis

ETIOLOGY/PATHOGENESIS

Etiology
- Eruptive syringomas may be due to autoimmune destruction of acrosyringium

CLINICAL ISSUES

Epidemiology
- Incidence
  - Relatively common tumors
- Age
  - Puberty to old age
- Gender
  - More common in females
- Ethnicity
  - More common in Asians

Site
- Commonly head and neck
  - Predilection for eyelids
  - Rare sites include: Vulva, penis, buttocks, hands, and feet

Presentation
- Often multiple, small, skin-colored to translucent papules
- Asymptomatic
  - Rarely pruritic, which is worse with perspiration
- Rare clinical variants
  - Giant, solitary, plaque, linear, disseminated, and eruptive
  - Clear cell variant associated with diabetes mellitus

- More common in Down syndrome patients
- Can be seen in Brooke-Spiegler syndrome

Treatment
- Treatment is not necessary
- If cosmetically bothersome: Cryotherapy, chemical peels, electrosurgical destruction, excision, and laser ablation are some options

Prognosis
- Benign; excellent prognosis
  - Malignant transformation is extremely rare, if it even exists
  - Syringoid eccrine carcinomas are likely de novo tumors, and not derived from syringomas

MICROSCOPIC PATHOLOGY

Histologic Features
- Small ducts, nests, cords, and cysts in superficial dermis
- Ducts and cysts lined by 1 or 2 layers of cuboidal cells
- Some ducts have "tadpole-like" appearance with comma-like tails
- Dilated ducts may have eosinophilic contents
- Horn cysts can rarely be present
- Fibrotic stroma
- Clear cell variant
  - Epithelial cells lining ducts with clear cytoplasm
  - Clear cell change might only be a focal finding
  - Clear cytoplasm is due to abundant glycogen
- Immunohistochemistry: Cells stain positive with CEA, EMA, and cytokeratins 1, 5, 10, 11, 19
- Rare variants
  - Syringoma admixed with benign melanocytes
  - Presence of dense plasmacytic inflammation within stroma

Cytologic Features
- Benign cuboidal cells

SYRINGOMA

Key Facts

Terminology
- Benign ductal proliferation in superficial dermis

Clinical Issues
- Predilection for eyelids
- Often multiple, small, skin-colored to translucent papules
- More common in Down syndrome patients
- More common in females
- More common in Asians

Microscopic Pathology
- Small ducts, nests, and cords in superficial dermis
- Ducts lined by 1 or 2 layers of cuboidal cells
- Tadpole-like pattern with comma-like tails
- Fibrotic stroma

Top Differential Diagnoses
- Desmoplastic trichoepithelioma
- Microcystic adnexal carcinoma
- Morpheaform basal cell carcinoma

DIFFERENTIAL DIAGNOSIS

Desmoplastic Trichoepithelioma
- Presents as single lesion rather than multiple, as is often seen with syringomas
- Often shows multiple basaloid islands, as well as superficial keratinizing horn cysts
- Usually shows focal papillary mesenchymal bodies
- Lacks true ductal differentiation
- Does not express CEA, unlike syringomas

Microcystic Adnexal Carcinoma (MAC)
- Often presents as single lesion
- Larger, more infiltrative tumor that extends into deep dermis or subcutaneous tissue
- Perineural invasion is common
- Superficial portion of tumor shows follicular differentiation, with keratinizing infundibulocystic structures
- May be difficult to differentiate MAC from syringoma in a superficial biopsy

Morpheaform Basal Cell Carcinoma (BCC)
- Often presents in sun-damaged skin of the elderly as single lesion that is indurated
  - Syringomas are often multiple and have skin-colored appearance
- Retraction of tumor cells from stroma is often seen
- Cytologic atypia and mitoses present
- Ductal differentiation only very rarely present in BCC

Metastatic Adenocarcinoma
- Scalp and trunk are most common sites
- Larger and more infiltrative tumors
- Cytologic atypia and mitosis are usually prominent

DIAGNOSTIC CHECKLIST

Pathologic Interpretation Pearls
- Proliferation of eccrine ducts in superficial dermis

SELECTED REFERENCES

1. Uede K et al: Brooke-Spiegler syndrome associated with cylindroma, trichoepithelioma, spiradenoma, and syringoma. J Dermatol. 31(1):32-8, 2004
2. Patrizi A et al: Syringoma: a review of twenty-nine cases. Acta Derm Venereol. 78(6):460-2, 1998
3. Wheeland RG et al: Carbon dioxide (CO2) laser vaporization of multiple facial syringomas. J Dermatol Surg Oncol. 12(3):225-8, 1986
4. Furue M et al: Clear-cell syringoma. Association with diabetes mellitus. Am J Dermatopathol. 6(2):131-8, 1984
5. Yung CW et al: Unilateral linear nevoidal syringoma. J Am Acad Dermatol. 4(4):412-6, 1981

IMAGE GALLERY

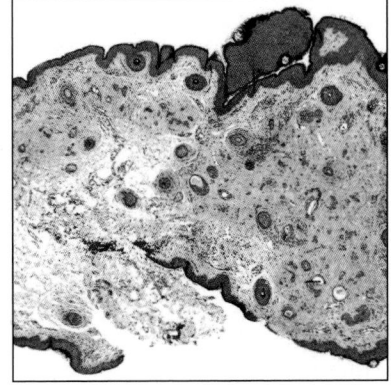 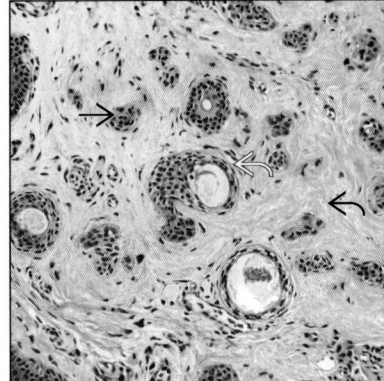 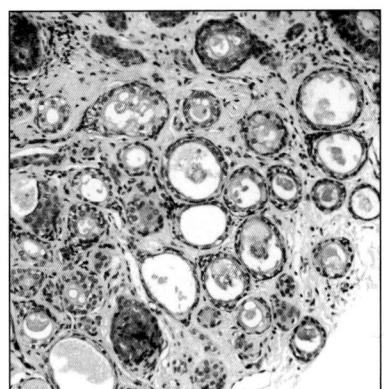

(Left) Low magnification shows basaloid nests and strands of epithelium admixed with small ducts. *(Center)* Higher magnification shows small ducts, one with tadpole-like shape ➜, solid nests ➜, and strands of epithelial cells in a fibrotic stroma ➜. *(Right)* This section shows a more cellular variant of an otherwise classic syringoma.

SYRINGOFIBROADENOMA

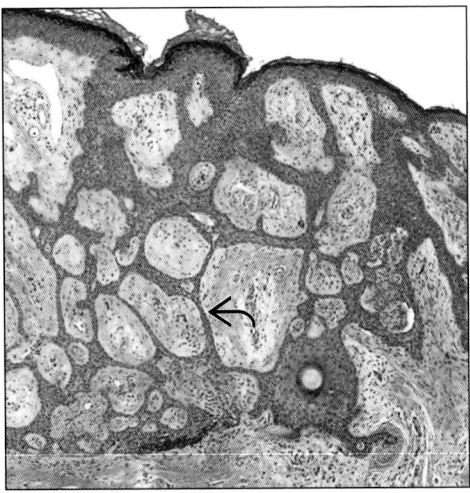

Arising from multiple points along the epidermis are anastomosing cords ➔ of uniform epithelial cells embedded in a fibrovascular stroma, findings typical of SFA.

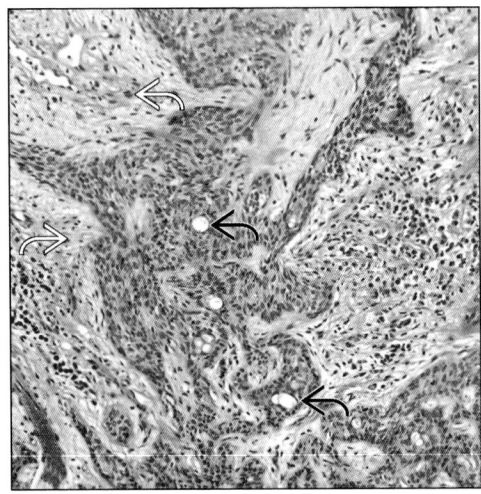

Epithelial strands of acrosyringeal cells with ductal formation ➔ in fibrovascular stroma ➔ is a characteristic finding of SFA.

TERMINOLOGY

Abbreviations
- Syringofibroadenoma (SFA)

Synonyms
- Eccrine syringofibroadenoma (of Mascaro), acrosyringeal adenomatosis

Definitions
- Rare benign tumor of eccrine ductal origin

CLINICAL ISSUES

Epidemiology
- Age
  o Commonly in elderly
- Gender
  o More common in women

Site
- Commonly on an extremity
- Rare locations include face, trunk, and nails

Presentation
- Clinical presentation
  o Usually solitary, hyperkeratotic plaque
  o Sometimes multiple, diffuse, or zosteriform
    ▪ Terms "acrosyringeal adenomatosis," "eccrine syringofibroadenomatosis," and "acrosyringeal nevus" are used to identify this clinical variation
  o Multiple SFA associated with hidrotic ectodermal dysplasia
  o Multiple SFA associated with Schöpf-Schulz-Passarge syndrome
    ▪ Rare ectodermal dysplasia
  o Multiple SFA associated with familial ophthalmologic abnormalities
  o Reactive eccrine syringofibroadenomatosis

    ▪ Rarely develop as reactive process in association with unrelated inflammatory conditions or tumors
    ▪ Usually on acral sites
    ▪ Lichen planus, bullous pemphigoid, burn scars, diabetic foot ulcer, leprosy, and squamous cell carcinoma are some of the associated conditions

Treatment
- Treatment is usually not necessary
- Some suggest simple excision or destruction due to rare possible risk of malignant transformation

Prognosis
- Excellent
- Rare reports of malignant transformation

MICROSCOPIC PATHOLOGY

Histologic Features
- Vertically oriented, slender, interconnected basaloid epithelial cords extending from epidermis into dermis
- Epithelial cords contain ducts and cystic structures
  o Ducts are lined with cuboidal cells resembling eccrine ducts
- Basaloid cells are smaller than adjacent keratinocytes
- Lesion is embedded in fibrovascular stroma
- Mild superficial lymphocytic infiltrate can be seen
  o Lacks prominent plasma cell infiltrate reported in acrosyringeal nevus
- Clear cell syringofibroadenoma is a rare variant

Cytologic Features
- Small cuboidal cells lacking atypia

ANCILLARY TESTS

Immunohistochemistry
- Luminal cells are highlighted by CEA

SYRINGOFIBROADENOMA

Key Facts

Clinical Issues
- Commonly on an extremity
- More common in women
- Usually solitary, hyperkeratotic plaque
- Multiple lesions might be associated with rare syndromes

Microscopic Pathology
- Vertically oriented, slender, interconnected basaloid epithelial cords extending from epidermis

- Lumina formation can be present
- Embedded in fibrovascular stroma

Top Differential Diagnoses
- Basal cell carcinoma (fibroepithelioma of Pinkus variant)
- Poroma
- Hidroacanthoma simplex
- Acrosyringeal nevus
- Syringofibroadenocarcinoma

- Cytokeratin stains have been inconsistent and not helpful

- Development of reactive SFA within carcinoma instead of malignant transformation is a possibility

DIFFERENTIAL DIAGNOSIS

Basal Cell Carcinoma (BCC): Fibroepithelioma of Pinkus Variant
- Thin anastomosing cords of basaloid cells
- Peripheral palisading, typical of BCC
- Tumor-stromal clefting artifact
- Loose myxoid stroma

Poroma
- Thicker anastomosing cords
- More uniform, smaller epithelial cells
- Loose stroma

Hidroacanthoma Simplex
- Intraepidermal proliferation that lacks anastomosing architecture of SFA
- Proliferation of basaloid and clear cells with ducts

Acrosyringeal Nevus
- Some consider this entity to be same as SFA
- Strong PAS positivity of acrosyringeal keratinocytes
- Prominent plasma cell infiltrate

Syringofibroadenocarcinoma
- Only a few reported cases
- Foci of malignant transformation in association with syringofibroadenoma

DIAGNOSTIC CHECKLIST

Pathologic Interpretation Pearls
- Thin, anastomosing, benign epithelial proliferation in fibrovascular stroma

SELECTED REFERENCES

1. Cho E et al: A case of reactive eccrine syringofibroadenoma. Ann Dermatol. 23(1):70-2, 2011
2. Poonawalla T et al: Clouston syndrome and eccrine syringofibroadenomas. Am J Dermatopathol. 31(2):157-61, 2009
3. Bjarke T et al: Carcinoma and eccrine syringofibroadenoma: a report of five cases. J Cutan Pathol. 30(6):382-92, 2003
4. Komine M et al: Eccrine syringofibroadenoma (Mascaro): an immunohistochemical study. Am J Dermatopathol. 22(2):171-5, 2000
5. Noguchi M et al: Eccrine syringofibroadenoma developing in a sebaceous naevus. Br J Dermatol. 142(5):1050-1, 2000

Differential Diagnosis

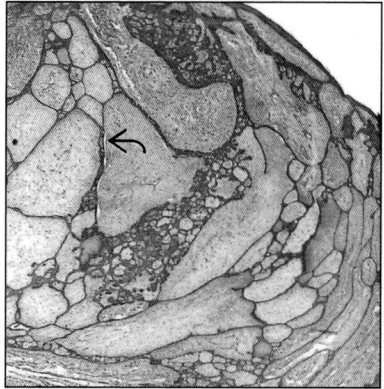 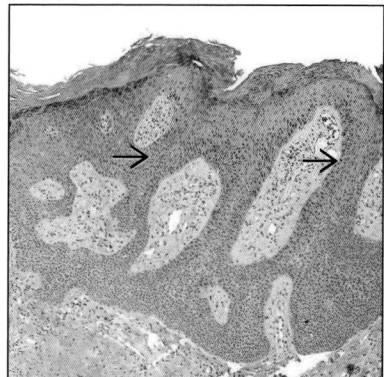 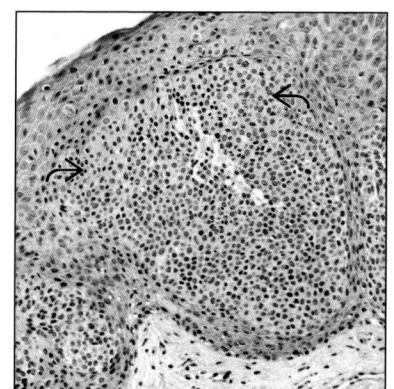

(Left) Fibroepithelioma of Pinkus shows thin strands of epithelial cells are arranged in a net-like pattern in a myxoid stroma. Focal tumor-stromal clefting ➔ is seen. (Center) Poroma shows anastomosing cords of epithelial cells extending from the epidermis ➔; the cells are generally smaller and more monotonous than in SFA. (Right) The intraepidermal proliferation of monotonous basaloid cells ➔ in hidroacanthoma simplex lacks the anastomosing architecture of SFA.

ECCRINE CARCINOMA

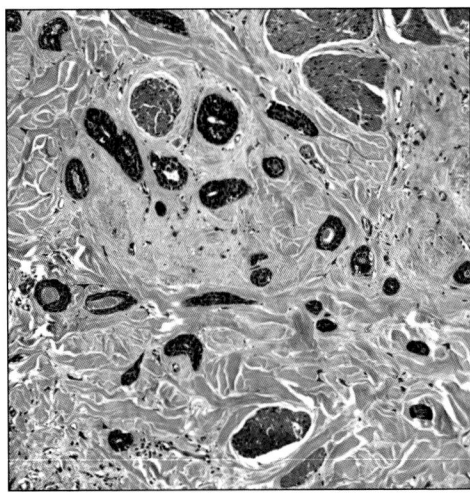

Eccrine carcinoma is characterized by an infiltrative growth pattern. The tumor forms glandular and duct-like structures that lack the organized appearance of normal eccrine glands.

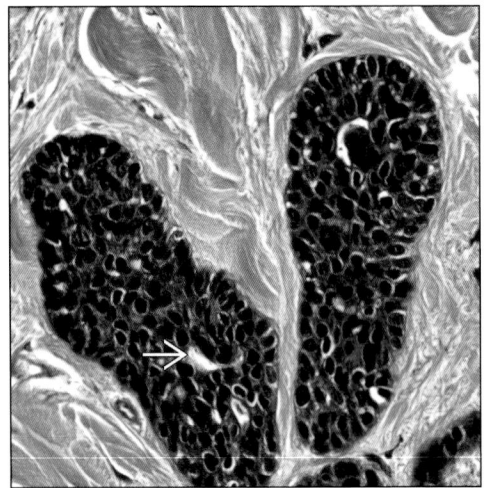

The neoplastic glands are lined by stratified epithelium with hyperchromatic nuclei with focal lumen ➡ formation. The tumor cells do not usually have prominent nuclear pleomorphism.

TERMINOLOGY

Synonyms
- Syringoid carcinoma, syringoid eccrine carcinoma, eccrine syringomatous carcinoma, eccrine epithelioma

Definitions
- Malignant adnexal tumor with eccrine differentiation somewhat resembling a syringoma
  - No evidence of association with or development from syringomas
- Some authorities group these tumors with microcystic adnexal carcinoma (MAC)

CLINICAL ISSUES

Epidemiology
- Incidence
  - Very rare tumors
- Age
  - Usually present in middle-aged patients
- Gender
  - More common in women (3:1)

Site
- Most common on scalp
- May also present on face, neck, trunk, or extremities

Presentation
- Typically present as plaque or nodule
  - May present as painful lesion ± alopecia
  - May be present for many years before diagnosis

Treatment
- Surgical approaches
  - Wide excision

Prognosis
- Locally aggressive
  - Multiple episodes of local recurrence common

- Rare lymph node metastasis

MICROSCOPIC PATHOLOGY

Histologic Features
- Based in dermis; attachment to epidermis is very rare
- Infiltrative growth pattern
  - May involve subcutis and underlying skeletal muscle
  - Perineural invasion common
- Tumor composed of basaloid epithelium
  - Tumor cells have relatively uniform hyperchromatic nuclei
    - Nuclear atypia usually relatively mild
  - Mitotic rate low
  - Occasionally have clear cytoplasm due to glycogen
    - Glycogen can be highlighted with PAS stain (without diastase)
- Tumor forms epithelial strands with lumen formation
  - May have "hand mirror" shape similar to syringoma
  - May also have cyst formation
- No keratocyst formation
- No squamous differentiation

ANCILLARY TESTS

Immunohistochemistry
- Immunohistochemistry may be useful to confirm diagnosis
  - Lumina highlighted by EMA &/or CEA
  - Tumor cells positive for high and low molecular weight cytokeratins
  - May show focal immunoreactivity for S100 protein

DIFFERENTIAL DIAGNOSIS

Microcystic Adnexal Carcinoma (MAC)
- MAC has similar growth pattern, and may be closely related to eccrine carcinoma

ECCRINE CARCINOMA

Key Facts

Clinical Issues
- Typically present as plaque on scalp
- Locally aggressive

Microscopic Pathology
- Infiltrative growth pattern, often with perineural invasion
- Tumor composed of basaloid epithelium with uniform hyperchromatic nuclei
- Tumor forms epithelial strands with lumen formation

- May have "hand mirror" shape similar to syringoma
- Lumina highlighted by EMA &/or CEA

Top Differential Diagnoses
- Microcystic adnexal carcinoma
  - Presence of keratocysts allows for distinction (absent in eccrine carcinoma)
- Adenoid cystic carcinoma
  - Cribriform architecture allows distinction (generally absent in eccrine carcinoma)

- Presence of keratocysts allows distinction (absent in eccrine carcinoma)

Squamoid Eccrine Ductal Carcinoma
- Very rare tumors with basaloid ductal elements and areas of squamous differentiation
- May actually represent an unusual variant of MAC

Adenoid Cystic Carcinoma
- Cribriform architecture (typically absent in eccrine carcinoma)
- Ductal lumina filled with mucinous and basement membrane-like material

Infiltrative Basal Cell Carcinoma (BCC)
- Lacks true lumen formation
- Often admixed with other BCC patterns
  - i.e., nodular, micronodular, or superficial-multicentric
- Connections to overlying epidermis often present

DIAGNOSTIC CHECKLIST

Pathologic Interpretation Pearls
- Infiltrative growth pattern of basaloid ductal structures key to diagnosis

SELECTED REFERENCES

1. Sidiropoulos M et al: Syringoid eccrine carcinoma: a clinicopathological and immunohistochemical study of four cases. J Clin Pathol. 64(9):788-92, 2011
2. Kavand S et al: "Squamoid eccrine ductal carcinoma": an unusual low-grade case with follicular differentiation. Are these tumors squamoid variants of microcystic adnexal carcinoma? Am J Dermatopathol. 31(8):849-52, 2009
3. Chhibber V et al: Ductal eccrine carcinoma with squamous differentiation: apropos a case. J Cutan Pathol. 34(6):503-7, 2007
4. Nishizawa A et al: Syringoid eccrine carcinoma with apparently aggressive transformation: case report and review of the literature. Int J Dermatol. 45(10):1218-21, 2006
5. Wildemore JK et al: Mohs surgery for malignant eccrine neoplasms. Dermatol Surg. 30(12 Pt 2):1574-9, 2004
6. Ramos D et al: Clear cell syringoid carcinoma: an ultrastructural and immunohistochemical study. Am J Dermatopathol. 22(1):60-4, 2000
7. Weber PJ et al: Syringoid eccrine carcinoma. J Dermatol Surg Oncol. 13(1):64-7, 1987
8. Wick MR et al: Adnexal carcinomas of the skin. I. Eccrine carcinomas. Cancer. 56(5):1147-62, 1985
9. Mehregan AH et al: Eccrine adenocarcinoma. A clinicopathologic study of 35 cases. Arch Dermatol. 119(2):104-14, 1983
10. Panet-Raymond G et al: Adenocarcinoma of the eccrine sweat gland. Arch Dermatol. 107(1):94-6, 1973
11. Dave VK: Eccrine sweat gland carcinoma with metastases. Br J Dermatol. 86(1):95-7, 1972

IMAGE GALLERY

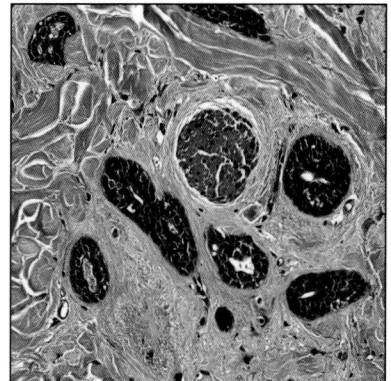 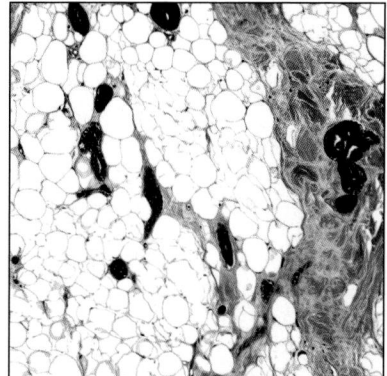 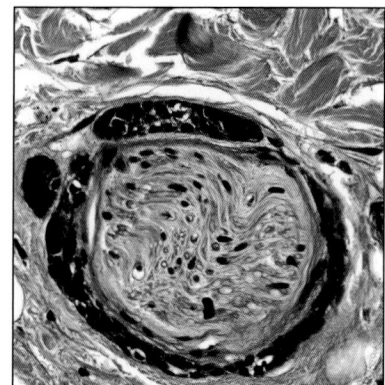

(Left) Eccrine carcinoma is characterized by a disorganized proliferation of atypical, neoplastic glands in the dermis. *(Center)* Eccrine carcinoma is very infiltrative and often extends into the underlying subcutaneous fat. *(Right)* Perineural invasion is a common and expected finding in many eccrine carcinomas.

SQUAMOID "ECCRINE" DUCTAL CARCINOMA

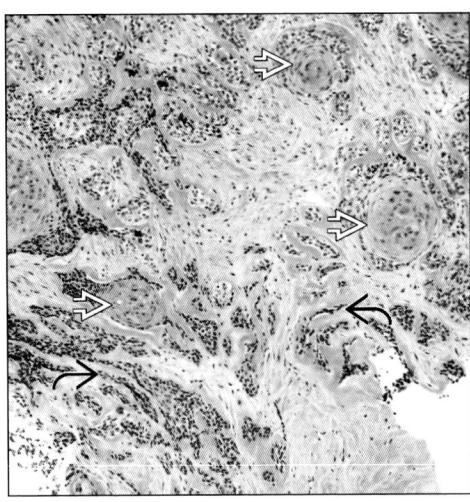

Squamoid eccrine ductal carcinoma shows a proliferation of both enlarged, squamoid cells forming islands ⊟ and smaller, more cord-like collections of basaloid cells ⊟.

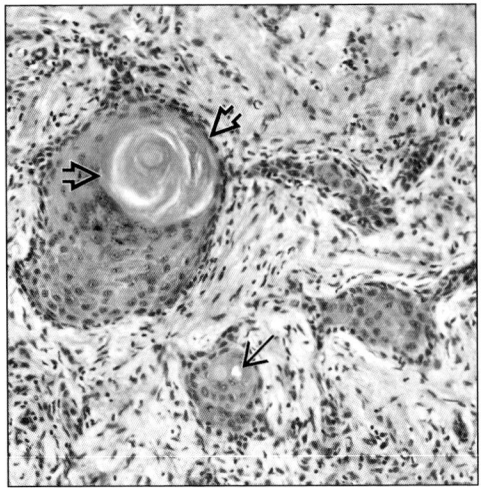

High magnification of a predominantly squamoid area shows collections of large cells with abundant eosinophilic cytoplasm surrounding keratinizing cystic spaces ⊟ and small ductal lumina ⊟.

TERMINOLOGY

Abbreviations
- Squamoid "eccrine" ductal carcinoma (SEDC)

Synonyms
- Ductal eccrine carcinoma with squamous differentiation

Definitions
- Rare adnexal carcinoma with ductal and squamous differentiation

ETIOLOGY/PATHOGENESIS

Unknown
- May be associated with solar damage or immunosuppression

CLINICAL ISSUES

Epidemiology
- Incidence
  - Very rare tumors; only 8 cases reported to date
- Age
  - Usually adult patients

Site
- Head and neck region or extremities

Presentation
- Nodular lesion

Treatment
- Surgical approaches
  - Wide local excision is recommended to ensure complete removal
  - Mohs micrographic surgery has also been reported to be effective in a few cases

Prognosis
- Aggressive local recurrences, but no metastases reported to date

MICROSCOPIC PATHOLOGY

Histologic Features
- Dermal-based invasive tumor
  - Composed of infiltrative-appearing lobules, nests, and cords of cells
  - Mixed population of smaller basaloid adnexal cells and larger squamoid cells
    - Adnexal cells show small hyperchromatic nuclei and scant amounts of cytoplasm
    - Squamoid cells show larger nuclei with prominent nucleoli and abundant eosinophilic-staining cytoplasm
    - Both cell types can surround ductal lumina
  - Evidence of follicular differentiation can be seen
    - Scattered infundibulocystic keratinizing structures can be present
    - Other evidence of follicular differentiation can include external root sheath (tricholemmal) differentiation
    - Suggests the possibility that these may represent squamoid variants of microcystic adnexal carcinoma
    - Many authorities now consider that microcystic adnexal carcinoma shows follicular and apocrine, rather than eccrine, differentiation

ANCILLARY TESTS

Immunohistochemistry
- Diffusely positive for cytokeratins (CK7, CK17, CK5/6), and p63
- Focally positive (ductal structures) for EMA and CEA

SQUAMOID "ECCRINE" DUCTAL CARCINOMA

Key Facts

Terminology
- Squamoid "eccrine" ductal carcinoma (SEDC)
- Rare carcinoma with ductal and squamous features

Clinical Issues
- Aggressive local recurrences, but no metastases

Microscopic Pathology
- Deeply infiltrative-appearing lobules, nests, and cords of cells

- Mixed population of smaller basaloid adnexal cells and larger squamoid cells
- Both cell types can surround ductal lumina
- Evidence of follicular differentiation can be seen
  - Suggests that these may represent squamoid variants of microcystic adnexal carcinoma

Top Differential Diagnoses
- Squamous cell carcinoma (SCC)
- Microcystic adnexal carcinoma (MAC)

DIFFERENTIAL DIAGNOSIS

Squamous Cell Carcinoma (SCC)
- Invasive tumor composed of large, atypical epithelioid cells with dense eosinophilic-staining cytoplasm
  - Degree of differentiation varies (well to moderately to poorly differentiated)
- SEDC lacks high-grade atypia and overlying AK or SCC in situ (present in majority of SCC cases)
- SCC lacks ductal differentiation

Microcystic Adnexal Carcinoma (MAC)
- Typically presents on the face of young adult patients
- More prominent superficial folliculocystic differentiation typically present
- SEDC may represent a squamoid variant of MAC; therefore, distinction may be academic

Eccrine (Syringoid/Syringomatous) Carcinoma
- Often regarded as a higher grade variant of MAC lacking superficial folliculocystic differentiation
- Monotonous proliferation of ductal structures deeply invading dermis and subcutis
- Lined by basaloid cells, not squamoid cells of SEDC

Porocarcinoma
- More common tumors, often occur in acral sites
- May show prominent squamous differentiation, however

  - Superficial portion of the tumor often shows attachments to the overlying epidermis and intraepidermal (pagetoid) involvement
  - Broad anastomosing cords and columns of tumor cells with focal ductal formation

DIAGNOSTIC CHECKLIST

Pathologic Interpretation Pearls
- Mixed population of smaller basaloid adnexal cells and larger squamoid cells
- Both can surround ductal lumina

SELECTED REFERENCES

1. Terushkin E et al: Squamoid eccrine ductal carcinoma: a case report and review of the literature. Am J Dermatopathol. 32(3):287-92, 2010
2. Kavand S et al: "Squamoid eccrine ductal carcinoma": an unusual low-grade case with follicular differentiation. Are these tumors squamoid variants of microcystic adnexal carcinoma? Am J Dermatopathol. 31(8):849-52, 2009
3. Cassarino DS et al: Cutaneous squamous cell carcinoma: a comprehensive clinicopathologic classification--part two. J Cutan Pathol. 33(4):261-79, 2006
4. Kim YJ et al: Mohs micrographic surgery for squamoid eccrine ductal carcinoma. Dermatol Surg. 31(11 Pt 1):1462-4, 2005
5. Herrero J et al: Squamoid eccrine ductal carcinoma. Histopathology. 32(5):478-80, 1998
6. Wong TY et al: Squamoid eccrine ductal carcinoma. Histopathology. 30(3):288-93, 1997

IMAGE GALLERY

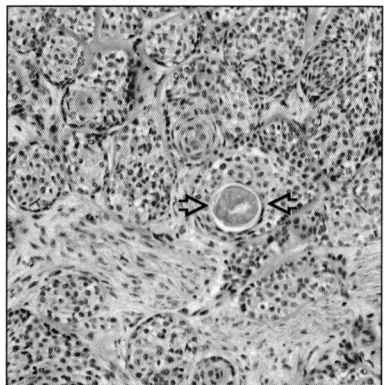 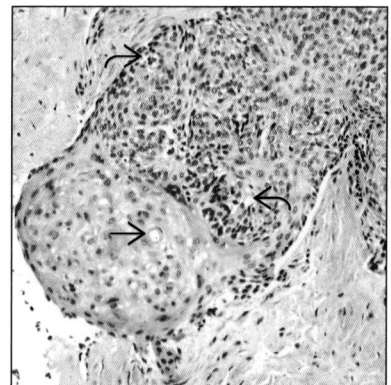 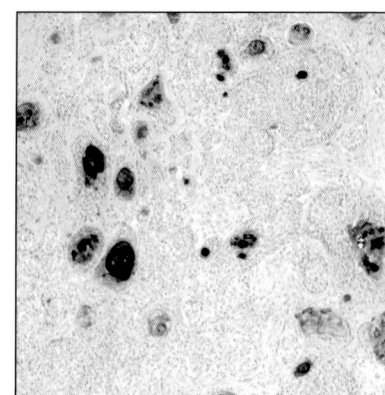

(Left) SEDC shows a nested proliferation of enlarged pale to clear squamoid cells surrounding a well-formed ductal lumina ⊵. (Center) Juxtaposition of a squamoid area with focal ductal lumina ⊵ and a more basaloid area composed of cells with hyperchromatic nuclei and pale to clear cytoplasm ⊵ is suggestive of follicular (external root sheath) differentiation. (Right) Immunohistochemistry for CEA shows strong and diffuse luminal staining in the ductal structures.

MICROCYSTIC ADNEXAL CARCINOMA

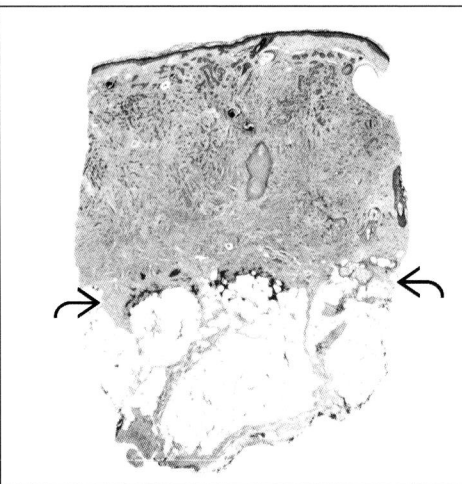

Scanning magnification of a microcystic adnexal carcinoma shows a diffusely infiltrative neoplasm in the dermis and extending into the dermal-subcutaneous interface ➢.

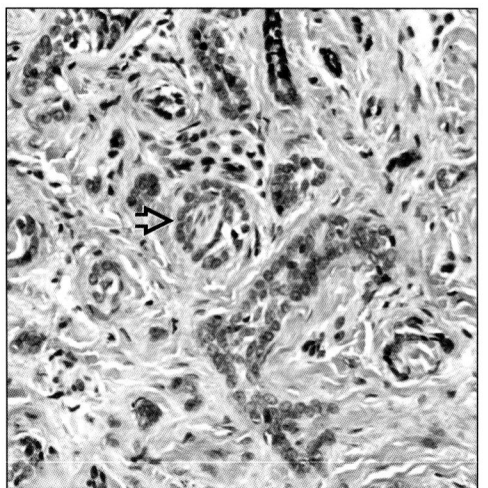

High magnification of MAC shows the relatively bland-appearing cells forming small cords in a desmoplastic stroma. Note the focal perineural invasion ➢.

TERMINOLOGY

Abbreviations
- Microcystic adnexal carcinoma (MAC)

Synonyms
- Sclerosing sweat duct carcinoma
- Syringoid carcinoma, malignant syringoma (older terms, should be avoided)

Definitions
- Low-grade malignant adnexal tumor with follicular and ductal differentiation

ETIOLOGY/PATHOGENESIS

Environmental Exposure
- Some cases may be related to solar damage (UV radiation) or radiation therapy
  - Higher incidence reported on left side of face, which receives greater solar exposure during driving

Unknown
- Most cases

CLINICAL ISSUES

Epidemiology
- Incidence
  - Uncommon adnexal tumors
- Age
  - Usually occur in middle-aged to older adults
- Gender
  - Slightly greater in females

Site
- Most common on the face
  - Upper lip is most common site

- Can also occur on scalp, trunk, extremities, axillae, and groin

Presentation
- Indurated, plaque-like, or nodular lesion

Treatment
- Surgical approaches
  - Complete excision with clear margins
  - Mohs excision is effective and likely the optimal approach in most cases
- Adjuvant therapy
  - Reports of effectiveness with adjuvant radiotherapy

Prognosis
- High incidence of local recurrence (up to 50%), but only very rare metastases
  - Metastases have been reported to local lymph nodes but may represent local, deep invasion, rather than true metastasis

MACROSCOPIC FEATURES

Size
- Typically measure > 1 cm in diameter

MICROSCOPIC PATHOLOGY

Histologic Features
- Bland-appearing dermal-based adnexal tumor
- Deeply invasive and not well-circumscribed
- Perineural invasion often present in deeper areas
- Superficially, typically consists of follicular elements
  - Well-differentiated infundibulocystic structures
  - Smaller basaloid nests and islands, similar to trichoepithelioma
- Deeply, consists of infiltrative cords and ductal structures

MICROCYSTIC ADNEXAL CARCINOMA

Key Facts

Terminology
- Microcystic adnexal carcinoma (MAC)
- Synonyms: Sclerosing sweat duct carcinoma, syringoid carcinoma
- Low-grade malignant adnexal tumor with follicular and ductal differentiation

Clinical Issues
- Most common on the face
- Indurated, plaque-like lesion
- Mohs excision is effective and likely the optimal approach in most cases
- High incidence of local recurrence, but only very rare metastases

Microscopic Pathology
- Bland-appearing dermal-based adnexal tumor

- Deeply invasive and not well-circumscribed
- Perineural invasion often present in deeper areas
- Superficially, typically consists of folliculocystic elements
- Deeply, consists of infiltrative cords and ductal structures lined by bland-appearing cells
- Lymph nodes only very rarely involved and likely represent local, deep invasion

Ancillary Tests
- Low proliferative rate by Ki-67 (high in BCC)
- Low levels of p53 and Bcl-2 (high in BCC)

Top Differential Diagnoses
- Desmoplastic trichoepithelioma
- Syringoma
- Desmoplastic basal cell carcinoma

- o Cells are small, cuboidal-shaped, and bland-appearing
- o Associated with desmoplastic stroma
- o Invade into subcutaneous adipose tissue, even fascia and skeletal muscle

Cytologic Features
- Bland-appearing small epithelioid cells

Lymphatic/Vascular Invasion
- Extremely rare

Lymph Nodes
- Only very rarely involved and likely represent local involvement by very deep invasion

ANCILLARY TESTS

Immunohistochemistry
- Positive for pancytokeratin, high molecular weight keratins, and often CK7
- Luminal cells often positive for EMA and CEA (negative in trichoepithelioma and basal cell carcinoma [BCC])
- Low proliferative rate by Ki-67 (high in BCC)
- Low levels of p53 and Bcl-2 (high in BCC)

DIFFERENTIAL DIAGNOSIS

Desmoplastic Trichoepithelioma (dTE)
- Histologically appears almost identical to superficial portion of MAC
- Typically shows more basaloid-appearing nests and islands
- Lacks deep subcutaneous and perineural invasion
  - o Therefore, it is virtually impossible to completely exclude MAC on a superficial shave biopsy

Syringoma
- Usually superficial and noninfiltrative ductal proliferation
  - o Ductal structures often show tadpole-like projections

- Lacks evidence of follicular differentiation (typical of MAC)
- No deep or perineural invasion

Desmoplastic Basal Cell Carcinoma (BCC)
- Infiltrative small nests and cords of atypical basaloid cells
- BCC usually shows multiple apoptotic and mitotic figures, which are absent in MAC
- Focal mucinous stroma and tumor-stromal retraction artifact may be present

DIAGNOSTIC CHECKLIST

Pathologic Interpretation Pearls
- Superficial folliculocystic structures and deeper infiltrative cords and ductal elements
- Perineural invasion often present in deeper areas
- Need deep biopsy or excision to distinguish from desmoplastic trichoepithelioma

SELECTED REFERENCES

1. Baxi S et al: Microcystic adnexal carcinoma of the skin: the role of adjuvant radiotherapy. J Med Imaging Radiat Oncol. 54(5):477-82, 2010
2. Kavand S et al: "Squamoid eccrine ductal carcinoma": an unusual low-grade case with follicular differentiation. Are these tumors squamoid variants of microcystic adnexal carcinoma? Am J Dermatopathol. 31(8):849-52, 2009
3. Gabillot-Carré M et al: Microcystic adnexal carcinoma: report of seven cases including one with lung metastasis. Dermatology. 212(3):221-8, 2006
4. Smith KJ et al: Microcystic adnexal carcinoma: an immunohistochemical study including markers of proliferation and apoptosis. Am J Surg Pathol. 25(4):464-71, 2001
5. Carroll P et al: Metastatic microcystic adnexal carcinoma in an immunocompromised patient. Dermatol Surg. 26(6):531-4, 2000
6. Goldstein DJ et al: Microcystic adnexal carcinoma: a distinct clinicopathologic entity. Cancer. 50(3):566-72, 1982

MICROCYSTIC ADNEXAL CARCINOMA

Clinical and Microscopic Features

(Left) Clinical photograph of a MAC on the cheek of a middle-aged female patient shows a flesh-colored papular to plaque-like lesion. (Right) Low magnification of MAC shows a dermal-based infiltrative basaloid neoplasm with focal calcifications and a large keratinizing cystic structure ⧁.

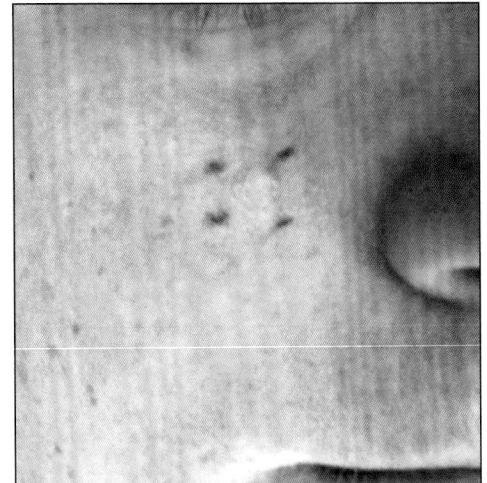
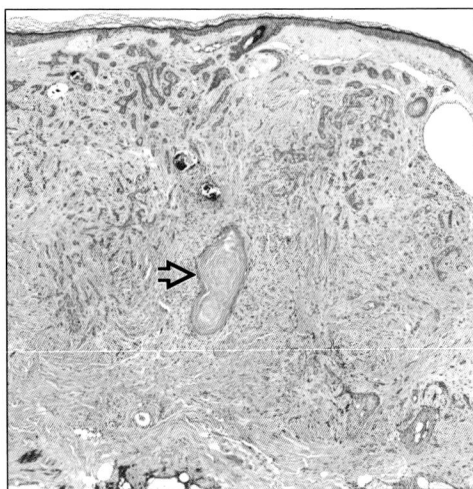

(Left) Superficial portion of MAC at higher magnification shows a proliferation of basaloid cords and nests in a sclerotic stroma. Prominent calcifications are present ⧁. (Right) High magnification of MAC shows the relatively bland appearance of the tumor cells, which show round to oval nuclei with uniform chromatin and inconspicuous to small nucleoli. Note the focal well-formed ductal lumen ⧁.

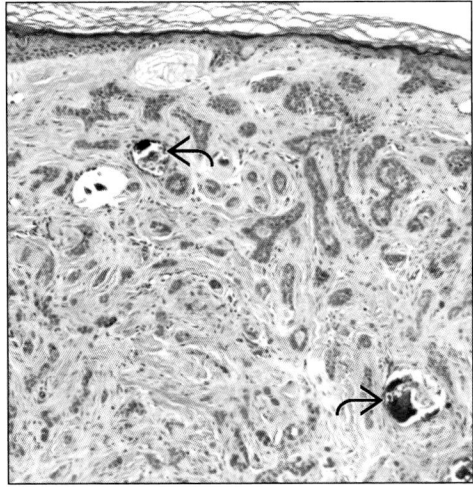
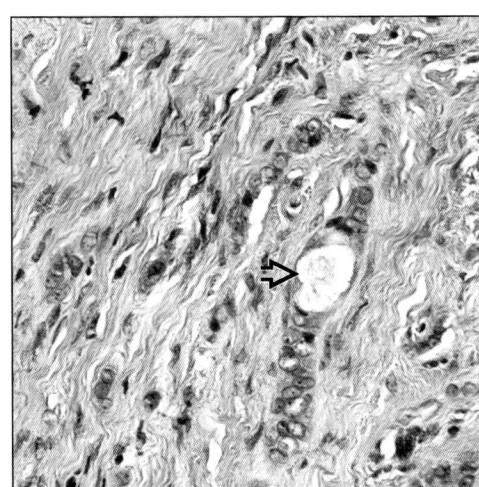

(Left) High magnification of a deep area of MAC shows infiltrative tumor nests ⧁ and cords invading into the adipose tissue. (Right) High magnification of a deep area of MAC shows tumor cell aggregates closely approaching a nerve ⧁.

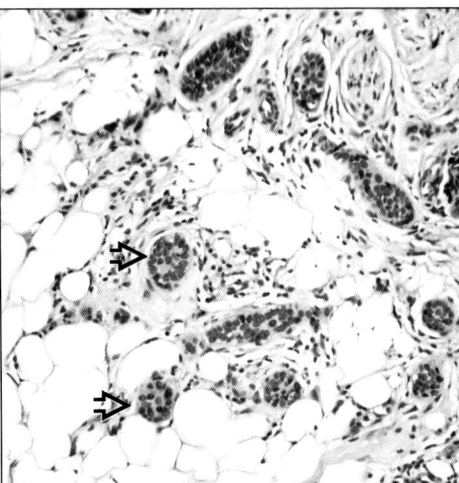
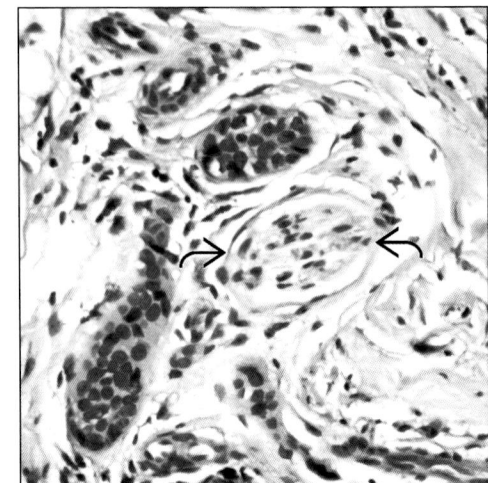

Differential Diagnosis

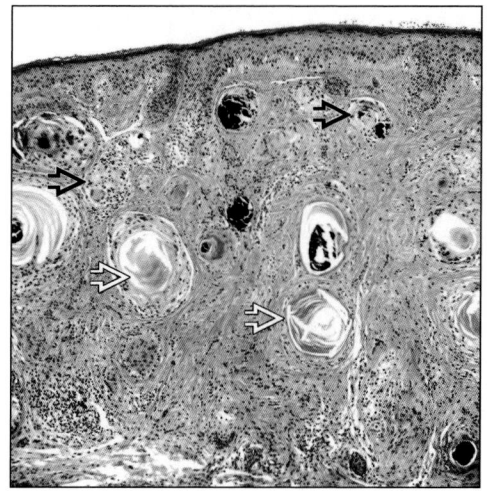

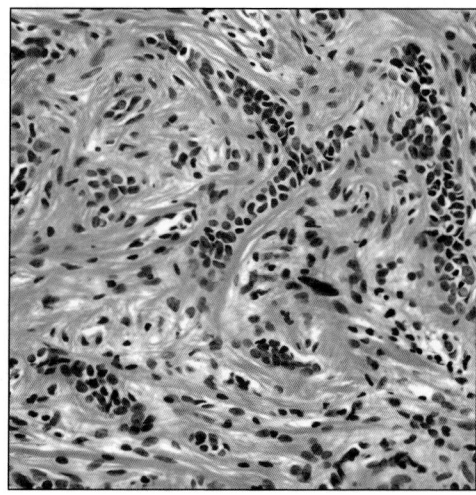

(Left) Low magnification of a desmoplastic trichoepithelioma shows multiple keratinizing cystic spaces ⬇ and calcifications with areas of granulomatous inflammation ⬇. **(Right)** High magnification of a desmoplastic trichoepithelioma shows the small, bland ductal structures in the deeper aspect of the tumor. The ductal structures in MAC are similar-appearing, but do not deeply invade the subcutis or show perineural invasion.

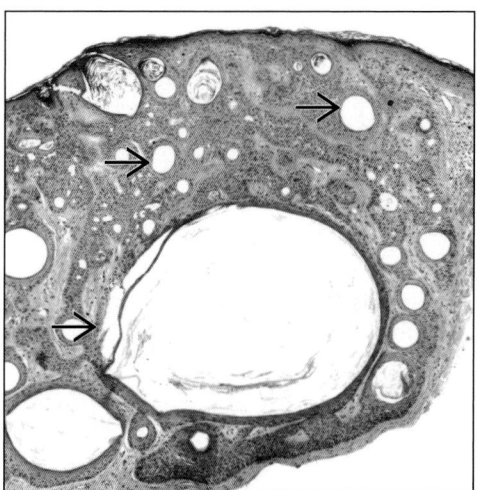

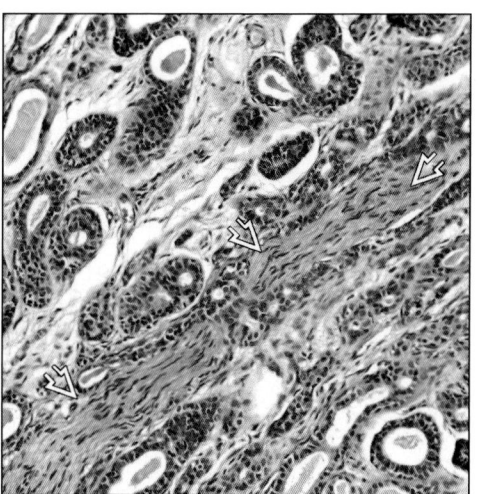

(Left) Low-magnification view of a trichoadenoma shows a dome-shaped lesion based in the dermis. There are numerous mature follicular cysts ➡ present, but there is no evidence of ductal differentiation identified. **(Right)** Adenoid cystic carcinoma frequently shows perineural invasion, similar to MAC; however, adenoid cystic carcinoma lacks follicular differentiation and shows a prominent cribriforming pattern. Here, a large central nerve ⬇ is surrounded by multiple tumor cords and ducts.

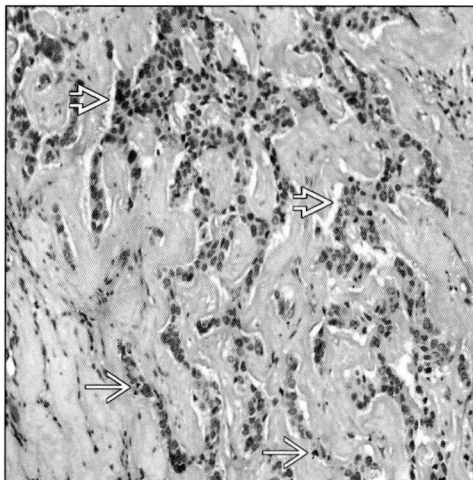

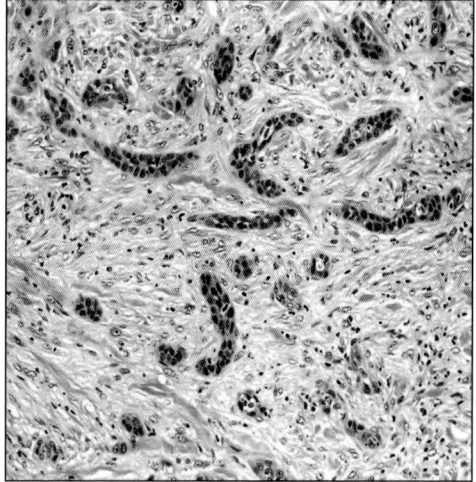

(Left) Desmoplastic basal cell carcinoma shows infiltrative cords of atypical cells with scattered apoptotic bodies ➡, which are usually absent in MAC. Note the focal mucinous stroma and tumor-stromal retraction artifact ⬇. **(Right)** Infiltrative squamous cell carcinoma with cord-like structures associated with a desmoplastic stroma can mimic desmoplastic/morpheaform basal cell carcinoma or, less likely, microcystic adnexal carcinoma.

CUTANEOUS MIXED TUMOR (CHONDROID SYRINGOMA)

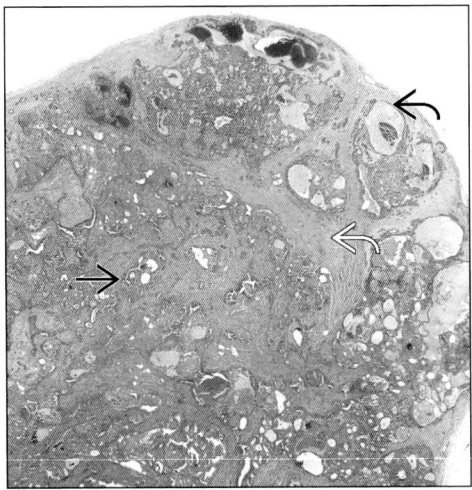

On low magnification, a well-circumscribed tumor composed of epithelial islands ➡ with easily identifiable ductal structures embedded in myxoid ➡ and hyaline ➡ stroma is seen.

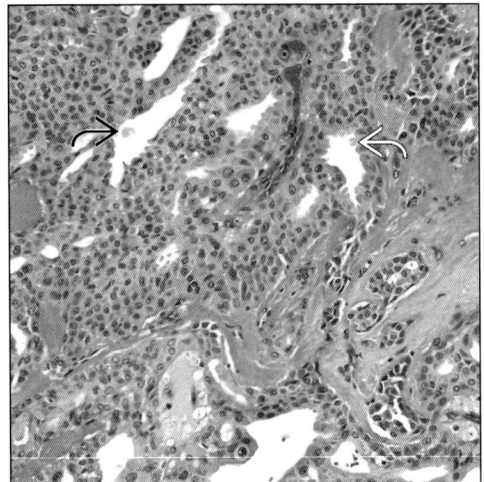

Ductal structures ➡ with some foci of decapitation secretion ➡ are present in the epithelial component.

TERMINOLOGY

Abbreviations
- Cutaneous mixed tumor (CMT)

Synonyms
- Apocrine mixed tumor
- Eccrine mixed tumor
- Mixed tumor of folliculosebaceous-apocrine complex

Definitions
- Well-circumscribed benign epithelial tumor in chondromyxoid matrix

CLINICAL ISSUES

Epidemiology
- Incidence
  - Rare
- Age
  - Middle-aged to elderly
- Gender
  - Male predominance
- Ethnicity
  - No ethnic predilection

Site
- Head and neck sites are most common
- Extremities and trunk

Presentation
- Skin-colored, asymptomatic, dermal to subcutaneous tumors

Natural History
- Slow growth

Treatment
- Surgical excision

Prognosis
- Excellent
  - Very rare malignant transformation

MACROSCOPIC FEATURES

Size
- 0.5-3.0 cm

Sections to Be Submitted
- Representative sections of grossly different-appearing areas should be submitted

MICROSCOPIC PATHOLOGY

Histologic Features
- Well-circumscribed dermal to subcutaneous tumor
- Composed of proliferation of epithelial cells embedded in a myxoid, chondroid, or fibrous stroma
- Apocrine ducts within tumor can be seen
  - Many authors consider CMT to be predominately a tumor of apocrine origin
- Differentiation toward different parts of folliculosebaceous-apocrine complex reported
  - Focal areas of matrical or sebaceous differentiation may rarely be seen
- Eccrine differentiation may be present in some cases
- Large amounts of adipose tissue are seen in what are called "lipomatous mixed tumors"
- Calcification and ossification are rare focal findings
- Due to shrinkage of stroma, fibroblasts and epithelial cells within stroma are surrounded by halos and appear similar to the cells of cartilage
- Epithelial component
  - Epithelial cells can be arranged singly, in small and large clusters, or in solid cords
  - Ductal structures are of variable size and shape

CUTANEOUS MIXED TUMOR (CHONDROID SYRINGOMA)

Key Facts

Terminology
- Well-circumscribed benign epithelial tumor in chondromyxoid matrix

Clinical Issues
- Head and neck
- Skin-colored, asymptomatic, dermal to subcutaneous tumors

Microscopic Pathology
- Epithelial cells embedded in a myxoid, chondroid or fibrous stroma
- Ductal structures of variable size and shape present
- Ducts lined by 2 layers of cuboidal cells and peripheral layer of myoepithelial cells
- Chondrocyte-like cells commonly seen

- Mucin is Alcian blue, mucicarmine, and aldehyde-fuchsin positive and hyaluronidase resistant
- Chondrocyte-like cells in lacunae secrete hyaline cartilage and are S100 protein positive
- Inner cuboidal cells express cytokeratin (CK), epithelial membrane antigen (EMA), and carcinoembryonic antigen (CEA)
- Outer myoepithelial cells express vimentin, S100 protein, and neuron-specific enolase (NSE)
- Tumor shows eccrine and apocrine differentiation
- Very rare malignant transformation

Top Differential Diagnoses
- Malignant chondroid syringoma
- Pleomorphic adenoma (mixed tumor of salivary gland)
- Chondroid lipoma

○ CMTs have been divided into 2 types according to ductal structures by some
  ■ Tumors with tubular, branching lumina
  ■ Tumors with small, tubular lumina
○ Cystic dilation and branching of ducts is common
○ PAS positive amorphous, eosinophilic material (collagenous spherulosis) can be seen in tubular lumina
○ Larger ducts lined by 2 layers of cuboidal cells and peripheral layer of myoepithelial cells
○ Some CMT composed predominately of small ducts and small epithelial clusters
○ Small ducts lined by single layer of cuboidal cells
○ Extension of epithelial cells of smaller ducts into the stroma may give a comma-like shape, similar to syringomas
○ Keratinous cysts are occasionally present
○ Epithelial cells in some CMT show "plasmacytoid" appearance
  ■ These cells have abundant hyalin in cytoplasm, which displaces nuclei to periphery
  ■ Tumors with predominately hyaline cells are termed hyaline-rich CMT
○ Epithelial component occasionally shows metaplastic changes
  ■ Squamous metaplasia is most common
  ■ Mucinous, oxyphilic, columnar, and hobnail metaplasia can be seen
  ■ Cytoplasmic vacuolization and clear cell changes may be present
○ Rare cases of intravascular involvement of tumor have been reported
  ■ This finding is currently considered to be a benign feature
  ■ Metastases were not observed on follow-up of these patients
- Stroma is abundant and may vary from myxoid to chondroid, hyalinized, fibroid, or a mixture of these
  ○ Stellate, fibroblast-like cells are present in stroma of early lesions
  ○ Older lesions show signet ring-like fat cells and cells that appear to be chondrocytes

○ Chondrocyte-like cells in lacunae secrete hyaline cartilage
- Rare histologic variants include tumors with clear cell changes, pseudorosette structures, prominent cribriform areas, osseous metaplasia, tyrosine crystals, and physaliphorous-like cells
- Atypical mixed tumor
  ○ This designation rarely given to tumors with borderline features between benign mixed tumor and malignant mixed tumor
  ○ Predominately of hyalin-rich cell type
  ○ Pushing border and epithelial cells with cytologic atypia seen
  ○ No lymph node or distant metastases on follow-up
- Electron microscopy
  ○ Ductal and secretory lumina present
  ○ Myoepithelial cells present

Cytologic Features
- Benign-appearing epithelial cells with hyperchromatic nuclei and scant cytoplasm
- Rare cases show abundant hyaline-rich cytoplasm
- Abundant fibroblasts are seen in myxoid stroma of younger lesions
- In older lesions, chondrocyte-like cells with lacunae that produce cartilaginous matrix are present

ANCILLARY TESTS

Immunohistochemistry
- Inner cuboidal cells express cytokeratin (CK), epithelial membrane antigen (EMA), and carcinoembryonic antigen (CEA)
- Myoepithelial cells express vimentin, S100 protein, smooth muscle markers (e.g., actin, calponin), CKs, EMA, and neuron-specific enolase (NSE)
- Chondrocyte-like cells are S100 protein positive
- Stromal mucin is Alcian blue, mucicarmine, and aldehyde-fuchsin positive and hyaluronidase resistant
  ○ It is mostly sulfated acid mucopolysaccharides or chondroitin sulfate

CUTANEOUS MIXED TUMOR (CHONDROID SYRINGOMA)

- Chondromyxoid matrix is positive for collagen IV, laminin, fibronectin, and tenascin
- Type II collagen, found in cartilage, may be positive in stromal or epithelial component

DIFFERENTIAL DIAGNOSIS

Malignant Mixed Tumor (Malignant Chondroid Syringoma)

- More common on extremities than head and neck
- More frequent in women
- Asymmetrical appearance at low magnification
- Infiltrative borders
- Atypia of epithelial component showing mitoses and nuclear pleomorphism
- Nuclear atypia is not a prominent feature in some tumors
- Tumor necrosis
- About 45% metastasize to regional lymph nodes, and 45% distant metastases are reported
- This tumor is not typically considered to arise from its benign CMT counterpart
  - Only in few cases have there been benign CMT adjacent to malignant chondroid syringoma

Myoepithelioma

- Rare primary cutaneous tumors considered closely related to chondroid syringomas
- Composed of a pure myoepithelial population
  - Lack epithelial elements with ductal differentiation of chondroid syringoma

Pleomorphic Adenoma (Mixed Tumor of Salivary Gland)

- Tumor arises in salivary glands and not the skin
- Most common tumor of parotid gland
- Although benign, tumor can recur after resection and can invade adjacent tissue
- Histology is essentially the same as CMT
- Chromosomal translocations between chromosomes 3 and 8 often found
- Radiographic studies in addition to tissue sampling are used in reaching diagnosis
  - Ultrasound, MR, and CT scans are helpful in areas difficult to biopsy
  - Fine needle aspiration used as diagnostic tool

Chondroid Lipoma

- Predominately occurs in females
- Frequently occurs on extremities
- Deep subcutaneous to intramuscular location
- Presents as a larger tumor than CMT
- No epithelial cells or glands present
- Lacks epithelial markers
- Mature lipocytes and multivacuolated lipoblast-like cells in chondromyxoid stroma

Extraskeletal Chondroma (Cutaneous Cartilaginous Tumor)

- Predominately occurs on hands and feet
- Largely composed of hypocellular mature hyaline cartilage
- Cystic degeneration is common
- Calcification is often present
- No epithelial or glandular component
- Lacks epithelial markers

DIAGNOSTIC CHECKLIST

Pathologic Interpretation Pearls

- Epithelial strands, cords with glandular spaces in a myxoid/cartilaginous stroma
- Small, medium-sized or large ductal structures
- Hyalinized stroma

SELECTED REFERENCES

1. Gupta N et al: Fine needle aspiration cytology in lesions of the nose, nasal cavity and paranasal sinuses. Acta Cytol. 55(2):135-41, 2011
2. Kazakov DV et al: Cutaneous apocrine mixed tumor with intravascular tumor deposits: a diagnostic pitfall. Am J Dermatopathol. Epub ahead of print, 2011
3. Sodhi KS et al: Role of high resolution ultrasound in parotid lesions in children. Int J Pediatr Otorhinolaryngol. 75(11):1353-8, 2011
4. Constantinescu MB et al: Chondroid syringoma with tyrosine crystals: case report and review of the literature. Am J Dermatopathol. 32(2):171-4, 2010
5. Bernaba BN et al: Myoepithelioma with melanocytic colonization (melanocytic myoepithelioma): a case report. J Cutan Pathol. 36(6):697-701, 2009
6. Kazakov DV et al: Apocrine mixed tumor of the skin ("mixed tumor of the folliculosebaceous-apocrine complex"). Spectrum of differentiations and metaplastic changes in the epithelial, myoepithelial, and stromal components based on a histopathologic study of 244 cases. J Am Acad Dermatol. 57(3):467-83, 2007
7. Ohata C et al: Lipomatous apocrine mixed tumor of the skin. Am J Dermatopathol. 25(2):138-41, 2003
8. Sheikh SS et al: Benign chondroid syringoma: report of a case clinically mimicking a malignant neoplasm. J Surg Oncol. 73(4):228-30, 2000
9. Chen AH et al: Chondroid syringoma of the head and neck: clinical management and literature review. Ear Nose Throat J. 75(2):104-8, 1996
10. Nakayama H et al: Hyaline cell-rich chondroid syringoma: epithelial nature of the hyaline cells. Jpn J Clin Oncol. 26(4):237-42, 1996
11. DelSignore JL et al: Extraskeletal chondroma of the hand. Case report and review of the literature. Clin Orthop Relat Res. (254):147-52, 1990
12. Argenyi ZB et al: Immunohistochemical characterization of chondroid syringomas. Am J Clin Pathol. 90(6):662-9, 1988
13. Mills SE: Mixed tumor of the skin: a model of divergent differentiation. J Cutan Pathol. 11(5):382-6, 1984

CUTANEOUS MIXED TUMOR (CHONDROID SYRINGOMA)

Microscopic and Immunohistochemical Features

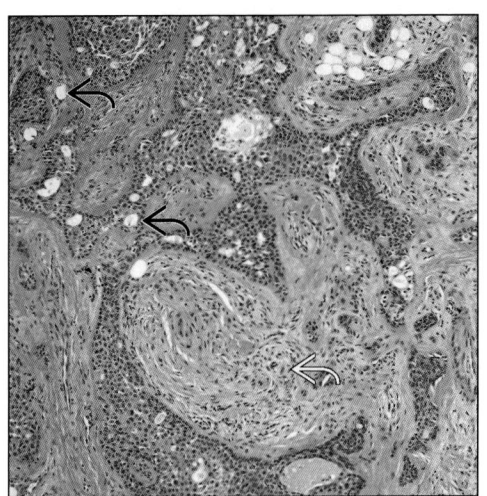

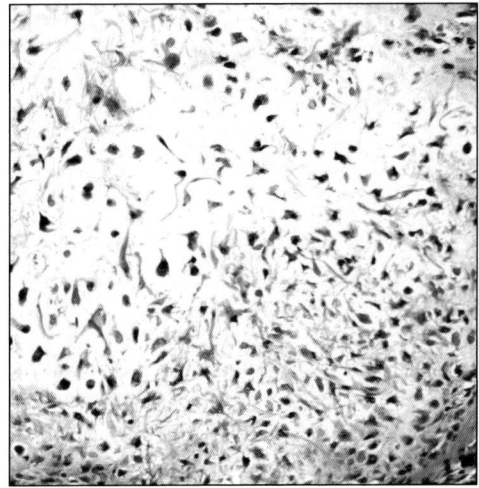

(Left) Small ducts ⊿ lined by cuboidal cells are a common finding. The classic abundant myxoid and cartilaginous stroma is seen ⊿. *(Right)* The stroma of CMT in earlier lesions shows abundant fibroblasts in a loose myxoid stroma.

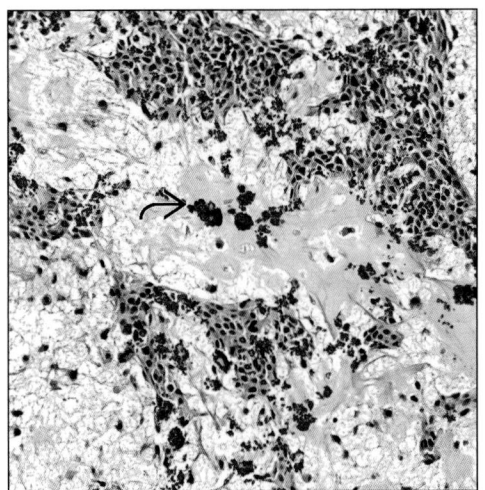

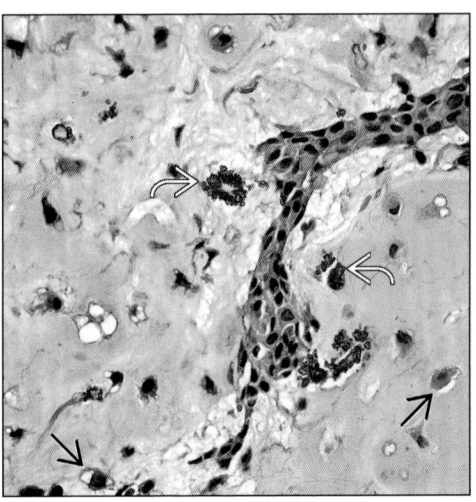

(Left) A CMT with basaloid epithelial cells in a myxoid and cartilaginous stroma with scattered tyrosine crystals ⊿ is a rare finding that may also be seen in salivary gland mixed tumors. *(Right)* Chondrocyte-like cells ⊿ with perinuclear halos are found within a cartilaginous stroma adjacent to a thin epithelial structure and tyrosine crystals ⊿.

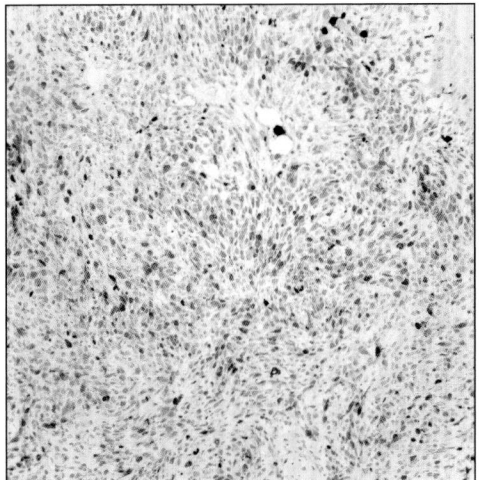

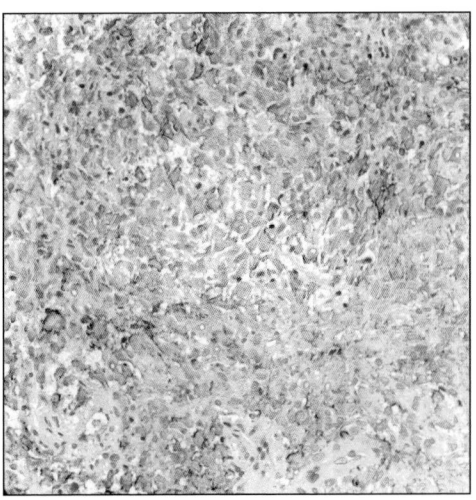

(Left) The myoepithelial component of CMT is strongly positive with S100 protein. *(Right)* CMT shows relatively weak to moderate positive staining with epithelial membrane antigen (EMA).

MALIGNANT MIXED TUMOR

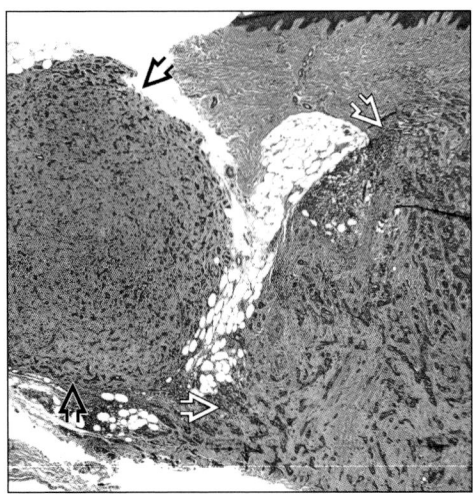

MMT ➤ arising in a longstanding benign mixed tumor ⮞ shows a large, asymmetrical, lobular, and infiltrative tumor invading from the dermis into the subcutaneous tissue.

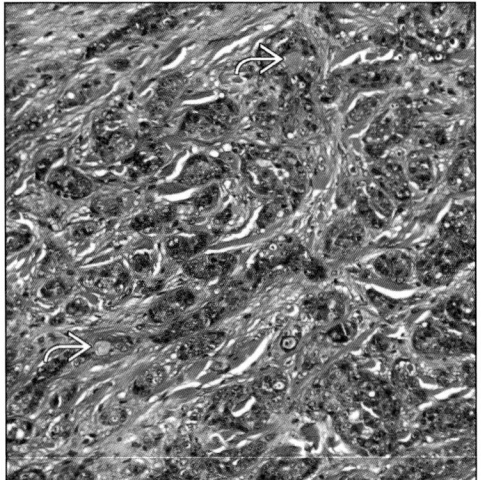

High magnification of an epithelial area shows infiltrative cords of cells, which demonstrate marked cytologic atypia with enlarged, hyperchromatic-staining nuclei surrounding small ductal lumina ➤.

TERMINOLOGY

Abbreviations
- Malignant mixed tumor (MMT)

Synonyms
- Malignant chondroid syringoma
- Malignant apocrine mixed tumor

Definitions
- Rare variant of a malignant tumor derived from adnexal ductal/gland and myoepithelial cells

CLINICAL ISSUES

Presentation
- Most often on extremities and trunk
- More common in women
  - Female:male ratio approximately 2:1
- Average age at time of diagnosis is 5th decade
- Slow-growing, skin-colored tumor
- Slow protracted growth phase followed by rapid growth
- Rarely, malignant transformation from mixed tumor of skin
  - Most tumors begin with anaplastic changes

Treatment
- Surgical approaches
  - Wide excision with broad margin is primary treatment
- Adjuvant therapy
  - Effectiveness of chemotherapy is not established
- Radiation
  - Effectiveness of radiotherapy is not established; however, it might be helpful since tumors have propensity to form satellite lesions

Prognosis
- Biologic behavior of MMT varies: Local recurrence, metastasis (regional lymph node to distant viscera)
- Bone and lung are most common sites for distant metastases
- Up to 39% of cases were found to have metastatic lesions, and 22% died of disease
- Tumor loses chondroid stroma and often metastasizes as an adenocarcinoma

MICROSCOPIC PATHOLOGY

Histologic Features
- Histologic appearances vary greatly
- It is often a large, lobulated tumor in dermis &/or subcutaneous tissue
- Composed of both an epithelial and a mesenchymal component
  - Epithelial component tends to be predominately at periphery of lesion
    - Irregular nests, cords, and sheets of cuboidal or polygonal cells
    - Glandular differentiation is often present; not as common as in benign mixed tumor of skin
    - Foci of highly atypical cells with hyperchromatic nuclei and numerous mitotic figures are often present
    - Areas with moderate nuclear atypia or lacking morphologic criteria of malignancy are also common
    - Infiltration of surrounding tissue, vascular invasion, and necrosis are helpful diagnostic features
- Stroma is myxoid, chondroid, or hyalinized and is most abundant at center of lesion
  - Spindled mesenchymal cells are observed in the stroma
  - Some cases may show frankly malignant stromal cells (i.e., true "carcinosarcoma")

MALIGNANT MIXED TUMOR

Key Facts

Clinical Issues
- Slow-growing tumor on extremities and trunk
- Local recurrence; regional and distant metastasis
- Wide excision with broad margin is primary treatment

Microscopic Pathology
- Histologic appearances vary greatly
- Composed of an epithelial and chondroid/myxoid stromal component

- Epithelial component shows carcinomatous features and benign-appearing islands
- Foci of highly atypical cells with hyperchromatic nuclei and numerous mitotic figures
- Infiltration of surrounding tissue, vascular invasion and necrosis are helpful diagnostic features

Top Differential Diagnoses
- Cutaneous mixed tumor
- Biphasic synovial sarcoma

- Satellite tumor nodules might be present
- Rarely, features of associated benign mixed tumor can be seen
- MMT can easily be misdiagnosed due to its rare occurrence

Cytologic Features
- Epithelial cells with glandular differentiation and carcinomatous features

ANCILLARY TESTS

Immunohistochemistry
- Epithelial cells express cytokeratins (CK-PAN, HMWCKs such as CK5/6) and p63
- Chondroid and myoepithelial areas are often S100 protein, actin, calponin, and vimentin positive

DIFFERENTIAL DIAGNOSIS

Benign Cutaneous Mixed Tumor
- Often small, symmetric, nodular dermal-based tumor
- Lacks features of malignancy
  - i.e., infiltration of surrounding tissue, cytologic atypia of epithelial cells, tumor necrosis, and perineural or vascular invasion
- Glandular areas are more abundant in benign lesions

Biphasic Synovial Sarcoma
- Commonly found in deep, intramuscular soft tissue

- Biphasic histology including epithelial and spindle cells
- S100 protein is rarely positive

DIAGNOSTIC CHECKLIST

Pathologic Interpretation Pearls
- Malignant epithelial tumor with glandular differentiation embedded in chondroid/myxoid stroma

SELECTED REFERENCES

1. Takahashi H et al: Malignant chondroid syringoma with bone invasion: a case report and review of the literature. Am J Dermatopathol. 26(5):403-6, 2004
2. Barnett MD et al: Recurrent malignant chondroid syringoma of the foot: a case report and review of the literature. Am J Clin Oncol. 23(3):227-32, 2000
3. Bates AW et al: Atypical mixed tumor of the skin: histologic, immunohistochemical, and ultrastructural features in three cases and a review of the criteria for malignancy. Am J Dermatopathol. 20(1):35-40, 1998
4. Trown K et al: Malignant mixed tumor of the skin (malignant chondroid syringoma). Pathology. 26(3):237-43, 1994
5. Steinmetz JC et al: Malignant chondroid syringoma with widespread metastasis. J Am Acad Dermatol. 22(5 Pt 1):845-7, 1990

IMAGE GALLERY

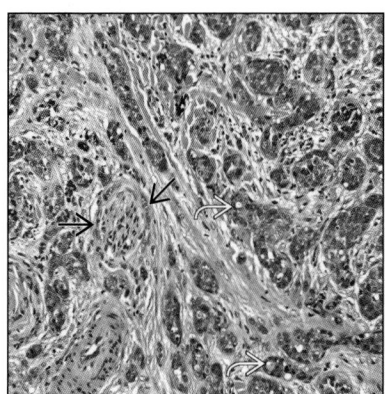 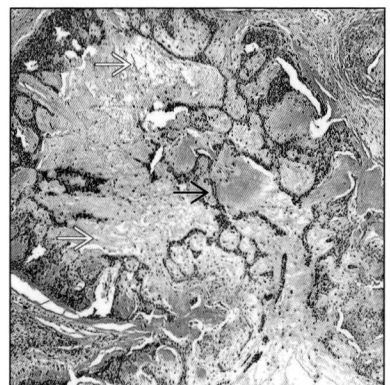 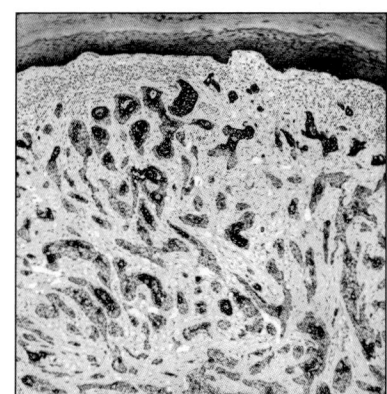

(Left) Cords and nests of epithelial cells with hyperchromatic nuclei and scant cytoplasm are present. Small foci of ductal differentiation ➡ are observed, and perineural invasion was also present ➡. *(Center)* This MMT shows a lace-like pattern of interconnecting tubuloalveolar epithelial structures ➡ in a myxoid and fibroid stroma ➡ that also included malignant stromal cells (i.e., a "carcinosarcoma"). *(Right)* The epithelial component of the tumor is strongly highlighted by a HMWCK (CK5/6) stain.

Metastatic Tumors

METASTATIC SKIN TUMORS

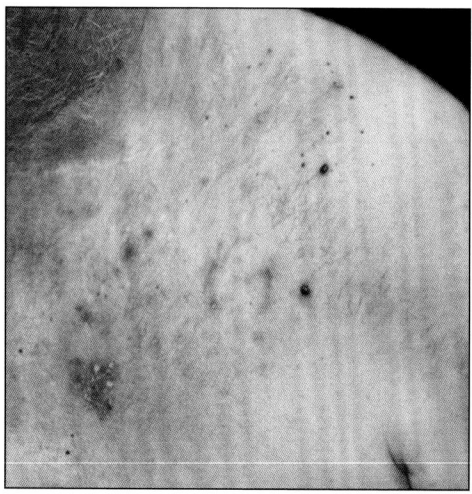

This patient with a history of melanoma on the chest has an unusual presentation of metastatic melanoma, with numerous 1-3 mm black-red papules.

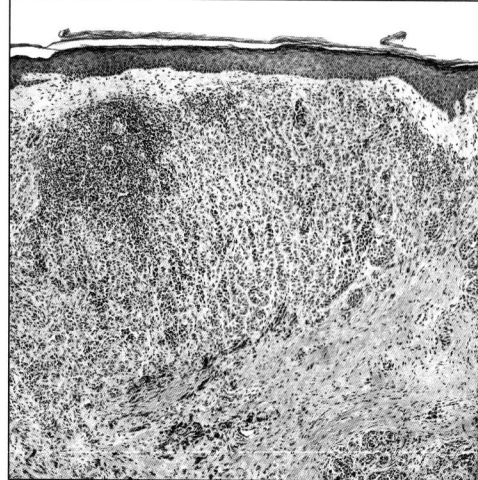

This metastatic melanoma shows a lack of epidermal involvement, and is composed of nests of atypical cells with melanin pigment in the dermis.

TERMINOLOGY

Definitions
- Metastatic tumor originating from skin

CLINICAL ISSUES

Presentation
- Melanoma
  - Cutaneous metastases
    - Nodule or papule, often pigmented, may be ulcerated, multiple or solitary
    - Rarely the presenting sign of disease
    - Occasionally primary tumor site cannot be determined
  - Nodal metastases
    - Most commonly in regional, draining lymph nodes
  - Distant metastases
    - Any site, including bone, gastrointestinal tract, lung, brain
  - Blue nevus-like melanoma
    - Blue macule/papule, often near original site of primary melanoma
- Merkel cell carcinoma
  - Spreads to lymph nodes in up to 50-75% of cases
  - Distant metastasis in up to 30-50% of cases
    - Other sites of metastasis include liver, lungs, bone, brain
- Squamous cell carcinoma (SCC)
  - Nonspecific nodules, often pink to red
  - Rarely zosteriform pattern
- Basal cell carcinoma (BCC)
  - Very rarely metastasizes to other sites (lymph nodes, bone, parotid, lungs, other internal organs)
- Dermatofibrosarcoma protuberans (DFSP)
  - Essentially only fibrosarcomatous cases
  - Often history of multiple local recurrences
  - Rarely metastasizes

- Lung most common site; also lymph nodes, bone, soft tissue
- Many other cutaneous malignancies may metastasize
  - Adnexal carcinomas
    - Sebaceous carcinoma: Relatively high incidence of metastasis
    - Microcystic adnexal carcinoma (extremely rare, with history of multiple recurrences)
    - Apocrine and eccrine carcinomas
    - Aggressive digital papillary adenocarcinoma (typically to lungs)
  - Sarcomas that involve dermis

Treatment
- Melanoma
  - Nodal metastasis
    - Excision if possible (lymph node dissection)
    - Observation, clinical trial, interferon-α, &/or radiation
  - Distant metastasis
    - Consider clinical trial, vemurafenib, ipilimumab, chemotherapy, IL-2, radiation, &/or palliative care
- Merkel cell carcinoma
  - Nodal metastasis
    - Nodal dissection &/or radiation treatment
    - Consider adjuvant chemotherapy (cisplatin or carboplatin ± etoposide)
  - Distant metastasis
    - Multidisciplinary tumor board consultation
    - Consider surgery, radiation treatment, chemotherapy (cisplatin or carboplatin ± etoposide; or topotecan or cyclophosphamide)
- SCC
  - Excision if possible
  - Radiation or chemotherapy (cisplatin ± another agents)
- BCC
  - Excision if possible
  - Chemotherapy (cisplatin ± another agent) or treatment with hedgehog inhibitors

Key Facts

Clinical Issues

- Melanoma
  - Nodule, often pigmented, may be ulcerated, multiple or solitary
  - Nodal metastases; most commonly in regional lymph nodes
  - Blue nevus-like melanoma: Blue macule/papule, often near original site of primary melanoma
  - Survival often < 3 years, but varies
- SCC and BCC: Nonspecific nodule(s), often pink to red
- Merkel cell carcinoma: Nodal &/or distant metastasis common
- DFSP: Essentially only the fibrosarcomatous variant

Microscopic Pathology

- Metastatic melanoma
  - Nodal metastases: Micrometastasis better detected with use of stains, i.e., S100, MART-1/Melan-A, HMB-45, MITF
  - Cutaneous metastases generally lack an epidermal component (only rare epidermotropism)
- Blue nevus-like metastatic melanoma: Virtually identical to blue nevus; history may be the key clue to diagnosis

Top Differential Diagnoses

- All metastatic skin tumors: Primary skin tumor (rather than metastasis to skin from primary focus elsewhere in skin)
- Nodal metastasis of melanoma: Nodal nevus (typically p16[+], low proliferation rate with Ki-67)
- Merkel cell carcinoma: Other metastatic small cell neuroendocrine tumors

---

- DFSP
  - Excision if possible
  - Consider imatinib, chemotherapy, radiation treatment

Prognosis

- Melanoma
  - Survival often < 3 years, but varies
- Merkel cell carcinoma
  - Survival at 5 years: 59% for regional metastasis, 25% for distant metastasis

MICROSCOPIC PATHOLOGY

Histologic Features

- Melanoma
  - Nodal metastases
    - Micrometastasis better detected with use of stains: S100, MART-1/Melan-A, HMB-45, MITF
  - Cutaneous metastases
    - Generally lack an epidermal component (only very rare epidermotropism)
    - Often similar histology to primary tumor, e.g., if primary tumor were spindle cell, metastasis would typically show spindle cell features
  - Distant metastases
    - Often similar histology to primary tumor
  - Blue nevus-like metastatic melanoma
    - Virtually identical to blue nevus; history may be the major clue to diagnosis
    - Histopathologic clues include mitoses, atypical epithelioid melanocytes, and peripheral inflammation
- Merkel cell carcinoma
  - Anastomosing bands/sheets of cells, often in lower dermis/subcutaneous
  - Cells with indistinct cytoplasmic borders, little cytoplasm, salt-and-pepper chromatin; numerous mitoses; CK20 positive, TTF-1 negative
  - Ultrastructural: Perinuclear whorls of intermediate filaments, peripheral dense core granules
- SCC
  - May be poorly differentiated; in such cases, staining with HMWCK &/or p63 is helpful
  - Aggressive variants such as desmoplastic SCC and adenosquamous carcinoma are more likely to metastasize
- BCC
  - Typical histologic features of BCC with peripheral palisading, retraction artifact, mucinous stroma
- DFSP
  - Often has a fibrosarcomatous component

DIFFERENTIAL DIAGNOSIS

DDx of Metastatic Cutaneous Tumors to the Skin

- Primary tumor needs to be considered; primary tumors often have epidermal connections &/or in situ component (for melanoma and SCC) or are located more superficially in dermis (for BCC and Merkel cell carcinoma)
- Clinical history and examination findings may be key for diagnosis

DDx of Nodal Metastasis of Melanoma

- Nodal nevus
  - Generally subcapsular, but rarely parenchymal; p16(+), low proliferation rate with Ki-67

DDx of Merkel Cell Carcinoma

- Metastatic small cell carcinoma of lung (TTF-1[+]) and other neuroendocrine tumors should be excluded

SELECTED REFERENCES

1. Hussein MR: Skin metastasis: a pathologist's perspective. J Cutan Pathol. 37(9):e1-20, 2010
2. Richmond HM et al: Primary and metastatic malignant tumors of the scalp: an update. Am J Clin Dermatol. 11(4):233-46, 2010
3. Lookingbill DP et al: Cutaneous metastases in patients with metastatic carcinoma: a retrospective study of 4020 patients. J Am Acad Dermatol. 29(2 Pt 1):228-36, 1993

Microscopic Features and Ancillary Techniques

(Left) This example of metastatic melanoma shows diffuse replacement of a lymph node by the tumor cells. (Right) This is a higher magnification view of metastatic melanoma replacing a lymph node. The cells are somewhat nested and show hyperchromatic nuclei with pleomorphism and large, purple nucleoli. Mitotic figures are present ➡.

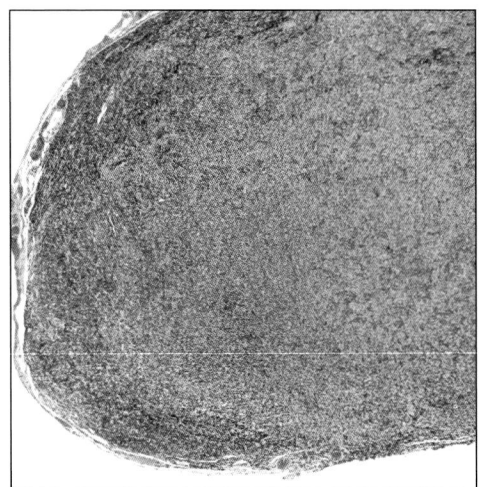
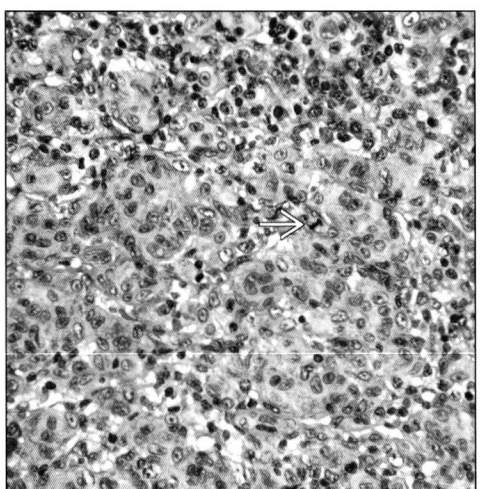

(Left) This is an S100 protein stain of metastatic melanoma replacing a lymph node. (Right) Other metastases of malignant melanoma are not as obvious. In this case, there is a micrometastasis of malignant melanoma in the lymph node. S100 protein staining is often very helpful to identify micrometastases, as it is the most sensitive melanocytic marker.

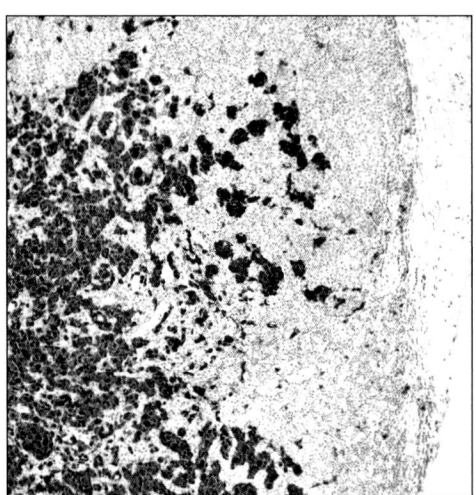
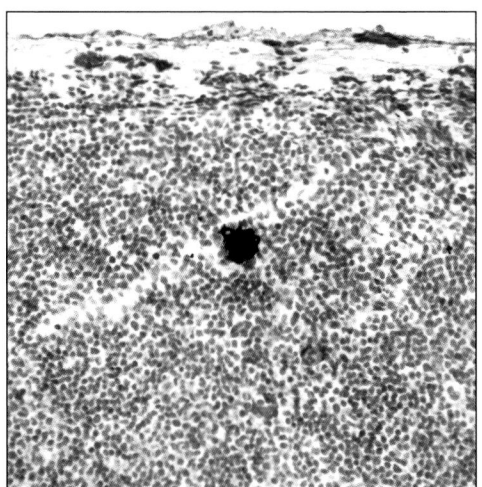

(Left) This is an example of a micrometastasis of melanoma in a lymph node. Immunohistochemical stains including HMB-45 (shown here) are helpful in identifying these collections of tumor cells. HMB-45 is less sensitive but more specific than S100, making use of a panel of immunostains the optimal approach. (Right) This micrometastasis is also strongly MART-1/Melan-A positive; this marker is slightly less sensitive than S100, but is more specific.

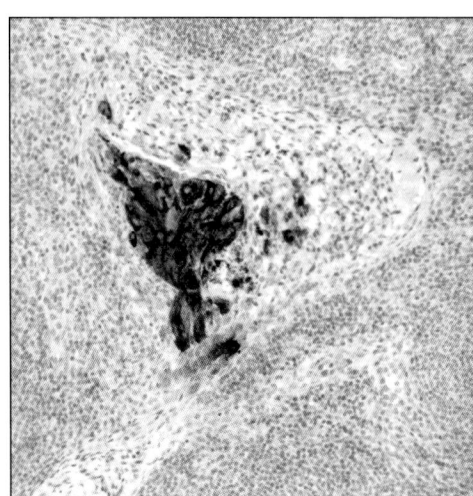
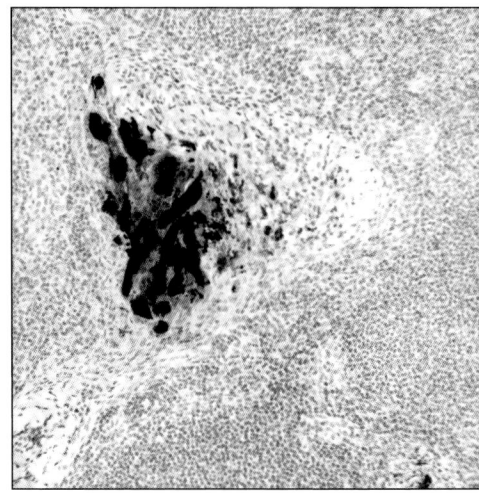

I

6

Microscopic Features and Ancillary Techniques

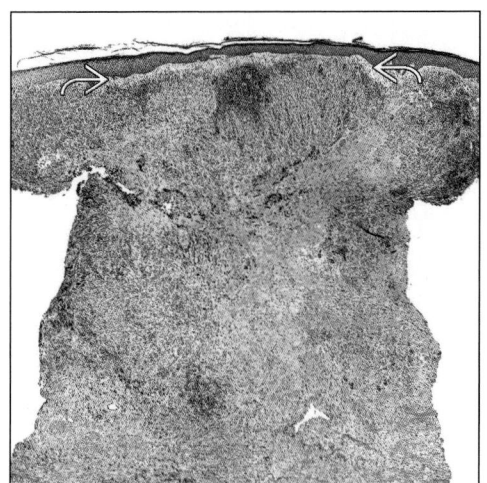

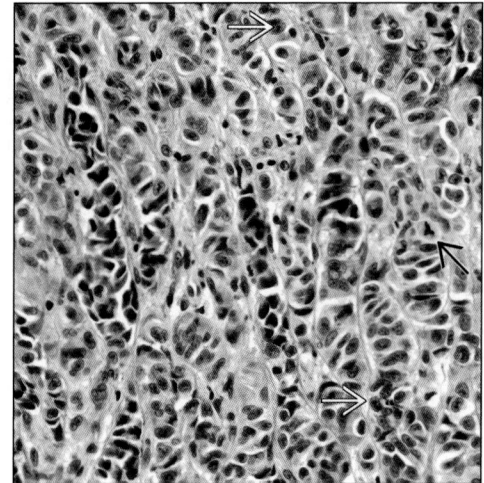

(Left) This metastatic melanoma shows extensive involvement of the dermis. There is a slight grenz zone ➡ and no evidence of epidermotropism. *(Right)* Higher magnification view of metastatic melanoma shows nests of atypical, hyperchromatic-staining cells with marked pleomorphism. There are enlarged nucleoli ➡ and mitoses ➡ are evident.

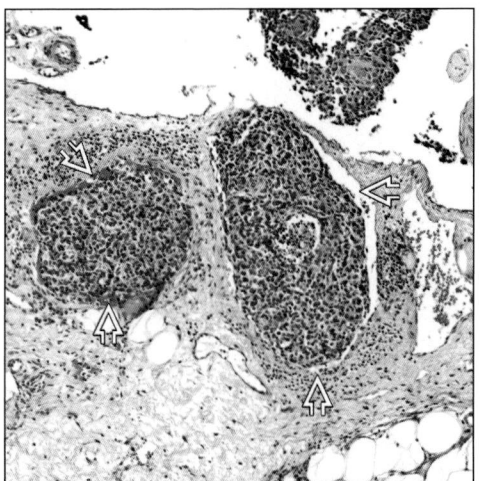

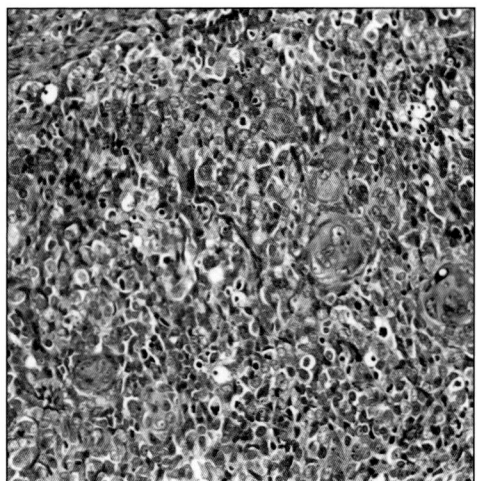

(Left) This is an example of a metastatic Merkel cell carcinoma ➡ to soft tissue with lymphovascular invasion. *(Right)* This is a higher magnification view of metastatic Merkel cell carcinoma showing cohesive clusters of cells with large nuclei and scant amounts of cytoplasm. The cells have salt-and-pepper chromatin, typical of neuroendocrine tumors.

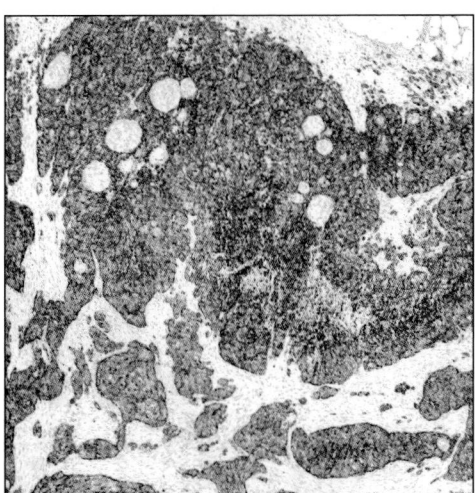

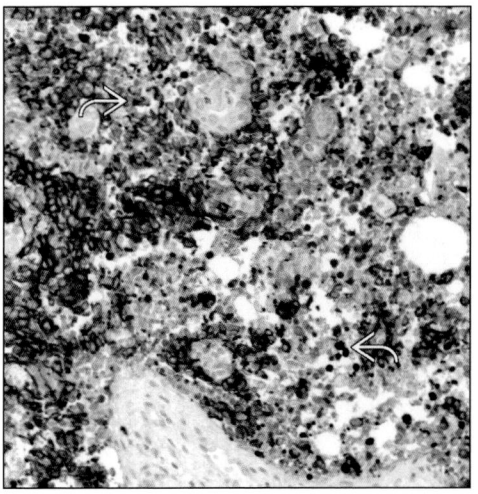

(Left) Metastatic Merkel cell carcinoma shows strong and diffuse positive staining for the neuroendocrine marker synaptophysin. *(Right)* Metastatic Merkel cell carcinoma shows strong and diffuse positivity with cytokeratin 20, with the presence of a perinuclear dot-like pattern ➡.

6

METASTATIC TUMORS TO THE SKIN

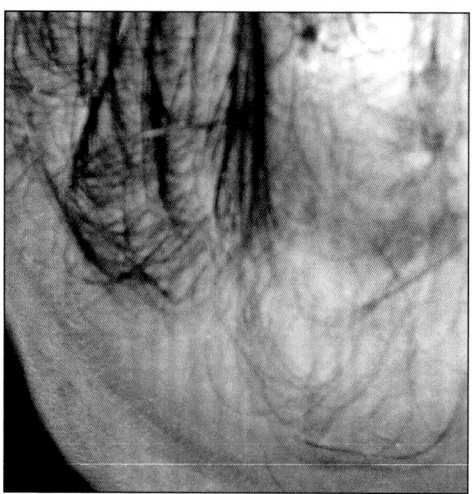

This patient presented with a pink nodule on the anterior scalp. Certain tumors, like renal cell carcinoma (RCC), have the tendency to metastasize to the scalp.

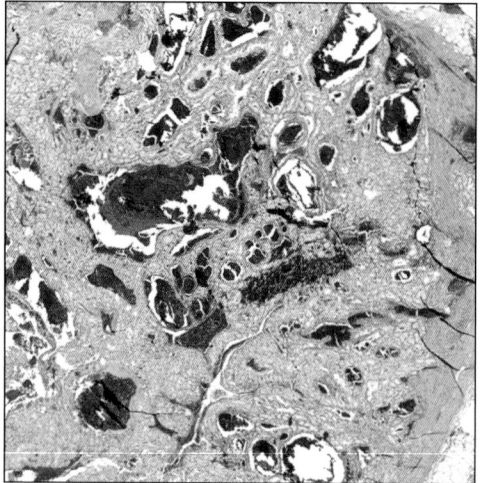

This low-power image shows collections of clear cells with pools of extravasated erythrocytes, consistent with metastatic RCC. These tumors are typically positive with CD10, EMA, and RCC-Ma.

ETIOLOGY/PATHOGENESIS

Mode of Metastasis
- Hematogenous spread
- Lymphatic spread
- Direct extension from primary tumor
- Accidental implantation during surgical procedure
  - Described with oral cavity, laryngeal, lung, mesothelioma, renal cell, colorectal cancers and others

CLINICAL ISSUES

Epidemiology
- Gender
  - Male: Primary tumor most often lung, colon
  - Female: Primary tumor most often breast, colon

Site
- Cutaneous metastases often located near primary tumor site
  - Breast carcinoma: Chest wall
  - Lung carcinoma: Chest wall
  - Genitourinary carcinoma: Abdominal wall, rarely genitalia
  - Oral cavity: Head and neck
- Scalp
  - Tumors with a predilection to metastasize to scalp
    - Thyroid
    - Breast
    - Kidney
    - Lung
- Umbilicus: Sister Mary Joseph nodule
  - Associated with adenocarcinoma of stomach, pancreas, ovary, and others

Presentation
- General points
  - Incidence rate of ~ 2-10% in patients with internal malignancy
  - Rare among skin tumors (~ 2% of all skin tumors)
  - Patients generally of age 60 or above, but exceptions occur
    - In neonates, neuroblastoma or other small round blue cell tumors may metastasize to skin
  - Skin metastases usually present within 2-3 years of diagnosis of primary
  - Breast cancer metastasizes to skin most frequently
  - Other internal cancers with not infrequent skin metastases include lung, colorectal, ovarian, head and neck, renal cell carcinoma, and gastrointestinal cancer
- Signs/symptoms
  - Appearance
    - Generally red-pink, 1-3 cm firm nodule
    - Deeper purple or "vascular" appearance has been described for renal cell carcinoma metastasis
    - Multiple or solitary
    - Clustered or randomly distributed
    - May be movable or fixed, sometimes ulcerated
    - Uncommon bullous or inflammatory patterns of metastasis
  - Asymptomatic or painful
- Special clinical variants
  - Inflammatory (erysipeloid) carcinoma
    - Lymphatic spread of carcinoma
    - Warm, red, tender plaque; resembles erysipelas
    - Most commonly associated with breast carcinoma, but also may be due to other carcinomas (i.e., colon, prostate) and melanoma
  - Carcinoma telangiectoides
    - Secondary to breast carcinoma
    - Plaque of coalescing telangiectasias and erythematous papules
  - Carcinoma en cuirasse
    - Secondary to breast carcinoma
    - Skin hardened and leathery
  - Superior vena cava syndrome

METASTATIC TUMORS TO THE SKIN

Key Facts

Clinical Issues
- Cutaneous metastases often located near primary tumor site
- Incidence rate of ~ 2-10% in patients with internal malignancy
- Breast cancer metastasizes to skin most frequently
- In most cases, skin metastases present after primary tumor has been diagnosed
- Very poor prognosis

Microscopic Pathology
- Many metastases represent adenocarcinoma
  - Irregular collections of cells, often with lumina

Ancillary Tests
- "Organ-specific" markers include PSA, TTF-1, CDX-2, and RCC

- Cytokeratin 7 (CK7) and cytokeratin 20 (CK20)
  - Traditionally, these stains helpful in narrowing down origin of metastatic carcinoma
- Cytokeratin 5/6, p63, podoplanin/D2-40
  - Positivity with these stains supports a primary cutaneous origin over a metastasis

Top Differential Diagnoses
- Metastatic adenocarcinoma
  - Primary adnexal tumors of skin: Generally positive with p63, cytokeratin 5/6, podoplanin
- Metastatic renal cell carcinoma
  - Clear cell hidradenoma and hidradenocarcinoma
- Metastatic small cell carcinoma of the lung
  - Main differential is with primary cutaneous Merkel cell carcinoma

---

    - Can be secondary to lung carcinoma
    - Obstruction of superior vena cava leads to edema, cyanosis, plethora of head/neck; subcutaneous vessels may be prominent
  - Sister Mary Joseph nodule
    - Classically described as red nodule on umbilicus, most commonly due to gastric carcinoma
  - Alopecia neoplastica
    - Localized patches of alopecia on scalp secondary to metastatic disease in dermis

Laboratory Tests
- Ovarian cancer
  - High CA-125 suggestive of advanced disease
  - CA 19-9 may be elevated
- Colon cancer
  - CEA may be used to monitor disease
- Hepatocellular and testicular cancer (and some others)
  - α-fetoprotein may be elevated
- Pancreatic cancer
  - CA 19-9 may be elevated
- Gastric cancer
  - CA 19-9 may be elevated
- Prostate cancer
  - Prostate-specific antigen (PSA) often elevated

Natural History
- Skin metastases are rarely presenting clue to internal malignancy
- In most cases, skin metastases present after primary tumor has been diagnosed

Treatment
- In advanced disease, excision of metastases may be palliative
- Other treatment options dependent on type of tumor and extent of disease (e.g., chemotherapy or radiation)
  - Chemotherapy
    - Traditional drugs (e.g., anthracyclines, taxanes)
    - Trend is to test tissue for molecular targets, and if positive, use targeted treatment (e.g., trastuzumab in Her2-neu positive breast cancer, tamoxifen in estrogen receptor positive cancers)

Prognosis
- Poor overall survival
  - One study cites range of 1-34 months

MICROSCOPIC PATHOLOGY

Histologic Features
- Many metastases represent adenocarcinoma: Irregular collections of cells in dermis, often forming lumina
  - Breast
    - Glandular differentiation may be virtually absent in high-grade cases
    - Cytologically atypical cells may be seen infiltrating in a single file ("Indian file") pattern between collagen bundles (lobular carcinoma)
    - Inflammatory carcinoma: Cytologically atypical cells in clusters within lymphatic vessels
    - Cells are often positive with GCDFP-15, CEA, CK7, mammaglobin, ER/PR
  - Colon
    - "Dirty" necrosis (neutrophils and degenerating cells in glandular lumina) may be evident
    - Glandular differentiation often obvious with columnar cells lining lumina
  - Gastric
    - Signet ring cells may be present
  - Ovarian
    - Psammoma bodies may be present
    - Papillations may be evident
- Mucinous carcinoma
  - Primary mucinous carcinoma of the skin can mimic metastatic mucinous carcinoma (typically of breast, colon)
  - Immunohistochemical stains may not be helpful (especially versus breast, i.e., ER, PR, GCDFP-15 often positive)
- Metastatic renal cell carcinoma (RCC)
  - Clear cells, often bland, in nests and forming ducts
  - Stroma with rich vascularity and numerous extravasated erythrocytes
- Metastatic squamous cell carcinoma (SCC)

- o Lacks epidermal connections
- o Often secondary to a primary of lung or head and neck
- o TTF-1 positivity rarely seen in metastases from lung
- Neuroblastoma and other small round blue cell tumors
  - o Small, hyperchromatic cells
  - o Rosettes may be present
  - o Positive with neuron-specific enolase &/or CD99 (Ewing/PNET)

ANCILLARY TESTS

Immunohistochemistry
- Markers suggestive of a particular primary
  - o Thyroid transcription factor-1 (TTF-1)
    - Positive in lung adenocarcinoma, small cell carcinoma, and rarely SCC
    - Positive in thyroid cancers
    - Negative in primary cutaneous Merkel cell carcinoma
  - o Prostate specific antigen (PSA)
    - Metastatic prostate cancer
  - o CDX-2
    - Positive in colonic carcinoma and mucinous carcinomas of pancreas, intestine, ovary
  - o Thyroglobulin
    - Positive in papillary and follicular thyroid carcinoma
  - o Calcitonin
    - Positive in medullary thyroid carcinoma
  - o RCC-antigen (PCRNA)
    - Positive in RCC
- Cytokeratin 7 (CK7) and cytokeratin 20 (CK20)
  - o Traditionally, these stains helpful in narrowing down origin of metastatic adenocarcinoma
  - o CK7 positive, CK20 negative
    - Breast carcinoma
    - Lung adenocarcinoma
    - Ovarian adenocarcinoma
  - o CK7 negative, CK20 positive
    - Colon carcinoma (although ~ 15% of primary colon cancer negative for CK20; also ~ 15% positive for CK7)
  - o CK7 positive, CK20 positive
    - Pancreatic carcinoma
    - Transitional renal cell carcinoma and bladder carcinoma
    - Some gastric carcinomas
- Cytokeratin 5/6 and p63
  - o Diffuse positivity with these 2 stains supports a primary adnexal cutaneous origin over metastatic adenocarcinoma
  - o Important exception: Primary mucinous carcinoma of the skin stains poorly with these markers
- Podoplanin (D2-40)
  - o Generally positive in primary cutaneous adnexal tumors
  - o Negative in metastatic adenocarcinomas
- CD10
  - o Staining with CD10 is supportive of RCC

- o Also positive in some sebaceous carcinomas, and, rarely, clear cell hidradenomas
- Other stains
  - o Useful stains reported in literature include calretinin, TAG72, WT1, BER-EP4, MUCs

DIFFERENTIAL DIAGNOSIS

Metastatic Adenocarcinoma
- Primary adnexal tumors of skin
  - o May show well-differentiated areas with characteristic features
  - o Generally diffusely positive with
    - p63 and CK 5/6
    - Podoplanin/D2-40

Lobular Breast Carcinoma
- Infiltrating cords of cells create a "busy dermis" pattern (can consider)
  - o Granuloma annulare
  - o Dermatofibroma
  - o Leukemia cutis

Metastatic RCC
- Main differential is with clear cell hidradenoma and hidradenocarcinoma
  - o Generally negative with CD10 and RCC-antigen
  - o Vessels and extravasated erythrocytes not prominent
  - o Hyalinized stroma
  - o Other clues
    - Ducts lined by eosinophilic cuticles
    - Squamoid differentiation
    - Poroid differentiation

Metastatic Small (Oat) Cell Carcinoma of the Lung
- Main differential is with primary cutaneous Merkel cell carcinoma
- Small cell carcinoma is TTF-1(+), CK20(-)

SELECTED REFERENCES

1. Nashan D et al: Cutaneous metastases from internal malignancies. Dermatol Ther. 23(6):567-80, 2010
2. Plaza JA et al: Value of p63 and podoplanin (D2-40) immunoreactivity in the distinction between primary cutaneous tumors and adenocarcinomas metastatic to the skin: a clinicopathologic and immunohistochemical study of 79 cases. J Cutan Pathol. 37(4):403-10, 2010
3. Ivan D et al: Use of p63 expression in distinguishing primary and metastatic cutaneous adnexal neoplasms from metastatic adenocarcinoma to skin. J Cutan Pathol. 34(6):474-80, 2007
4. Liang H et al: Podoplanin is a highly sensitive and specific marker to distinguish primary skin adnexal carcinomas from adenocarcinomas metastatic to skin. Am J Surg Pathol. 31(2):304-10, 2007
5. Ivan D et al: Expression of p63 in primary cutaneous adnexal neoplasms and adenocarcinoma metastatic to the skin. Mod Pathol. 18(1):137-42, 2005
6. Lookingbill DP et al: Cutaneous metastases in patients with metastatic carcinoma: a retrospective study of 4020 patients. J Am Acad Dermatol. 29(2 Pt 1):228-36, 1993

METASTATIC TUMORS TO THE SKIN

Microscopic and Immunohistochemical Features

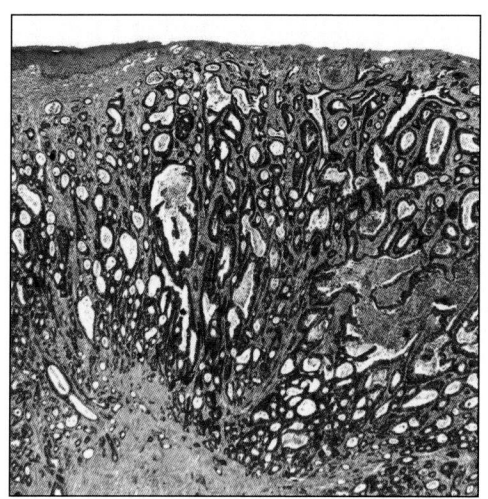
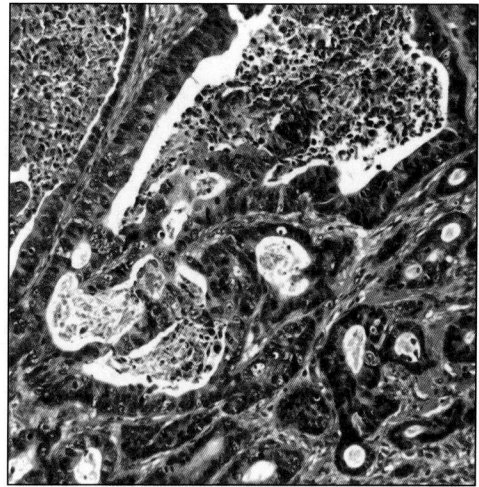

(Left) This is an example of a metastatic colon carcinoma with overlying ulceration. There are variably sized ductal and glandular structures with irregular lumina lined by columnar cells. *(Right)* This is a higher magnification of an example of metastatic colon carcinoma to the skin. There are atypical columnar cells lining lumina. There is evidence of "dirty necrosis," with scattered necrotic cells and neutrophils within the lumen.

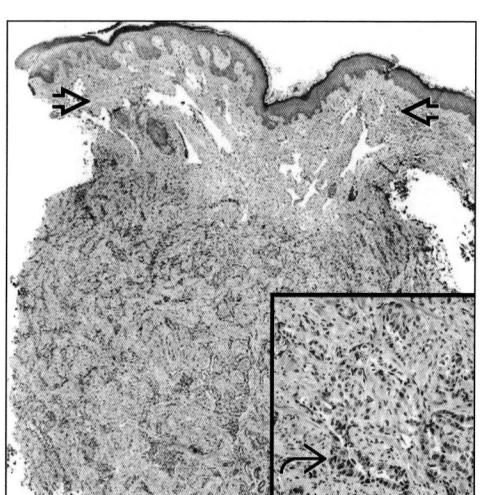
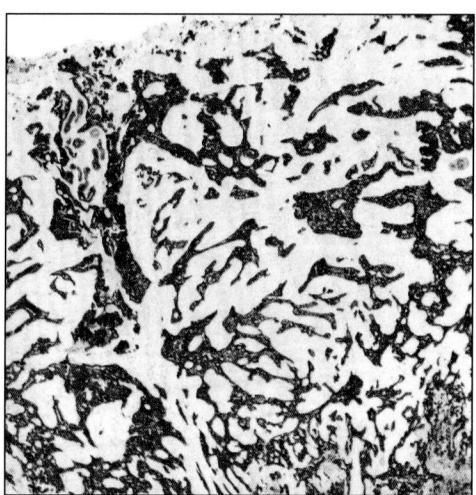

(Left) Metastatic lung adenocarcinoma to the skin is shown. Diffusely infiltrating the dermis are irregular, jagged islands of epithelial cells. Note the absence of epidermal or superficial dermal involvement ⊟. Higher magnification shows glandular lumina lined by markedly enlarged and atypical-appearing epithelial cells ⊟ with columnar features. *(Right)* The metastatic lung adenocarcinoma shows strong, diffuse positive cytoplasmic staining with CK7.

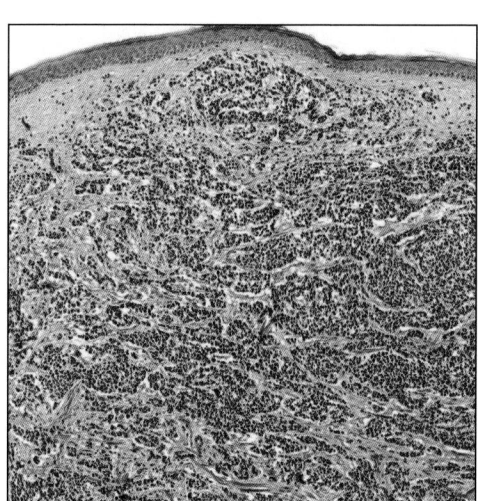
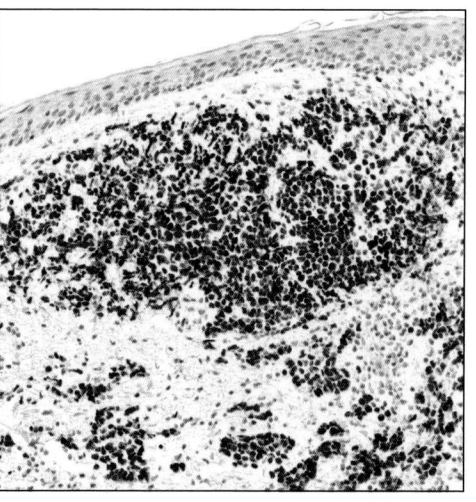

(Left) Metastatic small cell carcinoma of lung to the skin is shown. The cells show prominent nuclear hyperchromasia and a high N:C ratio, similar to Merkel cell carcinoma. *(Right)* Metastatic small cell carcinoma of the lung stains with TTF-1, distinguishing it from primary cutaneous Merkel cell carcinoma, which is uniformly TTF-1 negative. In general, metastatic adenocarcinoma of the lung shows nuclear positivity with TTF-1. Rarely, SCCs of the lung may also be positive with TTF-1.

Microscopic and Immunohistochemical Features

(Left) This example of carcinoma erysipelatoides (metastatic breast carcinoma) shows a perivascular lymphocytic inflammatory infiltrate ➡. Within one of the lymphatic vessels, there is a cluster of atypical cells ➡. *(Right)* High-magnification view of carcinoma erysipelatoides is shown. In this section, clustered atypical cells with multiple mitotic figures ➡ more prominently fill a superficial lymphatic vessel. Part of the epidermis is visible in the right upper corner.

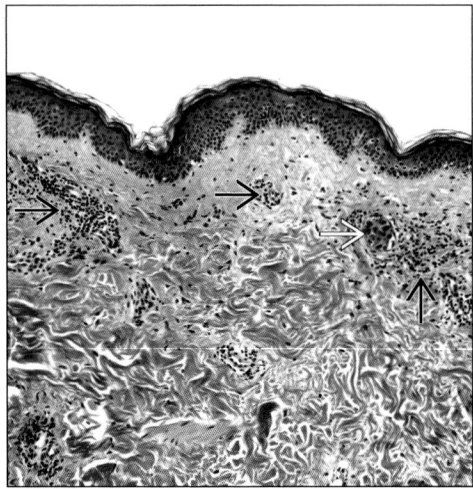
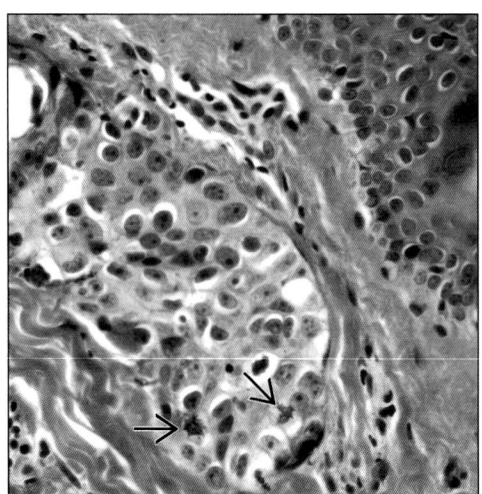

(Left) High magnification of a metastatic high-grade ductal breast carcinoma, with circular islands of cells forming central lumina ➡. The cells composing the islands are markedly atypical, with nuclear hyperchromasia and prominent nucleoli. *(Right)* Cases of metastatic breast carcinoma often show diffuse infiltration of the dermis with atypical, hyperchromatic, single cells ➡; the cells show an "Indian filing" pattern through the collagen. This pattern is most commonly associated with metastatic lobular carcinoma.

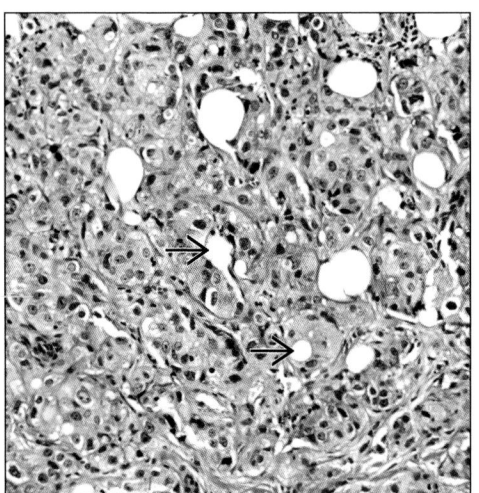
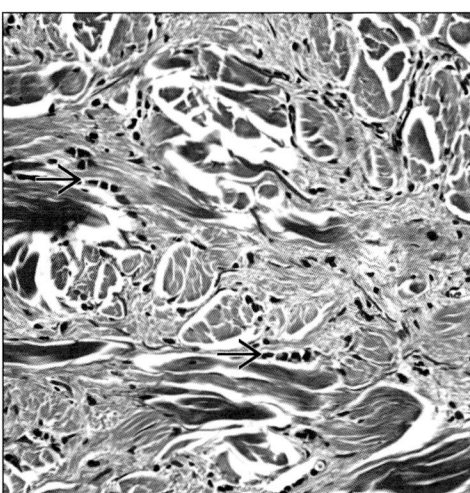

(Left) Metastatic ductal carcinoma of the breast at low magnification shows moderate positive staining with GCDFP-15. This case was also CK7 positive and positive for estrogen and progesterone receptors. *(Right)* This is an example of a metastatic poorly differentiated salivary gland carcinoma. There are irregular, jagged islands in a sclerotic stroma. There are focal areas suggestive of ductal lumina ➡.

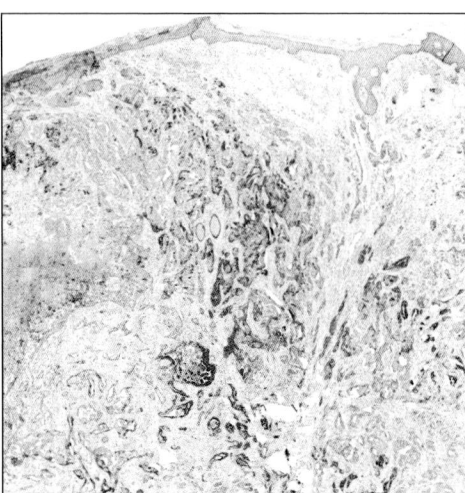
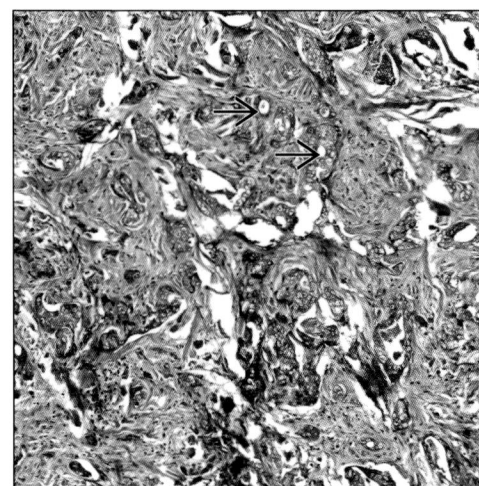

METASTATIC TUMORS TO THE SKIN

Microscopic and Immunohistochemical Features

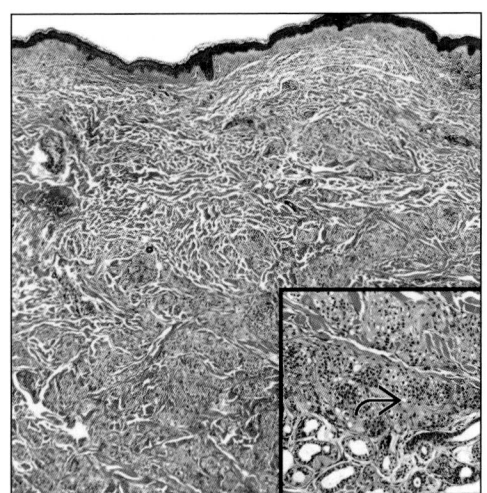

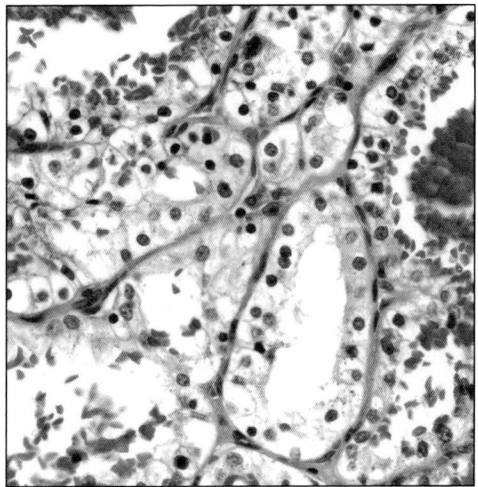

(Left) Metastatic urothelial (transitional cell) carcinoma of the bladder to the skin shows deep dermal infiltration by atypical eosinophilic-staining cells. High magnification (inset) shows marked cytologic atypia and occasional mitotic figures ➡. *(Right)* Higher magnification shows an example of metastatic renal cell carcinoma with clear cells forming lumina. Extravasated erythrocytes are prominent.

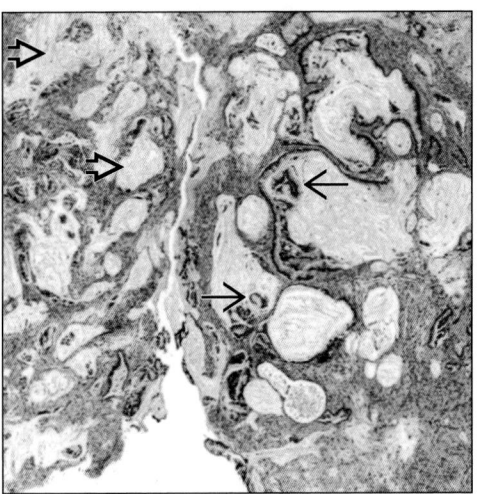

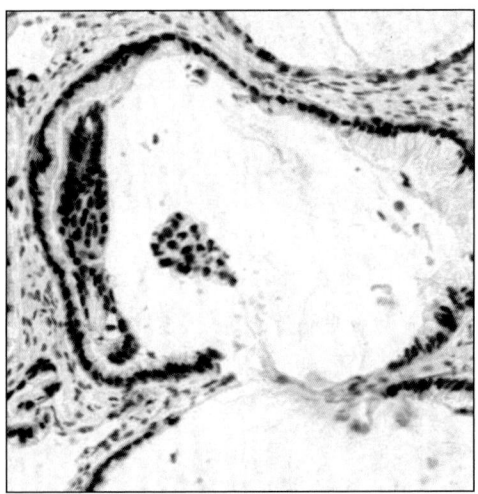

(Left) This is an example of metastatic mucinous pancreatic cancer. There are numerous pools of mucin ➡, within some of which are suspended epithelial islands ➡. Primary cutaneous mucinous carcinoma can appear identical to metastatic mucinous carcinomas, and immunohistochemistry and clinical history are critical in making the diagnosis. *(Right)* Immunohistochemistry shows that the mucinous pancreatic carcinoma stains strongly with CDX-2 (with nuclear staining).

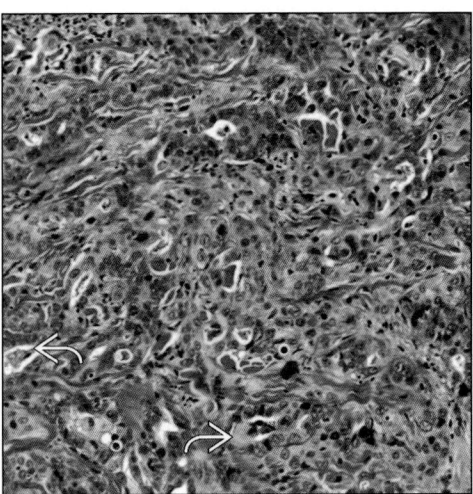

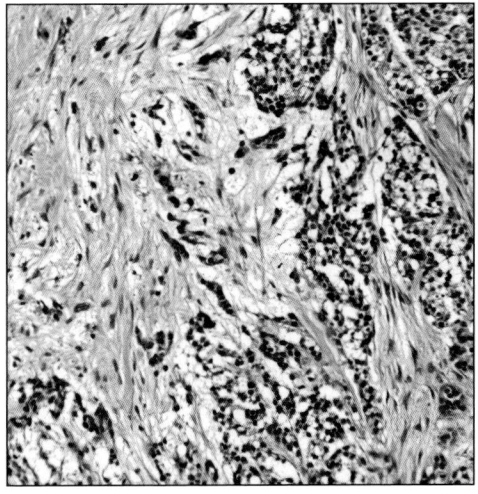

(Left) This is an example of metastatic high-grade pancreaticobiliary carcinoma. There are clusters and tubules of atypical cells forming glandular clusters with small lumina containing mucinous secretions ➡. The stroma is sclerotic. *(Right)* This is an example of a rare metastatic glioblastoma multiforme (GBM) to the skin of the scalp. Hyperchromatic oval to spindle-shaped cells show indistinct cytoplasmic borders with a fibrillary background. The cells typically stain with GFAP.

Fibrous and "Fibrohistiocytic" Tissue Tumors

FIBROEPITHELIAL POLYPS (ACROCHORDONS)

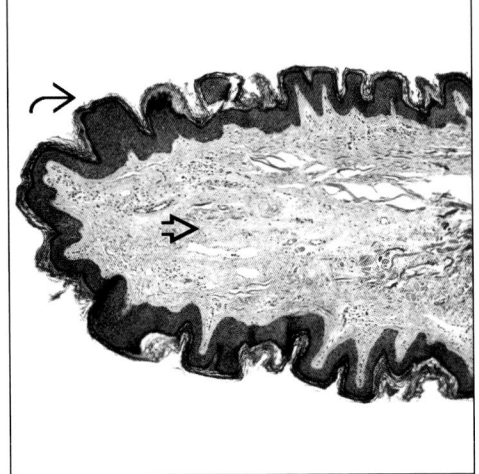

Acrochordon characterized by a core of loose connective tissue devoid of adnexal structures ⟹ is covered by squamous epithelium ➘.

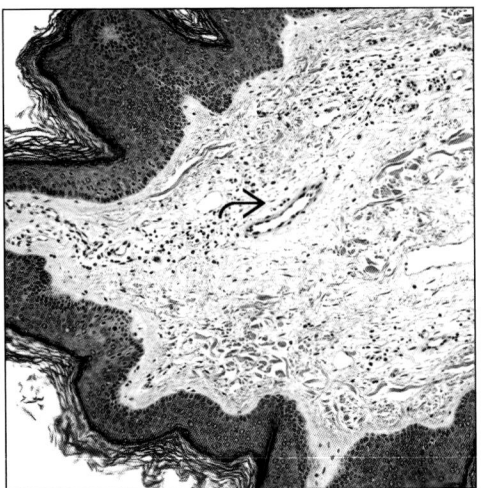

The fibrovascular core in this fibroepithelial polyp is composed of loose connective tissue with scattered vessels ➚ and a few inflammatory cells.

TERMINOLOGY

Synonyms
- Skin tag, soft fibroma, fibrolipoma (with adipose tissue)

ETIOLOGY/PATHOGENESIS

May Be Associated with
- Obesity
- Colonic polyps (controversial)
- Diabetes
- Acromegaly

CLINICAL ISSUES

Epidemiology
- Incidence
  - Very common
- Age
  - Adults
    - > 50 years old
- Gender
  - Predilection for females
    - Obese patients

Site
- Neck, axilla, eyelid
- Inguinal and perianal lesions are frequent
- Lymphedematous fibroepithelial polyps of the glans penis and prepuce have been described

Presentation
- Furrowed papules
  - 1-2 mm
  - Usually multiple
  - Especially on neck and axilla
- Filiform lesions
  - < 5 mm

- Solitary or multiple
- Variable location
- Pedunculated (bag-like) polyps
  - > 1 cm
  - Solitary
  - Lower trunk, buttocks
  - Some of these lesions represent fibrolipomas

Treatment
- Surgical approaches
  - Shave excision is curative

Prognosis
- Excellent

MACROSCOPIC FEATURES

General Features
- Papular
- Filiform
- Pedunculated

Size
- Ranges from a few millimeters to a few centimeters
  - Most measure < 1 cm

MICROSCOPIC PATHOLOGY

Histologic Features
- Squamous epithelium
  - Thin to acanthotic
  - Papillomatosis and horn pseudocysts may be present
    - Most such lesions likely represent seborrheic keratoses with polypoid/pedunculated features
- Connective tissue stalk
  - Loose to dense connective tissue with variable amount of blood vessels
  - Mature adipocytes may be present

FIBROEPITHELIAL POLYPS (ACROCHORDONS)

Key Facts

Terminology
- Skin tag, soft fibroma

Clinical Issues
- Very common lesions
- Usually affect adults
  - \> 50 years old
- Single or multiple
- Neck, axilla, groin
- Association with diabetes and obesity

Microscopic Pathology
- Squamous epithelium
- Loose to dense connective tissue with variable amount of blood vessels
- Mature adipocytes may be present (fibrolipoma)

Top Differential Diagnoses
- Seborrheic keratosis
- Nevus lipomatosus superficialis
- Pleomorphic fibroma

- ■ Such lesions represent fibrolipomas (similar to nevus lipomatosus superficialis)
- In special locations (e.g., eyelids, axillae, and neck) different lesions (e.g., nevi and seborrheic keratoses) may be polypoid and clinically present as skin tags
  - 30% of skin tag growths represent melanocytic nevi
- Rarely, malignant tumors (basal cell carcinoma, melanoma) may arise in a skin tag
  - Atypical lipomatous tumors (well-differentiated liposarcomas) presenting as skin tags have been described

DIFFERENTIAL DIAGNOSIS

Seborrheic Keratosis
- May show polypoid appearance, especially in sites such as axilla and groin
- Usually show more epidermal acanthosis and pseudohorn cysts

Nevus Lipomatosus Superficialis
- Fibroadipose tissue present in superficial dermis, but flatter lesion than fibrolipoma
- Usually present in hips &/or buttocks region

Pleomorphic Fibroma
- Acrochordon-like lesions containing atypical stromal cells
- May represent a variant of fibroepithelial polyp with ancient changes

Polypoid Melanocytic Nevus
- Acrochordon-like growths containing nevus cells
- Usually are intradermal nevi with congenital-like growth pattern

DIAGNOSTIC CHECKLIST

Pathologic Interpretation Pearls
- Skin polyp with thin squamous epithelium and fibrovascular core without adnexal structures

SELECTED REFERENCES

1. Aksoy B et al: Basal cell carcinoma in a skin tag. Eur J Dermatol. 18(5):605-6, 2008
2. Fetsch JF et al: Lymphedematous fibroepithelial polyps of the glans penis and prepuce: a clinicopathologic study of 7 cases demonstrating a strong association with chronic condom catheter use. Hum Pathol. 35(2):190-5, 2004
3. Chiritescu E et al: Acrochordons as a presenting sign of nevoid basal cell carcinoma syndrome. J Am Acad Dermatol. 44(5):789-94, 2001
4. Banik R et al: Skin tags: localization and frequencies according to sex and age. Dermatologica. 174(4):180-3, 1987
5. Kahana M et al: Skin tags: a cutaneous marker for diabetes mellitus. Acta Derm Venereol. 67(2):175-7, 1987
6. Chobanian SJ et al: Skin tags as a marker for adenomatous polyps of the colon. Ann Intern Med. 103(6 (Pt 1)):892-3, 1985
7. Field LM: A giant pendulous fibrolipoma. J Dermatol Surg Oncol. 8(1):54-5, 1982

Differential Diagnosis

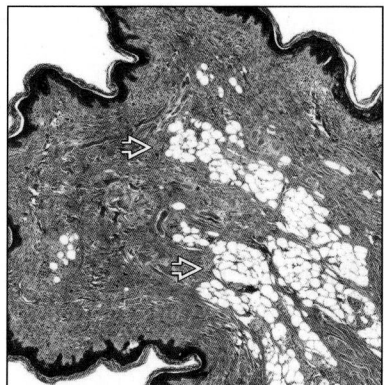 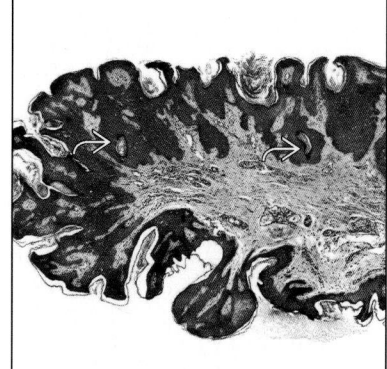 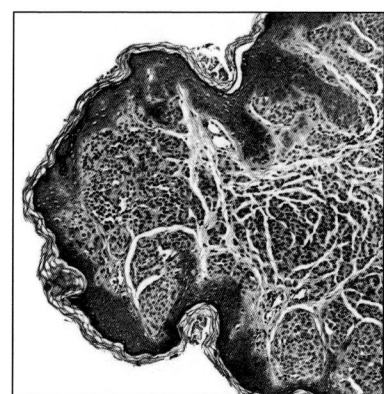

(Left) Fibrolipoma (nevus lipomatosus superficialis) with polypoid features is shown. Some would consider this a skin tag containing mature adipose tissue ➡️ in its fibrovascular core. *(Center)* Skin tag-like growth with acanthotic and papillomatous epithelium shows a few horn pseudocysts ➡️. Such lesions most likely represent seborrheic keratoses that, in special locations (e.g., axillae), have polypoid features. *(Right)* Compound nevus arising in a skin tag-like lesion is shown.

KELOID AND CELLULAR SCAR

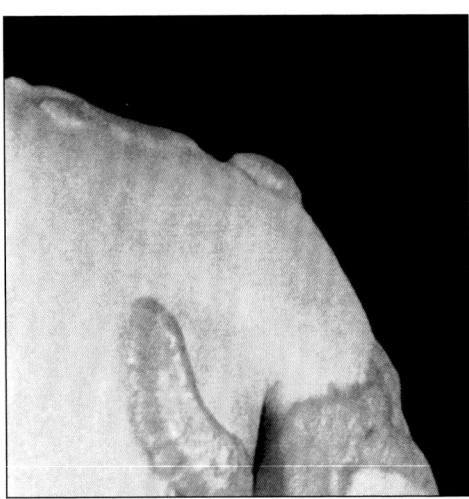

Clinical photograph shows multiple keloids on the shoulder and upper arm of this patient.

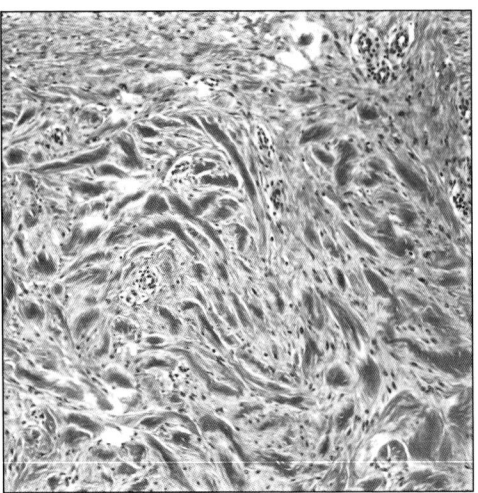

High-power examination of a keloid shows a proliferation of thickened, hyalinized eosinophilic collagen bundles with increased numbers of stromal fibroblasts. Collagen bundles are randomly oriented and unevenly distributed.

TERMINOLOGY

Synonyms
- Scar with keloidal collagen

Definitions
- Scar with prominent thickened and eosinophilic bundles of collagen extending beyond original wound

ETIOLOGY/PATHOGENESIS

Unknown, Possibly Genetic
- Fibroblasts from keloids show decreased apoptosis
- Many cytokines implicated in stimulating fibroblasts, including TGF-B and IL-15

CLINICAL ISSUES

Epidemiology
- Age
  - Most common in patients < 30 years
- Ethnicity
  - More common in African-American patients; least common in Caucasians

Site
- Earlobe is most common site
  - Typically follows ear piercing or other trauma

Presentation
- Nodule/mass lesion is most common
- Scar that grows beyond confines of original wound
- Often erythematous, pruritic lesions with predilection for earlobe

Treatment
- Options, risks, complications
  - Potentially disfiguring with high risk of recurrence
- Surgical approaches
  - Complete excision, accompanied by concurrent steroid injections or radiotherapy to decrease risk of recurrence
- Drugs
  - Direct injection of steroids is often first-line treatment

Prognosis
- Persistence and recurrence are common, but no risk of malignancy

MACROSCOPIC FEATURES

General Features
- Large, nodular, dermal-based lesion with firm, white cut surface

MICROSCOPIC PATHOLOGY

Histologic Features
- Dense proliferation of thickened, hyalinized collagen bundles in dermis
- May be background of conventional or hypertrophic scar with smaller collagen bundles and perpendicular vessels
- Decreased vessels compared to conventional and hypertrophic scars
  - Superficial telangiectatic vessels often present
  - Associated with mild chronic inflammation
- Overlying epidermis shows atrophy in most cases, may show hyperplasia in some cases
- Increased fibroblasts, lymphocytes, and mast cells usually present

Predominant Pattern/Injury Type
- Fibrosis, thickened collagen bundles

Predominant Cell/Compartment Type
- Fibroblast

KELOID AND CELLULAR SCAR

Key Facts

Terminology
- Scar with prominent thickened and eosinophilic bundles of collagen

Clinical Issues
- Persistence and recurrence are common, but no risk of malignancy
- Scar that grows beyond original wound
- Often erythematous, pruritic lesions with predilection for earlobe in African-American patients

Microscopic Pathology
- Dense proliferation of thickened, hyalinized collagen bundles in dermis
- Decreased vessels compared to conventional and hypertrophic scars
- Increased fibroblasts, lymphocytes, and mast cells usually present

Top Differential Diagnoses
- Hypertrophic scar

DIFFERENTIAL DIAGNOSIS

Hypertrophic Scar
- Lacks characteristic hyalinized collagen bundles of keloid
- Has more small, perpendicularly oriented vessels; lacks telangiectasia
- Overlapping cases may be seen and may be diagnosed as "hypertrophic scar with focal keloidal collagen"
- Clinically not as elevated as keloid

Nodular Fasciitis
- May rarely show focal keloidal collagen
- Background shows classic features of nodular fasciitis with loose, tissue culture appearance
- Zonation with cellular, myxoid, and more fibrous areas

Desmoplastic Melanoma
- Unlikely, but rarely may enter differential diagnosis if no history of trauma or previous biopsy/surgery
- Reexcision specimens of desmoplastic melanoma may show keloidal collagen
- S100 immunohistochemical stain should be positive
  - Increased numbers of dermal dendritic cells may be seen in scars
  - Should not show spindled morphology of desmoplastic melanoma cells

DIAGNOSTIC CHECKLIST

Pathologic Interpretation Pearls
- Nodular, elevated lesion compared to adjacent skin
- Thickened, hyalinized eosinophilic collagen bundles
- Often see background of hypertrophic scar

SELECTED REFERENCES

1. Wolfram D et al: Hypertrophic scars and keloids--a review of their pathophysiology, risk factors, and therapeutic management. Dermatol Surg. 35(2):171-81, 2009
2. Butler PD et al: Current progress in keloid research and treatment. J Am Coll Surg. 206(4):731-41, 2008
3. Köse O et al: Keloids and hypertrophic scars: are they two different sides of the same coin? Dermatol Surg. 34(3):336-46, 2008
4. Froelich K et al: Therapy of auricular keloids: review of different treatment modalities and proposal for a therapeutic algorithm. Eur Arch Otorhinolaryngol. 264(12):1497-508, 2007
5. Thompson LD: Skin keloid. Ear Nose Throat J. 83(8):519, 2004
6. Thompson LD et al: Nodular fasciitis of the external ear region: a clinicopathologic study of 50 cases. Ann Diagn Pathol. 5(4):191-8, 2001
7. Tuan TL et al: The molecular basis of keloid and hypertrophic scar formation. Mol Med Today. 4(1):19-24, 1998

IMAGE GALLERY

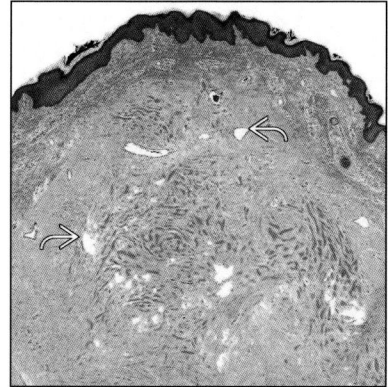 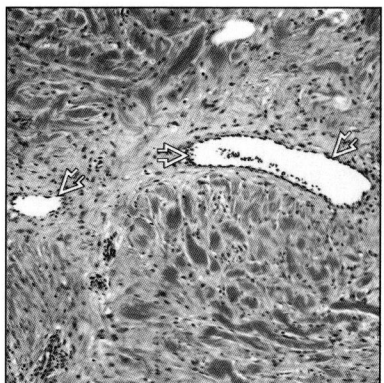 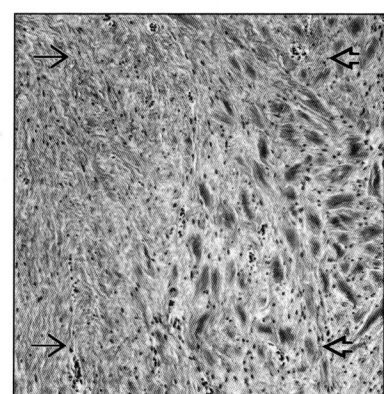

(Left) Scanning magnification of a keloid shows a polypoid skin lesion with dense dermal collagen. Note the mild epidermal hyperplasia and telangiectatic vessels ➡. *(Center)* Superficial portion of keloid shows telangiectatic vessels ➡ surrounded by thickened collagen bundles. *(Right)* Intermediate magnification shows comparison between an area of hypertrophic scar ➡ juxtaposed to an area of keloid ➡.

COLLAGENOUS FIBROMA

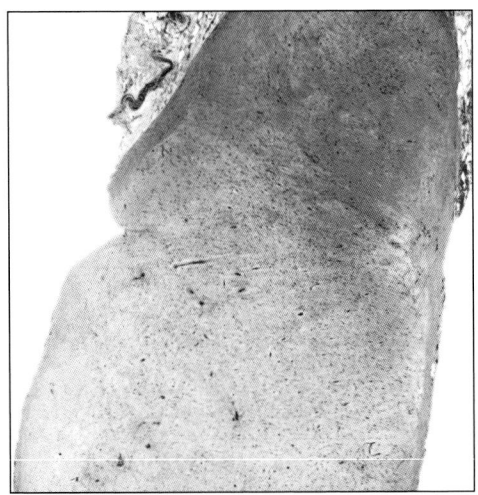

In this case of collagenous fibroma (desmoplastic fibroblastoma), the lesion is a well-circumscribed ovoid or fusiform mass. The hypocellularity is apparent at low power.

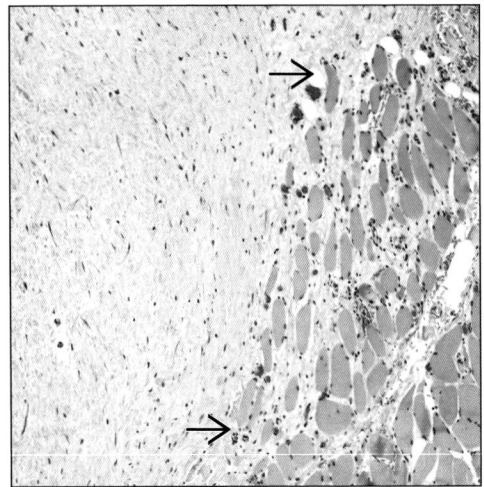

Although the tumor is largely circumscribed, focal infiltration of surrounding soft tissues may be seen ➔.

TERMINOLOGY

Synonyms
- Desmoplastic fibroblastoma (DF)

Definitions
- Rare, benign, fibrous soft tissue neoplasm occurring mainly in adult males and consisting of paucicellular arrays of stellate and spindled fibroblasts
- Reciprocal translocation t(2;11)(q31;q12) in some

ETIOLOGY/PATHOGENESIS

Developmental Anomaly
- Etiology unknown

CLINICAL ISSUES

Epidemiology
- Age
  - All ages; particularly older adults (5th-6th decades)
- Gender
  - M > F

Site
- Most occur in subcutaneous tissue
- Up to 25% involve skeletal muscle
- Rarely arise in dermis
  - 5-year history of preceding pemphigus vulgaris reported in 1 case
- Most common in upper extremity (shoulder, upper arm, forearm), followed by lower extremity
- Rare in head and neck

Presentation
- Slow growing
- Painless mass

Treatment
- Surgical approaches
  - Complete conservative excision

Prognosis
- Benign; does not recur locally or metastasize

MACROSCOPIC FEATURES

General Features
- Firm, circumscribed lobulated mass
- White or gray cut surface
- No necrosis or hemorrhage

Size
- Majority small (< 4 cm); range 1.5-20 cm

MICROSCOPIC PATHOLOGY

Histologic Features
- Usually located in subcutaneous tissues; rarely involves dermis
- Sparsely cellular, patternless distributions of bland spindled or stellate cells
- Hypovascular fibrous or fibromyxoid stroma
- Mitotic figures very rare; no necrosis
- Isolated cases show dystrophic calcification and metaplastic bone or small foci of floret-like multinucleated giant cells

Margins
- Generally circumscribed, although many infiltrate adjacent soft tissues

ANCILLARY TESTS

Immunohistochemistry
- Variable positivity for smooth muscle actin

COLLAGENOUS FIBROMA

Key Facts

Terminology
- Rare, benign, fibrous soft tissue neoplasm occurring mainly in adult males and consisting of paucicellular arrays of stellate and spindled fibroblasts

Clinical Issues
- Usually older adults
- Male preponderance
- Most in subcutaneous tissue; up to 25% involve skeletal muscle; more rarely involve dermis
- Most common in proximal extremity

Microscopic Pathology
- Sparsely cellular patternless distributions of bland spindle or stellate cells
- Hypovascular fibrous or fibromyxoid stroma
- Mitotic figures rare; no necrosis

Ancillary Tests
- Variable positivity for smooth muscle actin

- May show focal weak S100 protein and rare focal desmin or keratin; CD34 negative

Cytogenetics
- Reciprocal translocation t(2;11)(q31;q12) reported in 2 cases; translocation has also been reported in 1 case of fibroma of tendon sheath
- 11q12 breakpoint in 3 further cases

Electron Microscopy
- Features of fibroblasts and myofibroblasts

DIFFERENTIAL DIAGNOSIS

Fibromatosis
- More infiltrative and cellular than collagenous fibroma
- Loose fascicles; prominent vascular pattern

Neurofibroma
- Cell nuclei may be wavy or schwannian-appearing
- Strongly positive for S100 protein

Nodular Fasciitis (Late Stage)
- Foci of increased cellularity
- Chronic inflammation, extravasated red cells

Elastofibroma
- Typically located in subscapular region
- Fragmented elastic fibers

Fibroma of Tendon Sheath
- Peritendinous locations, particularly of hands

Calcifying Fibrous Pseudotumor
- Affects children and young adults
- Psammomatous calcifications
- Lymphoplasmacytic infiltrate

Low-Grade Fibromyxoid Sarcoma
- More cellular; may show rosette formation
- Characteristic translocations t(7;16) and t(11;16)

SELECTED REFERENCES

1. Sakamoto A et al: Desmoplastic fibroblastoma (collagenous fibroma) with a specific breakpoint of 11q12. Histopathology. 51(6):859-60, 2007
2. Bernal K et al: Translocation (2;11)(q31;q12) is recurrent in collagenous fibroma (desmoplastic fibroblastoma). Cancer Genet Cytogenet. 149(2):161-3, 2004
3. Huang HY et al: Superficial collagenous fibroma: immunohistochemical, ultrastructural, and flow cytometric study of three cases, including one pemphigus vulgaris patient with a dermal mass. APMIS. 110(4):283-9, 2002
4. Sciot R et al: Collagenous fibroma (desmoplastic fibroblastoma): genetic link with fibroma of tendon sheath? Mod Pathol. 12(6):565-8, 1999
5. Miettinen M et al: Collagenous fibroma (desmoplastic fibroblastoma): a clinicopathologic analysis of 63 cases of a distinctive soft tissue lesion with stellate-shaped fibroblasts. Hum Pathol. 29(7):676-82, 1998
6. Evans HL: Desmoplastic fibroblastoma. A report of seven cases. Am J Surg Pathol. 19(9):1077-81, 1995

IMAGE GALLERY

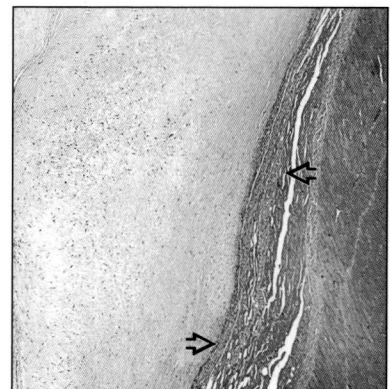 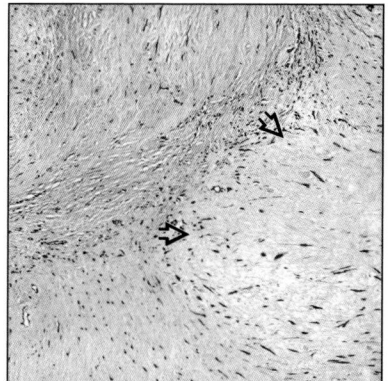 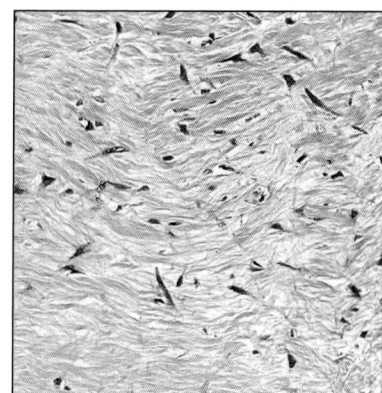

(Left) Collagenous fibroma at scanning magnification. Most tumors are subcutaneous, with rarer involvement of skin or skeletal muscle, shown here ⊵. *(Center)* The lesion is sparsely cellular. The stroma is densely collagenous to focally myxoid ⊵, and contains spindled and stellate-shaped fibroblasts in a patternless distribution. Vessels are inconspicuous. *(Right)* High magnification shows a collagenous fibroma. Although the cells may be plump, no true atypia is seen, and mitotic figures are rare or absent.

PLEOMORPHIC FIBROMA

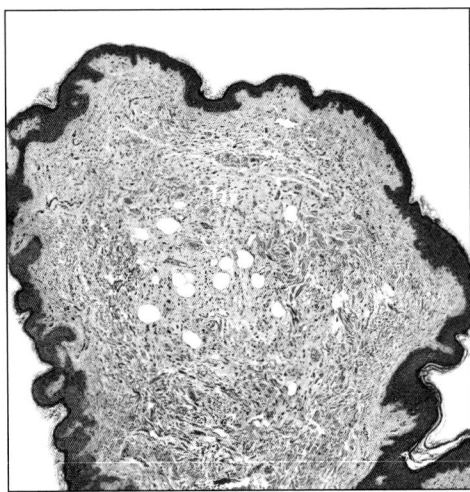

Scanning magnification shows a polypoid (skin tag-like) lesion with a fibromyxoid stroma. The lesion is usually solitary and occurs on the trunk, head and neck region, or extremities.

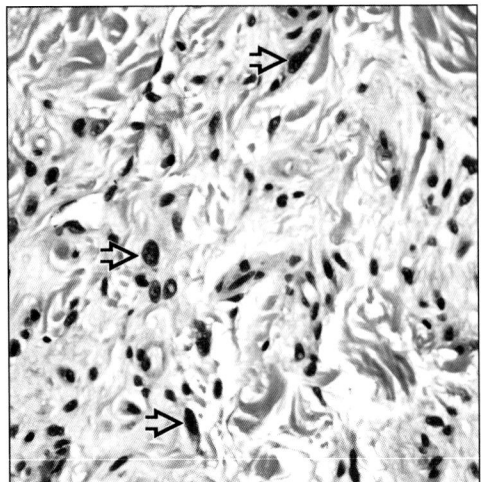

High-power examination shows a population of enlarged, hyperchromatic-staining spindled ➡, stellate, and multinucleated cells set in a fibromyxoid stroma. No mitoses are seen.

TERMINOLOGY

Abbreviations
- Pleomorphic fibroma (PF)

Definitions
- Benign dermal-based neoplasm composed of pleomorphic-appearing myofibroblasts

ETIOLOGY/PATHOGENESIS

Unknown
- Some cases may be related to ischemia, trauma, or degenerative changes

CLINICAL ISSUES

Presentation
- Slow-growing skin nodule
  - Usually dome-shaped or polypoid appearing
  - Flesh colored and nonulcerated
- Typically occur on trunk, extremities, or head and neck region

Treatment
- Surgical approaches
  - Complete conservative excision curative

Prognosis
- Benign tumors with excellent prognosis
- May show local recurrence if incompletely excised

MACROSCOPIC FEATURES

Size
- 0.4-1.6 cm

MICROSCOPIC PATHOLOGY

Histologic Features
- Well-circumscribed, dome-shaped or polypoid hypocellular proliferation of dermal spindle cells
- Lesional cells are predominantly spindle-shaped, also with stellate and multinucleated cells
- Cells show enlarged, hyperchromatic-staining nuclei with small nucleoli, scant amounts of eosinophilic cytoplasm
- Mitotic figures rare or absent
  - No atypical mitoses should be seen
- Stroma typically composed of hyalinized-appearing collagen fibers
  - Some cases show overlapping features with sclerotic fibroma
    - These cases show storiforming of hyalinized collagen bundles with collagen clefts
- Myxoid areas may be present
  - Can be prominent/diffuse in some cases (myxoid pleomorphic fibroma)

Cytologic Features
- Enlarged spindled to stellate-shaped cells with irregular, hyperchromatic-staining nuclei

Predominant Cell/Compartment Type
- Fibroblast/myofibroblast

ANCILLARY TESTS

Immunohistochemistry
- Typically positive for actin-sm, CD34, and vimentin
- FXIIIA variably positive

PLEOMORPHIC FIBROMA

Key Facts

Terminology

- Pleomorphic fibroma (PF)
- Benign dermal-based neoplasm composed of pleomorphic-appearing myofibroblasts

Clinical Issues

- Slow-growing skin nodule
- Usually dome-shaped or polypoid appearing
- May show local recurrence if incompletely excised

Ancillary Tests

- Cells typically positive for actin, CD34, and vimentin; variable positivity for FXIIIA reported

Diagnostic Checklist

- Cells appear pleomorphic and show hyperchromatic-staining nuclei, but lack mitotic activity
- Hypocellular dermal proliferation of spindled, stellate, and multinucleated cells

DIFFERENTIAL DIAGNOSIS

Fibrous Papule (Angiofibroma)

- Small, dome-shaped papule that shows dermal fibrosis and blood vessels with telangiectasia
- Scattered, enlarged, mildly pleomorphic-appearing fibroblasts may be present
- CD34(-), FXIIIA usually positive

Dermatofibroma (DF)

- Usually does not show degree of pleomorphism seen in PF, although rare cases may (atypical DF/"dermatofibroma with monster cells")
- More typical dermatofibroma areas should be present at periphery of tumor
  - Collagen trapping, histiocytoid cells, and overlying epidermal hyperplasia usually present
- CD34 typically negative, unlike PF

Sclerotic Fibroma

- Shows characteristic storiform pattern of thickened, hyalinized-appearing collagen bundles with clefts between them
- Some cases show overlapping features with PF, with population of enlarged, pleomorphic-appearing spindled cells
  - Therefore, some believe that PF is a variant of sclerotic fibroma, but this is not well accepted

Atypical Fibroxanthoma

- Highly cellular and atypical-appearing dermal-based tumor associated with solar elastosis
- Mitotic figures easily found in most cases, including atypical forms
- CD34(-); nonspecific markers, including CD68, CD10, and CD99, are usually positive

DIAGNOSTIC CHECKLIST

Pathologic Interpretation Pearls

- Hypocellular dermal proliferation of spindled, stellate, and multinucleated cells
- Cells appear pleomorphic and hyperchromatic, but lack mitotic activity

SELECTED REFERENCES

1. Mahmood MN et al: Solitary sclerotic fibroma of skin: a possible link with pleomorphic fibroma with immunophenotypic expression for O13 (CD99) and CD34. J Cutan Pathol. 30(10):631-6, 2003
2. García-Doval I et al: Pleomorphic fibroma of the skin, a form of sclerotic fibroma: an immunohistochemical study. Clin Exp Dermatol. 23(1):22-4, 1998
3. Pitt MA et al: Myxoid cutaneous pleomorphic fibroma. Histopathology. 25(3):300, 1994
4. Kamino H et al: Pleomorphic fibroma of the skin: a benign neoplasm with cytologic atypia. A clinicopathologic study of eight cases. Am J Surg Pathol. 13(2):107-13, 1989

IMAGE GALLERY

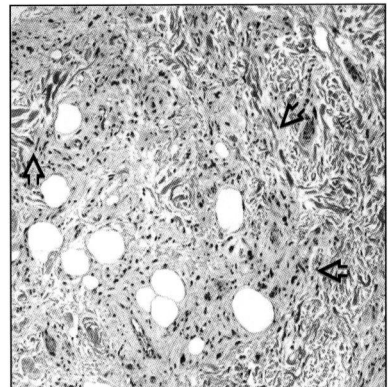 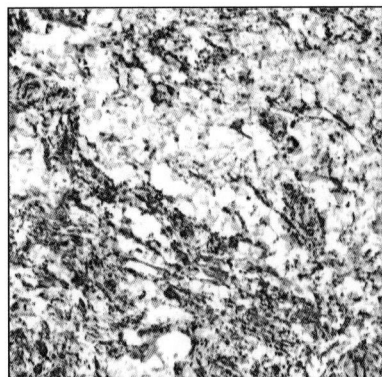 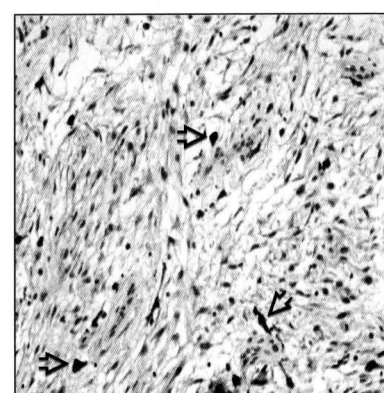

(Left) Intermediate-power examination shows areas of collagenous stroma alternating with more myxoid areas ⯈ containing the pleomorphic, hyperchromatic-staining cells. (Center) CD34 immunohistochemistry shows strong and diffuse staining of the spindled and multinucleated cells. (Right) FXIIIA staining shows more patchy positivity of a subset of the lesional cells ⯈.

SCLEROTIC FIBROMA

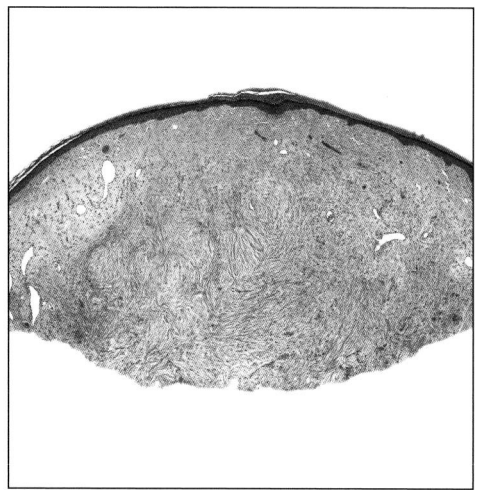

Scanning magnification view shows a dermal-based nodular fibroblastic proliferation with storiforming of collagen.

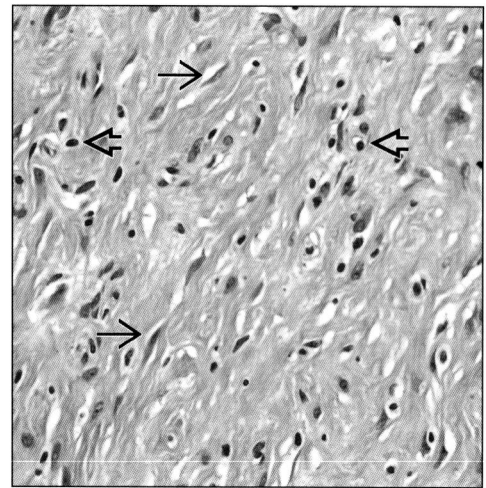

Higher power magnification shows bland fibroblasts ➡ and scattered inflammatory cells ⊳ in a dense fibrous stroma.

TERMINOLOGY

Synonyms
- Storiform collagenoma
- Pleomorphic sclerotic fibroma

Definitions
- Benign, dermal-based fibroblastic proliferation with storiforming bundles of collagen

ETIOLOGY/PATHOGENESIS

Unknown
- May be related to trauma
- Some cases may represent regressed dermatofibromas

Genetic Syndrome
- Multiple lesions are associated with Cowden syndrome, consistent with genetic influence

CLINICAL ISSUES

Epidemiology
- Age
  - May occur at any age, including in infants and elderly
- Gender
  - Roughly equal incidence in males and females

Site
- Presents most commonly on face, extremities, and trunk

Presentation
- Slow-growing, flesh-colored papule or nodule

Treatment
- Surgical approaches
  - Complete conservative excision is curative

Prognosis
- Excellent; may locally recur, but no metastatic potential

MACROSCOPIC FEATURES

General Features
- Dermal nodule with firm, yellow-tan surface

Size
- Typically 0.5-3 cm

MICROSCOPIC PATHOLOGY

Histologic Features
- Circumscribed, unencapsulated dermal nodule
- Composed of thickened, hyalinized-appearing collagen bundles in storiform/whorled pattern
  - Prominent clefts often seen between collagen bundles
- Cells are typically small, bland, spindled to stellate-shaped fibroblasts
- Occasional cases may show large, bizarre-appearing cells ("pleomorphic sclerotic fibroma" or "giant cell collagenoma"), similar to pleomorphic fibroma
  - These cells do not show infiltrative features or increased mitotic activity
- Pacinian collagenoma is rare variant with onion skinning, mimicking pacinian corpuscle

Predominant Cell/Compartment Type
- Fibroblast

ANCILLARY TESTS

Immunohistochemistry
- Generally not necessary, but cells will typically stain for FXIIIA, CD34 (focally), and vimentin

SCLEROTIC FIBROMA

Key Facts

Terminology
- Storiform collagenoma
- Benign, dermal-based fibroblastic proliferation

Microscopic Pathology
- Composed of thickened, hyalinized-appearing collagen bundles in storiform/whorled pattern
- Occasional cases may show large, bizarre-appearing cells ("pleomorphic sclerotic fibroma"), similar to pleomorphic fibroma

Ancillary Tests
- IHC generally not necessary, but cells should stain for FXIIIA, CD34 (focally), and vimentin

Top Differential Diagnoses
- Dermatofibroma
- Pleomorphic fibroma
- Collagenous fibroma
- Acral fibrokeratoma (subungual and periungual fibroma)

- Ki-67 staining may highlight a few scattered nuclei, but overall staining is low

DIFFERENTIAL DIAGNOSIS

Dermatofibroma (DF)
- Typically does not show prominent storiforming of collagen, although it may be focally present in rare cases
- Areas of conventional DF with collagen trapping and histiocytic cells should be present
  - Some cases may show overlapping features, leading some investigators to believe that sclerotic fibromas are involuting dermatofibromas

Pleomorphic Fibroma
- Clinically resembles skin tag
- Pleomorphic cells are more prominent, and storiforming pattern of collagen should be absent

Collagenous Fibroma
- Usually subcutaneous tumor with only rare dermal involvement
- Densely collagenous or fibromyxoid stroma; lacks prominent storiforming of collagen

Acral Fibrokeratoma (Subungual and Periungual Fibroma)
- Usually shows overlying hyperkeratosis and acanthosis
- Proliferation of thick collagen bundles, often vertically oriented

DIAGNOSTIC CHECKLIST

Pathologic Interpretation Pearls
- Dermal nodule of thickened, hyalinized-appearing collagen bundles in storiform/whorled pattern

SELECTED REFERENCES

1. Nakashima K et al: Solitary sclerotic fibroma of the skin: morphological characterization of the 'plywood-like pattern'. J Cutan Pathol. 35 Suppl 1:74-9, 2008
2. González-Vela MC et al: Sclerotic fibroma-like dermatofibroma: an uncommon distinctive variant of dermatofibroma. Histol Histopathol. 20(3):801-6, 2005
3. Chen TM et al: Pleomorphic sclerotic fibroma: a case report and literature review. Am J Dermatopathol. 24(1):54-8, 2002
4. Chang SN et al: Solitary sclerotic fibroma of the skin: degenerated sclerotic change of inflammatory conditions, especially folliculitis. Am J Dermatopathol. 22(1):22-5, 2000
5. Martín-López R et al: Pleomorphic sclerotic fibroma. Dermatology. 198(1):69-72, 1999
6. Pujol RM et al: Solitary sclerotic fibroma of the skin: a sclerotic dermatofibroma? Am J Dermatopathol. 18(6):620-4, 1996
7. Requena L et al: Multiple sclerotic fibromas of the skin. A cutaneous marker of Cowden's disease. J Cutan Pathol. 19(4):346-51, 1992
8. Rapini RP et al: Sclerotic fibromas of the skin. J Am Acad Dermatol. 20(2 Pt 1):266-71, 1989

IMAGE GALLERY

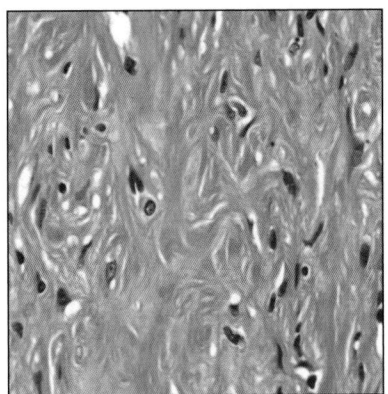 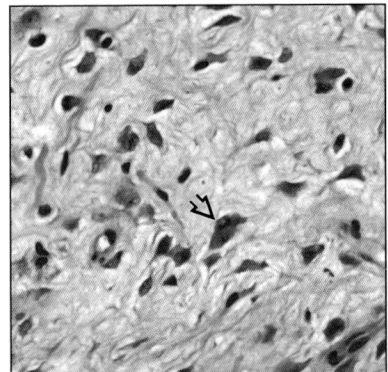 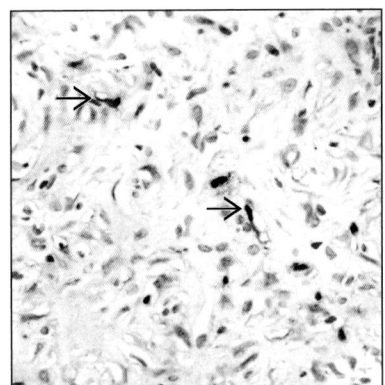

(Left) High-power magnification shows bland fibroblast cells in a dense fibrous stroma. *(Center)* An example of sclerotic fibroma with scattered, large, pleomorphic, stellate fibroblasts ⊵ shows features similar to pleomorphic fibroma (so-called "pleomorphic sclerotic fibroma" or "giant cell collagenoma"). *(Right)* FXIIIA immunohistochemistry shows staining of scattered spindle cells ⊡.

FIBROMATOSIS

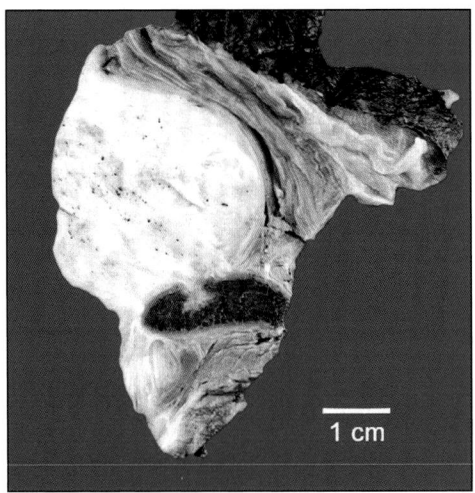

Gross photograph shows a large, deep fibromatosis of the shoulder that has eroded into the scapula. Superficial portions of such lesions can be encountered on skin biopsies.

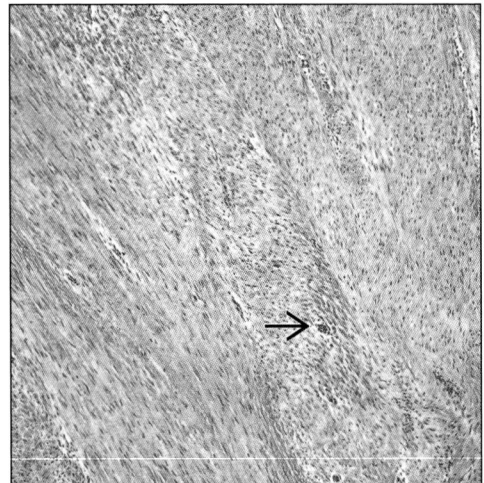

Hematoxylin & eosin shows sweeping fascicles of spindle cells separated by regularly spaced collagen. Even at this magnification, small vessels are readily apparent ⊞→.

TERMINOLOGY

Synonyms
- Deep fibromatosis: Aggressive fibromatosis, desmoid tumor
- Superficial fibromatoses: Palmar fibromatosis (Dupuytren contracture, Dupuytren disease), plantar fibromatosis (Ledderhose disease), penile fibromatosis (Peyronie disease), knuckle pads

Definitions
- **Palmar fibromatosis**: Nodular myofibroblastic proliferation of volar surface of hand that is prone to local persistence, but does not metastasize
- **Plantar fibromatosis**: Nodular myofibroblastic proliferation of plantar surface of foot that is prone to local persistence, but does not metastasize
- **Peyronie disease**: Penile fibrous lesion causing various deformities; initially pain with erection, erectile dysfunction
- **Knuckle pads**: Well-circumscribed thickening of skin over metacarpophalangeal and, more commonly, proximal interphalangeal joints
- **Deep fibromatosis**: Myofibroblastic proliferation of deep soft tissues with infiltrative growth pattern; prone to local recurrences, but does not metastasize

CLINICAL ISSUES

Epidemiology
- Incidence
  - Palmar fibromatosis
    - 4-6% of Caucasian adults > 50 years of age; reports of up to 75% of Celtic males
    - Uncommon in nonwhites; marked male predominance
  - Plantar fibromatosis
    - 1-2 per 100,000 persons per year (northern Europe)

- Most patients 30-50 years of age; slight male predominance
  - Penile fibromatosis
    - About 3.5% of white men > 50 years of age
  - Deep fibromatosis
    - 2.4-4.43 new cases per 100,000 persons per year (Scandinavian data)
  - Knuckle pads (rare)

Presentation
- Superficial fibromatoses present as nodular lesions on palms, soles, knuckles, or penis
- Deep fibromatoses present as firm large masses
  - Relationship to age and gender
    - In children and older adults, no gender predominance: Lesions of shoulders, chest wall, back, thigh, head, and neck
    - In women in childbearing years: Abdominal wall
- Familial adenomatous polyposis-associated (FAP) lesions
  - Risk of fibromatoses is 2.56/1,000 person-years; comparative risk is 852x that of general population
- Occasionally associated with scar ("cicatricial fibromatosis")

Treatment
- Superficial fibromatoses treated by excision
- Nonsurgical treatments for penile lesions: Verapamil, colchicine, Potaba, L-carnitine, and liposomal superoxide dismutase
- Deep fibromatoses treated by wide excision; for unresectable lesions, radiation, chemotherapy, hormone therapy

Prognosis
- Recurrences common for both superficial and deep fibromatoses; occasional deaths from deep fibromatoses

FIBROMATOSIS

Key Facts

Terminology
- Deep fibromatosis: Desmoid tumor
- Palmar fibromatosis: Dupuytren contracture
- Plantar fibromatosis: Ledderhose disease
- Penile fibromatosis: Peyronie disease
- Myofibroblastic proliferations with infiltrative growth pattern that show local recurrences but not metastasis

Clinical Issues
- Palmar fibromatosis
  - 4-6% of Caucasian adults > 50 years of age
- Deep fibromatosis
  - 2.4-4.43 new cases per 100,000 persons per year
- Recurrences common for both superficial and deep fibromatoses, but deaths only from deep fibromatoses
- Increased incidence in familial adenomatous polyposis (FAP)

Microscopic Pathology
- Sweeping fascicles of myofibroblasts
- Smooth nuclear membranes and small nucleoli in most cells
- Occasional cells with stellate cytoplasmic contours
- Occasional foci with storiform pattern similar to nodular fasciitis
- Some cases show keloid-like collagen
- Small but conspicuous vessels
- Gaping, thin-walled vessels with perivascular sclerosis often feature of mesenteric fibromatosis

Ancillary Tests
- β-catenin positive (nuclear), especially in deep lesions, SMA(+); desmin(-), keratins(-), CD117(+/-)

MICROSCOPIC PATHOLOGY

Histologic Features
- Sweeping fascicles of myofibroblasts
  - Smooth nuclear membranes, delicate nucleoli in most cells, occasional cells with stellate cytoplasmic contours
- Uniformly distributed collagen, some cases with keloid-like collagen
- Prominent vascular pattern
  - Small but conspicuous vessels
- Minimal background inflammation
- Scattered giant cells (plantar fibromatoses)

ANCILLARY TESTS

Immunohistochemistry
- β-catenin(+) (nuclear), especially in deep lesions, SMA(+), desmin(-), keratins(-), CD117 can be (+/-) (pitfall in mesenteric lesions)

DIFFERENTIAL DIAGNOSIS

Clear Cell Sarcoma
- Most involve hands and feet of young adults
- Packeted arrangement of spindle cells, scattered giant cells; S100 protein, HMB-45, Melan-A positive, *EWS-ATF1* gene fusion

Epithelioid Sarcoma
- Most involve distal upper extremity
- Epithelioid cells arranged around necrotic zones, reminiscent of granulomatous inflammation; cytokeratin, EMA, CD34 positive, loss of nuclear INI1

Tenosynovial Giant Cell Tumor (Giant Cell Tumor of Tendon Sheath)
- Usually involves fingers and toes of middle-aged women

- Rounded cells, giant cells, foamy macrophages, hemosiderin, CD68(+), clusterin(+)

Scar
- Disorganized myofibroblastic proliferation without nodular configuration; β-catenin negative

Leiomyoma and Leiomyosarcoma
- Perpendicularly oriented fascicles of spindle cells with brightly eosinophilic cytoplasm, blunt-ended nuclei, paranuclear vacuoles, none to few mitoses (leiomyoma), bland cytologic features (leiomyoma) or scattered mitoses (leiomyosarcoma), and atypical nuclei (leiomyosarcoma)
- Actin, desmin, calponin, H-caldesmon positive; S100 protein, CD34, β-catenin negative

Low-Grade Fibromyxoid Sarcoma
- Deep lesions without gender predilection
- Disorganized and swirled arrangement of fibroblastic cells with hyperchromatic nuclei, variable myxoid background, cellularity similar to that of fibromatosis
- S100 protein, desmin, CD34, β-catenin negative; occasionally actin(+), claudin-1(+), epithelial membrane antigen(+); pitfall with perineurioma, *FUS-CREB3L2* fusion

SELECTED REFERENCES

1. Bhattacharya B et al: Nuclear beta-catenin expression distinguishes deep fibromatosis from other benign and malignant fibroblastic and myofibroblastic lesions. Am J Surg Pathol. 29(5):653-9, 2005
2. Evans HL: Multinucleated giant cells in plantar fibromatosis. Am J Surg Pathol. 26(2):244-8, 2002
3. Montgomery E et al: Superficial fibromatoses are genetically distinct from deep fibromatoses. Mod Pathol. 14(7):695-701, 2001
4. Reitamo JJ et al: The desmoid tumor. I. Incidence, sex-, age- and anatomical distribution in the Finnish population. Am J Clin Pathol. 77(6):665-73, 1982

Microscopic Features

(Left) Plantar fibromatosis, such as this, can be fairly large and have pockets of enhanced cellularity, leading to misidentification as a sarcoma. Superficial fibromatoses can have β-catenin immunolabeling but lack β-catenin and APC gene mutations. *(Right)* High magnification shows a giant cell in plantar fibromatosis ⇨. Such cells can also occur in palmar lesions and can cause confusion with a tenosynovial giant cell tumor and clear cell sarcoma.

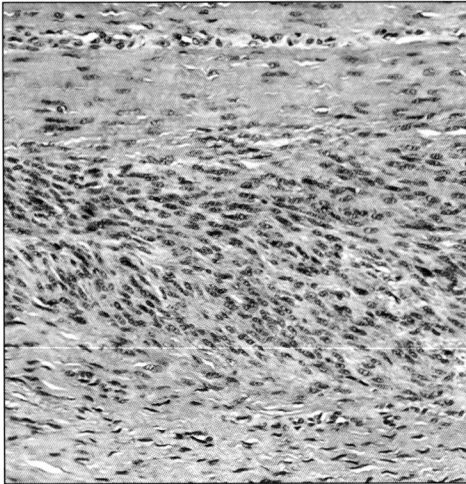
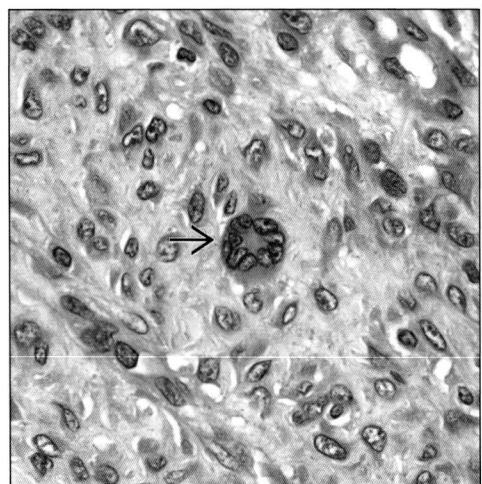

(Left) High magnification shows a mitosis in a palmar fibromatosis ⇨. Mitotic activity can be encountered in both palmar and plantar fibromatoses and should not lead to a concern for malignancy. *(Right)* This is an example of Peyronie disease (penile fibromatosis) that has ossified. Peyronie disease consists of a fibrous proliferation of the tunica albuginea, resulting in a palpable scar and penile curvature, hinging, narrowing, shortening, and painful erections.

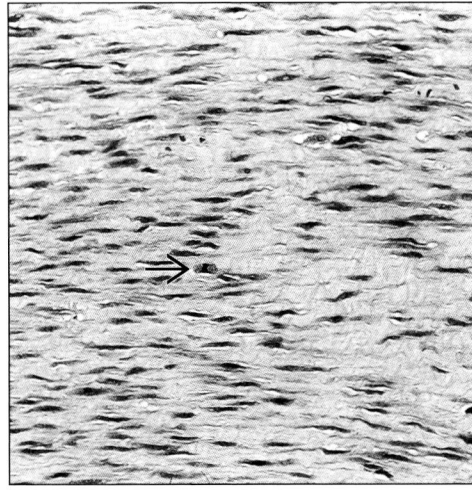
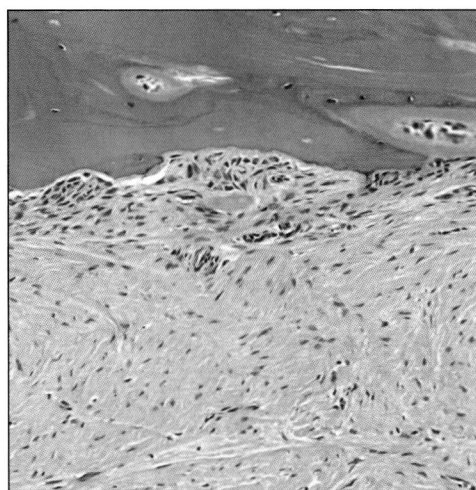

(Left) Histology examination shows a deep fibromatosis proliferating adjacent to a small vessel. The vascular smooth muscle appears more eosinophilic than the myofibroblastic appearance of the lesional cells. *(Right)* High magnification of a deep fibromatosis demonstrates cells that contain nuclei with single delicate nucleoli ⇨ and bipolar or stellate cytoplasm. Collagen is evenly distributed in most examples but is occasionally keloid-like.

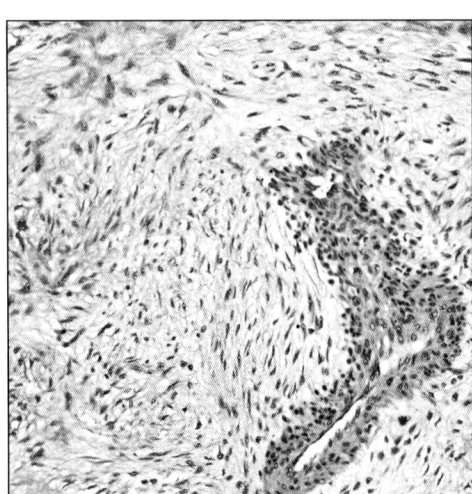
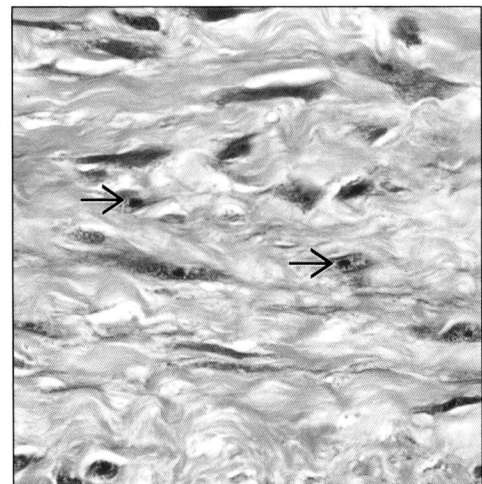

FIBROMATOSIS

Immunohistochemical Features and Differential Diagnosis

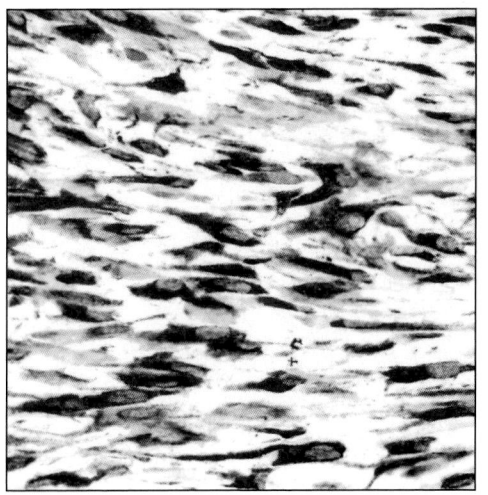

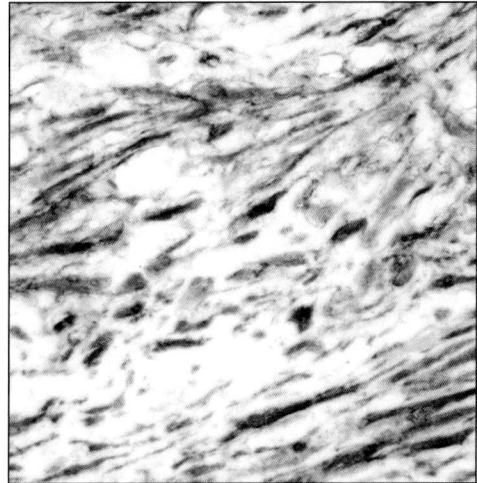

(Left) CD117 shows strong labeling in a deep fibromatosis. This particular example displays more prominent staining than most fibromatoses, and this finding can result in misdiagnosis as a (metastatic) gastrointestinal stromal tumor. Fibromatoses lack KIT mutations and have minimal response to imatinib. *(Right)* β-catenin shows nuclear staining in a fibromatosis, a reflection of either APC or β-catenin mutations in most fibromatoses.

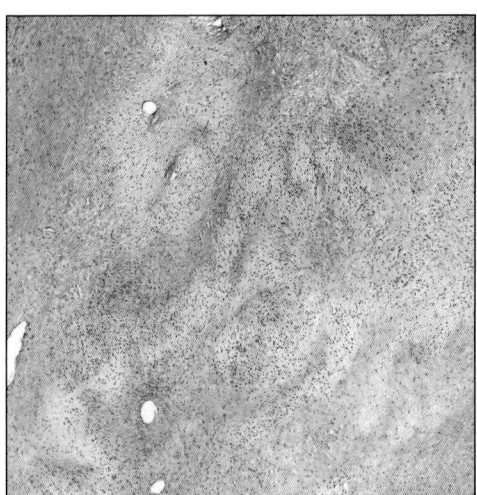

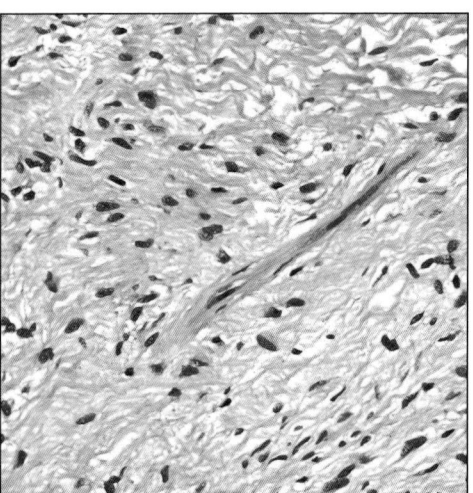

(Left) Low magnification shows a low-grade fibromyxoid sarcoma. Although the lesion appears similar to a fibromatosis at low magnification, it differs by featuring a less uniformly fascicular low-power appearance. *(Right)* High magnification shows a low-grade fibromyxoid sarcoma. The lesional cells are far more hyperchromatic than those of a fibromatosis. These lesions lack nuclear β-catenin and have a characteristic translocation, t(7;16) (q32-34;p11), with a FUS/CREB3L2 fusion gene.

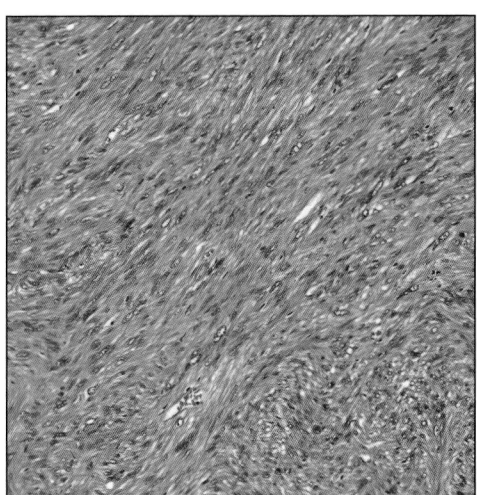

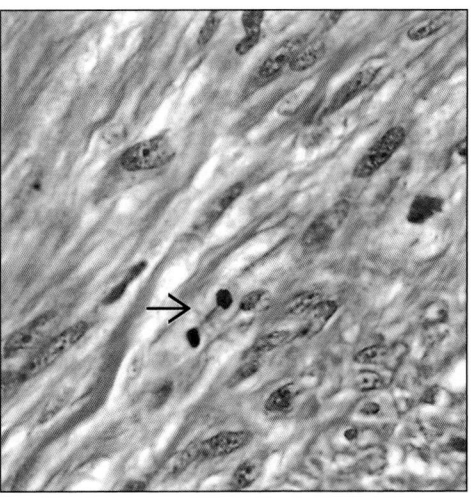

(Left) Histology examination shows a leiomyosarcoma. The lesional nuclei are larger and more hyperchromatic than those of fibromatoses, and the cytoplasm is strikingly eosinophilic. *(Right)* High magnification of a leiomyosarcoma demonstrates that the nuclear chromatin is coarser than that in fibromatoses. There is an anaphase bridge ➡, a feature of chromosomally unstable tumors (in contrast to the lack of anaphase bridges in tumors with characteristic mutations or translocations).

JUVENILE HYALINE FIBROMATOSIS

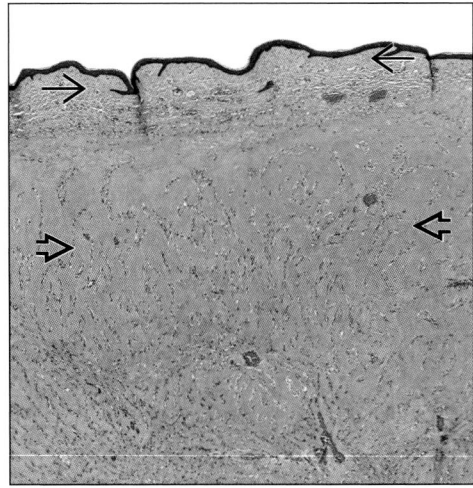

Low magnification shows juvenile hyaline fibromatosis of the face in the deep dermis ⊵. There is a tumor-free (grenz) zone ⇨ between the epidermis and the lesional tissue.

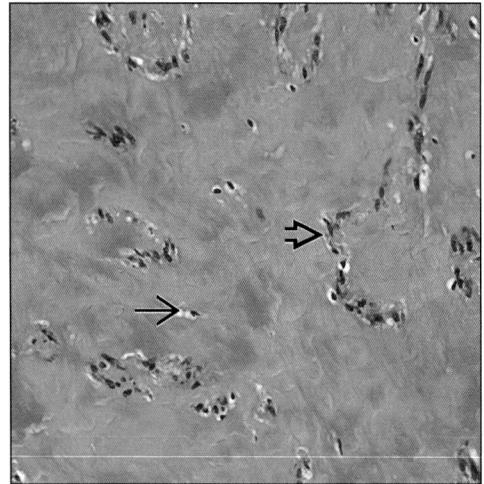

Higher magnification shows scattered lesional cells in homogeneous-appearing dense eosinophilic stroma. The cells are small and uniform, arranged in short curved cords ⊵. Some nuclei appear in spaces ⇨.

TERMINOLOGY

Abbreviations
- Juvenile hyaline fibromatosis (JHF)

Synonyms
- Related disorder: Infantile systemic hyalinosis (ISH)
  - Suggested synonym: Hyaline fibromatosis syndrome

Definitions
- Rare autosomal recessive disorder (often found in consanguineous populations) characterized by multiple skin papules and early onset

ETIOLOGY/PATHOGENESIS

Genetic Disorder
- Mutations in *ANTXR2* in both juvenile hyaline fibromatosis and infantile systemic hyalinosis
- Autosomal recessive transmission

CLINICAL ISSUES

Presentation
- Juvenile hyaline fibromatosis
  - Infantile presentation of lesions of scalp, face, neck, retroauricular areas, and perineal region, and gingival hypertrophy
  - Joint contractures and motion limitation
  - Osteolytic lesions, mainly in phalanges and distal portions of long bones; cortical defects in subset of patients
- Infantile systemic hyalinosis
  - More severe end of clinical spectrum of mutations in *ANTXR2*
    - Hyaline changes are seen in multiple viscera as well as in skin
    - More prominent than those described in JHF

- Affected individuals usually die in 1st years of life as result of complications of visceral involvement
  - Infiltration of intestines leads to malabsorption

MACROSCOPIC FEATURES

Skin and Gingival Lesions
- Plaques and papules of skin
- Larger lesions form soft tissue masses
- Gingival hyperplasia

Systemic Lesions
- Infiltration of small bowel and colon, forming masses

MICROSCOPIC PATHOLOGY

Histologic Features
- Histologic findings in both JHF and ISH are indistinguishable
  - Round to spindle cell proliferation composed of bland fibroblasts often lying in clear spaces and simulating chondrocyte lacunae
  - No significant cellular pleomorphism or mitoses
  - Homogeneous, hyalinized, dense eosinophilic intercellular matrix
  - PAS positive; diastase-resistant stromal material
  - Displaces normal components of dermis and lamina propria of gingival and intestinal mucosa
  - Early lesions can lack classic hyalinized stroma

DIFFERENTIAL DIAGNOSIS

Fibrodysplasia (Myositis) Ossificans Progressiva
- Rare, autosomal dominant disease
  - Characterized by soft tissue ossification at multiple sites and skeletal abnormalities of digits and cervical spine

JUVENILE HYALINE FIBROMATOSIS

Key Facts

Terminology
- Juvenile hyaline fibromatosis (JHF)
- Related disorder: Infantile systemic hyalinosis (ISH)

Clinical Issues
- Autosomal recessive transmission
- Infantile presentation of lesions of scalp, face, neck, retroauricular areas
  - Gingival hypertrophy
- Cutaneous papules and plaques

Microscopic Pathology
- Uniform round to spindle cells
  - Some in clear spaces
- No significant cellular pleomorphism
- No mitoses or necrosis
- Homogeneous, hyalinized, pale, eosinophilic intercellular matrix
  - PAS positive; diastase resistant
- Blood vessels sparse

  - Short great toes
- No gender predominance
- Trauma (accidental or surgical) results in painful soft tissue lesions
  - Progressive ossification of lesions over 2-3 months
- Lesions appear similar to those of myositis ossificans
  - Mitotically active myofibroblasts
  - Variable ossification depending on age of lesions

Infantile Myofibromatosis
- Multiple lesions presenting in infancy
  - Can involve bones, soft tissues, and viscera
    - Pulmonary involvement is poor prognostic feature
- Biphasic lobulated lesions
  - Central myoid nodules composed of short oval to spindle-shaped cells
  - Peripheral hemangiopericytoma-like zones

Desmoid-type Fibromatosis
- Large masses of deep soft tissues, usually solitary
- Cellular fascicular lesions
- Associated with familial adenomatous polyposis (FAP)
- Nuclear immunoreactivity for β-catenin (deep examples)

Calcifying Aponeurotic Fibroma
- Distal extremities of infants and children
- Solitary lesions
- Stippled calcifications and fibrous areas

Nuchal Fibrocartilaginous Tumor
- Solitary lesion of adults

- Associated with prior neck injury
- Posterior aspect of base of neck
  - Junction of nuchal ligament and deep cervical fascia
- Fibrocartilaginous tissue forming mass

SELECTED REFERENCES

1. Nofal A et al: Juvenile hyaline fibromatosis and infantile systemic hyalinosis: a unifying term and a proposed grading system. J Am Acad Dermatol. 61(4):695-700, 2009
2. Tanaka K et al: Abnormal collagen deposition in fibromas from patient with juvenile hyaline fibromatosis. J Dermatol Sci. 55(3):197-200, 2009
3. Al-Malik MI et al: Gingival hyperplasia in hyaline fibromatosis--a report of two cases. J Int Acad Periodontol. 9(2):42-8, 2007
4. Antaya RJ et al: Juvenile hyaline fibromatosis and infantile systemic hyalinosis overlap associated with a novel mutation in capillary morphogenesis protein-2 gene. Am J Dermatopathol. 29(1):99-103, 2007
5. Anadolu RY et al: Juvenile non-hyaline fibromatosis: juvenile hyaline fibromatosis without prominent hyaline changes. J Cutan Pathol. 32(3):235-9, 2005
6. Hanks S et al: Mutations in the gene encoding capillary morphogenesis protein 2 cause juvenile hyaline fibromatosis and infantile systemic hyalinosis. Am J Hum Genet. 73(4):791-800, 2003
7. Rahman N et al: The gene for juvenile hyaline fibromatosis maps to chromosome 4q21. Am J Hum Genet. 71(4):975-80, 2002

IMAGE GALLERY

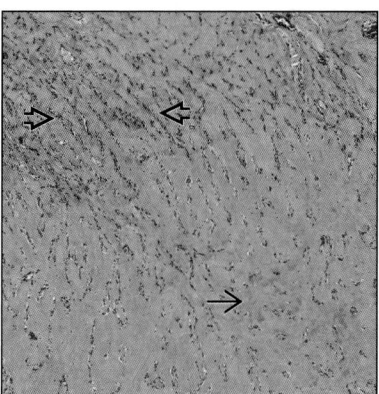 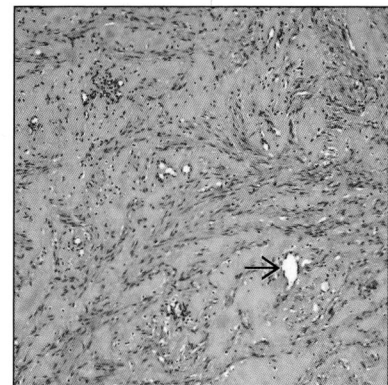 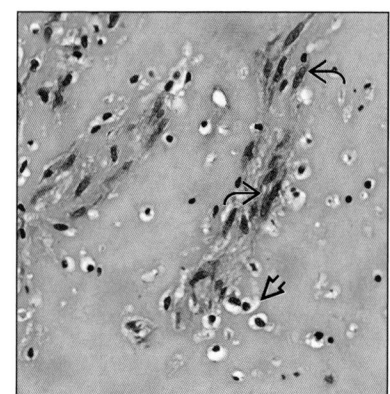

(Left) Low-magnification H&E stain shows cords of cells within characteristic sclerotic stroma. The cords show a vaguely parallel alignment ➡. Some parts of the tumor ➡ are less cellular. *(Center)* A cellular example of JHF with branching cords of spindle cells. Note the occasional thin-walled dilated blood vessel ➡. *(Right)* High magnification shows numerous cells with clear cytoplasm ➡ resembling chondrocytes, and small clusters of spindle cells ➡. Note the absence of pleomorphism and mitotic activity.

ANGIOFIBROMA AND RELATED LESIONS

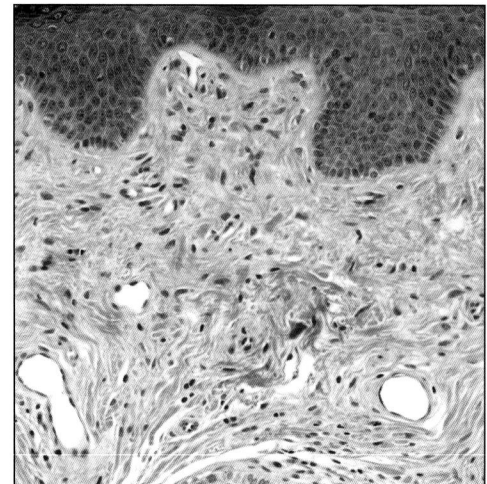

Fibrous papule is characterized by a dome-shaped lesion with ectatic thin-walled blood vessels ➨ and dense collagenous stroma.

This high-power image of a fibrous papule demonstrates the relatively hypocellular proliferation of bland spindled to stellate fibroblasts, small ectatic vessels, and dense collagenous stroma.

TERMINOLOGY

Synonyms
- Fibrous papule (FP), adenoma sebaceum, acral angiofibroma, pearly penile papule

Definitions
- Angiofibroma encompasses a group of benign mesenchymal tumors characterized by spindled to stellate fibroblasts, dense collagenous stroma, and ectatic blood vessels
  - May be related to a proliferation of papillary dermal elements

CLINICAL ISSUES

Presentation
- **Fibrous papule**
  - Middle-aged patients
  - Solitary dome-shaped flesh-colored papules on nose or central face
    - May clinically mimic basal cell carcinoma
- **Adenoma sebaceum**
  - Angiofibromas associated with tuberous sclerosis
    - Tuberous sclerosis: Autosomal dominant inheritance, but most cases sporadic
    - Mutation in *TSC1* or *TSC2*
  - Term is a misnomer, as there is no proliferation of sebaceous glands
  - Grouped papules or nodules with butterfly distribution on central face
- **Pearly penile papules**
  - Grouped or linear white papules on coronal margin &/or sulcus of penis

Treatment
- No treatment necessary
- Excision or laser can be used in selected cases

Prognosis
- Benign

MICROSCOPIC PATHOLOGY

Histologic Features
- Involves superficial dermis
- Scattered bland, spindle-shaped to stellate, and multinucleated fibroblasts
- Dense collagen
  - Elastic tissue absent in collagenous stroma
- Ectatic thin-walled blood vessels
  - May have concentric perivascular fibrosis, especially in fibrous papules
- Scant perivascular lymphocytic infiltrate may be present
- Variants
  - **Clear cell fibrous papule**
    - Tumor cells have abundant clear vacuolated cytoplasm
    - Otherwise resembles fibrous papule
  - **Epithelioid fibrous papule**
    - Sheets and small groups of epithelioid tumor cells
    - Increased small blood vessels
    - Collagenous stroma
  - **Granular cell fibrous papule**
    - Tumor cells have granular eosinophilic cytoplasm

ANCILLARY TESTS

Immunohistochemistry
- Plays little role in diagnosis, other than to exclude potential mimics
- Positive for vimentin; variably positive for CD34, factor XIIIA, CD68
  - Negative for cytokeratins, S100 protein, HMB-45, Melan-A

ANGIOFIBROMA AND RELATED LESIONS

Key Facts

Clinical Issues
- Fibrous papule
- Adenoma sebaceum: Angiofibromas associated with tuberous sclerosis
- Solitary dome-shaped flesh-colored papules on nose or central face
- May clinically mimic basal cell carcinoma

Microscopic Pathology
- Involves superficial dermis

- Scattered bland, spindled to stellate, and multinucleated fibroblasts
- Dense collagen
- Ectatic thin-walled blood vessels

Top Differential Diagnoses
- Dermatofibroma
- Scar
- Xanthogranuloma
- Epithelioid fibrous histiocytoma

DIFFERENTIAL DIAGNOSIS

Dermatofibroma
- Uncommon on face
- Storiform proliferation of spindled cells with overlying epidermal hyperplasia
- More cellular
  - Polymorphous population of spindled cells, histiocytes, multinucleated cells
- Peripheral collagen trapping

Scar
- More organized with horizontally oriented fibroblasts and vertically oriented blood vessels
- Effacement of rete peg architecture often present

Xanthogranuloma
- Clear cell and epithelioid fibrous papule variants can be confused with xanthogranuloma
  - Xanthogranuloma has foamy histiocytes, Touton giant cells, and an infiltrate that usually includes eosinophils

Epithelioid Fibrous Histiocytoma (Epithelioid Histiocytoma)
- Epithelioid fibrous papule resembles this entity
- Epithelioid fibrous histiocytoma rarely occurs on face; tumor population more polymorphous

Intradermal Nevus
- Cohesive nests of melanocytes

- Positive for S100 protein and other melanocytic markers

DIAGNOSTIC CHECKLIST

Pathologic Interpretation Pearls
- Dense collagenous stroma with absence of solar elastosis clue to diagnosis

SELECTED REFERENCES

1. Borkowska J et al: Tuberous sclerosis complex: tumors and tumorigenesis. Int J Dermatol. 50(1):13-20, 2011
2. Ma D et al: Histologic variants of periungual fibromas in tuberous sclerosis complex. J Am Acad Dermatol. 64(2):442-4, 2011
3. Chiang YY et al: Clear cell fibrous papule: report of a case mimicking a balloon cell nevus. J Cutan Pathol. 36(3):381-4, 2009
4. Jacyk WK et al: Fibrous papule of the face with granular cells. Dermatology. 216(1):56-9, 2008
5. Kucher C et al: Epithelioid fibrous papule - a new variant. J Cutan Pathol. 34(7):571-5, 2007
6. Bansal C et al: Histologic variants of fibrous papule. J Cutan Pathol. 32(6):424-8, 2005
7. Lee AN et al: Clear cell fibrous papule with NKI/C3 expression: clinical and histologic features in six cases. Am J Dermatopathol. 27(4):296-300, 2005
8. Shea CR et al: CD34-reactive fibrous papule of the nose. J Am Acad Dermatol. 35(2 Pt 2):342-5, 1996
9. Guitart J et al: Fibrous papule of the nose with granular cells: two cases. J Cutan Pathol. 18(4):284-7, 1991

IMAGE GALLERY

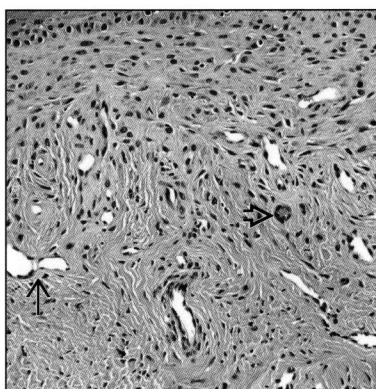 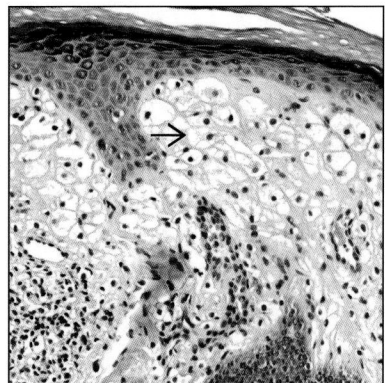 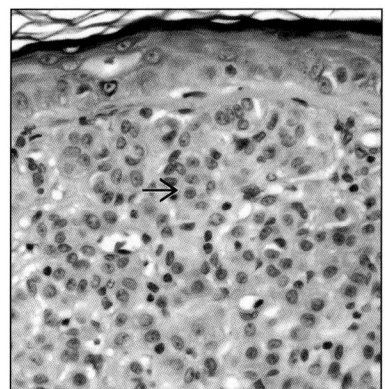

(Left) Higher power image of fibrous papule highlights the spindled cells, ectatic blood vessels ➡, and occasional multinucleated fibroblastic cells ➡. *(Center)* Clear cell fibrous papule is composed of epithelioid cells with abundant clear cytoplasm ➡. The lesion still has dense collagenous stroma and focal dilated vessels. *(Right)* Epithelioid fibrous papule is more cellular and shows a proliferation of round cells with eosinophilic cytoplasm ➡.

ACRAL FIBROKERATOMA

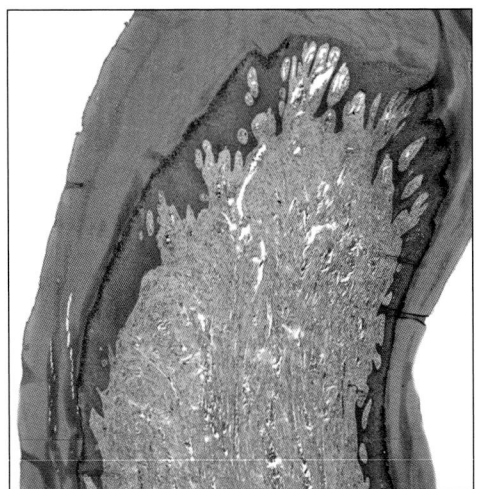

Acral fibrokeratoma is a protuberant, pedunculated lesion covered by a hyperkeratotic, variably acanthotic epidermis.

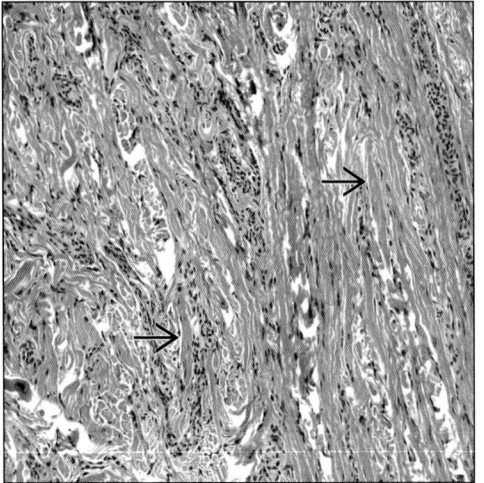

Acral fibrokeratoma is characterized by a relatively hypocellular fibroblastic proliferation and thickened, vertically oriented collagen bundles ➡.

TERMINOLOGY

Synonyms
- Acquired digital fibrokeratoma
- Acquired periungual fibrokeratoma
- Garlic clove fibroma
- Subungual fibroma of tuberous sclerosis

Definitions
- Benign, dome-shaped, relatively hypocellular mesenchymal tumor that usually presents on digits

ETIOLOGY/PATHOGENESIS

Genetic Syndrome
- Subset of cases associated with tuberous sclerosis
- Mutation of *TSC1* or *TSC2*

CLINICAL ISSUES

Epidemiology
- Incidence
  - Relatively rare lesions
- Age
  - Present in adults most commonly
- Gender
  - Men more commonly affected

Site
- Fingers or toes

Presentation
- Usually solitary
- Dome-shaped to elongated hyperkeratotic papule on digit
- Multiple lesions associated with tuberous sclerosis
  - Often in clusters
  - Ungual location
  - Develop in adolescence

Treatment
- Surgical approaches
  - Simple excision for solitary lesions

Prognosis
- Benign

MICROSCOPIC PATHOLOGY

Histologic Features
- Dome-shaped to elongated silhouette at lower magnification
- Epidermis is hyperkeratotic and acanthotic
- Relatively hypocellular proliferation of fibroblasts
- Vertically oriented, thickened collagen bundles
- May have dilated capillaries superficially
- Absence of adnexal structures in affected dermis

ANCILLARY TESTS

Immunohistochemistry
- Typically FXIIIA positive
- Usually CD34 negative

DIFFERENTIAL DIAGNOSIS

Cellular Digital Fibroma
- Polypoid lesion affecting digits
- More cellular with fascicles of bland spindled cells
- Lacks vertically oriented collagen bundles
- Immunohistochemistry shows CD34 positivity

Superficial Acral Fibromyxoma
- Toes are affected > fingers
- Loose storiform to fascicular growth pattern
- Myxoid to collagenous matrix
- Lacks vertically oriented collagen bundles
- CD34 positive

ACRAL FIBROKERATOMA

Key Facts

Microscopic Pathology
- Dome-shaped to elongated silhouette
- Epidermis is hyperkeratotic and acanthotic
- Relatively hypocellular proliferation of fibroblasts
- Vertically oriented thick collagen bundles

Top Differential Diagnoses
- Cellular digital fibroma
  - More cellular than acral fibrokeratoma
  - Fascicles of spindled cells

- Lacks vertically oriented collagen bundles
- CD34 positive
- Superficial acral fibromyxoma
  - More cellular
  - Loose storiform to fascicular growth pattern
  - Lacks vertically oriented collagen bundles
  - CD34 positive
- Supernumerary digit
  - Clinically resembles acral fibrokeratoma
  - Disorganized nerve bundles in dermis

- Often EMA positive

Accessory Digit
- a.k.a. supernumerary digit
- Polypoid lesion usually at ulnar base of 5th finger
- Clinical overlap with digital fibrokeratoma
- Disorganized nerves and Meissner corpuscles
  - Resembles traumatic neuroma

Infantile Digital Fibromatosis (Inclusion Body Fibromatosis)
- Presents in 1st 2 years of life
- Fascicles of fibroblasts
- Eosinophilic perinuclear inclusions classically present
  - Stain positively with PTAH, trichrome
  - Immunohistochemistry positive for actin, desmin

Dermatofibroma/Fibrous Histiocytoma
- Rarely presents on digits
- Storiform arrangement of fibroblastic and histiocytoid cells
- Peripheral collagen trapping
- Lacks vertically oriented collagen bundles
- Epidermis is acanthotic and shows basilar hyperpigmentation, but typically lacks prominent hyperkeratosis

- Hypocellular fibroblastic proliferation
- Vertically oriented collagen bundles
- Lacks storiform growth pattern

SELECTED REFERENCES

1. Baykal C et al: Acquired digital fibrokeratoma. Cutis. 79(2):129-32, 2007
2. Guitart J et al: Cellular digital fibromas: what about superficial acral fibromyxoma? J Cutan Pathol. 33(11):762-3; author reply 764, 2006
3. McNiff JM et al: Cellular digital fibromas: distinctive CD34-positive lesions that may mimic dermatofibrosarcoma protuberans. J Cutan Pathol. 32(6):413-8, 2005
4. Kakurai M et al: Giant acquired digital fibrokeratoma. J Am Acad Dermatol. 48(5 Suppl):S67-8, 2003
5. Fetsch JF et al: Superficial acral fibromyxoma: a clinicopathologic and immunohistochemical analysis of 37 cases of a distinctive soft tissue tumor with a predilection for the fingers and toes. Hum Pathol. 32(7):704-14, 2001
6. Kint A et al: Acquired (digital) fibrokeratoma. J Am Acad Dermatol. 12(5 Pt 1):816-21, 1985
7. Cahn RL: Acquired periungual fibrokeratoma. A rare benign tumor previously described as the garlic-clove fibroma. Arch Dermatol. 113(11):1564-8, 1977
8. Selmanowitz VJ: Acral fibrokeratoma. Int J Dermatol. 10(3):166-9, 1971
9. Hare PJ et al: Acquired (digital) fibrokeratoma. Br J Dermatol. 81(9):667-70, 1969

DIAGNOSTIC CHECKLIST

Pathologic Interpretation Pearls
- Acral location

IMAGE GALLERY

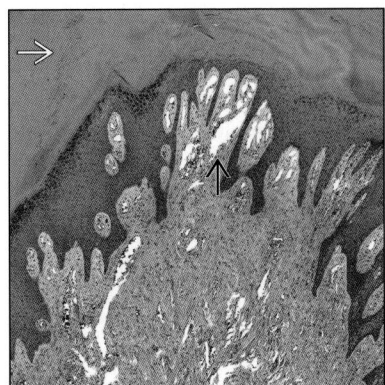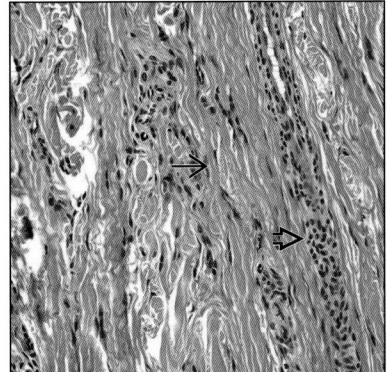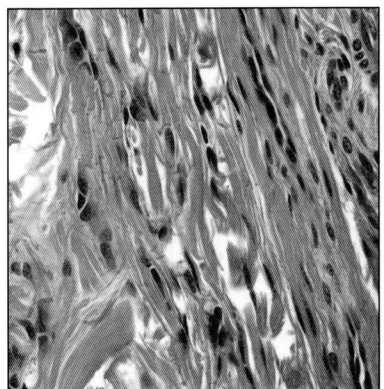

(Left) The epidermis overlying acral fibrokeratoma demonstrates thick, compact hyperkeratosis ➡. In the superficial dermis, there may be dilated blood vessels ➡. *(Center)* Thickened, vertically oriented collagen bundles ➡ and a hypocellular proliferation of fibroblasts are present. A scant perivascular lymphocytic infiltrate may be present ➡. *(Right)* High-power examination demonstrates the bland fibroblasts and vertically oriented, thickened collagen bundles.

DERMATOFIBROMA AND FIBROUS HISTIOCYTOMA

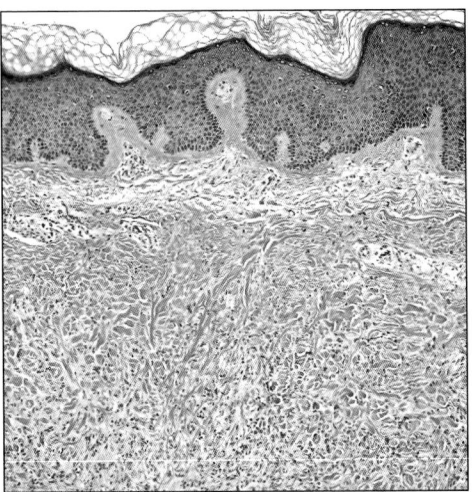

Classic dermatofibroma shows a dermal-based proliferation of bland spindled to histiocytic-appearing cells associated with a grenz zone and overlying epidermal hyperplasia and basilar pigmentation.

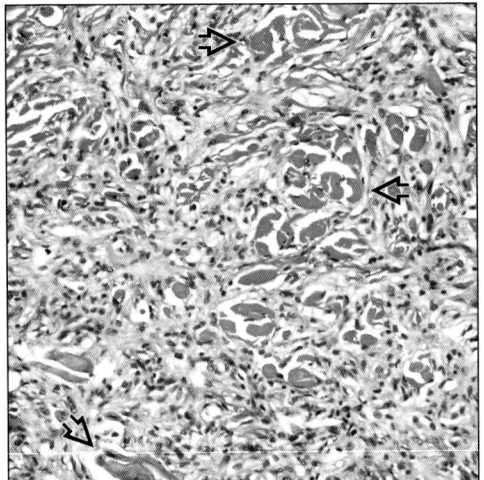

Higher power examination of a classic dermatofibroma shows a proliferation of bland, spindled to histiocytoid cells entrapping numerous hyalinized balls of collagen ⧐.

TERMINOLOGY

Abbreviations
- Dermatofibroma (DF)
- Fibrous histiocytoma (FH)

Synonyms
- Cutaneous fibrous histiocytoma
- Sclerosing hemangioma
- Histiocytoma
- Epithelioid cell histiocytoma

Definitions
- Common, benign, limited proliferation of mesenchymal cells in dermis
- Lineage not well defined, although commonly referred to as "fibrohistiocytic"

ETIOLOGY/PATHOGENESIS

Unknown
- Evidence supports both reactive and neoplastic pathogenesis
  - Histiocytic population may be clonal; fibroblast/myofibroblastic population may be polyclonal (reactive)
- Tumor may be preceded by local trauma, including insect bite in some cases
  - However, no inciting event identified in majority of cases

CLINICAL ISSUES

Epidemiology
- Incidence
  - Common tumors in most populations
- Age
  - All ages, but most common in 4th and 5th decades
- Gender
  - Affects males and females equally

Site
- Typically occur on distal extremities, but may present at any cutaneous site

Presentation
- Firm, isolated, flesh-colored subcutaneous papule or nodule
  - New DFs are typically pink (vascular); older DFs are brown (overlying epidermal hyperplasia with basilar pigmentation)
- Multiple DFs may occur in immunosuppressed populations
- "Dimpling" sign when in vivo DF is pinched by fingers

Treatment
- Complete excision is curative

Prognosis
- Excellent in vast majority of cases
  - Local recurrence potential significant (up to 30%) with cellular variant
  - Metastasis and death from rare cellular and atypical tumors reported
    - Usually large and deep lesions

MACROSCOPIC FEATURES

General Features
- Firm, circumscribed, but nonencapsulated dermal-based tumor
- White to yellow cut surface
- Can have cystic changes and hemorrhage

MICROSCOPIC PATHOLOGY

Histologic Features
- Dermal-based proliferation of typically bland, spindled to histiocytoid-appearing cells

DERMATOFIBROMA AND FIBROUS HISTIOCYTOMA

Key Facts

Terminology
- Benign, limited proliferation of histiocytic and fibroblastic cells in dermis

Etiology/Pathogenesis
- Evidence supports both neoplastic and reactive pathogenesis

Clinical Issues
- Affects all ages, but most common in young adults
- Excellent prognosis in vast majority of cases
- Metastasis and death in rare cases of cellular & atypical DF

Microscopic Pathology
- Dermal-based proliferation of typically bland, spindled to histiocytoid-appearing cells
- Collagen trapping at periphery

- Overlying epithelial basilar induction with hyperpigmentation

Ancillary Tests
- FXIIIA(+), CD163(+), CD68(+), CD34(-)

Top Differential Diagnoses
- Basal cell carcinoma
  - CD20(+) Merkel cells overlying DF
- Angiosarcoma and Kaposi sarcoma
  - CD31 and HHV8 are negative in aneurysmal DF
- Dermatofibrosarcoma protuberans
  - Deep subcutaneous extension and fat entrapment
  - CD34(+), CD163(-) and FXIIIA(-)
- Atypical fibroxanthoma (AFX)
  - Highly atypical spindled and epithelioid cells

- Either spindled (fibroblastic) or histiocytoid cells may predominate
- Early lesions typically show more histiocytes and lymphocytes
- Established lesions show greater cellularity and spindled cells
- Older lesions show more fibrosis
- Spindled cells show elongated eosinophilic cytoplasmic processes
- "Histiocytic" type cells are larger, epithelioid-shaped, and have abundant pale vacuolated cytoplasm
- Cytologic atypia and pleomorphism are usually minimal, but can be focally present
- Tumors are grossly circumscribed, but microscopically have irregular, often jagged borders
- Collagen trapping at periphery
  - Spheres of intensely eosinophilic collagen (so-called "collagen balls") separated by bands of pale fibrohistiocytic cells
- Grenz zone
  - Tumor often spares band of superficial papillary dermis
- Folliculosebaceous induction and basilar epidermal hyperplasia overlying DF
  - Can mimic basal cell carcinoma if basilar induction is marked
- Adjacent adnexal hyperplasia
- Overlying epidermal hyperplasia with basilar hyperpigmentation is common, occasional melanocytic hyperplasia
  - So-called "dirty feet" or "dirty sock" sign

Predominant Pattern/Injury Type
- Ill-defined borders
- Nodular proliferation
- Fibrous
- Histiocytic

Predominant Cell/Compartment Type
- "Fibrohistiocytic"

Histologic Subtypes
- Aneurysmal (hemosiderotic/sclerosing hemangioma variant)
  - Pseudovascular spaces, hemosiderin, reactive spindled and epithelioid cells
    - May mimic vascular tumor, including Kaposi sarcoma and angiosarcoma
  - Aneurysmal DF can show some cytologic atypia, but lacks high-grade atypia and shows only a few mitoses
- Cellular
  - Uncommon, often large, deeply penetrating tumors
    - May show overlap with atypical dermatofibroma
    - Occasional mitoses and multinucleated cells are seen
    - Up to 12% of cases may show focal central necrosis
  - Most likely subtype to recur (up to 30% in some studies)
    - Complete conservative excision should be recommended
- Epithelioid cell histiocytoma
  - Nodular to sheet-like, well-circumscribed proliferation in papillary dermis
    - Often has associated epidermal collarette
  - Clinical and histologic mimic of intradermal Spitz nevus, but negative for melanocytic markers
- Atypical/pseudosarcomatous/"DF with monster cells"
  - Shows population of atypical cells with nuclear hyperchromasia and prominent nucleoli, often with abundant cytoplasm
    - Mitotic figures are sparse, usually not atypical in appearance
  - Some cases have been reported to metastasize
    - Complete excision should be recommended
- Lipidized
  - Often large tumors, typically present in ankle region
  - Numerous large foamy cells are present, with a few hemosiderin-containing cells
  - Stromal hyalinization is typically present, which may be "wiry" or "keloidal" in appearance

DERMATOFIBROMA AND FIBROUS HISTIOCYTOMA

- Many other rare variants described, including granular cell, clear cell, histiocytic/xanthomatous, osteoclastic, myxoid, keloidal/scar-like, palisading, deep penetrating (may mimic DFSP), and lichenoid

ANCILLARY TESTS

Immunohistochemistry
- FXIIIA(+), CD163(+), HMGA1/HMGA2(+), MMP-11(+)
  - CD68 also often positive; typically highlights histiocytic-appearing cells
  - Actin-sm often positive; may indicate myofibroblastic differentiation
- CD34 typically negative but may show focal staining, especially at periphery of lesion
- Nestin(-), S100(-), MART-1/Melan-A(-), HMB-45(-), desmin(-)

DIFFERENTIAL DIAGNOSIS

Dermatofibrosarcoma Protuberans (DFSP)
- Shows monotonous proliferation of spindled cells
- Typically extends deeply along septae of subcutaneous fat with honeycombing fat entrapment
  - Typically CD34(+), nestin(+), CD163(-), HMGA1/HMGA2(-), FXIIIA(±)

Basal Cell Carcinoma (BCC)
- In superficial biopsies, BCC can be difficult to distinguish from benign follicular induction overlying DF
  - CK20 highlights Merkel cells in basal layer overlying DF; these cells are absent in BCC

Angiosarcoma
- Aneurysmal variant of DF can have atypical cells, pseudovascular spaces, and mitoses
  - Aneurysmal DF is negative for vascular markers, including CD31, CD34, and HHV8

Kaposi Sarcoma
- Nodular/tumor stage Kaposi sarcoma shows cellular spindle cell proliferation
- Slit-like vascular spaces and extravasated red blood cells are often present
  - Immunohistochemistry shows CD31 and HHV8 positivity

Atypical Fibroxanthoma (AFX)
- Dermal nodule composed of highly atypical spindled and pleomorphic epithelioid cells
- Typically occurs in heavily sun-damaged skin (especially head and neck area) of elderly patients
  - Both AFX and DF are positive for nonspecific markers, including CD68, CD10, and vimentin
  - FXIIIA may show greater positivity in DF

DIAGNOSTIC CHECKLIST

Clinically Relevant Pathologic Features
- Cellularity and atypia

- Tumor size (more aggressive cases typically large and deep)

Pathologic Interpretation Pearls
- "Collagen balls"
- Basilar epidermal induction with hyperpigmentation
- Occasional adnexal and melanocytic hyperplasia

SELECTED REFERENCES

1. Fernandez-Flores A et al: Mitosis in dermatofibroma: a worrisome histopathologic sign that does not necessarily equal recurrence. J Cutan Pathol. 35(9):839-42, 2008
2. Gleason BC et al: Deep "benign" fibrous histiocytoma: clinicopathologic analysis of 69 cases of a rare tumor indicating occasional metastatic potential. Am J Surg Pathol. 32(3):354-62, 2008
3. Mori T et al: Expression of nestin in dermatofibrosarcoma protuberans in comparison to dermatofibroma. J Dermatol. 35(7):419-25, 2008
4. Kim HJ et al: Stromelysin-3 expression in the differential diagnosis of dermatofibroma and dermatofibrosarcoma protuberans: comparison with factor XIIIa and CD34. Br J Dermatol. 157(2):319-24, 2007
5. Sachdev R et al: Expression of CD163 in dermatofibroma, cellular fibrous histiocytoma, and dermatofibrosarcoma protuberans: comparison with CD68, CD34, and Factor XIIIa. J Cutan Pathol. 33(5):353-60, 2006
6. Mahmoodi M et al: Anti-cytokeratin 20 staining of Merkel cells helps differentiate basaloid proliferations overlying dermatofibromas from basal cell carcinoma. J Cutan Pathol. 32(7):491-5, 2005
7. Li N et al: Differential expression of HMGA1 and HMGA2 in dermatofibroma and dermatofibrosarcoma protuberans: potential diagnostic applications, and comparison with histologic findings, CD34, and factor XIIIa immunoreactivity. Am J Dermatopathol. 26(4):267-72, 2004
8. Hui P et al: Clonal analysis of cutaneous fibrous histiocytoma (dermatofibroma). J Cutan Pathol. 29(7):385-9, 2002
9. Kaddu S et al: Atypical fibrous histiocytoma of the skin: clinicopathologic analysis of 59 cases with evidence of infrequent metastasis. Am J Surg Pathol. 26(1):35-46, 2002
10. Massone C et al: Multiple eruptive dermatofibromas in patients with systemic lupus erythematosus treated with prednisone. Int J Dermatol. 41(5):279-81, 2002
11. Nuovo M et al: Utility of HHV8 RNA detection for differentiating Kaposi's sarcoma from its mimics. J Cutan Pathol. 28(5):248-55, 2001
12. Chen TC et al: Dermatofibroma is a clonal proliferative disease. J Cutan Pathol. 27(1):36-9, 2000
13. Vanni R et al: Cytogenetic evidence of clonality in cutaneous benign fibrous histiocytomas: a report of the CHAMP study group. Histopathology. 37(3):212-7, 2000
14. Ammirati CT et al: Multiple eruptive dermatofibromas in three men with HIV infection. Dermatology. 195(4):344-8, 1997
15. Li DF et al: Dermatofibroma: superficial fibrous proliferation with reactive histiocytes. A multiple immunostaining analysis. Cancer. 74(1):66-73, 1994
16. Altman DA et al: Differential expression of factor XIIIa and CD34 in cutaneous mesenchymal tumors. J Cutan Pathol. 20(2):154-8, 1993
17. Santa Cruz DJ et al: Aneurysmal ("angiomatoid") fibrous histiocytoma of the skin. Cancer. 47(8):2053-61, 1981

Variant Microscopic Features

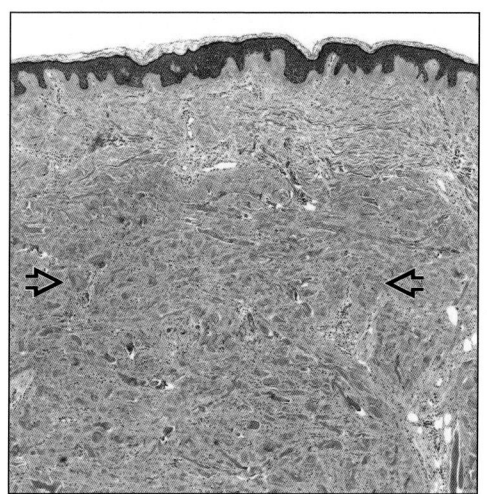
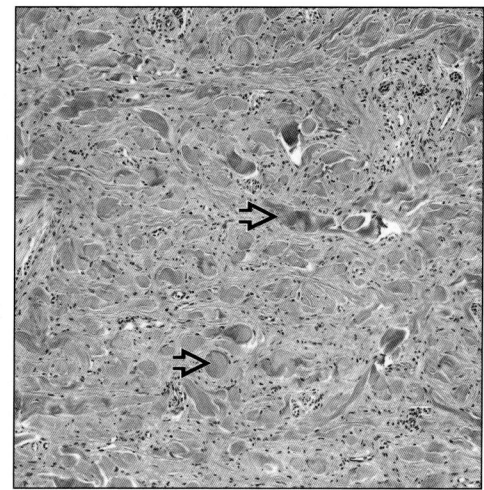

(Left) Scanning magnification of a scar-like dermatofibroma with prominent thickened, keloidal collagen bundles ⊳ is shown. *(Right)* Higher power view of scar-like dermatofibroma shows dense and glassy-appearing bundles of keloidal collagen ⊳.

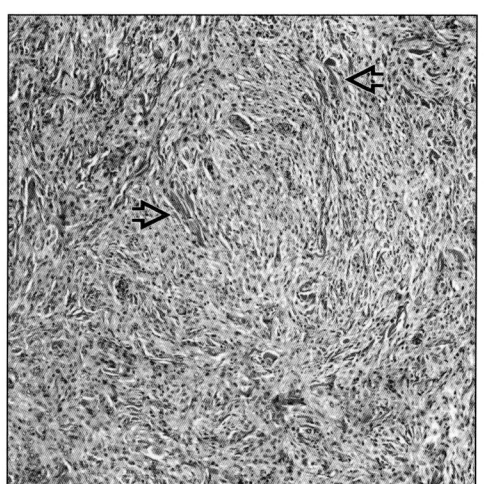
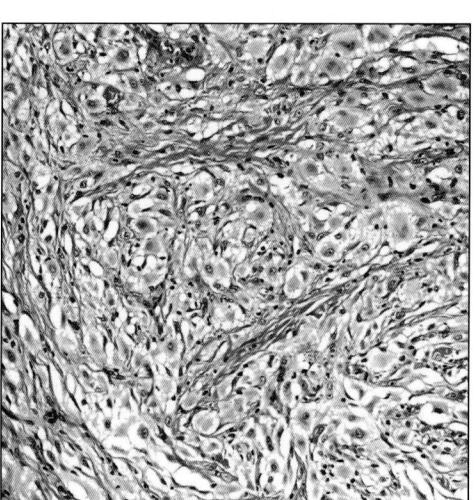

(Left) Histiocytic-predominant dermatofibroma shows a proliferation of large, epithelioid-appearing cells with abundant pale/vacuolated cytoplasm and scattered small entrapped collagen bundles ⊳. *(Right)* Higher power examination of histiocytic dermatofibroma shows a proliferation of large cells with abundant pale to vacuolated cytoplasm and bland-appearing nuclei.

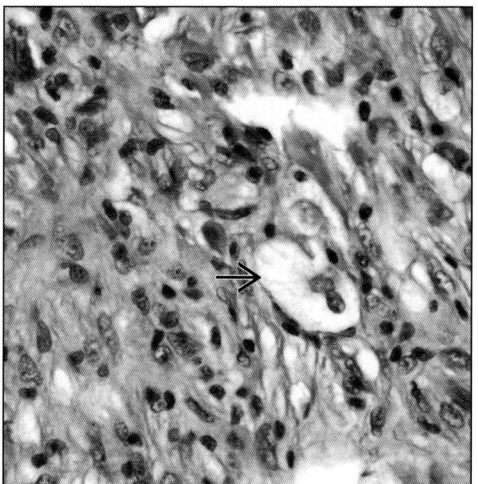
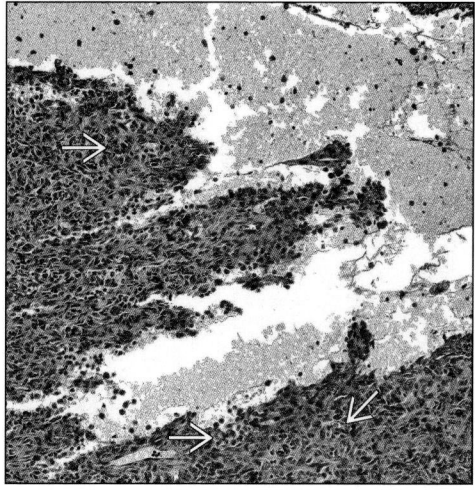

(Left) Lipidized DF shows proliferation of bland histiocytoid cells and scattered multivacuolated cells with nuclear indentation, simulating lipoblasts →. *(Right)* An example of an aneurysmal fibrous histiocytoma shows large, irregular, blood-filled spaces and prominent hemosiderin deposition →.

Variant Microscopic Features

(Left) Higher magnification of an aneurysmal fibrous histiocytoma shows bland spindled cells and scattered hemosiderin-laden macrophages ➡. *(Right)* Another area of aneurysmal fibrous histiocytoma shows numerous hemosiderin-laden macrophages.

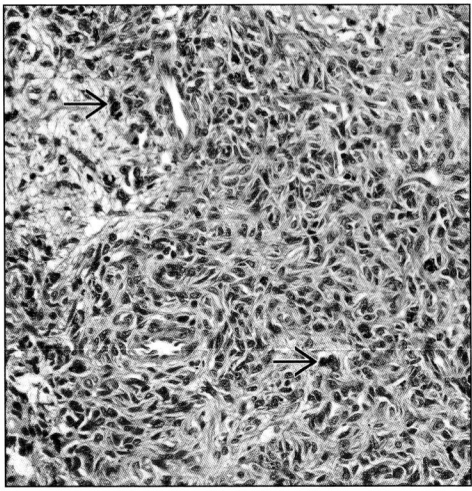
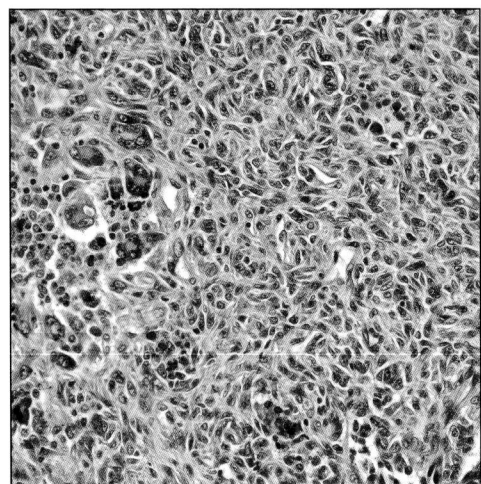

(Left) Scanning magnification shows an otherwise typical dermatofibroma with a small associated osteoma cutis ➡. *(Right)* Higher magnification shows an osteoma cutis surrounded by an otherwise typical-appearing dermatofibroma.

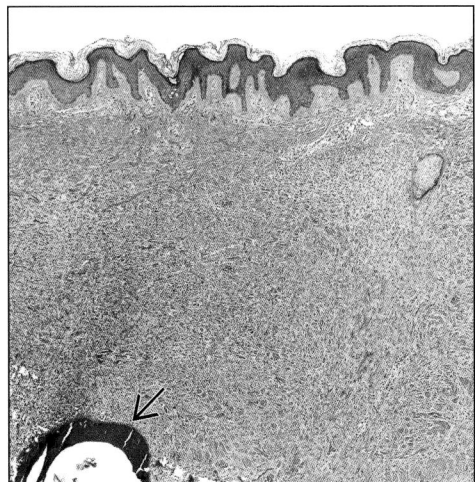
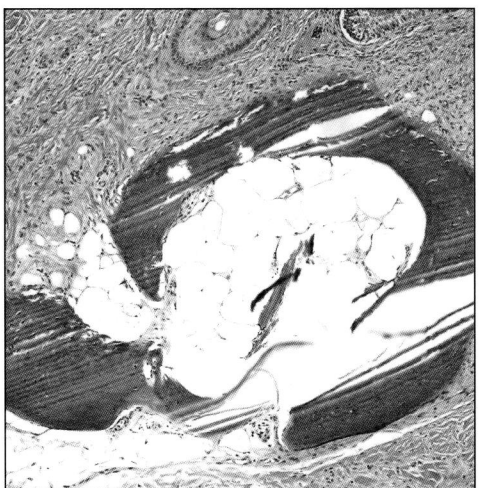

(Left) Low-power view of a cellular dermatofibroma shows a dense proliferation of spindled and histiocytic-appearing cells with mild atypia. *(Right)* Higher power view of a cellular dermatofibroma with focal atypia ("DF with monster cells") shows scattered bizarre-appearing cells with enlarged, irregular, hyperchromatic nuclei ➡.

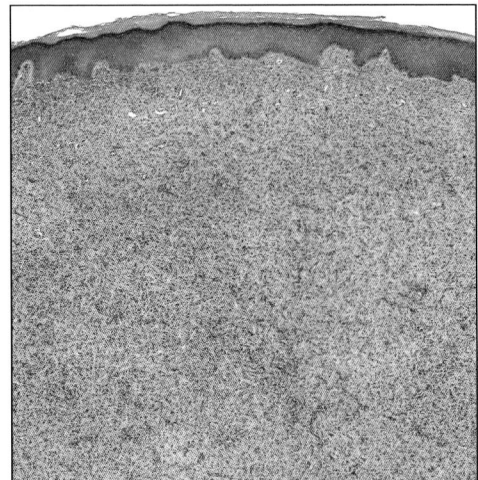
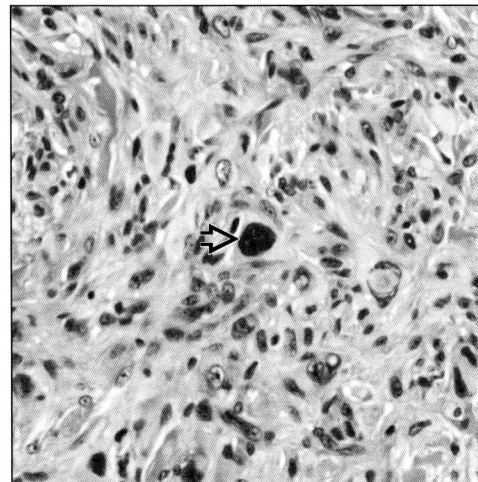

Microscopic and Immunohistochemical Features

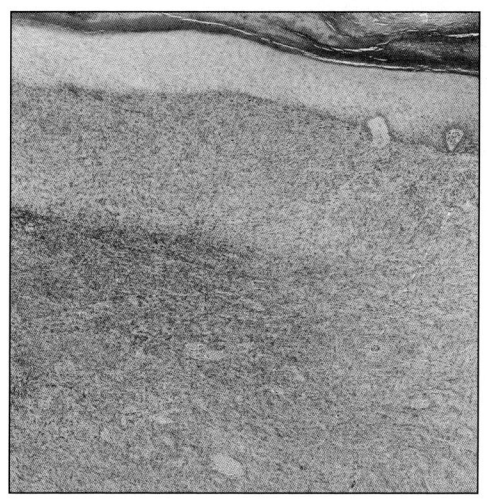
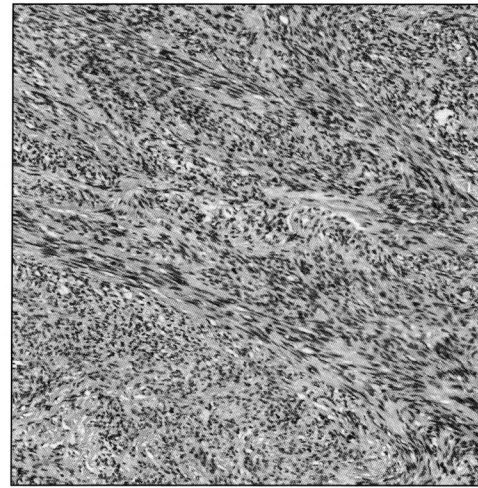

(Left) Low-power view of a large and highly cellular FH with atypia is shown. The tumor fills the dermis and presses directly against the epidermis (loss of the normal grenz zone). (Right) Higher power view shows quite marked atypia and a focal fascicular growth pattern, favoring a low-grade sarcoma (fibrosarcoma-like) arising in a cellular FH.

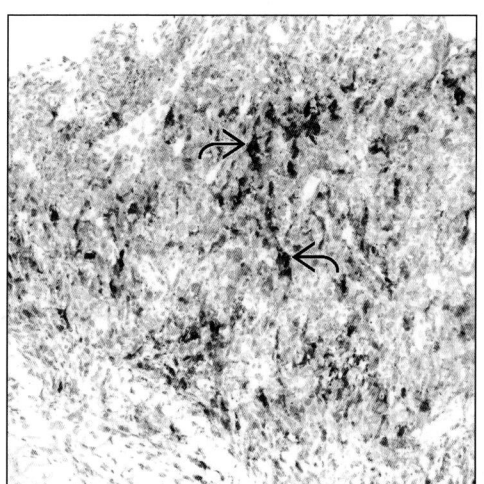
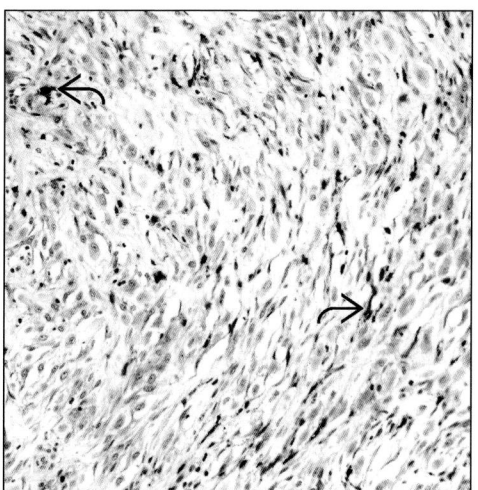

(Left) Positive FXIIIA shows strong staining of many of the spindled and dendritic-appearing tumor cells ⇨. (Right) Weakly positive FXIIIA stain in another case shows weak staining of the tumoral spindled cells and stronger staining of scattered dermal dendritic cells ⇨.

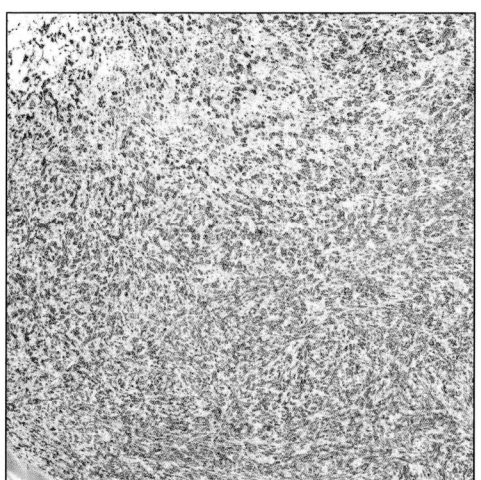
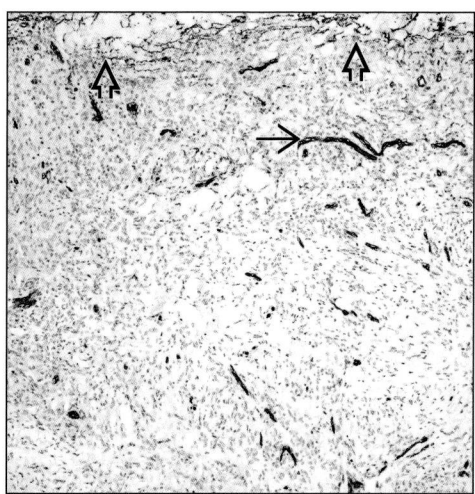

(Left) Positive CD163 shows strong and diffuse staining in a histiocytic-type DF. (Right) CD34 strongly highlights vessels ⇨ and shows weak background staining of peripheral stroma ⇨, but is negative within the tumoral cells.

EPITHELIOID CELL HISTIOCYTOMA

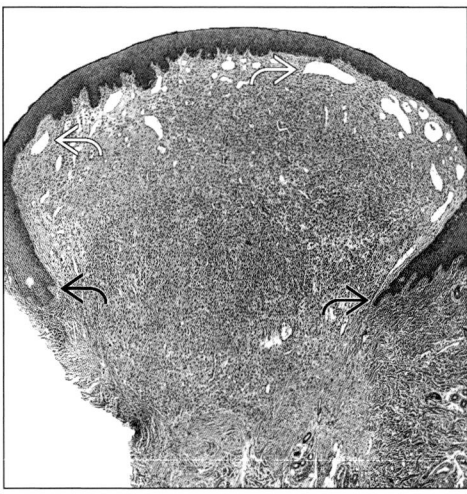

Low magnification of an epithelioid histiocytoma shows a nodular, dermal-based tumor surrounded by an epidermal collarette ➔. Note the prominent superficial blood vessels with telangiectasia ➔.

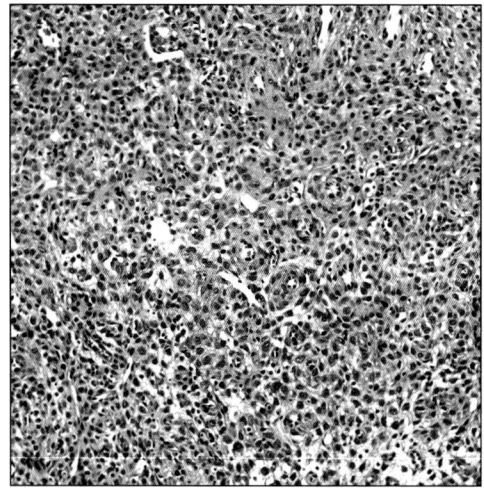

Higher magnification of epithelioid histiocytoma shows a proliferation of moderately enlarged, epithelioid-appearing cells with eosinophilic cytoplasm and oval to angulated, hyperchromatic nuclei.

TERMINOLOGY

Abbreviations
- Epithelioid cell histiocytoma (ECH)

Synonyms
- Epithelioid histiocytoma variant of dermatofibroma

Definitions
- Dermal-based benign fibrohistiocytic tumor, which can mimic melanocytic, vascular, epithelial, or other histiocytic lesions

ETIOLOGY/PATHOGENESIS

Unknown
- May arise from activated dermal dendrocytes

CLINICAL ISSUES

Epidemiology
- Incidence
  - Rare tumors
- Age
  - Usually occur in young adults (mean age ~ 40 years)
- Gender
  - Slightly more common in males

Site
- Most cases occur on extremities
  - Lower extremity > upper
- May also present on trunk, head, and neck region

Presentation
- Dermal nodule
- Erythematous

Treatment
- Surgical approaches
  - Conservative excision is curative

Prognosis
- Excellent; no malignant potential reported

MACROSCOPIC FEATURES

Size
- 0.5-2 cm in greatest diameter

MICROSCOPIC PATHOLOGY

Histologic Features
- Dermal-based nodular proliferation
  - Shows symmetry and relatively sharp circumscription
  - Often surrounded by an epidermal collarette
  - Typically centered in papillary dermis
  - Cellular versions based in reticular dermis
- Composed of a monomorphic proliferation of enlarged, epithelioid to polygonal-appearing cells
  - Show round to oval nuclei, uniform vesicular chromatin, small nucleoli, and abundant eosinophilic-staining cytoplasm
  - Lack of (or rare) giant cells, foamy, or hemosiderin-laden macrophages
- Prominent vascularity usually present
- Mild background inflammatory infiltrate

ANCILLARY TESTS

Immunohistochemistry
- Cells are positive for fibrohistiocytic markers including CD68, FXIIIA
- CD31 can be positive (reflecting histiocytic, rather than endothelial, differentiation)

EPITHELIOID CELL HISTIOCYTOMA

Key Facts

Terminology
- Dermal-based benign fibrohistiocytic tumor, which can mimic melanocytic, vascular, epithelial, or other histiocytic lesions

Clinical Issues
- Usually occur in young adults (mean age ~ 40 years)
- Most cases occur on extremities
- Dermal nodule
- Excellent; no malignant potential reported

Microscopic Pathology
- Dermal-based nodular proliferation
- Shows symmetry and relatively sharp circumscription
- May be surrounded by an epidermal collarette
- Composed of a monomorphic proliferation of enlarged, epithelioid to polygonal-appearing cells
- Show round to oval nuclei, uniform vesicular chromatin, small nucleoli, and abundant eosinophilic-staining cytoplasm

DIFFERENTIAL DIAGNOSIS

Spitz Nevus
- Often composed of a proliferation of mixed spindled and epithelioid cells, but purely epithelioid variants can mimic ECH
- Junctional and intradermal proliferation (ECH is purely dermal) in most cases
- Melanocytic markers including S100, HMB-45, and MART-1/Melan-A strongly positive

Dermatofibroma
- Conventional dermatofibroma shows a more diffuse, poorly demarcated proliferation
- Prominent collagen trapping and overlying epidermal hyperplasia
- More polymorphic population, often including giant cells, foamy, and hemosiderin-laden macrophages

Epithelioid Angiomatous Nodule
- Rare dermal-based nodular vascular proliferation
- May represent a variant of epithelioid hemangioma (angiolymphoid hyperplasia with eosinophilia)
- Composed of enlarged epithelioid endothelial cells and scattered small blood vessels
  - Cells show frequent intracytoplasmic vacuoles
- Positive for vascular markers including CD31 and CD34

SELECTED REFERENCES

1. Mitteldorf C et al: Sclerotic epithelioid dermatofibroma. Am J Dermatopathol. 33(1):98-101, 2011
2. Wilk M et al: Dermatofibroma with intracytoplasmic eosinophilic globules--another case with features overlapping between epithelioid cell histiocytoma and dermal nodular fasciitis. J Cutan Pathol. 38(2):254-5, 2011
3. Cangelosi JJ et al: Unusual presentation of multiple epithelioid cell histiocytomas. Am J Dermatopathol. 30(4):373-6, 2008
4. Lee J: Epithelioid cell histiocytoma with granular cells (another nonneural granular cell neoplasm). Am J Dermatopathol. 29(5):475-6, 2007
5. High WA et al: Epithelioid cell histiocytoma with hemangiopericytoma-like features. Am J Dermatopathol. 28(4):369-71, 2006
6. Busam KJ et al: Immunohistochemical distinction of epithelioid histiocytic proliferations from epithelioid melanocytic nevi. Am J Dermatopathol. 22(3):237-41, 2000
7. Glusac EJ et al: Epithelioid cell histiocytoma: a simulant of vascular and melanocytic neoplasms. Am J Dermatopathol. 21(1):1-7, 1999
8. Glusac EJ et al: Epithelioid cell histiocytoma. A report of 10 cases including a new cellular variant. Am J Surg Pathol. 18(6):583-90, 1994
9. Singh Gomez C et al: Epithelioid benign fibrous histiocytoma of skin: clinico-pathological analysis of 20 cases of a poorly known variant. Histopathology. 24(2):123-9, 1994
10. Jones EW et al: Epithelioid cell histiocytoma: a new entity. Br J Dermatol. 120(2):185-95, 1989

Microscopic Features

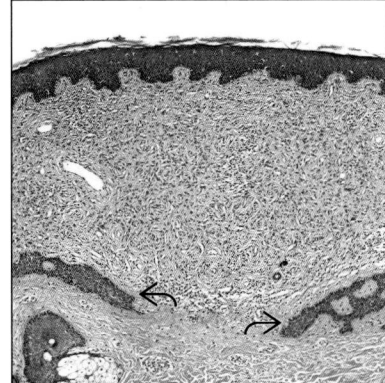 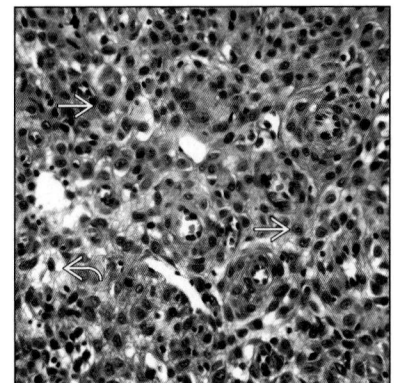 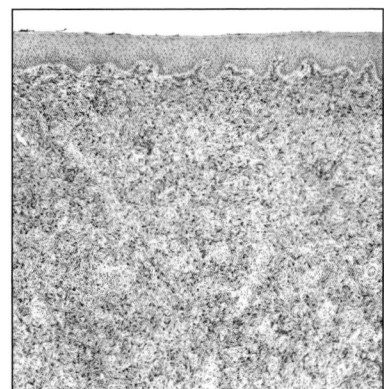

(Left) An example of ECH at low magnification shows a nodular, dermal-based tumor with a prominent enveloping epidermal collarette ➡. (Center) High magnification of ECH shows a population of moderately enlarged, epithelioid-appearing cells with eosinophilic-staining to focally vacuolated ➡ cytoplasm. Many of the cells show small nucleoli ➡. (Right) Immunohistochemical stain for FXIIIA is typically positive, similar to other variants of dermatofibroma.

DERMATOMYOFIBROMA

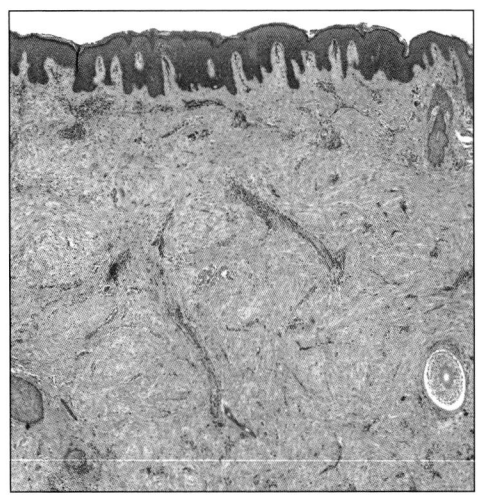

Scanning magnification of a dermatomyofibroma shows a dermal-based, plaque-like spindle proliferation with overlying epidermal hyperplasia, similar to a dermatofibroma.

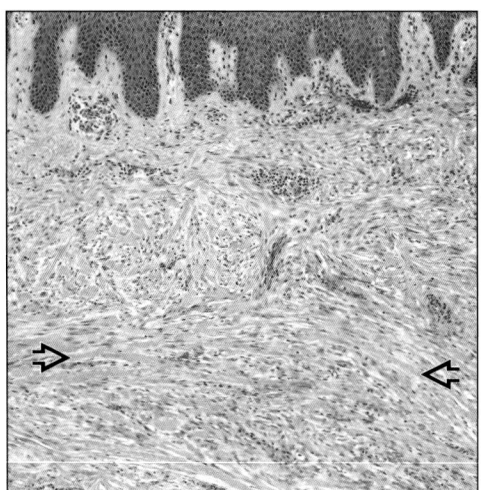

Higher magnification shows a proliferation of bland spindle cells arranged in fascicles, largely running parallel to the epidermis and associated with focal collagen trapping ▷.

TERMINOLOGY

Synonyms
- Plaque-like dermal fibromatosis

Definitions
- Myofibroblastic tumor with many features similar to dermatofibroma

ETIOLOGY/PATHOGENESIS

Unknown
- May be related to trauma in some cases

CLINICAL ISSUES

Epidemiology
- Incidence
  - Rare tumor
- Age
  - Usually occurs in young adults
- Gender
  - Typically females (M:F = 1:8)

Site
- Most cases present in shoulder and axillary regions
  - Also may occur in trunk, head, and neck

Presentation
- Slow-growing indurated plaque or nodule
  - Often red-brown in color
- Rarely, may present as multiple lesions

Treatment
- Surgical approaches
  - Complete surgical excision is curative

Prognosis
- Excellent

- No malignant potential but may continue to enlarge if not completely removed

MACROSCOPIC FEATURES

General Features
- Small, dermal-based nodule

Size
- Usually 1-2 cm in size, but occasionally much larger

MICROSCOPIC PATHOLOGY

Histologic Features
- Dermal-based, plaque-like spindle cell proliferation oriented parallel to epidermis
  - Usually located in reticular dermis but may show involvement of superficial subcutis
  - Adnexal structures are usually preserved
  - Overlying epidermal hyperplasia, similar to dermatofibroma, is often seen
- Tumor is composed of broad fascicles of elongated monomorphous spindle cells
  - Nuclei bland and tapered
  - Uniform chromatin
  - Small nucleoli
  - Cytoplasm eosinophilic, poorly delineated
- Mitotic figures are rare and not atypical
- Elastic fibers are typically increased in numbers and fragmented
  - Can highlight with elastic stains

Predominant Pattern/Injury Type
- Fibrous/spindle cell proliferation
- Parallel orientation to epidermis

Predominant Cell/Compartment Type
- Fibroblast, myofibroblast

DERMATOMYOFIBROMA

Key Facts

Terminology
- Myofibroblastic tumor with features overlapping with dermatofibroma

Clinical Issues
- Slow-growing plaque or nodule
- Most cases present in shoulder and axillary regions

Microscopic Pathology
- Dermal-based spindle cell proliferation

- Tumor is composed of broad fascicles of elongated monomorphous spindle cells oriented parallel to surface
- Elastic fibers are typically increased in numbers and fragmented, which may be highlighted with elastic stains

Top Differential Diagnoses
- Dermatofibroma
- Hypertrophic scar

ANCILLARY TESTS

Immunohistochemistry
- Tumor cells variably positive for smooth muscle actin (SMA)
- Cells are negative for muscle specific actin (MSA), desmin, S100, CD34, and FXIIIA

DIFFERENTIAL DIAGNOSIS

Dermatofibroma
- Lacks parallel orientation of tumor cells to epidermis
- Shows more prominent collagen trapping and overlying epidermal hyperplasia

Hypertrophic Scar
- Dense proliferation of thickened collagen with vertically oriented vessels
- Adnexal structures are lost, as opposed to preserved in dermatomyofibroma

Leiomyoma
- Shows strong smooth muscle differentiation with SMA, MSA, and desmin staining
- Fascicles of spindle cells not typically oriented parallel to epidermis

Dermatofibrosarcoma Protuberans
- Plaque-like variant can show histologic features similar to dermatomyofibroma

- In dermatofibrosarcoma protuberans, CD34 is typically strongly positive and SMA is negative

DIAGNOSTIC CHECKLIST

Pathologic Interpretation Pearls
- Dermal-based, plaque-like proliferation composed of broad fascicles of elongated monomorphous spindle cells oriented parallel to surface

SELECTED REFERENCES

1. Mentzel T et al: Dermatomyofibroma: clinicopathologic and immunohistochemical analysis of 56 cases and reappraisal of a rare and distinct cutaneous neoplasm. Am J Dermatopathol. 31(1):44-9, 2009
2. Viglizzo G et al: A unique case of multiple dermatomyofibromas. Clin Exp Dermatol. 33(5):622-4, 2008
3. Mortimore RJ et al: Dermatomyofibroma: a report of two cases, one occurring in a child. Australas J Dermatol. 42(1):22-5, 2001
4. Mentzel T et al: Dermatomyofibroma: additional observations on a distinctive cutaneous myofibroblastic tumour with emphasis on differential diagnosis. Br J Dermatol. 129(1):69-73, 1993
5. Cooper PH: Dermatomyofibroma: a case of fibromatosis revisited. J Cutan Pathol. 19(2):81-2, 1992
6. Kamino H et al: Dermatomyofibroma. A benign cutaneous, plaque-like proliferation of fibroblasts and myofibroblasts in young adults. J Cutan Pathol. 19(2):85-93, 1992

IMAGE GALLERY

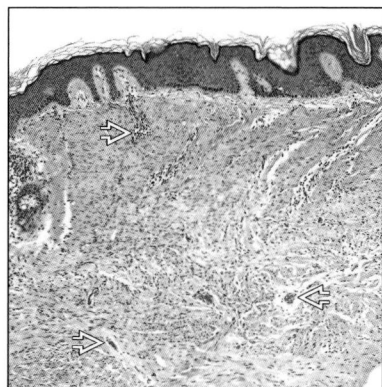 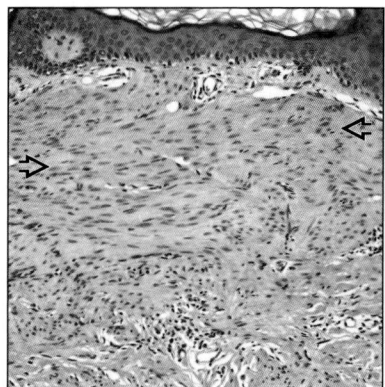 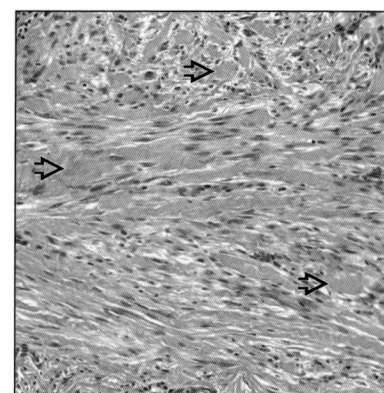

(Left) Another example of a dermatomyofibroma shows a scar-like plaque of spindle cells in the dermis associated with mild chronic inflammation and increased numbers of small blood vessels ➡. *(Center)* Higher magnification shows the superficial portion of the lesion with parallel arrays of spindle cells ➡ closely approaching the epidermis. *(Right)* High-power examination shows bland cytologic features of the elongated myofibroblastic cells. There is also associated collagen trapping ➡.

FIBROUS HAMARTOMA OF INFANCY

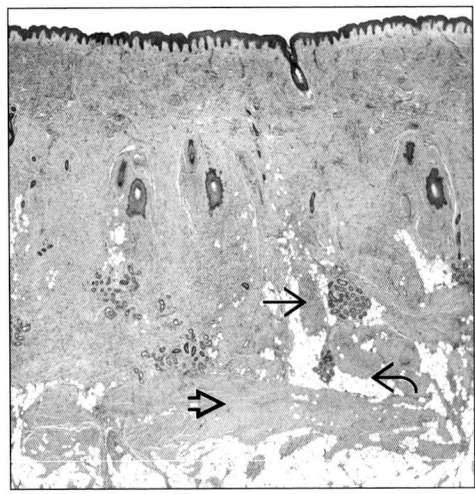

H&E shows fibrous hamartoma of infancy. The lesion expands the deep dermis and superficial submucosa consisting of eosinophilic fibrous zones ➤, more basophilic areas ➡, and fat ➘.

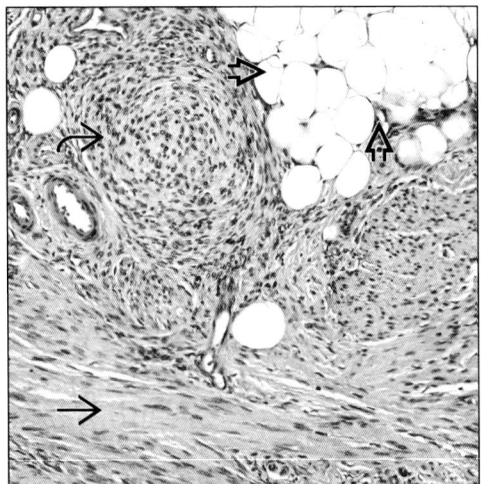

This field shows the 3 key components of fibrous hamartoma of infancy. The so-called "primitive cells" are on the upper left ➤, intimately admixed with the fibrous ➡ and fat ➤ elements.

TERMINOLOGY

Abbreviations
- Fibrous hamartoma of infancy (FHI)

Definitions
- Benign superficial fibrous lesion occurring in 1st 2 years of life

ETIOLOGY/PATHOGENESIS

Developmental Anomaly
- No conclusive familial or syndromic associations
  - Rare cases reported in tuberous sclerosis patients

CLINICAL ISSUES

Epidemiology
- Age
  - Infants and children up to 2 years
    - Up to 25% present at birth
  - Rarely in older children
- Gender
  - M > F

Site
- Deep dermis or subcutis
- Most occur in upper body, especially axillary fold
  - Other sites include upper arm, shoulder, forearm, groin, thigh, chest wall, back, neck, and scalp
- Usually solitary
  - Rarely multiple synchronous nodules

Presentation
- Suddenly enlarging mass
- Painless and often freely mobile

Natural History
- Rapid growth, which slows but does not regress

Treatment
- Complete local excision curative

Prognosis
- Excellent, but can recur if incompletely excised

MACROSCOPIC FEATURES

General Features
- Poorly defined, variegated surface
- Admixture of firm white tissue and fat
- Sometimes overlying skin changes (e.g., altered pigmentation)

Size
- Most up to 5 cm, but larger lesions reported

MICROSCOPIC PATHOLOGY

Histologic Features
- 3 distinct components in varying amounts
- "Organoid" growth pattern
  - Intersecting bands and trabeculae of mature fibrous tissue, comprising spindle-shaped myofibroblasts and fibroblasts
  - Nests and whorls of immature round, ovoid, or spindle cells in loose stroma
  - Interspersed mature fat
  - Lymphocytes and patent capillaries often within mesenchyme

ANCILLARY TESTS

Immunohistochemistry
- Vimentin in both fibrous and primitive areas
- Actin and rarely CD34 or desmin in fibrous areas

Cytogenetics
- Translocations reported in 2 cases

FIBROUS HAMARTOMA OF INFANCY

Key Facts

Terminology
- Benign superficial fibrous lesion occurring during 1st 2 years of life

Clinical Issues
- Congenital in up to 25% of cases
- M > F
- Occurs in deep dermis or subcutis
  - Typically in upper torso, but at variety of sites
- Complete excision curative

- Can recur if incompletely excised

Microscopic Pathology
- 3 components in organoid growth pattern
  - Intersecting bands of mature fibrous tissue, comprising spindle-shaped myofibroblasts and fibroblasts
  - Nests of immature round, ovoid, or spindle cells within loose stroma
  - Interspersed mature fat

- Reciprocal t(2;3)(q31;q21)
- Complex t(6;12;8)(q25;q24.3;q13)
- Raises possibility of FHI being neoplastic rather than hamartomatous

Electron Microscopy
- Transmission
  - Fibroblasts and myofibroblasts in fascicular areas
  - Primitive mesenchymal cells in immature areas
  - Irregular collagen fibers among mature fat

DIFFERENTIAL DIAGNOSIS

Fibromatosis
- No primitive oval cell component
- β-catenin(+) in nuclei

Infantile Fibromatosis/Lipofibromatosis
- Deep-seated lesions
- Predilection for distal extremities
- Can occur in older children (up to early 2nd decade)
- No primitive oval cell component

Lipoblastoma
- Lobulated architecture
- Immature adipocytes

Diffuse Myofibromatosis
- Nodular cell proliferations
- Hemangiopericytoma-like areas

Embryonal Rhabdomyosarcoma
- Occurs in older children
- Cytologic atypia and mitoses present
- Desmin(+), myogenin(+)

Infantile Fibrosarcoma
- Cells in sheets and intersecting fascicles
- Lack of organoid pattern

SELECTED REFERENCES

1. Rougemont AL et al: A complex translocation (6;12;8) (q25;q24.3;q13) in a fibrous hamartoma of infancy. Cancer Genet Cytogenet. 171(2):115-8, 2006
2. Lakshminarayanan R et al: Fibrous hamartoma of infancy: a case report with associated cytogenetic findings. Arch Pathol Lab Med. 129(4):520-2, 2005
3. Popek EJ et al: Fibrous hamartoma of infancy in the genital region: findings in 15 cases. J Urol. 152(3):990-3, 1994
4. Sotelo-Avila C et al: Subdermal fibrous hamartoma of infancy: pathology of 40 cases and differential diagnosis. Pediatr Pathol. 14(1):39-52, 1994
5. Efem SE et al: Clinicopathological features of untreated fibrous hamartoma of infancy. J Clin Pathol. 46(6):522-4, 1993
6. Michal M et al: Fibrous hamartoma of infancy. A study of eight cases with immunohistochemical and electron microscopical findings. Pathol Res Pract. 188(8):1049-53, 1992
7. Groisman G et al: Fibrous hamartoma of infancy: an immunohistochemical and ultrastructural study. Hum Pathol. 22(9):914-8, 1991

IMAGE GALLERY

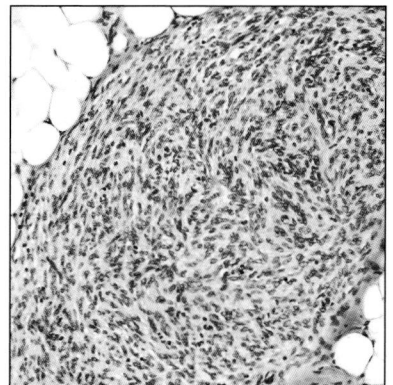 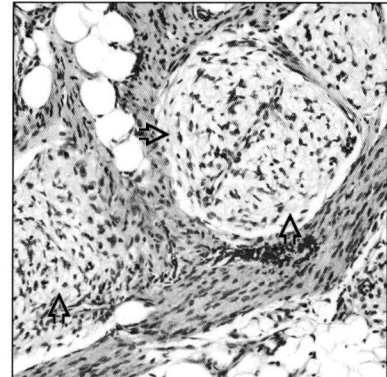 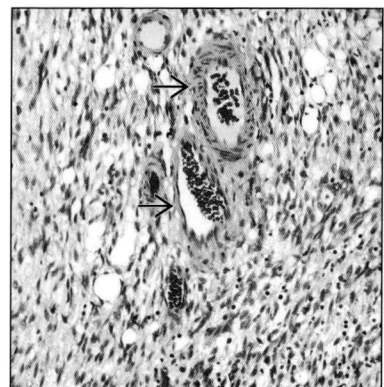

(Left) Histologic examination shows a fibrous hamartoma of infancy with a nodule comprising sheets of immature cells with bland, ovoid vesicular nuclei. Mitotic figures are absent. *(Center)* Higher magnification shows the 3 components of FHI. There is prominent myxoid stroma within the nodules ➡. No cellular atypia is seen in any of the elements. *(Right)* High magnification of a FHI shows that the myxoid zones are often oriented around small veins ➡.

DIGITAL FIBROMATOSIS (INFANTILE DIGITAL FIBROMATOSIS)

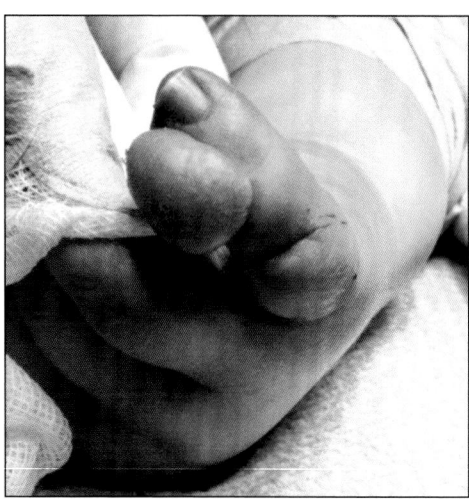

Clinical examination of infantile digital fibromatosis shows an exophytic, dome-shaped superficial neoplasm, which presents in infants and small children.

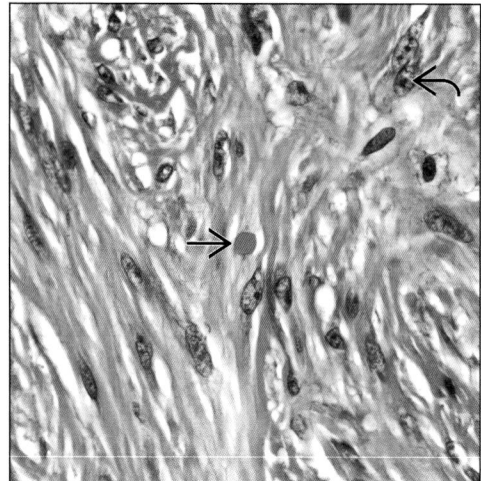

Eosinophilic-staining cytoplasmic inclusions ➔ are the morphologic hallmark of infantile digital fibromatosis. The proliferating myofibroblasts each contain a small to slightly enlarged nucleolus ➘.

TERMINOLOGY

Synonyms
- Infantile digital fibromatosis
- Digital fibrous tumor of childhood
- Inclusion body fibromatosis

Definitions
- Benign proliferation of fibroblasts and myofibroblasts, containing scattered eosinophilic spherical inclusions, that arises on the digits of young children

CLINICAL ISSUES

Epidemiology
- Incidence
  - Rare fibroblastic/myofibroblastic neoplasm
- Age
  - Most cases occur in 1st year of life
  - Very rare in adult patients
- Gender
  - M = F

Site
- Dorsal aspects of hands or feet most common
- Rarely synchronous or asynchronous involvement of more than 1 digit
- Thumb or great toe is only very rarely affected
- Extradigital soft tissues (i.e., arm, breast) are only extremely rarely affected

Presentation
- Digital enlargement
- Dome-shaped swelling overlying phalanges or interphalangeal joints
- Nontender nodules
- Rarely erosion of bone

Natural History
- May recur locally

- May regress spontaneously
- No progression
- No metastases

Treatment
- Surgical approaches
  - Local excision with preservation of function

Prognosis
- Excellent overall prognosis
- May recur locally
- May show spontaneous regression
- Main prognostic indicator is adequacy of primary excision

MACROSCOPIC FEATURES

General Features
- Ill-defined neoplasm
- Dermal-based neoplasm with gray-white, indurated cut surface covered by intact skin
- No areas of hemorrhage
- No areas of necrosis

Size
- Nodules of variable size
  - Usually measure < 2 cm

MICROSCOPIC PATHOLOGY

Histologic Features
- Infiltrating fascicles and sheets
- Uniform-appearing spindle-shaped fibroblasts and myofibroblasts
- No significant cytologic atypia
- Elongated spindled nuclei
- Pale eosinophilic, fibrillary cytoplasm
- Intracytoplasmic eosinophilic spherical inclusions
  - Often in perinuclear location

DIGITAL FIBROMATOSIS (INFANTILE DIGITAL FIBROMATOSIS)

Key Facts

Terminology
- Benign proliferation of fibroblasts and myofibroblasts containing scattered eosinophilic inclusion bodies that occur on digits of young children

Clinical Issues
- Rare fibroblastic/myofibroblastic neoplasm
- Occurs usually in 1st year of life
- Dorsal aspects of hands or feet
- Presents with digital enlargement
- Dome-shaped swelling overlying phalanges or interphalangeal joints
- Extradigital soft tissues (i.e., arm, breast) are extremely rarely affected
- May recur locally, but excellent prognosis
- May show spontaneous regression
- Local excision with preservation of function

Macroscopic Features
- Ill-defined neoplasms

Microscopic Pathology
- Infiltrating fascicles
- Uniform spindle-shaped tumor cells
- No significant cytologic atypia
- Pale eosinophilic, fibrillary cytoplasm
- Intracytoplasmic eosinophilic spherical inclusions
- Inclusions are trichrome positive

Ancillary Tests
- Spindled cells show features of myofibroblasts
- Expression of actins, desmin, calponin, and CD99
- Inclusions show granular &/or filamentous features by EM
- Cytoplasmic filaments extend onto inclusions

- o Lack of refringence helps in distinction from erythrocytes
- o Stain red with Masson trichrome
- o PAS negative
- Rare mitoses
- Variable amount of extracellular collagen

Predominant Pattern/Injury Type
- Fascicular
- Infiltrative

Predominant Cell/Compartment Type
- Myofibroblast

ANCILLARY TESTS

Electron Microscopy
- Spindled cells show features of myofibroblasts
- Tumor cells contain rough endoplasmic reticulum and cytoplasmic aggregates of filaments
- Scattered dense bodies
- Inclusions show granular &/or filamentous features
- Cytoplasmic filaments extend onto inclusions

DIFFERENTIAL DIAGNOSIS

Dermatofibroma
- Often presents on extremities, but not usually on digits
- Acanthotic, hyperpigmented epidermis
- Stellate appearance with irregular borders
- Storiform growth pattern
- Tumor cells grow around hyalinized collagen bundles
- Admixture of plump spindled and histiocytoid tumor cells
- May contain multinucleated giant cells
- May contain hemosiderin deposits
- Lack of cytoplasmic inclusions

Pilar Leiomyoma
- Adult patients, typically not on digits
- Lobules and bundles of spindled cells

- Bright eosinophilic, fibrillary cytoplasm with perinuclear vacuoles
- Spindle-shaped, blunt-ended nuclei
- Lack of cytoplasmic inclusions
- Actin and desmin positive

Neurofibroma
- Usually adult patients
- Elongated spindled tumor cells
- Spindled to wavy or wrinkled-appearing nuclei
- Lack of cytoplasmic inclusions
- S100 strongly positive
- Muscle markers negative

Extraneural Spindle Cell Perineurioma
- Usually adult patients
- Elongated spindled tumor cells
- May show perivascular accentuation
- Lack of cytoplasmic inclusions
- EMA positive
- Muscle markers negative

Dermatomyofibroma
- Does not occur in 1st years of life
- Does not occur on fingers and toes
- Plaque-like dermal neoplasms
- Bundles of spindle cells oriented parallel to epidermis
- Tumor cells grow around preexisting adnexal structures
- Lack of cytoplasmic inclusions
- Increased number of fragmented elastic fibers

Superficial Acral Fibromyxoma
- Usually in adults
- Typically involves fingers and toes
- Varying myxoid and collagenous stroma
- Lack of cytoplasmic inclusions
- No/focal expression of actins
- Frequent expression of EMA

Desmoid Fibromatosis
- Involves proximal extremities, trunk
- Occurs usually in deep soft tissues

DIGITAL FIBROMATOSIS (INFANTILE DIGITAL FIBROMATOSIS)

Immunohistochemistry

Antibody	Reactivity	Staining Pattern	Comment
Actin-sm	Positive	Cytoplasmic inclusion	Parallel positivity beneath cell membrane; eosinophilic globules are variably positive
Desmin	Positive	Cytoplasmic	
Calponin	Positive	Cytoplasmic	
CD99	Positive	Cytoplasmic	
Caldesmon	Negative		
S100	Negative		
EMA	Negative		
AE1/AE3	Negative		
β-catenin	Negative		Can display nonspecific cytoplasmic labeling, but no nuclear staining
CD34	Negative		

- Locally aggressive
- High rate of local recurrences
- Nuclear expression of β-catenin
- Numerous vessels
- Perivascular edema

Superficial Solitary Fibrous Tumor
- Typically adults
- Usually well-circumscribed, nodular neoplasms
- Varying cellularity
- Numerous hemangiopericytoma-like blood vessels
- No/focal expression of actins
- Usually homogeneous CD34 and Bcl-2 expression

Myofibroma
- Can affect children and adults
- Multinodular growth
- Biphasic growth
  o Small undifferentiated mesenchymal cells associated with hemangiopericytoma-like vessels
  o Mature, spindled, eosinophilic myofibroblasts
- Myxohyaline stroma
- Lack of cytoplasmic inclusions

DIAGNOSTIC CHECKLIST

Clinically Relevant Pathologic Features
- Gross appearance
- Organ distribution
- Age distribution

Pathologic Interpretation Pearls
- Ill-defined dermal neoplasms
- Proliferation of fibroblastic/myofibroblastic tumor cells
- Bland cytology of neoplastic cells
- Tumor cells contain characteristic cytoplasmic inclusions
- Expression of actins
- Coexpression of desmin may be present

SELECTED REFERENCES

1. Laskin WB et al: Infantile digital fibroma/fibromatosis: a clinicopathologic and immunohistochemical study of 69 tumors from 57 patients with long-term follow-up. Am J Surg Pathol. 33(1):1-13, 2009
2. Niamba P et al: Further documentation of spontaneous regression of infantile digital fibromatosis. Pediatr Dermatol. 24(3):280-4, 2007
3. Plusjé LG et al: Infantile-type digital fibromatosis tumour in an adult. Br J Dermatol. 143(5):1107-8, 2000
4. Kawaguchi M et al: A case of infantile digital fibromatosis with spontaneous regression. J Dermatol. 25(8):523-6, 1998
5. Hayashi T et al: Infantile digital fibromatosis: a study of the development and regression of cytoplasmic inclusion bodies. Mod Pathol. 8(5):548-52, 1995
6. Pettinato G et al: Inclusion body fibromatosis of the breast. Two cases with immunohistochemical and ultrastructural findings. Am J Clin Pathol. 101(6):714-8, 1994
7. Choi KC et al: Infantile digital fibromatosis. Immunohistochemical and immunoelectron microscopic studies. J Cutan Pathol. 17(4):225-32, 1990
8. Viale G et al: Infantile digital fibromatosis-like tumour (inclusion body fibromatosis) of adulthood: report of two cases with ultrastructural and immunocytochemical findings. Histopathology. 12(4):415-24, 1988
9. Yun K: Infantile digital fibromatosis. Immunohistochemical and ultrastructural observations of cytoplasmic inclusions. Cancer. 61(3):500-7, 1988
10. Fringes B et al: Identification of actin microfilaments in the intracytoplasmic inclusions present in recurring infantile digital fibromatosis (Reye tumor). Pediatr Pathol. 6(2-3):311-24, 1986
11. Mukai M et al: Infantile digital fibromatosis. An electron microscopic and immunohistochemical study. Acta Pathol Jpn. 36(11):1605-15, 1986
12. Purdy LJ et al: Infantile digital fibromatosis occurring outside the digit. Am J Surg Pathol. 8(10):787-90, 1984
13. Faraggiana T et al: Ultrastructural histochemistry of infantile digital fibromatosis. Ultrastruct Pathol. 2(3):241-7, 1981
14. Iwasaki H et al: Infantile digital fibromatosis. Ultrastructural, histochemical, and tissue culture observations. Cancer. 46(10):2238-47, 1980
15. Sarma DP et al: Infantile digital fibroma-like tumor in an adult. Arch Dermatol. 116(5):578-9, 1980
16. Bhawan J et al: A myofibroblastic tumor. Infantile digital fibroma (recurrent digital fibrous tumor of childhood). Am J Pathol. 94(1):19-36, 1979

DIGITAL FIBROMATOSIS (INFANTILE DIGITAL FIBROMATOSIS)

Microscopic and Immunohistochemical Features

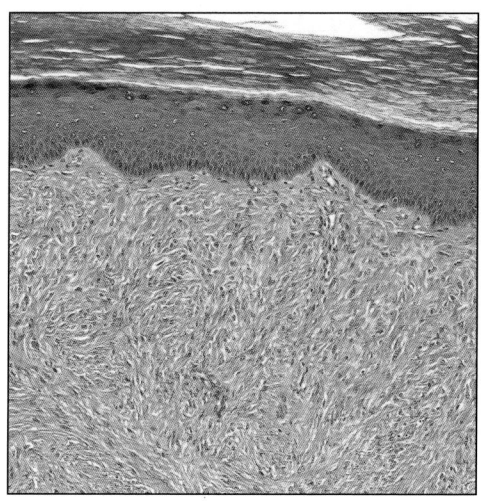

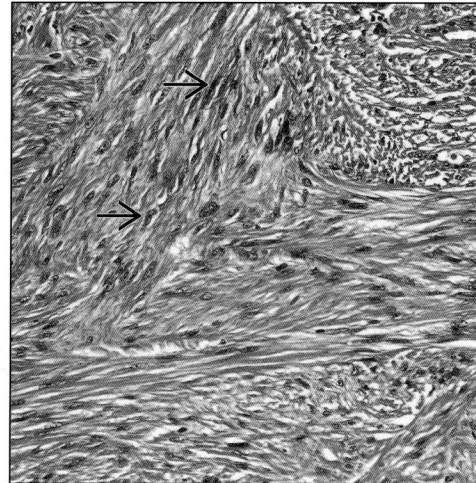

(Left) Histology of digital fibromatosis shows a moderately cellular spindle cell neoplasm of the superficial dermis. There is no grenz zone between the lesion and the overlying squamous epithelium. *(Right)* The neoplasm shows ill-defined fascicles composed of cytologically bland-appearing, spindled fibroblasts and myofibroblasts with pale eosinophilic cytoplasm and elongated, spindle-shaped nuclei ⇒.

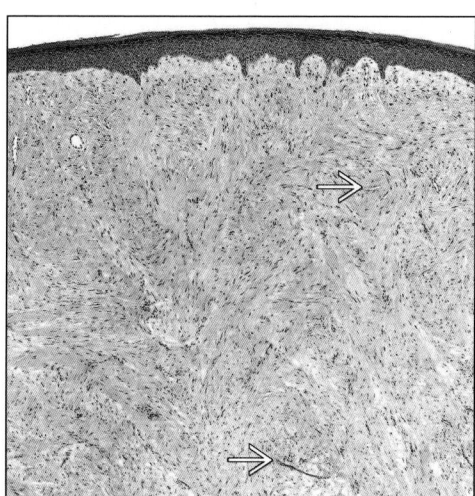

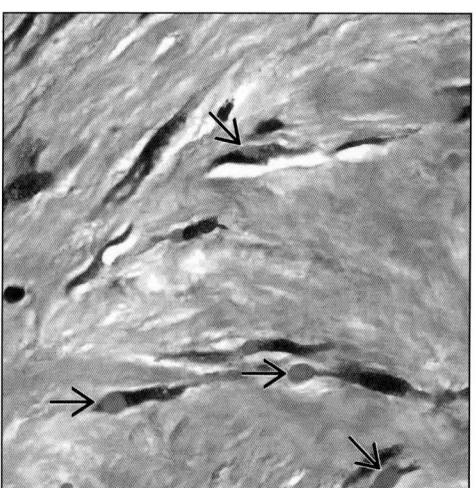

(Left) A relatively hypocellular spindle cell neoplasm is seen in this case. The neoplastic cells are set in a collagenous stroma. Since the proliferating cells are pale, the delicate stromal capillaries are readily identified ⇒. *(Right)* High magnification shows numerous cytoplasmic inclusions ⇒ in this case. The background in this field is heavily collagenized. The inclusions, believed in the past to reflect viral material, are now known to contain actin filaments.

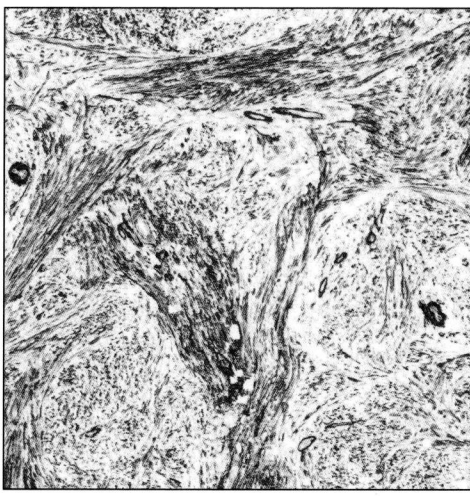

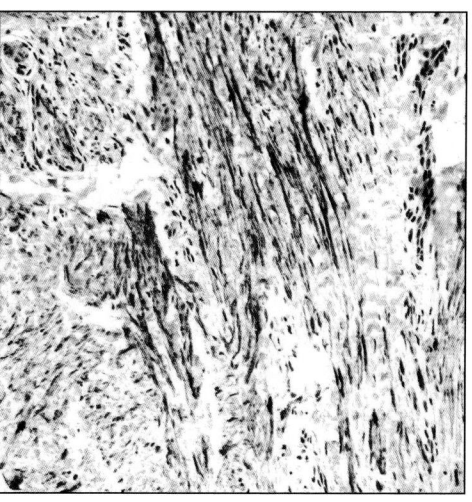

(Left) Neoplastic cells in digital fibromatosis stain positively for actin-sm in most cases. This feature indicates myofibroblastic differentiation rather than true smooth muscle differentiation. Desmin stains are usually, but not invariably, negative. In general, it is not necessary to perform immunostaining on these lesions, as their routine histologic features (with inclusion bodies) are diagnostic. *(Right)* In some cases, focal expression of desmin may be present.

ANGIOMYOFIBROBLASTOMA

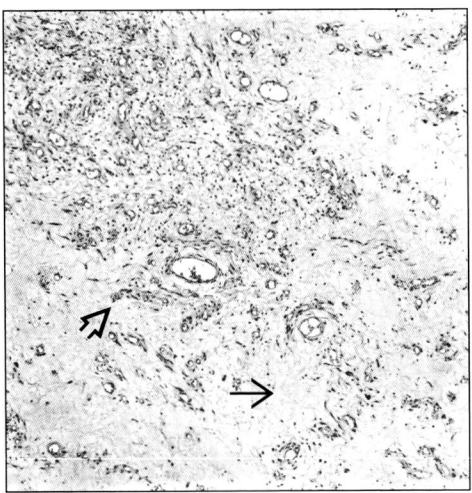

Angiomyofibroblastoma is characterized by numerous capillary-sized vessels ⊃, alternating zones of cellularity, and more fibrous areas ➔, without necrosis.

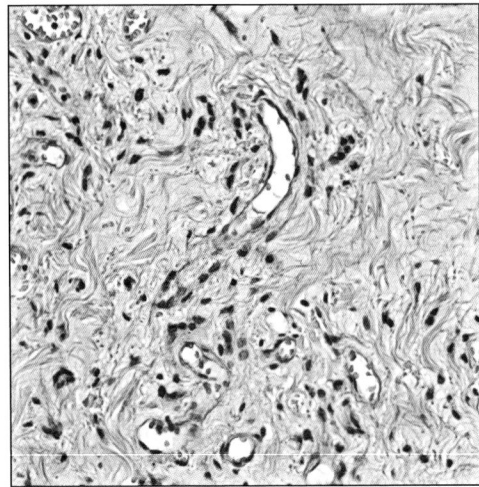

The stromal cells tend to cluster around the prominent yet delicate vascular component. The intervening tissue is sparsely cellular and contains slender collagen fibrils. The cells lack nuclear atypia.

TERMINOLOGY

Abbreviations
- Angiomyofibroblastoma (AMF)

Definitions
- Benign stromal tumor composed of numerous capillaries and myofibroblasts

ETIOLOGY/PATHOGENESIS

Cell of Origin
- Subepithelial mesenchyme of distal female genital tract

CLINICAL ISSUES

Epidemiology
- Age
  o Typically women of reproductive age

Site
- Vulva
- Vagina

Presentation
- Most common signs/symptoms
  o Painless mass
    ▪ Often thought to represent a cyst

Treatment
- Local excision

Prognosis
- Excellent
- No recurrent potential

MACROSCOPIC FEATURES

General Features
- Well circumscribed
- Tan-white
- Rubbery cut surface

Size
- Usually < 5 cm

MICROSCOPIC PATHOLOGY

Histologic Features
- Nonencapsulated
- Well demarcated
- Rich vascular component
  o Numerous thin-walled capillaries
- Alternating zones of cellularity
- Variably edematous to collagenous matrix
- Plump, ovoid (plasmacytoid) to spindle-shaped cells
  o Cells cluster around capillaries
- Less commonly may have lipomatous component
- No cytologic atypia
- Few mitoses
- Rarely, associated with sarcomatous transformation

Margins
- Well circumscribed

ANCILLARY TESTS

Immunohistochemistry
- Typically desmin(+)
- ER and PR usually positive
- S100 and CD34 variably positive
- Smooth muscle actin usually negative

ANGIOMYOFIBROBLASTOMA

Key Facts

Terminology

- Benign stromal tumor composed of numerous capillaries and myofibroblasts

Clinical Issues

- Women of reproductive age
- Arises in vulva or vagina
- Often thought to represent a cyst
- Local excision
- No recurrent potential

Microscopic Pathology

- Well demarcated
- Numerous thin-walled capillaries
- Alternating zones of cellularity
- Variably edematous to collagenous matrix
- Plump, ovoid (plasmacytoid) to spindle-shaped cells
- Cells cluster around capillaries

Ancillary Tests

- Typically desmin(+)

DIFFERENTIAL DIAGNOSIS

Deep Angiomyxoma

- Infiltrative (not circumscribed) margins
- Uniformly cellular
  - Lacks alternating zones of cellularity seen in AMF
- Less vascular; contains medium- to large-sized vessels

Cellular Angiofibroma

- More uniformly cellular
- Less vascular; contains medium-sized vessels, often with hyalinized walls
- Typically CD34(+)
- Genetic changes at 13q14

Fibroepithelial Stromal Polyp

- Typically polypoid
  - Overlying squamous epithelium
  - May have thin connecting stalk
- Vascular component tends to be central (vascular core)
  - Medium- to large-sized vessels
- Does not have distinct margin
- Stellate and multinucleate cells are characteristic
  - Often located beneath epithelial surface at epithelial-stromal interface
  - May be present around central vasculature
- Can be desmin(+)
- Can be pseudosarcomatous
  - Marked cellularity and increased mitotic activity
  - Pleomorphism
  - Atypical mitoses

DIAGNOSTIC CHECKLIST

Pathologic Interpretation Pearls

- Stromal cells tend to be spindled in tumors from postmenopausal women

SELECTED REFERENCES

1. McCluggage WG: Recent developments in vulvovaginal pathology. Histopathology. 54(2):156-73, 2009
2. Alameda F et al: Vulvar angiomyxoma, aggressive angiomyxoma, and angiomyofibroblastoma: an immunohistochemical and ultrastructural study. Ultrastruct Pathol. 30(3):193-205, 2006
3. Cao D et al: Lipomatous variant of angiomyofibroblastoma: report of two cases and review of the literature. Int J Gynecol Pathol. 24(2):196-200, 2005
4. Nucci MR et al: Vulvovaginal soft tissue tumours: update and review. Histopathology. 36(2):97-108, 2000
5. Fukunaga M et al: Vulval angiomyofibroblastoma. Clinicopathologic analysis of six cases. Am J Clin Pathol. 107(1):45-51, 1997
6. Laskin WB et al: Angiomyofibroblastoma of the female genital tract: analysis of 17 cases including a lipomatous variant. Hum Pathol. 28(9):1046-55, 1997
7. Nielsen GP et al: Angiomyofibroblastoma of the vulva and vagina. Mod Pathol. 9(3):284-91, 1996
8. Hisaoka M et al: Angiomyofibroblastoma of the vulva: a clinicopathologic study of seven cases. Pathol Int. 45(7):487-92, 1995
9. Fletcher CD et al: Angiomyofibroblastoma of the vulva. A benign neoplasm distinct from aggressive angiomyxoma. Am J Surg Pathol. 16(4):373-82, 1992

IMAGE GALLERY

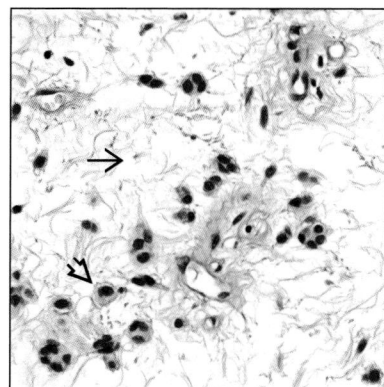 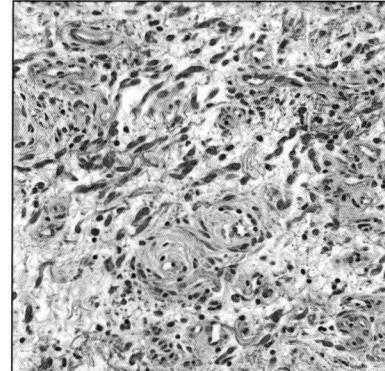 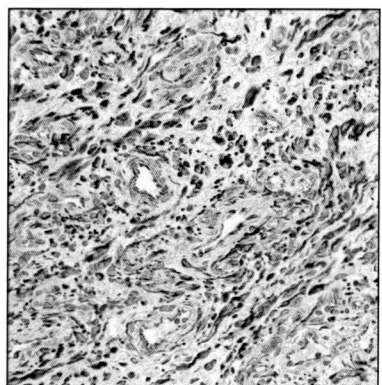

(Left) The plump plasmacytoid stromal cells ➡ surround thin-walled capillaries. Note edematous matrix ➡. *(Center)* The stromal cells are spindled in this tumor from a postmenopausal patient; however, the cells maintain their relationship to the vasculature. *(Right)* The tumor cells typically are diffusely immunoreactive for desmin, as seen here.

MULTINUCLEATE CELL ANGIOHISTIOCYTOMA

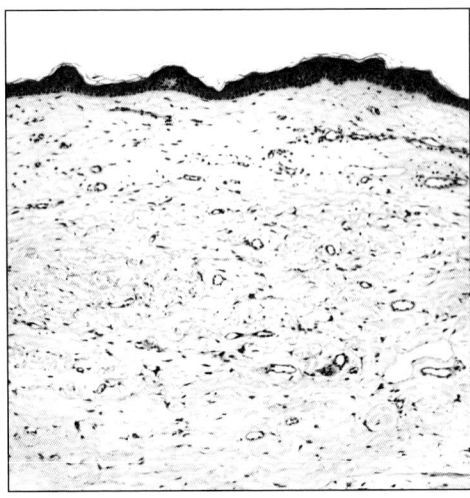

Low-power examination of multinucleate cell angiohistiocytoma shows a dermal-based proliferation of small vessels with focal telangiectasia and increased numbers of stromal cells.

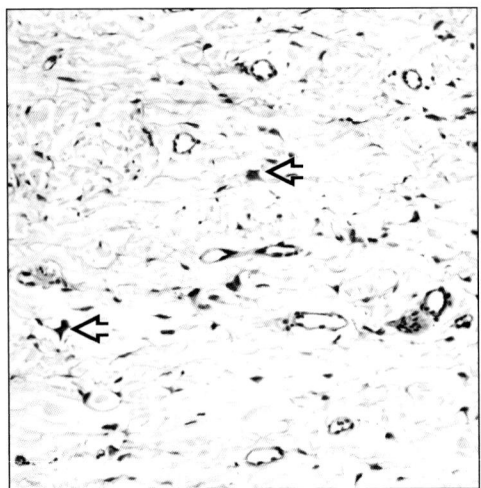

Higher power view shows a proliferation of numerous small blood vessels and scattered enlarged, angulated mononuclear and multinucleated ⧁ stromal cells.

TERMINOLOGY

Abbreviations
- Multinucleate cell angiohistiocytoma (MCAH)

Definitions
- Proliferation of vessels and multinucleated stromal cells

ETIOLOGY/PATHOGENESIS

Unknown
- May actually represent a nonneoplastic reactive process
- Some authors consider MCAH a variant of dermatofibroma

CLINICAL ISSUES

Epidemiology
- Age
  - Usually presents in patients > 40 years old
- Gender
  - Typically occurs in females

Site
- Most cases have been reported on legs (calves and thighs) or hands
  - Others sites rarely described, including oral mucosa

Presentation
- Multiple grouped round to oval papules
  - Usually described as red to violet lesions
  - May rarely be generalized
  - Rarely, may coalesce into 1 large annular lesion
- May be asymptomatic or pruritic

Prognosis
- Excellent, no malignant potential described

- Treatment not necessary; some lesions may regress spontaneously

MACROSCOPIC FEATURES

General Features
- Well-circumscribed, nonencapsulated dermal-based lesion

MICROSCOPIC PATHOLOGY

Histologic Features
- Increased numbers of superficial small to telangiectatic vessels in reticular dermis
  - Endothelial cells show hyperchromatic nuclei
  - Do not show slit-like spaces suggestive of Kaposi sarcoma
- Proliferation of enlarged, angulated multinucleated cells
  - Cells contain 3-10 nuclei, which may be arranged in a ring or aggregated together
  - Nuclear hyperchromasia and mild atypia present
    - However, no frank atypia or pleomorphism
  - Lack of, or only rare, mitotic figures
- No infiltrative features should be identified
- Surrounding stroma may show mild inflammatory infiltrate
  - Consists of lymphocytes, plasma cells, mast cells, and neutrophils

Predominant Pattern/Injury Type
- Vascular and fibrohistiocytic

ANCILLARY TESTS

Immunohistochemistry
- Multinucleated cells are typically positive for FXIIIA and vimentin

MULTINUCLEATE CELL ANGIOHISTIOCYTOMA

Key Facts

Terminology
- Proliferation of vessels and multinucleated stromal cells

Etiology/Pathogenesis
- May be nonneoplastic reactive process

Clinical Issues
- Usually occurs in patients > 40 years old
- Multiple grouped papules

- Typically in females

Microscopic Pathology
- Increased numbers of superficial small to telangiectatic vessels
- Proliferation of enlarged, angulated multinucleated cells
- No infiltrative features identified
- Nuclear hyperchromasia and mild atypia present

---

  o CD68 staining is variably positive
- Stromal cells are positive for FXIIIA, vimentin, and lysozyme
- Vessels are positive for CD31, CD34, and FVIIIRAg; HHV8 is negative

DIFFERENTIAL DIAGNOSIS

Kaposi Sarcoma
- Proliferation of atypical spindle cells and slit-like blood vessels
- Chronic infiltrate with plasma cells usually present
- Multinucleate cells not identified
- Immunoreactive for HHV8 (nuclear staining)

Giant Cell Angioblastoma
- Exceptionally rare tumor, present at birth or shortly thereafter
- Concentric arrays of spindle cells around small vessels

Pleomorphic Fibroma
- Polypoid lesion, likely related to fibroepithelial polyp
- Large, atypical-appearing multinucleated pleomorphic fibroblasts present
- Proliferation of small vessels not prominent, as in MCAH

DIAGNOSTIC CHECKLIST

Pathologic Interpretation Pearls
- Proliferation of enlarged, angulated multinucleated cells associated with numerous small vessels
  o Cells show 3-10 nuclei, which may be arranged in a ring or clumped together

SELECTED REFERENCES

1. Rawal YB et al: Multinucleate cell angiohistiocytoma: an uncommon mucosal tumour. Clin Exp Dermatol. 34(3):333-6, 2009
2. Puig L et al: Multinucleate cell angiohistiocytoma: a fibrohistiocytic proliferation with increased mast cell numbers and vascular hyperplasia. J Cutan Pathol. 29(4):232-7, 2002
3. Sass U et al: Multinucleate cell angiohistiocytoma: report of two cases with no evidence of human herpesvirus-8 infection. J Cutan Pathol. 27(5):258-61, 2000
4. Chang SN et al: Generalized multinucleate cell angiohistiocytoma. J Am Acad Dermatol. 35(2 Pt 2):320-2, 1996
5. Shapiro PE et al: Multinucleate cell angiohistiocytoma: a distinct entity diagnosable by clinical and histologic features. J Am Acad Dermatol. 30(3):417-22, 1994
6. Jones WE et al: Multinucleate cell angiohistiocytoma: an acquired vascular anomaly to be distinguished from Kaposi's sarcoma. Br J Dermatol. 122(5):651-63, 1990
7. Smolle J et al: Multinucleate cell angiohistiocytoma: a clinicopathological, immunohistochemical and ultrastructural study. Br J Dermatol. 121(1):113-21, 1989

IMAGE GALLERY

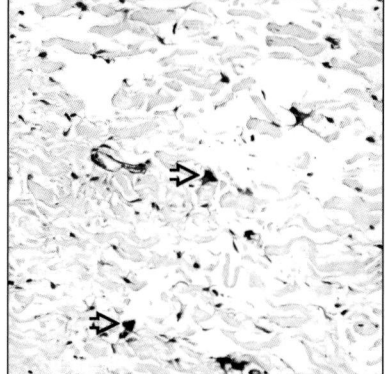 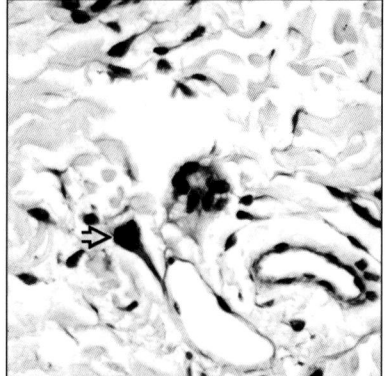 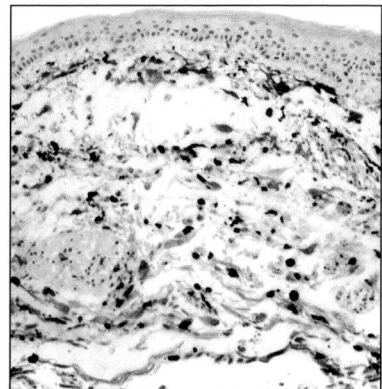

(Left) Histologic examination of MCAH shows scattered enlarged multinucleated cells ⊵ with nuclear hyperchromasia. *(Center)* High-power examination of the multinucleated cells shows clumping or a wreath-like arrangement of the hyperchromatic nuclei ⊵. *(Right)* FXIIIA immunohistochemistry shows strong cytoplasmic staining of most of the lesional cells.

GIANT CELL TUMOR OF TENDON SHEATH

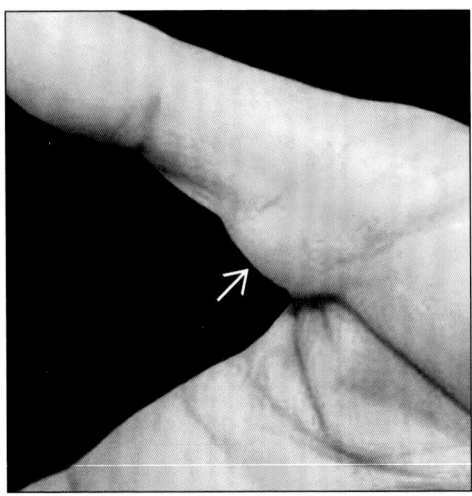

Giant cell tumor of tendon sheath presents as a painless, slow-growing mass that arises from a tendon sheath, most often on the volar aspect of a finger ➡. Secondary skin involvement is rare.

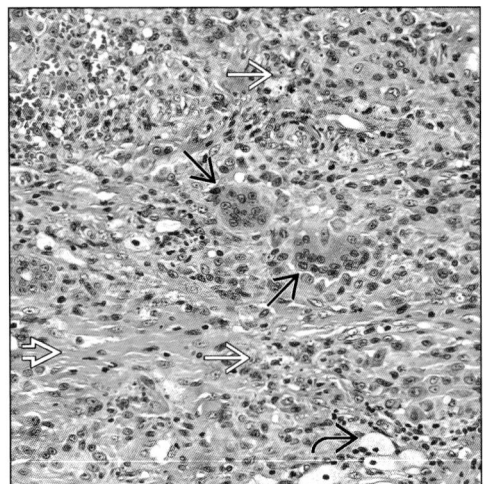

GCTTS has a mixture of mononuclear stromal cells, multinucleated giant cells ➡, and macrophages, including xanthoma cells ➡. Stromal fibrosis ➡ and hemosiderin deposits ➡ are very common.

TERMINOLOGY

Abbreviations
- Giant cell tumor of tendon sheath (GCTTS)

Synonyms
- Localized tenosynovial giant cell tumor, localized pigmented villonodular synovitis (PVNS), nodular tenosynovitis

Definitions
- Benign soft tissue tumor of synovial origin
  - Polymorphous population of neoplastic stromal cells, macrophages, and osteoclast-like giant cells
  - Well circumscribed, noninvasive

ETIOLOGY/PATHOGENESIS

Histogenesis
- Neoplastic growth
  - Balanced translocation involving 1p13 (CSF1 gene) in many tumors
    - CSF1 overexpression by neoplastic stromal cells
    - Recruitment and activation of intratumoral macrophages by CSF1R activation

CLINICAL ISSUES

Epidemiology
- Incidence
  - 2nd most common tumor of hand
- Age
  - Any age; peak 3rd-4th decade
- Gender
  - Women outnumber men 2:1

Site
- Digits (85%)
  - Especially fingers (75%)
  - Tendon sheath (usually volar) or interphalangeal joint
- Large joints (10%)
  - Ankle, knee, wrist, elbow
  - Bursa
  - Intraarticular tumors called localized PVNS
- Skin secondarily involved in < 5% of cases

Presentation
- Painless mass
- Slow growing
- Uncommon findings: Triggering, carpal and ulnar tunnel syndromes

Treatment
- Surgical approaches
  - Complete local excision

Prognosis
- Benign, but recurs locally (around 20%)
- Risk factors for recurrence: Degenerative joint disease, distal phalanx, interphalangeal joint of thumb, osseous erosion

IMAGE FINDINGS

Radiographic Findings
- Soft tissue mass
- Cortical bony erosion (10%)
  - Rarely invades bone to mimic primary bone tumor

MR Findings
- Lobulated mass with low T1 and T2 signals

MACROSCOPIC FEATURES

General Features
- Well-circumscribed mass
- Partially encapsulated
- Lobular configuration with surface clefting

GIANT CELL TUMOR OF TENDON SHEATH

Key Facts

Terminology
- Localized tenosynovial giant cell tumor, localized PVNS, nodular tenosynovitis

Etiology/Pathogenesis
- Balanced translocation involving 1p13 (*CSF1* gene) in many tumors
- Arises from tendon sheath, intraarticular site, or bursa

Clinical Issues
- 2nd most common tumor of hand
- Any age; peak 3rd-4th decade
- Digits (85%)
- Large joints (10%)
- Intraarticular tumors called localized PVNS
- Benign but recurs locally (around 20%)
- Rarely involves overlying skin

Macroscopic Features
- Average size: 1.1 cm (range: 0.5-6 cm)
- Well demarcated
- Multinodular with fibrous septa

Microscopic Pathology
- Polymorphous population of stromal cells, macrophages, and osteoclast-like giant cells
- Stromal fibrosis and hemosiderin deposits
- Mitotic rate: 1-20 mitoses per 10 high-power fields (average: 5/10)

Top Differential Diagnoses
- Dermatofibroma
- Giant cell tumor of soft tissue
- Diffuse-type tenosynovial giant cell tumor/PVNS

- Variegated cut surface: Tan, red-brown, yellow

Size
- Average size: 1.1 cm (range: 0.5-6 cm)
  - Large joint tumors are bigger (average: 2 cm)

MICROSCOPIC PATHOLOGY

Histologic Features
- Well-demarcated subcutaneous mass
- Multinodular with fibrous septa
- Stromal fibrosis
  - Can appear hyalinized, mimicking osteoid
  - Can be extensive
- Hemosiderin deposits
- Dyscohesive areas may be present, rendering a pseudoglandular pattern
- Cleft-like spaces lined by synoviocytes
- Can invade dermis usually with a sharp, pushing-type border

Cytologic Features
- Polymorphous population
  - Stromal cells with pale cytoplasm and round, spindle-shaped, or reniform nuclei
  - Large epithelioid macrophages with eosinophilic cytoplasm and vesicular nuclei
  - Osteoclast-like giant cells
    - Giant cells can be sparse in some tumors
  - Xanthoma cells and siderophages
- Mitotic rate: 1-20 mitoses per 10 high-power fields (average: 5/10)

ANCILLARY TESTS

Immunohistochemistry
- Stromal cells: CD68, few cells SMA, desmin in 50% of tumors
- Giant cells: CD68, CD45, TRAP

DIFFERENTIAL DIAGNOSIS

Dermatofibroma
- Spindle cells arranged in storiform pattern with collagen trapping
- Infiltrative growth pattern within dermis
- Touton-like giant cells

Giant Cell Tumor of Soft Tissue
- More uniform, less polymorphous mononuclear stromal cell population
- Less stromal fibrosis
- Often encased by shell of bone

Diffuse-type Tenosynovial Giant Cell Tumor
- Similar microscopically to GCTTS
- Diffuse intraarticular tumors form villonodular masses: Pigmented villonodular synovitis (PVNS)
  - Large joints, knee most common site
- Diffuse extraarticular tumors invade adjacent tissues
  - Often have fewer giant cells and less lobular architecture

SELECTED REFERENCES

1. Williams J et al: Recurrence of giant cell tumors in the hand: a prospective study. J Hand Surg Am. 35(3):451-6, 2010
2. Darwish FM et al: Giant cell tumour of tendon sheath: experience with 52 cases. Singapore Med J. 49(11):879-82, 2008
3. Cupp JS et al: Translocation and expression of CSF1 in pigmented villonodular synovitis, tenosynovial giant cell tumor, rheumatoid arthritis and other reactive synovitides. Am J Surg Pathol. 31(6):970-6, 2007
4. Nilsson M et al: Molecular cytogenetic mapping of recurrent chromosomal breakpoints in tenosynovial giant cell tumors. Virchows Arch. 441(5):475-80, 2002
5. Reilly KE et al: Recurrent giant cell tumors of the tendon sheath. J Hand Surg Am. 24(6):1298-302, 1999
6. Ushijima M et al: Giant cell tumor of the tendon sheath (nodular tenosynovitis). A study of 207 cases to compare the large joint group with the common digit group. Cancer. 57(4):875-84, 1986

Radiographic, Gross, and Microscopic Features

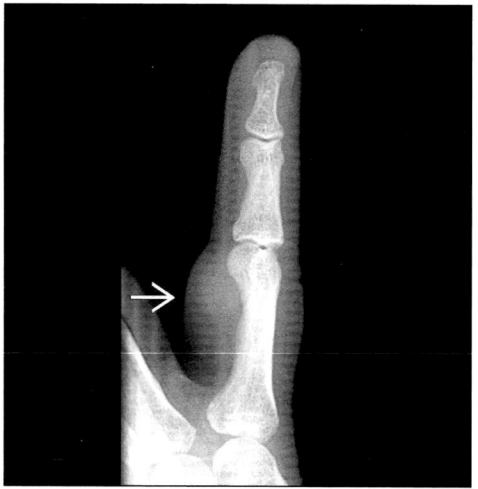
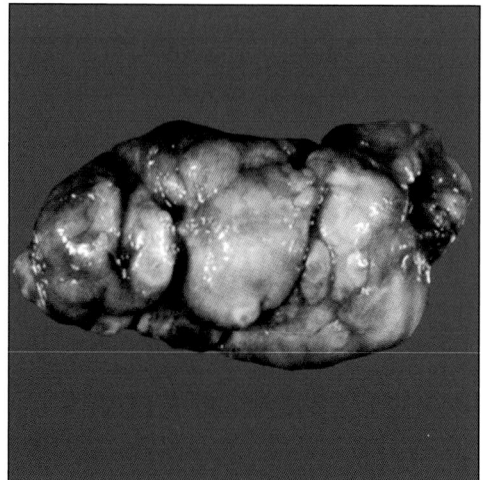

(Left) *Radiographically, GCTTS presents as a soft tissue mass* ➡ *most frequently located on the palmar side of a finger as depicted. Around 10% erode the cortex of adjacent bone, as in this example.* **(Right)** *Grossly, GCTTS is well demarcated, yellow to red-brown, and typically has a lobular configuration with surface clefting as depicted. Average size is 1.1 cm, ranging from 0.5-6 cm.*

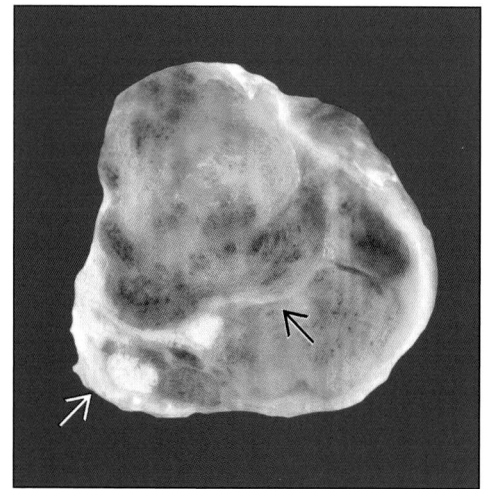
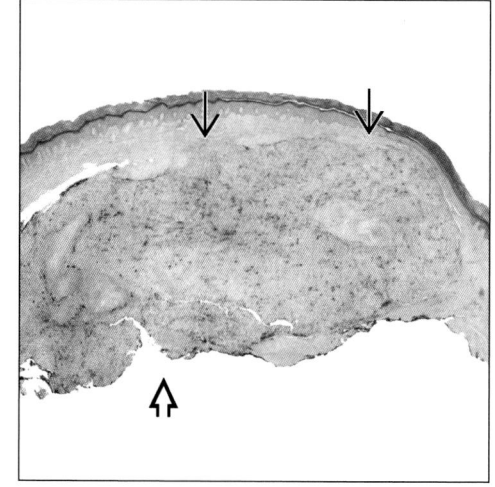

(Left) *GCTTS is well circumscribed, partially encapsulated, and has a multinodular, variegated appearance on cut surface. In this example, fibrous septa* ➡ *divide and surround tumor nodules. Mottled areas of tan, gold, red-brown, and yellow are present. The bright yellow areas* ➡ *represent xanthoma cells.* **(Right)** *GCTTS secondarily involves skin in < 5% of cases. This GCTTS extends into dermis with sharp demarcation* ➡ *and ragged undersurface where it was excised off a tendon* ➡.

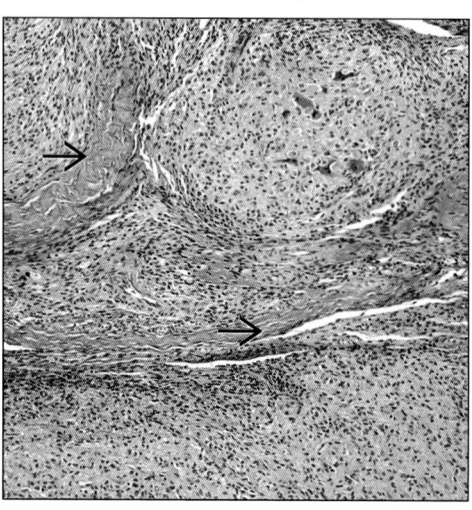
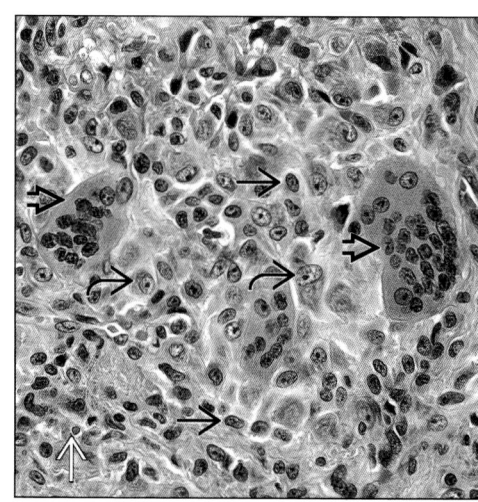

(Left) *The lobular/multinodular architecture of GCTTS is highlighted by this low-power micrograph. Note the long, thick fibrous septa* ➡ *that divide the tumor into nodules.* **(Right)** *GCTTS is composed of a polymorphous population of mononuclear stromal cells with small round, spindled, or reniform nuclei* ➡, *epithelioid macrophages with abundant eosinophilic cytoplasm and larger vesicular nuclei* ➡, *and osteoclast-like giant cells* ➡. *Note the hemosiderin deposits* ➡.

Microscopic Features

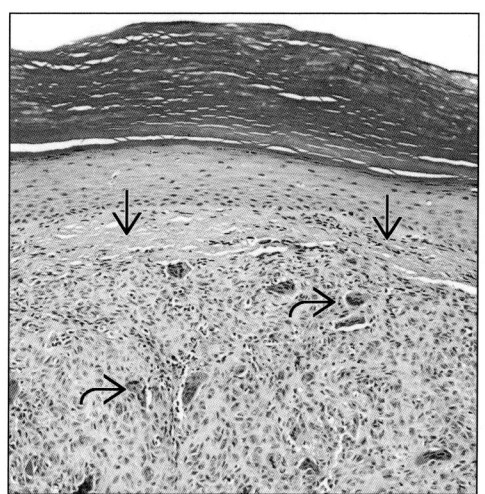

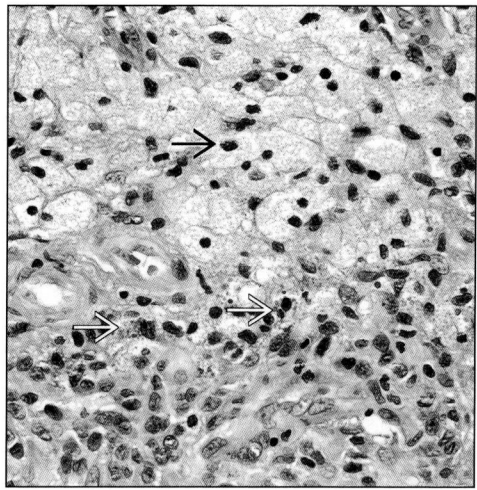

(Left) Unlike dermatofibroma, GCTTS has a sharp, noninfiltrative border with the dermis ➡ and numerous osteoclast-like giant cells ➡, which are rarely seen in dermatofibromas, and more often contain Touton-like giant cells. (Right) Sheets & clusters of xanthoma cells are very frequent in GCTTS. Xanthoma cells (foamy macrophages) have copious finely vacuolated cytoplasm and small central nuclei ➡. Siderophages (hemosiderin-laden macrophages) ➡ are also common.

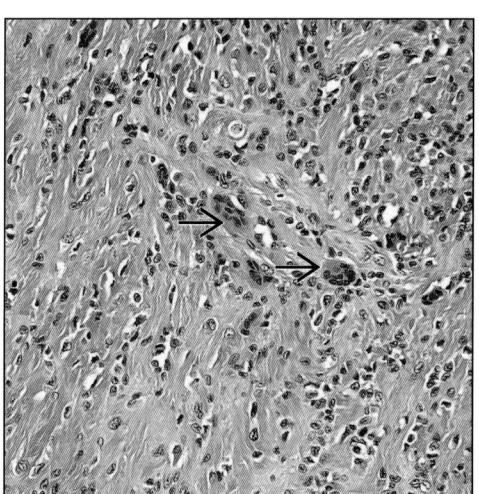

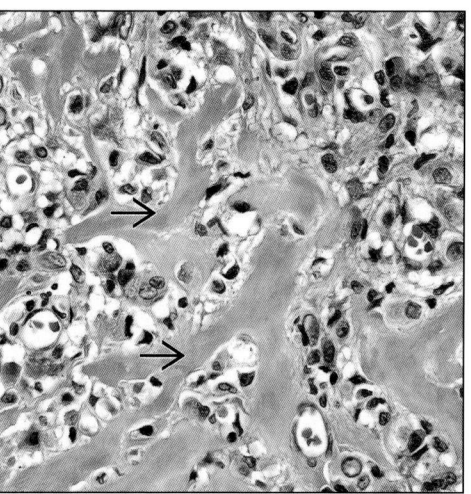

(Left) Occasionally, fibrosis can be very extensive, affecting large areas of a tumor. This low-power micrograph shows diffuse stromal fibrosis that entraps mononuclear cells and multinucleated giant cells ➡. (Right) Stromal fibrosis is invariably present in GCTTS, but highly variable in its extent. In some instances it consists of lace-like, hyalinized collagen that resembles osteoid ➡.

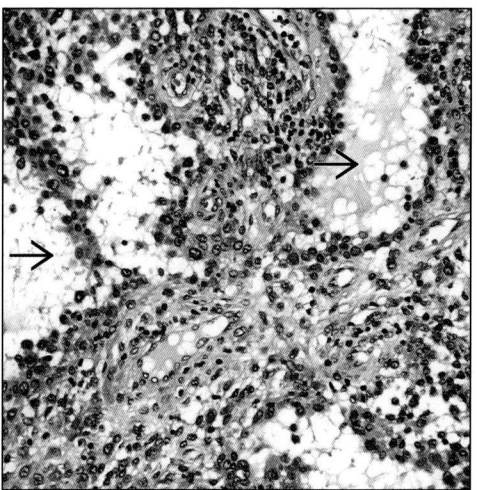

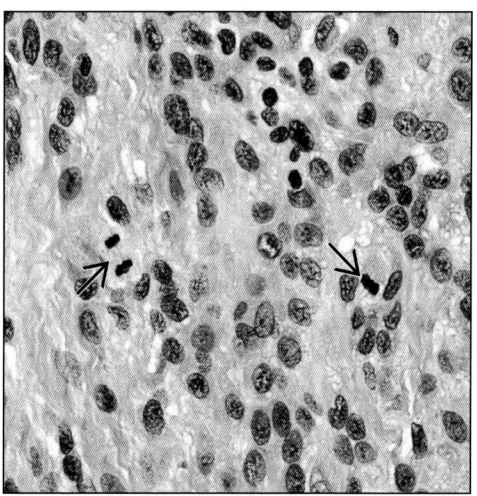

(Left) Areas of cellular dyscohesion are not uncommon in GCTTS. In some tumors, it can be so pronounced as to form cystic spaces ➡, creating a pseudoglandular pattern. (Right) Mitotic activity ranges from 1-20 mitoses per 10 HPF (average: 5/10). Brisk mitotic activity therefore is not uncommon, as in this example that shows 2 mitotic figures in a single field ➡.

MYOFIBROMA AND MYOFIBROMATOSIS

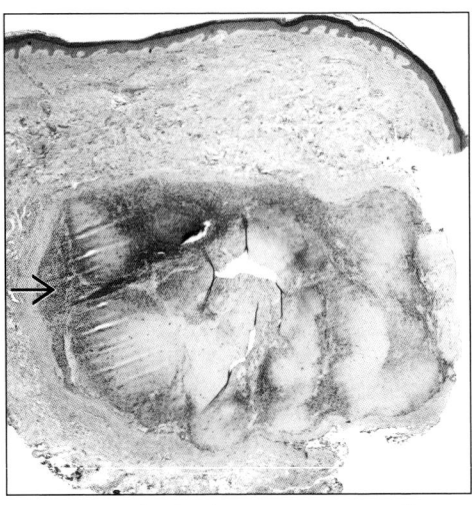

Scanning magnification shows a cutaneous myofibroma. Note the multilobulated appearance. In this example, the darker hemangiopericytoma-like component is at the periphery ⊒ of the tumor.

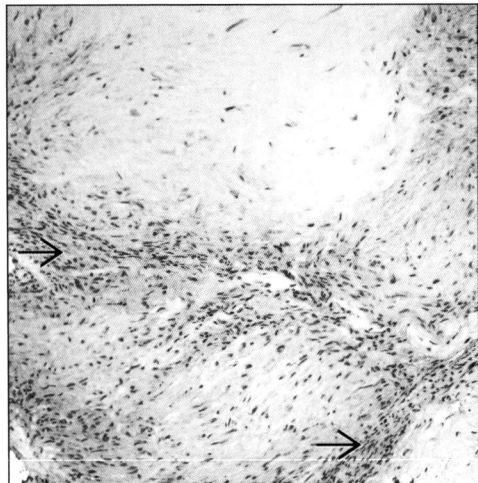

Higher magnification shows myoid lobules separated by more cellular areas. The myoid cells show cytoplasmic eosinophilia ⊒.

TERMINOLOGY

Synonyms
- Infantile myofibromatosis, congenital generalized fibromatosis
  - Continuum with lesions termed "myopericytoma" and "infantile hemangiopericytoma"

Definitions
- Benign neoplasms composed of lobules of myoid cells separated by vascularized zones (biphasic pattern)
  - Solitary form (myofibroma)
  - Multicentric form (myofibromatosis)

CLINICAL ISSUES

Epidemiology
- Incidence
  - Solitary form rare, but more common than multicentric form
  - Multicentric form extremely rare
  - Rare familial cases
- Age
  - Wide age range (neonates to elderly)
  - Most common from birth to 2 years
- Gender
  - Male predominance

Site
- Most solitary examples in subcutaneous tissues of head and neck
  - Trunk, extremities
  - Occasional skeletal example, especially skull
- Multicentric form usually involves soft tissue and bone
  - Usually long bones
  - Visceral sites
    - Gastrointestinal tract
    - Liver, kidney, pancreas

Presentation
- Asymptomatic skin nodules with purplish color (solitary form)
- Visceral lesions with site specific presentations
- Bone lesions seen as multiple elongated radiolucencies in metaphysis

Treatment
- Simple excision for solitary lesions
- Selective excisions for multicentric form

Prognosis
- Excellent for solitary form
- Outcome for multicentric form is function of involved sites
  - Extensive lung involvement poor prognostic factor

MICROSCOPIC PATHOLOGY

Histologic Features
- Most lesions well marginated
  - Can be locally infiltrative with intravascular and osseous extension and foci of necrosis
- Biphasic pattern
  - Myoid nodules separated by cellular pockets with hemangiopericytoma-like vascular pattern
  - Variable amounts of each component
  - Most cases have minimal atypia and mitotic activity
- Spindle cell areas
  - Prominent beneath ulcerated mucosal surfaces
- Myoid nodules
  - Pink cytoplasm and round to tapered nuclei
  - Myxoid change or hyalinization
- Hemangiopericytoma-like areas
  - Cellular but with minimal mitotic activity
  - Round cells similar to glomus cells

MYOFIBROMA AND MYOFIBROMATOSIS

Key Facts

Terminology

- Benign neoplasms composed of lobules of myoid cells separated by vascularized zones (biphasic pattern)
  - Solitary form (myofibroma)
  - Multicentric form (myofibromatosis)
- Synonyms: Infantile myofibromatosis, congenital generalized fibromatosis
  - Continuum with lesions termed "myopericytoma, infantile hemangiopericytoma"

Clinical Issues

- Most common from birth to 2 years
- Most solitary examples in subcutaneous tissues of head and neck
- Simple excision for solitary lesions
- Outcome for multicentric form is function of involved sites
  - Extensive lung involvement poor prognostic factor

Microscopic Pathology

- Biphasic pattern classic
- Myoid nodules separated by cellular pockets with hemangiopericytoma-like vascular pattern
- Variable amounts of each component may be present
- Most cases have minimal atypia and mitotic activity
- Spindle cell areas
  - Often prominent beneath ulcerated mucosal surfaces

Ancillary Tests

- Usually label with α-actin and calponin, but negative to focal desmin, caldesmon
- Negative S100 protein and keratin
- No characteristic alterations or mutations

Immunohistochemistry

Antibody	Reactivity	Staining Pattern	Comment
α-1-antichymotrypsin	Positive	Cytoplasmic	Strong labeling in myoid component, minimal in vascular portion
Vimentin	Positive	Cytoplasmic	All components label
S100	Negative		
CD34	Negative		Occasional focal labeling
CK-PAN	Negative		
Desmin	Equivocal	Cytoplasmic	Usually focal and weak (or negative)
Caldesmon	Equivocal	Cytoplasmic	Focal in myofibroma; more labeling in myopericytoma

ANCILLARY TESTS

Immunohistochemistry

- Usually label with α-actin and calponin, but not desmin or caldesmon
- Negative S100 protein and keratin

Cytogenetics

- No characteristic alterations or mutation

DIFFERENTIAL DIAGNOSIS

Smooth Muscle Tumors

- Not lobulated
- Perpendicularly oriented fascicles, cigar-shaped nuclei
- Express actins, desmin, caldesmon

Fibromatosis

- Highly infiltrative growth pattern; sweeping fascicles of myofibroblasts
- Express actins, usually not desmin; nuclear β-catenin labeling
- β-catenin and APC mutations

Hemangiopericytoma

- No myoid areas
- Infantile form on continuum with myofibroma

SELECTED REFERENCES

1. Dray MS et al: Myopericytoma: a unifying term for a spectrum of tumours that show overlapping features with myofibroma. A review of 14 cases. J Clin Pathol. 59(1):67-73, 2006
2. Gengler C et al: Solitary fibrous tumour and haemangiopericytoma: evolution of a concept. Histopathology. 48(1):63-74, 2006
3. Mentzel T et al: Myopericytoma of skin and soft tissues: clinicopathologic and immunohistochemical study of 54 cases. Am J Surg Pathol. 30(1):104-13, 2006
4. Montgomery E et al: Myofibromas presenting in the oral cavity: a series of 9 cases. Oral Surg Oral Med Oral Pathol Oral Radiol Endod. 89(3):343-8, 2000
5. Granter SR et al: Myofibromatosis in adults, glomangiopericytoma, and myopericytoma: a spectrum of tumors showing perivascular myoid differentiation. Am J Surg Pathol. 22(5):513-25, 1998
6. Coffin CM et al: Congenital generalized myofibromatosis: a disseminated angiocentric myofibromatosis. Pediatr Pathol Lab Med. 15(4):571-87, 1995
7. Smith KJ et al: Cutaneous myofibroma. Mod Pathol. 2(6):603-9, 1989
8. Jennings TA et al: Infantile myofibromatosis. Evidence for an autosomal-dominant disorder. Am J Surg Pathol. 8(7):529-38, 1984
9. Chung EB et al: Infantile myofibromatosis. Cancer. 48(8):1807-18, 1981

Microscopic Features

(Left) Histologic examination shows a prominent lobular configuration in a myofibroma. Note the biphasic appearance; the upper portion of the field shows a prominent hemangiopericytomatous vascular pattern ⇨. *(Right)* Many vessels are typically present at the periphery of a myoid nodule in a myofibroma. The stroma has a chondromyxoid appearance.

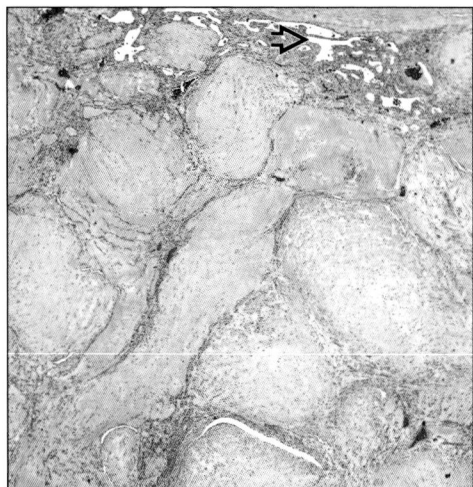
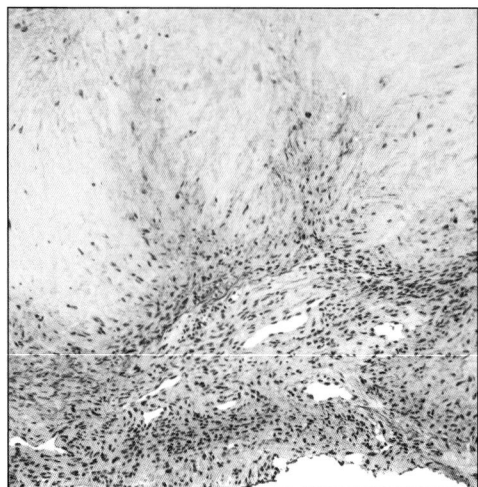

(Left) Higher magnification shows the hemangiopericytoma-like component of a myofibroma. *(Right)* High magnification shows the myoid cells in a myofibroma. Many of the cells have prominent cytoplasmic eosinophilia ⇨, and there are delicate amphophilic cytoplasmic processes ⇨.

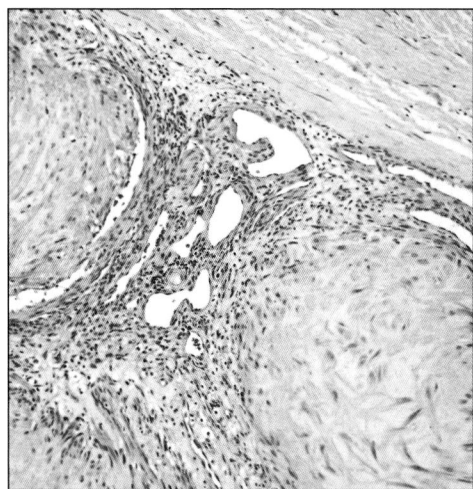
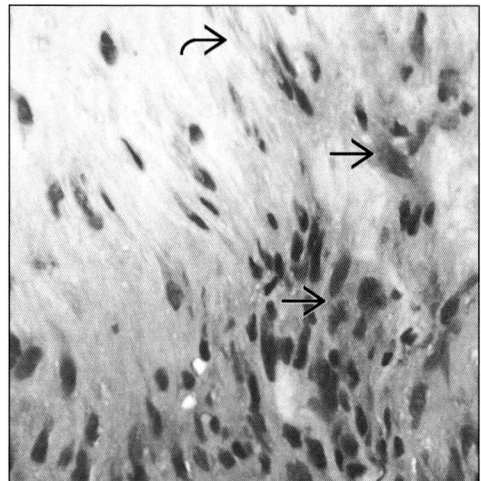

(Left) This is an example of a skeletal myofibroma. There is a vaguely lobulated appearance, and the tumor is infiltrative at the periphery. There is also focal necrosis ⇨. *(Right)* High magnification shows a myofibroma of the parotid region of a child. The spindle cells are arranged in nodules.

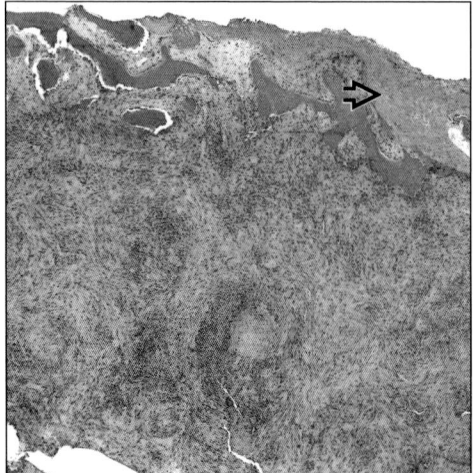
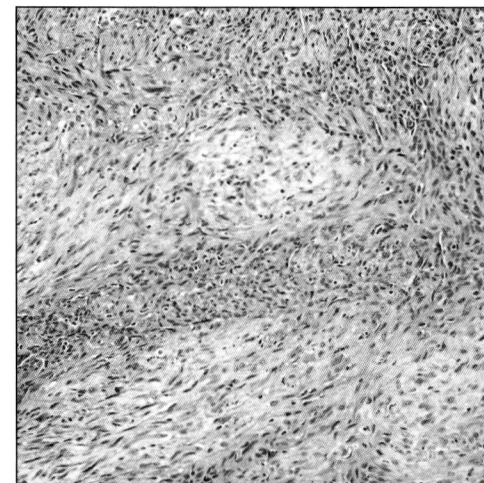

Variant Microscopic Features

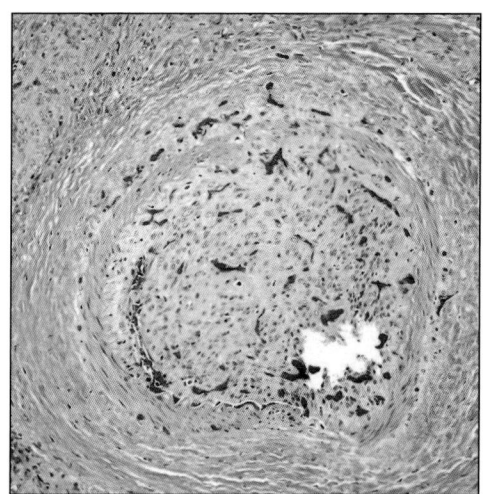
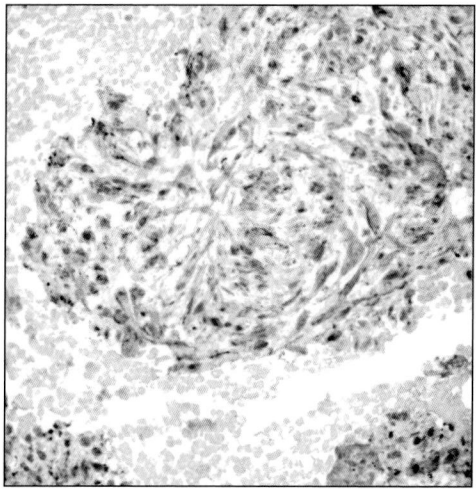

(Left) Histologic examination shows vascular space invasion in a myofibroma. This feature can lead to an erroneous interpretation of malignancy. (Right) Actin-HHF-35 shows cytoplasmic labeling in a myofibroma.

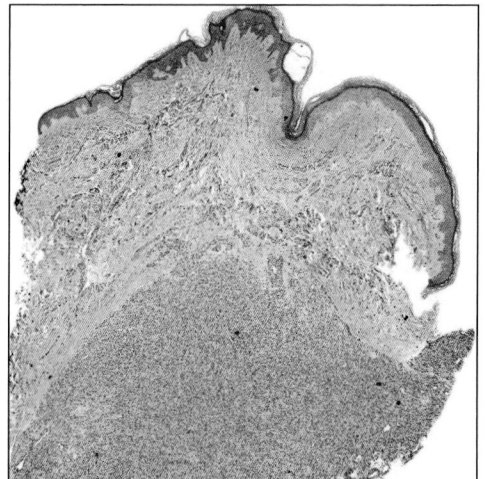
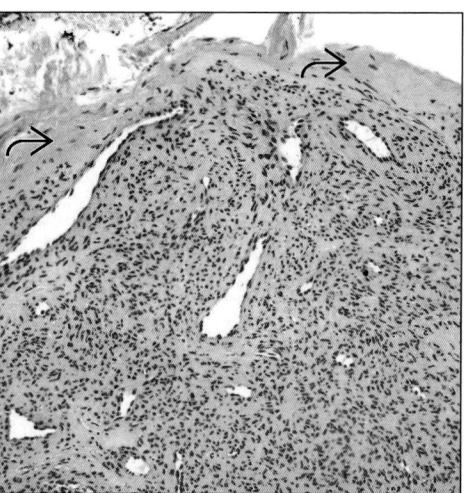

(Left) Low magnification shows a lesion that has a predominance of hemangiopericytoma-like areas. This lesion should be regarded as "myopericytoma," a tumor that is on a continuum with myofibroma. (Right) Higher magnification shows a cutaneous myopericytoma. Subtle myoid features can be appreciated, particularly at the edge of the nodule ➘.

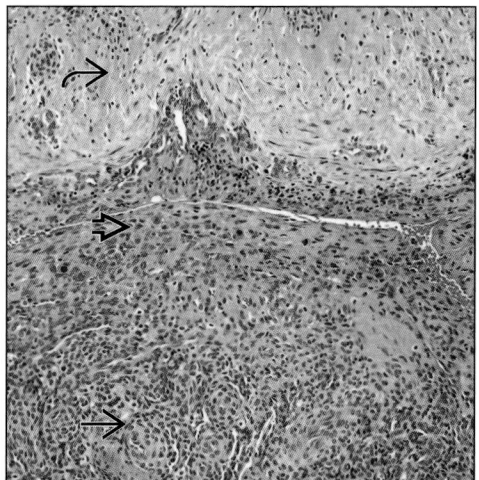
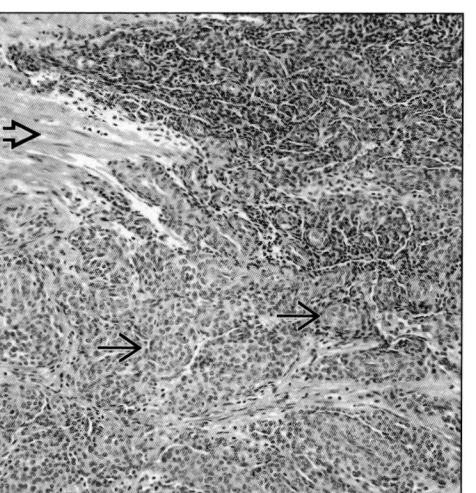

(Left) A lesion with myoid ➘, whorled hemangiopericytomatous ➘, and glomus cell ➘ areas is shown. Such a lesion would be classified as a myopericytoma. (Right) Another field from a myopericytoma shows cellular areas that are alarming but have negligible mitotic activity. Note the myoid area ➘ and whorled areas ➘.

CUTANEOUS MYXOMA AND ANGIOMYXOMA

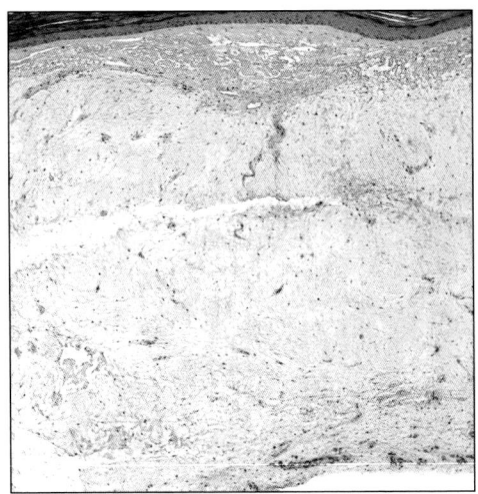

Cutaneous myxomas are dermal-based tumors characterized by a hypocellular proliferation of bland spindled cells and abundant myxoid stroma.

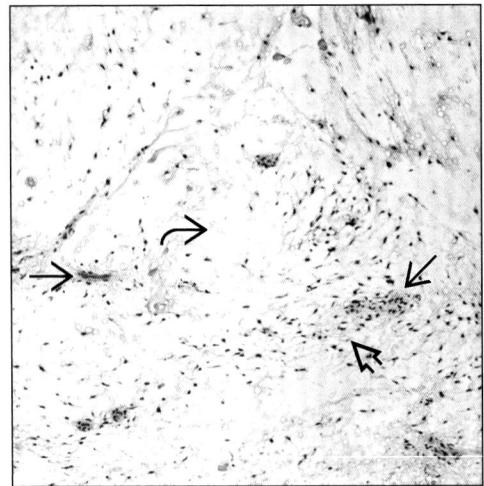

Intermediate magnification shows that the spindled cells are associated with a capillary vasculature ➡. Often there are subtly more cellular ➡ and less cellular ➡ areas.

TERMINOLOGY

Synonyms
- Superficial angiomyxoma

Definitions
- Benign mesenchymal proliferation of spindled to stellate fibroblasts in abundant myxoid stroma

ETIOLOGY/PATHOGENESIS

Some Cases Associated with Carney Complex
- Carney complex
  - Also known as NAME (nevi, atrial myxomas, myxoid neurofibromas, and ephelides) and LAMB (lentigines, atrial myxomas, and blue nevi) syndromes
  - Multiple cutaneous myxomas
  - Endocrine overactivity
  - Psammomatous melanotic schwannoma

CLINICAL ISSUES

Epidemiology
- Incidence
  - Relatively uncommon lesions
- Age
  - Present in adults

Presentation
- Papule, nodule, or polypoid lesion

Treatment
- Surgical approaches: Simple excision is curative

Prognosis
- Benign
  - Local recurrence common (up to ~ 20%)
  - No risk of metastasis

MICROSCOPIC PATHOLOGY

Histologic Features
- Dermal-based tumor that may extend into subcutis
- Poorly circumscribed, multinodular growth pattern
- Relatively hypocellular proliferation of bland spindled to stellate-shaped fibroblasts
  - Cellularity is not uniform
    - Subtle variations in cellularity with relatively more and less cellular areas
- Abundant myxoid stroma
- Thin-walled blood vessels
- Stromal neutrophils common
- May have associated epithelial proliferation
  - May demonstrate basaloid proliferation in overlying epidermis (similar to dermatofibroma)
  - Rarely associated with benign adnexal tumors
  - Usually the result of proliferation of entrapped adnexal tumors

DIFFERENTIAL DIAGNOSIS

Focal Cutaneous Mucinosis
- Dermal mucin between collagen bundles of the reticular dermis
- Lacks multinodular growth pattern
- Lacks tumor-associated vasculature
- Lacks secondary epithelial proliferation

Myxoid Dermatofibrosarcoma Protuberans (DFSP)
- Randomly arranged spindled to stellate cells in myxoid stroma
- More uniform cellularity
- Areas of conventional DFSP present in > 60% of cases

CUTANEOUS MYXOMA AND ANGIOMYXOMA

Key Facts

Etiology/Pathogenesis

- May be associated with Carney complex (also known as NAME and LAMB syndromes)
  - If patient has multiple cutaneous myxomas, consider the possibility of Carney complex

Microscopic Pathology

- Relatively hypocellular proliferation of bland spindled to stellate fibroblasts
- Abundant myxoid stroma

- Thin-walled blood vessels
- Perivascular neutrophils common
- May have associated epithelial proliferation, usually resulting from entrapped adnexal structures

Top Differential Diagnoses

- Focal dermal mucinosis
  - Lacks associated vasculature
- Myxoid dermatofibrosarcoma protuberans
  - More uniformly cellular

- Areas with fat infiltration always at least focally present
- Stromal neutrophils less common than in angiomyxoma
- Usually strongly CD34(+) by immunohistochemistry

Perineurioma

- Swirling growth pattern
- Spindled cells with delicate, elongated cytoplasmic processes
- Positive for EMA

Myxoid Neurofibroma

- Sometimes have abundant myxoid stroma, but areas of collagenous stroma also invariably present
- Tumor cells have wavy/comma-shaped nuclei
- S100 strongly positive

Myxoid Neurothekeoma (Dermal Nerve Sheath Myxoma)

- Distinctly nested growth of spindled cells in myxoid stroma
- Nests separated by fibrous septae
- Positive for S100

Superficial Acral Fibromyxoma

- Stroma fibrous and myxoid, rather than purely myxoid
- Spindled cells may have vaguely storiform pattern
- Almost exclusively occurs on acral surfaces

DIAGNOSTIC CHECKLIST

Pathologic Interpretation Pearls

- Hypocellular tumor with abundant myxoid stroma
  - Subtle variations in cellularity present
- Tumor-associated vasculature
- Associated stromal neutrophils can be clue

SELECTED REFERENCES

1. Al-Brahim N et al: Cutaneous angiomyxoma and pilomatricoma: a new combination. Ann Diagn Pathol. 14(5):328-30, 2010
2. Satter EK: Solitary superficial angiomyxoma: an infrequent but distinct soft tissue tumor. J Cutan Pathol. 36 Suppl 1:56-9, 2009
3. Pérez Tato B et al: Superficial angiomyxoma with trichofolliculoma. Ann Diagn Pathol. 12(5):375-7, 2008
4. Mentzel T et al: Myxoid dermatofibrosarcoma protuberans: clinicopathologic, immunohistochemical, and molecular analysis of eight cases. Am J Dermatopathol. 29(5):443-8, 2007
5. Calonje E et al: Superficial angiomyxoma: clinicopathologic analysis of a series of distinctive but poorly recognized cutaneous tumors with tendency for recurrence. Am J Surg Pathol. 23(8):910-7, 1999
6. Fetsch JF et al: Superficial angiomyxoma (cutaneous myxoma): a clinicopathologic study of 17 cases arising in the genital region. Int J Gynecol Pathol. 16(4):325-34, 1997
7. Allen PW et al: Superficial angiomyxomas with and without epithelial components. Report of 30 tumors in 28 patients. Am J Surg Pathol. 12(7):519-30, 1988

IMAGE GALLERY

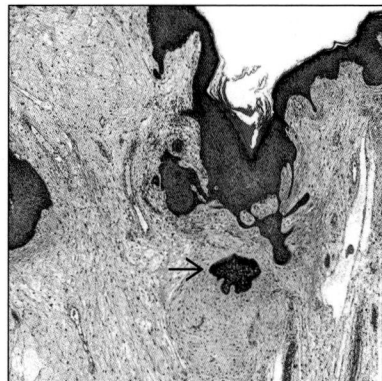 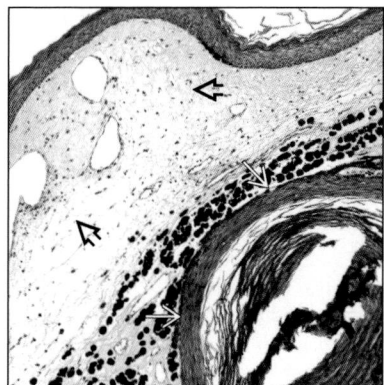 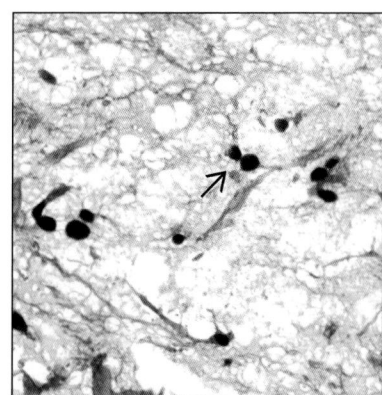

(Left) Angiomyxomas may induce a superficial proliferation of basaloid epithelium ⊉, similar to dermatofibroma. *(Center)* Entrapped adnexal structures in angiomyxomas may undergo secondary proliferation. In this case, this has resulted in the formation of an epidermoid cyst ⊉ with surrounding pigment incontinence. Note the angiomyxoma in the upper left portion of the image ⊉. *(Right)* Stromal neutrophils ⊉ are often present within cutaneous myxomas.

SUPERFICIAL ACRAL FIBROMYXOMA

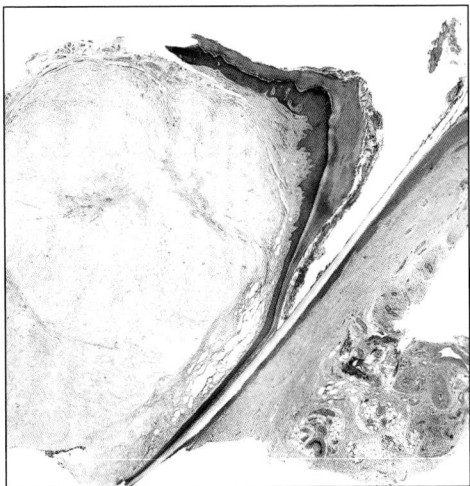

Hematoxylin & eosin at scanning magnification shows a hypocellular dermal-based myxoid neoplasm in the nail bed region.

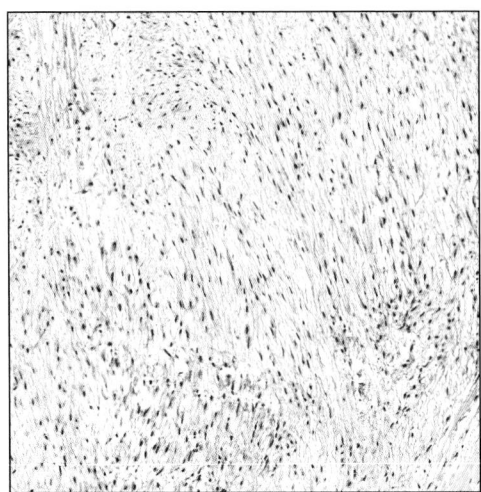

High magnification of superficial acral fibromyxoma shows a predominantly myxoid spindle cell neoplasm with variable cellularity.

TERMINOLOGY

Abbreviations
- Superficial acral fibromyxoma (SAF)

Definitions
- Benign fibroblastic neoplasm with predilection for hands and feet, especially nail bed region

ETIOLOGY/PATHOGENESIS

Environmental Exposure
- Previous trauma reported only rarely

CLINICAL ISSUES

Epidemiology
- Incidence
  - Rare
- Age
  - Mainly adults

Presentation
- Solitary mass
- Usually painless lesion

Treatment
- Surgical approaches
  - Complete excision

Prognosis
- Recurrences have been reported in up to 22%; no metastasis reported to date

MACROSCOPIC FEATURES

General Features
- Superficial lesions
- May appear dome-shaped, polypoid, or verrucoid

Size
- Usually < 5 cm

MICROSCOPIC PATHOLOGY

Histologic Features
- Nodular, lobular, or infiltrative growth
- Dermal neoplasms with involvement of deeper structures in some cases
- Myxoid, myxocollagenous, or predominantly collagenous stroma with numerous blood vessels
- May contain inflammatory cells (mast cells)
- Minimal cytologic atypia and rare mitoses
- Increased cellularity and atypia may be present, but have no prognostic influence

Predominant Pattern/Injury Type
- Storiform
- Fascicular

Predominant Cell/Compartment Type
- Spindle
  - Spindled and stellate fibroblast-like cells
  - Multinucleated stromal cells may be present

DIFFERENTIAL DIAGNOSIS

Dermatofibroma
- Hyperplastic epidermis with basilar hyperpigmentation
- Mixture of fibrous and histiocytoid cells
- Hyalinized collagenous stroma with collagen trapping
- Rarely myxoid stroma

Dermatofibrosarcoma Protuberans
- Exophytic neoplasms on trunk or proximal parts of extremities
- Infiltrating, locally destructive lesions
- Monotonous storiform growth pattern

SUPERFICIAL ACRAL FIBROMYXOMA

Key Facts

Terminology

- Benign fibroblastic neoplasm with predilection for hands and feet

Clinical Issues

- Rare tumor
- Dermal &/or subcutaneous neoplasm
- Mainly adults
- Biologically benign neoplasm with recurrences, but no metastases

Microscopic Pathology

- Dermal neoplasms with involvement of deeper structures in some cases
- Loose storiform &/or fascicular growth pattern
- Rare infiltrative growth
- Spindled and stellate fibroblast-like cells
- Minimal cytologic atypia and rare mitoses
- Scattered inflammatory cells (mast cells)
- CD34 and EMA often positive

- Diffuse infiltration of subcutaneous tissue
- Rarely myxoid
- Usually strong CD34 expression

Acral Fibrokeratoma

- Hyperkeratotic lesion often with acanthosis
- Dense connective tissue core with stellate fibroblasts

Superficial Angiomyxoma

- Lobular growth pattern
- Blood vessels with slightly fibrosed walls
- Prominent myxoid stroma
- Perivascular neutrophils

Myxoid Neurofibroma

- Elongated wrinkled nuclei
- Diffuse growth
- S100 protein positive
- Axons sometimes detectable by immunostaining for neurofilaments

DIAGNOSTIC CHECKLIST

Clinically Relevant Pathologic Features

- Organ distribution
  - Often involvement of nail bed region

Pathologic Interpretation Pearls

- Spindled and stellate fibroblast-like tumor cells
- Absence of significant nuclear pleomorphism
- Fascicular or loose storiform growth pattern

- Varying myxoid/collagenous stroma
- CD34 and EMA often positive

SELECTED REFERENCES

1. Al-Daraji WI et al: Superficial acral fibromyxoma: a clinicopathological analysis of 32 tumors including 4 in the heel. J Cutan Pathol. 35(11):1020-6, 2008
2. Misago N et al: Superficial acral fibromyxoma on the tip of the big toe: expression of CD10 and nestin. J Eur Acad Dermatol Venereol. 22(2):255-7, 2008
3. Tardío JC et al: Superficial acral fibromyxoma: report of 4 cases with CD10 expression and lipomatous component, two previously underrecognized features. Am J Dermatopathol. 30(5):431-5, 2008
4. Mentzel T et al: Myxoid dermatofibrosarcoma protuberans: clinicopathologic, immunohistochemical, and molecular analysis of eight cases. Am J Dermatopathol. 29(5):443-8, 2007
5. McNiff JM et al: Cellular digital fibromas: distinctive CD34-positive lesions that may mimic dermatofibrosarcoma protuberans. J Cutan Pathol. 32(6):413-8, 2005
6. Perret AG et al: [Superficial angiomyxoma: report of four cases, including two subungueal tumors] Ann Pathol. 25(1):54-7, 2005
7. André J et al: Superficial acral fibromyxoma: clinical and pathological features. Am J Dermatopathol. 26(6):472-4, 2004
8. Fetsch JF et al: Superficial acral fibromyxoma: a clinicopathologic and immunohistochemical analysis of 37 cases of a distinctive soft tissue tumor with a predilection for the fingers and toes. Hum Pathol. 32(7):704-14, 2001

IMAGE GALLERY

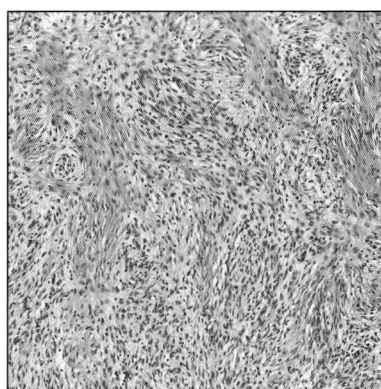 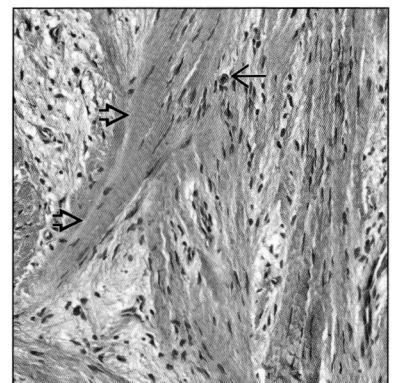 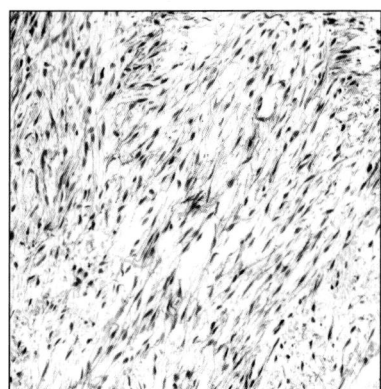

(Left) Hematoxylin & eosin of SAF shows a more cellular lesion composed of spindled tumor cells set in a varying myxoid and collagenous stroma. *(Center)* High-power view shows bland spindled tumor cells with ill-defined, pale eosinophilic cytoplasm and elongated nuclei. Note the scattered mast cells ⊐ and fibrous bands ⊳. *(Right)* Positive EMA immunohistochemistry shows moderate diffuse cytoplasmic staining.

DISTINCTIVE DERMAL CLEAR CELL MESENCHYMAL TUMOR

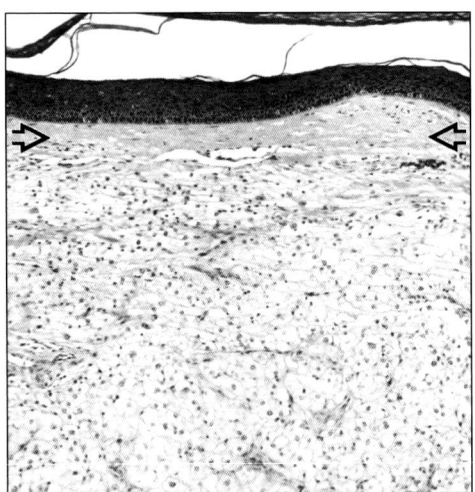

Low-power examination shows a dermal-based clear cell tumor with a thin grenz zone ⊵ separating it from the overlying epidermis. (Courtesy A. Lazar, MD, PhD.)

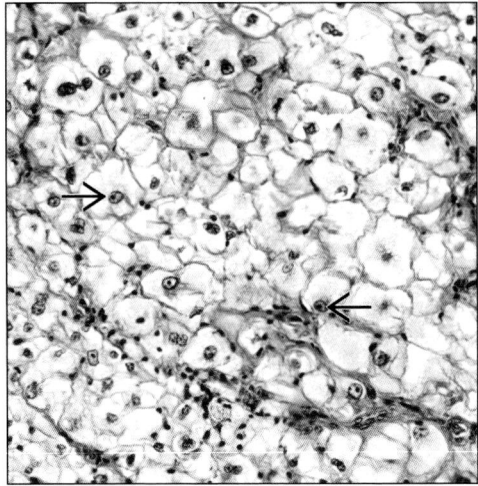

Higher magnification shows the relatively bland cytologic features of the large clear cells with vesicular nuclei, focally enlarged nucleoli ⊡, and abundant clear cytoplasm. (Courtesy A. Lazar, MD, PhD.)

TERMINOLOGY

Abbreviations
- Distinctive dermal clear cell mesenchymal tumor (DDCCMT)

Synonyms
- Distinctive dermal clear cell mesenchymal neoplasm

Definitions
- Rare, dermal-based clear cell tumor of unclear derivation

ETIOLOGY/PATHOGENESIS

Unknown
- Very rare tumors of unknown etiology

CLINICAL ISSUES

Epidemiology
- Incidence
  - Extremely rare
- Age
  - Reported in adults over age 35

Site
- Most cases have occurred on lower extremities

Presentation
- Cutaneous nodule

Treatment
- Surgical approaches
  - Complete conservative excision should be encouraged

Prognosis
- Uncertain, given rarity of this tumor, but appear to be benign or low-grade tumors

MACROSCOPIC FEATURES

General Features
- Nonencapsulated, poorly circumscribed reticular dermal-based nodule

Size
- 0.5-3 cm in greatest dimension

MICROSCOPIC PATHOLOGY

Histologic Features
- Dermal-based tumor composed of nodules of large clear cells
  - Tumors may focally infiltrate subcutaneous adipose tissue
  - Lateral borders are typically poorly circumscribed, but deep border is smooth and rounded
- Cytologically, cells are usually bland-appearing with vesicular nuclei and abundant clear cytoplasm
  - Some cases may show cytologic atypia and pleomorphism with increased numbers of mitoses

Predominant Pattern/Injury Type
- Clear cell

Predominant Cell/Compartment Type
- Mesenchymal

ANCILLARY TESTS

Immunohistochemistry
- Reportedly positive for NKI-C3/CD63 in all cases
- Variable positivity for CD68 and vimentin
- Negative for CD34, FXIIIA, and melanocytic (S100, HMB-45, MART-1/Melan-A), smooth muscle (actin-sm, desmin), and epithelial (cytokeratins) markers

DISTINCTIVE DERMAL CLEAR CELL MESENCHYMAL TUMOR

Key Facts

Terminology
- Rare, dermal-based clear cell tumor of unknown derivation

Clinical Issues
- Cutaneous nodule
- Most cases have been reported on lower extremities
- Prognosis uncertain, given rarity of this tumor, but appear to be benign or low-grade tumors

Microscopic Pathology
- Clear cell proliferation
- Cytologically, cells are usually bland-appearing, with vesicular nuclei and abundant clear cytoplasm

Top Differential Diagnoses
- Clear cell sarcoma
- Clear cell squamous cell carcinoma and tricholemmal carcinoma
- Clear cell fibrous papule

DIFFERENTIAL DIAGNOSIS

Clear Cell Sarcoma
- Packets of atypical spindled clear cells surrounded by fibrous stroma
- S100 and other melanocytic markers, such as HMB-45, MART-1/Melan-A, &/or tyrosinase typically positive
- Usually deep soft tissue tumor, may rarely involve dermis

Clear Cell Squamous Cell Carcinoma and Tricholemmal Carcinoma
- Should show more cytologic atypia and abundant mitoses than DDCCMT
- Focal epidermal attachments and areas of keratinization and dyskeratotic cells often present
- Positive for cytokeratins, especially high molecular weight (CK5/6, CK903, etc.), and p63

Clear Cell Fibrous Papule
- More superficial, often in papillary dermis with dome-shaped appearance
- Cells may show staining for CD68 and FXIIIA

Paraganglioma-like Dermal Melanocytic Tumor
- Packets of cells with clear to eosinophilic-staining cytoplasm
- Melanocytic markers, including S100, HMB-45, and MART-1/Melan-A are positive

Perivascular Epithelioid Cell Tumor (PEComa)
- Rare soft tissue tumor, which may occasionally present in skin
- Tumor cells typically show clear, palely eosinophilic, or granular cytoplasm
- Immunoreactivity for melanocytic markers, especially HMB-45, as well as actin-sm

DIAGNOSTIC CHECKLIST

Pathologic Interpretation Pearls
- Dermal-based proliferation composed of nodules of large clear cells with relatively bland cytologic features

SELECTED REFERENCES

1. Gavino AC et al: Atypical distinctive dermal clear cell mesenchymal neoplasm arising in the scalp. J Cutan Pathol. 35(4):423-7, 2008
2. Liegl B et al: Primary cutaneous PEComa: distinctive clear cell lesions of skin. Am J Surg Pathol. 32(4):608-14, 2008
3. Cassarino DS et al: Cutaneous squamous cell carcinoma: a comprehensive clinicopathologic classification--part two. J Cutan Pathol. 33(4):261-79, 2006
4. Lee AN et al: Clear cell fibrous papule with NKI/C3 expression: clinical and histologic features in six cases. Am J Dermatopathol. 27(4):296-300, 2005

IMAGE GALLERY

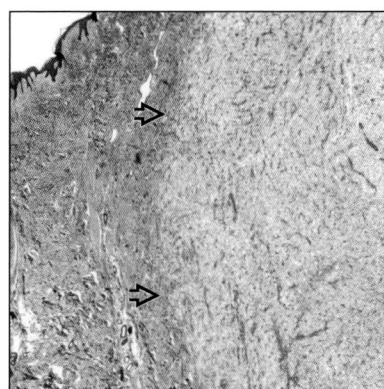 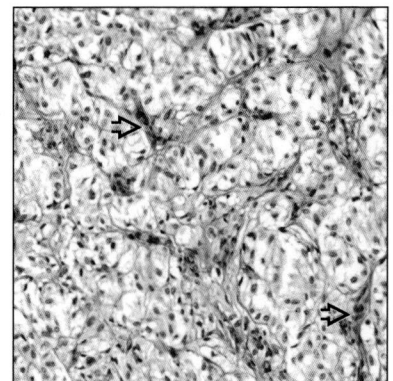 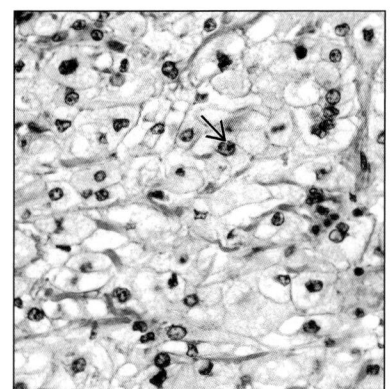

(Left) Low-power examination shows nonencapsulated lateral border ⊡ of the tumor. *(Courtesy A. Lazar, MD, PhD.)* *(Center)* Intermediate magnification shows vaguely nested appearance & numerous small caliber blood vessels ⊡ surrounding tumor cells. *(Courtesy A. Lazar, MD, PhD.)* *(Right)* Higher magnification shows relatively bland cytologic features of large clear cells, which show enlarged nuclei with vesicular chromatin & focally prominent nucleoli ⊒. Cytoplasm is predominantly clear to focally granular-appearing. *(Courtesy A. Lazar, MD, PhD.)*

PSEUDOSARCOMATOUS FIBROBLASTIC PROLIFERATIONS

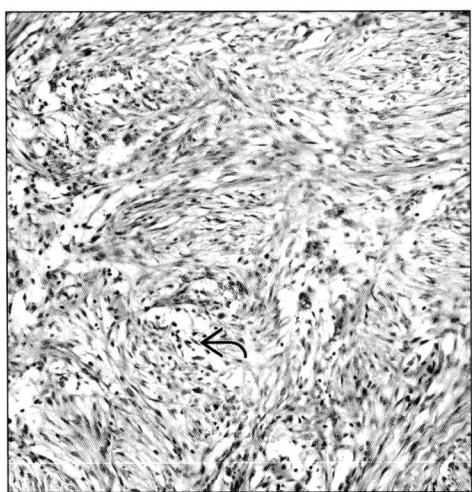

This classic image of nodular fasciitis shows a myofibroblastic lesion with a storiform pattern, cystic spaces, scattered lymphocytes ➘, and extravasated erythrocytes.

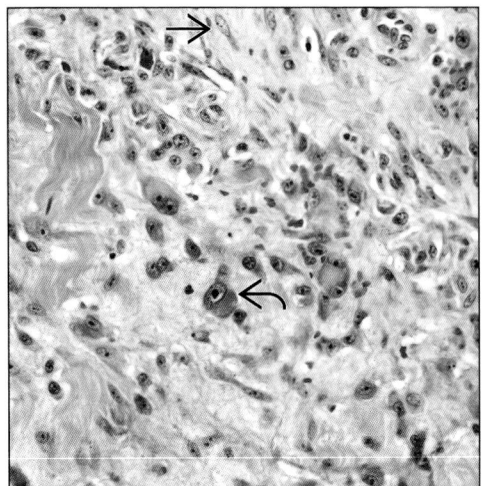

Proliferative fasciitis features the same background myofibroblastic cells as nodular fasciitis ➔, with the addition of ganglion cell-like fibroblasts ➔. The latter are not true ganglion cells.

TERMINOLOGY

Abbreviations
- Nodular fasciitis (NF)

Synonyms
- Pseudosarcomatous fasciitis (nodular fasciitis)
- Subcutaneous pseudosarcomatous fibromatosis (nodular fasciitis)
- Atypical decubital fibroplasia (ischemic fasciitis)

Definitions
- **Nodular fasciitis**: Rapidly growing myofibroblastic mass-forming proliferation that is often cellular and mitotically active, but behaves in a benign fashion
- **Intravascular fasciitis**: Rare variant of nodular fasciitis arising in association with small- and medium-sized vessels
- **Cranial fasciitis**: Variant of nodular fasciitis involving soft tissues of scalp and underlying skull in infants
- **Proliferative fasciitis/myositis**: Tumefactive subcutaneous (fasciitis) or intramuscular (myositis) proliferation featuring ganglion-like fibroblasts in a background of myofibroblasts similar to those seen in nodular fasciitis
- **Ischemic fasciitis**: Pseudosarcomatous proliferation composed of zones of fat and fibrinoid necrosis with zonal ingrowth of capillaries, fibroblasts, and myofibroblasts
  - Initially described as tumefactive pressure sore arising over bony prominences in debilitated patients, but some examples do not fit this profile

CLINICAL ISSUES

Epidemiology
- Incidence
  - All are uncommon; nodular fasciitis is most common among them

- Age
  - Nodular fasciitis: Most patients are in their 3rd and 4th decades
  - Intravascular fasciitis: Most patients are in their 3rd and 4th decades
  - Cranial fasciitis: Infants in peripartum period
  - Proliferative fasciitis: Middle-aged and older adults; rare in children
  - Ischemic fasciitis: Elderly patients
- Gender
  - No predilection

Site
- Nodular fasciitis: Classic site is forearm
- Intravascular fasciitis: Classic sites are distal extremities (especially fingers) and head and neck
- Cranial fasciitis: Head
- Proliferative fasciitis: Classic site is forearm
- Ischemic fasciitis: Classic sites are overlying sacral promontory or greater trochanter

Presentation
- All of these pseudosarcomatous processes present as mass lesions, usually painless
  - Most lesions: 1-3 cm
  - Ischemic fasciitis lesions can be large

Treatment
- Simple excision is curative

Prognosis
- Excellent; all of these lesions are benign and typically do not recur
- Recurrence should prompt review of prior sample to ensure that initial diagnosis was correct

PSEUDOSARCOMATOUS FIBROBLASTIC PROLIFERATIONS

Key Facts

Terminology

- Nodular fasciitis: Rapidly growing myofibroblastic proliferation that is often cellular and mitotically active, but behaves in a benign fashion
- Intravascular fasciitis: Rare variant of nodular fasciitis arising in association with small- and medium-sized vessels
- Cranial fasciitis: Variant of nodular fasciitis involving soft tissues of scalp and underlying skull in infants
- Proliferative fasciitis/myositis: Subcutaneous (fasciitis) or intramuscular (myositis) proliferation of ganglion-like cells in a background of myofibroblasts similar to those seen in nodular fasciitis
- Ischemic fasciitis: Proliferation composed of zones of fat and fibrinoid necrosis with ingrowth of capillaries, fibroblasts, and myofibroblasts

Clinical Issues

- Excellent prognosis: All these lesions are benign and typically do not recur even after incomplete excision
- Recurrence should prompt re-review of prior sample to ensure initial diagnosis was correct

Microscopic Pathology

- Myofibroblastic differentiation results in expression of "smooth muscle" immunohistochemical markers

Top Differential Diagnoses

- Fibrous histiocytoma (dermatofibroma)
- Neurofibroma
- Fibromatosis
- Malignant fibrous histiocytoma (undifferentiated pleomorphic sarcoma)
- Leiomyosarcoma

IMAGE FINDINGS

General Features

- Imaging generally shows well-marginated subcutaneous process
  - Exception: Proliferative fasciitis tracks along connective tissue septa

MACROSCOPIC FEATURES

General Features

- Well-marginated but unencapsulated lesions
- White to gelatinous cross section
- Ischemic fasciitis can feature areas of hemorrhage

Size

- Most 2-3 cm (exception is ischemic fasciitis, which can attain large sizes)

MICROSCOPIC PATHOLOGY

Histologic Features

- Nodular fasciitis
  - Loose storiform pattern with tissue culture appearance, variable myxoid stroma, cystic spaces, strands of keloid-like collagen
  - Osteoclast-like giant cells common (see in most lesions if sought; can be enhanced by CD68 staining)
  - Scattered lymphocytes but negligible plasma cells
  - Extravasated erythrocytes unassociated with hemosiderin deposition
  - 3 reported forms: Myxoid, cellular, fibrous
    - Loose correlation with duration of lesions
    - Myxoid lesions often have been resected within 10 days of coming to clinical attention
    - Cellular and fibrous forms more longstanding
    - Some lesions show mixed patterns
  - Myofibroblastic differentiation results in expression of "smooth muscle" immunohistochemical markers
    - Lesions can thus be mistaken for leiomyosarcoma when mitotically active
- Intravascular fasciitis
  - Similar features to nodular fasciitis, except has intravascular component
    - Often associated extravascular component encountered
  - Abundant osteoclast-like giant cells
  - Prominent mitotic activity can result in an incorrect diagnosis of intravascular leiomyosarcoma
- Cranial fasciitis
  - Lesion of infancy sometimes attributed to birth trauma
  - Similar morphology to that of nodular fasciitis, but more myxoid
  - Some reported lesions are probably instead fibromatoses
- Proliferative fasciitis
  - Predominantly plump stellate to spindled fibroblasts and myofibroblasts
  - Extravasated erythrocytes
  - Background myofibroblasts
  - Large ganglion-like fibroblasts
    - Macronucleoli, abundant amphophilic cytoplasm
    - Not true ganglion cells; no Nissl substance
  - Pediatric examples
    - Ganglion-like cells predominate
    - Exuberant mitotic activity
    - Mistaken for rhabdomyosarcomas in the past
    - Lack skeletal muscle markers (MYOD1, myogenin)
- Ischemic fasciitis
  - Ill-defined focally myxoid masses
  - Lobular configuration
  - Most centered in deep subcutis
  - A few extend into skeletal muscle or tendon/aponeurosis
  - Overlying skin typically intact
  - Zones of fibrinoid necrosis and myxoid stroma
  - Necrotic zones rimmed by ingrowing ectatic thin-walled vessels

PSEUDOSARCOMATOUS FIBROBLASTIC PROLIFERATIONS

○ Atypical enlarged degenerating fibroblasts with abundant basophilic cytoplasm, large hyperchromatic nuclei, prominent nucleoli
○ Occasional mitoses, including atypical forms

DIFFERENTIAL DIAGNOSIS

Fibrous Histiocytoma (Dermatofibroma)
- Mostly in differential diagnosis of nodular fasciitis
- Typically small superficial lesions
- Storiform pattern
- Collagen trapping
- Abundant background changes (foamy histiocytes, hemosiderin, plasma cells)
- Overlying dermal hyperplasia
- Factor VIII reactive; variable actin expression
- Tend to recur locally when incompletely excised

Neurofibroma
- Small superficial lesions
- Serpentine nuclei
- Shredded-appearing collagen, nuclei "plastered" against collagen fibrils
- Myxoid change, mast cells
- S100 protein(+), variable CD34(+)
- Benign behavior

Fibromatosis
- Large, deep, infiltrative lesions
- Shoulder girdle, abdomen (in women in childbearing years), head and neck
- Sweeping fascicles of myofibroblasts
- Uniform collagen deposition
- Prominent vascular pattern
- Highly infiltrative
- Express actin (myofibroblastic), show nuclear β-catenin labeling
- Prone to local recurrences

Kaposi Sarcoma
- Immunocompromised patients and elderly patients
- In setting of AIDS/HIV, often in skin and mucosal surfaces of upper half of body
- In elderly, in distal lower extremity
- All examples associated with HHV8
- Hyperchromatic spindle cells
- Extravasated erythrocytes, hemosiderin, plasma cells, hyaline globules
- Immunoreactivity: CD34, CD31, HHV8
- Most behave indolently
- Quasineoplastic: Can regress if immunosuppression is reduced

Malignant Fibrous Histiocytoma (Undifferentiated Pleomorphic Sarcoma)
- Deep lesions in 6th, 7th decade
- Storiform pattern
- Pleomorphic nuclei
- Outcome related to stage; overall 5-year survival about 60%

Embryonal Rhabdomyosarcoma
- Mostly in differential diagnosis of proliferative fasciitis in children
- Genital region/head and neck of young children
- Enhanced cellularity beneath mucous membranes (cambium layer)
- Atypical nuclei often without prominent nucleoli
- Expresses skeletal muscle markers on immunolabeling
- Responds to chemotherapy (70-80% 5-year survival)

Well-Differentiated Liposarcoma
- Mostly in differential diagnosis for ischemic fasciitis
- Large, deep lesions of proximal extremities and retroperitoneum
- Mature-appearing adipose tissue lesion with relatively homogeneous low-power appearance
- Lobules of fat separated by fibrous bands containing enlarged hyperchromatic nuclei
- Occasional lipoblasts (not required for diagnosis)
- Minimal mitotic activity
- Low-grade sarcoma

Leiomyosarcoma
- Wide range of clinical presentations
- Perpendicularly oriented fascicles
- Brightly eosinophilic cytoplasm
- Hyperchromatic nuclei with blunt ends
- Paranuclear vacuoles
- Immunolabeling: Actin, desmin, calponin, and caldesmon all reactive
- Outcome relates to stage and site

Pleomorphic Rhabdomyosarcoma
- In differential diagnosis of proliferative fasciitis in adults
- Highly aggressive tumors of deep proximal extremities of older adults
- Markedly pleomorphic cells
- Skeletal muscle immunophenotype
- Poor outcome

SELECTED REFERENCES

1. Liegl B et al: Ischemic fasciitis: analysis of 44 cases indicating an inconsistent association with immobility or debilitation. Am J Surg Pathol. 32(10):1546-52, 2008
2. Perosio PM et al: Ischemic fasciitis: a juxta-skeletal fibroblastic proliferation with a predilection for elderly patients. Mod Pathol. 6(1):69-72, 1993
3. Meis JM et al: Proliferative fasciitis and myositis of childhood. Am J Surg Pathol. 16(4):364-72, 1992
4. Montgomery EA et al: Atypical decubital fibroplasia. A distinctive fibroblastic pseudotumor occurring in debilitated patients. Am J Surg Pathol. 16(7):708-15, 1992
5. Montgomery EA et al: Nodular fasciitis. Its morphologic spectrum and immunohistochemical profile. Am J Surg Pathol. 15(10):942-8, 1991
6. Shimizu S et al: Nodular fasciitis: an analysis of 250 patients. Pathology. 16(2):161-6, 1984
7. Chung EB et al: Proliferative fasciitis. Cancer. 36(4):1450-8, 1975

PSEUDOSARCOMATOUS FIBROBLASTIC PROLIFERATIONS

Microscopic Features

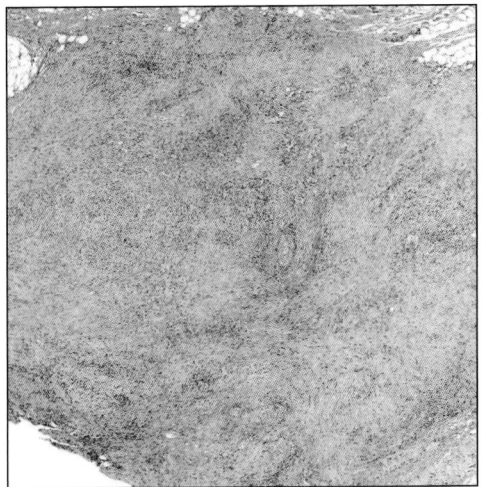

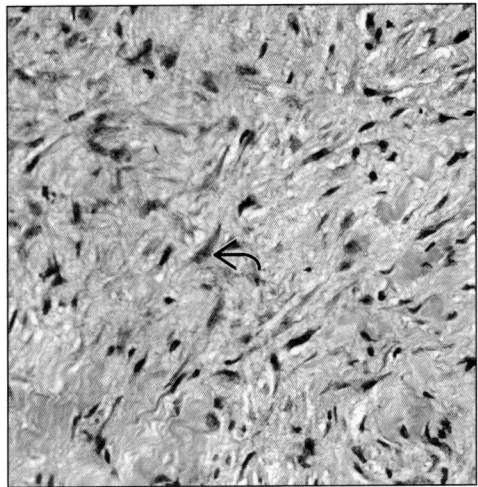

(Left) The appearance of many examples of nodular fasciitis is similar to that of granulation tissue, although there is not a consistent history of trauma. Overall, most examples are small. (Right) Note the stellate appearance of the myofibroblastic cells. There are interspersed fragments of keloid-like collagen. Each myofibroblastic nucleus features a delicate nucleolus ➢. This lesion was from the forearm of a 20-year-old male patient.

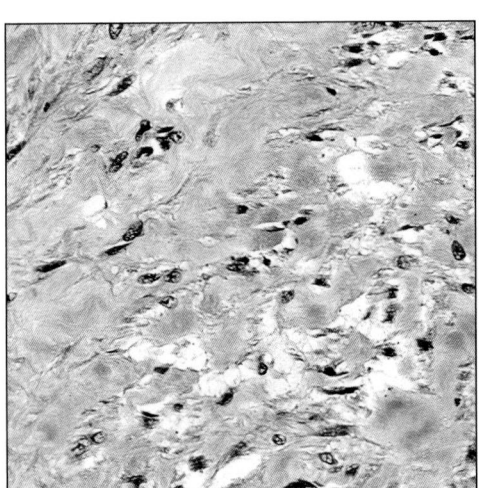

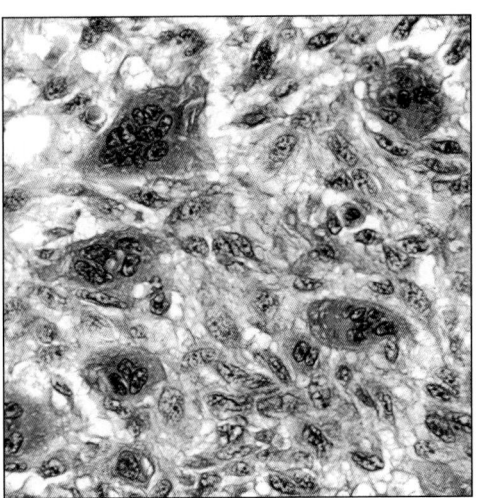

(Left) This field shows an example with striking keloid-like collagen. Some observers believe this suggests that the lesion has been present for months. (Right) Some examples contain numerous osteoclast-like giant cells. This appearance is reminiscent of that of tenosynovial giant cell tumor (giant cell tumor of tendon sheath). In contrast to tenosynovial giant cell tumor, hemosiderin deposition is not a feature of nodular fasciitis.

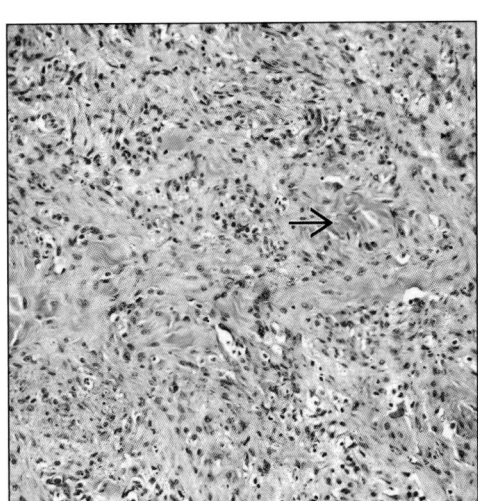

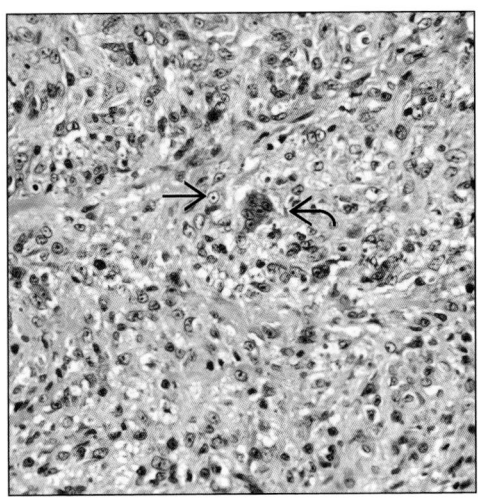

(Left) This example is relatively cellular and expressed strong actin, but not desmin, a profile typical of nodular fasciitis. This example also shows keloid-like collagen ➢ and scattered lymphocytes, but no hemosiderin or plasma cells. (Right) An osteoclast-like giant cell is present in the center of the field ➢. Otherwise, the tumor is composed of uniform spindle cells with delicate chromatin. Most of the cells contain delicate nucleoli ➢.

Microscopic Features

(Left) This field shows the typical constellation of features of nodular fasciitis: An osteoclast-like giant cell, keloid-like collagen, numerous myofibroblasts with pale chromatin, and extravasated erythrocytes ➡. *(Right)* At low magnification, proliferative fasciitis is striking for tracking along fibrous connective tissue septa in the subcutaneous tissue. The center of the lesion shows some thickened, keloid-like collagen ⇨.

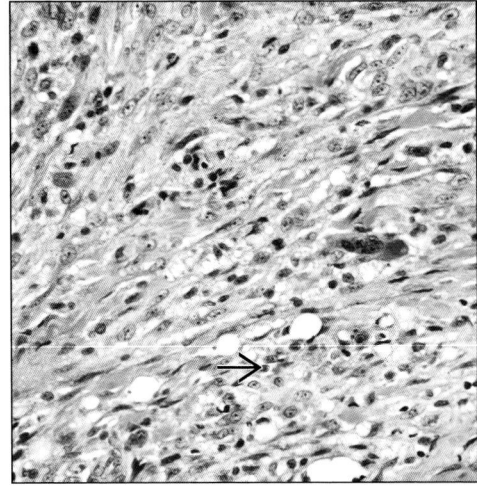
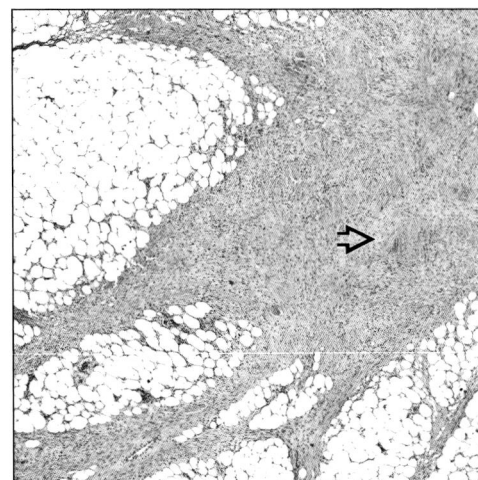

(Left) At this magnification of proliferative fasciitis, a background of cells similar to those of nodular fasciitis is present, but larger ganglion-like fibroblasts ➡ can also be seen. Note the paucicellular appearance at the center of the lesion ⇨. *(Right)* This image shows several ganglion-like cells of proliferative fasciitis ➡ in a background of other cells that are more like those seen in nodular fasciitis ➡. There are also extravasated erythrocytes ⇨.

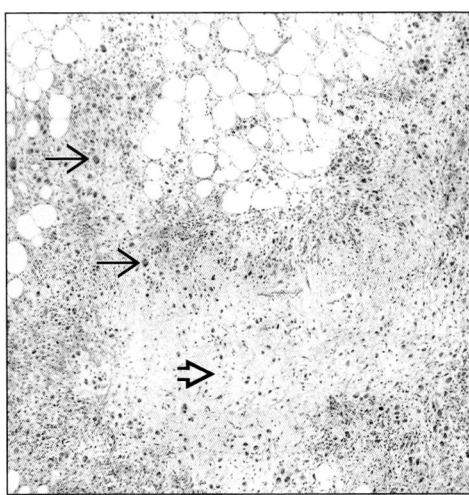
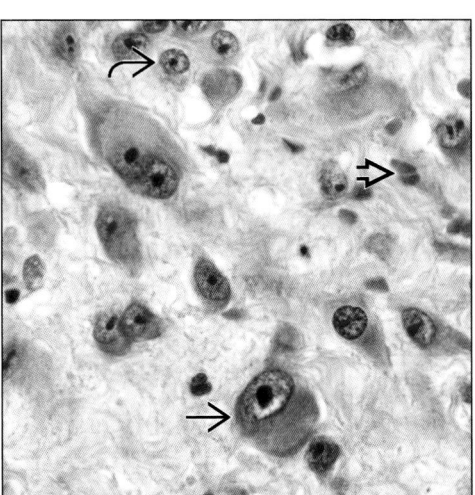

(Left) Proliferative myositis is exactly akin to proliferative fasciitis, but is centered in skeletal muscle ➡. Ganglion-like cells ⇨ are apparent at this magnification. Like nodular fasciitis, proliferative fasciitis/myositis displays a backdrop of lymphocytes ➡. *(Right)* Ganglion-like cells ⇨ are the key element of proliferative myositis, but the background cells ➡ are identical to those of nodular fasciitis. Scattered lymphocytes ➶ are present.

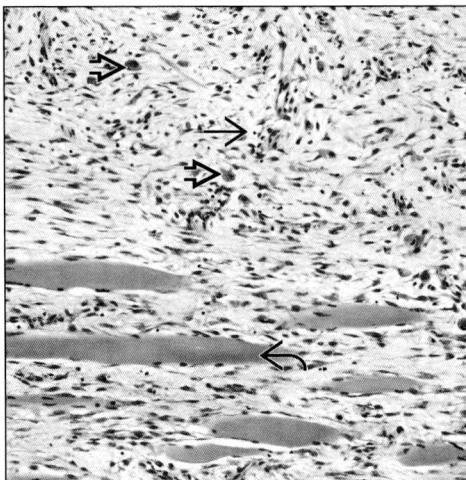
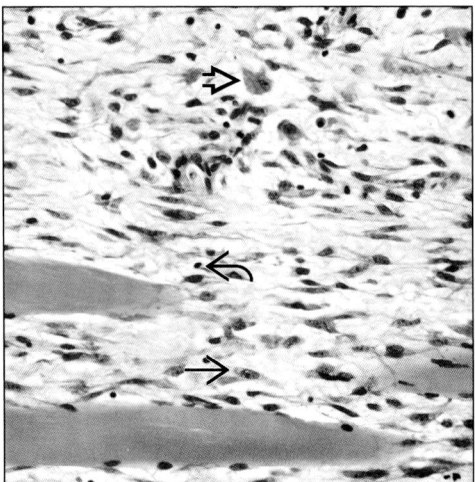

PSEUDOSARCOMATOUS FIBROBLASTIC PROLIFERATIONS

Gross and Microscopic Features

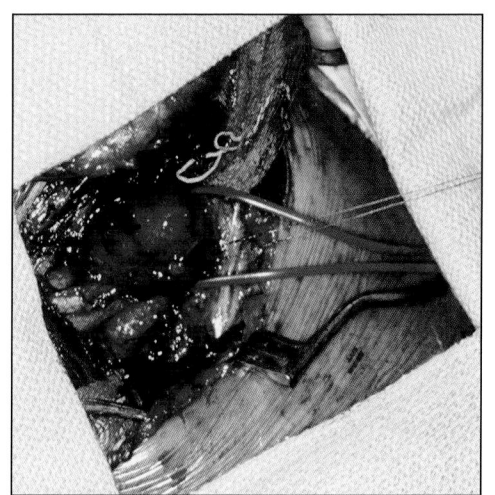

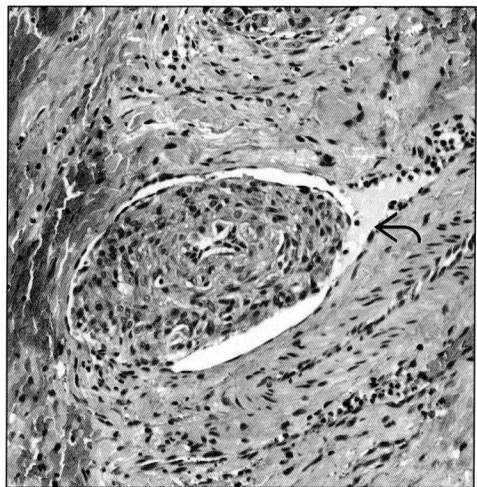

(Left) This intraoperative image is of an example of intravascular fasciitis obstructing the brachial artery. The patient gave a history of falling asleep slumped over a wooden chair. Intraoperatively, the surgeon interpreted this 3 cm mass as a sarcoma. (Right) Note that the nuclei of intravascular fasciitis are paler than those of the endothelial cells ➔ in the involved capillary. This feature is a clue that the process is pseudosarcomatous rather than sarcomatous.

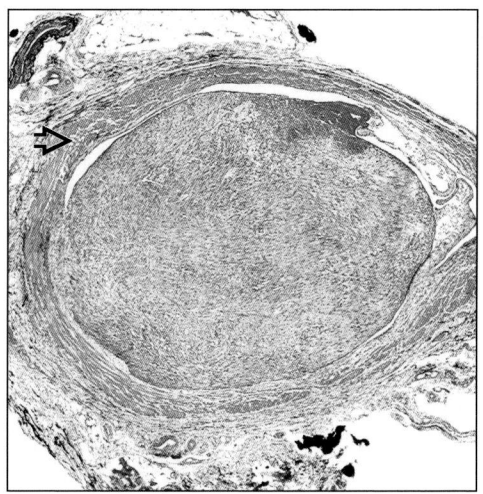

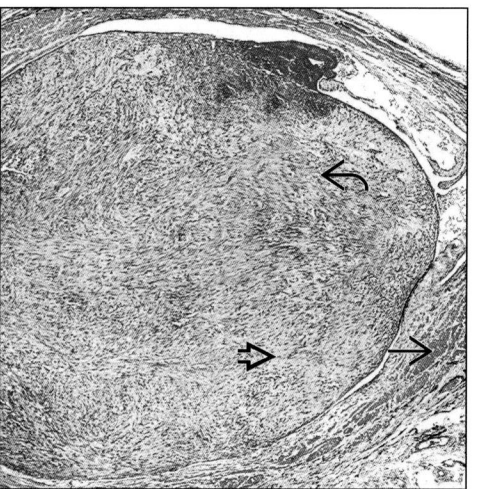

(Left) Low magnification Movat stain shows an investing vessel ➔ containing intravascular fasciitis. (Right) Higher magnification Movat stain, intravascular fasciitis shows a reddish color ➔ that is less striking than the color of the vessel containing the process ➔ accompanied by more clearly fibroblastic zones that appear bluish ➔. These tinctorial qualities on the Movat indicate that the lesion is myofibroblastic. This stain also confirms nicely that the tumor is indeed within a vessel.

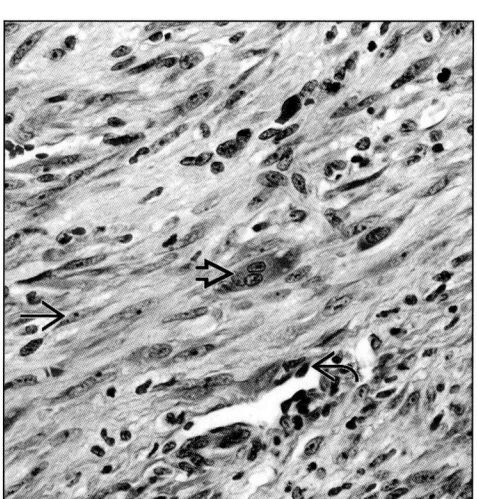

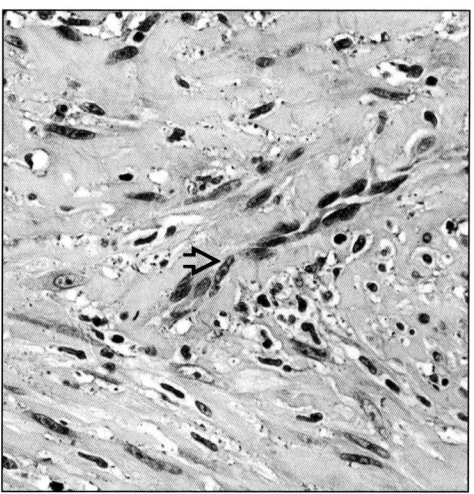

(Left) Osteoclast-like giant cells ➔ are often a prominent feature of intravascular fasciitis. The background cells are paler than the internal control endothelial cells ➔. As in nodular fasciitis, the individual cells have uniform delicate nucleoli ➔. (Right) This image demonstrates the comparison between endothelial cells and lesional cells of intravascular fasciitis. The benign endothelial cells ➔ are darker.

Immunohistochemical, Gross, and Microscopic Features

(Left) This smooth muscle actin stain is strongly reactive since nodular fasciitis is a myofibroblastic lesion. This feature can lead to misinterpretation as leiomyosarcoma. Actin staining highlights the stellate appearance of the cytoplasm ➡ of lesional cells, which differs from the bipolar cytoplasm of smooth muscle tumors. *(Right)* Ischemic fasciitis (atypical decubital fibroplasia) generally involves subcutaneous fat ⇨ and has a hemorrhagic center ➡.

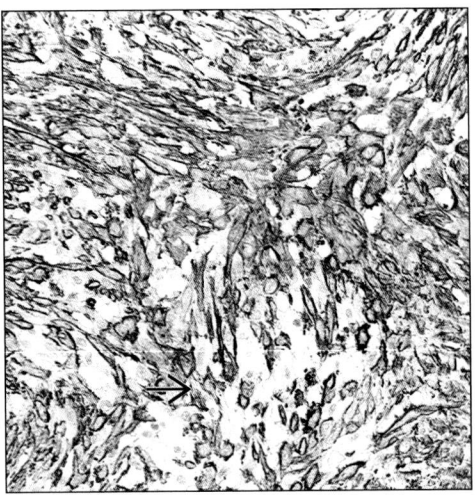
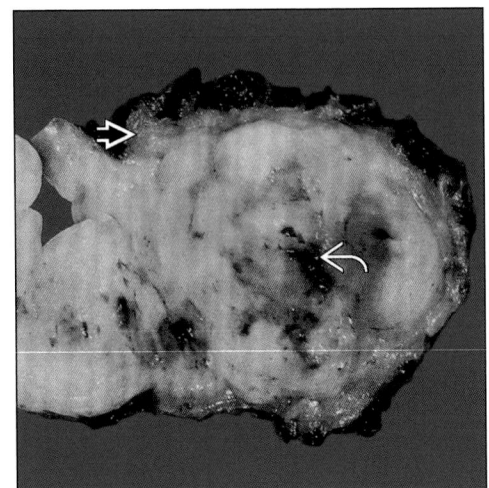

(Left) In this example of ischemic fasciitis (atypical decubital fibroplasia), the top of the field ➡ and the right side ➡ show zones of fibrinoid necrosis. A more cellular area containing ingrowing fibroblasts and vessels is at the left of the field ⇨. Even at this low magnification, there appear to be enlarged nuclei ➡. *(Right)* This example of ischemic fasciitis shows fibrinoid necrosis ➡. Enlarged fibroblasts are found in the viable portion ➡.

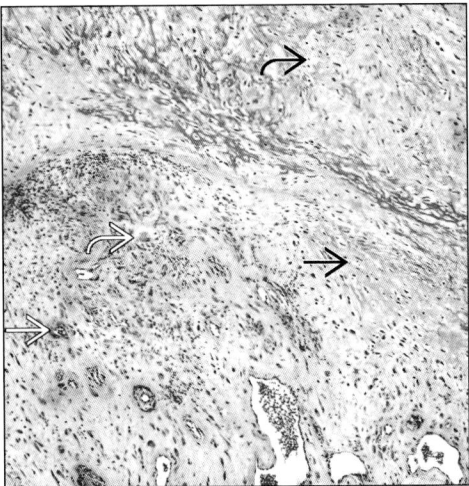
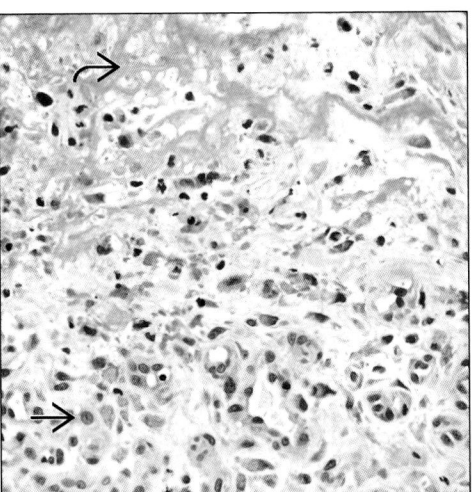

(Left) This image from a case of ischemic fasciitis is from the interface between an area of fibrinoid necrosis and a viable area. There are prominent capillaries ➡ as well as enlarged fibroblasts ⇨ with appearances similar to those encountered in proliferative fasciitis. *(Right)* Note the enlarged fibroblast in this example of ischemic fasciitis (atypical decubital fibroplasia). The cell has a conspicuous nucleolus ➡ and is seen in a background of fat with fibrinoid necrosis.

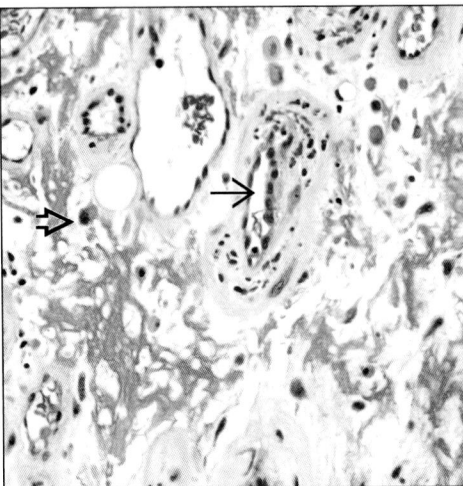
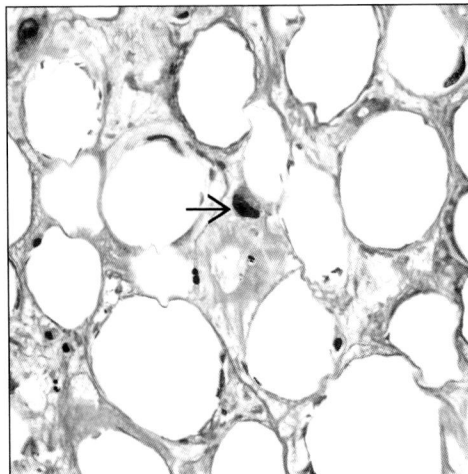

PSEUDOSARCOMATOUS FIBROBLASTIC PROLIFERATIONS

Differential Diagnosis

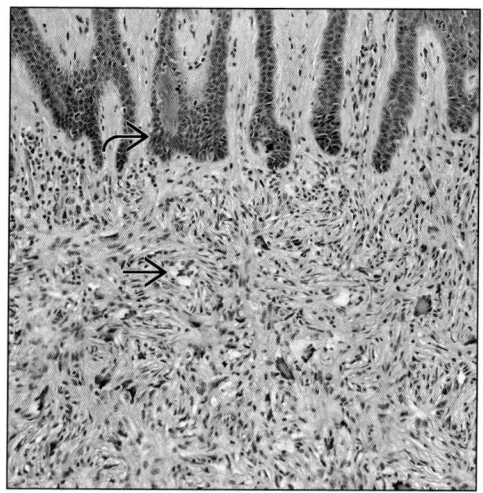
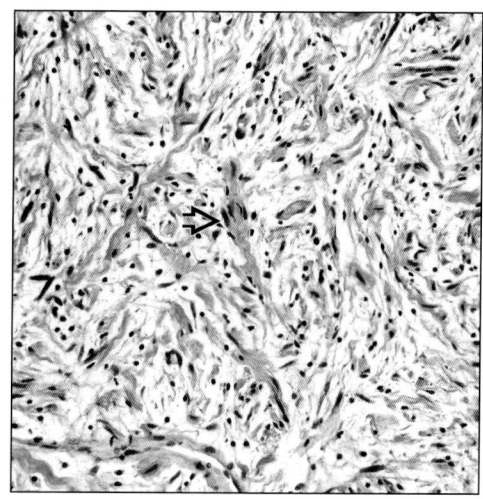

(Left) Fibrous histiocytoma/ dermatofibroma shows overlying epidermal hyperplasia with basilar hyperpigmentation ➡, and the lesion contains foamy histiocytes ➡, in contrast to the osteoclast-like giant cells in nodular fasciitis. (Right) Neurofibromas feature prominent wiry collagen, and the lesional cell nuclei appear tightly plastered against the collagen ➡. This pattern of collagen is very different from the keloid-like collagen in nodular fasciitis.

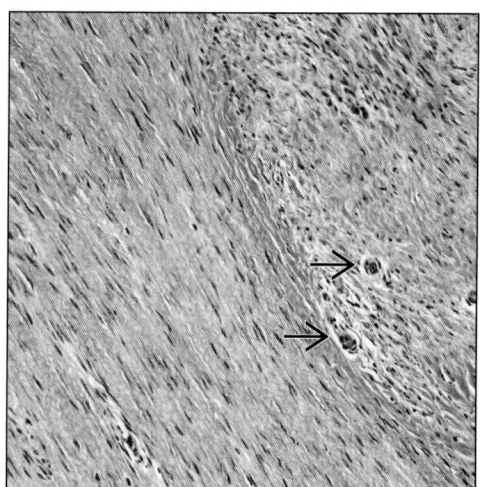
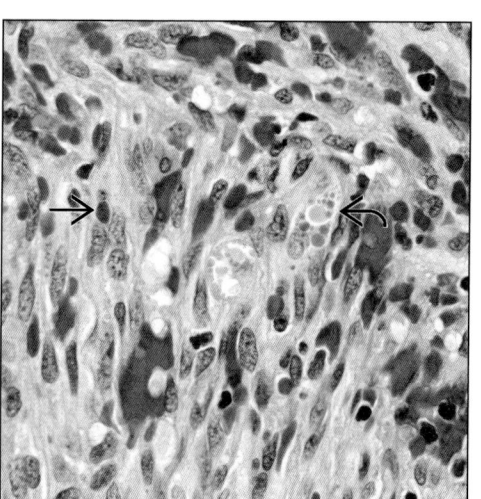

(Left) This field shows an example of fibromatosis (aggressive fibromatosis, desmoid tumor). Pale nuclei are separated evenly by collagen. The blood vessels ➡, while small, appear prominent, as they are darker than the surrounding lesion. Compare this to the storiform pattern of nodular fasciitis. (Right) There are extravasated erythrocytes ➡ in Kaposi sarcoma, just as in nodular fasciitis, but these are accompanied by hyaline globules ➡ (erythrophagolysosomes).

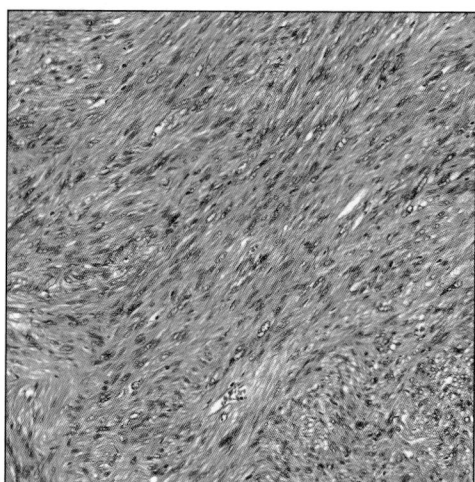
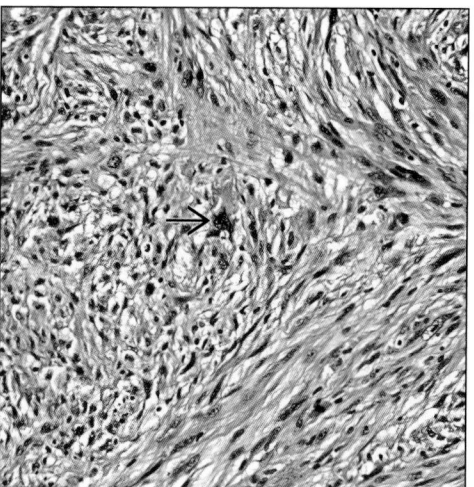

(Left) Leiomyosarcomas are arranged in fascicles, and the cytoplasm of the cells is brightly eosinophilic. Compare this to fibromatosis, which has much paler cytoplasm. Most leiomyosarcomas lack the background lymphocytes seen in nodular fasciitis. (Right) Like nodular fasciitis, pleomorphic undifferentiated sarcoma (malignant fibrous histiocytoma) has a storiform pattern, but contains pleomorphic nuclei ➡.

ANGIOMATOID FIBROUS HISTIOCYTOMA

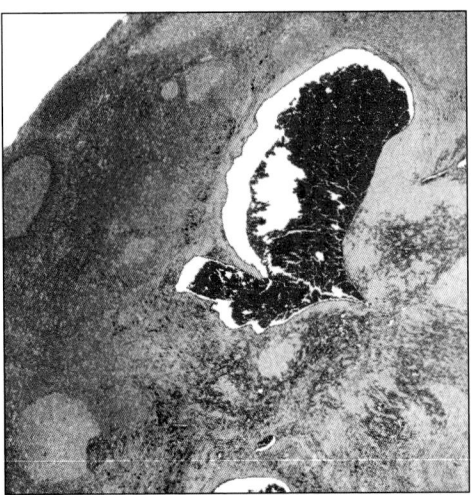

Angiomatoid fibrous histiocytoma is a circumscribed lesion with a pronounced lymphoid cuff, including prominent germinal centers. This appearance may mimic that of a tumor metastatic to a lymph node.

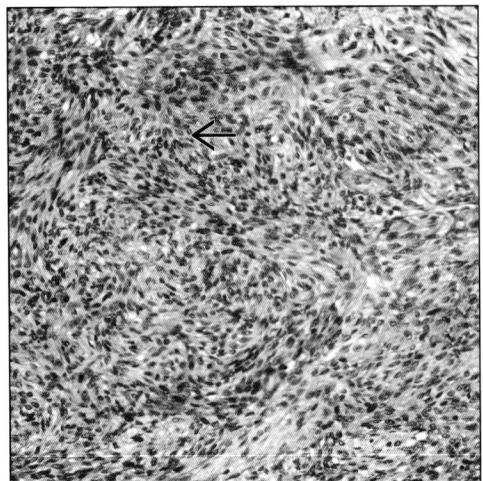

The tumor is composed of a cellular proliferation of spindle cells in loose fascicles and other areas ➔ with a storiform pattern. The cells have relatively bland ovoid nuclei.

TERMINOLOGY

Abbreviations
- Angiomatoid fibrous histiocytoma (AFH)

Synonyms
- Originally termed "angiomatoid malignant fibrous histiocytoma"
  - Term "malignant" removed due to indolent behavior
  - Unrelated to malignant fibrous histiocytoma (MFH)/ pleomorphic sarcoma group of neoplasms

Definitions
- Rare neoplasm of intermediate biologic potential with 3 characteristic translocations

ETIOLOGY/PATHOGENESIS

Lineage Unknown
- Desmin expression
  - Suggests myoid or myofibroblastic differentiation
- Endothelial or histiocytic differentiation unlikely
- Postulated nodal fibroblastic reticulum cell differentiation

CLINICAL ISSUES

Epidemiology
- Incidence
  - Rare
  - Accounts for approximately 0.3% of all soft tissue neoplasms
- Age
  - Infancy to 8th decade
  - Predominantly in children and young adults
- Gender
  - Slight female predilection

Site
- Extremities
- Trunk
- Head and neck
  - 1 primary intracerebral case reported
- Very rarely other sites
  - Lung, mediastinum, retroperitoneum, ovary, vulva
- Usually superficial
  - Deep dermis and subcutis
  - Few arise deeply

Presentation
- Slowly growing, painless mass
  - Usually small
    - Most often 2-4 cm
- Constitutional symptoms in subset
  - Malaise
  - Pyrexia
  - Anemia
  - Due to possible tumoral cytokine production

Treatment
- Surgical approaches
  - Wide excision
    - Usually curative
  - Radiotherapy and chemotherapy
    - For rare metastatic or unresectable tumors

Prognosis
- Excellent in most cases
  - Majority of lesions indolent
- Regional recurrence rate up to 15%
- Metastasis rate of approximately 1%
- No firm morphologic or clinical indicators of behavior
  - Infiltrative margin and deep location can predict recurrence

ANGIOMATOID FIBROUS HISTIOCYTOMA

Key Facts

Terminology
- Rare neoplasm of intermediate biologic potential
- Most often arises in extremities of children and young adults
- Histologically often confused with both benign and malignant lesions
- 3 characteristic translocations

Clinical Issues
- Slowly growing
- Mostly indolent
- 15% recur, 1% metastasize

Microscopic Pathology
- Fibrous and lymphoplasmacytic cuff
  - Dense peripheral lymphoplasmacytic cuff in up to 80%

- Histiocyte-like and spindle cells
  - In sheets, short fascicles, occasional storiform distributions
- Cells with bland, vesicular, ovoid to spindled nuclei
- Blood-filled spaces
- Some show marked pleomorphism and mitotic activity

Ancillary Tests
- Desmin positivity in 1/2 of cases
- Specific translocations

Top Differential Diagnoses
- Aneurysmal benign fibrous histiocytoma
- Spindle cell hemangioma
- Kaposi sarcoma
- Pleomorphic sarcoma (MFH)

MACROSCOPIC FEATURES

General Features
- Firm
- Circumscribed
- Blood-filled cystic cavities

Sections to Be Submitted
- Lesion should be thoroughly sampled
- Small lesions should be submitted in entirety

MICROSCOPIC PATHOLOGY

Histologic Features
- Circumscribed, lobulated mass
- Fibrous pseudocapsule
  - Dense peripheral lymphoplasmacytic cuff
    - Present in up to 80%
    - Mixture of B- and T cells
    - Germinal center formation may be present
- Cells with bland, vesicular, ovoid to spindled nuclei
  - Sheets
  - Short fascicles
  - Occasional storiform patterns
  - Ovoid or spindle forms may predominate
  - Mitoses infrequent
- Hemorrhagic cavities
  - Lack endothelial lining
- Some show marked pleomorphism and mitotic activity
  - Not shown to be associated with outcome
- Giant cells in some cases
- Clear cells and reticular and pulmonary edema-like patterns are rarely described

Predominant Pattern/Injury Type
- Circumscribed
- Cystic, macroscopic

Predominant Cell/Compartment Type
- Mesenchymal

ANCILLARY TESTS

Cytogenetics
- 3 characteristic translocations identified
  - (2;22)(q33;q12) EWSR1-CREB1
    - Most common gene fusion
  - (12;16)(q13;p11) FUS-ATF1
  - (12;22)(q13;q12) EWSR1-ATF1
  - Fusion type not thought to be related to tumor site
- No correlation between type of fusion gene and clinicopathologic features
- All these translocations also seen in clear cell sarcomas
  - Clear cell sarcoma (of tendons and aponeuroses)
  - Clear cell sarcoma-like tumor of the gastrointestinal tract
  - Morphologically and clinically distinct neoplasms

In Situ Hybridization
- Translocated chromosomes can be identified by FISH

PCR
- Fusion gene transcripts can be identified by RT-PCR
  - Frozen or paraffin-embedded material

Electron Microscopy
- No diagnostic ultrastructural findings

DIFFERENTIAL DIAGNOSIS

Aneurysmal Dermatofibroma (Benign Fibrous Histiocytoma)
- Usually intradermal
- Epidermal hyperplasia overlying lesion
- Tumor is not well-circumscribed
- Peripheral collagen bundles
- Mixed cell population
  - Giant cells
  - Siderophages
- Desmin negative

Spindle Cell Hemangioma
- Poorly circumscribed

ANGIOMATOID FIBROUS HISTIOCYTOMA

- Cavernous vascular spaces
  - Endothelial lining
- Epithelioid endothelial cells with vacuoles
- Spindle cells
  - SMA positive
  - Desmin and CD34 negative

Nodular Kaposi Sarcoma
- Predisposing factors (e.g., HIV[+])
- Endothelial-lined spaces
- CD34, CD31, and podoplanin positive
- HHV8 positivity in nuclei

Nodular Fasciitis
- Short history
- Spindle and stellate fibroblasts
- Loose, tissue culture-like appearance
- Related phenomena
  - e.g., extravasated erythrocytes
  - Giant cells
- Smooth muscle actin (+)

Pleomorphic Sarcoma (MFH)
- Older age group
- Deep soft tissue
- Marked diffuse pleomorphism
  - Spindled cells
  - Polygonal cells
  - Giant cells
- Atypical mitoses
- Necrosis

Rhabdomyosarcoma
- Rare in superficial sites
- Embryonal rhabdomyosarcoma
  - Urogenital region
  - Head and neck
- Alveolar rhabdomyosarcoma
  - Small round cells
  - At least focal alveolar pattern
  - Specific gene fusions
    - *PAX3/7* and *FOXO1*
- Pleomorphic rhabdomyoblasts may be present
- Nuclear expression of skeletal markers
  - Myogenin
  - MYOD1

Epithelioid Sarcoma
- Subcutaneous or deep
- Multinodular
- Epithelioid cells
  - Eosinophilic cytoplasm
  - Mitoses
  - Spindle cells at periphery of nodule
- Central necrosis
- Lacks fibrous or lymphoid cuff
- Desmin(-)
- CK(+) and EMA(+)
- CD34(+)
  - 50% of cases
- SNF(-)
  - 90% of cases

Smooth Muscle Tumors
- Not lobulated
- Characteristic architecture
  - Perpendicularly orientated fascicles
  - Intersecting fascicles
- Blunt-ended nuclei
- Eosinophilic cytoplasm
- Express actins and H-caldesmon
- May express ER/PR

Granulomatous Lesions
- Granulomas are usually dispersed and discrete
- Lack solid pattern of AFH
- Lack cystic hemorrhage
- CD68(+)
- Desmin(-)

Palisaded (Intranodal) Myofibroblastoma
- In lymph node
  - Majority in inguinal region in males
  - Occasionally in submandibular node
- Delicate spindle cells in fascicles
- Palisading
- Amianthoid fibers
- SMA(+)
- Desmin(-)

Inflammatory Pseudotumor of Lymph Node
- Lacks pseudovascular spaces
- Myofibroblastic differentiation
- Desmin negative

Nodal Metastasis
- Primary tumor site may be evident clinically
- True nodal architecture present
  - e.g., subcapsular and medullary sinuses
  - Well-organized germinal centers

Myofibroma/Myofibromatosis
- May be multicentric
- Most common from birth to 2 years
- Most solitary examples in subcutaneous tissues of head and neck
- Biphasic pattern
- Myoid nodules
- Cellular areas with hemangiopericytic vascular pattern
- Spindle cell areas
- Desmin usually negative or focal

DIAGNOSTIC CHECKLIST

Clinically Relevant Pathologic Features
- Age distribution
- Gross appearance

Pathologic Interpretation Pearls
- Features that may be absent or only present focally
  - Lymphoid cuff
  - Fibrous capsule
  - Hemorrhagic cavities
- Several tumor blocks should be sampled in tumors with appropriate clinical setting
- Desmin positive

ANGIOMATOID FIBROUS HISTIOCYTOMA

Immunohistochemistry

Antibody	Reactivity	Staining Pattern	Comment
Desmin	Positive	Cytoplasmic	50% of cases; scattered desmin(+) cells may also be present in the lymphoid population
EMA/MUC1	Positive	Cell membrane	Almost 50% of cases
CD68	Positive	Cytoplasmic	Focal, nonspecific
CD99	Positive	Cell membrane	Nonspecific
Actin-HHF-35	Positive	Cytoplasmic	Focal in 14% of cases
Actin-sm	Positive	Cytoplasmic	Focal in 14% of cases
CD34	Negative	Not applicable	Very occasional "intermediate" staining
CD31	Negative	Not applicable	
HCAD	Negative	Not applicable	Positive in about 3% of cases
MYOD1	Negative	Not applicable	
Myogenin	Negative	Not applicable	
CK8/18/CAM5.2	Negative	Not applicable	
CD45	Negative	Not applicable	
CD30	Negative	Not applicable	
S100P	Negative	Not applicable	
Calponin	Equivocal	Cytoplasmic	Occasional

- H-caldesmon and myogenin negative
- Ancillary diagnostic tests are useful in providing a definitive diagnosis in the appropriate histological context
  - RT-PCR for fusion transcripts
  - FISH for identifying chromosomal rearrangements

SELECTED REFERENCES

1. Chen G et al: Angiomatoid fibrous histiocytoma: unusual sites and unusual morphology. Mod Pathol. 24(12):1560-70, 2011
2. Ren L et al: Angiomatoid fibrous histiocytoma: first report of primary pulmonary origin. Am J Surg Pathol. 33(10):1570-4, 2009
3. Dunham C et al: Primary intracerebral angiomatoid fibrous histiocytoma: report of a case with a t(12;22)(q13;q12) causing type 1 fusion of the EWS and ATF-1 genes. Am J Surg Pathol. 32(3):478-84, 2008
4. Thway K: Angiomatoid fibrous histiocytoma: a review with recent genetic findings. Arch Pathol Lab Med. 132(2):273-7, 2008
5. Hallor KH et al: Fusion genes in angiomatoid fibrous histiocytoma. Cancer Lett. 251(1):158-63, 2007
6. Rossi S et al: EWSR1-CREB1 and EWSR1-ATF1 fusion genes in angiomatoid fibrous histiocytoma. Clin Cancer Res. 13(24):7322-8, 2007
7. Antonescu CR et al: EWS-CREB1: a recurrent variant fusion in clear cell sarcoma--association with gastrointestinal location and absence of melanocytic differentiation. Clin Cancer Res. 12(18):5356-62, 2006
8. Huang W et al: Osteoclast-rich tumor of the gastrointestinal tract with features resembling those of clear cell sarcoma of soft parts. Virchows Arch. 448(2):200-3, 2006
9. Zambrano E et al: An osteoclast-rich tumor of the gastrointestinal tract with features resembling clear cell sarcoma of soft parts: reports of 6 cases of a GIST simulator. Int J Surg Pathol. 11(2):75-81, 2003
10. Raddaoui E et al: Fusion of the FUS and ATF1 genes in a large, deep-seated angiomatoid fibrous histiocytoma. Diagn Mol Pathol. 11(3):157-62, 2002
11. Fanburg-Smith JC et al: Angiomatoid "malignant" fibrous histiocytoma: a clinicopathologic study of 158 cases and further exploration of the myoid phenotype. Hum Pathol. 30(11):1336-43, 1999
12. Morgan MB et al: Angiomatoid malignant fibrous histiocytoma revisited. An immunohistochemical and DNA ploidy analysis. Am J Dermatopathol. 19(3):223-7, 1997
13. Smith ME et al: Evaluation of CD68 and other histiocytic antigens in angiomatoid malignant fibrous histiocytoma. Am J Surg Pathol. 15(8):757-63, 1991
14. Costa MJ et al: Angiomatoid malignant fibrous histiocytoma. A follow-up study of 108 cases with evaluation of possible histologic predictors of outcome. Am J Surg Pathol. 14(12):1126-32, 1990
15. Pettinato G et al: Angiomatoid malignant fibrous histiocytoma: cytologic, immunohistochemical, ultrastructural, and flow cytometric study of 20 cases. Mod Pathol. 3(4):479-87, 1990
16. Kanter MH et al: Angiomatoid malignant fibrous histiocytoma. Cytology of fine-needle aspiration and its differential diagnosis. Arch Pathol Lab Med. 109(6):564-6, 1985
17. Kay S: Angiomatoid malignant fibrous histiocytoma. Report of two cases with ultrastructural observations of one case. Arch Pathol Lab Med. 109(10):934-7, 1985
18. Leu HJ et al: Angiomatoid malignant fibrous histiocytoma. Case report and electron microscopic findings. Virchows Arch A Pathol Anat Histol. 395(1):99-107, 1982
19. Sun CC et al: An ultrastructural study of angiomatoid fibrous histiocytoma. Cancer. 49(10):2103-11, 1982
20. Enzinger FM: Angiomatoid malignant fibrous histiocytoma: a distinct fibrohistiocytic tumor of children and young adults simulating a vascular neoplasm. Cancer. 44(6):2147-57, 1979

ANGIOMATOID FIBROUS HISTIOCYTOMA

Microscopic Features

(Left) Angiomatoid fibrous histiocytoma shows a circumscribed nodular lesion with prominent cavernous blood-filled spaces, adjacent to solid cellular lesional areas. This is a typical appearance of this tumor. *(Right)* A thick fibrous capsule is apparent in this example. The lymphoid cuff may be sparse ⇲ (as shown here) or entirely absent. While angiomatoid fibrous histiocytoma is usually encapsulated, a small number of cases are focally infiltrative.

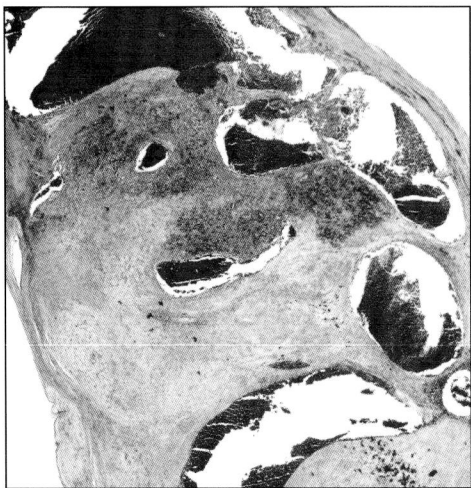
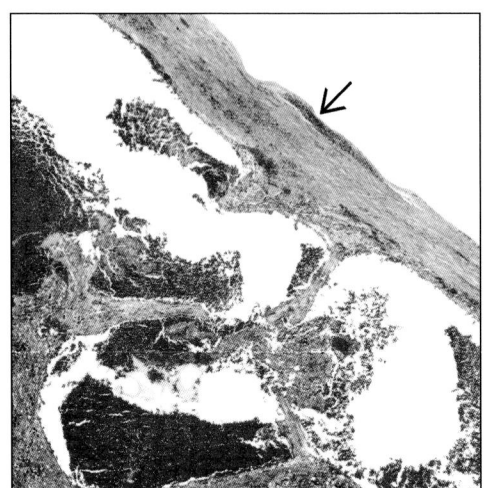

(Left) This tumor shows both a more prominent lymphoid cuff ⇲ and a fibrous capsule. This example has a predominantly solid growth pattern, but there is hemorrhage seen in the lower left corner of this image. *(Right)* This tumor has a solid morphology with tightly packed sheets of cells. Note the absence of a peripheral lymphoid cuff and hemorrhagic cavity formation. These variants of AFH may be difficult to distinguish from other neoplasms, and a high index of clinical suspicion is required for diagnosis.

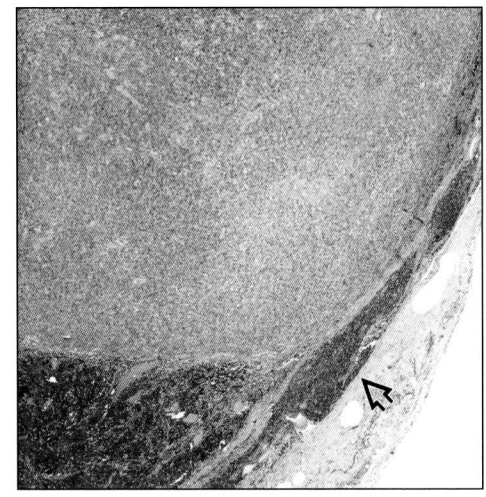
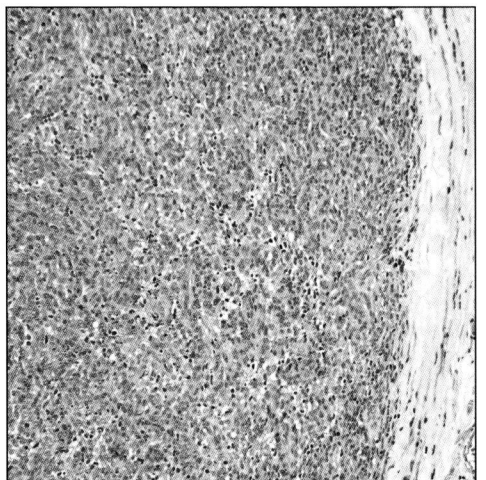

(Left) Multiple cellular nodules of spindle and ovoid cells are arranged next to irregularly shaped foci of hemorrhage and fibrin deposition ⇲. *(Right)* High magnification shows prominent hemosiderin deposition ⇲ and a lymphoplasmacytic infiltrate. The hemorrhagic cavities ⇲ are lined by tumoral cells and lack a vascular endothelial layer, making immunostaining for CD34 or CD31 negative, in contrast to a vascular neoplasm.

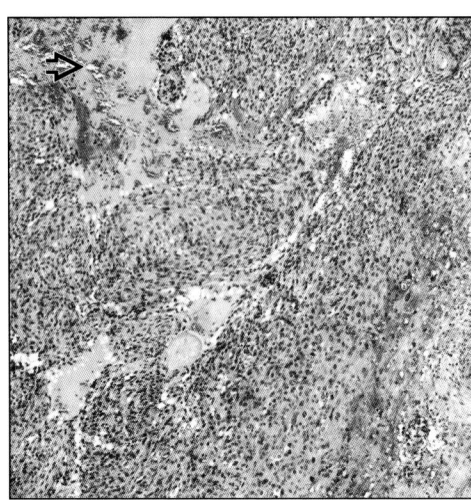
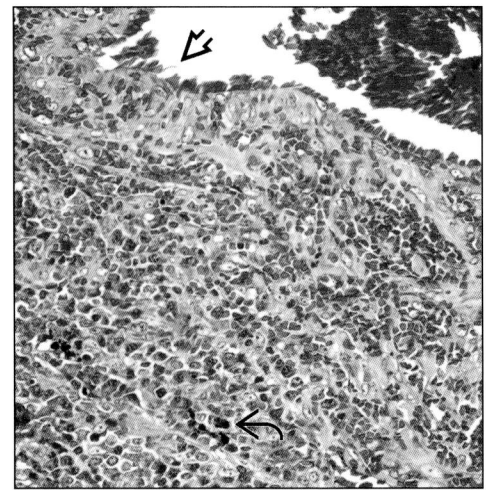

Microscopic Features and Ancillary Techniques

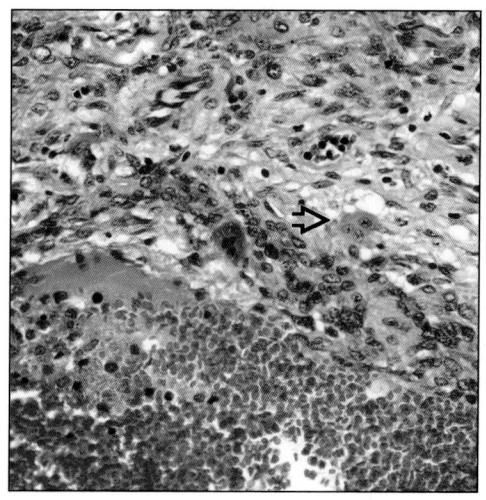

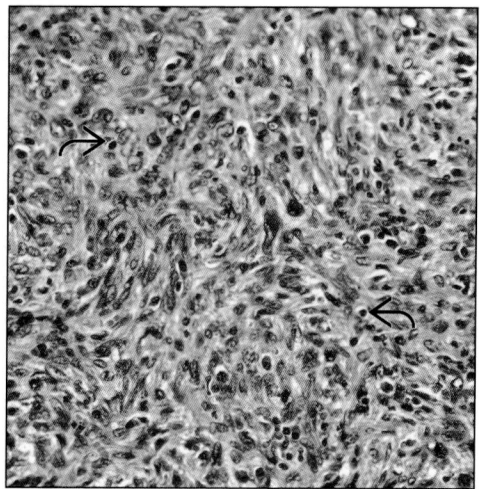

(Left) Higher power view shows the cavity-tumoral interface of an angiomatoid fibrous histiocytoma. Occasional multinucleate giant cells ⊵ are dispersed among the lesional cells. These are present in a small number of cases. *(Right)* High magnification shows dense storiform fascicles of plump spindle cells. Pleomorphism is minimal. Note the infiltrate of lymphocytes ⊰ scattered throughout. The appearances here somewhat resemble those of cutaneous fibrous histiocytoma.

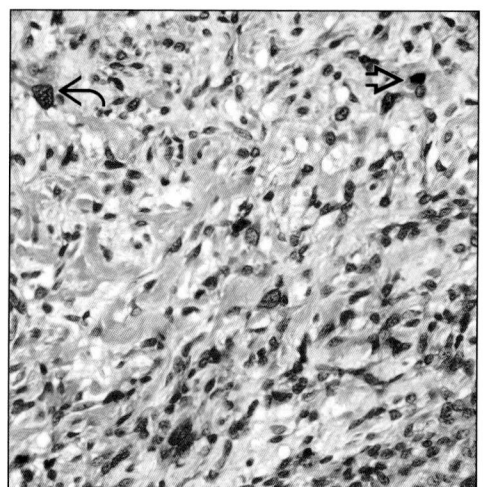

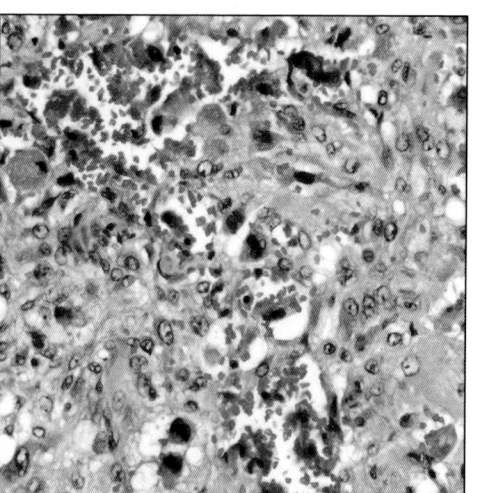

(Left) This example of angiomatoid fibrous histiocytoma shows a tumor of moderate cellularity in which there are occasional atypical nuclei ⊰, as well as a mitotic figure ⊵. Note the stromal fibrosis. *(Right)* This tumor displays focal but pronounced cellular atypia, seen in a number of cases. Lesional cells show enlarged hyperchromatic nuclei. The hemorrhagic channels are irregular, and the appearances can mimic vascular neoplasms such as Kaposi sarcoma or angiosarcoma.

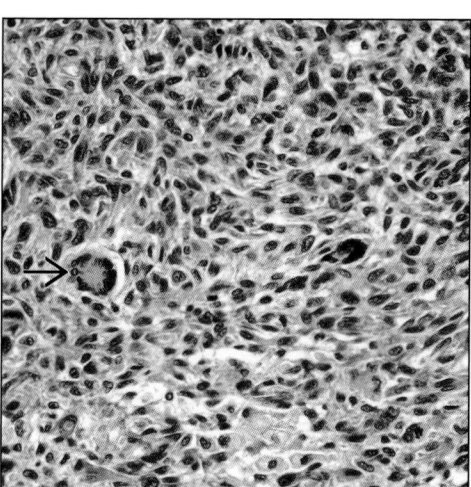

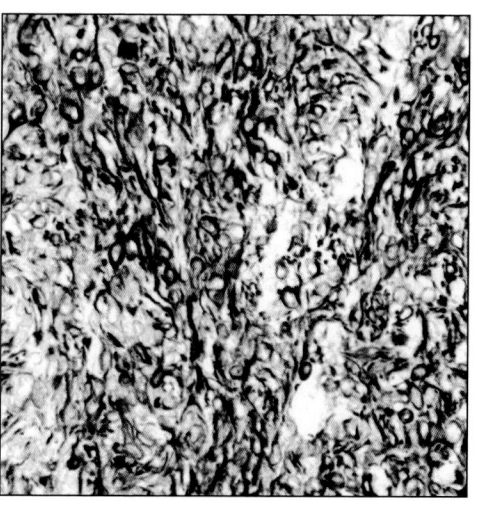

(Left) This example of angiomatoid fibrous histiocytoma shows prominent multinucleated giant cells. One has a Touton giant cell-like appearance ⊰. The morphologic features suggest that these giant cells are likely neoplastic rather than reactive osteoclast-like cells. *(Right)* Desmin shows strong cytoplasmic positivity in this case. This can be diffuse (as shown here), but is more often focal. Desmin immunoreactivity is found in about 50% of cases and is a useful diagnostic finding.

PLEXIFORM FIBROHISTIOCYTIC TUMOR

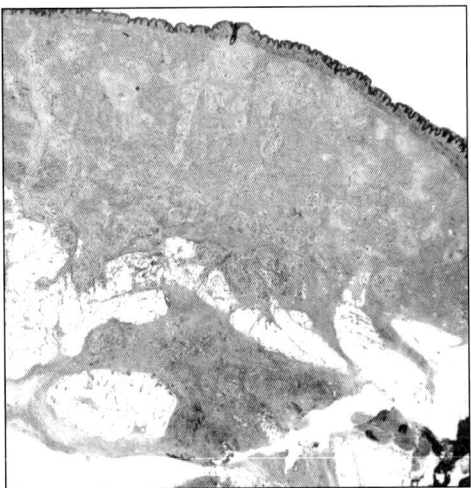

Low magnification shows plexiform fibrohistiocytic tumor (PFHT) at the dermal-subcutaneous interface with a plexiform appearance. Note the extensions into the dermis and subcutis.

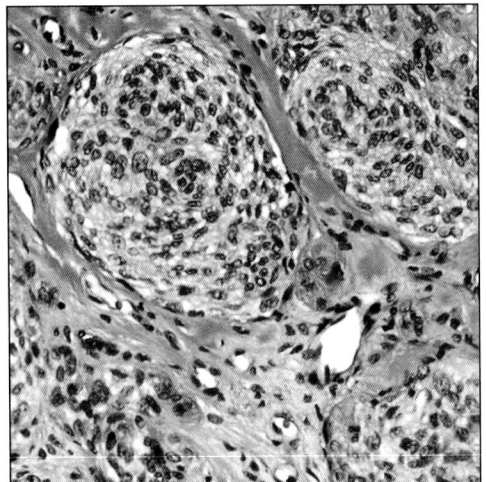

Higher magnification shows a dermal ball-like (plexiform) growth pattern of histiocytoid cells as part of a histiocytic-type of PFHT.

TERMINOLOGY

Abbreviations
- Plexiform fibrohistiocytic tumor (PFHT)

Synonyms
- Possibly represents deep form of cellular neurothekeoma

Definitions
- Fibrohistiocytic tumor of intermediate malignant potential (rarely metastasizing)
- Plexiform pattern
  o Cellular nodules; interlacing bands of fibroblasts

CLINICAL ISSUES

Epidemiology
- Incidence
  o Rare
- Age
  o Children and young adults
    ▪ Range: 1-77 years; median: 20 years
- Gender
  o Slight male predominance

Site
- Arises at dermal-subcutaneous junction
  o Extends into dermis and subcutis
- Upper extremity is most common site
- Followed by lower extremities and trunk
- Rare in head and neck region

Presentation
- Subcutaneous mass

Treatment
- Wide excision with follow-up
  o Examination of regional lymph nodes, possibly chest imaging

Prognosis
- Low metastatic potential
  o Rare examples involving regional lymph nodes
- Usually no systemic metastases
  o 1 reported case metastatic to lung

MACROSCOPIC FEATURES

General Features
- Often nodular protuberant lesions involving dermis and subcutis

MICROSCOPIC PATHOLOGY

Histologic Features
- Tumor located at dermal-subcutaneous interface
- Infiltrative growth pattern, no circumscription
- Morphologically 3 patterns
  o Fibroblastic
  o Histiocytic with osteoclast type giant cells
  o Mixed
- Cannonball-like or plexiform arrangement of cells
- Occasional metaplastic bone formation
- Low mitotic activity, rare nuclear pleomorphism
- Hemorrhage, hemosiderin, and lymphocytes
- Variable fibrosis in nodules
  o Sometimes dense hyalinization
- Rare myxoid change

ANCILLARY TESTS

Immunohistochemistry
- Positive for SMA in fibroblasts, CD68 & CD163 in histiocytes
- S100, CD34, desmin, cytokeratin, FXIIIA, and lysozyme negative
- Nonspecific markers PGP9.5, S100-A6, MITF, NKI/C3 (CD63) may be positive

PLEXIFORM FIBROHISTIOCYTIC TUMOR

Key Facts

Terminology

- Fibrohistiocytic tumor of intermediate malignant potential

Microscopic Pathology

- Tumor based at dermal-subcutaneous junction
- Infiltrative, plexiform, or multinodular growth pattern
- 3 histological patterns: Histiocyte-like with osteoclast type giant cells, fibroblastic and spindled, mixed

- SMA(+) fibroblasts, CD68/CD163(+) histiocyte-like cells

Top Differential Diagnoses

- Giant cell tumor of soft parts
- May be on spectrum with cellular neurothekeoma
  - PFHT involves subcutis, not only dermis
  - PFHT usually presents on extremities and trunk rather than face
  - PFHT less often myxoid or atypical

DIFFERENTIAL DIAGNOSIS

Giant Cell Tumor of Soft Parts

- Multinodular proliferation of bland histiocytic cells
- More osteoclast-type giant cells
- Less infiltrative, lacks spindled pattern

Cellular Neurothekeoma

- Related or possibly identical lesion to PFHT
- Typically dermal only
- Usually present in head and neck in younger children
- Myxoid areas common, giant cells rare

Nodular Fasciitis

- Typically fascial-based
- Myxoid degeneration, extravasation of erythrocytes
- Not plexiform

Fibromatosis

- Infiltrative fibroblastic proliferation
- Superficial or deep location
- Parallel-aligned uniform myofibroblasts
- β-catenin positive in nuclei (more often in deep fibromatoses)

Myofibromatosis

- Biphasic proliferation: Peripheral cellular, fascicular areas, and central hemangiopericytoma-like areas
- Lacks plexiform pattern

Fibrous Hamartoma of Infancy

- Presents in axillae of newborns

- Spindled component infiltrates fat
- Also has immature mesenchymal and collagenous components

Cutaneous Pilar Leiomyoma

- Plexiform pattern of spindled cells
- Intersecting smooth muscle bundles
- Desmin and H-caldesmon positive

SELECTED REFERENCES

1. Jaffer S et al: Neurothekeoma and plexiform fibrohistiocytic tumor: mere histologic resemblance or histogenetic relationship? Am J Surg Pathol. 33(6):905-13, 2009
2. Moosavi C et al: An update on plexiform fibrohistiocytic tumor and addition of 66 new cases from the Armed Forces Institute of Pathology, in honor of Franz M. Enzinger, MD. Ann Diagn Pathol. 11(5):313-9, 2007
3. Remstein ED et al: Plexiform fibrohistiocytic tumor: clinicopathologic analysis of 22 cases. Am J Surg Pathol. 23(6):662-70, 1999
4. Fisher C: Atypical plexiform fibrohistiocytic tumour. Histopathology. 30(3):271-3, 1997
5. Enzinger FM et al: Plexiform fibrohistiocytic tumor presenting in children and young adults. An analysis of 65 cases. Am J Surg Pathol. 12(11):818-26, 1988

IMAGE GALLERY

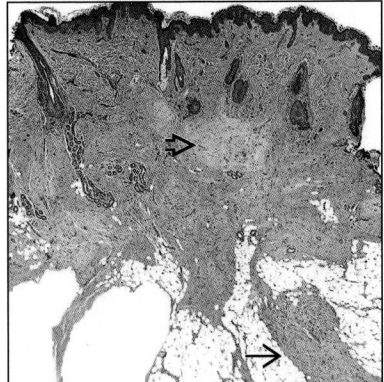
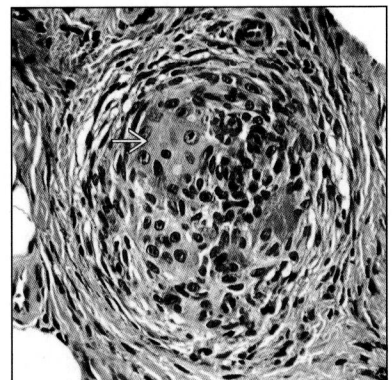
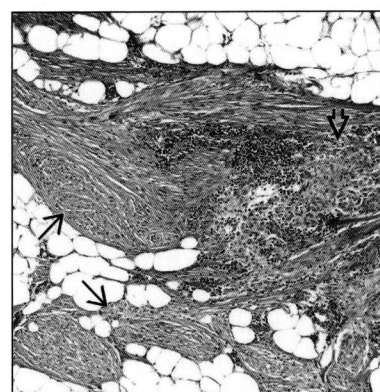

(Left) Low magnification shows the lesion is based at dermal-subcutaneous interface, with nodular ⊵ and infiltrative growth pattern, the latter being fibroblastic ➡. *(Center)* High magnification shows histiocytoid cells with osteoclast-type giant cells ➡. Giant cell tumor of soft parts has more giant cells and is less infiltrative. *(Right)* Subcutaneous area of a mixed-type PFHT shows histiocytic nodules ⊵ merging with sheets of fibroblastic cells ➡.

DERMATOFIBROSARCOMA PROTUBERANS

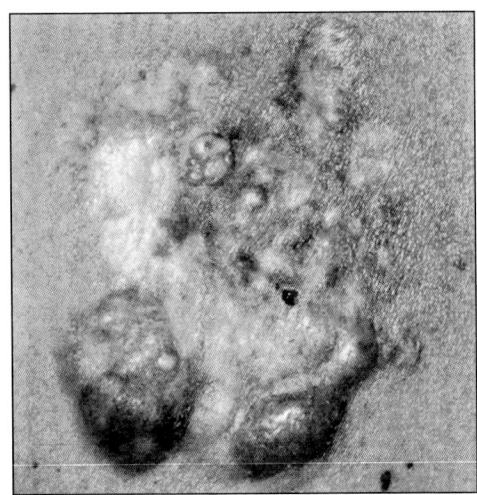

Dermatofibrosarcoma protuberans (DFSP) is often characterized clinically by an exophytic, multinodular growth with areas of interposed flattening or atrophy.

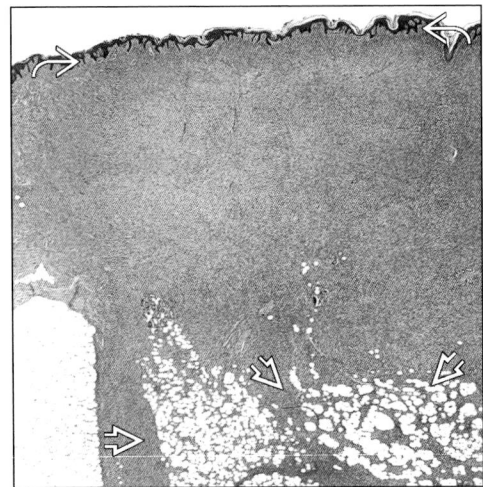

Low magnification of a DFSP shows deep dermal and subcutaneous ➡ involvement by a cellular spindle cell tumor with fat entrapment. Epidermis is separated from tumor by thin grenz zone ➡. (Courtesy T. Mentzel, MD.)

TERMINOLOGY

Abbreviations
- Dermatofibrosarcoma protuberans (DFSP)

Synonyms
- Bednar tumor (pigmented DFSP)

Definitions
- Low-grade malignant spindle cell tumor of skin characteristically showing prominent storiforming

ETIOLOGY/PATHOGENESIS

Unknown in Most Cases
- Rare cases reportedly associated with previous trauma, burns, or arsenic exposure

Genetics
- Rearrangements of collagen 1A1 (COL1A1)/platelet-derived growth factor B (PDGFB)
- Characteristic t(17;22) detected in most cases
  - Can be detected by FISH or PCR studies for the fusion protein

CLINICAL ISSUES

Epidemiology
- Incidence
  - Uncommon tumors
- Age
  - Typically occurs in young adults
  - Rare congenital cases reported
- Gender
  - Male predominance

Site
- Most often present on trunk or extremities
- Rarely occur on head and neck

Presentation
- Dermal and subcutaneous nodular/multinodular or plaque-like mass

Natural History
- Slowly progressive, locally aggressive tumor

Treatment
- Optimal treatment is complete surgical excision
- Imatinib has been used for locally extensive and metastatic disease
  - Complete response reported in up to 50% of cases

Prognosis
- Excellent in most cases
- Local recurrences in up to 30% of cases
- Very low metastatic potential (and essentially only in cases with fibrosarcomatous transformation)

MACROSCOPIC FEATURES

General Features
- Polypoid, multinodular, or bosselated-appearing tumor
  - Rare cases may be atrophic appearing
- Cut surface usually gray-white
- May show hemorrhage and cystic changes

Size
- Range: 1-10 cm

MICROSCOPIC PATHOLOGY

Histologic Features
- Dermal and subcutaneous involvement
- Proliferation of monomorphic spindle-shaped cells
- Arrayed in storiform or cartwheel patterns
- Lesional cells typically lack significant pleomorphism
  - Elongated spindle-shaped nuclei

DERMATOFIBROSARCOMA PROTUBERANS

Key Facts

Terminology
- Low-grade malignant spindle cell tumor of skin characteristically showing prominent storiforming
- Variant: Bednar tumor (pigmented DFSP)

Clinical Issues
- Typically occurs in young adults
- Excellent prognosis in most cases
- Relatively low recurrence rate
- Very low metastatic rates (usually only in cases with fibrosarcomatous transformation)

Microscopic Pathology
- Dermal and subcutaneous involvement
- Cells arrayed in storiform or cartwheel patterns
- Proliferation of monomorphic spindle-shaped cells
- Lesional cells lack significant pleomorphism

- Mitoses usually infrequent (< 4/10 HPF)
  - Atypical mitoses usually absent

Ancillary Tests
- CD34 is most reliable marker, typically strongly and diffusely positive
  - May be weak and focal in some cases
- FXIIIA is typically negative
  - Focal staining, usually at periphery or in scattered dendritic cells

Top Differential Diagnoses
- Cellular dermatofibroma/fibrous histiocytoma
- Indeterminate fibrohistiocytic lesion
- Fibrosarcoma (including transformation in DFSP)
- Leiomyosarcoma
- Spindle cell/desmoplastic melanoma

- Mild nuclear hyperchromasia, small to inconspicuous nucleoli
- Moderate amounts of eosinophilic cytoplasm
- Mitoses are usually infrequent (< 4/10 HPF) and not atypical
  - Increased mitoses and atypical forms are seen with fibrosarcomatous change
- Necrosis is usually absent
- Adnexal structures entrapped but not obliterated
- Subcutaneous areas typically show "honeycombing" fat entrapment
- Myxoid stromal change may be prominent in some cases

Cytologic Features
- Elongated spindle-shaped cells with hyperchromatic-staining nuclei, small or absent nucleoli, and eosinophilic-staining cytoplasm

Variants
- **Bednar tumor**
  - Pigmented DFSP due to intratumoral population of benign melanocytes
  - No prognostic significance
- **Giant cell fibroblastoma (GCFB)**
  - Clinical: Occurs in children and young adults
  - Histologic features are distinctive
    - Proliferation of spindled cells and giant cells with nuclear hyperchromasia
    - Pseudovascular spaces lined by the giant cells
  - Mutations involving COL1A1/PDGFR (same as in DFSP)

ANCILLARY TESTS

Immunohistochemistry
- Useful to confirm diagnosis, although often not necessary
  - CD34 is most reliable marker
    - Typically, strongly and diffusely positive
    - May be weak and focal in some cases

- FXIIIA is usually negative (positive in dermatofibroma [DF])
  - May show focal staining, usually at periphery or in scattered dendritic cells
- CD68, CD10, lysozyme, and chymotrypsin are typically negative
  - These markers are relatively nonspecific (but positive in DF and atypical fibroxanthoma)
- S100 can rarely be positive in a few (dendritic) cells
  - Will highlight pigmented cells in Bednar tumor

Cytogenetics
- t(17;22): Rearrangement of collagen 1A1 (COL1A1)/platelet-derived growth factor B (PDGFB)

DIFFERENTIAL DIAGNOSIS

Cellular Dermatofibroma/Fibrous Histiocytoma
- More pleomorphic cell types
  - Both small spindle-shaped fibroblastic cells and larger, histiocytoid-appearing cells
- No prominent storiforming
- May show superficial, jagged involvement of fat
  - No deep, honeycombing fat entrapment as in DFSP
- FXIIIA(+), CD68(+), CD163(+), and CD10(+); CD34(-)
  - CD34 may be focally positive, usually at periphery

Indeterminate Fibrohistiocytic Lesion
- Cellular fibrohistiocytic tumor with features intermediate between dermatofibroma and DFSP
- Often shows at least focal involvement of subcutis with fat entrapment
- CD34 and FXIIIA both usually positive
  - CD34 may only be weak/focal
- Lack COL1A/PDGFB translocation

Fibrosarcoma (Including Transformation in DFSP)
- Areas of increased cellularity, atypia, and mitoses (> 5/10 HPF)

DERMATOFIBROSARCOMA PROTUBERANS

Immunohistochemistry

Antibody	Reactivity	Staining Pattern	Comment
CD34	Positive	Cell membrane & cytoplasm	Usually strongly and diffusely positive
FXIIIA	Negative		May see focal staining of scattered single cells
CD68	Negative		May see focal staining of entrapped histiocytes
CD163	Negative		Strongly positive in dermatofibroma
S100	Negative		Rarely positive in pigmented cells (Bednar tumor)

- Spindle cells typically arrayed in prominent fascicles with "herringbone" appearance
  - Intersecting fascicles at 45° angles
- Usually see loss of CD34 expression in fibrosarcomatous areas

Fibromatosis
- Proliferation of elongated spindle cells associated with dense collagenous stroma
- Small blood vessels associated with extravasated red blood cells
- Often deeply infiltrates soft tissues but lacks honeycombing fat entrapment of DFSP
- β-catenin(+) and actin (SMA)(+); CD34(-)

Solitary Fibrous Tumor
- CD34(+) spindle cell proliferation but lacks storiforming of DFSP
- More common in soft tissues; only rarely occurs in the skin
- Composed of patternless proliferation of spindle cells associated with thickened, ropey collagen bundles and "staghorn" vessels

Leiomyosarcoma
- Long fascicles of enlarged, atypical, eosinophilic-staining spindle cells
- Usually shows more cytologic atypia, pleomorphism, and multiple mitoses
- Lacks storiforming pattern of DFSP
- Actin and desmin positive; CD34 typically negative

Atypical Fibroxanthoma (AFX)
- Occurs in sun-damaged skin of the elderly (typically head and neck region)
- Dermal-based proliferation of markedly atypical and pleomorphic-appearing tumor cells
- Usually shows a mixture of spindle-shaped and epithelioid cells with tumor giant cells
  - However, some cases can be mostly composed of spindle cells
    - But cells show higher grade atypia and lack the storiforming pattern of DFSP

Spindle Cell/Desmoplastic Melanoma
- Typically shows greater atypia, pleomorphism, and nuclear hyperchromasia
- Lacks areas of storiforming
- Overlying melanoma in situ present in majority of cases (> 70%)
- S100 positive; other melanocytic markers often negative

DIAGNOSTIC CHECKLIST

Clinically Relevant Pathologic Features
- Fibrosarcomatous transformation
- Margin status: Tumors with positive margins much more likely to recur

Pathologic Interpretation Pearls
- Dermal/subcutaneous proliferation of monomorphic spindle-shaped cells arrayed in storiform or cartwheel patterns

SELECTED REFERENCES

1. Wang WL et al: COL1A1:PDGFB chimeric transcripts are not present in indeterminate fibrohistiocytic lesions of the skin. Am J Dermatopathol. 32(2):149-53, 2010
2. Llombart B et al: Dermatofibrosarcoma protuberans: clinical, pathological, and genetic (COL1A1-PDGFB) study with therapeutic implications. Histopathology. 54(7):860-72, 2009
3. Sundram UN: Review: Dermatofibrosarcoma protuberans: histologic approach and updated treatment recommendations. Clin Adv Hematol Oncol. 7(6):406-8, 2009
4. Paradisi A et al: Dermatofibrosarcoma protuberans: wide local excision vs. Mohs micrographic surgery. Cancer Treat Rev. 34(8):728-36, 2008
5. Maire G et al: A clinical, histologic, and molecular study of 9 cases of congenital dermatofibrosarcoma protuberans. Arch Dermatol. 143(2):203-10, 2007
6. Mentzel T et al: Myxoid dermatofibrosarcoma protuberans: clinicopathologic, immunohistochemical, and molecular analysis of eight cases. Am J Dermatopathol. 29(5):443-8, 2007
7. Abrams TA et al: Targeted therapy for dermatofibrosarcoma protuberans. Curr Oncol Rep. 8(4):291-6, 2006
8. Terrier-Lacombe MJ et al: Dermatofibrosarcoma protuberans, giant cell fibroblastoma, and hybrid lesions in children: clinicopathologic comparative analysis of 28 cases with molecular data--a study from the French Federation of Cancer Centers Sarcoma Group. Am J Surg Pathol. 27(1):27-39, 2003
9. Horenstein MG et al: Indeterminate fibrohistiocytic lesions of the skin: is there a spectrum between dermatofibroma and dermatofibrosarcoma protuberans? Am J Surg Pathol. 24(7):996-1003, 2000
10. Wang J et al: Detection of COL1A1-PDGFB fusion transcripts in dermatofibrosarcoma protuberans by reverse transcription-polymerase chain reaction using archival formalin-fixed, paraffin-embedded tissues. Diagn Mol Pathol. 8(3):113-9, 1999
11. Mopper C et al: Dermatofibrosarcoma protuberans. Am J Clin Pathol. 20(2):171-6, 1950

DERMATOFIBROSARCOMA PROTUBERANS

Clinical and Microscopic Features

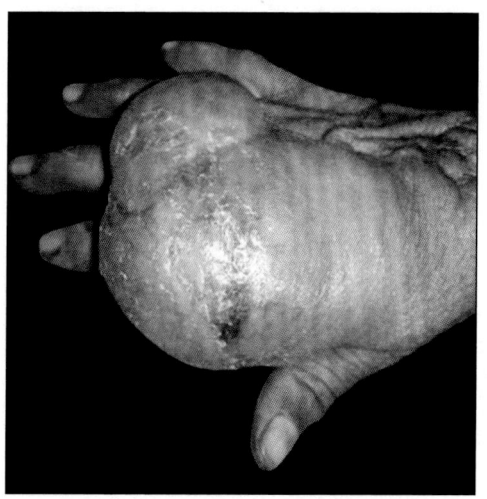

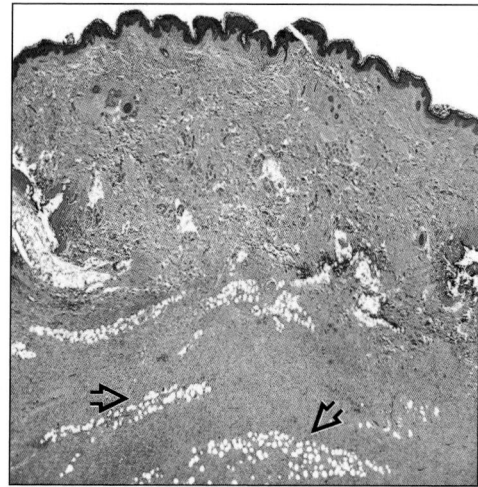

(Left) Clinical photograph shows a case of a recurrent DFSP with diffuse, nodular involvement of the distal hand. (Courtesy T. Mentzel, MD.) *(Right)* Scanning magnification view of a DFSP shows deep dermal and subcutaneous involvement by a cellular spindle cell tumor with fat entrapment ⇒. The epidermis and superficial dermis are unremarkable.

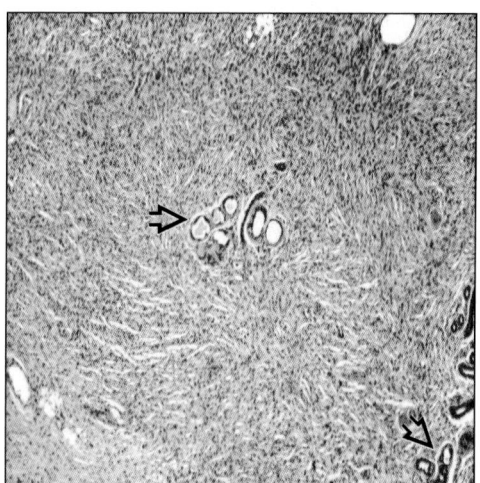

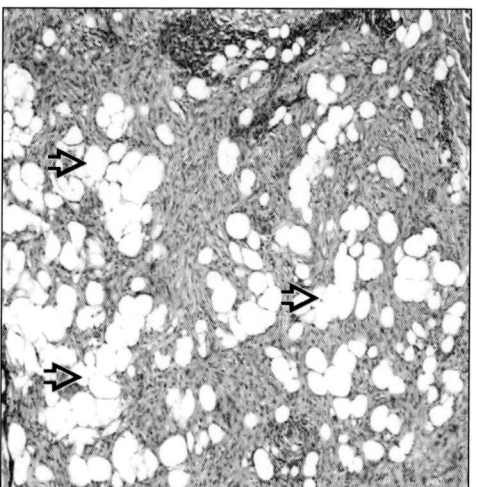

(Left) On low power, there are a number of adnexal glands that are entrapped ⇒ by the cellular, vaguely storiform neoplastic proliferation. However, there is no destruction of these adnexal structures by the tumor. *(Right)* The deep subcutaneous tissues of this DFSP highlight the significant fat entrapment ⇒. The neoplastic cells are cytologically bland, and mitotic figures are not easily identified.

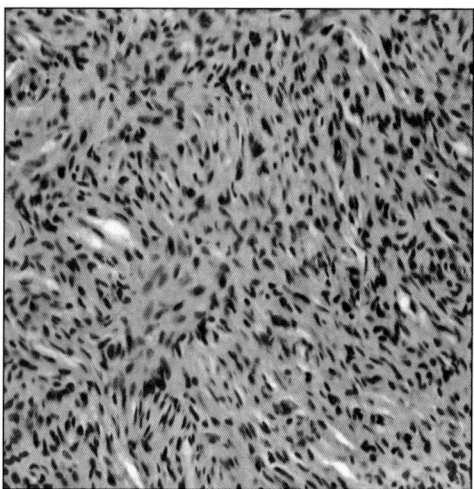

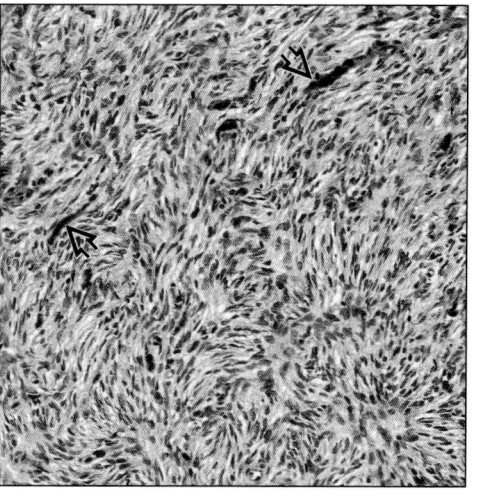

(Left) High power of DFSP shows a proliferation of bland spindled cells, lacking marked pleomorphism or anaplasia. Mitotic figures are often difficult to identify. *(Right)* In addition to spindled fibroblastic tumor cells, scattered elongated pigmented (melanin-containing) cells are seen ⇒ in the variant known as Bednar tumor. The finding is of no prognostic significance, and similar cells can be found in fibrosarcomatous DFSP and in giant cell fibroblastoma. (Courtesy T. Mentzel, MD.)

Variant Microscopic Features

(Left) Areas of myxoid stromal change may be seen in a minority of cases of DFSP. The myxoid changes give a lighter stromal appearance ⇉ to a tumor that is otherwise usually quite densely cellular. *(Right)* High magnification of a myxoid DFSP shows stellate and spindle cells in a myxoid stroma. There is a residual storiform pattern, although the cells are widely separated by the stromal material. A blood vessel is seen with a mildly thickened wall ➡. *(Courtesy T. Mentzel, MD.)*

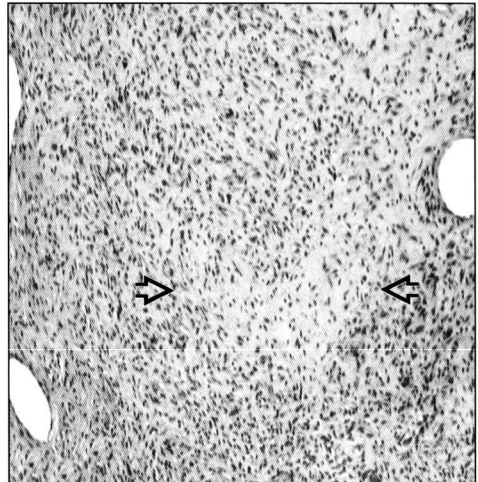
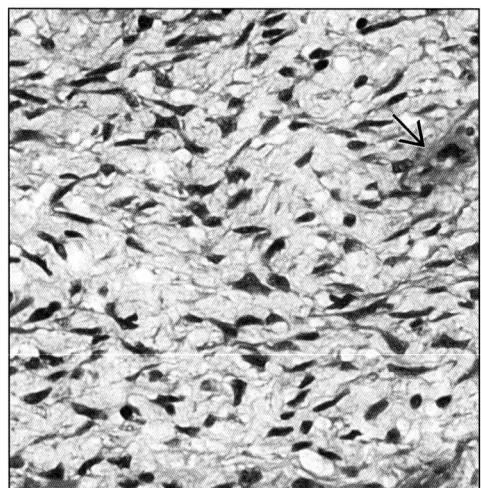

(Left) Diffuse infiltration of subcutaneous tissue is seen in many examples of giant cell fibroblastoma, such as this case, which shows honeycombing fat entrapment, similar to DFSP. *(Right)* Higher magnification of GCFB shows diffuse infiltration of subcutaneous tissue by spindle-shaped to multinucleated cells ➡ with nuclear hyperchromasia. Note the pseudovascular spaces ➡, which are typical of this tumor. *(Courtesy T. Mentzel, MD.)*

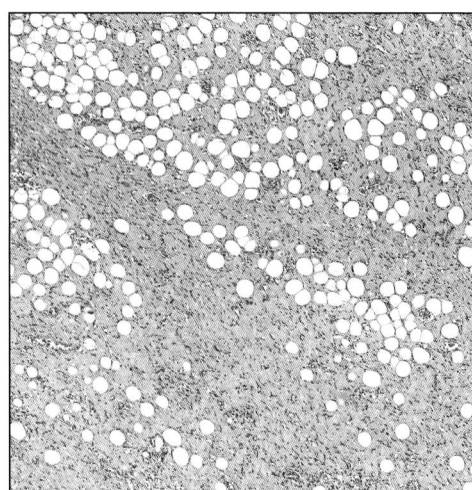
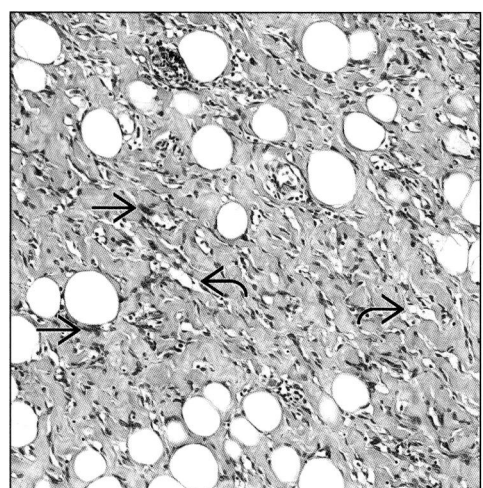

(Left) Cellular and more atypical area of DFSP shows a proliferation of densely packed atypical spindle cells with storiforming. A few adipocytes ➡ are surrounded (entrapped) by the neoplastic population. *(Right)* Fibrosarcomatous transformation in a DFSP is diagnosed when there is increased cellularity, increased cytologic atypia, and multiple mitotic figures ➡. The tumor is also arranged in a much more fascicular or "herringbone" architecture than a typical DFSP.

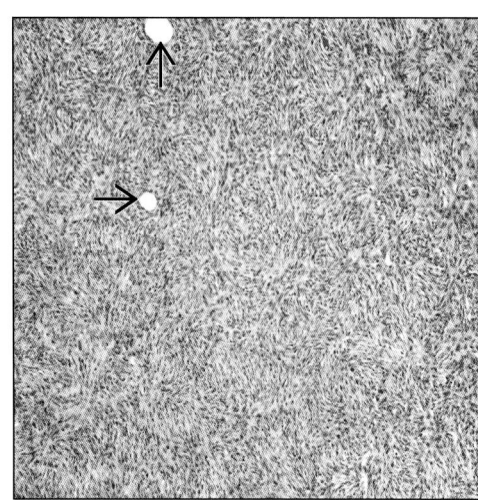
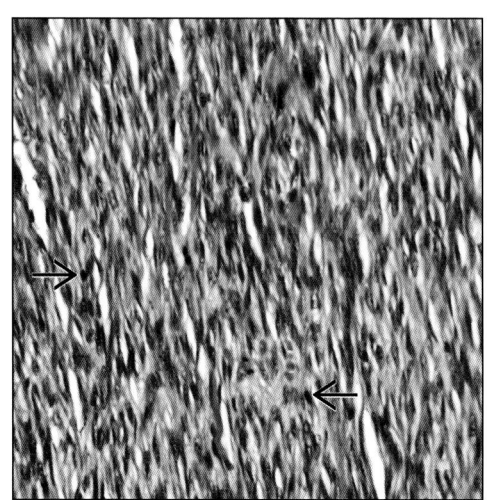

Ancillary Techniques and Differential Diagnosis

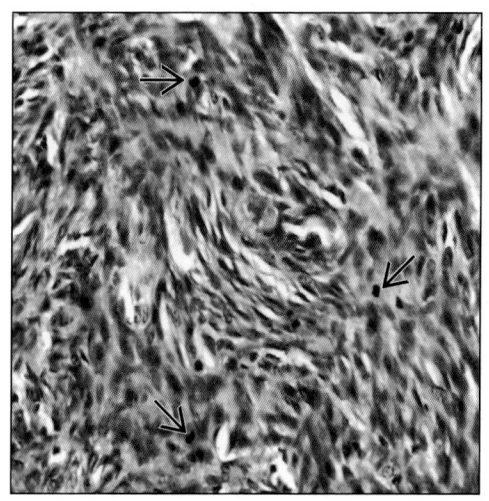

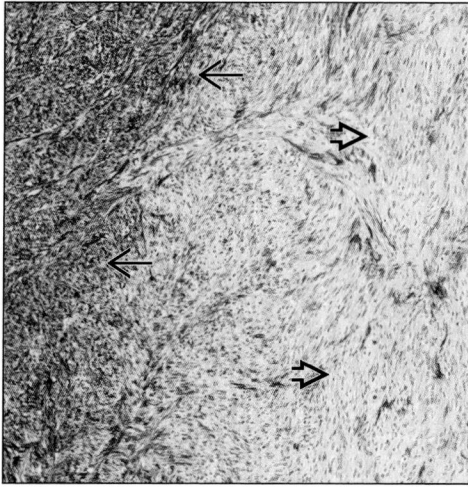

(Left) High-power view of fibrosarcomatous transformation in a DFSP shows residual vague storiforming by atypical hyperchromatic-staining spindle cells with numerous mitoses ➡. *(Right)* Loss of CD34 expression ▷ is seen in areas of fibrosarcomatous DFSP, compared with the residual adjacent dermatofibrosarcoma ➡. However, some cases retain diffuse CD34 immunoreactivity. (Courtesy T. Mentzel, MD.)

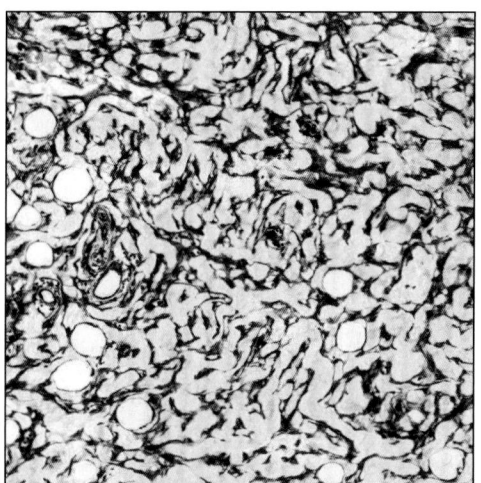

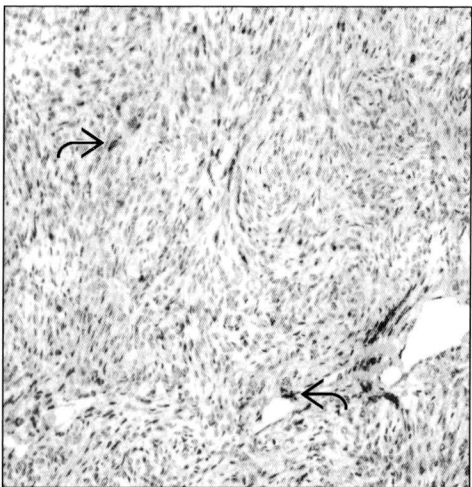

(Left) Giant cell fibroblastoma shows strong and diffuse CD34 staining in the spindle cells and multinucleated giant cells. (Courtesy T. Mentzel, MD.) *(Right)* Immunohistochemistry for FXIIIA typically shows only scattered positive entrapped fibroblasts or dendritic cells ➢, but the majority of the spindle cells are negative. The stain highlights the cytoplasm of these cells.

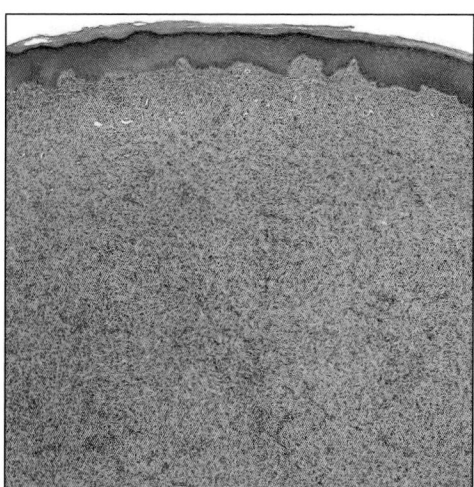

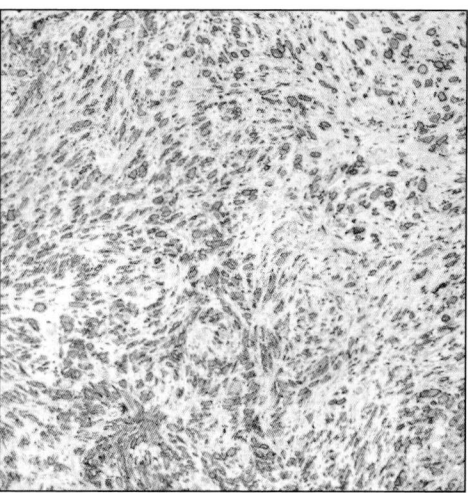

(Left) Scanning magnification view of a cellular and atypical DF shows deep dermal involvement by a cellular spindle cell tumor without prominent collagen trapping typical of conventional DF. *(Right)* CD163 shows strong and diffuse staining of the histiocytic and spindled cells in a cellular DF. This marker is typically negative in DFSP.

ATYPICAL FIBROXANTHOMA

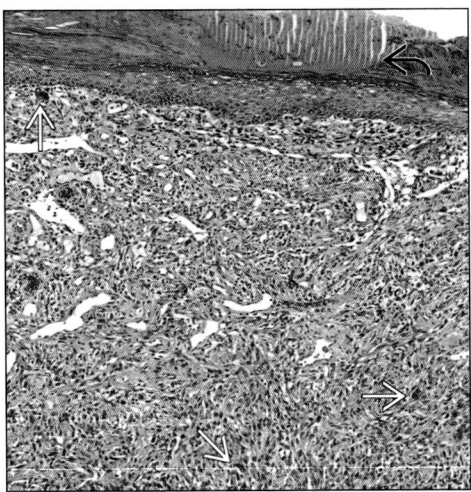

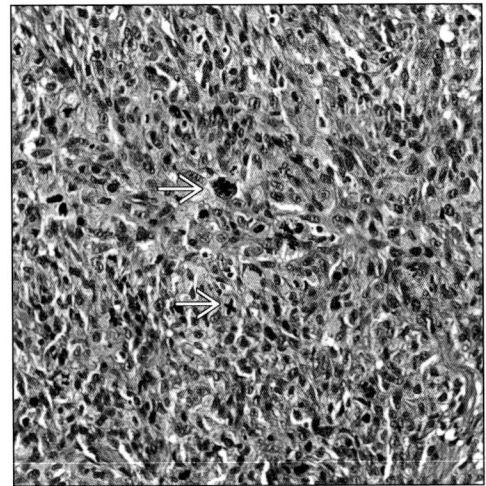

Low magnification of AFX shows a cellular and sheet-like, atypical dermal-based proliferation of spindle-shaped and pleomorphic ➡ cells. The epidermis shows dense overlying serum crusting ➔.

Higher magnification of an AFX shows a proliferation of markedly atypical and pleomorphic-appearing enlarged, epithelioid to spindle-shaped cells, with several frankly atypical mitotic figures ➡.

TERMINOLOGY

Abbreviations
- Atypical fibroxanthoma (AFX)

Synonyms
- Superficial malignant fibrous histiocytoma (MFH)
- Superficial pleomorphic sarcoma

Definitions
- Dermal-based, low-grade mesenchymal neoplasm showing no specific lineage of differentiation
  o Should be negative for markers of melanocytic (i.e., S100) and epithelial (i.e., cytokeratins and p63) differentiation

ETIOLOGY/PATHOGENESIS

Environmental Exposure
- Likely related to UV exposure, as most cases occur in sun-damaged skin
- Some cases reported following radiation therapy
- May also be increased in immunosuppressed patients (i.e., renal transplant patients)

CLINICAL ISSUES

Epidemiology
- Age
  o Typically occurs in elderly patients
  o Rare cases in children with xeroderma pigmentosum
- Gender
  o May have slight male predominance

Site
- Head and neck in general is most commonly affected area
  o Scalp is most common location
- Uncommonly occur on trunk or extremities

o May present in younger adult patients

Presentation
- Skin nodule, asymptomatic in most cases
  o Often rapidly growing lesion
  o Dermal-based lesion
  o May show overlying ulceration or bleeding/crusting
- Regional lymph node metastases may be found in small number of cases

Natural History
- Progressive lesion; does not regress without treatment

Treatment
- Surgical approaches
  o Complete and wide surgical excision
    ▪ Mohs surgery is also effective
  o Unresectable or metastatic cases may be treated with chemoradiation

Prognosis
- Very good
- Rate of local recurrence is low (< 10% reported)
- Vast majority of cases do not metastasize
  o Cases with subcutaneous involvement are considered MFH and can metastasize

MACROSCOPIC FEATURES

General Features
- Large, nodular, unencapsulated, dermal-based tumor

Size
- < 2 cm in most cases

MICROSCOPIC PATHOLOGY

Histologic Features
- Nodular, dermal-based proliferation of atypical, pleomorphic spindled and epithelioid-appearing cells

ATYPICAL FIBROXANTHOMA

Key Facts

Terminology

- Atypical fibroxanthoma (AFX)
- Dermal-based, low-grade mesenchymal neoplasm showing no specific lineage of differentiation

Clinical Issues

- Mass lesion, may be ulcerated or bleeding

Microscopic Pathology

- Highly atypical and pleomorphic proliferation of spindled to epithelioid-appearing cells
- Scattered large, bizarre-appearing multinucleated cells

Ancillary Tests

- Immunohistochemistry is key in confirming diagnosis
  - Essentially excluding other, more specific diagnoses

- Negative for melanocytic markers, cytokeratins (especially HMWCKs), p63, muscle and vascular markers
- Positive for nonspecific markers including CD68, CD10, CD99, and vimentin

Top Differential Diagnoses

- Sarcomatoid carcinoma (typically SCC)
  - Metastatic carcinoma should be considered
- Spindle cell melanoma
- Leiomyosarcoma

Diagnostic Checklist

- Depth of involvement: Subcutaneous extension implies more aggressive behavior
- Poorly differentiated malignancies often showing bizarre tumor cells and nonspecific IHC findings

---

- Cells are markedly enlarged and often bizarre-appearing
- Show irregular-appearing, hyperchromatic-staining nuclei
  - Irregular nuclear borders and prominent nucleoli
- Cytoplasm of tumor cells is abundant, eosinophilic, and sometimes foamy appearing
- Variants include spindle cell, clear cell, granular, chondroid, and osteoid
- Scattered large, bizarre-appearing multinucleated giant cells typically present
- Numerous mitoses, including highly atypical forms easily found
- No evidence of associated/overlying carcinoma or melanoma in situ
  - Often separated from epidermis by a thin grenz zone
- No evidence of epithelial (squamous, ductal, or glandular) or melanocytic differentiation

Cytologic Features

- Frankly atypical and pleomorphic spindle-shaped to epithelioid cells
- Multinucleated tumor giant cells with prominent nuclear atypia

Predominant Pattern/Injury Type

- Spindled
- Epithelioid

Predominant Cell/Compartment Type

- Mesenchymal

ANCILLARY TESTS

Immunohistochemistry

- Negative for melanocytic markers, cytokeratins (especially HMWCKs), p63, muscle and vascular markers
- IHC is key in confirming diagnosis
  - Essentially excluding other, more specific diagnoses
- Positive for nonspecific markers, including CD68, CD10, CD99, and vimentin

Electron Microscopy

- Transitional forms from fibroblasts to large giant cells, with intermediate forms exhibiting features of both

DIFFERENTIAL DIAGNOSIS

Sarcomatoid Carcinoma

- Typically squamous cell carcinoma (SCC), but poorly differentiated adnexal carcinoma and metastatic poorly differentiated carcinoma should also be considered
- Positive: High molecular weight cytokeratins (CK5/6, CK903/34βE12) and p63 (especially primary cutaneous tumors)
  - May or may not show staining for pancytokeratin, AE1/AE3, EMA, and CAM5.2 (low molecular weight CK)

Pleomorphic, Spindle Cell, and Desmoplastic Melanoma

- Junctional component is present in majority of cases (> 70%)
- Positive: S100; ± MART-1/Melan-A, HMB-45, tyrosinase, and MITF
  - S100 often the only positive marker in spindle cell and desmoplastic melanoma
  - Scattered S100(+) dendritic cells are present in AFX and should not be misinterpreted as melanoma

Leiomyosarcoma

- Proliferation of atypical spindle cells with elongated, blunt-ended, or "cigar-shaped" nuclei
- Cells show abundant eosinophilic-staining cytoplasm and perinuclear vacuoles
- Positive: MSA, actin-sm, desmin (most cases, although up to 30% can be desmin negative)
  - Focal/weak actin-sm in some AFXs, likely indicating myofibroblastic differentiation

ATYPICAL FIBROXANTHOMA

Immunohistochemistry

Antibody	Reactivity	Staining Pattern	Comment
CD10	Positive	Cell membrane & cytoplasm	Usually strongly and diffusely positive
CD68	Positive	Cell membrane & cytoplasm	Usually positive, may be weak/focal
CK-PAN	Negative		Positive control staining of epidermis and adnexal structures
CK-HMW-NOS	Negative		Positive control staining of epidermis and adnexal structures
p63	Negative		Rare cases reportedly positive; must be CK negative
S100	Negative		Entrapped dendritic cells positive
melan-A103	Negative		Junctional melanocytes serve as positive control
HMB-45	Negative		Junctional melanocytes serve as positive control
Desmin	Negative		
CD34	Negative		Highlights stromal vessels
CD31	Negative		Highlights stromal vessels
Actin-sm	Equivocal	Cytoplasmic	May be weakly positive in some cases, likely indicating myofibroblastic differentiation
MITF	Equivocal	Nuclear	Rare cases may be weakly/focally positive
CD99	Equivocal	Cell membrane & cytoplasm	Some cases positive, but often weak or negative

Other Sarcomas

- Much less likely consideration (but differential can include both primary and metastatic sarcomas)
- Angiosarcoma: CD31(+), CD34(+)
  - Other vascular neoplasms such as Kaposi sarcoma are even less likely
- Malignant peripheral nerve sheath tumor (MPNST)
  - Usually deep-seated lesions, but can rarely involve dermis
  - Focal to weak S100(+) in 50-70% of cases, may show CD56(+), nestin(+)
- Fibrosarcoma (FS)
  - Usually arises in dermatofibrosarcoma protuberans (DFSP) in skin
  - Prominent herringbone pattern in FS areas, storiforming in DFSP areas
  - DFSP shows strong CD34(+) (may be negative in fibrosarcoma areas)

DIAGNOSTIC CHECKLIST

Clinically Relevant Pathologic Features

- Depth of involvement (subcutaneous extension implies more aggressive behavior)

Pathologic Interpretation Pearls

- Poorly differentiated malignancy often shows bizarre tumor cells and nonspecific IHC findings

SELECTED REFERENCES

1. Kanner WA et al: CD10, p63 and CD99 expression in the differential diagnosis of atypical fibroxanthoma, spindle cell squamous cell carcinoma and desmoplastic melanoma. J Cutan Pathol. 37(7):744-50, 2010
2. New D et al: Atypical fibroxanthoma with regional lymph node metastasis: report of a case and review of the literature. Arch Dermatol. 146(12):1399-404, 2010
3. Ang GC et al: More than 2 decades of treating atypical fibroxanthoma at mayo clinic: what have we learned from 91 patients? Dermatol Surg. 35(5):765-72, 2009
4. Gleason BC et al: Utility of p63 in the differential diagnosis of atypical fibroxanthoma and spindle cell squamous cell carcinoma. J Cutan Pathol. 36(5):543-7, 2009
5. Hultgren TL et al: Immunohistochemical staining of CD10 in atypical fibroxanthomas. J Cutan Pathol. 34(5):415-9, 2007
6. Ríos-Martín JJ et al: Granular cell atypical fibroxanthoma: report of two cases. Am J Dermatopathol. 29(1):84-7, 2007
7. Farley R et al: Diagnosis and management of atypical fibroxanthoma. Skinmed. 5(2):83-6, 2006
8. Hartel PH et al: CD99 immunoreactivity in atypical fibroxanthoma and pleomorphic malignant fibrous histiocytoma: a useful diagnostic marker. J Cutan Pathol. 33 Suppl 2:24-8, 2006
9. Murali R et al: Clear cell atypical fibroxanthoma - report of a case with review of the literature. J Cutan Pathol. 33(5):343-8, 2006
10. Seavolt M et al: Atypical fibroxanthoma: review of the literature and summary of 13 patients treated with mohs micrographic surgery. Dermatol Surg. 32(3):435-41; discussion 439-41, 2006
11. Mirza B et al: Atypical fibroxanthoma: a clinicopathological study of 89 cases. Australas J Dermatol. 46(4):235-8, 2005
12. Leong AS et al: Atypical fibroxanthoma of the skin: a clinicopathological and immunohistochemical study and a discussion of its histogenesis. Histopathology. 11(5):463-75, 1987
13. Alguacil-Garcia A et al: Atypical fibroxanthoma of the skin: an ultrastructural study of two cases. Cancer. 40(4):1471-80, 1977
14. Fretzin DF et al: Atypical fibroxanthoma of the skin. A clinicopathologic study of 140 cases. Cancer. 31(6):1541-52, 1973
15. Kroe DJ et al: Atypical fibroxanthoma of the skin. Report of ten cases. Am J Clin Pathol. 51(4):487-92, 1969

ATYPICAL FIBROXANTHOMA

Clinical and Microscopic Features

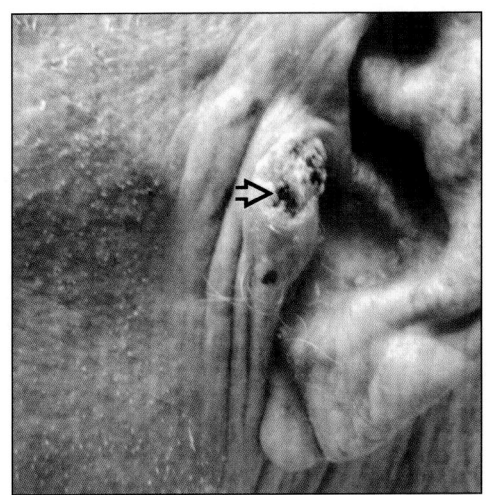

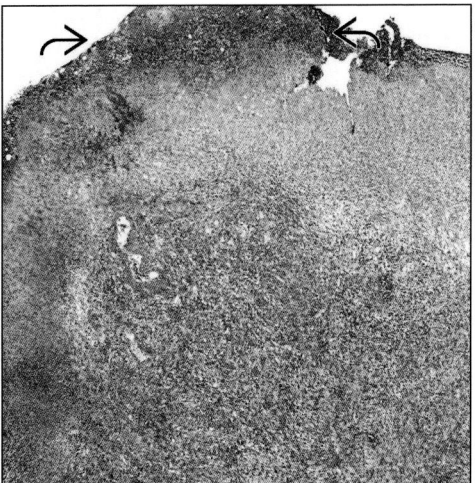

(Left) Clinical photograph shows an AFX on the ear of an elderly patient. Note that the surface is ulcerated and shows focal serum crusting ⮞. (Right) Histologic section of AFX at low magnification shows a large, dermal-based atypical nodular to sheet-like collection of tumor cells with overlying ulceration and serum crusting ⮞.

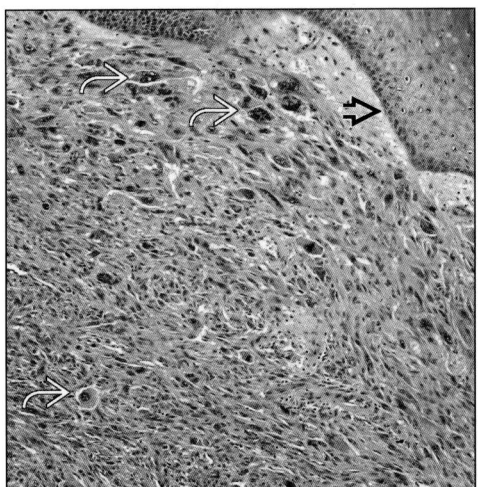

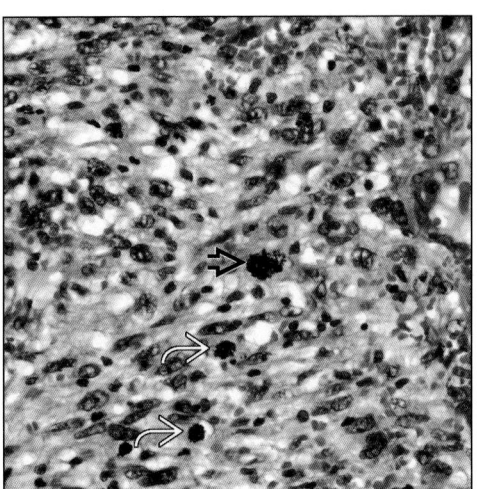

(Left) Histologic examination of the superficial portion of an AFX shows a proliferation of markedly atypical spindled cells, epithelioid cells, and numerous multinucleated tumor cells ⮞. The tumor closely abuts, but does not involve, the overlying epidermis ⮞. (Right) High magnification of AFX shows highly atypical cells with numerous mitoses ⮞, including frankly atypical forms ⮞.

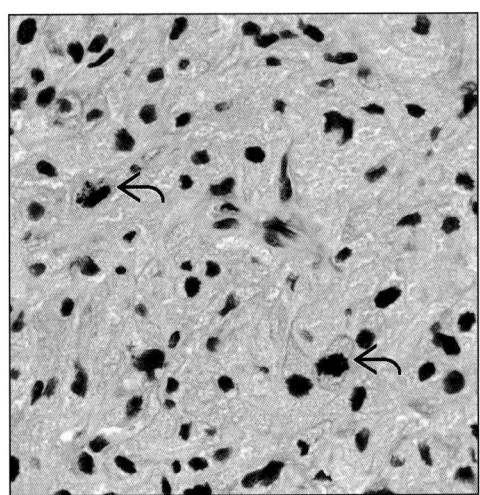

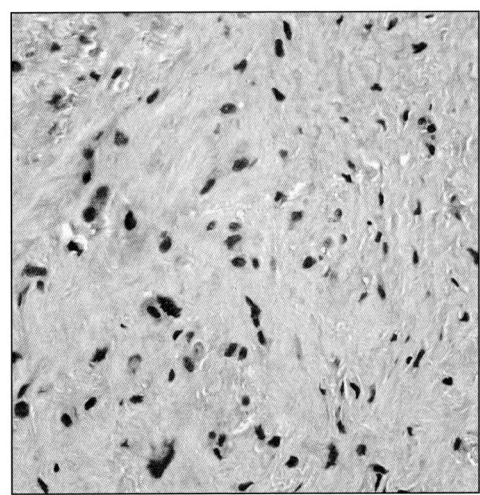

(Left) High magnification of an example of the granular cell variant of AFX shows large, bizarre-appearing histiocytoid cells containing abundant granular cytoplasm, similar to a malignant granular cell tumor. Mitoses ⮞ are easily found. (Right) An example of the chondroid variant of AFX shows an unusual hypocellular tumor with atypical, hyperchromatic-staining cells scattered in a chondromyxoid-appearing stroma.

Ancillary Techniques

(Left) High molecular weight cytokeratin (CK) stain shows positivity within the epidermis and adnexal ducts ⇒, but is negative within the tumor cells. *(Right)* S100 immunohistochemistry shows no staining of the tumor cells, but highlights a few intradermal dendritic cells ➡.

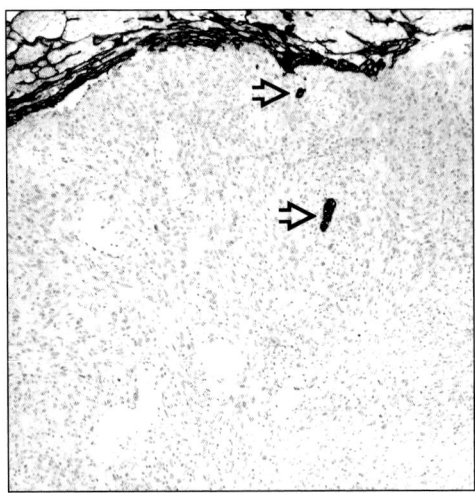
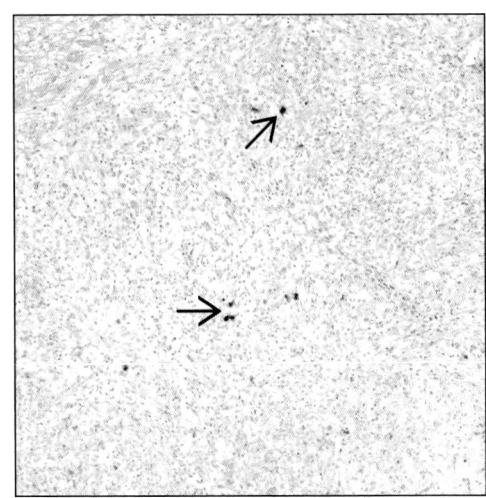

(Left) Smooth muscle actin stain shows scattered weakly positive cytoplasmic staining ➡, likely indicating myofibroblastic differentiation. *(Right)* CD34 immunohistochemical stain shows strong positive staining of small blood vessels, but is negative within the tumor cells (CD31 shows an identical pattern).

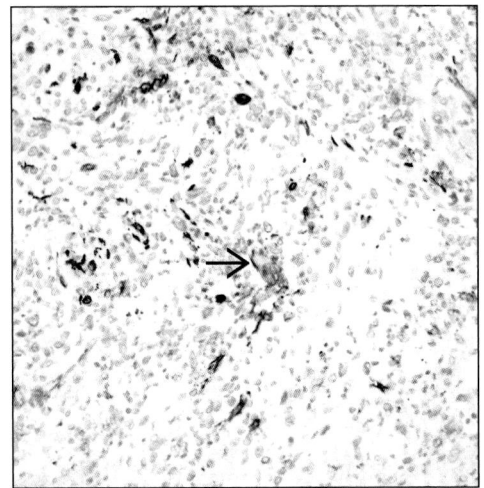
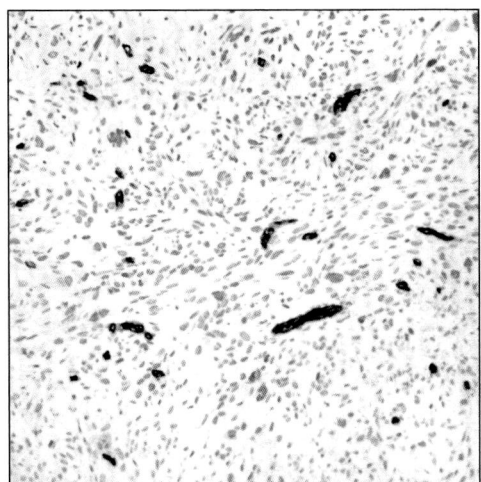

(Left) CD10 stain shows strong and diffuse staining of the tumor cells, a finding that is not very specific, but is helpful, as it is typically seen in AFX. *(Right)* CD68 is a nonspecific marker, but is typically positive in AFX. This example shows moderate to strong cytoplasmic staining of most of the tumor cells, especially the large multinucleated tumor giant cells ➡.

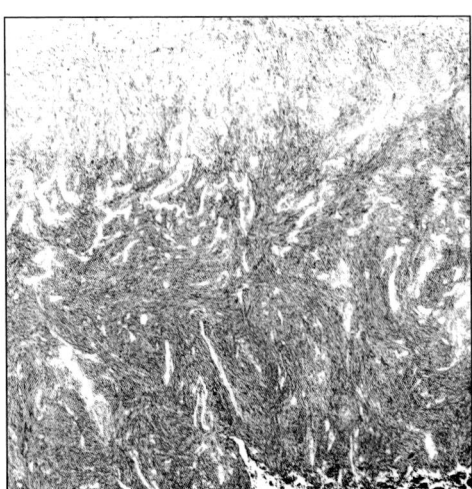
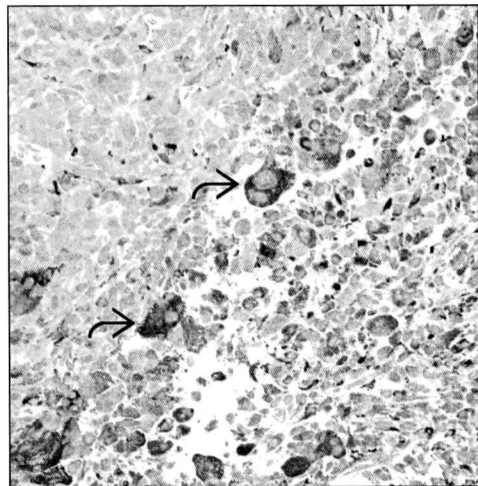

Differential Diagnosis

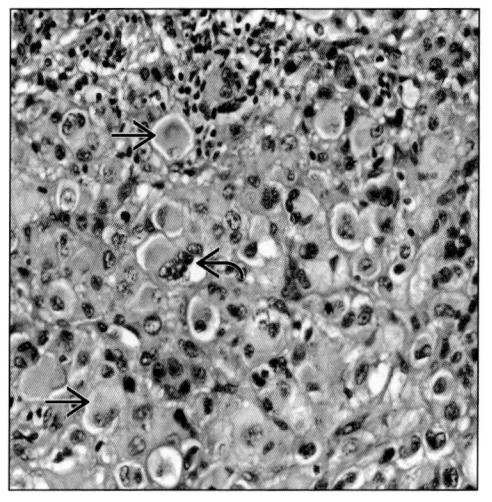 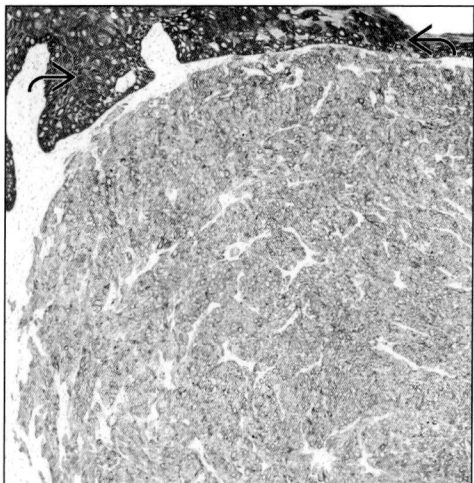

(Left) Poorly differentiated squamous cell carcinoma (SCC) is composed of atypical epithelioid cells with abundant pale to eosinophilic-staining cytoplasm ➡️. Scattered pleomorphic multinucleated tumor cells ➡️ can be seen in some cases of SCC. *(Right)* High molecular weight cytokeratins such as CK5/6 and CK903 are typically diffusely positive in most carcinomas, including poorly differentiated SCC. Note the strong positive internal control staining of the epidermis ➡️.

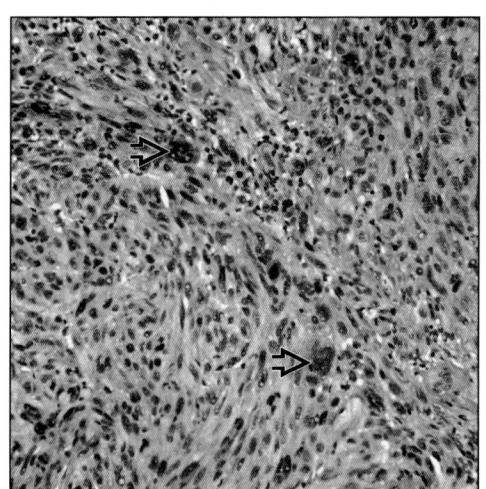 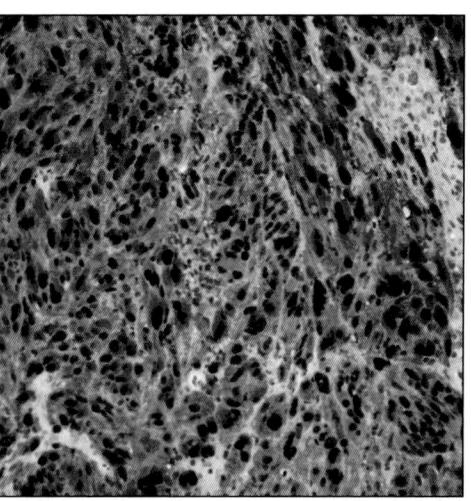

(Left) Melanoma should always be considered in the differential diagnosis with AFX, especially spindle cell/desmoplastic and metastatic melanomas, which can lack epidermal attachments and show striking atypia and pleomorphism, including multinucleated tumor giant cells ➡️. This is a rare case that lacks pigmentation. *(Right)* S100 immunohistochemistry shows diffuse, strong nuclear and cytoplasmic staining in a pleomorphic melanoma. This finding would exclude the possibility of AFX.

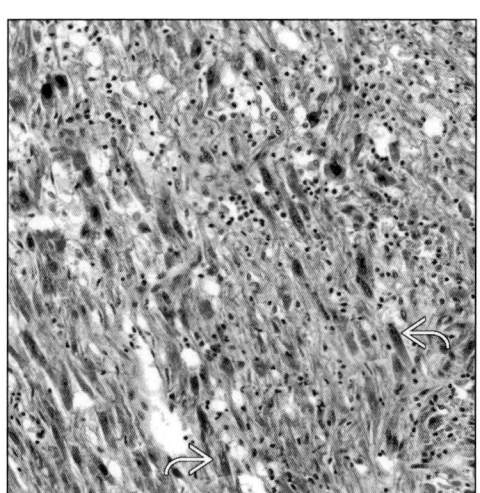 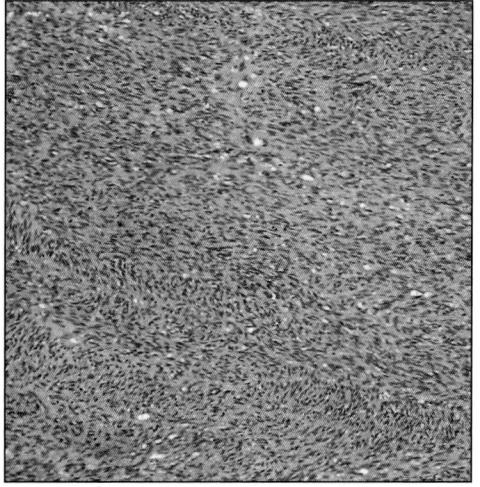

(Left) Leiomyosarcoma is composed of highly atypical spindle-shaped cells with oval to elongated, cigar-shaped nuclei ➡️ and abundant eosinophilic-staining cytoplasm. Actin is typically strongly positive, although desmin can be negative in up to 30% of cases. *(Right)* Fibrosarcoma (arising in a DFSP) displays dense cellularity, prominent cytologic atypia, and multiple mitotic figures. The tumor is arranged in a fascicular or "herringbone" architecture, which is not seen in AFX.

CUTANEOUS MALIGNANT FIBROUS HISTIOCYTOMA/PLEOMORPHIC SARCOMA

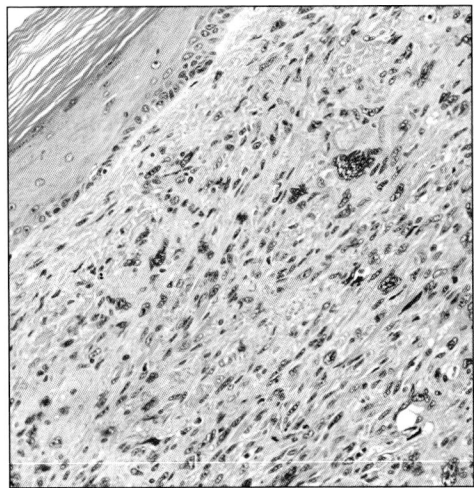

This cutaneous pleomorphic sarcoma is seen in the papillary dermis. Note the normal overlying epidermis without atypia or junctional activity, helping to exclude squamous cell carcinoma and melanoma.

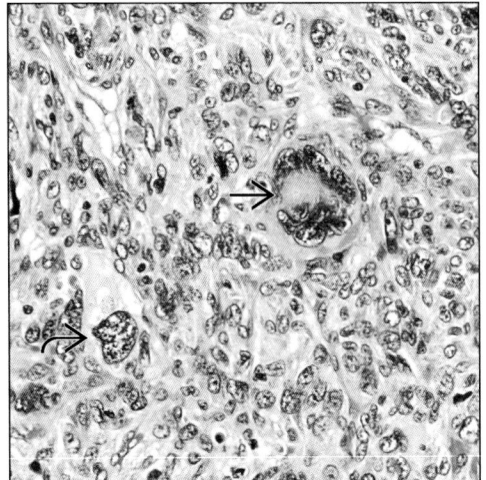

Microscopically, pleomorphic undifferentiated sarcoma is hypercellular with sheets of markedly anaplastic spindled and epithelioid cells, including bizarre ⊐ and multinucleated ⊐ forms.

TERMINOLOGY

Synonyms
- Pleomorphic sarcoma
- Undifferentiated high-grade sarcoma
- Malignant fibrous histiocytoma (MFH)

Definitions
- Anaplastic sarcoma composed of pleomorphic spindle and polygonal cells
  - No other definable differentiation, other than fibroblastic or myofibroblastic
- Morphologic pattern shared by poorly differentiated or anaplastic tumors of different lineages
  - Diagnosis of pleomorphic sarcoma is therefore one of exclusion

ETIOLOGY/PATHOGENESIS

Environmental Exposure
- Can occur at site of previous irradiation
- Rarely secondary to chronic ulceration or scarring

CLINICAL ISSUES

Epidemiology
- Incidence
  - Most common adult soft tissue sarcoma
  - Incidence increases with age
- Age
  - Older adults
  - Very rare in adolescents and young adults
- Gender
  - Slight male predominance

Site
- Most are in deep soft tissue
- Smaller numbers occur superficially in subcutaneous tissue
  - Dermal lesions are considered atypical fibroxanthoma (AFX) and have much better prognosis
- Most in extremities (lower limb > upper limb)
- May also arise on trunk

Presentation
- Enlarging mass
- Small proportion of patients have metastases at presentation

Prognosis
- Usually high-grade tumors
- Propensity for local recurrence and metastasis
- Superficial tumors have better prognosis than deep ones
- Myoid differentiation is prognostically adverse, with earlier metastasis
  - Applies whether differentiation is morphologic (leiomyosarcoma, myofibrosarcoma, rhabdomyosarcoma) or only immunohistochemical (actin, desmin)

MACROSCOPIC FEATURES

General Features
- Lobulated
- Generally circumscribed
- Heterogeneous cut surface
  - Firm, solid, and softer myxoid areas
- Necrosis and hemorrhage

Sections to Be Submitted
- Thorough sampling required to demonstrate any possible line of differentiation
  - e.g., lipoblastic, muscle, epithelial

Size
- Often large at presentation

CUTANEOUS MALIGNANT FIBROUS HISTIOCYTOMA/PLEOMORPHIC SARCOMA

Key Facts

Terminology
- Anaplastic sarcoma composed of pleomorphic spindle and polygonal cells
- No other definable differentiation, other than fibroblastic or myofibroblastic

Etiology/Pathogenesis
- Small proportion of cases occur post irradiation or secondary to chronic ulceration/scarring

Clinical Issues
- Most common adult soft tissue sarcoma
- Older adults
- Most frequent in deep soft tissue of extremities
- Usually high-grade tumors
  - Superficial tumors have better prognosis than deep ones

Macroscopic Features
- Thorough sampling required to demonstrate any possible line of differentiation
- Heterogeneous cut surface
- Necrosis and hemorrhage

Microscopic Pathology
- Diagnosis of exclusion
- Morphology shared by many tumors of different lineages
- Storiform pattern, loose fascicles or sheets
- Markedly atypical cells
- Abundant mitoses and necrosis
- No discernible microscopic features of differentiation
- Immunohistochemical panel required to exclude tumors with specific differentiation

MICROSCOPIC PATHOLOGY

Histologic Features
- Storiform or loose fascicles and sheets
- Markedly atypical cells
  - Spindle or polygonal-shaped
  - Bizarre and multinucleate forms frequent
  - Can have abundant foamy cytoplasm
- Abundant and atypical mitoses
- Necrosis often present
- Stroma ranges from fibrous to focally myxoid
- Chronic inflammation, including macrophages
- No discernible microscopic differentiation

ANCILLARY TESTS

Immunohistochemistry
- Use panel to exclude tumors with specific differentiation
- Focal smooth muscle actin (+) can be seen
  - Often in subplasmalemmal distribution
    - Indicates myofibroblastic differentiation
- May express CD34
- No evidence of true histiocytic differentiation

Cytogenetics
- Complex nonspecific cytogenetic abnormalities

DIFFERENTIAL DIAGNOSIS

Atypical Fibroxanthoma (AFX)
- Typically elderly patients, sun-damaged skin
- Most common on head and neck
- Histologically identical
- Dermal-based lesion (no subcutaneous invasion)

Melanoma
- Cells often have nested architecture
- Overlying skin may show junctional activity
- Expresses S100 protein, melanocytic markers

Anaplastic Carcinoma
- At least focal expression of epithelial antigens
- Epithelium may show dysplastic or in situ changes

Anaplastic Large Cell Lymphoma
- Sheets of large, atypical cells with abundant cytoplasm
- Variably positive for CD45, CD30, ALK1, EMA

Myxofibrosarcoma
- Subcutaneous or deep soft tissue origin
- Lobulated architecture, myxoid stroma
- Higher grades resemble pleomorphic sarcoma

Pleomorphic Leiomyosarcoma
- Focal fascicular architecture
- Focal smooth muscle cytology, e.g., blunt-ended nuclei
- Immunoreactive for desmin, SMA, and H-caldesmon

Pleomorphic Rhabdomyosarcoma
- Pleomorphic rhabdomyoblasts
- Expresses desmin and myogenin

Pleomorphic Liposarcoma
- Pleomorphic, multivacuolated lipoblasts

Dedifferentiated Liposarcoma
- Most frequent in internal trunk
- Can have adjacent well-differentiated liposarcoma
- Amplification of MDM2, CDK4 (by IHC or FISH)

SELECTED REFERENCES

1. Deyrup AT et al: Myoid differentiation and prognosis in adult pleomorphic sarcomas of the extremity: an analysis of 92 cases. Cancer. 98(4):805-13, 2003
2. Fletcher CD et al: Clinicopathologic re-evaluation of 100 malignant fibrous histiocytomas: prognostic relevance of subclassification. J Clin Oncol. 19(12):3045-50, 2001
3. Le Doussal V et al: Prognostic factors for patients with localized primary malignant fibrous histiocytoma: a multicenter study of 216 patients with multivariate analysis. Cancer. 77(9):1823-30, 1996
4. Weiss SW et al: Malignant fibrous histiocytoma: an analysis of 200 cases. Cancer. 41(6):2250-66, 1978

CUTANEOUS MALIGNANT FIBROUS HISTIOCYTOMA/PLEOMORPHIC SARCOMA

Microscopic Features

(Left) Cutaneous malignant fibrous histiocytoma/pleomorphic sarcoma. This tumor is present extensively within the dermis and extends into the subcutis. Here it is seen focally abutting skin adnexal structures ⊟. The atypia within many of the enlarged spindle cells is discernible even at low power. *(Right)* This example of cutaneous malignant fibrous histiocytoma is fairly well demarcated and predominantly located in the deep dermis and subcutis, although it is also seen focally abutting skeletal muscle ⊟.

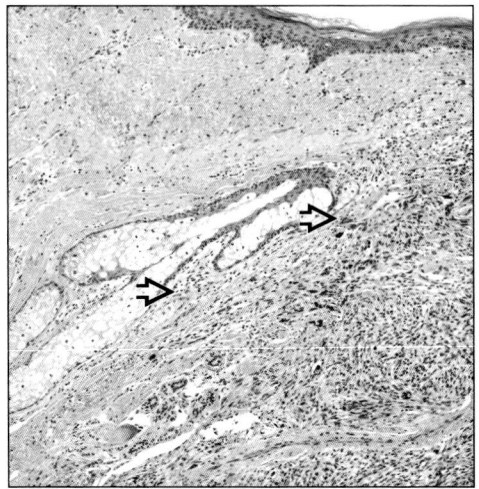
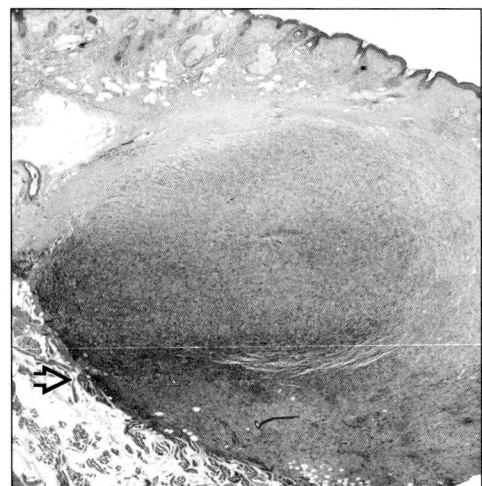

(Left) The cells are spindled in this field and are arranged in loosely fascicular distributions within collagenous stroma. Nuclear pleomorphism and cellular hyperchromasia are often discernible even at low-power magnification. *(Right)* The cellularity is high, and the architecture can vary from loosely fascicular to storiform to sheet-like. This case shows a more storiform or short fascicular pattern. Tumor giant cells ⇗ are interspersed and can be a prominent feature.

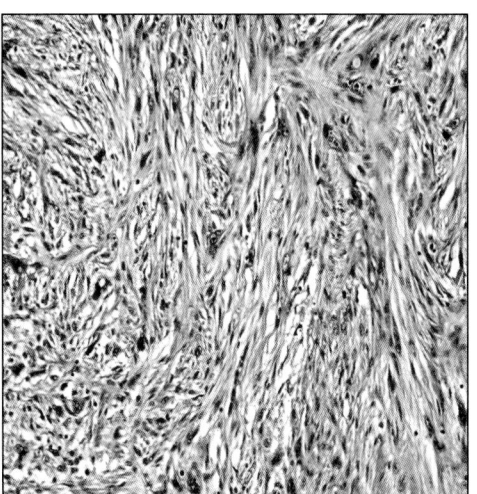
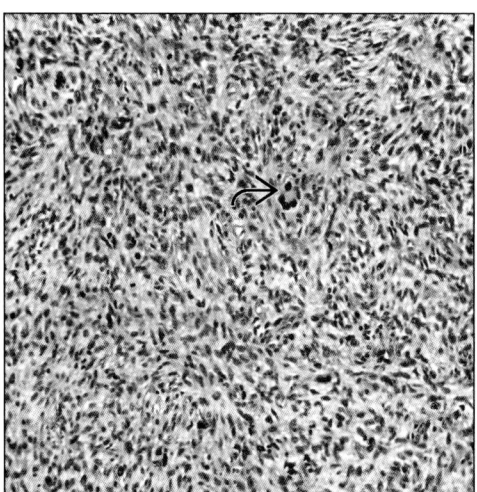

(Left) This pleomorphic undifferentiated sarcoma is composed of streams and fascicles of cells, many of which are epithelioid, with vesicular nuclei and prominent large nucleoli. Mitotic figures are readily identified ⇗. *(Right)* The anaplasia in this example is striking, with polygonal cells that vary greatly in size. Note the huge, often bizarre nuclei, macronucleoli ⇗, and abundant amphophilic cytoplasm. There is also a markedly atypical mitotic figure ⊟.

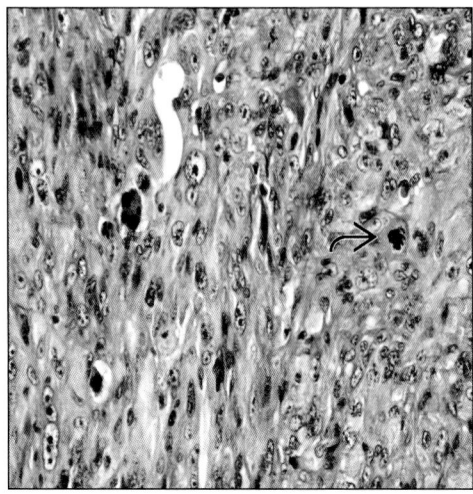
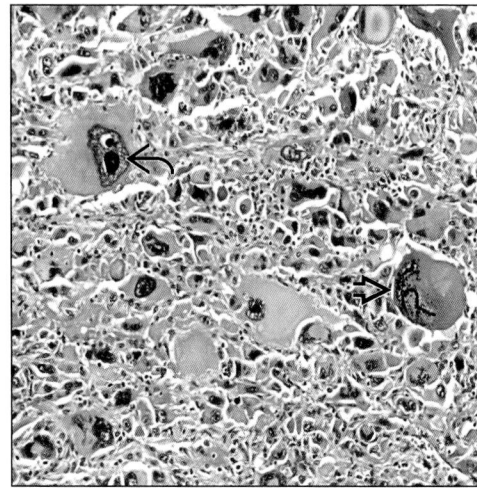

CUTANEOUS MALIGNANT FIBROUS HISTIOCYTOMA/PLEOMORPHIC SARCOMA

Microscopic Features and Ancillary Techniques

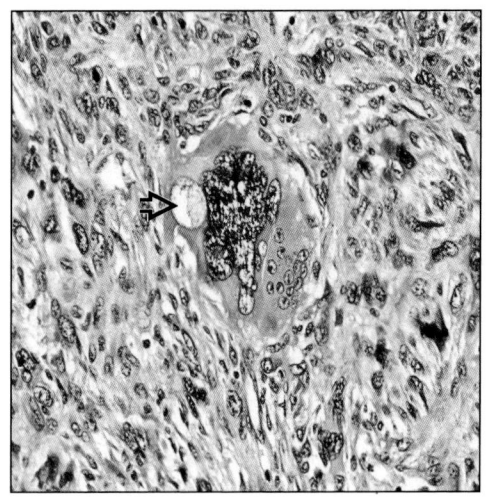

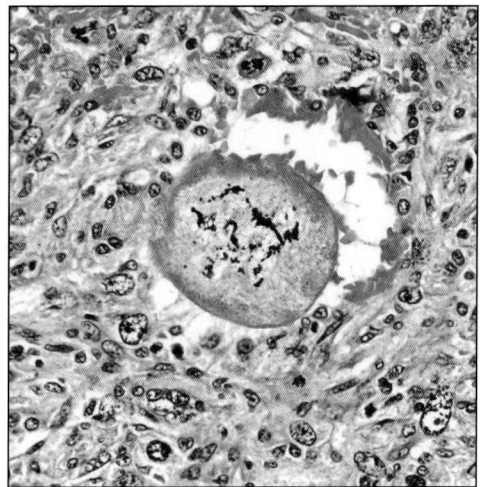

(Left) This cell is both bizarre and multinucleated and is several times the size of its neighbors, which are themselves enlarged. A cytoplasmic inclusion ⊵ is also seen within the large cell, and its nuclear chromatin is coarse and irregular. These differ from osteoclast-like giant cells, which have multiple uniform nuclei. *(Right)* A similarly enlarged neoplastic cell shows a large, fragmented atypical mitotic figure. Stromal hemorrhage and inflammation may also be features.

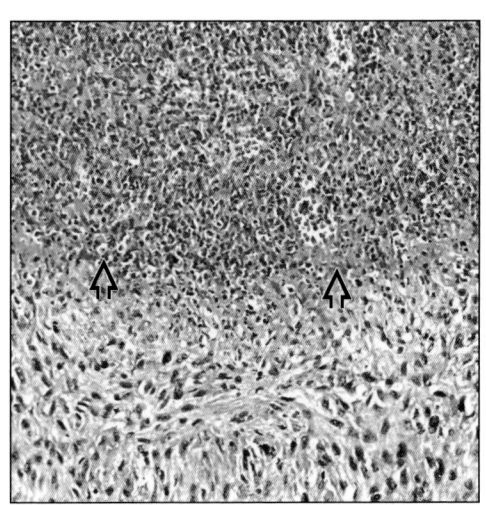

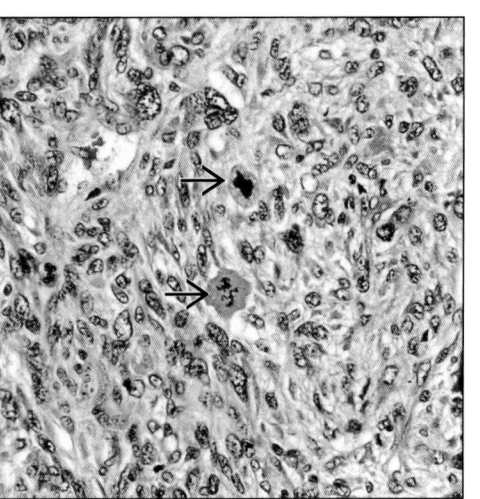

(Left) Necrosis ⊵ is a common finding in pleomorphic undifferentiated sarcoma and is often seen on gross examination. It can sometimes account for most of the tumor. *(Right)* This example is hypercellular, and atypical mitoses are easily discernible ⊡. This tumor shows no morphologically identifiable line of differentiation. A wide immunohistochemical panel is therefore required to exclude any specific mesenchymal lineage, carcinoma, or melanoma.

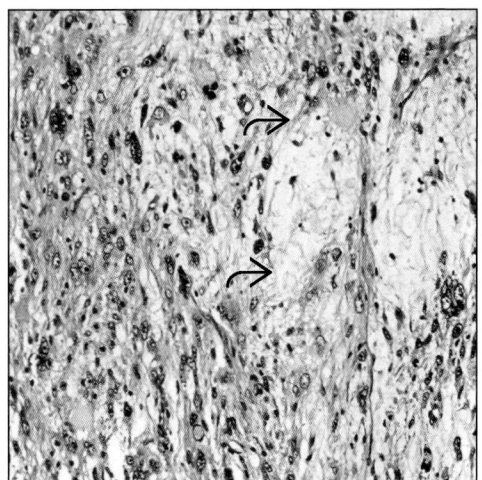

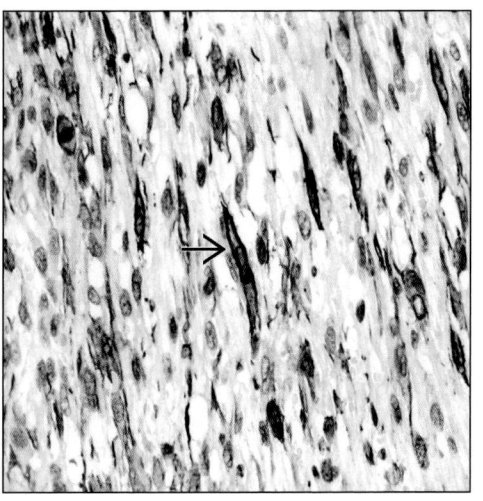

(Left) This pleomorphic undifferentiated sarcoma developed as recurrence of previous myxofibrosarcoma. Residual myxofibrosarcomatous zones are apparent ⊡; they are less cellular, with prominent myxoid stroma and a lobulated architecture. *(Right)* With immunohistochemistry, polygonal and spindled tumor cells may show focal expression of SMA, with subplasmalemmal linear distribution ⊡, typical of myofibroblastic differentiation.

FIBROSARCOMA

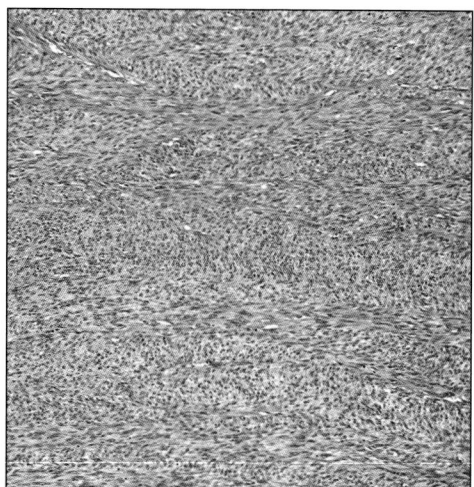

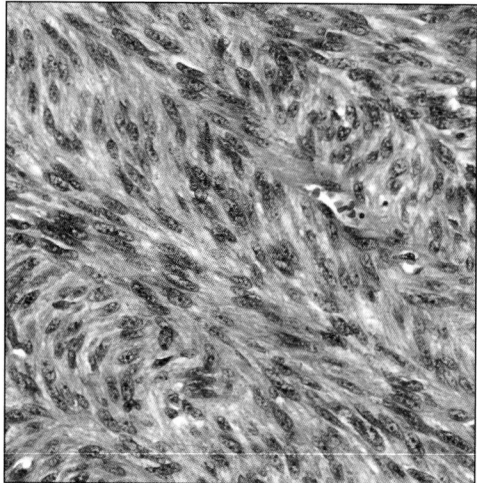

Low magnification shows a typically cellular low-grade fibrosarcoma with uniform spindle cells arranged in long intersecting fascicles in a so-called herringbone pattern. No necrosis is seen.

This well-differentiated fibrosarcoma shows uniform tapered spindle cells. The nuclei are elongated, and some have a small nucleolus.

TERMINOLOGY

Definitions

- Soft tissue sarcoma of adults composed of fibroblasts
- Lacks features of specific fibrosarcoma subtypes, which may be found in dermis/subcutis
  - Low-grade fibromyxoid sarcoma
  - Myxofibrosarcoma
  - Infantile fibrosarcoma
    - Has t(12;15)(p13;q26) with *ETV6-NTRK3* fusion
- Now very rare; mostly a diagnosis of exclusion
- Pleomorphic variants are currently classified as undifferentiated sarcoma/malignant fibrous histiocytoma
- Conclusive diagnosis can require electron microscopy

ETIOLOGY/PATHOGENESIS

De Novo

- Exceptionally rare if strictly defined

Arising in Association with Other Tumors

- Fibrosarcoma in dermatofibrosarcoma protuberans (DFSP)
  - Probable origin of many dermal or subcutaneous adult fibrosarcomas
- Malignant solitary fibrous tumor

Post Irradiation

- Usually therapeutic
- More often in deep soft tissue
- Long-time interval before sarcoma develops

CLINICAL ISSUES

Site

- Proximal limbs, head and neck

Presentation

- Painful or painless mass
  - Can ulcerate

Treatment

- Surgical approaches
  - Complete local excision
  - Pulmonary metastasectomy in selected cases

Prognosis

- Few modern studies
  - Older series represent a mixture of sarcoma types
- Relates to grade
- Local recurrence, especially if incompletely excised
- Metastasis in a small number of cases
  - To lungs, bone, and rarely, lymph node

MACROSCOPIC FEATURES

General Features

- Circumscribed, pseudoencapsulated
- Some subcutaneous, most deep (intramuscular)
- Firm, white, focal necrosis in some

Size

- Variable, can exceed 20 cm

MICROSCOPIC PATHOLOGY

Histologic Features

- Fascicular architecture
  - Characteristic "herringbone" or "chevron" pattern
- Elongated spindle cells
  - Slender, tapered, sometimes wavy nuclei
  - Variable hyperchromasia and pleomorphism
  - Variable mitotic activity; can include abnormal forms
- Scanty cytoplasm
- Variable stromal collagen

FIBROSARCOMA

Key Facts

Terminology
- Soft tissue sarcoma composed of fibroblasts
- Lacks features of specific types of fibrosarcoma

Etiology/Pathogenesis
- Exceptionally rare if strictly defined

Microscopic Pathology
- Fascicular architecture
- Characteristic "herringbone" or "chevron" pattern

- Elongated spindle cells; slender, tapered, sometimes wavy nuclei
- Scanty cytoplasm

Ancillary Tests
- Most cases negative for all immunohistochemical markers except vimentin
- Some express CD34 focally or diffusely
- Some superficial examples have *COL1A1-PDGFB* fusion transcripts as in dermatofibrosarcoma

---

  o Delicate intercellular network
  o Focal sclerosis or hyalinization
- Rare focal myxoid change
- Rare multinucleated tumor cells

ANCILLARY TESTS

Immunohistochemistry
- Most cases negative except for very focal SMA
- Some express CD34 focally or diffusely

Cytogenetics
- Some superficial examples have *COL1A1-PDGFB* fusion transcripts like dermatofibrosarcoma

Electron Microscopy
- Abundant rough endoplasmic reticulum
- No external lamina, junctions, or organized filaments

DIFFERENTIAL DIAGNOSIS

Low-Grade Fibromyxoid Sarcoma
- Less cellular
- Myxoid and fibrous areas with whorling
- Pleomorphism usually absent at 1st occurrence
- Nuclei less elongated, more rectangular
- Specific translocation: t(7;16)(q34;p11)

Low-Grade Myofibrosarcoma
- Cells have more cytoplasm
- Multifocal positivity for SMA

Synovial Sarcoma
- Younger age, any location, most common around knee
- Biphasic pattern with gland formation in 1/3 of cases
- Shorter, ovoid uniform cells, overlapping nuclei
- Mast cells frequent
- EMA or CK positive in 95%, CD34 negative in 95%
- Specific translocation: t(X;18)(p11;q11)

Malignant Peripheral Nerve Sheath Tumor
- Association with neurofibromatosis type 1
- Often originates in neurofibroma or large nerve
- Alternating myxoid and cellular areas
- Spindle cells with wavy or bullet-shaped nuclei
- S100 protein positive in 2/3 of cases

Fibromatosis
- Less cellular; cells evenly dispersed in mature collagen
- Myofibroblasts; punctate nucleoli
- Nuclear immunoreactivity for β-catenin

SELECTED REFERENCES

1. Bahrami A et al: Adult-type fibrosarcoma: A reevaluation of 163 putative cases diagnosed at a single institution over a 48-year period. Am J Surg Pathol. 34(10):1504-13, 2010
2. Sheng WQ et al: Expression of COL1A1-PDGFB fusion transcripts in superficial adult fibrosarcoma suggests a close relationship to dermatofibrosarcoma protuberans. J Pathol. 194(1):88-94, 2001
3. Scott SM et al: Soft tissue fibrosarcoma. A clinicopathologic study of 132 cases. Cancer. 64(4):925-31, 1989

IMAGE GALLERY

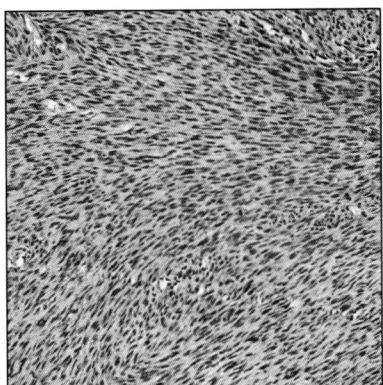 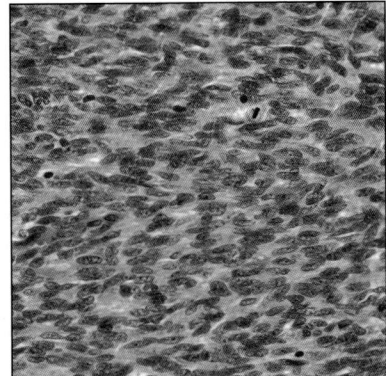 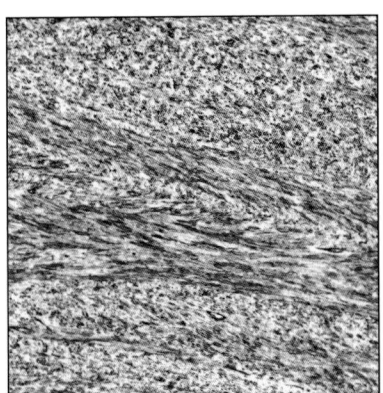

(Left) This higher grade fibrosarcoma displays nuclear hyperchromasia and focal pleomorphism. The fascicular architecture is retained. *(Center)* Moderately differentiated fibrosarcoma displays marked cellularity, nuclear variation, and mitotic figures. *(Right)* CD34 positivity can be seen in fibrosarcoma arising in DFSP or solitary fibrous tumor and in some fibrosarcomas without antecedent tumor. Other markers are absent, apart from very focal SMA in some.

MYXOFIBROSARCOMA

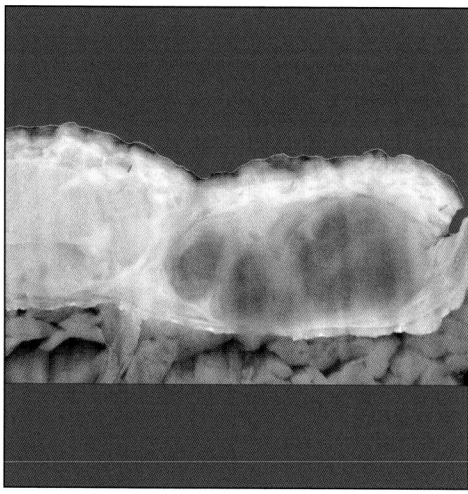

Grossly, myxofibrosarcoma often shows a multinodular growth pattern with gelatinous-appearing cut surfaces. (Courtesy T. Mentzel, MD.)

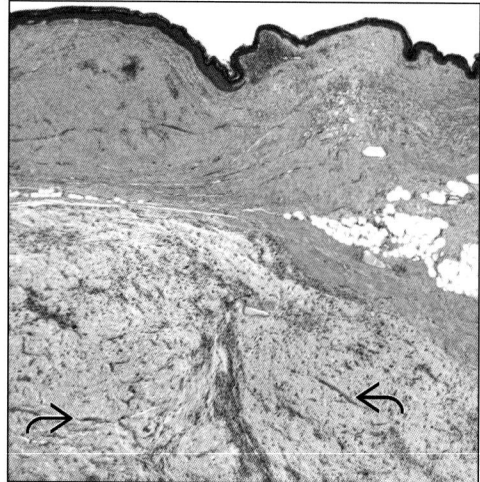

Scanning magnification view shows a superficial low-grade myxofibrosarcoma involving the subcutis and deep dermis. Numerous elongated, thin vessels ⟹ are easily identified in a prominent myxoid stroma.

TERMINOLOGY

Abbreviations
- Myxofibrosarcoma (MFS)

Synonyms
- Myxoid malignant fibrous histiocytoma (MFH)

Definitions
- MFS represents a spectrum of malignant fibroblastic neoplasms with variably myxoid stroma and characteristic elongated curvilinear vessels

CLINICAL ISSUES

Epidemiology
- Incidence
  - One of most common sarcomas in elderly patients
- Age
  - Affects mainly patients in 6th to 8th decade
  - Exceptionally rare in patients < 20 years old
- Gender
  - Slight male predominance

Site
- Majority arise in limbs and limb girdles
  - Lower > upper extremities
- Rarely on trunk, head and neck region
- Very rarely on hands and feet
- 2/3 of cases arise in dermal/subcutaneous tissues

Presentation
- Painless mass
- Slow growing

Treatment
- Surgical approaches
  - Complete and wide excision

Prognosis
- Local, often repeated, recurrences in up to 50-60% of cases (unrelated to histologic grade)
- Low-grade MFS usually does not metastasize
- Low-grade MFS may show tumor progression in subsequent recurrences
- Intermediate- and high-grade MFS may develop metastases in 30-35% of cases
- Overall 5-year survival is 60-70%

MACROSCOPIC FEATURES

General Features
- Superficially located neoplasms consist of multiple variably gelatinous or firmer nodules
- Deep-seated neoplasms often present as single mass with myxoid cut surfaces
- Areas of tumor necrosis may be seen in high-grade neoplasms

MICROSCOPIC PATHOLOGY

Histologic Features
- Broad spectrum of cellularity, cytologic atypia, and proliferative activity
- Multinodular growth with prominent myxoid stroma
- Elongated, curvilinear, thin-walled blood vessels
- Foci of inflammatory cells may be present
- Low-grade MFS
  - Hypocellular neoplasms
  - Scattered spindle-shaped tumor cells
  - Ill-defined eosinophilic cytoplasm
  - Enlarged hyperchromatic nuclei
- Intermediate-grade MFS
  - More cellular and pleomorphic than low-grade MFS
  - No solid areas or necrosis
- High-grade MFS
  - Large areas of solid sheets and cellular fascicles

MYXOFIBROSARCOMA

Key Facts

Terminology

- Myxofibrosarcoma represents a spectrum of malignant fibroblastic neoplasms with variably myxoid stroma and characteristic elongated curvilinear vessels

Clinical Issues

- One of most common sarcomas in elderly patients
- Majority arises in limbs, including limb girdles
  - Lower > upper extremities
- 2/3 of cases arise in dermal/subcutaneous tissues
- Local, often repeated, recurrences in up to 50-60% of cases (unrelated to histologic grade)
- Intermediate- and high-grade malignant neoplasms may develop metastases in 30-35% of cases

Macroscopic Features

- Superficially located neoplasms consist of multiple variably gelatinous or firmer nodules
- Deep-seated neoplasms often present as single mass with myxoid cut surfaces

Microscopic Pathology

- Broad spectrum of cellularity, cytologic atypia, and proliferative activity reflected by 3 grades of malignancy
- Multinodular growth, spindled and stellate atypical fibroblastic cells
- Myxoid stroma with elongated, curvilinear, thin-walled vessels
- Often pseudolipoblasts are present

- Spindled and pleomorphic tumor cells
- Bizarre, multinucleated tumor giant cells
- Numerous, often atypical mitoses
- Areas of tumor necrosis may be present
- At least focally, areas of lower grade neoplasm with prominent myxoid stroma and numerous curvilinear vessels

ANCILLARY TESTS

Cytogenetics

- Complex karyotypes
- Often triploid and tetraploid chromosome numbers

DIFFERENTIAL DIAGNOSIS

Myxoid Dermatofibrosarcoma Protuberans

- Often diffuse infiltration of dermis and subcutis
- No prominent cytologic atypia
- Homogeneous expression of CD34

Myxoid Liposarcoma

- Frequently in deep soft tissues of lower extremity
- Small, undifferentiated round tumor cells and vacuolated lipoblasts
- Usually lack prominent cytologic atypia
- Delicate, plexiform vascular pattern

Low-Grade Fibromyxoid Sarcoma (Evans Tumor)

- Mainly in deep soft tissues
- Bland spindled tumor cells in alternating myxoid and fibrous stroma
- May show expression of EMA/MUC1

Myxoinflammatory Fibroblastic Sarcoma

- Frequently arises in subcutaneous tissues of hands, wrists, feet, and ankles
- Spindled, polygonal, and bizarre ganglion-like tumor cells with huge inclusion-like nucleoli
- Prominent mixed inflammatory infiltrate

Myxoid Malignant Peripheral Nerve Sheath Tumor

- Fascicular arrangement of spindle-shaped tumor cells
- Often perivascular whorling of tumor cells
- In about 1/2 of cases, focal expression of S100

DIAGNOSTIC CHECKLIST

Pathologic Interpretation Pearls

- Spectrum of variably cellular atypical fibroblastic neoplasms
- Myxoid stromal changes with characteristic elongated curvilinear blood vessels

SELECTED REFERENCES

1. Nascimento AF et al: Epithelioid variant of myxofibrosarcoma: expanding the clinicomorphologic spectrum of myxofibrosarcoma in a series of 17 cases. Am J Surg Pathol. 31(1):99-105, 2007
2. Willems SM et al: Local recurrence of myxofibrosarcoma is associated with increase in tumour grade and cytogenetic aberrations, suggesting a multistep tumour progression model. Mod Pathol. 19(3):407-16, 2006
3. Mansoor A et al: Myxofibrosarcoma presenting in the skin: clinicopathological features and differential diagnosis with cutaneous myxoid neoplasms. Am J Dermatopathol. 25(4):281-6, 2003
4. Mentzel T et al: The association between tumour progression and vascularity in myxofibrosarcoma and myxoid/round cell liposarcoma. Virchows Arch. 438(1):13-22, 2001
5. Mentzel T et al: Myxofibrosarcoma. Clinicopathologic analysis of 75 cases with emphasis on the low-grade variant. Am J Surg Pathol. 20(4):391-405, 1996
6. Angervall L et al: Myxofibrosarcoma. A study of 30 cases. Acta Pathol Microbiol Scand A. 85A(2):127-40, 1977
7. Weiss SW et al: Myxoid variant of malignant fibrous histiocytoma. Cancer. 39(4):1672-85, 1977

Gross and Microscopic Features

(Left) A case of low-grade myxofibrosarcoma is shown with myxoid, gelatinous cut surfaces. (Courtesy T. Mentzel, MD.) *(Right)* Low-power view of a low-grade myxofibrosarcoma shows a deep-seated intramuscular tumor. Note the characteristic multinodular growth and the presence of thin fibrous septa. (Courtesy T. Mentzel, MD.)

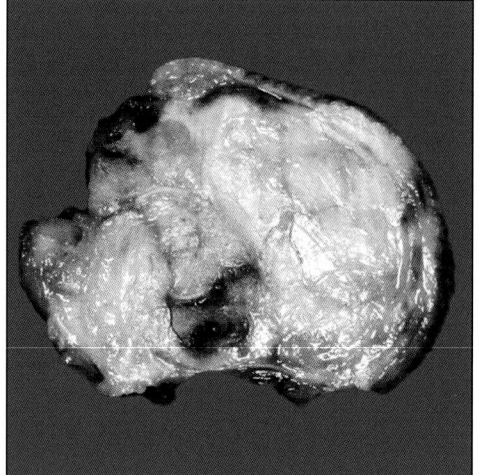 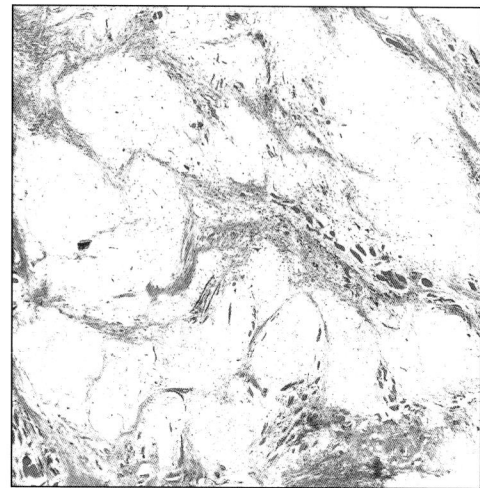

(Left) Despite low cellularity, cases of low-grade myxofibrosarcoma are composed of atypical fibroblastic tumor cells showing enlarged and hyperchromatic-staining nuclei ⇗. (Courtesy T. Mentzel, MD.) *(Right)* Higher magnification of a low-grade myxofibrosarcoma shows prominent elongated, thin-walled blood vessels ⇗ with scattered atypical spindle-shaped cells in a background of prominent mucinous stroma.

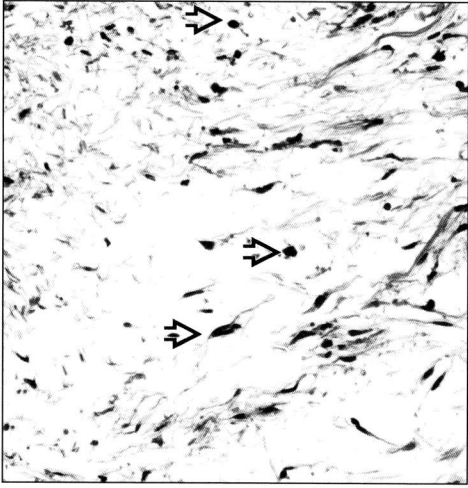 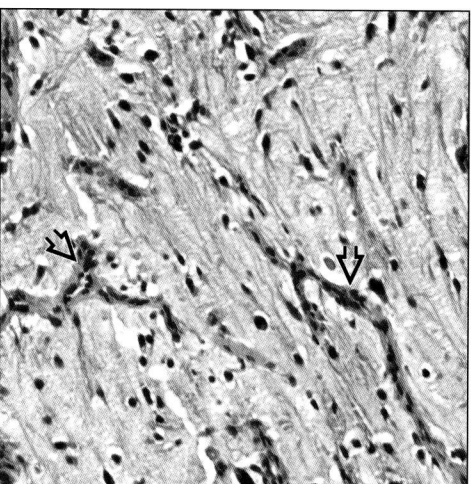

(Left) Alcian blue staining reveals the presence of abundant mucin in the stroma and also in the cytoplasm of the neoplastic cells in this case of low-grade myxofibrosarcoma. (Courtesy T. Mentzel, MD.) *(Right)* Cases of intermediate-grade myxofibrosarcoma show increased cellularity with numerous atypical spindle-shaped fibroblastic tumor cells that demonstrate nuclear hyperchromasia ⇒. (Courtesy T. Mentzel, MD.)

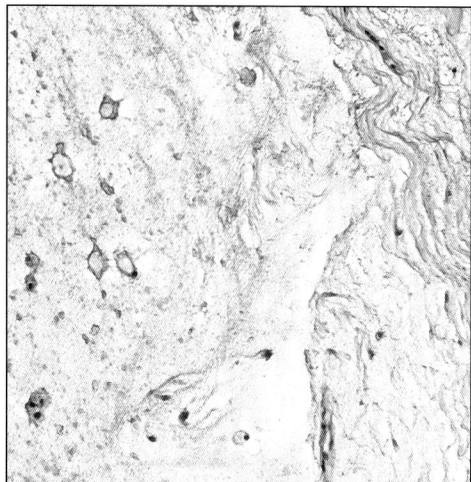 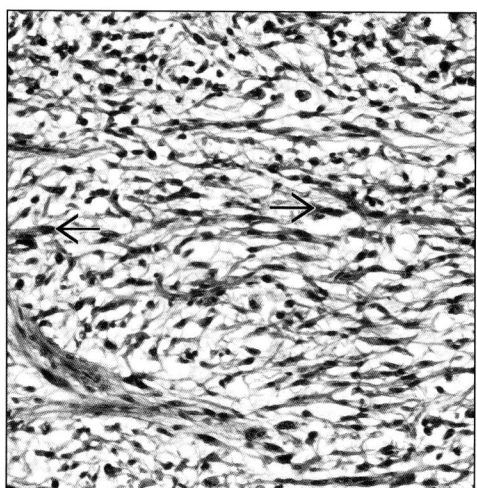

MYXOFIBROSARCOMA

Microscopic and Immunohistochemical Features

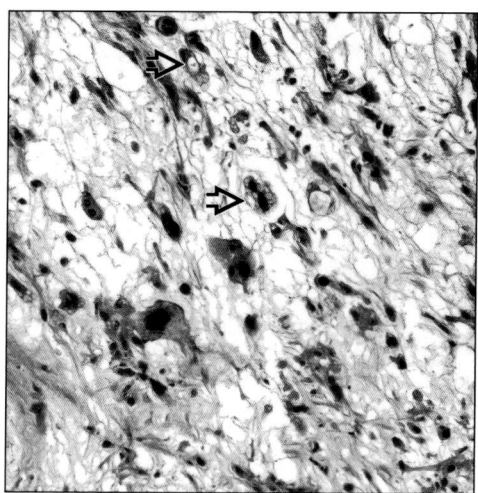

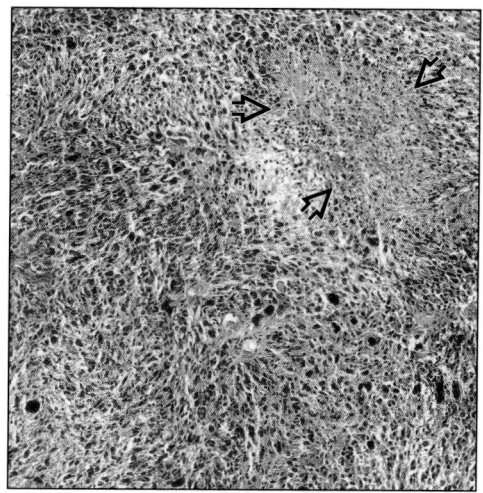

(Left) High-power view of an intermediate-grade myxofibrosarcoma shows atypical tumor cells with enlarged hyperchromatic-staining nuclei. Note the scattered multivacuolated pseudolipoblasts ⊅. (Courtesy T. Mentzel, MD.) (Right) Cases of high-grade myxofibrosarcoma show features of a high-grade pleomorphic sarcoma with increased proliferative activity and areas of tumor necrosis ⊅. (Courtesy T. Mentzel, MD.)

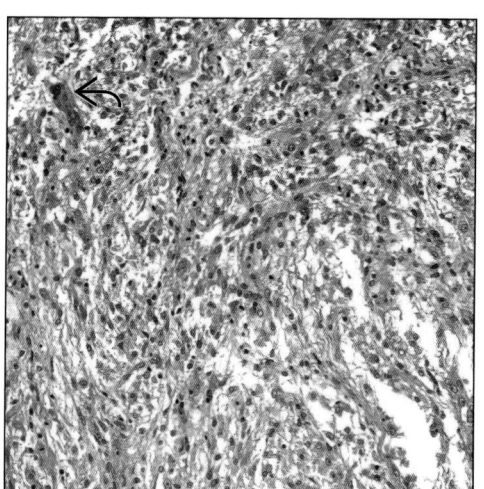

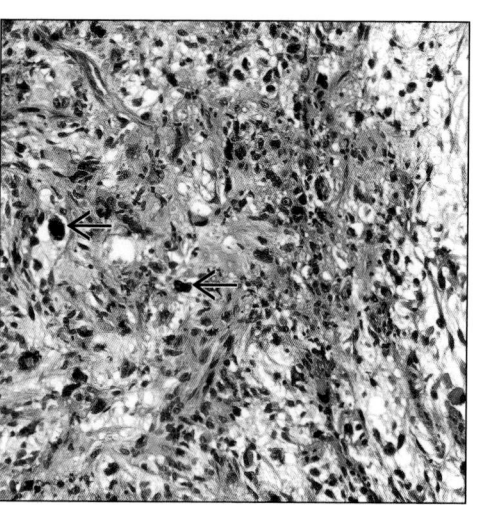

(Left) Multinucleated tumor giant cells containing abundant eosinophilic cytoplasm, mimicking a myogenic neoplasm, are seen in this example of a high-grade malignant myxofibrosarcoma ⊅. (Courtesy T. Mentzel, MD.) (Right) High magnification of a high-grade malignant myxofibrosarcoma shows prominent cytologic atypia with enlarged, hyperchromatic-staining nuclei ⊅. (Courtesy T. Mentzel, MD.)

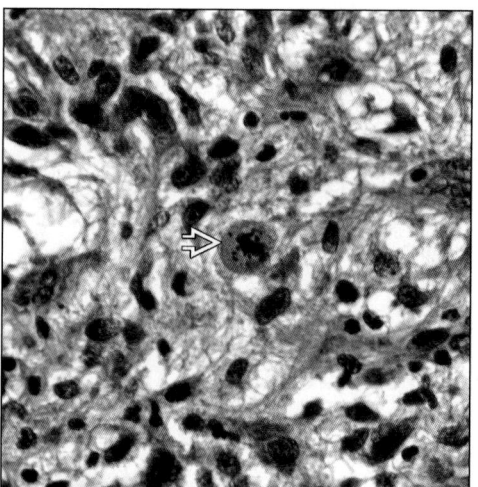

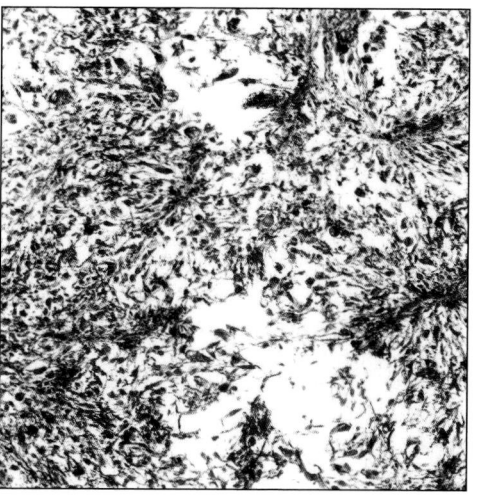

(Left) Higher magnification of a high-grade myxofibrosarcoma shows prominent cytologic atypia, nuclear hyperchromasia, irregular nuclear contours, and mitotic activity ⊅. (Right) The immunohistochemical expression of CD34 in some cases confirms the fibroblastic line of differentiation in these neoplasms. (Courtesy T. Mentzel, MD.)

LOW-GRADE FIBROMYXOID SARCOMA (EVANS TUMOR)

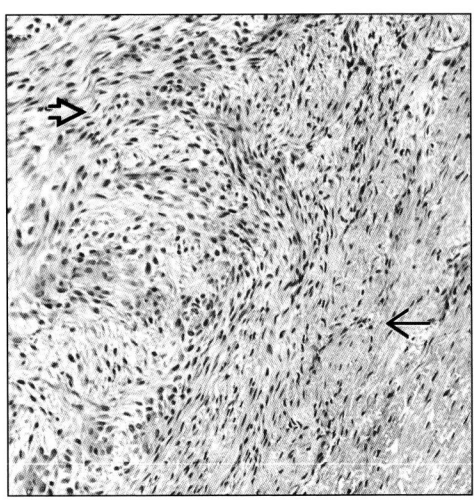

Low-grade fibromyxoid sarcoma (LGFMS) (hematoxylin & eosin) shows the interface between the myxoid areas ⇨ and the collagenous areas ➡ of the tumor.

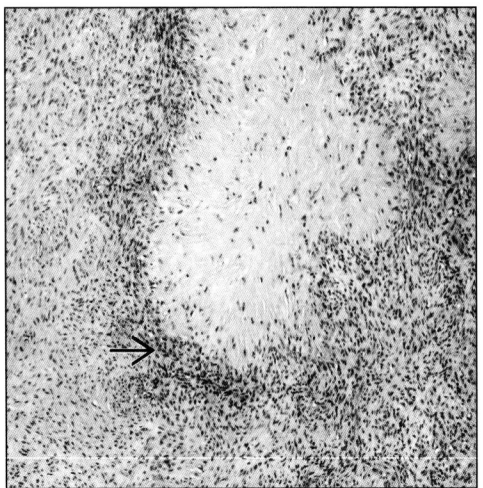

LGFMS displays a giant rosette composed of sparsely cellular collagenous tissue cuffed by a markedly cellular distribution of bland tumor cells ➡.

TERMINOLOGY

Abbreviations
- Low-grade fibromyxoid sarcoma (LGFMS)

Synonyms
- Fibrosarcoma, fibromyxoid type; hyalinizing spindle cell tumor with giant rosettes

Definitions
- Malignant fibroblastic neoplasm composed of bland spindle cells in collagenous and myxoid matrix, often with prominent collagenous nodules
- Characterized by specific translocations producing fusion oncogenes
- Despite histologically low-grade morphology, up to 30% can metastasize

ETIOLOGY/PATHOGENESIS

Characteristic Translocations
- Produce chimeric fusion genes
- Cellular origin still unknown, but mesenchymal neoplasm with fibroblastic-like cells

CLINICAL ISSUES

Epidemiology
- Incidence
  - True incidence unknown
  - Tumor probably underreported in literature due to its morphologic resemblance to other benign and malignant tumors
- Age
  - Adults (typically in 4th decade), but wide age distribution
    - Significant proportion in patients < 18 years old
- Gender
  - M > F

Site
- Mainly deep-seated, but a smaller proportion occurs in dermis and subcutis
- Proximal extremities (especially lower limbs) and trunk; rarely other sites including viscera
- Superficial lesions have higher incidence in childhood

Presentation
- Painless mass
  - Many are of long duration

Treatment
- Surgical approaches
  - Wide excision
  - Long-term follow-up is mandatory, in view of potential for late metastases

Prognosis
- Recurrence rates of up to 21%
  - Recurrence is lower in superficial cases
- Metastatic rate of approximately 30% in genetically confirmed cases
  - > 80% of metastases appeared after 9 years
  - No reported metastases in superficial tumors

MACROSCOPIC FEATURES

General Features
- Well-defined mass
- White cut surface, often with glistening myxoid areas
- Sometimes cystic foci, but necrosis rare

MICROSCOPIC PATHOLOGY

Histologic Features
- Lobulated and partially circumscribed, but frequent microscopic infiltration into adjacent soft tissue
- Sparsely to moderately cellular arrays of bland fibroblasts

LOW-GRADE FIBROMYXOID SARCOMA (EVANS TUMOR)

Key Facts

Terminology

- Malignant fibroblastic neoplasm composed of bland spindle cells in collagenous matrix, often with prominent collagenous nodules
- Characterized by specific translocations producing fusion oncogenes

Clinical Issues

- Adults (typically in 4th decade)
- Mainly deep-seated, but can also occur superficially in dermis and subcutis
- Proximal extremities (especially lower limbs) and trunk; rarely other sites
- Recurrence rates of up to 21%
- Recurrence lower in superficial cases
- Metastatic rate of approximately 30% in genetically confirmed cases

Microscopic Pathology

- Whorled distributions of bland fibroblasts
- Collagenous or myxoid matrix, often in distinct zones
- Owing to bland morphology, tumors often mistaken for variety of benign or low-grade neoplasms

Ancillary Tests

- MUC4 immunohistochemistry is sensitive and specific
- CD34 positivity in some cases
- Occasional EMA and claudin-1 positivity, which can make distinction from perineurioma difficult
- Balanced translocations
- t(7;16)(q32-34;p11) *FUS, CREB3L2*
- t(11;16)(p11;p11) *FUS, CREB3L1*

- Whorled or loosely fascicular distributions
- Collagenous or myxoid matrix, often in distinct zones
  - Abrupt transition to myxoid foci is characteristic
- Cells display angulated, slightly squared nuclei with pale even chromatin and indistinct fibrillary cytoplasm
- Pleomorphism is unusual
- Mitoses rare
- Owing to bland morphology, tumors often mistaken for variety of benign or low-grade neoplasms
- Approximately 10% show greater cellularity and atypia, more similar to usual intermediate-grade fibrosarcomas
- **Hyalinizing spindle cell tumor with giant rosettes**
  - Morphologic variant of LGFMS, though term is now used infrequently
  - Prominent paucicellular hyalinized rosette-like nodules, bordered by more rounded tumor cells
  - Similar to typical LGFMS in cytogenetic abnormalities and behavior
- Recurrences of LGFMS frequently show increased cellularity, pleomorphism, and mitotic activity
  - May show transition to frank high-grade spindle cell sarcoma
  - Foci of higher grade sarcoma at presentation, however, is not thought to be prognostically adverse
- Relationship between LGFMS and sclerosing epithelioid fibrosarcoma is also suggested

ANCILLARY TESTS

Immunohistochemistry

- Diffuse MUC4 expression in most tumors
  - Sensitive and specific marker for LGFMS
  - From gene expression profiling: *MUC4* (Mucin 4) gene differentially upregulated in LGFMS compared with histologically similar tumors
- Almost always negative for desmin, actin-sm, S100, and CK-PAN

- Occasional CD34, EMA/MUC1, and claudin-1 positivity make distinction from perineurioma more difficult

Cytogenetics

- Balanced translocations
- t(7;16)(q32-34;p11) *FUS, CREB3L2*
- t(11;16)(p11;p11) *FUS, CREB3L1*
- Frequency of *FUS* rearrangement in superficial LGFMS similar to that seen in deeper lesions
- Relationship between genetic findings and histology or clinical outcome not as yet established

Electron Microscopy

- Transmission
  - Cells show features of primitive fibroblasts, with paucity of organelles, but abundant vimentin-type intermediate filaments

DIFFERENTIAL DIAGNOSIS

Nodular Fasciitis

- Spindle and stellate fibroblasts with "tissue culture"-like appearance
- Related phenomena (e.g., extravasated erythrocytes, giant cells)
- Mitoses may be frequent
- Smooth muscle actin positive

Perineurioma

- Elongated spindle cells with bipolar processes
- Perivascular whorls
- CD34, EMA/MUC1, GLUT1, and claudin-1 positivity

Neurofibroma (Myxoid Neurofibroma)

- Cells with elongated, wavy-appearing nuclei
- Usually strong S100 positivity

Cellular Myxoma

- More prominent, diffuse myxoid stroma
- Lack of pronounced fibrous zones

LOW-GRADE FIBROMYXOID SARCOMA (EVANS TUMOR)

Immunohistochemistry

Antibody	Reactivity	Staining Pattern	Comment
MUC4	Positive	Cytoplasmic	Usually strong and diffuse; sensitive and specific for LGFMS
CD34	Positive	Cytoplasmic	Occasional
EMA	Positive	Cell membrane	Occasional
Claudin-1	Positive	Cell membrane & cytoplasm	Occasional
Desmin	Negative		
Actin-sm	Negative		
AE1/AE3	Negative		
S100	Negative		
β-catenin	Negative		Helps distinguish from fibromatosis

Superficial Angiomyxoma
- Lobular growth pattern
- Vessels with slightly fibrosed walls
- Perivascular neutrophils

Superficial Acral Fibromyxoma
- Predilection for hands and feet
- Scattered inflammatory cells (mast cells)
- CD34 and EMA often positive

Myxoid Dermatofibrosarcoma Protuberans
- Tight storiform fascicular growth pattern
- Diffuse, usually strong CD34 positivity

Fibromatosis
- Sweeping fascicles of myofibroblasts with elongated nuclei and small nucleoli
- Characteristic vascular pattern
- Nuclear β-catenin positivity

Myxofibrosarcoma
- Subcutaneous locations, in elderly patients
- Atypical hyperchromatic nuclei
- More prominent myxoid stroma
- Stromal vascularity with curvilinear vessels

Malignant Peripheral Nerve Sheath Tumor
- Elongated cells with angulated to spindled nuclei
- Nuclear atypia
- Variable, often focal S100 protein

SELECTED REFERENCES

1. Doyle LA et al: MUC4 is a highly sensitive and specific marker for low-grade fibromyxoid sarcoma. Am J Surg Pathol. 35(5):733-41, 2011
2. Patel RM et al: FUS (16p11) gene rearrangement as detected by fluorescence in-situ hybridization in cutaneous low-grade fibromyxoid sarcoma: a potential diagnostic tool. Am J Dermatopathol. 33(2):140-3, 2011
3. Fisher C: Soft tissue sarcomas with non-EWS translocations: molecular genetic features and pathologic and clinical correlations. Virchows Arch. 456(2):153-66, 2010
4. Thway K et al: Utility of sarcoma-specific fusion gene analysis in paraffin-embedded material for routine diagnosis at a specialist centre. J Clin Pathol. 63(6):508-12, 2010
5. Thway K et al: Claudin-1 is expressed in perineurioma-like low-grade fibromyxoid sarcoma. Hum Pathol. 40(11):1586-90, 2009
6. Jakowski JD et al: Primary intrathoracic low-grade fibromyxoid sarcoma. Hum Pathol. 39(4):623-8, 2008
7. Matsuyama A et al: DNA-based polymerase chain reaction for detecting FUS-CREB3L2 in low-grade fibromyxoid sarcoma using formalin-fixed, paraffin-embedded tissue specimens. Diagn Mol Pathol. 17(4):237-40, 2008
8. Saito R et al: Low-grade fibromyxoid sarcoma of intracranial origin. J Neurosurg. 108(4):798-802, 2008
9. Guillou L et al: Translocation-positive low-grade fibromyxoid sarcoma: clinicopathologic and molecular analysis of a series expanding the morphologic spectrum and suggesting potential relationship to sclerosing epithelioid fibrosarcoma: a study from the French Sarcoma Group. Am J Surg Pathol. 31(9):1387-402, 2007
10. Matsuyama A et al: Molecular detection of FUS-CREB3L2 fusion transcripts in low-grade fibromyxoid sarcoma using formalin-fixed, paraffin-embedded tissue specimens. Am J Surg Pathol. 30(9):1077-84, 2006
11. Billings SD et al: Superficial low-grade fibromyxoid sarcoma (Evans tumor): a clinicopathologic analysis of 19 cases with a unique observation in the pediatric population. Am J Surg Pathol. 29(2):204-10, 2005
12. Mertens F et al: Clinicopathologic and molecular genetic characterization of low-grade fibromyxoid sarcoma, and cloning of a novel FUS/CREB3L1 fusion gene. Lab Invest. 85(3):408-15, 2005
13. Reid R et al: Low-grade fibromyxoid sarcoma and hyalinizing spindle cell tumor with giant rosettes share a common t(7;16)(q34;p11) translocation. Am J Surg Pathol. 27(9):1229-36, 2003
14. Storlazzi CT et al: Fusion of the FUS and BBF2H7 genes in low grade fibromyxoid sarcoma. Hum Mol Genet. 12(18):2349-58, 2003
15. Bejarano PA et al: Hyalinizing spindle cell tumor with giant rosettes--a soft tissue tumor with mesenchymal and neuroendocrine features. An immunohistochemical, ultrastructural, and cytogenetic analysis. Arch Pathol Lab Med. 124(8):1179-84, 2000
16. Folpe AL et al: Low-grade fibromyxoid sarcoma and hyalinizing spindle cell tumor with giant rosettes: a clinicopathologic study of 73 cases supporting their identity and assessing the impact of high-grade areas. Am J Surg Pathol. 24(10):1353-60, 2000
17. Lane KL et al: Hyalinizing spindle cell tumor with giant rosettes: a distinctive tumor closely resembling low-grade fibromyxoid sarcoma. Am J Surg Pathol. 21(12):1481-8, 1997
18. Evans HL: Low-grade fibromyxoid sarcoma. A report of 12 cases. Am J Surg Pathol. 17(6):595-600, 1993

LOW-GRADE FIBROMYXOID SARCOMA (EVANS TUMOR)

Microscopic Features

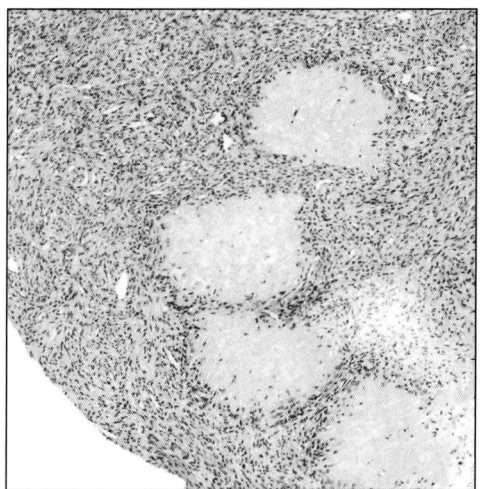

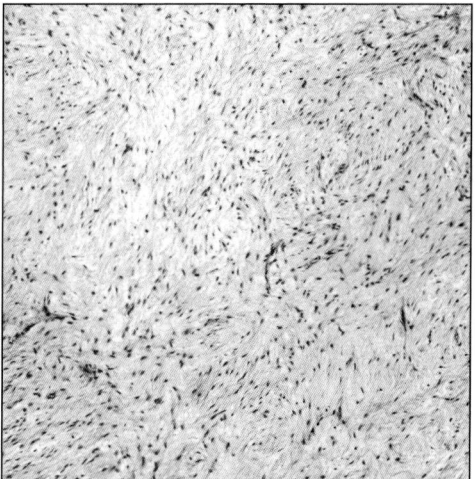

(Left) This needle core biopsy of low-grade fibromyxoid sarcoma shows prominent collagenous rosette formation. Rosettes, if present, often vary in distribution within the tumor and may not be sampled, making the diagnosis difficult. *(Right)* This low-power view shows vaguely fascicular distributions of bland spindle cells within a loosely collagenous stroma. Cellularity is frequently only sparse to moderate, and the morphology can be reminiscent of benign spindle cell lesions.

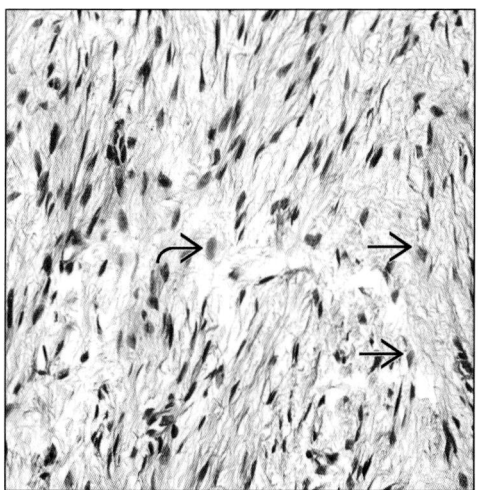

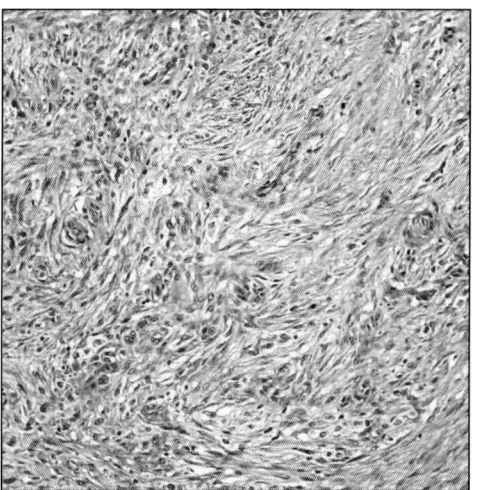

(Left) The cells of LGFMS have ovoid ⟳ or slightly angulated and squared nuclei ➔, with delicate, even chromatin and inconspicuous nucleoli, and fibrillary cytoplasm. Note the lack of atypia. The stroma is myxoid and delicately collagenous. *(Right)* This example shows prominent collagenous stroma with a loosely fascicular pattern. Small and medium-sized vessels can be seen interspersed, and the architecture may be mistaken for fibromatosis.

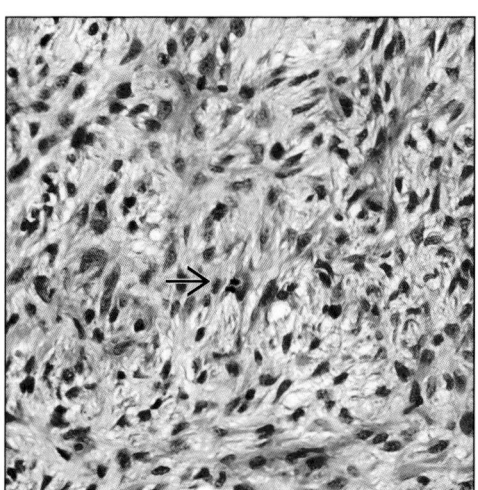

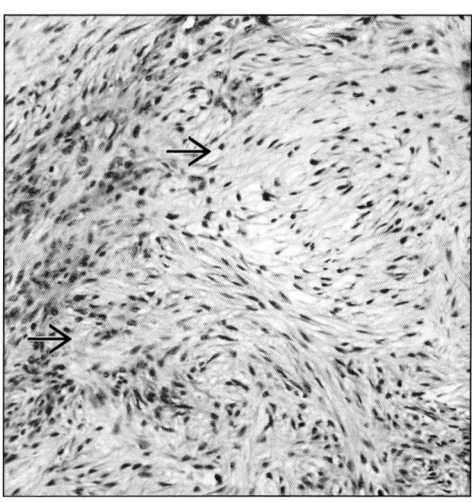

(Left) This example of recurrent low-grade fibromyxoid sarcoma shows high cellularity with occasional mitoses ➔, and a typical myxocollagenous background. *(Right)* There are prominent nodular formations of cells within a myxoid stroma ➔, and the appearances are reminiscent of myxofibrosarcoma, but the cells are uniform and no cellular atypia is apparent.

MYXOINFLAMMATORY FIBROBLASTIC SARCOMA

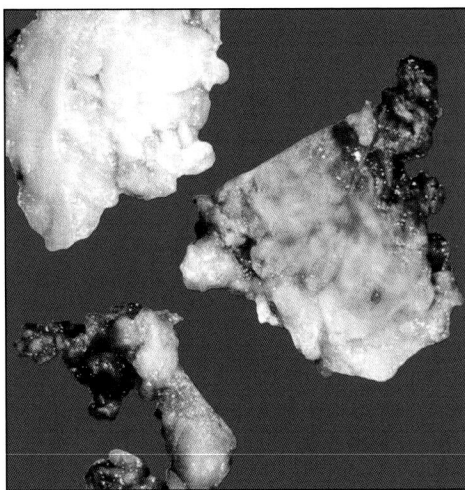

This is a gross specimen of a myxoinflammatory fibroblastic sarcoma. This lesion was highly infiltrative and clinically mistaken for pigmented villonodular tenosynovitis.

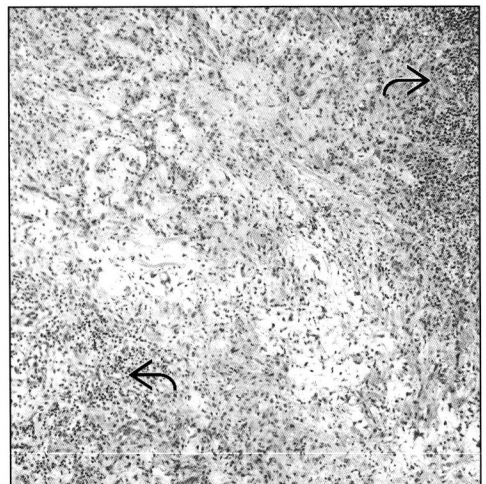

At scanning magnification, myxoinflammatory fibroblastic sarcoma displays a generous inflammatory background and scattered myxoid zones. Lymphoid cells are prominent at the edges of the field ➡.

TERMINOLOGY

Synonyms
- Acral myxoinflammatory fibroblastic sarcoma (MIFS), inflammatory myxohyaline tumor

Definitions
- Low-grade fibroblastic sarcoma characterized by typical acral presentation and inflammatory background, often rich in eosinophils

CLINICAL ISSUES

Presentation
- Slow-growing infiltrative mass usually affecting distal extremities (hands and feet) of adults

Prognosis
- Recurrences are common, but metastases are rare

MACROSCOPIC FEATURES

General Features
- Infiltrative masses

Size
- 1-10 cm, usually 3-4 cm

MICROSCOPIC PATHOLOGY

Histologic Features
- Poorly marginated tumor with fibrosis, hyalinization, myxoid stroma, and inflammatory components
  - Various lesions have different proportions of each component
- Inflammatory component shows variable mixture of lymphoplasmacytic cells, eosinophils, neutrophils, and histiocytes

- Lesional cells are fibroblasts ultrastructurally
- Scattered enlarged atypical fibroblasts, some with macronucleoli
- Areas with prominent myxoid change
  - Fibroblasts often vacuolated ("pseudolipoblasts")
- Low mitotic rate
  - Low proliferative index by Ki-67

ANCILLARY TESTS

Immunohistochemistry
- Variable expression of CD34, CD68, EGFR, CD163, CD117, EMA
- Negative CD15, CD30, CD45 in cells with macronucleoli
- No demonstration of various viral agents

Cytogenetics
- t(1;10) and amplification of 3p11-12, which myxoinflammatory fibroblastic sarcoma shares with hemosiderotic fibrolipomatous tumor
- t(2;6)(q31;p21.3) reported

DIFFERENTIAL DIAGNOSIS

Extranodal Hodgkin Disease
- Patients usually have history of nodal disease
- Usually no myxoid areas
- Background mostly lymphoid cells; neutrophils not common
- Reed-Sternberg cells label with CD15 and CD30, and are lymphoid rather than fibroblastic

Pigmented Villonodular Tenosynovitis
- Also termed tenosynovial giant cell tumor, diffuse type
- Often presents in knee joint area of young women
- Proliferated around joint space
- Proliferation of uniform rounded cells

MYXOINFLAMMATORY FIBROBLASTIC SARCOMA

Key Facts

Clinical Issues
- Slow-growing infiltrative mass usually affecting distal extremities (hands and feet) of adults
- Recurrences are common, but metastases are rare

Microscopic Pathology
- Poorly marginated tumor with fibrosis, hyalinization, myxoid stroma, and inflammatory components
  - Inflammatory component shows variable mixtures of lymphoplasmacytic cells, eosinophils, neutrophils, and histiocytes
- Scattered enlarged atypical fibroblasts, some with macronucleoli
- Areas with prominent myxoid change
- Low mitotic rate
- Lesional cells are fibroblasts ultrastructurally

Ancillary Tests
- Variable expression of CD34, CD68, EGFR, CD163, CD117, EMA
- t(1;10) and amplification of 3p11-12, which MIFS shares with hemosiderotic fibrolipomatous tumor
- Negative CD15, CD30, CD45 in cells with macronucleoli

Top Differential Diagnoses
- Extranodal Hodgkin disease
- Pigmented villonodular tenosynovitis
- Hemosiderotic fibrohistiocytic lipomatous lesion
- Viral infection
- Myxofibrosarcoma
- Epithelioid sarcoma

- Background of hemosiderin, histiocytes, lymphoplasmacytic cells
- Eosinophils and neutrophils not a feature
- Not myxoid
- No enlarged atypical cells

Hemosiderotic Fibrohistiocytic Lipomatous Lesion
- Classically involves the feet
- May form spectrum with both myxoinflammatory fibroblastic sarcoma and with pleomorphic hyalinizing angiectatic tumor
  - However, no metastases have been recorded for either hemosiderotic fibrohistiocytic lipomatous lesion or pleomorphic hyalinizing angiectatic tumor
  - Shares t(1;10) and amplification of 3p11-12
- Tracks along connective tissue septa
- Spindle cells, abundant hemosiderin, histiocytes
- Strongly CD34(+)

Viral Infection
- Usually involves internal organs and lymph nodes
- Viral cytopathic effect consists of nuclear (Cytomegalovirus [CMV] and herpes simplex virus [HSV]) or cytoplasmic (CMV) inclusions
- CMV effect best seen in stromal cells
- HSV effect often seen in epithelial cells
- Agents can be demonstrated by immunohistochemistry or molecular testing

Myxofibrosarcoma
- Usually in proximal extremities of older persons
- Typically superficial and lobulated rather than infiltrative
- Richly vascular
- Abundance of myxoid stroma
- No hyalinized zones
- Inflammatory cells a minor component

Epithelioid Sarcoma
- Distal extremities of adults
- Neoplastic cells surround zones of necrosis
  - Appearance mimics granulomatous process

- Minimal inflammation
- Pankeratin, EMA(+), CK5/6(-), CD34(+/-), loss of nuclear INI1
- Aggressive: Metastases to regional nodes as well as systemic metastases and death

Clear Cell Sarcoma ("Melanoma of Soft Parts")
- Distal extremities of adults
- Often centered in tendons or aponeuroses
- Packeted groups of uniform cells with macronucleoli
- S100 protein(+), HMB-45(+), Melan-A(+), MITF1(+)
- Characteristic translocation and gene fusion
  - t(12;22)(q13;q12) that results in fusion of *EWS* and *ATF1* genes

SELECTED REFERENCES
1. Hallor KH et al: Two genetic pathways, t(1;10) and amplification of 3p11-12, in myxoinflammatory fibroblastic sarcoma, haemosiderotic fibrolipomatous tumour, and morphologically similar lesions. J Pathol. 217(5):716-27, 2009
2. Kovarik CL et al: Acral myxoinflammatory fibroblastic sarcoma: case series and immunohistochemical analysis. J Cutan Pathol. 35(2):192-6, 2008
3. Ida CM et al: Myxoinflammatory fibroblastic sarcoma showing t(2;6)(q31;p21.3) as a sole cytogenetic abnormality. Cancer Genet Cytogenet. 177(2):139-42, 2007
4. Jurcić V et al: Myxoinflammatory fibroblastic sarcoma: a tumor not restricted to acral sites. Ann Diagn Pathol. 6(5):272-80, 2002
5. Lambert I et al: Acral myxoinflammatory fibroblastic sarcoma with unique clonal chromosomal changes. Virchows Arch. 438(5):509-12, 2001
6. Meis-Kindblom JM et al: Acral myxoinflammatory fibroblastic sarcoma: a low-grade tumor of the hands and feet. Am J Surg Pathol. 22(8):911-24, 1998
7. Montgomery EA et al: Inflammatory myxohyaline tumor of distal extremities with virocyte or Reed-Sternberg-like cells: a distinctive lesion with features simulating inflammatory conditions, Hodgkin's disease, and various sarcomas. Mod Pathol. 11(4):384-91, 1998

Microscopic Features

(Left) This image shows a myxoinflammatory fibroblastic sarcoma (MIFS) at low magnification. This lesion is characterized by myxoid areas alternating with fibrous areas, and it also has prominent cleft-like spaces ⇗. **(Right)** This MIFS is superficial and shows a myxoinflammatory expansion of the subcutaneous fat. Such neoplasms can also be associated with tendons and have an infiltrative appearance. A prominent lymphoid infiltrate ⇗ is present throughout the neoplasm.

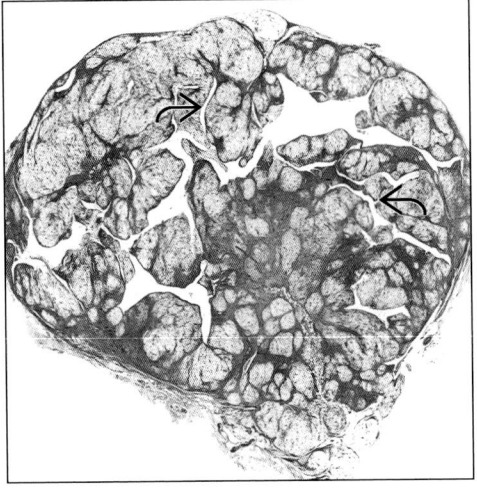 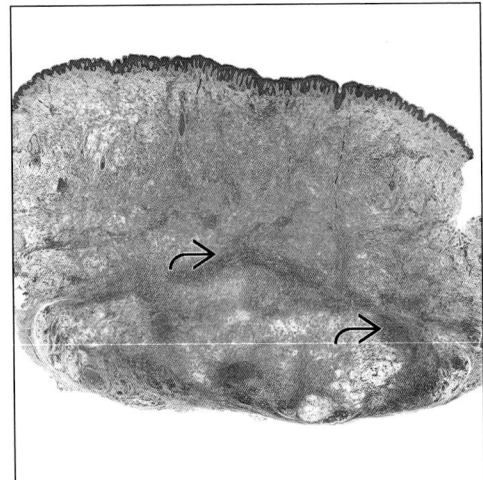

(Left) This myxoinflammatory fibroblastic sarcoma has pockets of myxoid matrix interspersed with more solid fibroinflammatory zones. **(Right)** Higher power of myxoinflammatory fibroblastic sarcoma shows the junction of a myxoid area with an inflammatory area. The cells suspended in the myxoid matrix are enlarged and hyperchromatic. Note the lymphocytes in the lower right portion of the image ⇗.

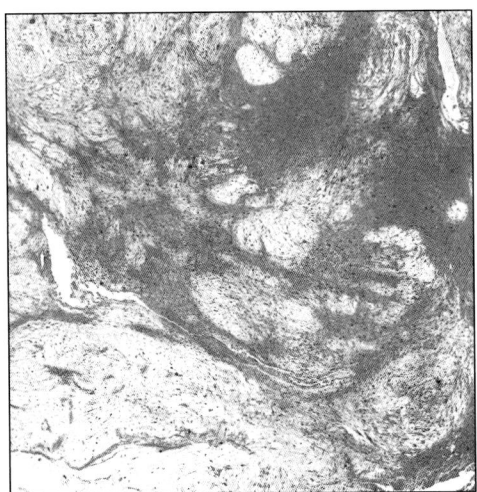 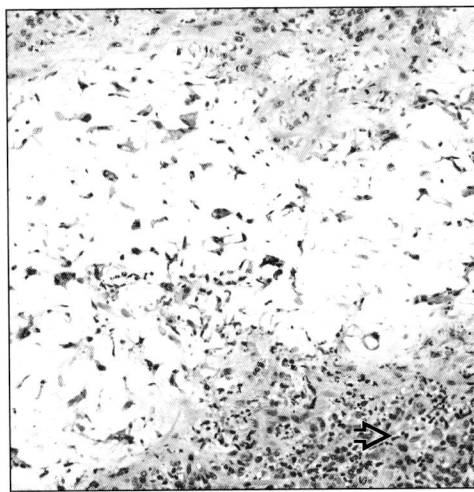

(Left) High magnification shows markedly atypical enlarged epithelioid cells. In this field, the cells also display a granular cytoplasmic appearance. The cell in the center has a striking macronucleolus ⇗. **(Right)** This myxoinflammatory fibroblastic sarcoma shows abundant myxoid matrix. In this field, the neoplasm appears similar to myxofibrosarcoma (myxoid malignant fibrous histiocytoma), but lacks the rich vascular pattern of myxofibrosarcoma and has inflammatory cells.

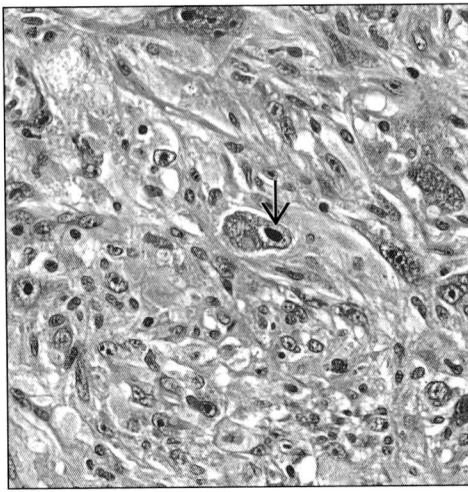 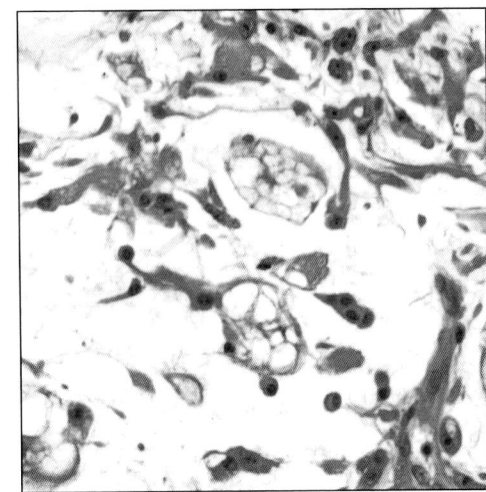

MYXOINFLAMMATORY FIBROBLASTIC SARCOMA

Microscopic and Immunohistochemical Features

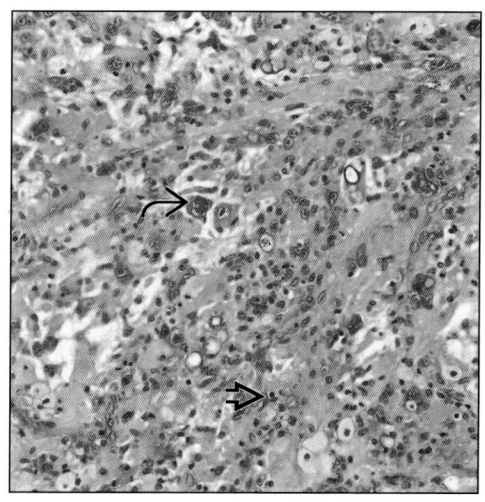

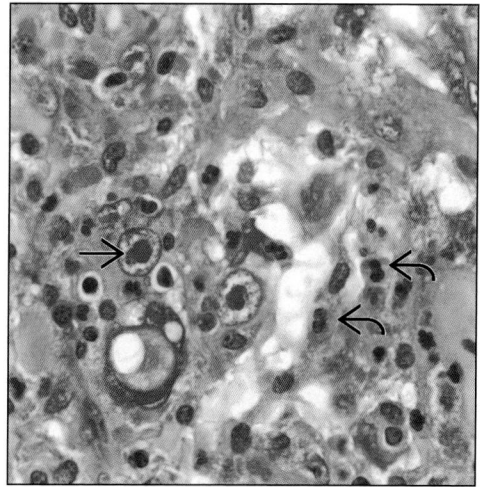

(Left) This is a hyalinized portion of a MIFS. Based on areas such as this, these neoplasms were initially described as "inflammatory myxohyaline tumors." Note the cells with macronucleoli ➔ and the scattered lymphoid cells in the background ➔. (Right) The fibroblasts in MIFS often have macronucleoli ➔. Paired with the frequent eosinophils in many examples ➔, the presence of the prominent nucleoli in many cells can lead to a misinterpretation of Hodgkin disease.

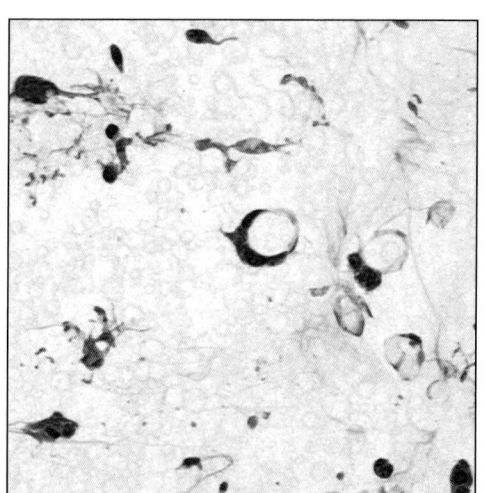

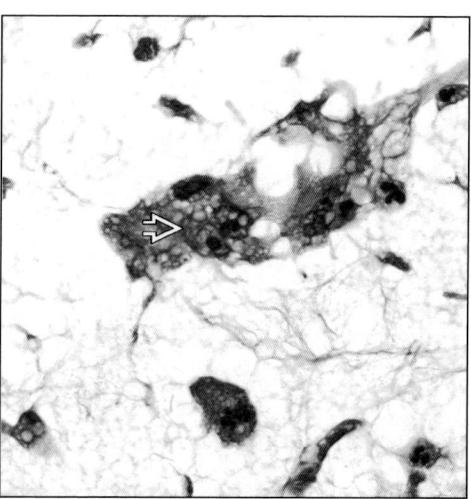

(Left) This myxoinflammatory fibroblastic sarcoma is characterized by hyperchromatic nuclei embedded in a myxoid mucopolysaccharide matrix. (Right) H&E shows a myxoid focus in a myxoinflammatory fibroblastic sarcoma. The cell in the center ➔, with a pair of nuclei with macronucleoli, is reminiscent of a Reed-Sternberg cell.

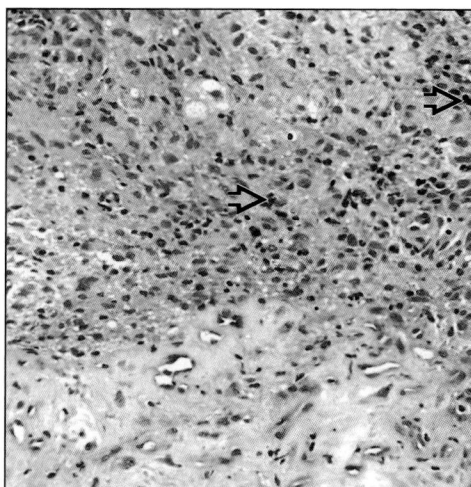

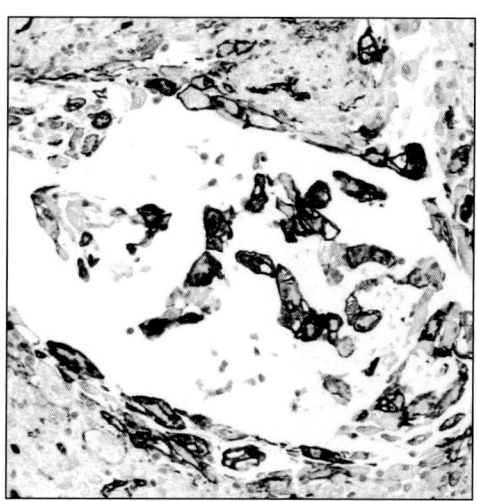

(Left) This particular example of myxoinflammatory fibroblastic sarcoma has fairly abundant hemosiderin deposition ➔. The lower portion of the field has a hyalinized appearance. (Right) CD34 expression is commonly found in myxoinflammatory fibroblastic sarcoma. Focal keratin expression in myxoinflammatory fibroblastic sarcoma can suggest epithelioid sarcoma as well, but there is retention of INI1.

Differential Diagnosis

(Left) This is a myxofibrosarcoma (myxoid malignant fibrous histiocytoma). This superficial lesion arose in the thigh. It appears similar to myxoinflammatory fibroblastic sarcoma, but differs by being richly vascular and by lacking prominent inflammation. **(Right)** This atypical fibroblast from a myxofibrosarcoma appears similar to the cells in myxoinflammatory fibroblastic sarcoma and contains abundant mucopolysaccharides, which are also present in the stroma surrounding the cell.

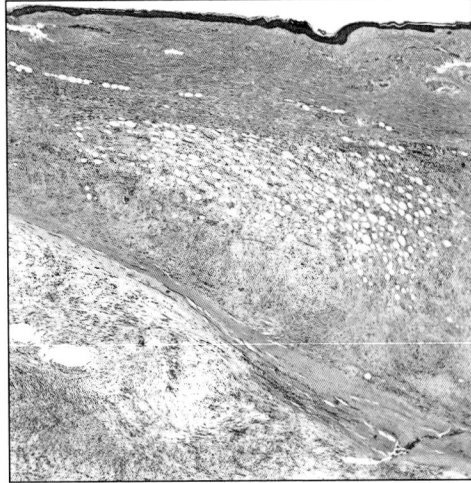
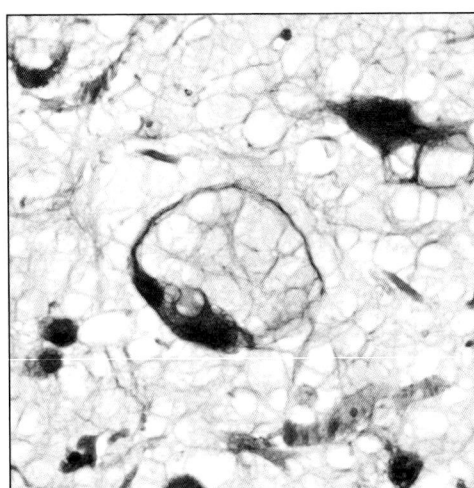

(Left) Pigmented villonodular tenosynovitis appears similar to myxoinflammatory fibroblastic sarcoma clinically, but differs histologically, consisting of giant cells and uniform mononucleate cells. Note the layer of pigmented synovium on the surface ➡. **(Right)** At high magnification, pigmented villonodular tenosynovitis features multinucleated giant cells, uniform cells with single nuclei, and hemosiderin. These lesions often affect the knee joint.

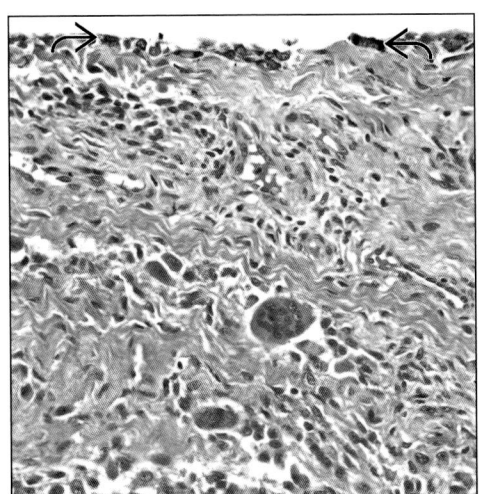
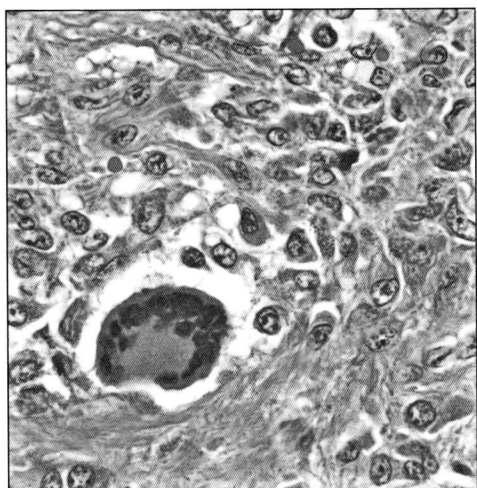

(Left) Hemosiderotic fibrohistiocytic lipomatous lesion, shown here, may form a spectrum with both myxoinflammatory fibroblastic sarcoma and with pleomorphic hyalinizing angiectatic tumor. It typically arises on the foot and consists of CD34(+) reactive spindle cells, fat, and abundant hemosiderin, which is often inconspicuous on routine H&E stains, but readily apparent on iron staining. **(Right)** Hemosiderotic fibrohistiocytic lipomatous lesion often shows abundant iron on iron stains.

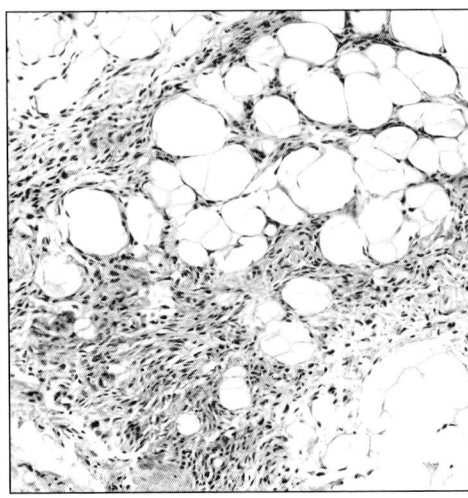
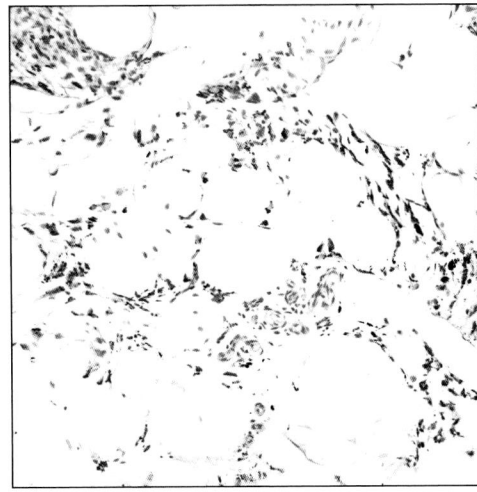

MYXOINFLAMMATORY FIBROBLASTIC SARCOMA

Differential Diagnosis

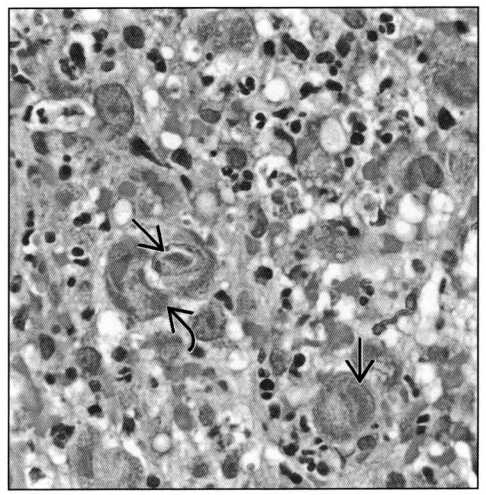 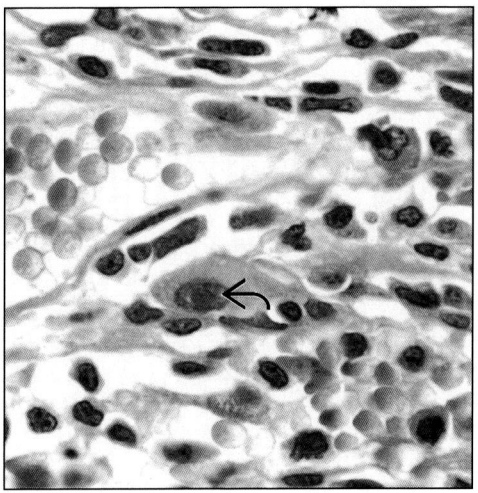

(Left) This example of Cytomegalovirus infection comes from a colon biopsy specimen, although stromal rather than epithelial cells show the classic viral cytopathic effect. The nuclei contain inclusions rather than macronucleoli ➡. There are also cytoplasmic inclusions ➡. *(Right)* This image shows a Cytomegalovirus nuclear inclusion in an endothelial cell ➡, a typical pattern for Cytomegalovirus viral cytopathic effect.

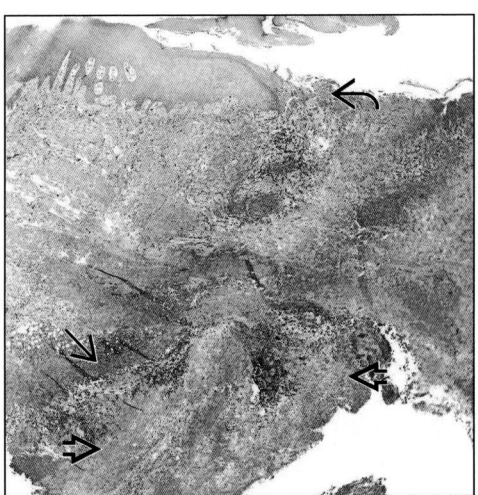 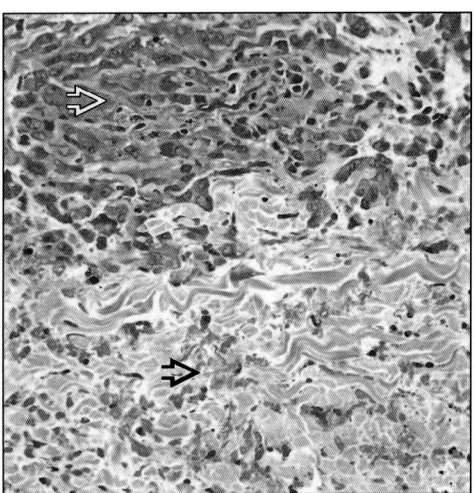

(Left) This image is from an epithelioid sarcoma that affected the distal forearm of a young adult. The lesion involved an aponeurosis but invaded the overlying skin with ulceration ➡. A rim of lesional cells ➡ surrounds a zone of necrosis ➡, an overall pattern reminiscent of granulomatous inflammation. *(Right)* High magnification of an epithelioid sarcoma shows atypical lesional cells ➡ adjacent to a confluent area of necrosis ➡. There is essentially no inflammation.

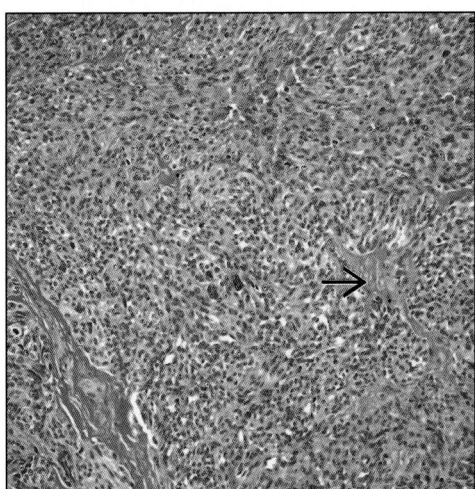 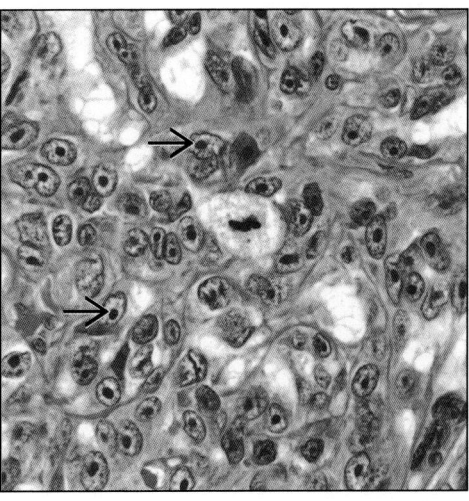

(Left) This is a clear cell sarcoma that arose in the foot of a young adult. The lesion infiltrated a tendon ➡. At this magnification, there is no myxoid change and no inflammation. *(Right)* Clear cell sarcomas have very uniform cells (a feature of sarcomas associated with characteristic translocations) and normal mitoses. Each cell has a uniform large nucleolus ➡. These tumors typically harbor an EWS-ATF1 fusion gene (or an alternate EWS-CREB1 fusion gene).

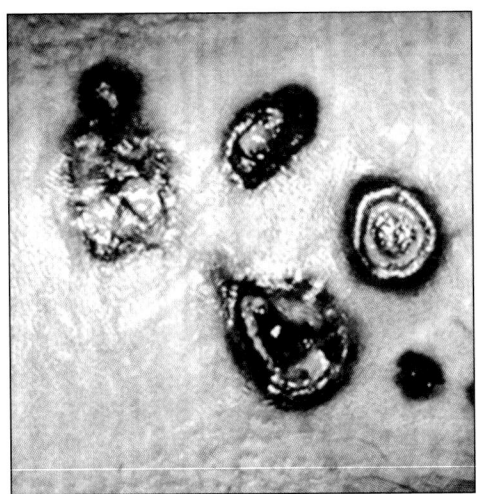

Clinical photograph shows several rounded lesions with raised red margins and central "targetoid" ulceration on the forearm of a 23-year-old man. Nonhealing ulcers are typical of epithelioid sarcoma.

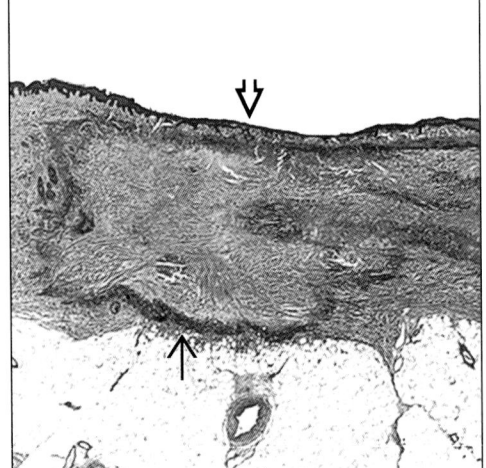

Scanning magnification shows skin with an irregularly shaped dermal lesion. Note the cellular rim ➡ and the necrobiotic central zone. The epidermis shows thinning and ulceration ⊡ over the lesion.

TERMINOLOGY

Abbreviations
- Epithelioid sarcoma (ES)

Synonyms
- Epithelioid cell sarcoma (no longer recommended)

Definitions
- Malignant mesenchymal tumor resembling carcinoma or granuloma, which shows predominantly epithelial, but also mesenchymal, differentiation
- ES occurs in classical and proximal (aggressive, large cell, or rhabdoid) forms

ETIOLOGY/PATHOGENESIS

Genetic Factors
- Some cases have abnormalities of chromosome 22q
- Rare association with neurofibromatosis type 2

CLINICAL ISSUES

Epidemiology
- Incidence
  - Rare
    - Accounts for about 1% of all soft tissue sarcomas
  - Classic ES
    - Most common in distal extremities, especially hand and forearm
    - Head and neck
    - Penis, vulva
  - Proximal ES
    - Proximal limb girdle
    - Axial locations: Perineum, pelvis, mediastinum
    - Trunk: Chest wall
- Age
  - Usually young, but may occur at any age
  - Classic ES
    - Mostly 2nd to 4th decades
  - Proximal ES
    - Median age: 40 years (range: 13-80 years)
- Gender
  - More frequent in males

Presentation
- 1 or more slow-growing lesions
- Subcutaneous mass
  - Classic ES
    - Dermal or subcutaneous nodule
  - Proximal ES
    - Subcutaneous or deeper mass
    - Can appear more rapidly
- Ulcer
  - Nonhealing ulcer with raised margin

Natural History
- Classic ES
  - Persistent and multiple recurrences
    - Successive lesions often recur and extend more proximally in limb
  - Eventual metastasis to regional lymph nodes
    - Via blood to lungs, bone, brain, and soft tissue, notably scalp
- Proximal ES
  - Rapidly growing, locally aggressive tumor with high mortality

Treatment
- Surgical approaches
  - Adequate local excision
    - Amputation for intractable recurrences
- Adjuvant therapy
  - No specific effective therapy

Prognosis
- Classic ES
  - > 70% recur
  - 30-50% metastasize
  - 5-year survival: 70%; 10-year survival: 40%

EPITHELIOID SARCOMA

Key Facts

Terminology
- Malignant mesenchymal tumor resembling carcinoma or granuloma
  - Classical and proximal aggressive forms

Etiology/Pathogenesis
- Some have abnormalities of chromosome 22q

Clinical Issues
- Most common in distal extremities, especially hand and forearm
- More frequent in males
- Subcutaneous nonhealing ulcer or deep mass
- Aggressive sarcoma
  - Persistent and multiple recurrences
  - > 70% recur
  - ~ 50% metastasize

Microscopic Pathology
- Central necrosis
- Epithelioid cells with transition to spindle cells at periphery
- Nuclei bland or mildly atypical, often resembles granuloma

Ancillary Tests
- CKs and EMA positive
- CD34 positive in 50% of cases
- INI1 negative in 80-90% of cases
- S100 and desmin negative

Top Differential Diagnoses
- Granuloma annulare
- Invasive carcinoma
- Melanoma

- Proximal ES
  - 65% local recurrence
  - 45-75% metastasize
  - 5-year survival: 35-65%
- Favorable prognostic factors
  - Young age at 1st diagnosis
  - Female sex
  - Primary tumor < 2 cm diameter
- Adverse prognostic factors
  - Proximal location
  - Greater degree of necrosis
  - Vascular invasion
  - Inadequate local excision

MACROSCOPIC FEATURES

General Features
- Classic ES
  - Ulcerated skin nodule
  - Raised "sealing-wax" margins
- Proximal ES
  - Multinodular mass
  - Hemorrhage and necrosis

Size
- Classic ES: 0.2 cm to > 5 cm diameter
- Proximal ES: Up to 20 cm diameter

MICROSCOPIC PATHOLOGY

Histologic Features
- Classic ES
  - Small dermal/subcutaneous nodules with central necrosis
  - Epithelioid cells, spindled at periphery
  - Mildly atypical nuclei, eosinophilic cytoplasm
  - Rare multinucleated osteoclast-like cells
  - Rare myxoid change
  - Calcification in 20%, rare stromal bone formation
  - Occasional hemorrhage ("angiomatoid" or angiosarcoma-like variant)

- Proximal ES
  - Multiple large nodules with necrosis
  - Larger, more atypical polygonal cells
  - Vesicular nuclei, prominent eosinophilic nucleoli
  - Abundant cytoplasm, rhabdoid cytomorphology
- Rare fibroma-like variant
  - Hypocellularity, fibrous stroma
  - Storiform pattern
  - Spindle or polygonal cells with indistinct cell boundaries and occasional hyperchromatic nuclei
  - Affinity for involving bone

Lymphatic/Vascular Invasion
- In 10% of ES

Margins
- Irregular, infiltrative

Lymph Nodes
- 30% of metastases are to lymph nodes

ANCILLARY TESTS

Flow Cytometry
- Can be diploid or polyploid

Cytogenetics
- Chromosome 22q deletions
  - Classical ES: Inconsistent t(8;22)(q22;q11)
  - Proximal ES: t(10;22) in 2 cases
- Abnormalities in 18q11 region also described

Electron Microscopy
- Transmission
  - Varies between cases; not all features in any 1 tumor
    - Surface microvilli
    - Intercellular junctions
    - Tonofilaments
    - Subplasmalemmal thin filaments

EPITHELIOID SARCOMA

Immunohistochemistry

Antibody	Reactivity	Staining Pattern	Comment
CK-PAN	Positive	Cytoplasmic	In 95% of cases; diffuse
CK7	Positive	Cytoplasmic	In 22% of cases; focal
CK8/18/CAM5.2	Positive	Cytoplasmic	In 94% of cases
CK19	Positive	Cytoplasmic	In 72% of cases
CK5/6	Positive	Cytoplasmic	In 20% of cases; focal
EMA/MUC1	Positive	Cell membrane	In 98% of cases; diffuse
CD34	Positive	Cell membrane	In 52% of cases
CD99	Positive	Cell membrane & cytoplasm	In 25% of cases
Actin-sm	Positive	Cytoplasmic	In 25% of cases in spindle cells
Cyclin-D1	Positive	Nuclear	In 96% of cases
INI1	Negative	Nuclear	Negative in 80-90% of cases
CK20	Negative	Cytoplasmic	Positive in 13% of cases; focal
CD31	Negative	Cell membrane & cytoplasm	Very rare cytoplasmic positivity
S100	Negative	Nuclear & cytoplasmic	
Desmin	Negative	Cytoplasmic	Very rarely, proximal variant is positive
FLI-1	Negative	Nuclear	

DIFFERENTIAL DIAGNOSIS

Granuloma Annulare
- Cells are smaller and bland-appearing, cytoplasm less eosinophilic
- No spindle cells at periphery of nodule
- Histiocytic markers positive; epithelial markers absent

Invasive Carcinoma
- Overlying in situ component usually present
- Usually more pleomorphic than classical ES
- CK5/6, p63, and INI1 positive; CD34 negative

Melanoma
- Junctional component usually present
- Variable cell types may be present, including epithelioid, spindled, and rhabdoid cells
  o Cells are usually larger and more pleomorphic than classic ES
- S100, HMB-45, MART-1/Melan-A, and INI1 typically positive

Rhabdomyosarcoma
- More infiltrative than nodular in the skin
- Desmin, myogenin, myoD1 positive

Epithelioid Hemangioendothelioma
- Nodules and cords of epithelioid cells
- Intracytoplasmic lumina present
- Myxoid/chondromyxoid stroma
- CD31, CD34, FVIIIRAg, INI1 positive

Epithelioid Sarcoma-like Hemangioendothelioma
- Sheets of bland cells with intracytoplasmic lumina
- Keratin positive, but EMA negative
- CD31 positive, but CD34 negative

Epithelioid Angiosarcoma
- Anastomosing vascular spaces and sheets of atypical pleomorphic epithelioid cells
- Foci of vasoformation and hemorrhage
- Positive CD31, FLI1, FVIIIRAg, INI1; variable for CD34

Clear Cell Sarcoma
- Deep subcutis, related to tendon sheaths
- Nests of uniform polygonal cells
- Clear or granular cytoplasm
- Round uniform nuclei, basophilic nucleoli
- Positive for S100, HMB-45, and MART-1/Melan-A in most cases
- Specific translocation t(11;22)(EWS;ATF1)

DIAGNOSTIC CHECKLIST

Clinically Relevant Pathologic Features
- Ulcerated granulomatous lesion with CK positivity

Pathologic Interpretation Pearls
- Coexpression of CK, EMA, and CD34; absence of INI1

GRADING

High Grade
- Formal grading not recommended, as all cases considered high-grade sarcoma

SELECTED REFERENCES

1. Chbani L et al: Epithelioid sarcoma: a clinicopathologic and immunohistochemical analysis of 106 cases from the French sarcoma group. Am J Clin Pathol. 131(2):222-7, 2009
2. Fisher C: Epithelioid sarcoma of Enzinger. Adv Anat Pathol. 13(3):114-21, 2006

EPITHELIOID SARCOMA

Microscopic Features

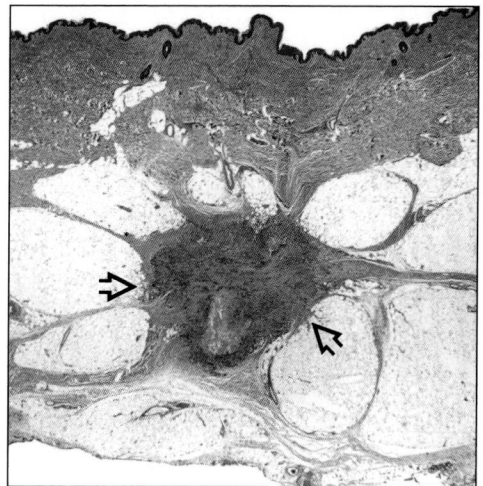

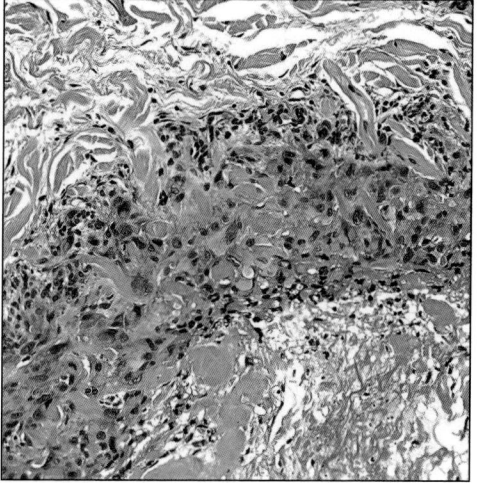

(Left) Scanning magnification shows a subcutaneous nodule of epithelioid sarcoma ➲. Note the lack of circumscription, incipient extension along the interlobular septa, and the central focus of necrosis. The overlying skin is intact. (Right) High magnification shows the cellular rim of the tumor nodule. The cells show distinctive cytoplasmic eosinophilia and uneven distribution of nuclei. Spindle cells are often seen at the periphery of tumor nodules in epithelioid sarcoma, but are not prominent here.

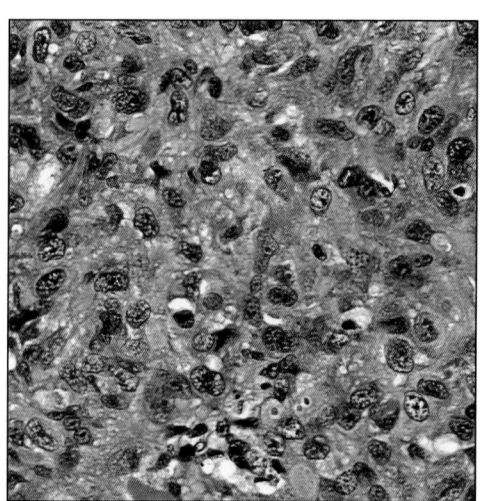

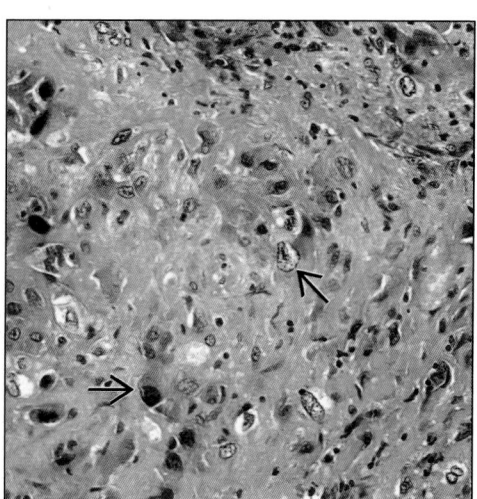

(Left) High magnification shows the cytomorphology of epithelioid sarcoma. The cells have mildly pleomorphic vesicular nuclei, focally prominent nucleoli, moderate amounts of cytoplasm, and indistinct margins. (Right) Recurrent epithelioid sarcoma at the site of a previous surgery is shown. The neoplastic cells ➲ are scattered within the fibrous tissue. Knowledge of the history and high suspicion are needed to identify the tumor. Cytokeratin immunostaining is diagnostic.

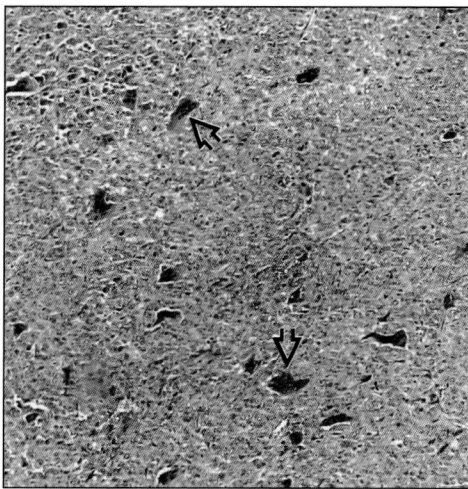

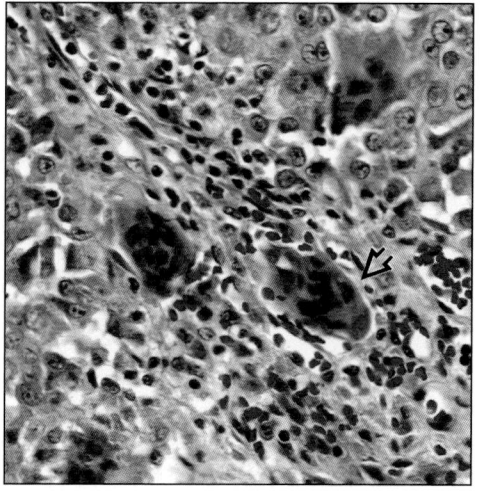

(Left) Low magnification shows an unusual example of epithelioid sarcoma containing osteoclast-like giant cells ➲ scattered within a sheet of tumor cells. This is usually a focal finding. (Right) Higher magnification shows the multinucleated (osteoclast-like) cells ➲ that are reactive, not neoplastic, and show immunohistochemical staining for CD68. The tumor cells express CK, EMA, and CD34, unlike tendon sheath-type giant cell tumor.

Variant Microscopic Features

(Left) Low magnification shows a proximal-type epithelioid sarcoma. The tumor is lobulated and highly cellular with irregular margins and geographic central necrosis. The tumor ulcerates at skin surface. *(Right)* Intermediate magnification shows a tumor composed of large polygonal cells in dyscohesive nodules with a focus of necrosis ⇨. Note that this deposit of tumor is circumscribed, but not encapsulated. There is scant adjacent inflammation.

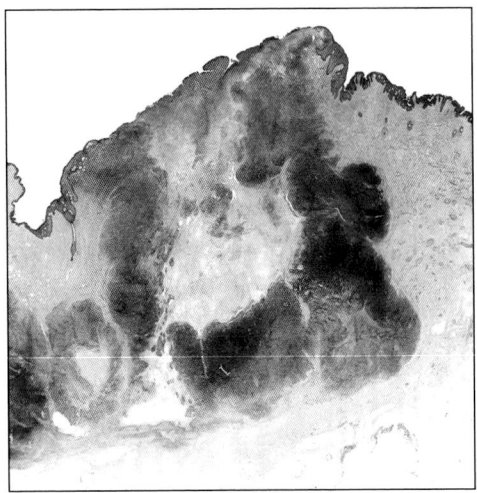
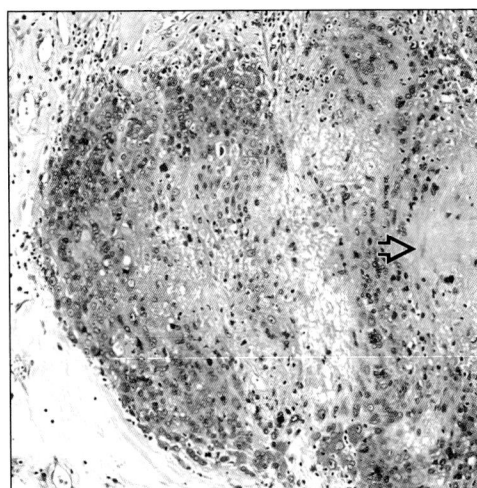

(Left) High magnification shows unevenly distributed cells in proximal-type ES with rounded, vesicular nuclei and prominent eosinophilic nucleoli ⇨. The cells are larger than those of classic epithelioid sarcoma. *(Right)* Another example of the proximal type of ES shows prominent rhabdoid morphology ⇨. The cells have abundant eosinophilic cytoplasm and eccentric displaced nuclei. The cytoplasm contains vimentin and cytokeratin intermediate filaments.

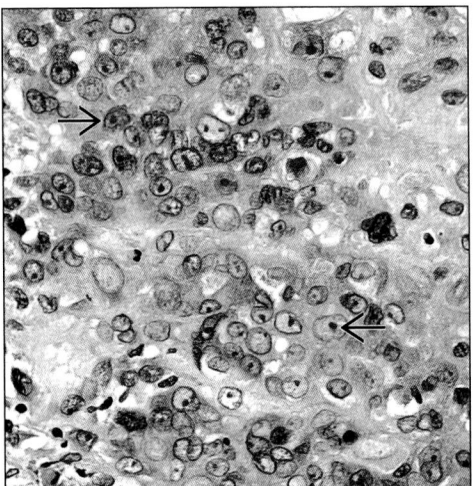
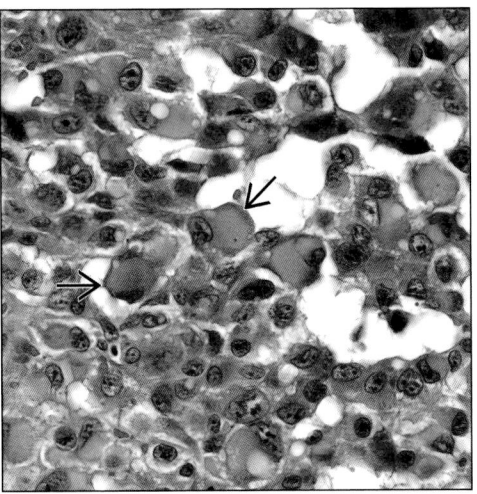

(Left) This example of ES shows dilated vascular spaces with hemorrhage, imparting an angiosarcoma-like appearance. This change is usually focal rather than diffuse, but can cause diagnostic difficulty in a biopsy specimen, especially when it is CD34 positive. *(Right)* This is an unusual example of ES that shows the very rare finding of prominent stromal myxoid change. Unlike in mucinous adenocarcinoma, the mucin is stromal and extracellular.

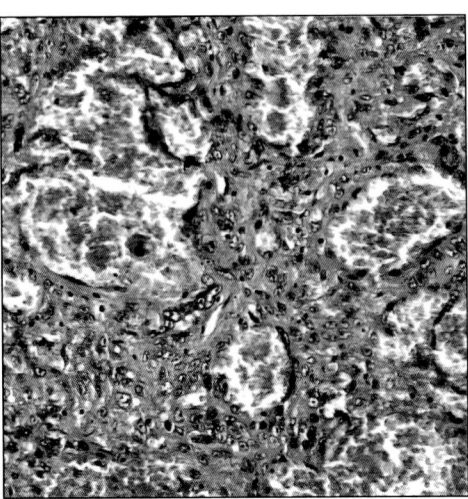
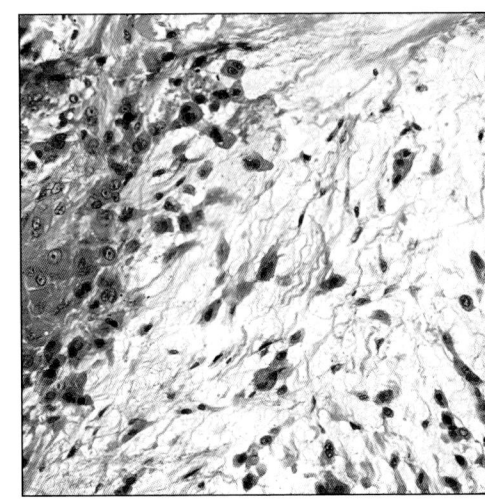

EPITHELIOID SARCOMA

Variant Microscopic Features and Ancillary Techniques

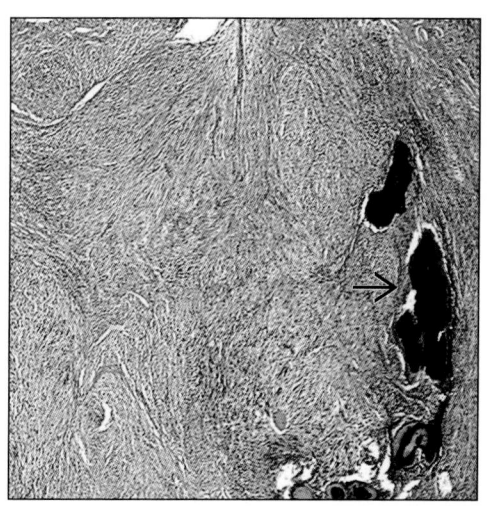

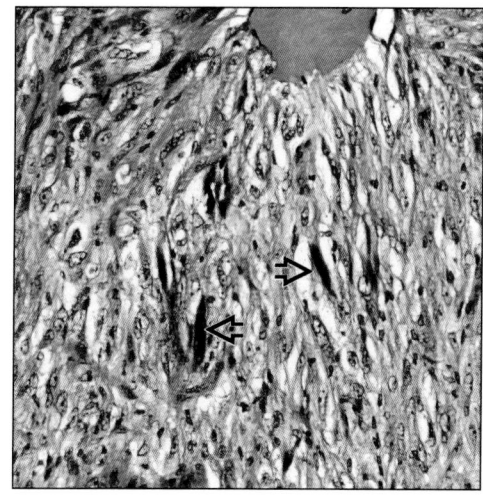

(Left) Histologic section shows the fibroma-like variant of ES with peripheral foci of metaplastic bone formation ➡. This rare feature is also occasionally found in typical ES. *(Right)* High magnification shows the fibroma-like variant of epithelioid sarcoma with spindle cells in a fibrous stroma. Note focal nuclear enlargement and hyperchromasia ➡. This variant can have a storiform pattern resembling fibrous histiocytoma, but differs in expressing CK and EMA.

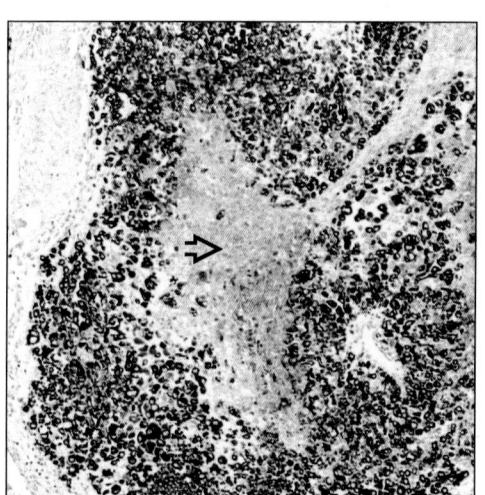

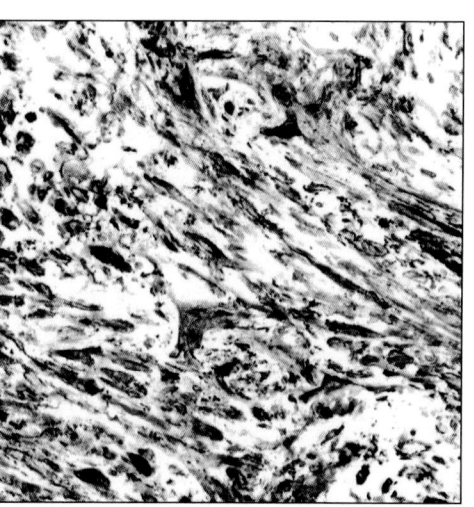

(Left) AE1/AE3 staining in a classic ES shows diffuse positivity in lesional cells surrounding a necrotic zone ➡. This staining pattern is typical of ES and excludes nonneoplastic granulomatous lesions. *(Right)* AE1/AE3 immunohistochemistry shows strong positivity in the spindle cells of fibroma-like variant of ES. These cells also express EMA and are often CD34 positive (50%). Principal differential diagnosis is spindle cell carcinoma, which is CD34 negative.

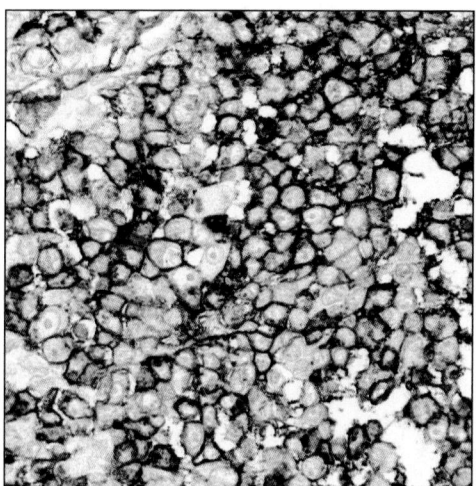

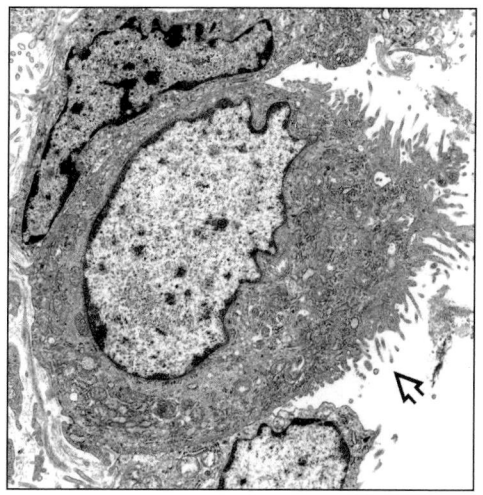

(Left) CD34 shows membranous immunoreactivity in the lesional cells and is found in about 1/2 of cases. The distribution of staining is diffuse in this classical ES, but it is often focal. Absence of CD31 and FLI1 help to exclude angiosarcoma. *(Right)* Transmission EM shows a tumor cell with numerous surface microvillous projections ➡. This is a feature of epithelial differentiation. Other features sometimes seen are intercellular junctions and cytoplasmic tonofilaments.

Vascular and Perivascular Tumors and Pseudotumors

VASCULAR HAMARTOMAS

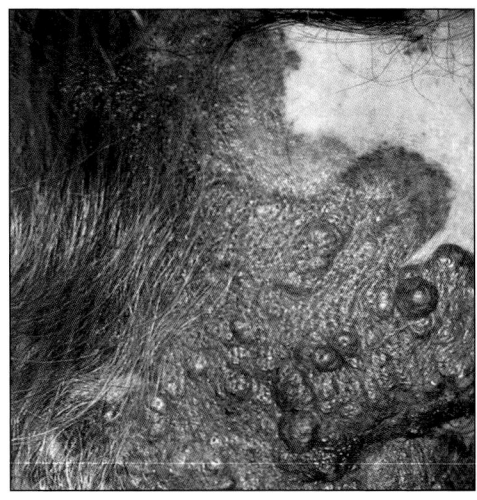

Port-wine stain is a vascular hamartoma that usually presents on the head and neck. As the patient ages, it often becomes thicker and more nodular. (Courtesy A. Vidimos, MD.)

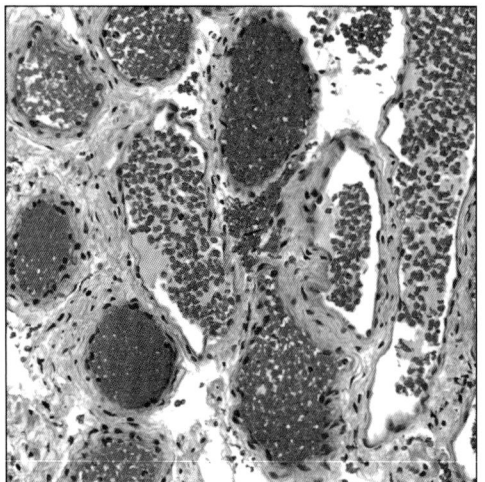

Vascular hamartomas are usually characterized by closely packed, dilated, thin-walled blood vessels.

TERMINOLOGY

Synonyms
- Congenital vascular malformations
- Sturge-Weber syndrome: Encephalotrigeminal angiomatosis
- Klippel-Trenaunay-Weber syndrome: Angioosteohypertrophy, hemangiectatic hypertrophy

Definitions
- Nevus flammeus: Group of congenital vascular malformations

ETIOLOGY/PATHOGENESIS

Developmental Anomaly
- Vascular malformations present at birth
  - Klippel-Trenaunay-Weber syndrome may be associated with t(8;14)(q22.3;q13)

CLINICAL ISSUES

Presentation
- Present at birth usually in the head and neck area, but may involve extremities or trunk
- Port-wine stain (PWS)
  - Present in 0.3% of all births
  - Usually involves head and neck, but any location may be affected
  - May be segmental
  - Usually starts as flat, pink lesions
  - Typically does not become apparent histologically until patients are about 10 years old
  - Grows with patient and becomes darker and thicker with time
- Salmon patch
  - Present in about 40% of population at birth
  - Presents as pink macule on head and neck
  - Majority fade within 1st year of life
- Sturge-Weber syndrome
  - Port-wine stain involving ophthalmic branch of trigeminal nerve and one of the following features
    - Ipsilateral vascular abnormality of leptomeninges
    - Ipsilateral vascular abnormality of choroid
- Klippel-Trenaunay-Weber syndrome
  - Men and women equally affected
  - Port-wine stain usually involving extremity
  - Underlying venous and lymphatic malformations
  - Limb overgrowth with hypertrophy of soft tissue and bone
  - Varicose veins
  - May be associated with high output cardiac failure
- Cobb syndrome
  - Present at birth, but may not be recognized initially
  - Port-wine stain in dermatomal distribution
  - Port-wine stain or verrucous hemangioma associated with underlying spinal arteriovenous hemangioma or venous hemangioma
  - May be associated with neurologic symptoms (e.g., weakness) from underlying spinal vascular tumor
- Blue rubber bleb nevus syndrome
  - Presents at birth or early childhood
  - Multiple blue-colored, rubbery hemangiomas of skin
  - Usually resemble cavernous hemangiomas
  - Gastrointestinal tract frequently involved
  - Sometimes painful
  - Lesions do not regress
  - May develop iron deficiency anemia from gastrointestinal hemorrhage
- Mafucci syndrome
  - Presents in childhood
  - Sporadic disease
  - Multiple "hemangiomas" of dermis and subcutis
  - Usually resembles cavernous hemangiomas
  - Capillary hemangiomas and spindle cell hemangiomas may also be present
  - Multiple enchondromas, most commonly affecting metacarpals and phalanges

VASCULAR HAMARTOMAS

Key Facts

Clinical Issues
- Port-wine stain
  - Usually involves head and neck
- Sturge-Weber syndrome
  - Port-wine stain involving ophthalmic branch of trigeminal nerve
- Klippel-Trenaunay-Weber syndrome
  - Port-wine stain usually involving extremity
- Blue rubber bleb nevus syndrome

- Multiple blue-colored rubbery hemangiomas of skin
- Mafucci syndrome
  - Multiple hemangiomas of dermis and subcutis and enchondromas

Microscopic Pathology
- Dilated blood-filled capillaries
  - Confined to papillary dermis in salmon patch
  - Involve deeper dermis in port-wine stain

- May have associated skeletal deformities
- Chondrosarcomas develop in 15-30%
- Associated with increased risk of pancreatic, ovarian, and central nervous system malignancies

Treatment
- Surgical approaches
  - Variable surgical approaches that depend on individual case
  - Laser treatment

Prognosis
- Benign, but some forms associated with increased risk of secondary malignancy or high output cardiac failure

MICROSCOPIC PATHOLOGY

Histologic Features
- All show similar features
  - Dilated blood-filled capillaries
    - Confined to papillary dermis in salmon patch
    - Involve deeper dermis in port-wine stain
  - May have cavernous vessels
    - In Maffucci syndrome and blue rubber bleb nevus
    - Often present in deep dermis and involving subcutis
  - May resemble arteriovenous malformation
  - Cobb syndrome lesion resembles verrucous hemangioma
  - Immunohistochemistry

- Positive for CD31, CD34; negative for WT1

DIFFERENTIAL DIAGNOSIS

Acquired Hemangiomas, Arteriovenous Hemangioma, Verrucous Hemangioma
- Histology may be indistinguishable; key difference is clinical presentation

SELECTED REFERENCES

1. Piram M et al: Sturge-Weber syndrome in patients with facial port-wine stain. Pediatr Dermatol. Epub ahead of print, 2011
2. Redondo P et al: Diagnosis and management of extensive vascular malformations of the lower limb Part I. Clinical diagnosis. J Am Acad Dermatol. 65(5):893-906, 2011
3. Dilmé-Carreras E et al: Cobb syndrome: case report and review of the literature. Dermatology. 221(2):110-2, 2010
4. Wong CH et al: Blue rubber bleb nevus syndrome: a clinical spectrum with correlation between cutaneous and gastrointestinal manifestations. J Gastroenterol Hepatol. 18(8):1000-2, 2003
5. Fanburg JC et al: Multiple enchondromas associated with spindle-cell hemangioendotheliomas. An overlooked variant of Maffucci's syndrome. Am J Surg Pathol. 19(9):1029-38, 1995
6. Paller AS: Vascular disorders. Dermatol Clin. 5(1):239-50, 1987

IMAGE GALLERY

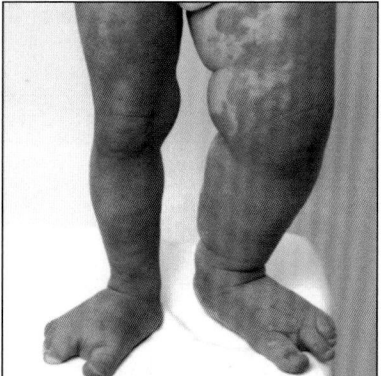 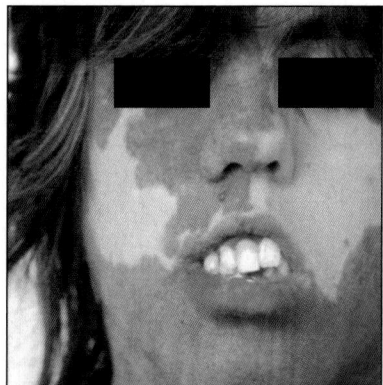 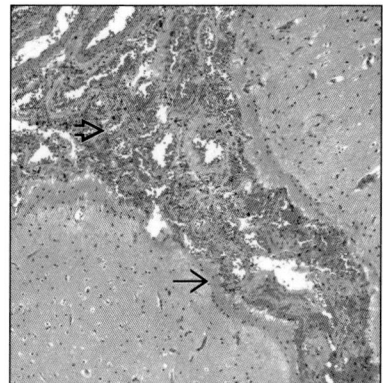

(Left) Klippel-Trenaunay syndrome is an extensive port-wine stain affecting an extremity associated with limb overgrowth. *(Courtesy A. Vidimos, MD.)* *(Center)* Sturge-Weber syndrome is a port-wine stain involving the distribution of the trigeminal nerve. *(Courtesy A. Vidimos, MD.)* *(Right)* In Sturge-Weber syndrome, an associated vascular hamartoma ➣ involving the ipsilateral meninges ➣ may be present.

ARTERIOVENOUS HEMANGIOMA (MALFORMATION)

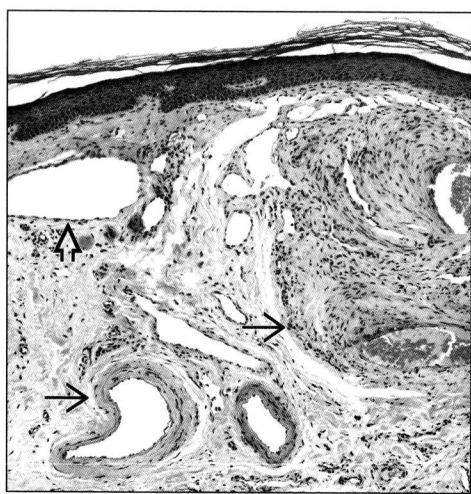

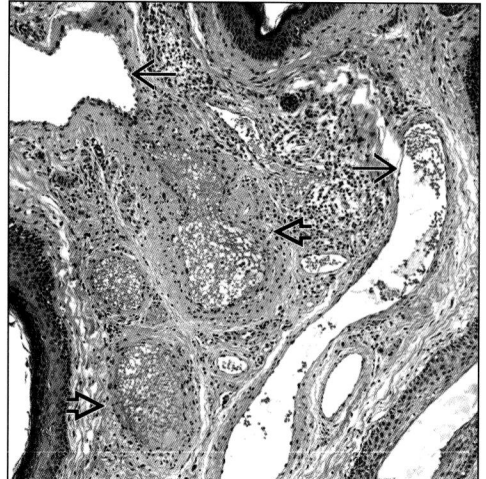

Arteriovenous hemangioma is composed of a circumscribed proliferation of thick-walled muscular vessels that resemble arteries ➡ and thin-walled ectatic veins ▷.

This higher power image of arteriovenous hemangioma demonstrates the ectatic thin-walled veins ➡ and the thicker walled vessels resembling arteries ▷. The vessels have flattened endothelium.

TERMINOLOGY

Synonyms
- Cirsoid aneurysm
- Cirsoid hemangioma
- Acral arteriovenous tumor

Definitions
- Benign vascular tumor composed of thick- and thin-walled blood vessels

CLINICAL ISSUES

Epidemiology
- Incidence
  - Uncommon lesions
- Age
  - Presents in adults
    - Usually in 5th-6th decades
- Gender
  - Women and men affected equally

Site
- Usually involves face
  - Especially lip
  - Rarely oral cavity
- Extremities: Acral arteriovenous tumors

Presentation
- Solitary dark red papule or nodule

Natural History
- Stable vascular proliferations that do not regress

Treatment
- Surgical approaches
  - Simple excision

Prognosis
- Benign

MACROSCOPIC FEATURES

Size
- Small (< 1 cm in most cases)

MICROSCOPIC PATHOLOGY

Histologic Features
- Circumscribed vascular tumor in dermis
  - Vessels closely aggregated together
- Ectatic thin- and thick-walled blood vessels
  - Thick-walled blood vessels have thick muscular walls resembling arteries
    - Most of the thick-walled vessels lack a true internal elastic lamina on elastic stains, indicating that they are more likely veins
    - Some of the thick-walled vessels likely represent "arterialized" veins
- Vessels lined by single layer of flattened endothelial cells
- May have thrombi
- Dystrophic calcification occasionally present in vascular walls

Cytologic Features
- Bland endothelial cells lacking nuclear atypia or pleomorphism

DIFFERENTIAL DIAGNOSIS

Deep Arteriovenous Malformation
- Usually presents on extremities in children
- Similar histologic appearance
- Involves deeper soft tissue than arteriovenous hemangioma

Capillary Hemangioma
- Clustered proliferation of capillary-like blood vessels
- Large "feeder" vessel supplies each lobule

ARTERIOVENOUS HEMANGIOMA (MALFORMATION)

Key Facts

Terminology
- Acral arteriovenous tumor
- Cirsoid aneurysm
- Benign vascular tumor composed of thick- and thin-walled blood vessels

Microscopic Pathology
- Circumscribed tumor in dermis
- Vessels closely aggregated together
- Ectatic thin- and thick-walled blood vessels

- Thicker blood vessels have muscular walls resembling arteries

Top Differential Diagnoses
- Deep arteriovenous malformation
- Capillary hemangioma
- Cavernous hemangioma
- Venous hemangioma
- Venous lake
- Angioleiomyoma

- Lacks thick-walled vessels
- Mitotic figures may be present, especially in juvenile and pyogenic granuloma forms

Cavernous Hemangioma
- Ectatic blood vessels
- Blood vessels have thin walls, not thick and thin walls

Venous Hemangioma
- Proliferation composed of enlarged, thick-walled vascular spaces
- Dilated lumen with thrombi or phleboliths
- Cystically dilated vessels may mimic cavernous hemangioma

Venous Lake
- Solitary ectatic vessel rather than aggregated vessels
- Thin vascular wall
- No thick-walled blood vessels

Angioleiomyoma
- Well-circumscribed nodular tumor composed of vascular smooth muscle punctuated by focal vascular lumina
- Smooth muscle of angioleiomyomas blends together in a syncytial manner, rather than just being part of discrete vessels
- Lacks distinctly separate vessels

Acquired Digital Arteriovenous Malformation
- Presents on fingertips

- Composed of superficial thick- and thin-walled vessels, but less aggregated than arteriovenous hemangioma

Angiosarcoma
- Architecturally complex vessels with anastomosing network of neoplastic vessels
- Cytologic atypia and mitotic activity present

SELECTED REFERENCES

1. Bekhor PS et al: Acquired digital arteriovenous malformation: ultrasound imaging and response to long-pulsed neodymium:yttrium-aluminum-garnet treatment. J Am Acad Dermatol. 56(5 Suppl):S122-4, 2007
2. Park CO et al: Treatment of unusual vascular lesions: usefulness of sclerotherapy in lymphangioma circumscriptum and acquired digital arteriovenous malformation. Dermatol Surg. 31(11 Pt 1):1451-3, 2005
3. Kadono T et al: Acquired digital arteriovenous malformation: a report of six cases. Br J Dermatol. 142(2):362-5, 2000
4. Rothstein MS: Cirsoid aneurysm. Int J Dermatol. 19(1):45-6, 1980
5. Chatterji P et al: Cirsoid aneurysm of the auricle and adjoining scalp. J Laryngol Otol. 91(11):997-1002, 1977
6. Poyton HG et al: Cirsoid aneurysm secondary to an arteriovenous fistula of the facial artery and vein. Oral Surg Oral Med Oral Pathol. 37(3):474-9, 1974
7. Biberstein HH et al: A cirsoid aneurysm in the skin; a case report. Dermatologica. 113(3):129-41, 1956
8. Burston H: Recurrent swelling of the tongue due to cirsoid aneurysm (angioma). AMA Arch Otolaryngol. 62(1):90-2, 1955

IMAGE GALLERY

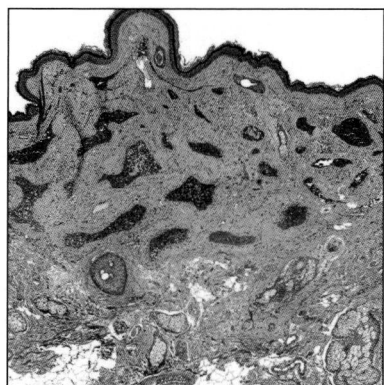
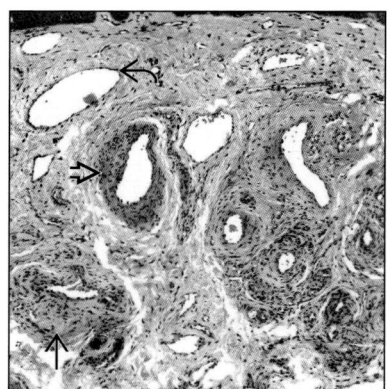
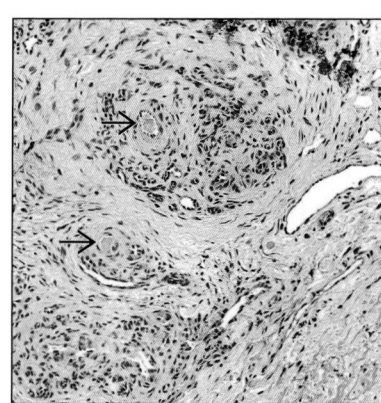

(Left) Low magnification of a superficial arteriovenous hemangioma shows a tumor that is mostly composed of thick-walled vessels. *(Center)* Arteriovenous hemangioma is classically composed of a combination of thick- ➡ and thin-walled vessels ➡. The thick-walled vessels often have degenerative changes resulting in myxoid stroma ➡ surrounding the vessel. *(Right)* Fibrin thrombi are sometimes present in the lumina of some of the thick-walled vessels ➡.

CAPILLARY, VENOUS, AND CAVERNOUS HEMANGIOMAS

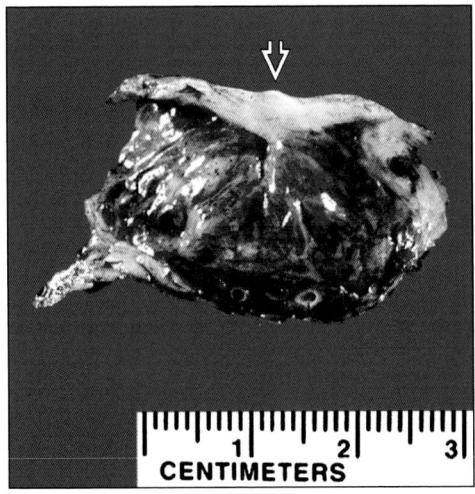

Capillary hemangiomas present as small, superficial, well-circumscribed, red-purple nodules. The overlying skin is intact in this example ⇒ but may be ulcerated (especially in pyogenic granulomas).

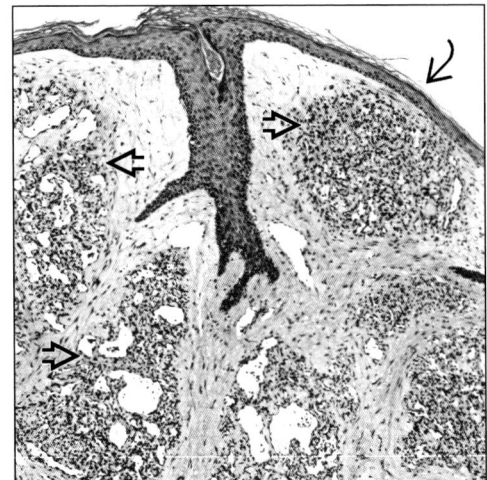

The lobular configuration of capillary hemangiomas is apparent at low-power examination ⇒. Multiple distinct lobules of capillaries are centered in the dermis, and the overlying skin is intact ⇗.

TERMINOLOGY

Abbreviations
- Pyogenic granuloma (PG)

Synonyms
- Capillary hemangioma = lobular hemangioma

Definitions
- Benign vascular tumors composed of blood vessels of various size lined by plump to flattened endothelial cells with no atypia

ETIOLOGY/PATHOGENESIS

Developmental Anomaly
- Juvenile (infantile) capillary hemangiomas may be congenital
- Venous hemangiomas may represent vascular malformations

CLINICAL ISSUES

Epidemiology
- Age
  - Depends on subtype
- Gender
  - Capillary and cavernous hemangiomas in adults occur more commonly in women

Site
- Depends on subtype

Presentation
- Painless mass
- Red elevated papule(s)

Natural History
- Juvenile capillary hemangiomas regress spontaneously with time

Treatment
- Surgical approaches
  - Surgical excision is curative, but usually not necessary unless affecting vital structures
- Drugs
  - Glucocorticoids or interferon-α therapy for large or symptomatic juvenile hemangiomas
- Watchful waiting for juvenile hemangiomas that regress with time

Prognosis
- Recurrences are rare; only occur in some incompletely excised lesions

MACROSCOPIC FEATURES

General Features
- Elevated nodular red-purple lesions
- Usually involve skin or subcutaneous tissue
- Discoloration may not be obvious in deep-seated lesions
- Recurrences may be sessile

Size
- Variable size

Capillary (Lobular) Hemangioma
- Most common type of hemangioma
- Variants
  - **Juvenile (infantile) hemangioma**
    - Occurs in infancy; 1:200 births
    - About 1/5 multiple; rarely familial (associated with several syndromes)
    - Flat red lesion in early stage
  - **Pyogenic granuloma (PG)**
    - Occurs on skin and mucosal surfaces
    - Gingiva, fingers, lips, face, and tongue are most common sites of involvement
    - Polypoid friable lesions that bleed easily and are often ulcerated

CAPILLARY, VENOUS, AND CAVERNOUS HEMANGIOMAS

Key Facts

Terminology
- Benign vascular tumors composed of blood vessels lined by plump to flattened endothelial cells with no atypia

Etiology/Pathogenesis
- May be congenital (infantile/juvenile hemangiomas)

Clinical Issues
- Capillary hemangioma is commonest subtype of hemangioma
- Juvenile hemangiomas occur in infancy
- Capillary and cavernous hemangiomas in adults occur more commonly in women
- Pyogenic granuloma occurs on skin and mucosal surfaces and is often ulcerated
- Cavernous hemangiomas present as birthmarks

- Venous hemangiomas are rare and present in adulthood
- Juvenile capillary hemangiomas regress spontaneously with time

Microscopic Pathology
- Nodules of small capillary-sized vessels in lobular pattern in capillary hemangioma
- Large, cystically dilated vessels filled with blood in cavernous hemangioma
- Large, thick-walled veins in venous hemangioma
- Lining endothelium in all lesions does not typically show atypia
- Thrombosis (± Masson tumor/change), hemorrhage, and calcifications may be present
  - Especially in venous and cavernous hemangiomas

- Intravenous pyogenic granuloma
  - Neck and upper extremities are common sites
  - Red-brown intravascular polyp
  - May be mistaken for organizing thrombus
- Pregnancy-related pyogenic granuloma
  - Gingiva commonest site
  - Regress after delivery
- Senile angioma (cherry angioma)
  - Trunk and extremity
  - Ruby red papule with halo around it

Venous Hemangioma
- Rare, presents in adulthood, predilection for limbs

Cavernous Hemangioma
- Common symptomatic birthmark
- Soft, compressible, purple lesions

MICROSCOPIC PATHOLOGY

Histologic Features
- Capillary hemangioma
  - Nodules of small capillaries arranged in lobular architecture
  - Large "feeder" vessel supplies each lobule
  - Vascular lumen may be inconspicuous in early lesions
  - Flat to plump endothelial cells with little or no atypia
  - Mitotic figures may be present, especially in juvenile and PG forms
  - Surface epithelium may be atrophic or ulcerated in PG
  - Marked acute and chronic inflammation present in PG
- Venous hemangioma
  - Large, thick-walled blood vessels
  - Dilated lumen with thrombi or phleboliths
  - Cystically dilated vessels may mimic cavernous hemangioma
- Cavernous hemangioma
  - Large, cystically dilated vessels filled with blood

- Lined by flat endothelium without atypia
- Organizing thrombi and Masson tumor-like change may be present
- Recanalizing thrombi may create sinusoidal pattern ("sinusoidal hemangioma")

DIFFERENTIAL DIAGNOSIS

Arteriovenous Malformation (AVM)
- May mimic venous hemangioma
- Unlike AVMs, elastic stain shows absence of internal elastic lamina in venous hemangioma

Kaposi Sarcoma (KS)
- Angiomatous form of KS may be mistaken for PG
  - PG is well-circumscribed and shows lobular arrangement
- Spindle cell proliferation with slit-like spaces
- Nuclear immunoreactivity for HHV8

Reactive Granulation Tissue
- Lacks lobular architecture of capillaries seen in PG

DIAGNOSTIC CHECKLIST

Pathologic Interpretation Pearls
- Lobular architecture of blood vessels is typical of capillary hemangiomas
- Cavernous hemangiomas may show Masson tumor-like changes

SELECTED REFERENCES

1. Jackson R: The natural history of strawberry naevi. J Cutan Med Surg. 2(3):187-9, 1998
2. Coffin CM et al: Vascular tumors in children and adolescents: a clinicopathologic study of 228 tumors in 222 patients. Pathol Annu. 28 Pt 1:97-120, 1993
3. Mills SE et al: Lobular capillary hemangioma: the underlying lesion of pyogenic granuloma. A study of 73 cases from the oral and nasal mucous membranes. Am J Surg Pathol. 4(5):470-9, 1980

CAPILLARY, VENOUS, AND CAVERNOUS HEMANGIOMAS

Clinical and Microscopic Features

(Left) Facial infantile hemangioma is seen in a patient with PHACES (posterior fossa malformations, hemangiomas, arterial and cardiac anomalies, eye abnormalities, and sternal cleft raphe). (Courtesy S. Yashar, MD.) **(Right)** The skin overlying capillary hemangiomas may ulcerate ⮕ and appear similar to inflamed granulation tissue, especially in cases referred to as "pyogenic granulomas." The sharp separation ⮕ between the 2 nodules of proliferating capillaries is a useful diagnostic clue.

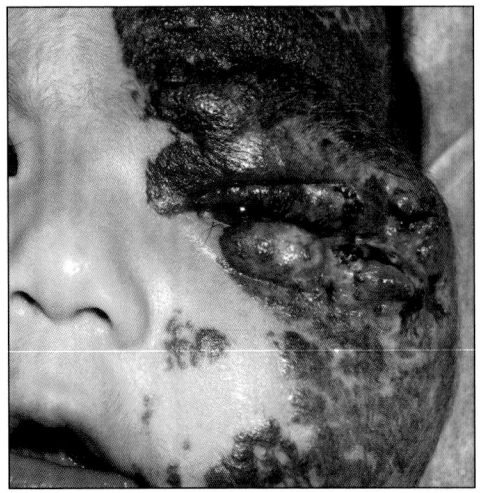
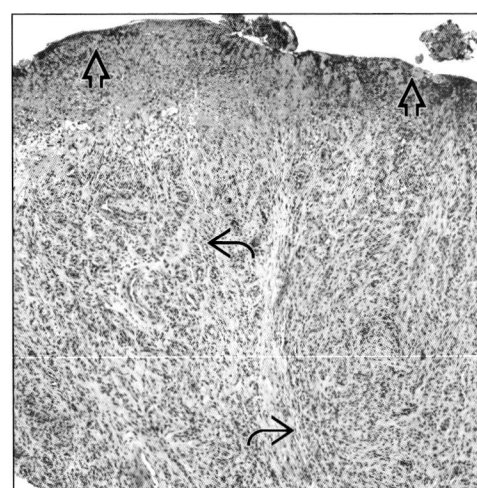

(Left) Capillary hemangiomas are well-circumscribed lesions composed of nodules of capillary-sized vessels with variable luminal size. **(Right)** Each lobule in lobular capillary hemangioma is supplied by a large "feeder vessel" ⮕. The capillary lumina may be inconspicuous in early lesions, but become more apparent as the lesion matures.

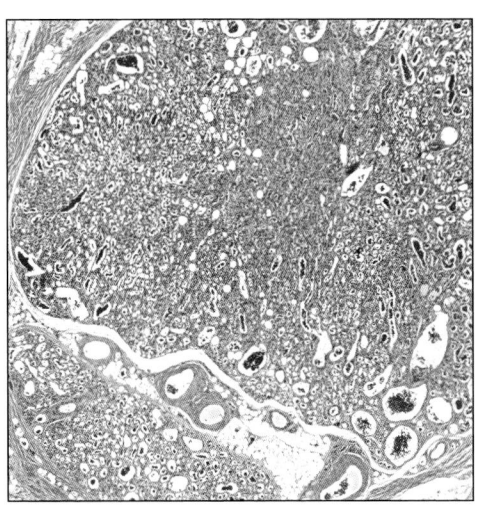
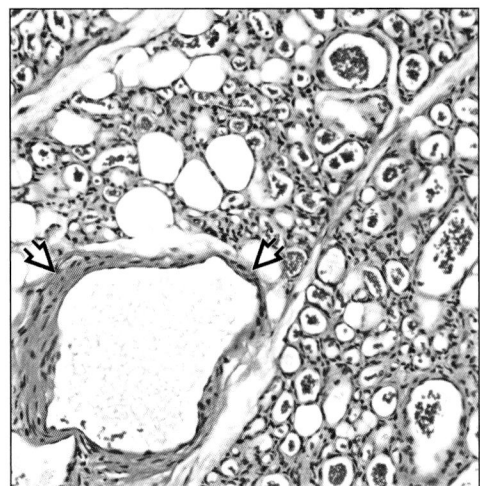

(Left) Capillary hemangiomas are composed of proliferating endothelial cells, pericytes, and a component of inflammatory cells. Endothelial cells lining the capillaries may be flattened ⮕ or plump ⮕ in appearance. **(Right)** Mitotic figures may be present ⮕ in capillary hemangiomas. The well-circumscribed, lobular architecture at low power as well as the lack of nuclear hyperchromasia and atypia in the lining endothelial cells are helpful in ruling out malignancy.

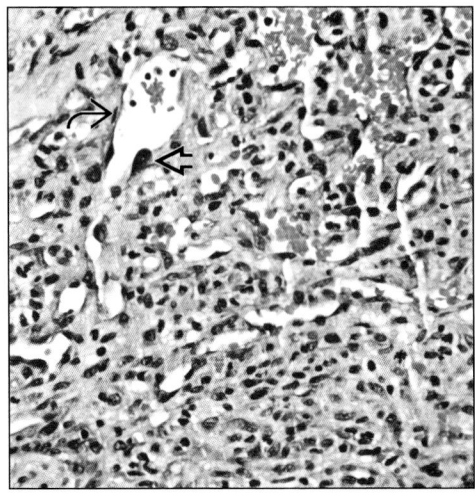
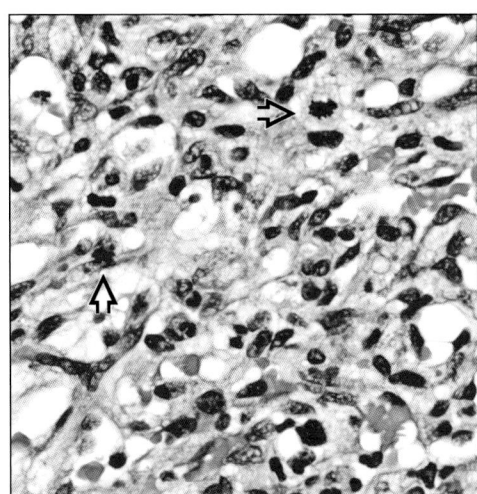

CAPILLARY, VENOUS, AND CAVERNOUS HEMANGIOMAS

Gross and Microscopic Features

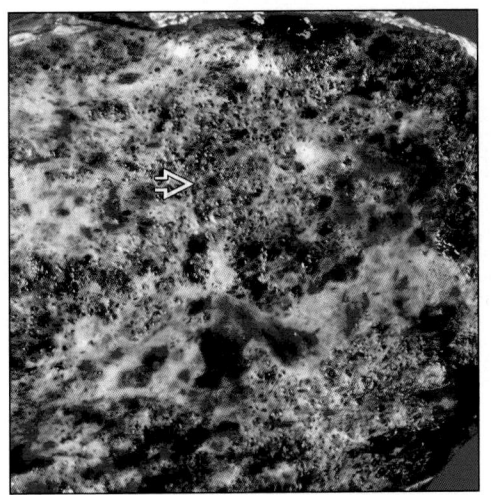 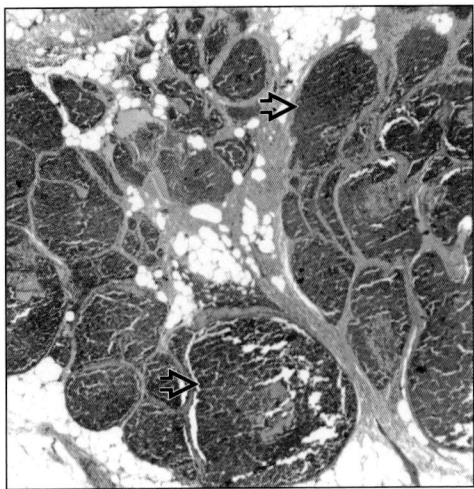

(Left) The cut surface of cavernous hemangiomas is typically spongy in appearance ➡ with cystic spaces of variable size filled with blood. (Right) Cavernous hemangiomas are well-circumscribed nodular lesions composed of lobules of cystically dilated ➡ vascular spaces filled with blood.

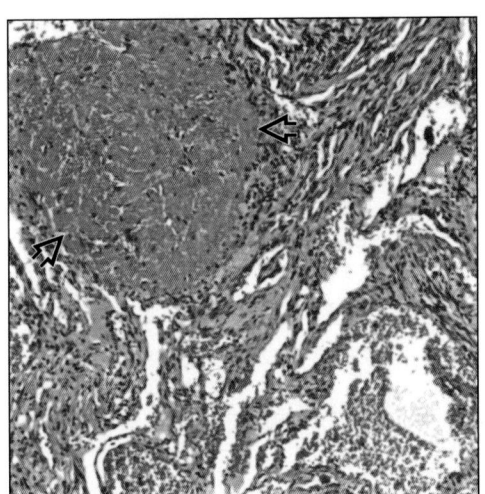 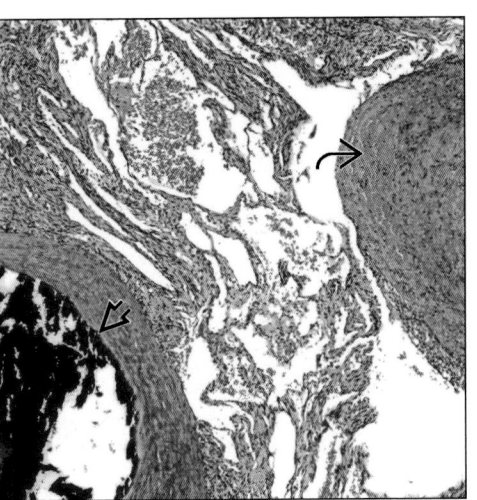

(Left) Large collections of blood within these cavernous spaces increases predisposition to thrombus formation ➡, which may undergo reorganization to Masson tumor (intravascular papillary endothelial hyperplasia)-like changes. (Right) Large intralesional thrombi may also undergo calcification ➡ and be apparent on imaging studies as phleboliths. A noncalcified thrombus ➡ is also present in this example of cavernous hemangioma.

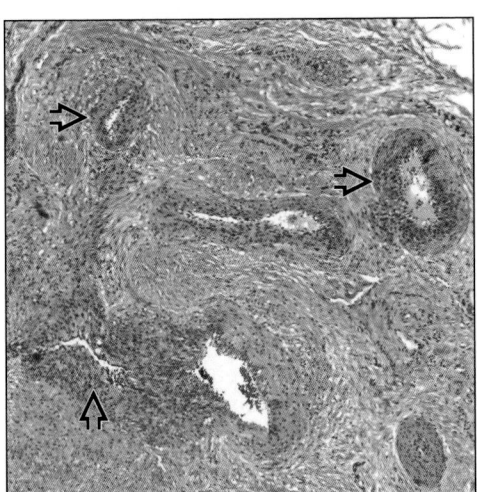 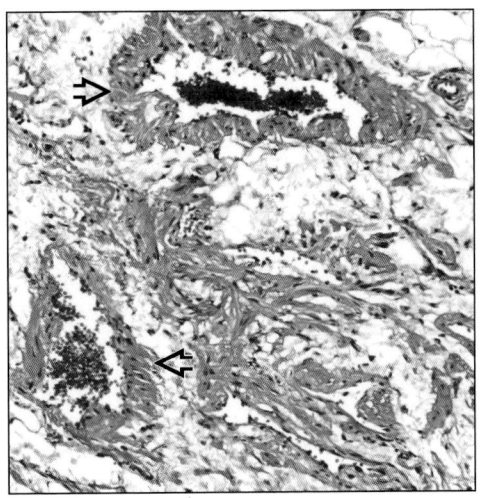

(Left) Venous hemangiomas are composed of circumscribed, nodular collections of thick-walled blood vessels ➡. The lack of an internal elastic lamina in these proliferating vessels is helpful in distinguishing venous hemangiomas from arteriovenous malformations. (Right) The smooth muscle layer surrounding the veins in venous hemangioma may be variable in thickness ➡ and not well formed. Cystically dilated veins in venous hemangiomas may mimic a cavernous hemangioma.

INFANTILE (JUVENILE) HEMANGIOMA

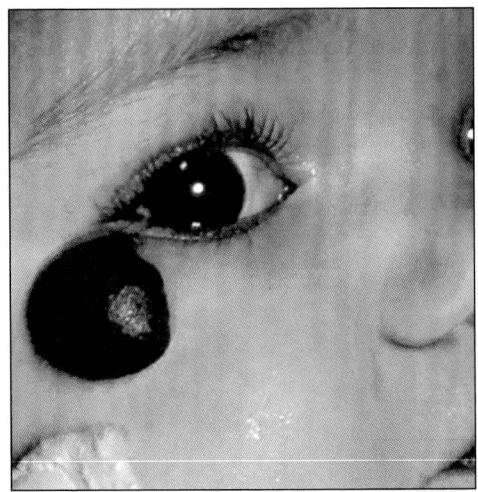

Clinical photograph of a medium-sized hemangioma in a female infant. Most of these lesions are located in the head and neck region. (Courtesy J. Hall, MD.)

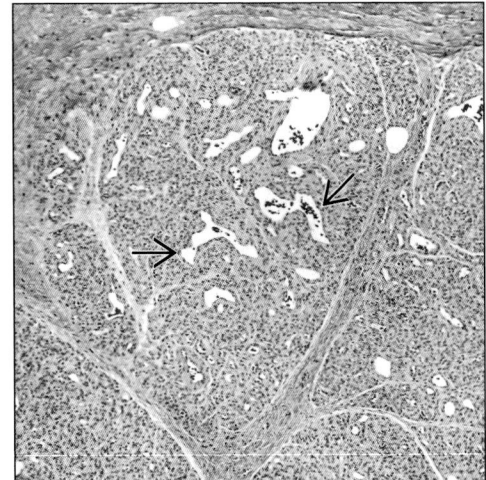

Multiple lobules composed of tightly packed small capillaries separated by fibroconnective tissue are shown in this hemangioma of infancy. Note the scattered centrally located "feeding" vessels ➡.

TERMINOLOGY

Synonyms
- Hemangioma of infancy
- Juvenile hemangioma
- Cellular hemangioma of infancy
- Strawberry nevus/hemangioma

Definitions
- Vascular neoplasm of infancy with characteristic onset, rapid growth, and spontaneous involution

CLINICAL ISSUES

Epidemiology
- Incidence
  - Most common tumor of infancy
  - Affects ~ 4% of children
- Gender
  - M < F
- Ethnicity
  - Caucasians more frequently affected

Site
- Skin and subcutis
  - Head and neck (60%)
  - Extremities, trunk, and genitals
- Viscera

Presentation
- Appear within a few weeks after birth
  - Blanched telangiectatic area

Natural History
- Rapidly enlarge over several months
  - Maximum size usually achieved by 6-12 months
- Regress over several years
  - 75-90% involute by age 7 years

Treatment
- Options, risks, complications
  - Corticosteroids
  - Pulsed dye laser
  - Surgical excision
  - Watchful waiting
    - Small innocuous lesions
  - Interferon-α
    - Restricted to life-threatening lesions
  - Topical imiquimod

Prognosis
- Excellent; all eventually spontaneously regress

MACROSCOPIC FEATURES

General Features
- Crimson-colored multinodular mass

MICROSCOPIC PATHOLOGY

Histologic Features
- Multiple lobules composed of tightly packed small to moderate-sized capillaries
- Early lesions
  - Plump endothelial cells that line small vascular spaces
  - Inconspicuous vascular lumina
  - Distinct lobules separated by normal stroma
  - Moderate mitotic activity and scattered mast cells
- Mature lesions
  - Small vessels lined by flattened endothelial cells
  - Zonal maturation begins at periphery
- Regressing lesions
  - Progressive and diffuse interstitial fibrosis
  - Increased apoptotic bodies and mast cells
- End-stage lesions
  - Scattered residual vessels

INFANTILE (JUVENILE) HEMANGIOMA

Key Facts

Clinical Issues
- Most common tumor of infancy
- Appear within 1st few weeks of life
- Rapidly enlarge over several months
- All eventually spontaneously regress

Microscopic Pathology
- Multiple lobules composed of tightly packed small to moderate-sized capillaries
- Lobules are separated by normal stroma

- Plump endothelial cells that line small vascular spaces in early lesions
- Progressive interstitial fibrosis in older lesions

Ancillary Tests
- GLUT1 is most useful marker for diagnosis

Top Differential Diagnoses
- Pyogenic granuloma
- Arteriovenous malformation
- Tufted angioma

Immunohistochemistry

Antibody	Reactivity	Staining Pattern	Comment
VEGF	Positive	Cytoplasmic	Intense staining in early lesions
CD31	Positive	Cell membrane	Lost after fully involuted
CD34	Positive	Cell membrane	Lost after fully involuted
Actin-sm	Positive	Cytoplasmic	
FVIIIRAg	Positive	Cell membrane & cytoplasm	Lost after fully involuted
GLUT1	Positive	Cell membrane	Not expressed in other vascular neoplasms
IGF-2	Positive	Cell membrane	Not expressed in other vascular neoplasms

    o Fibrofatty background

Predominant Cell/Compartment Type
- Endothelial cell
- Pericytic cell

DIFFERENTIAL DIAGNOSIS

Pyogenic Granuloma
- Another type of lobular capillary hemangioma
- Polypoid red mass surrounded by epidermal collarette
- Nodules of small capillaries subserved by "feeder" vessel

Arteriovenous Malformation
- Dilated, often thick-walled vessels within papillary and reticular dermis

Tufted Angioma
- Small capillaries in prominent clustered or "cannonball" pattern

Granulation Tissue
- Fibroblastic stromal cells and collagenous matrix with small capillaries and inflammatory cells

Kaposiform Hemangioendothelioma
- Infiltrating sheets of slender spindled endothelial cells

SELECTED REFERENCES

1. North PE et al: Vascular tumors of infancy and childhood: beyond capillary hemangioma. Cardiovasc Pathol. 15(6):303-17, 2006
2. North PE et al: GLUT1: a newly discovered immunohistochemical marker for juvenile hemangiomas. Hum Pathol. 31(1):11-22, 2000

IMAGE GALLERY

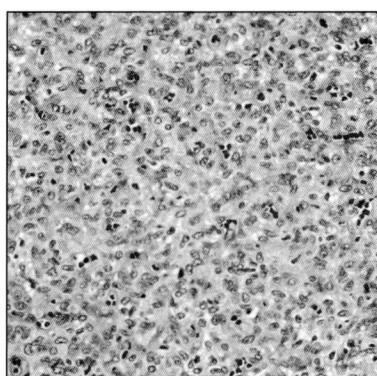 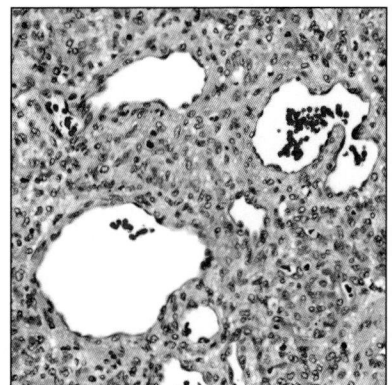 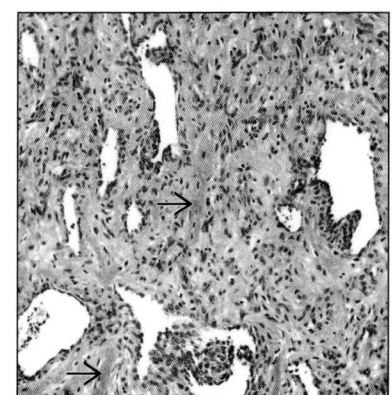

(Left) Hemangioma of infancy is shown at high power. Early lesions, as illustrated, are composed of plump endothelial cells with inconspicuous vascular lumina. Numerous mitoses may also be present. *(Center)* The central "feeding" vessels with dilated lumina lined by flattened endothelial cells are shown. *(Right)* An older, involuting lesion composed of scattered dilated vessels in a background of progressive and diffuse interstitial fibrosis ➔ is shown.

SINUSOIDAL HEMANGIOMA

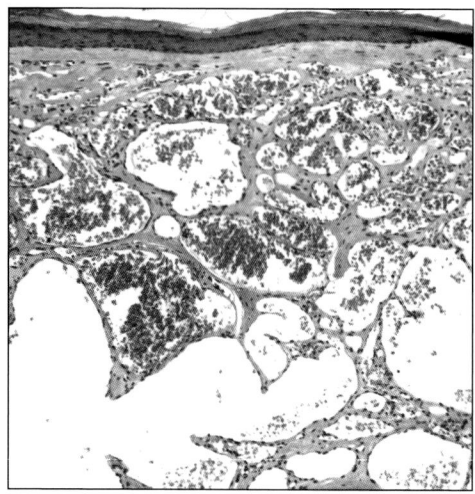

Low magnification histologic examination shows the superficial portion of a cutaneous sinusoidal hemangioma involving the papillary and reticular dermis with large dilated vascular spaces.

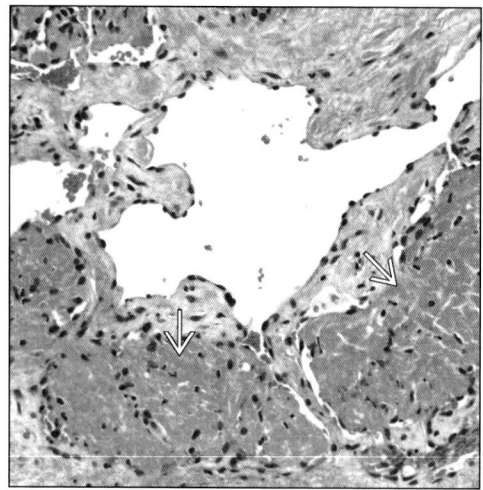

Histologic section shows sinusoidal vascular spaces with large areas of thrombosis ➡️, a finding often seen in SH.

TERMINOLOGY

Abbreviations
- Sinusoidal hemangioma (SH)

Synonyms
- Cavernous hemangioma (variant)

Definitions
- Acquired vascular lesion in adults; features similar to cavernous hemangioma/venous malformation

ETIOLOGY/PATHOGENESIS

Unknown
- May represent reactive vascular proliferation rather than true neoplastic process

CLINICAL ISSUES

Epidemiology
- Incidence
  - Rare
- Age
  - Typically occurs in adults
- Gender
  - More common in females

Site
- Often occurs on extremities, trunk, or breast

Presentation
- Subcutaneous or dermal mass
  - Solitary, painless, bluish (deep) or red (superficial) nodule
    - Freely movable

Treatment
- Surgical approaches

- Complete excision is curative, but not necessary given benign nature of lesions

Prognosis
- Excellent, no malignant potential

MACROSCOPIC FEATURES

Size
- Typically < 2.0 cm

MICROSCOPIC PATHOLOGY

Histologic Features
- Proliferation of numerous thin-walled anastomosing vessels
  - Well-circumscribed proliferation of vessels in sinusoidal pattern
  - Vessels are thin-walled and closely packed, with little intervening stroma
    - Occasional cases may show smooth muscle in vessel walls
    - Pseudopapillary pattern may be seen (due to tangential sectioning)
    - Thrombosis may occur and be associated with intravascular papillary endothelial hyperplasia (Masson tumor)
  - Lining cells are small endothelial cells with nuclear hyperchromasia
  - Mitotic figures typically not seen
  - Calcifications may rarely be present

Cytologic Features
- Nuclei are hyperchromatic but show regular borders and uniform chromatin

Predominant Pattern/Injury Type
- Vascular proliferation

Key Facts

Terminology

- Acquired vascular lesion in adults; features similar to venous malformation

Clinical Issues

- Painless bluish or red nodule
- Complete excision is curative, but not necessary given benign nature of lesions
- Excellent prognosis, no malignant potential

Microscopic Pathology

- Well-circumscribed vascular proliferation
- Vessels are thin-walled and closely packed, with little intervening stroma
- Lining cells are small endothelial cells with nuclear hyperchromasia
- Pseudopapillary pattern may be seen (due to tangential sectioning)

Predominant Cell/Compartment Type

- Endothelial

DIFFERENTIAL DIAGNOSIS

Arteriovenous Hemangioma (Malformation)

- Typically occurs on lips, perioral skin, or nose of older adult males
- Proliferation of large, thick-walled blood vessels with smooth muscle in their walls, which mostly represent veins
- "Feeder" vessel (ascending muscular artery) may be present in some cases

Venous Malformation (Cavernous Hemangioma)

- Occurs in children, usually present at birth
- Often larger and more poorly circumscribed than sinusoidal hemangioma
- Does not show as closely packed vessels or ramified pattern

Cherry Angioma

- Very common small papular lesions occurring in adults
- Superficial papillary dermal lesions, as opposed to sinusoidal hemangioma (which is typically deep dermal or subcutaneous)

Glomeruloid Hemangioma

- Associated with Castleman syndrome and polyneuropathy, organomegaly, endocrinopathy, monoclonal paraproteinemia, and skin lesions (POEMS) syndrome
- Typically present as multiple, eruptive lesions on trunk and limbs
- Dilated vascular spaces filled by grape-like clusters of capillaries, reminiscent of renal glomeruli

DIAGNOSTIC CHECKLIST

Pathologic Interpretation Pearls

- Closely packed lobular proliferation of vessels in deep dermis or subcutis

SELECTED REFERENCES

1. Nakamura M et al: Calcifying sinusoidal haemangioma on the back. Br J Dermatol. 141(2):377-8, 1999
2. Ruck P et al: Diffuse sinusoidal hemangiomatosis of the spleen. A case report with enzyme-histochemical, immunohistochemical, and electron-microscopic findings. Pathol Res Pract. 190(7):708-14; discussion 715-7, 1994
3. Calonje E et al: New entities in cutaneous soft tissue tumours. Pathologica. 85(1095):1-15, 1993
4. Calonje E et al: Sinusoidal hemangioma. A distinctive benign vascular neoplasm within the group of cavernous hemangiomas. Am J Surg Pathol. 15(12):1130-5, 1991

IMAGE GALLERY

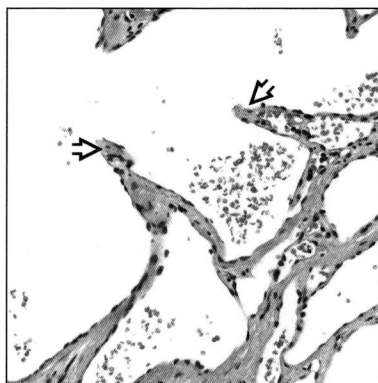 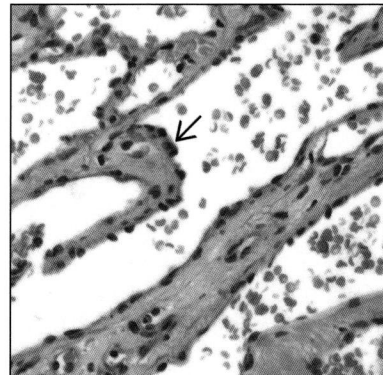 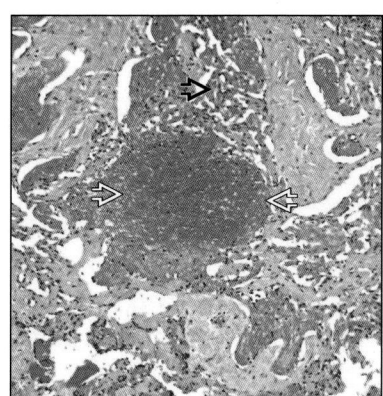

(Left) Histologic section shows pseudopapillary areas ⊳ with projections of thin endothelial-lined stroma into dilated vascular spaces. *(Center)* Histologic section shows the cytologic features of the endothelial cells, which show small, uniform nuclei with hyperchromasia ⊳. *(Right)* Another example of a sinusoidal hemangioma shows hemorrhage and thrombosis ➤ with adjacent areas of papillary endothelial hyperplasia (Masson change) ⊳.

TUFTED ANGIOMA

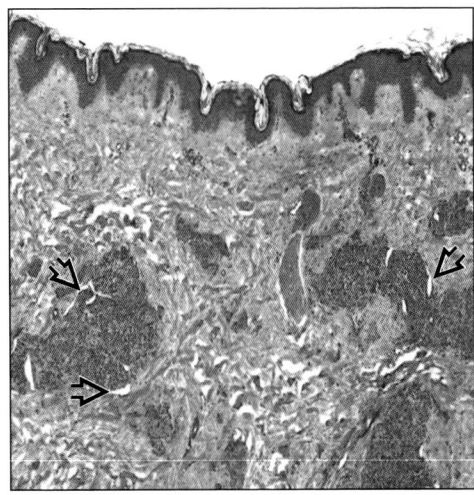

Scanning magnification of a tufted angioma shows scattered dermal lobular collections of vessels. The lobules bulge into dilated vessels, with a few peripheral semilunar spaces identified ⇒.

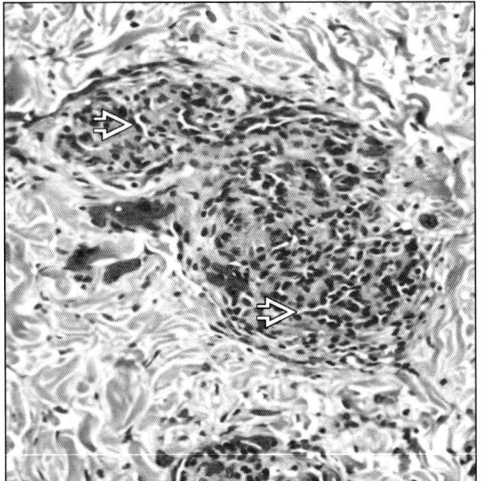

Higher magnification of a lobule shows a proliferation of small, slit-like vascular spaces ⇒ lined by bland oval to spindle-shaped endothelial cells.

TERMINOLOGY

Synonyms
- Acquired tufted angioma (ATA)
- Angioblastoma (of Nakagawa)
- Progressive capillary hemangioma
- Tufted hemangioma

Definitions
- Multiple cannonball-like, scattered cellular collections of small vessels in dermis

ETIOLOGY/PATHOGENESIS

Unknown
- Most cases sporadic; rare familial case described
- Some cases associated with pregnancy or liver transplantation

CLINICAL ISSUES

Epidemiology
- Incidence
  - Rare tumors
- Age
  - Children and young adults

Site
- Neck, shoulders, and upper trunk most common

Presentation
- Slow growing
  - Erythematous macules and plaques

Prognosis
- Excellent; completely benign behavior
- May be associated with Kasabach-Merritt syndrome (consumptive coagulopathy)

MACROSCOPIC FEATURES

General Features
- Reddish-brown nonencapsulated dermal lesion

Size
- Typically small papules, but may be large plaque

MICROSCOPIC PATHOLOGY

Histologic Features
- Multiple scattered lobular collections of small capillary-type vessels throughout dermis
  - Have typical "cannonball" appearance at low-power examination
  - Collections are larger in mid- and lower dermis
  - Cleft-like lumina often present around capillary tufts; may impart glomerular-like appearance
  - Capillaries may be so closely packed that lumina can be inconspicuous
  - Cells are oval to spindle-shaped
  - May show nuclear hyperchromasia, but lack significant cytologic atypia
  - A few mitoses may be present
- Hemosiderin deposition may be seen
- Inflammation typically not present
- Subcutaneous tissue typically not involved

DIFFERENTIAL DIAGNOSIS

Lobular Capillary Hemangioma
- Shows exophytic appearance and epidermal collarette, often ulcerated and acutely inflamed
- Proliferation of small capillary-type blood vessels typically arranged in a few larger nodular collections, rather than multiple smaller dispersed collections seen in ATA

TUFTED ANGIOMA

Key Facts

Terminology
- Acquired tufted angioma (ATA)
- Angioblastoma (of Nakagawa)
- Multiple cannonball-like cellular collections of small vessels in dermis

Clinical Issues
- Children and young adults
- Rare tumors
- Slowly growing erythematous macules and plaques

- May be associated with Kasabach-Merritt syndrome

Microscopic Pathology
- Scattered lobular collections of small capillary-type vessels throughout dermis; may involve subcutis
- Cleft-like lumina often present around capillary tufts; may impart glomeruloid appearance
- Cells are oval to spindle-shaped
- Mitoses may be present, but cells lack significant cytologic atypia

Infantile (Juvenile) Hemangioma
- Cellular dermal nodules composed of lobular collections of oval endothelial cells
- Vascular lumina often small and slit-like, become larger later-stage lesions

Glomeruloid Hemangioma
- Usually associated with Castleman disease or polyorganomegaly, endocrinopathy, M-protein, skin changes (POEMS syndrome)
- Smaller capillary-like collections inside vascular spaces with clefts around them
- Cytoplasmic globules, which are PAS(+) (immunoglobulin aggregates)

Targetoid Hemosiderotic Hemangioma ("Hobnail" Hemangioma)
- Superficial dilated vessels and smaller, narrow deeper vessels lined by plump ("hobnailed") cells
- Extravasated red blood cells and prominent stromal hemosiderin deposition

Kaposi Sarcoma
- Proliferation of interlacing bundles of spindle cells forming slit-like vascular spaces
- Cytoplasmic hyalinized globules, plasma cells, and hemosiderin deposits typically present
- HHV8(+) by immunohistochemistry

DIAGNOSTIC CHECKLIST

Pathologic Interpretation Pearls
- Scattered cannonball-like lobular collections of small capillary-type vessels throughout dermis

SELECTED REFERENCES
1. Arai E et al: Usefulness of D2-40 immunohistochemistry for differentiation between kaposiform hemangioendothelioma and tufted angioma. J Cutan Pathol. 33(7):492-7, 2006
2. Lee B et al: Adult-onset tufted angioma: a case report and review of the literature. Cutis. 78(5):341-5, 2006
3. Ishikawa K et al: The spontaneous regression of tufted angioma. A case of regression after two recurrences and a review of 27 cases reported in the literature. Dermatology. 210(4):346-8, 2005
4. Wong SN et al: Tufted angioma: a report of five cases. Pediatr Dermatol. 19(5):388-93, 2002
5. Igarashi M et al: The relationship between angioblastoma (Nakagawa) and tufted angioma: report of four cases with angioblastoma and a literature-based comparison of the two conditions. J Dermatol. 27(8):537-42, 2000
6. Padilla RS et al: Acquired "tufted" angioma (progressive capillary hemangioma). A distinctive clinicopathologic entity related to lobular capillary hemangioma. Am J Dermatopathol. 9(4):292-300, 1987
7. Scott OL: Tufted haemangioma. Proc R Soc Med. 70(4):283, 1977

IMAGE GALLERY

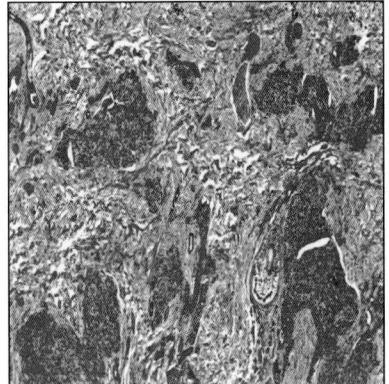 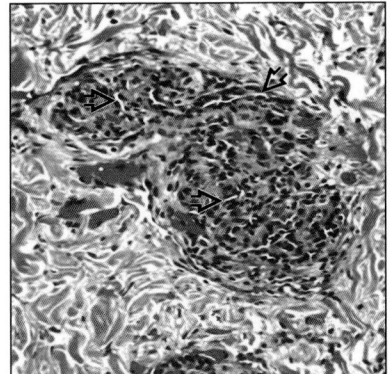 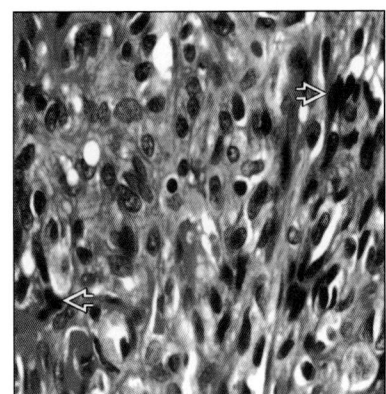

(Left) Low-magnification examination of a tufted angioma shows a diffuse dermal proliferation of clustered blood vessels. (Center) Higher magnification shows a lobular cluster of blood vessels lined by small, oval to spindle-shaped cells. Lumina are collapsed and slit-like. (Right) High-power view shows bland cytologic features of the tufted angioma endothelial cells. Some of the cells show mild nuclear hyperchromasia, but no significant cytologic atypia is identified.

GLOMERULOID HEMANGIOMA

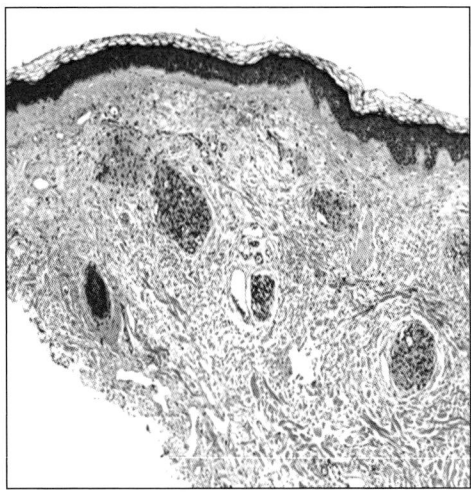

Low magnification shows a superficial dermal proliferation of small clusters of vessels with a glomeruloid pattern.

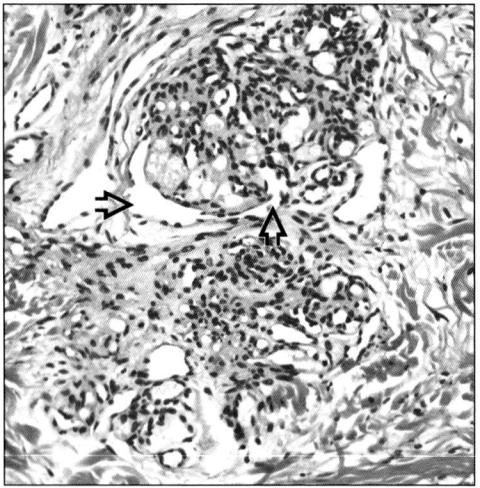

High-power view of a glomeruloid hemangioma shows small, grape-like clusters of vessels projecting into vascular lumina (with peripheral crescentic spaces ⊳).

TERMINOLOGY

Abbreviations
- Glomeruloid hemangioma (GH)

Synonyms
- Glomeruloid angioma

Definitions
- Benign proliferation of small vessels mimicking renal glomeruli

ETIOLOGY/PATHOGENESIS

Paraneoplastic Syndrome
- Association with POEMS syndrome (polyneuropathy, organomegaly, endocrinopathy, M-protein, skin changes) or multicentric Castleman disease in almost all cases

Unknown
- Rare cases not associated with POEMS syndrome

CLINICAL ISSUES

Epidemiology
- Incidence
  - Rare tumors
- Gender
  - More common in females
- Ethnicity
  - More common in Asians (Japanese)

Site
- Trunk and extremities

Presentation
- Multiple red to purple eruptive papules (POEMS syndrome)

  - Most patients also have diffuse skin hyperpigmentation
- Single lesions reported in patients without POEMS

Treatment
- Surgical approaches
  - Excision is curative, but not necessary in most cases
- Adjuvant therapy
  - Treatment of underlying plasma cell disorder may lead to regression of lesions

Prognosis
- Excellent, no malignant potential

MACROSCOPIC FEATURES

General Features
- Dermal-based, well-circumscribed unencapsulated lesions

Size
- Small, typically only a few millimeters

MICROSCOPIC PATHOLOGY

Histologic Features
- Dermal-based proliferation of dilated spaces containing small capillary-type vessels
- Vessels show distinctive grape-like clusters projecting into lumina, mimicking renal glomeruli
- Endothelial cells are mildly enlarged, and many show cytoplasmic eosinophilic globules
  - Cytoplasmic globules (secondary lysosomes containing immunoglobulins) are PAS(+)
- Endothelial cells may show nuclear hyperchromasia, but do not show significant cytologic atypia
- Few mitoses, no necrosis or infiltrative features

GLOMERULOID HEMANGIOMA

Key Facts

Terminology
- Glomeruloid angioma

Etiology/Pathogenesis
- Association with polyneuropathy, organomegaly, endocrinopathy, M-protein, skin changes (POEMS) or multicentric Castleman syndrome in most cases

Clinical Issues
- More common in Asians (especially Japanese)

- Multiple red to purple eruptive papules (POEMS syndrome)

Microscopic Pathology
- Vessels show distinctive grape-like clusters, mimicking renal glomeruli
- Endothelial cells are mildly enlarged and many show cytoplasmic eosinophilic globules
- Cytoplasmic globules (immunoglobulins) are PAS(+)

DIFFERENTIAL DIAGNOSIS

Acquired Tufted Hemangioma (Angioblastoma)
- Slowly spreading macules and plaques in young children and adults
- Multiple dermal and subcutaneous vascular lobules composed of spindled and polygonal-shaped cells
- Some cases may show overlapping features with glomeruloid hemangioma

Lobular Capillary Hemangioma (Pyogenic Granuloma)
- Often shows polypoid configuration with epidermal collarette
- Lobular proliferation typically associated with ulceration, edema, and acute inflammation

Targetoid Hemosiderotic Hemangioma ("Hobnail" Hemangioma)
- Superficial dilated vessels and smaller, narrow, deeper vessels lined by plump ("hobnailed") cells
- Extravasated red blood cells and prominent stromal hemosiderin deposition

Kaposi Sarcoma
- Clinical history distinctive (HIV[+] with multiple lesions or lower extremity lesion in elderly Mediterranean male)

- Cords or fascicles of spindled cells with slit-like lumina associated with hemosiderin deposition and plasma cells
- HHV8(+) (not reported in glomeruloid hemangioma)

DIAGNOSTIC CHECKLIST

Pathologic Interpretation Pearls
- Dermal proliferation of vessels showing distinctive glomeruloid groups or clusters mimicking renal glomeruli

SELECTED REFERENCES

1. Forman SB et al: Glomeruloid hemangiomas without POEMS syndrome: series of three cases. J Cutan Pathol. 34(12):956-7, 2007
2. Perdaens C et al: POEMS syndrome characterized by glomeruloid angioma, osteosclerosis and multicentric Castleman disease. J Eur Acad Dermatol Venereol. 20(4):480-1, 2006
3. Uthup S et al: Renal involvement in multicentric Castleman disease with glomeruloid hemangioma of skin and plasmacytoma. Am J Kidney Dis. 48(2):e17-24, 2006
4. Rongioletti F et al: Glomeruloid hemangioma. A cutaneous marker of POEMS syndrome. Am J Dermatopathol. 16(2):175-8, 1994
5. Chan JK et al: Glomeruloid hemangioma. A distinctive cutaneous lesion of multicentric Castleman's disease associated with POEMS syndrome. Am J Surg Pathol. 14(11):1036-46, 1990

IMAGE GALLERY

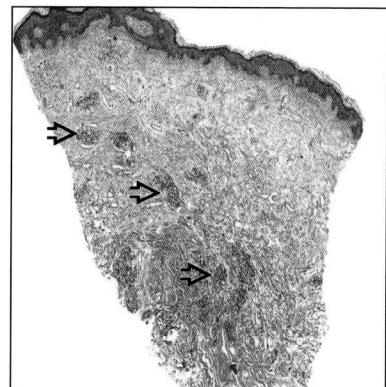 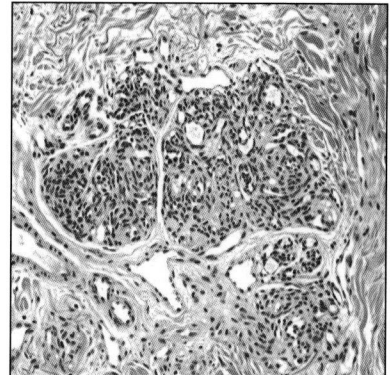 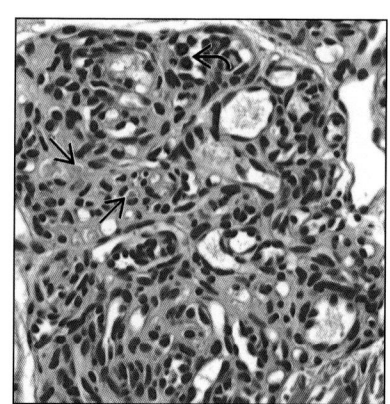

(Left) Scanning magnification view of a glomeruloid hemangioma shows small clusters of vessels in the mid to deep dermis ⊅. (Center) Higher magnification shows the grape-like pattern of clustered small vessels, mimicking renal glomeruli. (Right) High magnification of the vessels in a glomeruloid hemangioma shows endothelial cells with oval- to spindle-shaped nuclei. Cytoplasmic eosinophilic globules are present focally ⊅. A few intraluminal eosinophils are also present ⊅.

ANGIOLYMPHOID HYPERPLASIA WITH EOSINOPHILIA

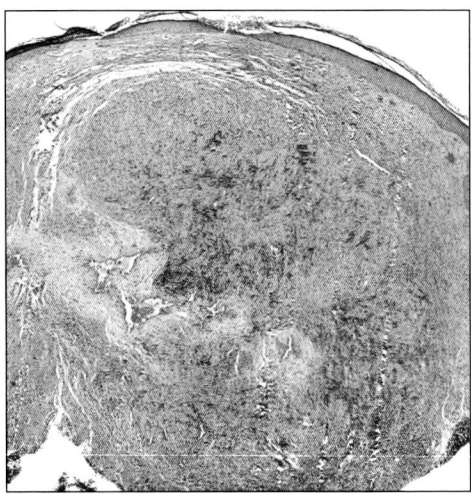

Histology at scanning magnification shows an intact surface epithelium with a richly vascularized stroma containing inflammatory cells.

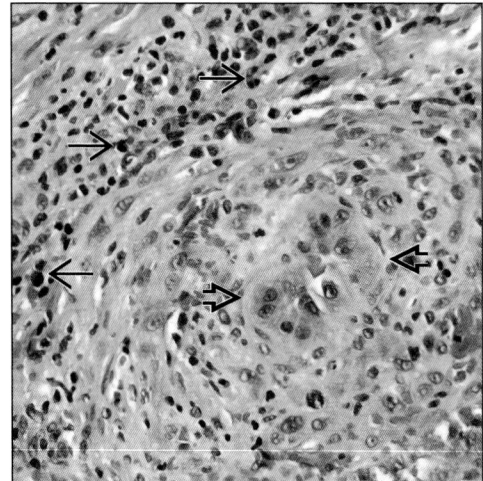

High magnification shows endothelial hyperplasia with a thickened vessel wall ➡, and numerous inflammatory cells, including eosinophils ➡, in the surrounding tissue. Note the extravasated erythrocytes.

TERMINOLOGY

Abbreviations
- Angiolymphoid hyperplasia with eosinophilia (ALHE)

Synonyms
- Epithelioid hemangioma
- Nodular, angioblastic hyperplasia with eosinophilia and lymphofolliculosis

Definitions
- Benign vascular tumor with well-formed, immature blood vessels, most of which are lined by plump, epithelioid (histiocytoid) endothelial cells
- Most cases have prominent inflammatory component in which eosinophils are conspicuous feature

ETIOLOGY/PATHOGENESIS

Reactive
- History of trauma; larger vessels show damage with prominent inflammatory component

Neoplastic
- May represent benign neoplasm

CLINICAL ISSUES

Epidemiology
- Age
  o Wide range
    ▪ Mean: 3rd to 5th decades
- Gender
  o Female > Male
- Ethnicity
  o **Not** increased in Asian patients
    ▪ **Not** synonymous with Kimura disease

Site
- Head (scalp, ears) most commonly affected
  o Digits next most common
  o Mucous membranes rare

Presentation
- Nodule or mass in dermal &/or subcutaneous tissues (**not** lymph nodes), present for up to 12 months
- Pain &/or pruritus
- Often excoriated or bleeding
- Pink to red-brown (hyperpigmented)
- Nodules may be multiple, ultimately coalescing
- Rarely may spontaneously regress/involute

Laboratory Tests
- Peripheral blood eosinophilia in some patients
- **Absent** raised IgE levels

Treatment
- Excision, but recurrence, regrowth, or persistence after surgery requires follow-up

Prognosis
- Excellent, although with frequent local recurrences

MACROSCOPIC FEATURES

General Features
- May resemble lymph node due to circumscription and peripheral inflammation

Size
- Mean: 0.5-2 cm; rarely > 5 cm

MICROSCOPIC PATHOLOGY

Histologic Features
- Multiple lobules of inflammatory elements with increased vascularity on low power
- Surface usually intact, but can be excoriated

ANGIOLYMPHOID HYPERPLASIA WITH EOSINOPHILIA

Key Facts

Terminology

- Benign vascular tumor with well-formed, immature blood vessels associated with prominent inflammatory component, rich in eosinophils

Clinical Issues

- Head most commonly affected; nodule in dermal/subcutaneous tissues
- Nodules may be multiple, ultimately coalescing

Microscopic Pathology

- Multiple lobules composed of inflammatory cells within rich vascularity
- Proliferation of small immature capillary-type vessels, lined by enlarged endothelial cells
- Endothelial cells are epithelioid or histiocytic with cytoplasmic vacuolization

Top Differential Diagnoses

- Kimura disease, papillary endothelial hyperplasia

- Dermal &/or subcutaneous proliferation of small immature capillary-type to medium vessels, usually without lumina
  - May be attached to or associated with larger vessels
  - May have solid appearance
  - Endothelial cells are enlarged with epithelioid or histiocytic appearance
  - May have cytoplasmic vacuolization
  - Endothelial nuclei are enlarged
- Many eosinophils and lymphocytes are typically present, but eosinophil numbers can vary greatly
- Lymphoid follicles sparse and poorly formed

ANCILLARY TESTS

Immunohistochemistry

- Endothelial cells positive for CD31, CD34, FVIIIRAg
- Actin(+) vascular muscle walls
- IgE positive mast cells, but no IgE on follicular dendritic cells
  - Mast cells have IgE receptors, but are distinct from follicular dendritic cells

DIFFERENTIAL DIAGNOSIS

Kimura Disease

- Asian men with large disfiguring preauricular lymph node masses
- Peripheral eosinophilia

- Reactive lymphoid follicles with follicular lysis, eosinophilic abscesses, polykaryocytes, and IgE expression

Papillary Endothelial Hyperplasia (Masson Tumor)

- Reactive process limited to intravascular space(s)
- Papillary projections of enlarged endothelial cells

Epithelioid Hemangioendothelioma

- Epithelioid cells with cytoplasmic lumina
- Myxohyaline stroma lacking eosinophils
- Vessels not well formed

Epithelioid Angiosarcoma

- Highly atypical, infiltrative, mitotically active, anastomosing endothelial proliferation
- Usually shows necrosis and hemorrhage

SELECTED REFERENCES

1. Sun ZJ et al: Epithelioid hemangioma in the oral mucosa: a clinicopathological study of seven cases and review of the literature. Oral Oncol. 42(5):441-7, 2006
2. Martín-Granizo R et al: Epithelioid hemangiomas of the maxillofacial area. A report of three cases and a review of the literature. Int J Oral Maxillofac Surg. 26(3):212-4, 1997
3. Tosios K et al: Intravascular papillary endothelial hyperplasia of the oral soft tissues: report of 18 cases and review of the literature. J Oral Maxillofac Surg. 52(12):1263-8, 1994

IMAGE GALLERY

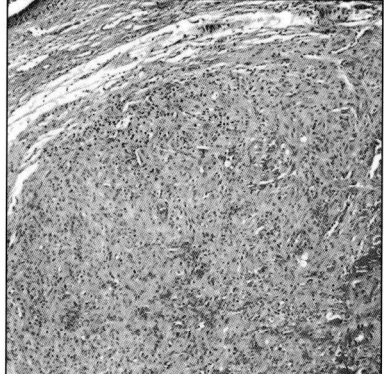 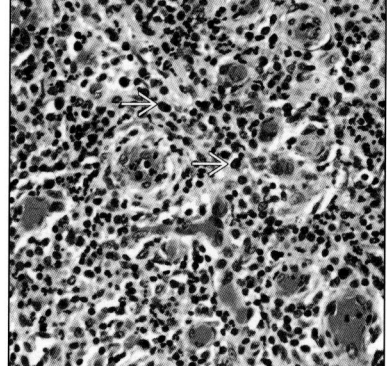 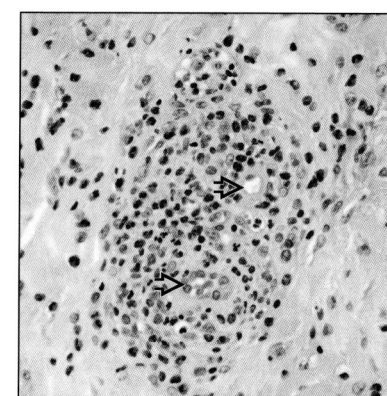

(Left) Low magnification shows a rich vascular proliferation, increased numbers of endothelial cells, with extravasated erythrocytes, eosinophils, and lymphocytes. *(Center)* Higher magnification shows lymphocytes and plasma cells ➡ with isolated acute inflammatory cells adjacent to the small vessels. *(Right)* Another area shows the mixture of eosinophils and lymphocytes around small vessels ⇒ with high endothelial cells.

HOBNAIL (TARGETOID HEMOSIDEROTIC) HEMANGIOMA

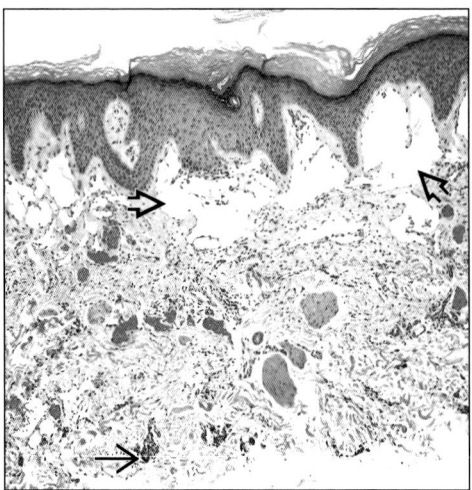

Low-magnification view of a hobnail hemangioma demonstrates superficial dilated vascular spaces ⊡ in the papillary dermis with deeper small blood vessels and stromal hemosiderin deposits ➡.

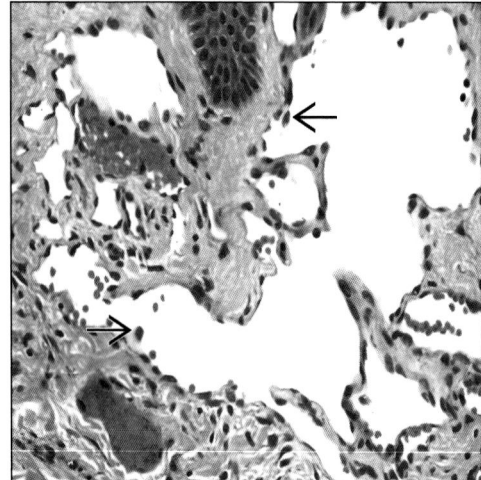

Higher power examination shows a hobnail hemangioma with superficial dilated vessels lined by small endothelial cells protruding into the lumina ➡ and showing nuclear hyperchromasia.

TERMINOLOGY

Abbreviations
- Hobnail hemangioma (HH)

Synonyms
- Targetoid hemosiderotic hemangioma (clinical term)

Definitions
- Benign vascular proliferation, typically wedge-shaped, showing intravascular papillae and hobnailed endothelial cells

ETIOLOGY/PATHOGENESIS

Unknown
- Trauma has been implicated in some cases
  - Postulated to represent traumatized lymphangioma or hemangioma

CLINICAL ISSUES

Epidemiology
- Incidence
  - Uncommon tumors
- Age
  - Young to middle-aged adults
- Gender
  - More common in males

Site
- Typically presents on lower extremities; also may occur on upper extremities, rarely in oral cavity

Presentation
- Skin papule or nodule
  - Often pigmented due to hemosiderin deposition
  - May show a halo ("targetoid" appearance) in minority of cases

Treatment
- Surgical approaches
  - Complete excision is curative but not necessary, given benign nature

Prognosis
- Excellent, with no tendency for local recurrence

MACROSCOPIC FEATURES

General Features
- Dermal-based reddish brown lesion with hemorrhage

Size
- Small, usually < 2 cm

MICROSCOPIC PATHOLOGY

Histologic Features
- Vascular proliferation with wedge-shaped appearance
- Superficial vessels are dilated and thin-walled
  - Some vessels may resemble lymphatics
  - Focal papillary projections with fibrous cores may be present
  - Vessels are lined by small, bland-appearing endothelial cells with hobnail appearance
    - Nuclei project into lumina
  - Mitoses should not be present
- Deeper vessels are progressively smaller and show narrow lumina
- Hemorrhage and hemosiderin deposition are typically prominent
- Inflammation is usually minimal

Cytologic Features
- Bland, plump endothelial cells with uniform-appearing nuclei

HOBNAIL (TARGETOID HEMOSIDEROTIC) HEMANGIOMA

Key Facts

Terminology
- Targetoid hemosiderotic hemangioma
- Benign vascular proliferation, typically wedge-shaped, showing intravascular papillae and hobnailed endothelial cells

Etiology/Pathogenesis
- Postulated to represent traumatized lymphangioma or hemangioma

Clinical Issues
- Typically presents on lower extremities; also may occur on upper extremities, rarely in oral cavity

Microscopic Pathology
- Superficial vessels are dilated and thin-walled
- Deeper vessels are progressively smaller
- Vessels are lined by small, bland-appearing endothelial cells with hobnail appearance

---

Predominant Pattern/Injury Type
- Vascular

Predominant Cell/Compartment Type
- Endothelial

DIFFERENTIAL DIAGNOSIS

Progressive Lymphangioma
- Thin-walled, dilated superficial vascular spaces with narrower deeper vessels
- Lacks hobnail endothelial cell morphology and hemosiderin deposition of HH

Kaposi Sarcoma
- Shows proliferation of slit-like spaces lined by atypical spindle cells
- Typically lacks superficial dilated vascular spaces and hobnail cells of HH
- HHV8(+) by immunohistochemistry

Microvenular Hemangioma
- Proliferation of small, round to slit-like, thin-walled vessels involving reticular dermis
- Lacks superficial dilated vascular spaces, hobnail cells, and hemosiderin deposition of HH

Retiform Hemangioendothelioma
- Dermal and subcutaneous tumor characterized by proliferation of arborizing vessels lined by hobnailed endothelial cells

- Typically prominent lymphoid infiltrate, which is lacking in HH
- HH is typically more superficial, and deeper vessels are smaller and compact

DIAGNOSTIC CHECKLIST

Pathologic Interpretation Pearls
- Wedge-shaped vascular proliferation
- Dilated superficial vessels, deeper small/collapsed vessels
- Intravascular papillae and hobnailed endothelial cells
- Prominent hemosiderin deposition

SELECTED REFERENCES

1. Fernandez-Flores A et al: Clinical changes in "true" hobnail hemangioma during menstruation. Bratisl Lek Listy. 109(3):141-3, 2008
2. Franke FE et al: Hobnail hemangiomas (targetoid hemosiderotic hemangiomas) are true lymphangiomas. J Cutan Pathol. 31(5):362-7, 2004
3. Pabuccuoğlu U et al: Hobnail haemangioma occurring on the nasal dorsum. Br J Dermatol. 146(1):162-4, 2002
4. Guillou L et al: Hobnail hemangioma: a pseudomalignant vascular lesion with a reappraisal of targetoid hemosiderotic hemangioma. Am J Surg Pathol. 23(1):97-105, 1999
5. Santonja C et al: Hobnail hemangioma. Dermatology. 191(2):154-6, 1995

IMAGE GALLERY

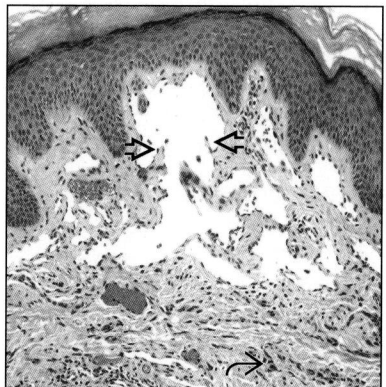 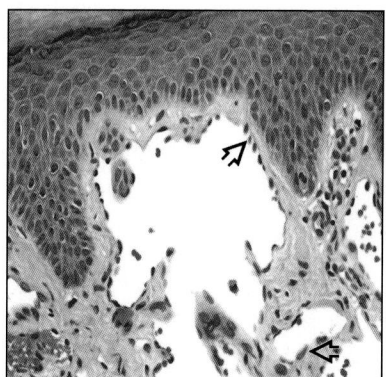 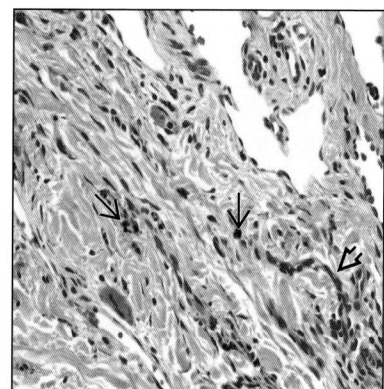

(Left) Low magnification shows the superficial portion of a hobnail hemangioma with dilated vascular spaces, papillary endothelial structures ➡, and stromal hemosiderin deposits ➡. *(Center)* Higher magnification of the tumor shows the bland cytologic features of the endothelial cells lining the vascular spaces ➡. *(Right)* Histologic examination of the deeper aspect of the lesion shows small, thin-walled blood vessels ➡ and prominent hemosiderin deposition in the stroma ➡.

SPINDLE CELL HEMANGIOMA

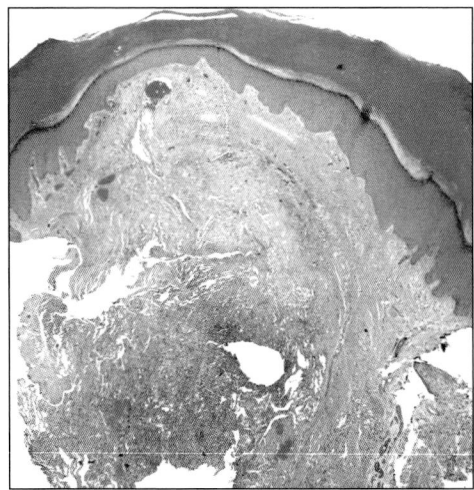

Low magnification shows a noncircumscribed lesion in the dermis and subcutis composed of an admixture of thin-walled dilated blood vessels and sheets of spindle cells.

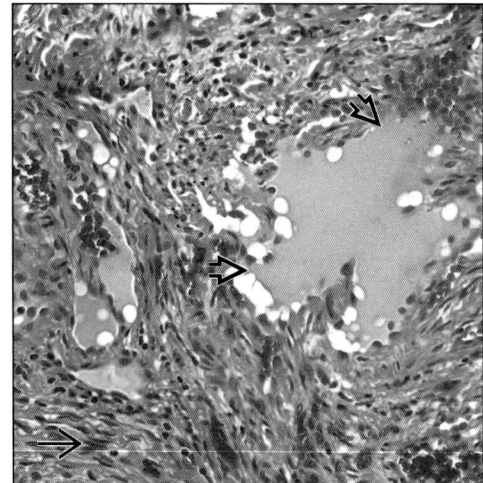

High magnification of spindle cell hemangioma shows straight/curved fascicles of uniform spindle cells ⇨ with irregularly shaped vascular spaces ⊠ and small areas of hemorrhage.

TERMINOLOGY

Synonyms
- Formerly known as spindle cell hemangioendothelioma

Definitions
- Benign vascular tumor characterized by cavernous vascular spaces and spindled cell areas

ETIOLOGY/PATHOGENESIS

Unknown
- Some cases associated with Mafucci syndrome, Klippel-Trenaunay syndrome, varicosities, and congenital lymphedema

CLINICAL ISSUES

Epidemiology
- Age
  - Young adults

Site
- Distal extremities
  - Acral location most common

Presentation
- Subcutaneous mass
  - Sometimes multifocal

Treatment
- Surgical approaches
  - Excision

Prognosis
- Local recurrence in 50-60%
- No metastatic potential

MICROSCOPIC PATHOLOGY

Histologic Features
- Dilated vessels often with focal thrombi
  - Cavernous thin-walled vascular spaces
- Solid spindled cell areas
  - May resemble Kaposi sarcoma
- Vacuolated endothelial cells, so-called "blister cells"
- ~ 50% are intravascular tumors

Cytologic Features
- Oval to spindle-shaped hyperchromatic-staining nuclei

Predominant Pattern/Injury Type
- Circumscribed dermal/subcutaneous nodular spindle cell tumor

Predominant Cell/Compartment Type
- Endothelial cell

DIFFERENTIAL DIAGNOSIS

Kaposi Sarcoma
- Patch stage
  - Irregular vessels and atypical spindle cells dissecting through collagen
- Plaque/tumor stage
  - More cellular areas with fascicles of spindled cells and slit-like vascular lumina
- Immunoreactive for HHV8 latent nuclear antigen

Kaposiform Hemangioendothelioma
- Almost exclusively in children
- Dilated vessels
- Solid spindled cell areas
- Glomeruloid nests of rounded endothelial cells
- Associated with Kasabach-Merritt phenomenon

SPINDLE CELL HEMANGIOMA

Key Facts

Terminology
- Formerly called spindle cell hemangioendothelioma

Clinical Issues
- Subcutaneous mass
- Usually acral location
- Sometimes multifocal
- Local recurrence in 50-60% of cases
- No metastatic potential
- Associated with Mafucci syndrome in some cases

Microscopic Pathology
- Dilated vessels often with focal thrombi
- Solid spindled cell areas
- Vacuolated endothelial cells, so-called "blister cells"
- Negative for HHV8 nuclear antigen

Top Differential Diagnoses
- Kaposi sarcoma
- Kaposiform hemangioendothelioma
- Epithelioid hemangioendothelioma

Immunohistochemistry

Antibody	Reactivity	Staining Pattern	Comment
CD31	Positive	Cell membrane & cytoplasm	In endothelial cells
CD34	Positive	Cell membrane & cytoplasm	In endothelial cells
FVIIIRAg	Positive	Cell membrane & cytoplasm	In endothelial cells (of historical interest only)
Actin-sm	Positive	Cytoplasmic	In spindle cells focally
S100	Negative		
HHV8	Negative		

Epithelioid Hemangioendothelioma
- Nodules and cords of epithelioid endothelial cells
- Vacuolated endothelial cells
- Myxohyaline-hyaline stroma
- Lacks cavernous vascular spaces

Organizing Thrombus/Intravascular Papillary Endothelial Hyperplasia (Masson Tumor)
- Less prominent spindle cell proliferation
- Lacks so-called "blister cells"
- Papillary architecture of endothelial cells overlying fibrin cores

DIAGNOSTIC CHECKLIST

Pathologic Interpretation Pearls
- Combination of ectatic vessels, spindled cells, and vacuolated endothelial cells ("blister cells") are key features

- At least partially intravascular in ~ 1/2 of cases

SELECTED REFERENCES

1. Lyons LL et al: Kaposiform hemangioendothelioma: a study of 33 cases emphasizing its pathologic, immunophenotypic, and biologic uniqueness from juvenile hemangioma. Am J Surg Pathol. 28(5):559-68, 2004
2. Perkins P et al: Spindle cell hemangioendothelioma. An analysis of 78 cases with reassessment of its pathogenesis and biologic behavior. Am J Surg Pathol. 20(10):1196-204, 1996
3. Fletcher CD et al: Spindle cell haemangioendothelioma: a clinicopathological and immunohistochemical study indicative of a non-neoplastic lesion. Histopathology. 18(4):291-301, 1991
4. Weiss SW et al: Spindle cell hemangioendothelioma. A low-grade angiosarcoma resembling a cavernous hemangioma and Kaposi's sarcoma. Am J Surg Pathol. 10(8):521-30, 1986

IMAGE GALLERY

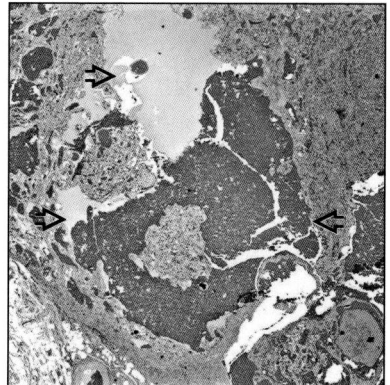 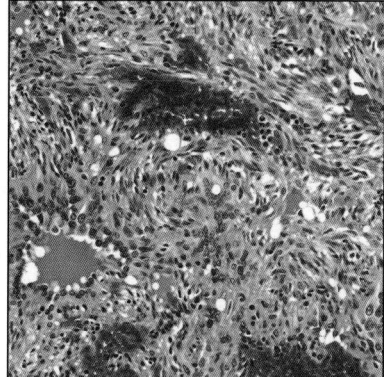 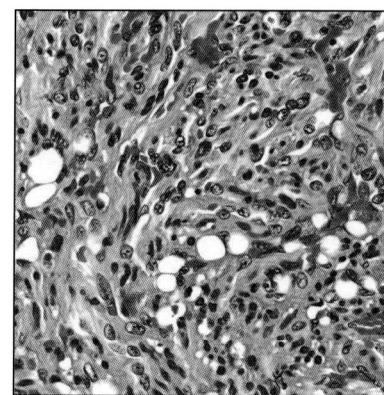

(Left) Low magnification of a spindle cell hemangioma shows a well-circumscribed intravascular tumor with ectatic vascular spaces ⇒ and a cellular spindle cell proliferation. (Center) Higher magnification shows a more solid area of a spindle cell hemangioma that mimics Kaposi sarcoma. However, nuclear atypia and significant mitotic activity are lacking. (Right) High magnification shows the spindled tumor cells and the characteristic vacuolated endothelial cells (so-called "blister cells").

MICROVENULAR HEMANGIOMA

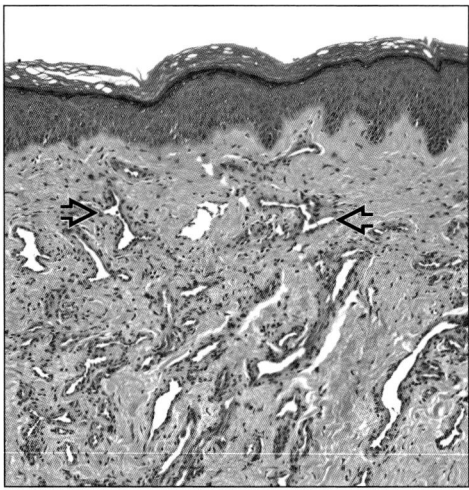

Histologic section shows increased numbers of small blood vessels in the superficial dermis with irregular branching ⊵ and narrow lumina.

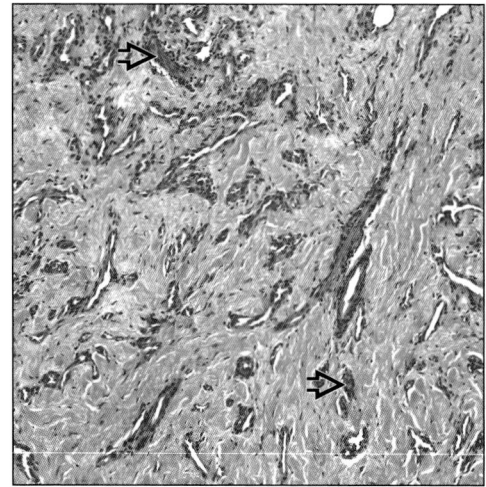

Higher magnification shows a proliferation of small blood vessels with thin walls and small to collapsed lumina ⊵ associated with a dense, sclerotic stroma.

TERMINOLOGY

Abbreviations
- Microvenular hemangioma (MVH)

Synonyms
- Microcapillary angioma

Definitions
- Slowly growing benign vascular proliferation composed of small, collapsed vessels

ETIOLOGY/PATHOGENESIS

Unknown
- Most cases

Hormonal Influence
- Some cases reportedly related to pregnancy or contraceptives

CLINICAL ISSUES

Epidemiology
- Age
  - Young to middle-aged adults
- Gender
  - Occurs in both males and females about equally

Site
- Typically occurs on trunk or upper extremities, especially forearms

Presentation
- Slow-growing papule or nodule

Natural History
- Often present for only a few weeks to months at presentation

Treatment
- Surgical approaches
  - Simple excision is curative, but not necessary, as these are benign lesions

Prognosis
- Excellent

MACROSCOPIC FEATURES

Size
- Small, typically < 1 cm

MICROSCOPIC PATHOLOGY

Histologic Features
- Poorly circumscribed dermal proliferation of small blood vessels that diffusely involve reticular dermis
  - Branching vessels typically present
  - Most vessels show narrow or collapsed lumina
    - Few erythrocytes may be present within lumina
  - Endothelial cells may be slightly enlarged, but lack significant cytologic atypia
  - Some cases may show large epithelioid cells resembling those seen in epithelioid (histiocytoid) hemangiomas
- Tufted groups of vessels may be seen in deep dermis
- Background of dermal sclerosis
- Inflammation and hemosiderin deposition typically lacking

Cytologic Features
- Endothelial cells may be enlarged, but show bland nuclei without significant atypia or pleomorphism

MICROVENULAR HEMANGIOMA

Key Facts

Terminology
- Microvenular hemangioma (MVH)
- Microcapillary angioma
- Slowly growing benign vascular proliferation composed of small, collapsed vessels

Clinical Issues
- Young to middle-aged adults
- Typically occur on upper extremities, especially forearms

Microscopic Pathology
- Poorly circumscribed dermal proliferation of small blood vessels that diffusely involve reticular dermis
- Most vessels show narrow or collapsed lumina
- Endothelial cells may be slightly enlarged but lack significant cytologic atypia
- Tufted groups of vessels may be seen in deep dermis
- Background of dermal sclerosis
- Usually lacks inflammation and hemosiderin

DIFFERENTIAL DIAGNOSIS

Kaposi Sarcoma
- May show thin-walled vessels, but typically also has irregular slit-like vascular spaces lined by atypical spindle cells
- Plasma cells and hyaline globules are lacking in MVH
- HHV8(+) by immunohistochemistry

Targetoid Hemosiderotic Hemangioma (Hobnail Hemangioma)
- While deeper small vessels are similar to those in MVH, superficial vessels are larger and more dilated
- Hobnailed endothelial cells project into vascular lumina
- Hemosiderin deposition is typically very prominent

Stasis Changes and Stasis Dermatitis
- Superficial proliferation of small, thick-walled blood vessels
- Show prominent hemosiderin deposition throughout dermis (lacking in MVH)
- Often show more inflammation and overlying spongiosis (stasis dermatitis)
- Clinical presentation distinctive: Lower extremities of elderly adults

Early Scar
- Angiogenesis in early scars may mimic MVH
  - But vessels more vertically oriented

- Typically greater fibrosis, inflammation, extravasated red blood cells, and hemosiderin deposition in scars

DIAGNOSTIC CHECKLIST

Pathologic Interpretation Pearls
- Benign vascular proliferation composed of small, collapsed vessels
- Branching vessels typically present
- Endothelial cells may be enlarged, but lack cytologic atypia
- Background of dermal sclerosis

SELECTED REFERENCES

1. Chang SE et al: Microvenular hemangioma in a boy with acute myelogenous leukemia. Pediatr Dermatol. 20(3):266-7, 2003
2. Kim YC et al: Microvenular hemangioma. Dermatology. 206(2):161-4, 2003
3. Rikihisa W et al: Microvenular haemangioma in a patient with Wiskott-Aldrich syndrome. Br J Dermatol. 141(4):752-4, 1999
4. Hunt SJ et al: Acquired benign and "borderline" vascular lesions. Dermatol Clin. 10(1):97-115, 1992
5. Hunt SJ et al: Microvenular hemangioma. J Cutan Pathol. 18(4):235-40, 1991
6. Bantel E et al: [Understanding microcapillary angioma, observations in pregnant patients and in females treated with hormonal contraceptives.] Z Hautkr. 64(12):1071-4, 1989

IMAGE GALLERY

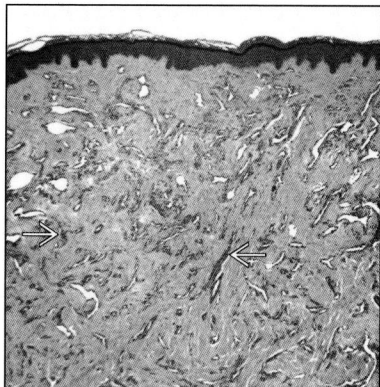 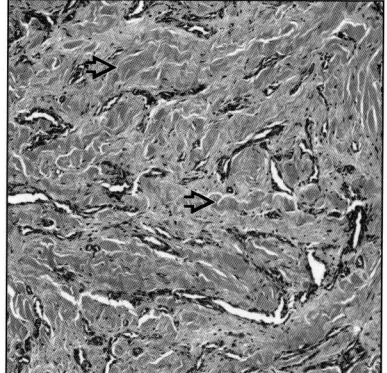 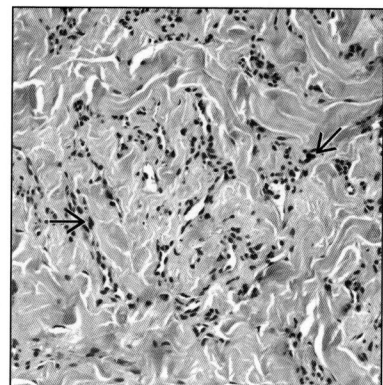

(Left) Scanning magnification of skin shows a diffuse dermal proliferation of small, elongated blood vessels with narrow to collapsed ➡ lumina and a background of dermal sclerosis. *(Center)* Higher magnification of MVH shows small, thin branching vessels associated with sclerotic collagen bundles ➡. *(Right)* High-power examination shows bland cytologic features of the endothelial cells, with small, hyperchromatic-staining nuclei ➡. No necrosis or mitoses are present.

VERRUCOUS HEMANGIOMA

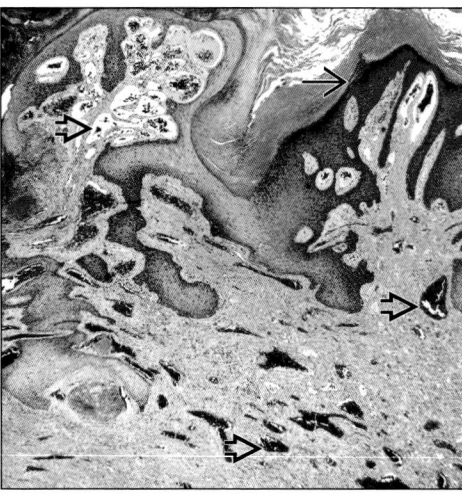

Verrucous hemangioma has an acanthotic papillomatous epidermis ➡ and ectatic dermal blood vessels ⇥ involving both the superficial and deep dermis.

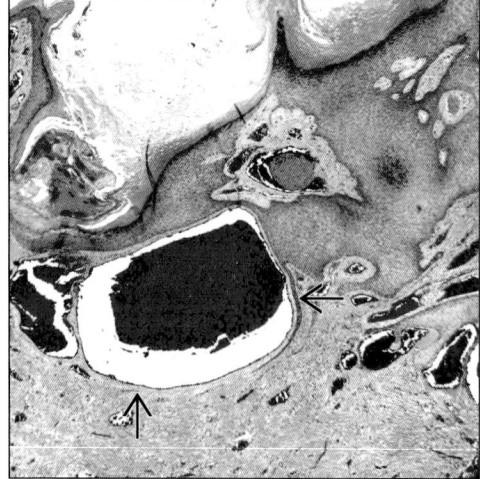

In addition to the verrucous-like epidermal changes, this case demonstrates cavernous vascular spaces ➡ in close apposition to the epidermis, resembling an angiokeratoma.

TERMINOLOGY

Definitions
- Vascular tumor with superficial verrucous appearance

ETIOLOGY/PATHOGENESIS

Developmental Anomaly
- Most likely a congenital lymphovascular malformation

CLINICAL ISSUES

Epidemiology
- Incidence
  - Very rare lesion
- Age
  - Present in children
    - At birth or early childhood
    - Only very rare cases present in adults
- Gender
  - No gender predilection

Presentation
- Dark blue papule or nodule
  - Usually solitary
  - May develop satellite lesions over time
  - Rare linear form
- Surface has warty appearance
  - Becomes more verrucous-appearing over time
- Most common on extremities
  - Lower extremities > upper extremities
- Cobb syndrome
  - Verrucous hemangioma on midline of back
  - Associated with spinal cord vascular malformation

Treatment
- Surgical approaches
  - Simple excision

- Radiologic examination should be performed on midline back lesions to help exclude Cobb syndrome
  - Laser removal

Prognosis
- Benign
  - Local recurrence common
    - Related to involvement of deep dermis

MICROSCOPIC PATHOLOGY

Histologic Features
- Epidermis is acanthotic and papillomatous
  - Early lesions may be less verrucous in appearance
- Composed of dilated capillaries
- Cavernous vascular spaces present superficially
  - May appear to extend into epidermis due to very superficial location in dermal papillae, similar to angiokeratoma
- Vascular proliferation involves superficial and deep dermis
  - Vascular spaces lined by bland, flattened endothelial cells
  - Deeper spaces include a mixture of small capillary-type and larger, cavernous, thin-walled vessels

ANCILLARY TESTS

Immunohistochemistry
- Positive for CD31, CD34
- Negative for WT1

DIFFERENTIAL DIAGNOSIS

Angiokeratoma
- Superficial resemblance is striking
- Key difference is distribution of vascular proliferation

VERRUCOUS HEMANGIOMA

Key Facts

Clinical Issues
- Presents in children
- Dark blue nodule
- Surface has warty appearance
- Most common on the extremities

Microscopic Pathology
- Epidermis is acanthotic and papillomatous
- Cavernous vascular spaces
- Dilated capillaries

- Vascular proliferation involves superficial and deep dermis

Top Differential Diagnoses
- Angiokeratoma
  - In angiokeratoma, vascular proliferation restricted to superficial dermis
- Lymphangioma
- Hamartomatous vascular lesions
- Pyogenic granuloma (lobular capillary hemangioma)

- In angiokeratoma, restricted to superficial dermis
- In verrucous hemangioma, extends into deep dermis

Lymphangioma
- May be superficial and deep
- Lacks verrucous epidermal changes of verrucous hemangioma
- Lymphatic valves present

Hamartomatous Vascular Lesions
- Usually lack verrucous epidermal changes
- Different clinical presentations, often associated with syndromes and present in head and neck region

Pyogenic Granuloma (Lobular Capillary Hemangioma)
- Polypoid lesion, but lacks verrucous epidermal changes
- Often ulcerated and inflamed with numerous lymphocytes and neutrophils present
- Lobular proliferation of closely packed capillaries with less ectatic vessels
- Epidermal collarette not seen in verrucous hemangioma

DIAGNOSTIC CHECKLIST

Pathologic Interpretation Pearls
- Verrucous epidermal appearance
- Capillaries and cavernous vascular spaces
- Involvement of superficial and deep dermis

SELECTED REFERENCES

1. Al Dhaybi R et al: Differentiation of vascular tumors from vascular malformations by expression of Wilms tumor 1 gene: evaluation of 126 cases. J Am Acad Dermatol. 63(6):1052-7, 2010
2. Lara-Corrales I et al: Verrucous hemangioma: a challenging vascular lesion. J Cutan Med Surg. 14(3):144-6, 2010
3. Brown A et al: Verrucous lymphovascular malformation versus verrucous hemangioma: controversial nomenclature. Cutis. 81(5):390-6, 2008
4. Tennant LB et al: Verrucous hemangioma revisited. Pediatr Dermatol. 23(3):208-15, 2006
5. Hayashi H et al: Linear verrucous haemangioma on the abdomen. Acta Derm Venereol. 84(1):79-80, 2004
6. Clinton TS et al: Cobb syndrome associated with a verrucous (angiokeratomalike) vascular malformation. Cutis. 71(4):283-7, 2003
7. Rossi A et al: Verrucous hemangioma and angiokeratoma circumscriptum: clinical and histologic differential characteristics. J Dermatol Surg Oncol. 15(1):88-91, 1989
8. Imperial R et al: Verrucous hemangioma. A clinicopathologic study of 21 cases. Arch Dermatol. 96(3):247-53, 1967

IMAGE GALLERY

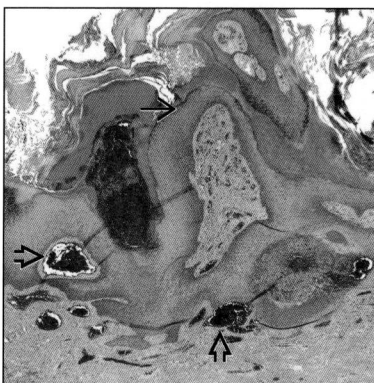 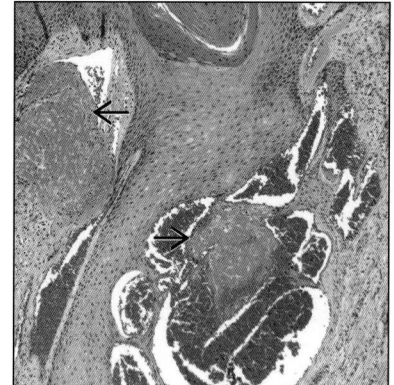 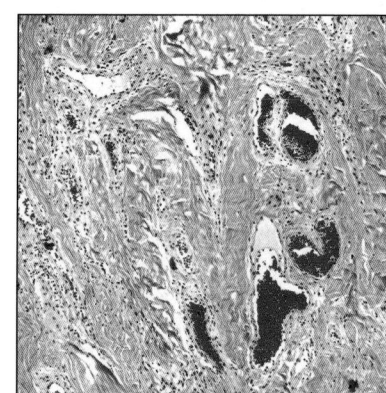

(Left) This low-power image demonstrates the prominent acanthosis and papillomatosis of the epidermis ➡ typical of verrucous hemangioma. Dilated vessels are present in the dermis ➡. *(Center)* The superficial cavernous vascular spaces may undergo thrombosis ➡. *(Right)* In addition to involvement of the superficial dermis, verrucous hemangioma has a vascular proliferation of small to dilated vessels extending into the deep dermis.

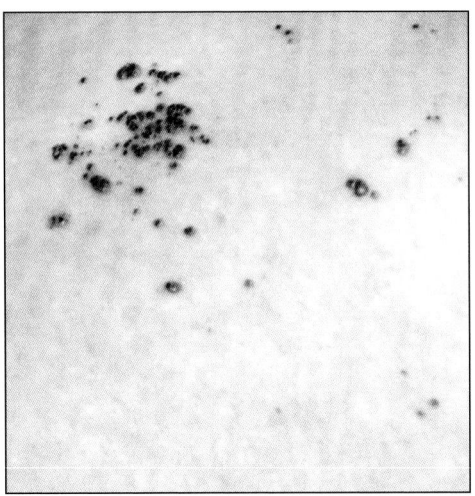

This clinical image demonstrates numerous grouped angiokeratomas in a patient with Anderson-Fabry disease.

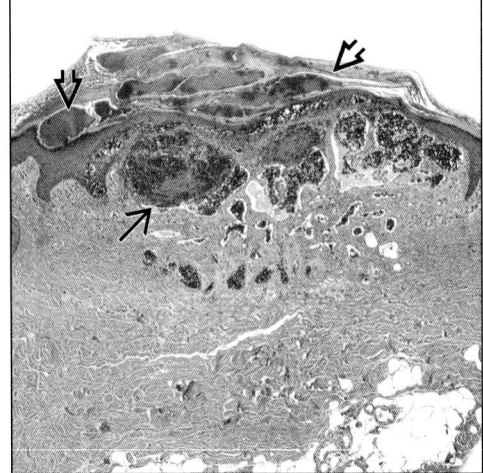

Angiokeratomas are characterized by ectatic vessels ⮕ in the superficial dermis that herniate into the epidermis ⮕ in association with epidermal acanthosis and frequently compact hyperkeratosis.

TERMINOLOGY

Definitions
- Ectatic superficial dermal blood vessels associated with reactive epidermal hyperplasia

CLINICAL ISSUES

Presentation
- 5 clinical variants
  - Solitary and multiple angiokeratoma
    - Usually solitary
    - Multiple lesions may have zosteriform presentation
    - Wide age range
    - Usually on extremities
  - Angiokeratoma of Fordyce
    - Elderly men
    - Solitary or multiple papules on scrotum
  - Angiokeratoma of Mibelli
    - Presents in childhood and adolescence
    - Warty lesions over bony prominences of acral locations
  - Angiokeratoma corporis diffusum
    - Multiple, often clustered papules
    - Bathing suit distribution
    - Associated with Anderson-Fabry disease: X-linked recessive disorder of α-galactosidase A
    - Male > female
    - May also be associated with deficiency of α-L-fucosidase, β-galactosidase, β-mannosidase, α-N-acetylgalactosaminidase, or neuraminidase
  - Angiokeratoma circumscriptum
    - Least common variant
    - Usually presents in children
    - Plaque composed of grouped papules &/or nodules
    - Trunk or extremities

Treatment
- Surgical approaches
  - Simple excision in solitary lesions
  - Excision may not be practical for multiple lesions
  - Laser treatment
- Drugs
  - Enzyme replacement therapy for patients with Anderson-Fabry disease or other heritable enzyme deficiencies
- May follow clinically

Prognosis
- Benign, no risk for transformation to malignancy

MACROSCOPIC FEATURES

General Features
- Red to blue superficial dermal papules or plaques

MICROSCOPIC PATHOLOGY

Histologic Features
- Marked ectasia of papillary dermal blood vessels
  - Blood vessels lined by flattened, bland-appearing endothelial cells
  - May have evidence of thrombosis and intravascular papillary endothelial hyperplasia (Masson tumor/change)
  - Blood vessels herniate into overlying epidermis
    - This can result in appearance that vessels are within epidermis
- Reactive epidermal changes
  - Irregular acanthosis
  - Variable hyperkeratosis
  - Elongation of rete pegs that encircle dermal blood vessels
  - May have epidermal collarette

ANGIOKERATOMA

Key Facts

Terminology
- Ectatic superficial dermal blood vessels associated with reactive epidermal hyperplasia

Clinical Issues
- Solitary and multiple angiokeratomas
- Angiokeratoma of Fordyce
- Angiokeratoma of Mibelli
- Angiokeratoma corporis diffusum
  - Associated with Anderson-Fabry disease

- Angiokeratoma circumscriptum

Microscopic Pathology
- Marked ectasia of papillary dermal blood vessels, which may appear to extend into epidermis
- May have evidence of thrombosis and intravascular papillary endothelial hyperplasia
- Reactive epidermal changes: Acanthosis, hyperkeratosis, and elongation of rete ridges around ectatic vessels

- Angiokeratomas associated with Anderson-Fabry disease
  - May have lipid vacuoles in endothelial cells, pericytes, and fibroblasts
  - PAS positive, Sudan black positive granules may be seen in endothelial cells on frozen section
  - Electron microscopy may show characteristic lamellar cytoplasmic granules

DIFFERENTIAL DIAGNOSIS

Verrucous Hemangioma
- Verrucous epidermal hyperplasia
- Superficial and deep vascular proliferation, which is not limited to papillary dermis, as in angiokeratoma

Pyogenic Granuloma (Lobular Capillary Hemangioma)
- Polypoid lesion with epidermal collarette
- Granulation tissue-like dermal vascular proliferation
- Lacks acanthosis and hyperkeratosis
- Vascular proliferation more florid than angiokeratoma

DIAGNOSTIC CHECKLIST

Clinically Relevant Pathologic Features
- Ectatic vessels limited to superficial dermis
- Acanthotic epidermis, vessels may appear to extend into epidermis, often with surrounding collarette

SELECTED REFERENCES

1. Albano LM et al: Angiokeratoma: a cutaneous marker of Fabry's disease. Clin Exp Dermatol. 35(5):505-8, 2010
2. Oni G et al: Treatment of angiokeratoma of the vulva with pulsed dye laser therapy. J Cosmet Laser Ther. 12(1):51-2, 2010
3. Goldman L et al: Thrombotic angiokeratoma circumscriptum simulating melanoma. Arch Dermatol. 117(3):138-9, 1981
4. Kornfeld M et al: Fucosidosis with angiokeratoma. Electron microscopic changes in the skin. Arch Pathol Lab Med. 101(9):478-85, 1977
5. Derblay PR: Angiokeratoma circumscriptum. Br J Dermatol. 82(6):633, 1970
6. Kint JA: Fabry's disease: alpha-galactosidase deficiency. Science. 167(922):1268-9, 1970
7. Perrelet A et al: A study of Fabry's disease. II. Light and electron microscopy. Dermatologica. 138(4):222-37, 1969
8. Burda CD et al: Angiokeratoma corporis diffusum universale (Fabry's disease) in female subjects. Am J Med. 42(2):293-301, 1967
9. Imperial R et al: Angiokeratoma. A clinicopathological study. Arch Dermatol. 95(2):166-75, 1967
10. Haye KR et al: Angiokeratoma of Mibelli. Acta Derm Venereol. 41:56-60, 1961
11. Ruiter M: Angiokeratoma corporis diffusum. AMA Arch Derm Syphilol. 68(1):21-7, 1953
12. Klaber R: Angiokeratoma (Mibelli). Proc R Soc Med. 28(11):1535, 1935

Microscopic Features

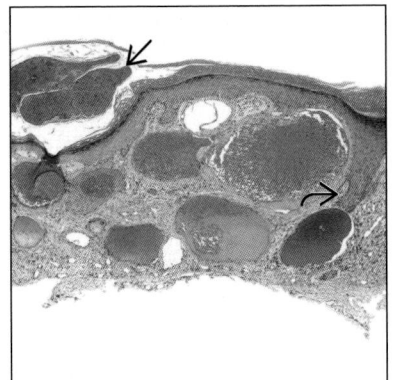 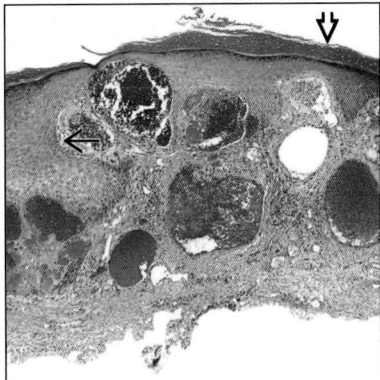 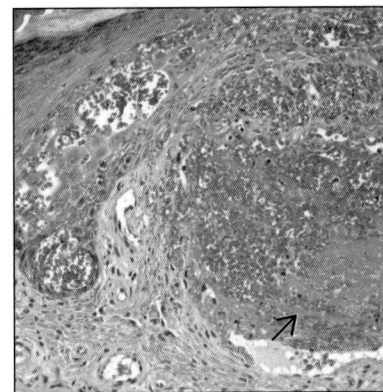

(Left) The herniation of the blood vessels into the epidermis often results in collections of erythrocytes in the stratum corneum ➡. This angiokeratoma also has a partial epidermal collarette ➡. *(Center)* The epidermis of angiokeratomas typically demonstrate acanthosis ➡ and compact hyperkeratosis ➡. *(Right)* The vessels in angiokeratoma frequently undergo thrombosis. This case demonstrates an early thrombus characterized by fibrin ➡ admixed with erythrocytes.

VENOUS LAKE

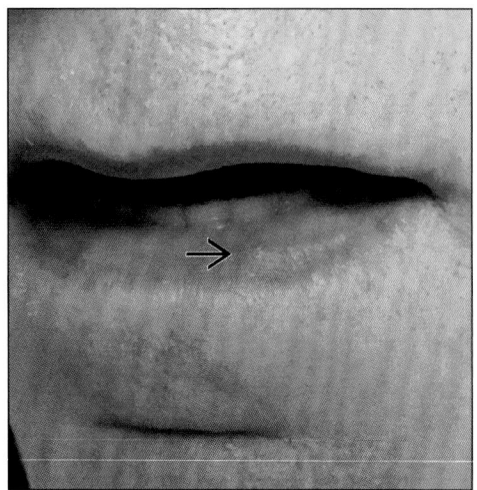

Venous lake presents as a dark-blue papule ⇨ on sun-damaged skin of elderly patients. It is especially common on the lip.

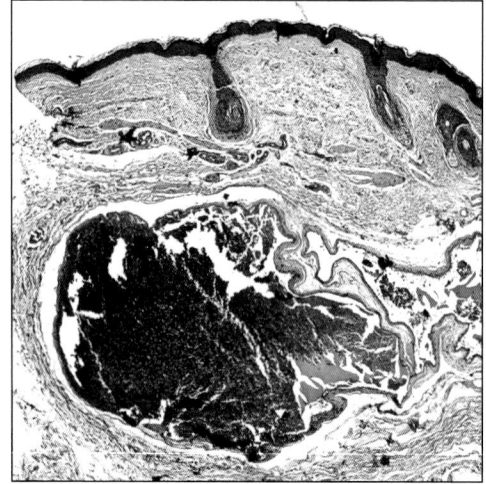

Venous lake is characterized by a single large, ectatic vessel in actinically damaged skin.

TERMINOLOGY

Synonyms
- Capillary aneurysm

Definitions
- Type of telangiectasia characterized by ectatic superficial blood vessel in superficial dermis

ETIOLOGY/PATHOGENESIS

Chronic Sun Damage
- Chronic sun damage results in inadequate stromal support for the affected vessel, resulting in marked ectasia

CLINICAL ISSUES

Epidemiology
- Incidence
  - Relatively common lesions
- Age
  - Usually in elderly patients
- Ethnicity
  - More common in Caucasians

Presentation
- Usually presents in sun-damaged skin of elderly patients
- Dark blue papules
- Often multiple
- Head and neck
  - Especially common on lip
- Can mimic melanoma clinically

Treatment
- Surgical approaches
  - Laser treatment
  - Simple excision

- Can be managed expectantly

Prognosis
- Benign

MICROSCOPIC PATHOLOGY

Histologic Features
- Ectatic vessel in upper dermis
  - Usually single, large dilated vessel with relatively thin, muscular wall
  - Vessel may collapse after biopsy and not appear ectatic
  - Vessel lined by flattened endothelial cells
  - Vessel may be thrombosed and show papillary endothelial hyperplasia (Masson change/tumor)
- Solar elastosis typically present

Cytologic Features
- Bland endothelial cells with uniform round to oval nuclei, inconspicuous nucleoli

DIFFERENTIAL DIAGNOSIS

Hemangioma
- Capillary hemangiomas are composed of multiple small, capillary-type vessels
- Cavernous hemangiomas are composed of multiple large, thin-walled dilated vessels
- Venous hemangiomas are similar to cavernous hemangiomas, but are composed of large, thick-walled dilated vessels

Pyogenic Granuloma
- 1 type of lobular capillary hemangioma
- Epidermal collarette and ulceration with acute inflammation often present (absent in venous lake)
- Lobular proliferation of capillaries resembling granulation tissue, rather than single dilated vessel

VENOUS LAKE

Key Facts

Clinical Issues
- Usually presents in elderly patients
- More common in Caucasians
- Head and neck
- Especially common on lip
- Can clinically mimic melanoma

Microscopic Pathology
- Ectatic vessel in upper dermis
- Usually single dilated vessel

- Vessel may collapse after biopsy and not appear ectatic
- Vessel may be thrombosed
- Background of solar elastosis

Top Differential Diagnoses
- Hemangioma
- Pyogenic granuloma
- Angiokeratoma
- Lymphangioma

Angiokeratoma
- Superficial dilated, thin-walled vessels
- Appear to extend into epidermis on low-power examination
- Show overlying epidermal acanthosis and hyperkeratosis

Arteriovenous Hemangioma
- May mimic venous hemangioma, with large, thick-walled vessels
- Elastic stain shows presence of elastic lumina in some of the vessels

Lymphangioma
- Ectatic lymphatic channels
  ○ Often larger spaces superficially, progressing to narrower channels deeper in dermis (absent in venous lake)
  ○ Lymphatic vessels of superficial dermis have valves, unlike venous lake

Angiosarcoma
- Usually composed of multiple large, irregularly shaped, anastomosing vessels, unlike venous lake, which is a single dilated vessel
- Lined by enlarged, atypical epithelioid or spindle-shaped cells
- Pleomorphism and mitoses often prominent (lacking in venous lake)

Kaposi Sarcoma
- Proliferation of small, irregular vascular spaces lined by spindle-shaped endothelial cells (absent in venous lake)
- Stroma often shows hemosiderin deposition and plasma cells
- Positive for HHV8 by immunohistochemistry

DIAGNOSTIC CHECKLIST

Pathologic Interpretation Pearls
- Single dilated blood vessel in upper dermis of sun-damaged skin

SELECTED REFERENCES

1. Astner S et al: Preliminary evaluation of benign vascular lesions using in vivo reflectance confocal microscopy. Dermatol Surg. 36(7):1099-110, 2010
2. Bekhor PS: Long-pulsed Nd:YAG laser treatment of venous lakes: report of a series of 34 cases. Dermatol Surg. 32(9):1151-4, 2006
3. Requena L et al: Cutaneous vascular anomalies. Part I. Hamartomas, malformations, and dilation of preexisting vessels. J Am Acad Dermatol. 37(4):523-49; quiz 549-52, 1997

IMAGE GALLERY

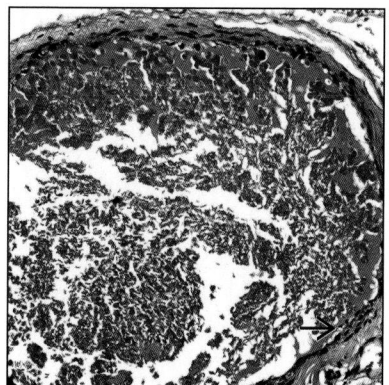
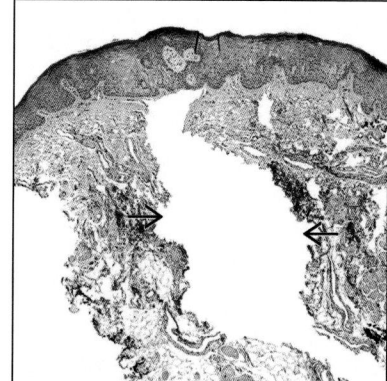
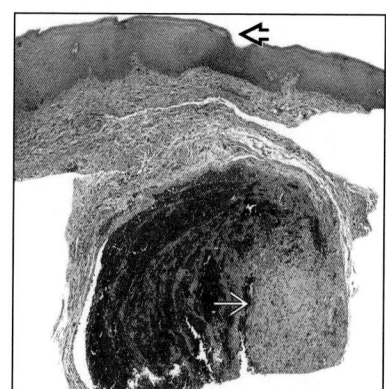

(Left) The vessel of venous lake is lined by flattened endothelial cells ➡ that lack atypia. *(Center)* In some cases of venous lake, the blood is lost from the vessel during processing creating an empty space in the dermis ➡. *(Right)* This is an example of a venous lake presenting on the lip (note the squamous mucosa ➡ overlying the lesion), one of the most common locations. The venous lake has a partial thrombus ➡ filling its lumen.

PAPILLARY ENDOTHELIAL HYPERPLASIA (MASSON TUMOR)

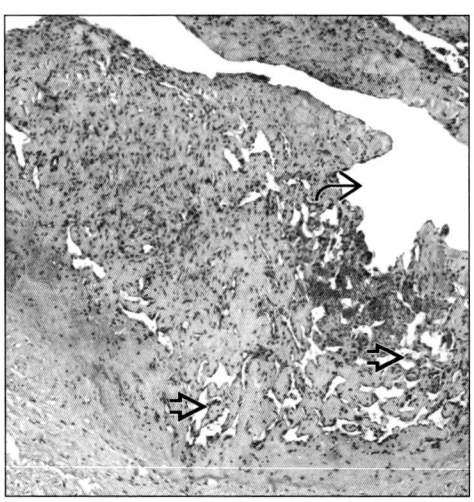

PEH is a well-circumscribed reactive lesion in which papillary fronds ⊵ lined by a single layer of endothelial cells proliferate within a vascular lumen ⊅.

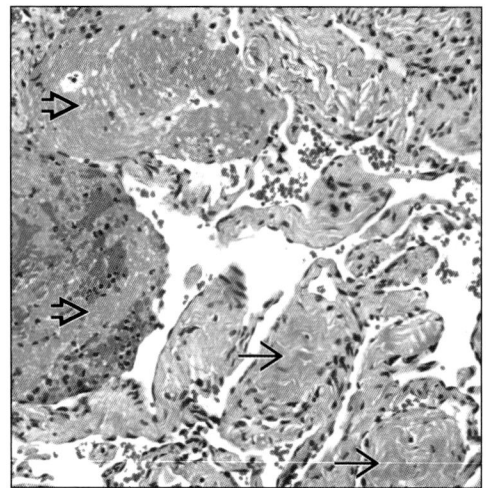

Fibrin thrombi ⊵ are apparent in early stages, and with time are replaced by papillary fronds with a fibrous core ⊃ characteristic of PEH.

TERMINOLOGY

Abbreviations
• Papillary endothelial hyperplasia (PEH)

Synonyms
• Masson tumor
• Vegetant intravascular hemangioendothelioma
• Intravascular angiomatosis

Definitions
• Benign, reactive, intravascular papillary endothelial proliferation

ETIOLOGY/PATHOGENESIS

Reactive Vascular Proliferation
• Manifestation of organizing intravascular thrombus
• PEH-like changes may be present in preexisting hemangiomas or vascular malformations

CLINICAL ISSUES

Site
• Wide distribution
• Common sites include
  ○ Head & neck, fingers, trunk

Presentation
• Painless mass
• Located in deep dermis &/or subcutaneous tissue

Treatment
• Excision is not necessary, but is curative

Prognosis
• Excellent
• Cases with underlying hemangioma or vascular malformation may recur

MACROSCOPIC FEATURES

General Features
• Cystic mass with red-purple discoloration
• Often surrounded by pseudocapsule

Size
• Mostly small (< 2 cm)

MICROSCOPIC PATHOLOGY

Histologic Features
• Circumscribed lesion with pseudocapsule
  ○ Residual smooth muscle or elastic lamina of preexisting vessel may be apparent
• Fibrin thrombus
• Papillary structures lined by endothelial cells
  ○ Endothelial cells in single layer
  ○ Papillae form anastomosing network
• Papillary cores may consist of fibrin or fibrous connective tissue
• Vessel rupture may lead to extension of papillary endothelial proliferation into adjacent soft tissue
• Rare examples of extravascular variant in soft tissue have been reported
  ○ Represent reactive endothelial proliferation in organizing hematoma

Cytologic Features
• Nuclei lining papillae may appear plump or hobnailed in appearance
  ○ However, significant nuclear pleomorphism is absent

ANCILLARY TESTS

Electron Microscopy
• Transmission
  ○ Differentiated endothelial cells line papillae

PAPILLARY ENDOTHELIAL HYPERPLASIA (MASSON TUMOR)

Key Facts

Terminology
- Benign, reactive, intravascular papillary endothelial proliferation

Clinical Issues
- Wide site distribution; located in deep dermis or subcutaneous tissue

Macroscopic Features
- Small, cystic lesions with red-purple discoloration

Microscopic Pathology
- Circumscribed lesion with pseudocapsule
- Papillary structures lined by endothelial cells
- Significant nuclear pleomorphism is absent

Top Differential Diagnoses
- Angiosarcoma
  - PEH lacks nuclear atypia, tumor cell necrosis, and mitotic activity present in angiosarcoma
- Hemangioma

- ■ Luminal micropinocytotic vesicles
- ■ Tight junctions and basal lamina
- ■ Weibel-Palade bodies
- ○ Undifferentiated &/or pericytic cells present within papillary cores

DIFFERENTIAL DIAGNOSIS

Angiosarcoma
- PEH is intraluminal process, unlike angiosarcoma, which is infiltrative
- Even PEH cases with soft tissue extension have bulk of the lesion confined to vascular lumen
- PEH lacks nuclear atypia, tumor cell necrosis, and mitotic activity present in angiosarcoma

Hemangioma
- PEH-like changes may occur in hemangiomas complicated by thrombosis

Arteriovenous Malformation (AVM)
- PEH-like changes may occur in background of AVM
- Important to recognize since these may recur

Hematoma
- Soft tissue hematomas may have foci of PEH
- May be mistaken for angiosarcoma

DIAGNOSTIC CHECKLIST

Clinically Relevant Pathologic Features
- Tissue distribution
  - Intravascular process

Pathologic Interpretation Pearls
- Intravascular papillary proliferation lined by endothelial cells without significant nuclear atypia

SELECTED REFERENCES

1. Pins MR et al: Florid extravascular papillary endothelial hyperplasia (Masson's pseudoangiosarcoma) presenting as a soft-tissue sarcoma. Arch Pathol Lab Med. 117(3):259-63, 1993
2. Hashimoto H et al: Intravascular papillary endothelial hyperplasia. A clinicopathologic study of 91 cases. Am J Dermatopathol. 5(6):539-46, 1983
3. Barr RJ et al: Intravascular papillary endothelial hyperplasia. A benign lesion mimicking angiosarcoma. Arch Dermatol. 114(5):723-6, 1978
4. Clearkin KP et al: Intravascular papillary endothelial hyperplasia. Arch Pathol Lab Med. 100(8):441-4, 1976
5. Kuo T et al: Masson's "vegetant intravascular hemangioendothelioma:" a lesion often mistaken for angiosarcoma: study of seventeen cases located in the skin and soft tissues. Cancer. 38(3):1227-36, 1976
6. Salyer WR et al: Intravascular angiomatosis: development and distinction from angiosarcoma. Cancer. 36(3):995-1001, 1975

IMAGE GALLERY

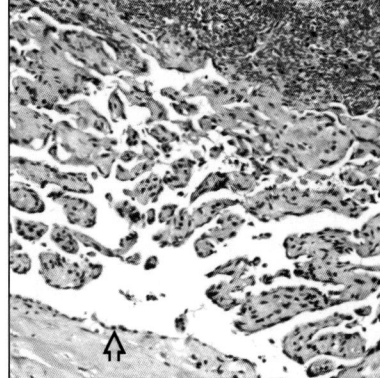 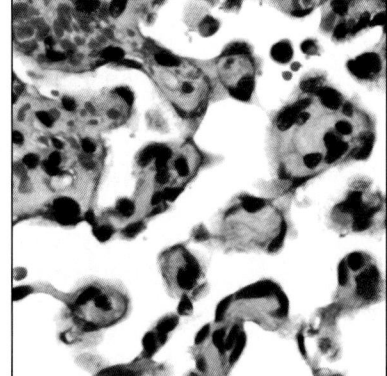 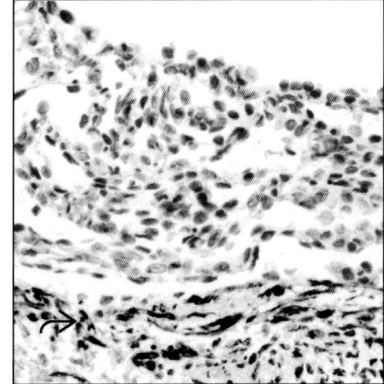

(Left) PEH can be mistaken for the dissecting vascular spaces seen in low-grade angiosarcoma. Note the bland endothelial lining ➡ of the blood vessel lumen. *(Center)* A single layer of endothelial cells line the papillary fronds in PEH. The endothelial cells may be plump and swollen, but do not show significant nuclear atypia. *(Right)* A desmin immunostain highlights remnants of smooth muscle in the blood vessel wall ➘ and confirms the intravascular location of PEH.

GLOMUS TUMORS

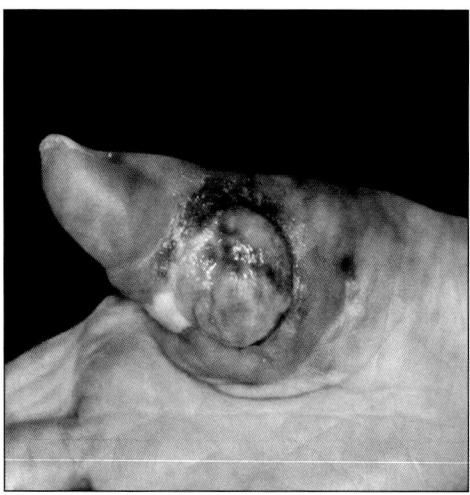

Clinical photograph shows a rare malignant glomus tumor.

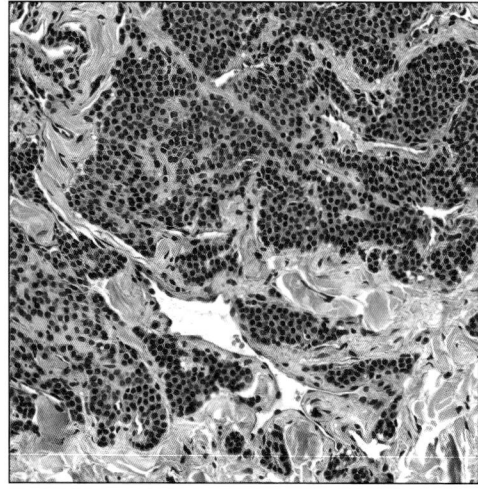

Hematoxylin & eosin shows perivascularly arranged myogenic tumor cells that contain uniform round nuclei in a benign glomus tumor.

TERMINOLOGY

Abbreviations
- Glomus tumor (GT)

Definitions
- Perivascular myogenic mesenchymal neoplasm composed of cells closely resembling smooth muscle cells of normal glomus body

CLINICAL ISSUES

Epidemiology
- Incidence
  - Rare
  - Account for < 2% of soft tissue neoplasms
- Age
  - Predominantly occur in young adults
  - May occur at any age
- Gender
  - No sex predilection

Site
- Distal extremities
- Often in subungual location
- Rare in other anatomic locations (visceral organs, bone, mediastinum, nerve)
- Skin, subcutis
- Rare in deep soft tissue

Presentation
- Typically small, red-blue nodules
- Painful mass; long history of pain
- Pain with exposure to cold &/or tactile stimulation
- Usually solitary lesions
- Rarely, may be multiple neoplasms
- Multiple lesions more common in children

Natural History
- < 10% recur locally

- Malignant glomus tumors highly aggressive
- Metastases and death of patients in up to 40% of cases

Treatment
- Surgical approaches
  - Complete excision

Prognosis
- Benign behavior in most cases

MACROSCOPIC FEATURES

General Features
- Red-blue nodular lesions

MICROSCOPIC PATHOLOGY

Histologic Features
- Perivascular myoid tumor cells
- Small, uniform, round tumor cells
- Centrally placed, sharply punched-out, round nuclei
- Eosinophilic cytoplasm
- Each cell surrounded by basal lamina

Predominant Pattern/Injury Type
- Circumscribed

Predominant Cell/Compartment Type
- Smooth muscle

Solid Glomus Tumor
- Most common variant
- Well-circumscribed nodular neoplasm
- Contains numerous capillary-sized vessels
- Nest of tumor cells surrounding capillaries
- Stroma may show hyalinization
- Stroma may show myxoid changes
- Rare degenerative cytologic atypia
- Rare vascular invasion may be identified
- Peripheral rim of collagen (fibrous pseudocapsule)

GLOMUS TUMORS

Key Facts

Terminology
- Perivascular myogenic mesenchymal neoplasm composed of cells closely resembling smooth muscle cells of normal glomus body

Clinical Issues
- Distal extremities, especially in subungual location
- Typically small, red-blue, painful nodules
- < 10% recur locally
- Malignant glomus tumors highly aggressive

Macroscopic Features
- Red-blue nodular lesions

Microscopic Pathology
- Solid glomus tumor
  - Most common variant
  - Well-circumscribed nodular neoplasm

- Small, uniform, round tumor cells
- Centrally placed, sharply punched-out, round nuclei
- Glomangioma
  - Comprises up to 20% of glomus tumor
- Glomangiomyoma
  - Solid glomus tumor or glomangioma and elongated, spindled smooth muscle cells
- Glomangiomatosis
  - Extremely rare variant
- Malignant glomus tumor (glomangiosarcoma)
  - Exceedingly rare neoplasms
  - Enlarged size (> 2 cm) &/or subfascial/visceral location
  - Marked nuclear atypia
  - Increased number of mitoses

- May contain numerous hemangiopericytoma-like vessels
- Rare oncocytic changes
- Rare epithelioid variant

Glomangioma
- Comprises up to 20% of glomus tumors
- Most common type in patients with multiple lesions
- Less well-circumscribed
- Dilated veins surrounded by clusters of glomus cells
- Secondary thrombosis may occur

Glomangiomyoma
- Rare subtype
- Solid glomus tumor or glomangioma with elongated, spindled smooth muscle cells

Glomangiomatosis
- Extremely rare variant
- Infiltrative growth
- Multiple nodules of solid glomus tumor
- Biologically benign lesions

Symplastic Glomus Tumor
- Cells show prominent degenerative atypia
- Multinucleated giant cells
- Enlarged nuclei
- No increased proliferative activity
- No tumor necrosis

Malignant Glomus Tumor (Glomangiosarcoma)
- Exceedingly rare neoplasms
- Criteria for malignancy include
  - Enlarged size (> 2 cm)
  - Subfascial/visceral location
  - Marked nuclear atypia
  - Mitoses
  - Necrosis
  - Intravascular growth
- Preexisting benign-appearing glomus tumor may be present
- Spindle cell subtype

- Atypical spindled tumor cells
- Increased number of mitoses
- Round cell subtype
  - Sheets of atypical round tumor cells
  - Increased number of mitoses

Glomus Tumor of Uncertain Malignant Potential
- Nuclear pleomorphism
- One additional atypical feature

ANCILLARY TESTS

Cytogenetics
- Gene for inherited glomangiomas localized at 1p21-22
- Multiple familial glomus tumors may have autosomal dominant pattern of inheritance

Electron Microscopy
- Short interdigitating cytoplasmic processes
- Bundles of cytoplasmic actin-like filaments
- Dense bodies
- External lamina

DIFFERENTIAL DIAGNOSIS

Myopericytoma
- Distinction can be problematic because of overlapping morphologic features
- Perivascular, onion-like growth pattern
- Round and plump spindled tumor cells
- Nuclei usually not so sharply punched out

Myofibroma
- Biphasic pattern
- Spindled tumor cells in more mature component
- Small, undifferentiated cells associated with hemangiopericytoma-like vessels
- Usually H-caldesmon (HCAD) negative

GLOMUS TUMORS

Immunohistochemistry

Antibody	Reactivity	Staining Pattern	Comment
Actin-sm	Positive	Cytoplasmic	
HCAD	Positive	Cytoplasmic	
Collagen IV	Positive	Cell membrane	
CD34	Negative		May be positive in myxoid glomus tumor
Desmin	Negative		
CK-PAN	Negative		
S100P	Negative		

Hidradenoma (Solid Form)
- Often focal stromal hyalinization
- Ductal differentiation
- Poroid and cuticular tumor cells
- Pancytokeratin and EMA/CEA (ductal structures) positive
- Actin negative

Paraganglioma
- Clinical features
- Expression of neuroendocrine markers
- Sustentacular S100 protein positive cells
- Zellballen of tumor cells

Dermal Melanocytic Nevus
- Nests of melanocytic cells
- Pigmentation of tumor cells
- Intranuclear pseudoinclusions
- Expression of S100 protein
- Expression of MART-1/Melan-A

Angioleiomyoma
- Thick-walled blood vessels
- Bundles of spindled tumor cells
- Eosinophilic spindled tumor cells
- Expression of desmin

DIAGNOSTIC CHECKLIST

Clinically Relevant Pathologic Features
- Organ distribution
- Nuclear features
- Symptom complex
- Often painful neoplasms
- Biologically benign neoplasms in most cases

Pathologic Interpretation Pearls
- Perivascular myogenic mesenchymal neoplasm
- Varying number of blood vessels
- Uniform round tumor cells
- Round, sharply punched-out nuclei
- Expression of actins and HCAD
- No expression of cytokeratin, desmin, S100 protein

SELECTED REFERENCES

1. Semaan MT et al: Current assessment and management of glomus tumors. Curr Opin Otolaryngol Head Neck Surg. 16(5):420-6, 2008
2. Brouillard P et al: Four common glomulin mutations cause two thirds of glomuvenous malformations ("familial glomangiomas"): evidence for a founder effect. J Med Genet. 42(2):e13, 2005
3. De Chiara A et al: Malignant glomus tumour: a case report and review of the literature. Sarcoma. 7(2):87-91, 2003
4. Brouillard P et al: Mutations in a novel factor, glomulin, are responsible for glomuvenous malformations ("glomangiomas"). Am J Hum Genet. 70(4):866-74, 2002
5. Mentzel T et al: CD34-positive glomus tumor: clinicopathologic and immunohistochemical analysis of six cases with myxoid stromal changes. J Cutan Pathol. 29(7):421-5, 2002
6. Calvert JT et al: Additional glomangioma families link to chromosome 1p: no evidence for genetic heterogeneity. Hum Hered. 51(3):180-2, 2001
7. Folpe AL et al: Atypical and malignant glomus tumors: analysis of 52 cases, with a proposal for the reclassification of glomus tumors. Am J Surg Pathol. 25(1):1-12, 2001
8. Takata H et al: Treatment of subungual glomus tumour. Hand Surg. 6(1):25-7, 2001
9. Boon LM et al: A gene for inherited cutaneous venous anomalies ("glomangiomas") localizes to chromosome 1p21-22. Am J Hum Genet. 65(1):125-33, 1999
10. Hiruta N et al: Malignant glomus tumor: a case report and review of the literature. Am J Surg Pathol. 21(9):1096-103, 1997
11. Van Geertruyden J et al: Glomus tumours of the hand. A retrospective study of 51 cases. J Hand Surg [Br]. 21(2):257-60, 1996
12. Pulitzer DR et al: Epithelioid glomus tumor. Hum Pathol. 26(9):1022-7, 1995
13. Haque S et al: Multiple glomus tumors of the stomach with intravascular spread. Am J Surg Pathol. 16(3):291-9, 1992
14. Gould EW et al: Locally infiltrative glomus tumors and glomangiosarcomas. A clinical, ultrastructural, and immunohistochemical study. Cancer. 65(2):310-8, 1990
15. Hulsebos TJ et al: Inheritance of glomus tumours. Lancet. 335(8690):660, 1990
16. Slater DN et al: Oncocytic glomus tumour: a new variant. Histopathology. 11(5):523-31, 1987
17. Miettinen M et al: Glomus tumor cells: evaluation of smooth muscle and endothelial cell properties. Virchows Arch B Cell Pathol Incl Mol Pathol. 43(2):139-49, 1983

Microscopic and Immunohistochemical Features

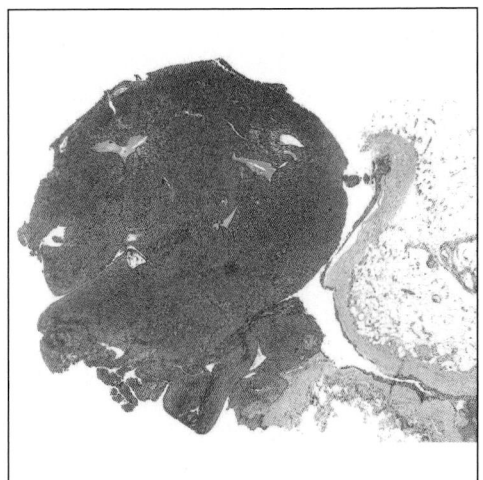

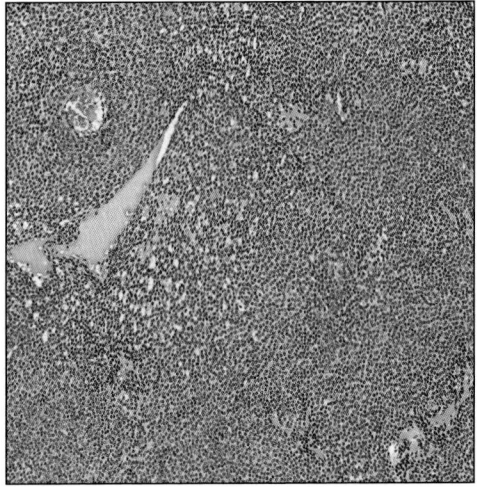

(Left) Low-magnification examination shows a solid glomus tumor. Note the nodular growth of a well-circumscribed neoplasm. *(Right)* Intermediate-power examination shows a solid growth of uniform round tumor cells, mimicking an adnexal cutaneous neoplasm.

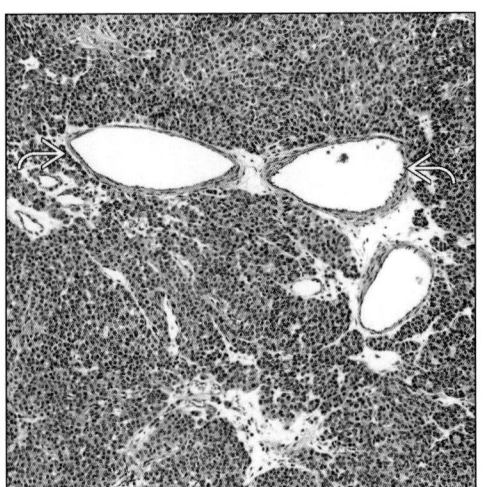

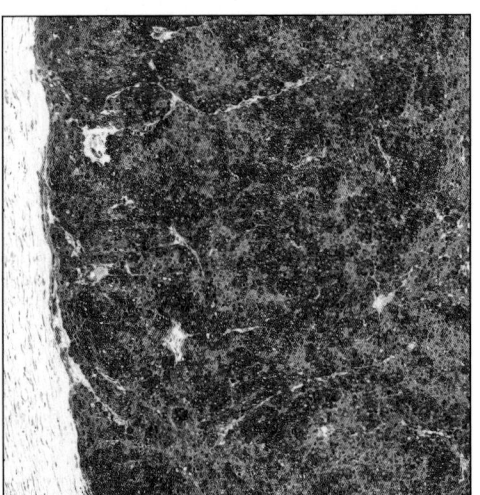

(Left) Intermediate-power examination shows sheets of myogenic tumor cells with slightly enlarged nuclei surrounding dilated vascular spaces ➤. *(Right)* Actin-sm immunohistochemistry shows homogeneous, strong expression in this glomus tumor.

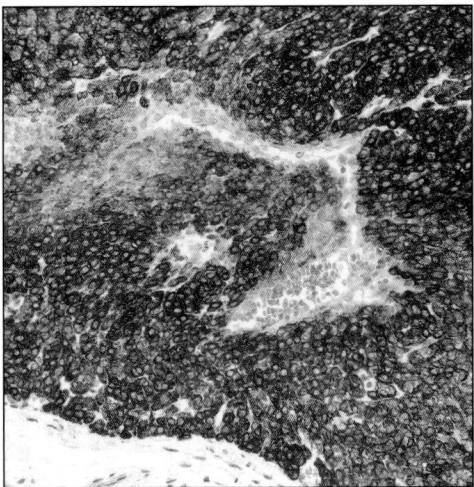

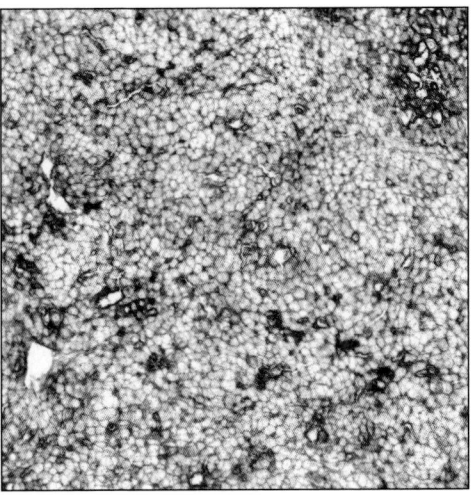

(Left) Caldesmon shows strong and diffuse expression. *(Right)* Collagen IV highlights clear membranous staining of the tumor cells.

Nonmelanocytic Tumors of the Skin: Vascular and Perivascular Tumors and Pseudotumors

Microscopic and Immunohistochemical Features

(Left) Histologic section at scanning magnification shows a deep dermally located, well-circumscribed ➡ glomangioma. *(Right)* Higher magnification shows a perivascular arrangement of glomus cells in this example of glomangioma.

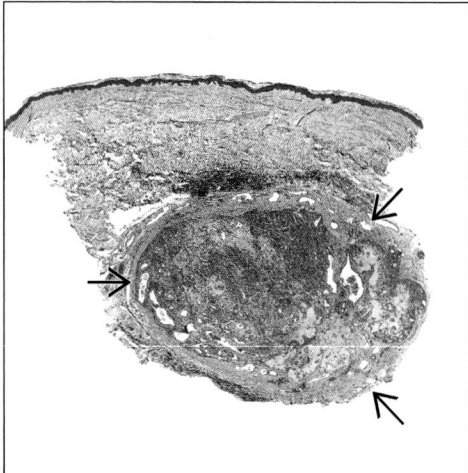
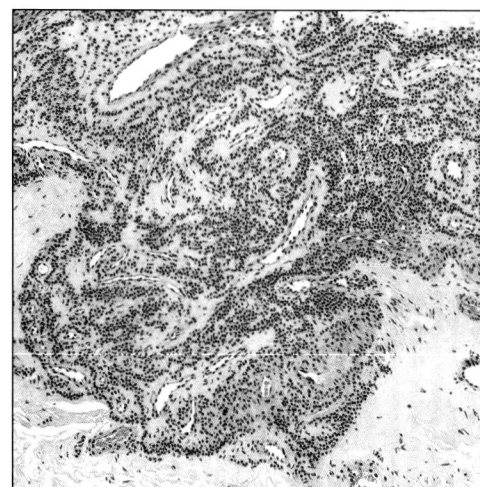

(Left) Higher magnification shows the bland cytology of round glomus cells containing sharply demarcated, round nuclei ➡. *(Right)* Actin-sm staining shows the perivascular arrangement of round, myogenic tumor cells.

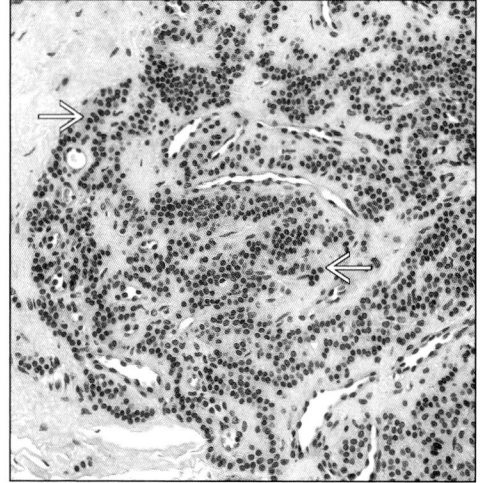
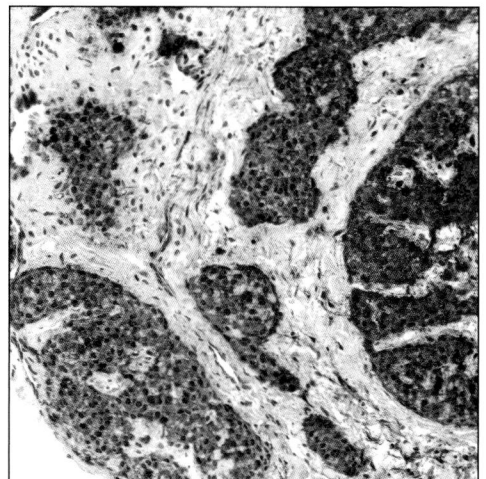

(Left) This is a rare example of a glomus tumor with myxoid stromal changes. *(Right)* This example shows a "transition" of an ordinary glomus tumor (left upper corner ➤) to a glomus tumor with myxoid stromal changes.

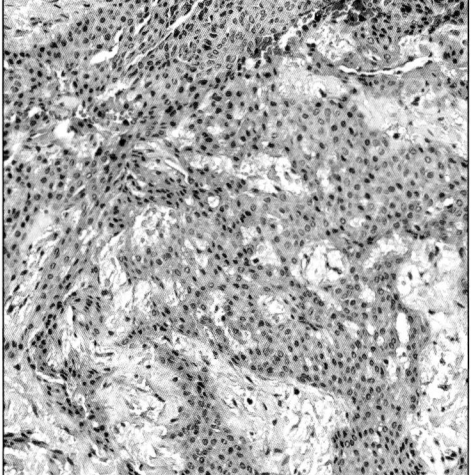
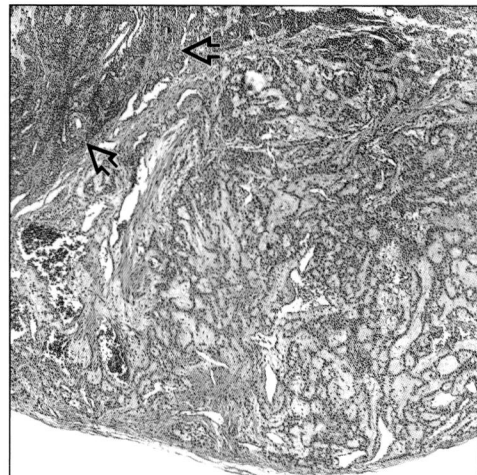

GLOMUS TUMORS

Microscopic and Immunohistochemical Features

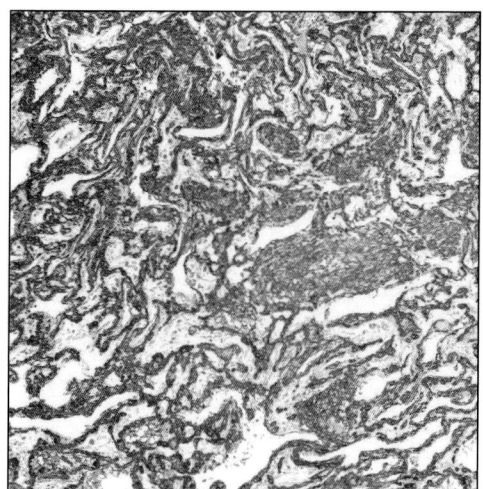

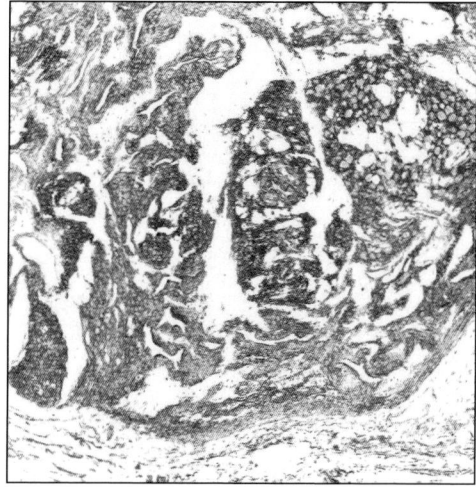

(Left) Actin-sm shows strong, homogeneous expression in this example of a rare myxoid glomus tumor. *(Right)* CD34 immunohistochemistry shows strong expression in this example of a myxoid glomus tumor. All CD34 positive glomus tumors were characterized by myxoid changes.

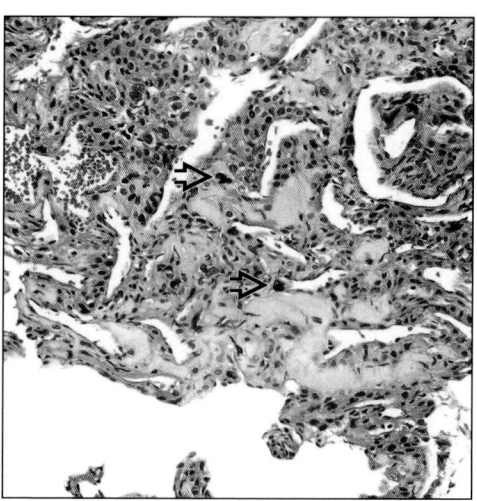

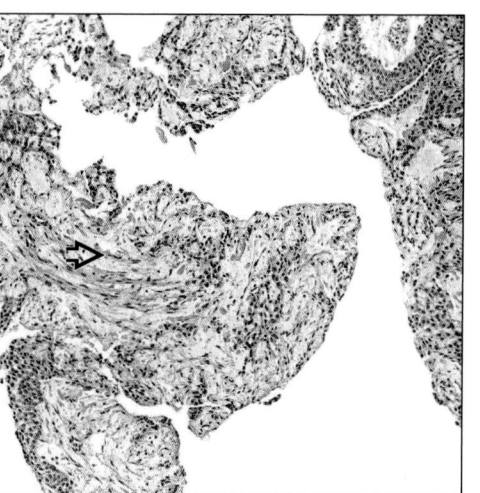

(Left) Histologic examination shows a rare case of symplastic glomus tumor. Note the enlarged tumor cells containing enlarged and irregular-shaped nuclei ➢. *(Right)* This is a rare example of glomangiomyoma with myxoid stromal changes. Note the presence of elongated spindle-shaped tumor cells containing abundant eosinophilic cytoplasm and elongated nuclei ➢.

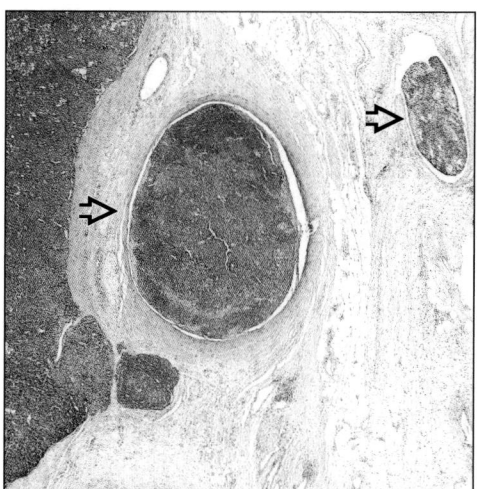

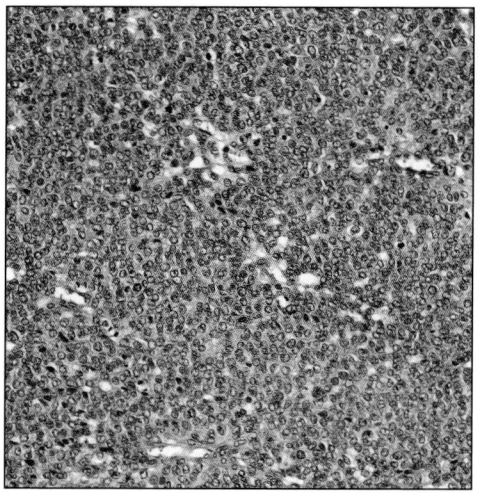

(Left) Low magnification shows a very rare malignant glomus tumor with widespread vascular invasion ➢. *(Right)* This is a high-power view of a malignant glomus tumor with prominent cytologic atypia and numerous mitoses.

LYMPHANGIOMA AND SUPERFICIAL LYMPHANGIOMA

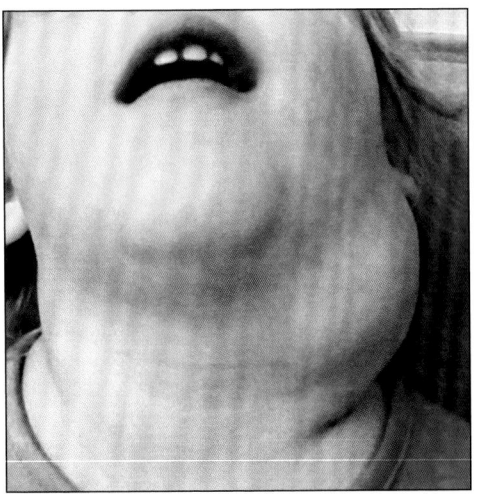

Clinical photograph shows a large deep lymphangioma (cystic hygroma) on the lateral neck of a child.

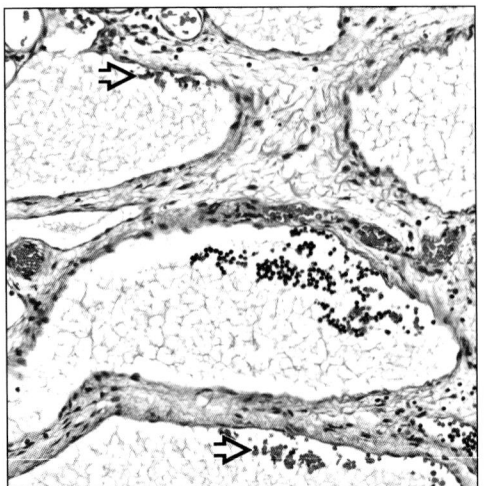

Deep lymphangioma shows large vascular channels filled with proteinaceous material, a few lymphocytes, and scattered erythrocytes ⇨.

TERMINOLOGY

Synonyms

- Lymphangioma circumscriptum (superficial cutaneous lymphangioma) (LAC)
- Lymphangiomatosis (generalized lymphangioma, systemic angiomatosis) (LAS)
- Cystic lymphangioma (cystic hygroma)
- Deep lymphangioma (cavernous lymphangioma)
- Lymphatic malformation

Definitions

- Proliferation of lymphatic vessels; may be
  - Superficial (lymphangioma circumscription)
  - Deep (cavernous lymphangioma)
  - Diffusely involve most organ systems (lymphangiomatosis)

ETIOLOGY/PATHOGENESIS

Developmental Anomaly

- Most cases are considered developmental or congenital malformations/hamartomas, **not** true neoplasms
  - Maldevelopment during embryonic lymphangiogenesis most likely etiology
    - Leads to sequestered lymphatics that fail to communicate with normal lymphovascular system
  - May be due to maternal infections or substance abuse
  - LAS considered congenital in most cases

Genetics

- Associated with genetic syndromes including Turner syndrome (cystic hygroma), Noonan syndrome, Maffucci syndrome, trisomies 13, 18, 21
- Mutations in *VEGFR-C*, *VEGFR3*, *PROX1*, *FOXC2*, and *SOX18* genes implicated

Acquired

- Rare acquired cases occur in adults
  - Likely associated with infection or trauma

CLINICAL ISSUES

Epidemiology

- Incidence
  - More common in children: Estimated 6% of benign childhood tumors
- Age
  - Often present at birth or within 1st 2 years of life (approximately 90% of cases)
  - LAS usually presents within 1st 2 decades of life
- Gender
  - Intraabdominal lymphangiomas have slight male predominance
  - LAS has no gender predilection

Site

- Head and neck most common site for cystic lymphangiomas
  - Usually posterior triangle, but can occur in anterior triangle
  - Also occur in axillae, abdomen, and internal organs
- Cavernous type more frequent in oral cavity, upper trunk, limbs, and abdominal sites
  - Intraabdominal lymphangiomas occur in mesentery, omentum, and retroperitoneum
- LAC: Axillary folds, neck, and trunk are most common sites
- LAS: Can affect any organ system, but often involves bones, soft tissues, and skin

Presentation

- Cystic mass lesion; may be superfical or deep
  - Typically presents as large, slow-growing, painless mass (deep lymphangioma) or as multiple small, grouped, superficial vesicular lesions (LAC)

LYMPHANGIOMA AND SUPERFICIAL LYMPHANGIOMA

Key Facts

Terminology
- Lymphangioma circumscriptum (superficial lymphangioma) (LAC)
- Lymphangiomatosis (systemic angiomatosis) (LAS)
- Cystic lymphangioma (cystic hygroma)
- Deep lymphangioma (cavernous lymphangioma)

Etiology/Pathogenesis
- Most cases considered developmental malformations/hamartomas, **not** true neoplasms
- Associated with trisomies and other genetic syndromes, including Turner (cystic hygroma), Noonan, and Maffucci

Clinical Issues
- More common in children (6% of benign childhood tumors); present at birth or within 1st 2 years of life

- Typically presents as large, slow-growing, painless mass (deep lymphangioma) or as multiple small, grouped, superficial vesicular lesions (LAC)
- Excellent prognosis in most cases, although may be fatal if involving mediastinum or internal organs
- Recurrence rate high if removal incomplete

Microscopic Pathology
- Variably sized anastomosing vascular spaces lined by small, bland endothelial cells
- Often contain abundant proteinaceous debris, scattered lymphocytes, and erythrocytes
- Walls show stromal fibrosis (older lesions) and may contain smooth muscle
- Endothelial cells are small with uniform, bland-appearing, oval to flattened, hyperchromatic nuclei

---

- ○ Lymphangiomatosis presents with numerous cystic lesions, both superficial and deep
- Soft and fluctuant swellings on palpation
- Intraabdominal cases may present with abdominal distension, mass on palpation
  - ○ May also develop abdominal obstruction, volvulus, and infarction
- Generalized lymphangiomatosis: Depends on affected site
  - ○ Bone: Pathologic fractures
  - ○ Lungs: Dyspnea, wheezing due to chylothorax, chylous ascites
  - ○ Spleen: Splenomegaly, left upper quadrant pain

Treatment
- Surgical approaches
  - ○ May be indicated in large, deep lesions, especially if symptomatic
  - ○ LAS not amenable to surgical excision
- Drugs
  - ○ Intralesional injection of sclerosing agents, including bleomycin and OK-432 (Picibanil)

Prognosis
- Excellent in most cases, although lymphangiomatosis may be fatal if involving mediastinum or internal organs, especially lungs
- Recurrence rate high with incomplete removal
- No malignant transformation reported

IMAGE FINDINGS

Ultrasonographic Findings
- Unilocular or multilocular anechoic mass
- Can be used in utero to detect cystic lymphangioma (associated with hydrops fetalis, Turner syndrome, and high death rate)

CT Findings
- Nonenhancing cystic lesions with homogeneous attenuation

- Visceral and osseous lesions often show contrast enhancement
- May displace surrounding organs

MACROSCOPIC FEATURES

General Features
- Multiple cystic spaces with clear to whitish fluid

MICROSCOPIC PATHOLOGY

Histologic Features
- Variably sized anastomosing vascular spaces lined by small, bland endothelial cells
- Dilated lumina
  - ○ Often contain abundant proteinaceous debris, scattered lymphocytes, and erythrocytes
- Walls show stromal fibrosis (older lesions) and occasional myxoid change
  - ○ Often contain lymphoid infiltrates
    - ■ May show occasional reactive germinal centers
  - ○ Mast cells are common
  - ○ Hemosiderin deposition in stroma may be seen
- Large vessels may contain smooth muscle in their walls
- Cavernous hemangiomas have infiltrative margins and often extend into surrounding tissues

Cytologic Features
- Endothelial cells are small with uniform, bland-appearing, oval to flattened, hyperchromatic nuclei

Predominant Pattern/Injury Type
- Cystic, macroscopic

Predominant Cell/Compartment Type
- Lymphatics

ANCILLARY TESTS

Immunohistochemistry

- Endothelial lining cells show variable positivity with vascular markers CD31, CD34, and FVIIIRAg
- Newer lymphatic markers, including podoplanin (D2-40), VEGFR-3, and LYVE-1, typically positive

DIFFERENTIAL DIAGNOSIS

Hemangiomas

- Most cases show smaller vascular spaces with more red blood cells, less proteinaceous material, and fewer lymphocytes
- Often well-circumscribed, noninfiltrative borders

Progressive Lymphangioma

- Form of cutaneous lymphangioma with distinct clinical findings
  - Typically presents on lower extremities of adults as slow-growing patches or plaques
- Histologic findings very similar to other forms of lymphangioma
  - Superficially dilated spaces that become progressively smaller with deep extension

Secondary Lymphangiectasia

- May be due to local factors, such as obstruction (e.g., due to tumor), scarring, or previous radiation therapy
- Identical histologic findings; can only be distinguished by clinical history or other findings (if present)

Atypical Vascular Proliferation

- Radiation-induced lesion; most frequent in breast
- Clinically, presents as multiple small vesicles in radiation field
- Irregularly dilated vascular spaces lined by atypical endothelial cells

Lymphangioma-like Kaposi Sarcoma

- Usually shows at least focal areas of more typical Kaposi sarcoma
  - Infiltrative slit-like spaces lined by hyperchromatic spindle-shaped cells
  - Stromal hemosiderin deposition and inflammatory infiltrate containing plasma cells
- HHV8(+) is diagnostic

Angiosarcoma/Lymphangiosarcoma

- Atypical vascular proliferation showing irregular, anastomosing vascular spaces
- Poorly circumscribed, infiltrative neoplasm
- Endothelial cells typically show epithelioid or spindle cell features, prominent nuclear enlargement, and atypia with enlarged nucleoli
  - Endothelial multilayering often present
  - Mitotic figures easily identified

DIAGNOSTIC CHECKLIST

Clinically Relevant Pathologic Features

- Margins
  - High recurrence rate with positive margins

Pathologic Interpretation Pearls

- Proliferation of superficial &/or deep dilated vascular spaces lined by bland oval or flattened endothelial cells

SELECTED REFERENCES

1. Ji RC et al: Multiple expressions of lymphatic markers and morphological evolution of newly formed lymphatics in lymphangioma and lymph node lymphangiogenesis. Microvasc Res. 80(2):195-201, 2010
2. Kim DH et al: Lymphangiomatosis involving the inferior vena cava, heart, pulmonary artery and pelvic cavity. Korean J Radiol. 11(1):115-8, 2010
3. Chen EY et al: Similar histologic features and immunohistochemical staining in microcystic and macrocystic lymphatic malformations. Lymphat Res Biol. 7(2):75-80, 2009
4. Gedikbasi A et al: Multidisciplinary approach in cystic hygroma: prenatal diagnosis, outcome, and postnatal follow up. Pediatr Int. 51(5):670-7, 2009
5. Patel GA et al: Cutaneous lymphangioma circumscriptum: frog spawn on the skin. Int J Dermatol. 48(12):1290-5, 2009
6. Patel GA et al: Zosteriform lymphangioma circumscriptum. Acta Dermatovenerol Alp Panonica Adriat. 18(4):179-82, 2009
7. Rattan KN et al: Pediatric chylolymphatic mesenteric cyst - a separate entity from cystic lymphangioma: a case series. J Med Case Reports. 3:111, 2009
8. Richmond B et al: Adult presentation of giant retroperitoneal cystic lymphangioma: case report. Int J Surg. 7(6):559-60, 2009
9. Edwards JR et al: Lymphatics and bone. Hum Pathol. 39(1):49-55, 2008
10. François M et al: Sox18 induces development of the lymphatic vasculature in mice. Nature. 456(7222):643-7, 2008
11. Santo S et al: Prenatal ultrasonographic diagnosis of abdominal cystic lymphangioma: a case report. J Matern Fetal Neonatal Med. 21(8):565-6, 2008
12. Norgall S et al: Elevated expression of VEGFR-3 in lymphatic endothelial cells from lymphangiomas. BMC Cancer. 7:105, 2007
13. Wilting J et al: Embryonic development and malformation of lymphatic vessels. Novartis Found Symp. 283:220-7; discussion 227-9, 238-41, 2007
14. Wilting J et al: The transcription factor Prox1 is a marker for lymphatic endothelial cells in normal and diseased human tissues. FASEB J. 16(10):1271-3, 2002
15. Prevo R et al: Mouse LYVE-1 is an endocytic receptor for hyaluronan in lymphatic endothelium. J Biol Chem. 276(22):19420-30, 2001

Gross and Microscopic Features

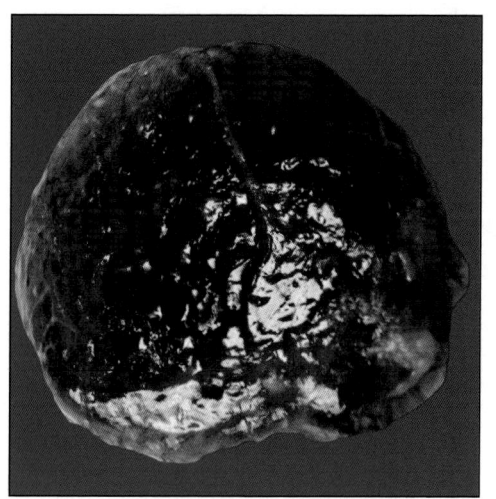

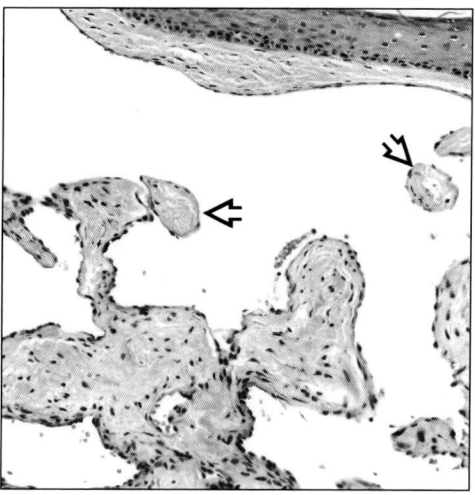

(Left) *Macroscopic view of a lymphangioma shows a reddish brown translucent cystic mass. Small vessels are noted within the lining; the cyst was filled with clear, watery fluid.* **(Right)** *Low-magnification examination of a superficial lymphangioma shows widely dilated spaces in the superficial dermis. The lumina show several papillary projections ⮕ with slightly fibrinous cores lined by small, hyperchromatic-staining endothelial cells.*

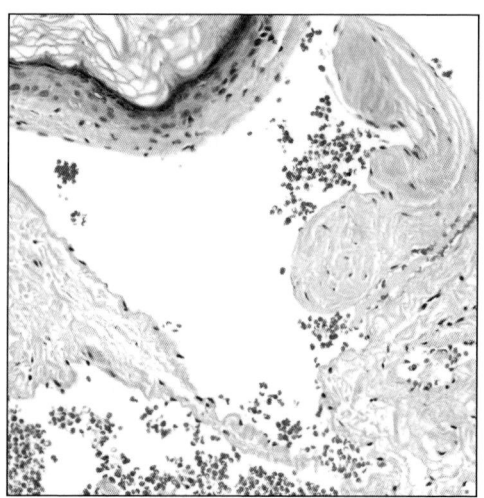

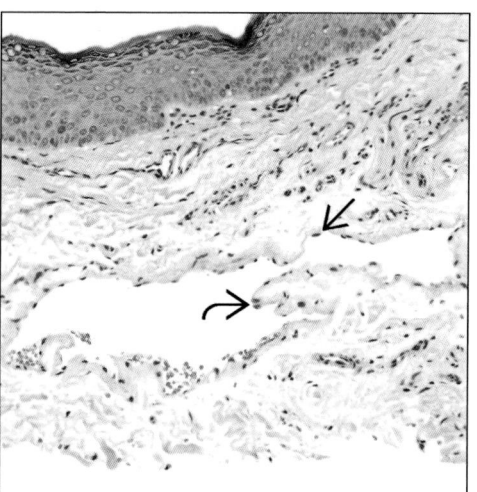

(Left) *Examination of a superficial lymphangioma shows a large, irregularly dilated space lined by thin endothelial cells containing scattered red blood cells in the superficial dermis.* **(Right)** *Higher magnification examination of a superficial lymphangioma shows the dilated spaces lined by small, bland endothelial cells with uniform, hyperchromatic-staining oval ⮕ to flattened ⮕ nuclei.*

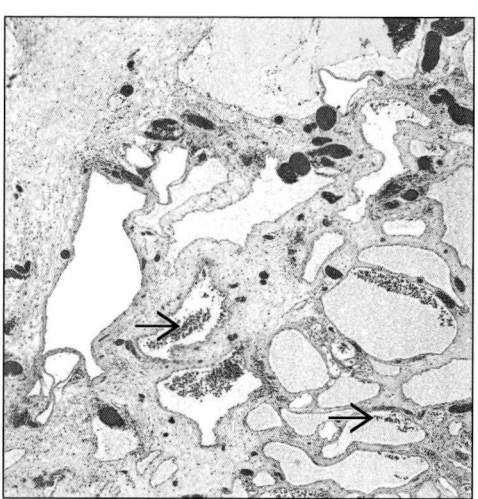

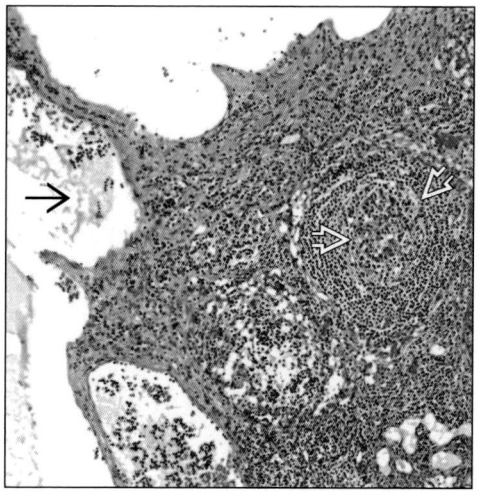

(Left) *This example of a deep lymphangioma shows multiple dilated endothelial-lined channels with small collections of lymphocytes ⮕ within the lumina, along with fluid and erythrocytes.* **(Right)** *Another deep lymphangioma shows a lumen lined by flattened endothelium and containing proteinaceous fluid ⮕. There is a lymphocytic aggregate with a germinal center ⮕ in the surrounding connective tissue.*

PROGRESSIVE LYMPHANGIOMA

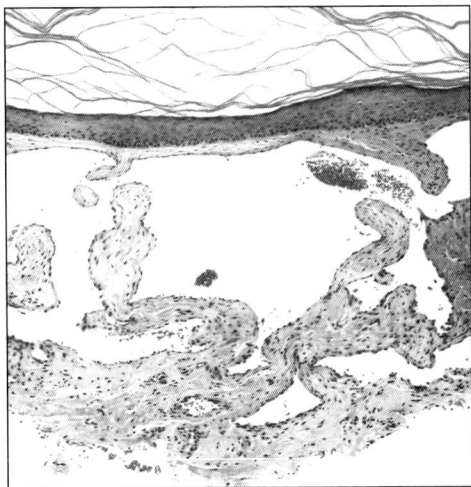

Low-magnification histologic examination of a progressive lymphangioma shows widely dilated lymphatic spaces in the superficial dermis.

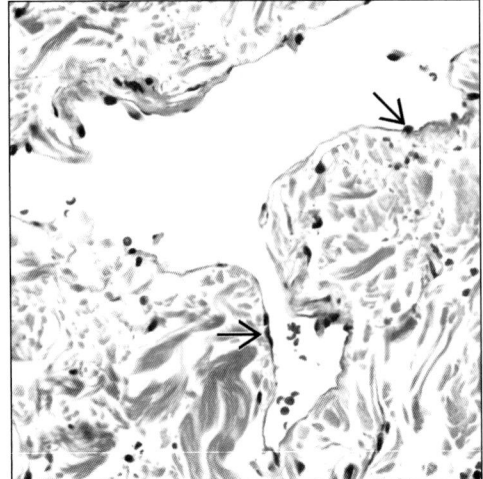

High-power examination shows irregular contours of lymphatic spaces and small, bland-appearing lining endothelial cells ➡.

TERMINOLOGY

Synonyms
- Acquired progressive lymphangioma
- Benign lymphangioendothelioma

Definitions
- Benign, localized proliferation of lymphatic vessels

ETIOLOGY/PATHOGENESIS

Unknown
- May be related to trauma in some cases

CLINICAL ISSUES

Epidemiology
- Age
  - Middle-aged or older adults
- Gender
  - No predilection

Site
- Usually presents on lower extremities, but may occur anywhere

Presentation
- Slow-growing lesion
- Patches or plaques

Treatment
- Surgical approaches
  - Complete surgical excision is curative, but not necessary, given the benign nature of this lesion
- Drugs
  - Corticosteroids have been reported to induce complete regression in some cases

Prognosis
- Excellent; local recurrences are rare, metastases do not occur

MACROSCOPIC FEATURES

General Features
- Dermal-based mass lesion with cystic spaces and hemorrhage

Size
- May measure up to several centimeters

MICROSCOPIC PATHOLOGY

Histologic Features
- Dermal and subcutaneous proliferation of dilated vascular channels
- Spaces are often widely dilated superficially, but become narrower with deep extension
  - Vascular channels are lined by monomorphous, bland-appearing endothelial cells
  - Endothelial cells may show mild hyperchromasia, but no significant atypia is present
- Endothelial-lined papillary projections with mild fibrosis may be present

Predominant Pattern/Injury Type
- Vascular proliferation

Predominant Cell/Compartment Type
- Endothelial

ANCILLARY TESTS

Immunohistochemistry
- Usually not necessary for diagnosis
- Endothelial cells positive for CD31, CD34, and podoplanin (D2-40)

PROGRESSIVE LYMPHANGIOMA

Key Facts

Terminology
- Benign, localized proliferation of lymphatic vessels
- Also known as
  - Acquired progressive lymphangioma and benign lymphangioendothelioma

Clinical Issues
- Usually presents on lower extremities, but may occur anywhere
- Prognosis excellent; local recurrences rare

Microscopic Pathology
- Dermal and subcutaneous proliferation of dilated vascular channels
- Spaces are often widely dilated superficially, but become narrower with deep extension
- Endothelial-lined papillary projections with mild fibrosis may be present
- Endothelial cells may show mild hyperchromasia, but no significant atypia

DIFFERENTIAL DIAGNOSIS

Lymphangioma Circumscriptum
- Presents at birth or in early childhood as multiple small vesicular lesions grouped together
- Superficial dermis is involved; may be deep dilated lymphatics as well

Lymphangiomatosis
- Clinically very distinctive, with diffuse involvement of many organ systems, including skin, soft tissues, bone, and internal organs

Atypical Vascular Lesion (Radiotherapy-related)
- Clinically, presents as multiple tiny vesicles in radiation field, usually on breast
- Histologically, greater endothelial atypia in most cases, and lymphatic spaces are more widely dilated

Lymphangioma-like Kaposi Sarcoma (KS)
- Usually shows more typical areas of KS and inflammatory infiltrate including plasma cells
- HHV8 immunohistochemistry positive

Angiosarcoma
- Highly atypical vascular proliferation with dissection throughout dermis and subcutis in most cases
- Significant cytologic atypia, endothelial multilayering, and mitoses are present

DIAGNOSTIC CHECKLIST

Pathologic Interpretation Pearls
- Proliferation of dilated lymphatic channels lined by bland endothelial cells
- Widely dilated spaces superficially; narrower spaces with deep extension

SELECTED REFERENCES

1. Paik AS et al: Acquired progressive lymphangioma in an HIV-positive patient. J Cutan Pathol. 34(11):882-5, 2007
2. Hwang LY et al: Acquired progressive lymphangioma. J Am Acad Dermatol. 49(5 Suppl):S250-1, 2003
3. Guillou L et al: Benign lymphangioendothelioma (acquired progressive lymphangioma): a lesion not to be confused with well-differentiated angiosarcoma and patch stage Kaposi's sarcoma: clinicopathologic analysis of a series. Am J Surg Pathol. 24(8):1047-57, 2000
4. Cossu S et al: Lymphangioma-like variant of Kaposi's sarcoma: clinicopathologic study of seven cases with review of the literature. Am J Dermatopathol. 19(1):16-22, 1997
5. Rosso R et al: Acquired progressive lymphangioma of the skin following radiotherapy for breast carcinoma. J Cutan Pathol. 22(2):164-7, 1995
6. Meunier L et al: Acquired progressive lymphangioma. Br J Dermatol. 131(5):706-8, 1994

Microscopic Features

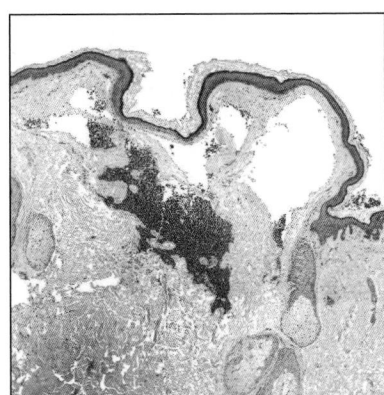 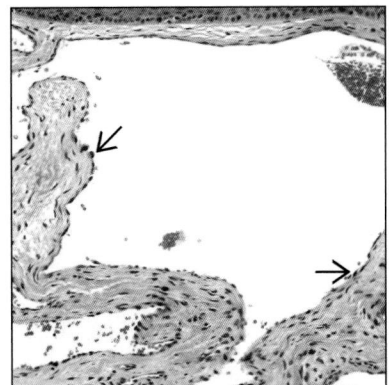 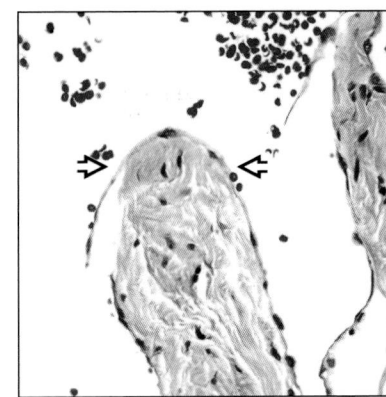

(Left) Low-power examination of a progressive lymphangioma shows superficial dermal dilated lymphatic spaces, some of which contain numerous red blood cells. (Center) Higher magnification shows the widely dilated lymphatic spaces lined by a single layer of small, flattened, hyperchromatic-staining bland endothelial cells ➡. (Right) High-power examination of another section shows a large papillary projection ➢ protruding into the lymphatic space.

BACILLARY ANGIOMATOSIS

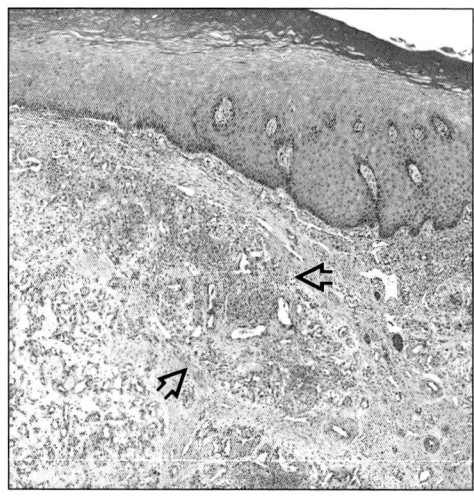

Low-power examination of bacillary angiomatosis demonstrates a superficial dermal proliferation of blood vessels in a lobular configuration ➡ associated with edema and inflammation.

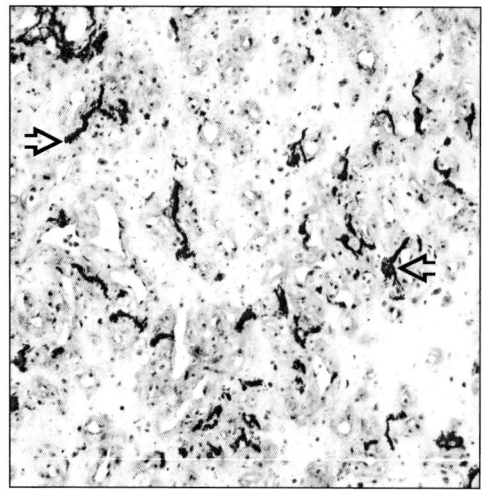

Warthin-Starry silver stain preparation shows numerous clusters of bacterial organisms ➡ around blood vessels.

TERMINOLOGY

Abbreviations
- Bacillary angiomatosis (BA)

Synonyms
- Epithelioid angiomatosis

Definitions
- Reactive vascular proliferation associated with *Bartonella* species bacterial infection

ETIOLOGY/PATHOGENESIS

Infectious Agents
- Caused by infection with *Bartonella* (gram-negative coccobacilli) species, usually *B. henselae* or *B. quintana*
  - Most patients have a history of cat exposure (and may have preceding scratch or bite)
- Most patients are immunosuppressed, especially due to HIV/AIDS
  - Also associated with organ transplantation, systemic steroids, and leukemia

CLINICAL ISSUES

Epidemiology
- Age
  - May occur in adults and children

Site
- Can involve any cutaneous site; uncommonly may involve mucosal sites and deep soft tissues
  - Internal organ involvement rare, but may affect liver (peliosis hepatis)

Presentation
- Skin nodules or, less likely, plaques
  - Typically present with multiple lesions, often pyogenic granuloma-like

Treatment
- Drugs
  - Antibiotics typically lead to resolution of lesions

Prognosis
- Typically good, but depends on patient's immune status and sites involved

MACROSCOPIC FEATURES

General Features
- Reddish brown, dermal-based nodular, hemorrhagic lesion

MICROSCOPIC PATHOLOGY

Histologic Features
- Typically a nodular to dome-shaped/polypoid dermal-based vascular proliferation
  - May have overlying epidermal ulceration and collarette (similar to pyogenic granuloma)
- Vessels are arranged in loose lobular configuration
  - Endothelial cells show mild enlargement and oval to epithelioid shape
  - Deeper parts of lesion may show greater cellularity and crowding of vessels
  - No significant cytologic atypia or atypical mitotic activity
- Background stroma shows fibrosis, edema, and mixed inflammatory infiltrate
  - Infiltrate is rich in neutrophils with nuclear dust, macrophages, and may show focal collections of basophilic granular material (clumps of bacteria)
    - Neutrophils are more plentiful in deeper lesions

BACILLARY ANGIOMATOSIS

Key Facts

Terminology
- Reactive vascular proliferation associated with *Bartonella* (gram-negative coccobacilli) bacterial infection

Etiology/Pathogenesis
- Most patients are immunosuppressed, especially HIV/AIDS
- Also associated with organ transplantation, systemic steroids, and leukemia

Clinical Issues
- Can involve any cutaneous site; uncommonly involves mucosal sites, deep soft tissues

Microscopic Pathology
- Nodular to dome-shaped/polypoid dermal-based vascular proliferation
- Infiltrate of neutrophils with nuclear dust, macrophages, focal clumps of basophilic granular material (bacteria)

ANCILLARY TESTS

Histochemistry
- Warthin-Starry
  - Reactivity: Positive
  - Staining pattern
    - Granular (coccobacillary organisms)
- GMS (Gomori methenamine silver)
  - Reactivity: Positive
  - Staining pattern
    - Granular (coccobacillary organisms)

PCR
- PCR for *Bartonella* species may be ordered if organisms are not identified on histochemical stains

DIFFERENTIAL DIAGNOSIS

Pyogenic Granuloma
- Polypoid dermal-based lesion composed of lobular collection of capillary-type vessels
- Overlying ulceration and peripheral epidermal collarette are typically present, similar to BA
- No evidence of organisms identified on H&E or special stains

Kaposi Sarcoma
- Plaque-like or nodular collection of slit-like vessels lined by atypical spindle cells

- Inflammatory infiltrate is typically composed of lymphocytes and plasma cells, not neutrophils
- No bacterial organisms identified
- HHV8(+) is diagnostic

DIAGNOSTIC CHECKLIST

Clinically Relevant Pathologic Features
- Organ distribution

Pathologic Interpretation Pearls
- Proliferation of vessels associated with neutrophils and clumps of bacterial organisms

SELECTED REFERENCES

1. Amsbaugh S et al: Bacillary angiomatosis associated with pseudoepitheliomatous hyperplasia. Am J Dermatopathol. 28(1):32-5, 2006
2. Tucci E et al: Localized bacillary angiomatosis in the oral cavity: observations about a neoplasm with atypical behavior. Description of a case and review of the literature. Minerva Stomatol. 55(1-2):67-75, 2006
3. Maurin M et al: Bartonella infections: diagnostic and management issues. Curr Opin Infect Dis. 11(2):189-93, 1998
4. LeBoit PE et al: Bacillary angiomatosis. The histopathology and differential diagnosis of a pseudoneoplastic infection in patients with human immunodeficiency virus disease. Am J Surg Pathol. 13(11):909-20, 1989

IMAGE GALLERY

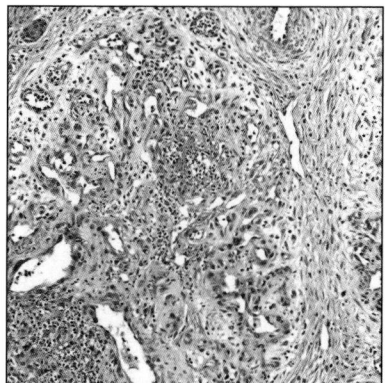 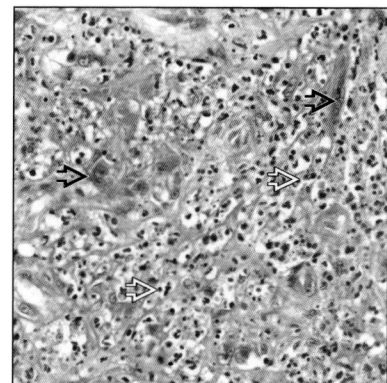 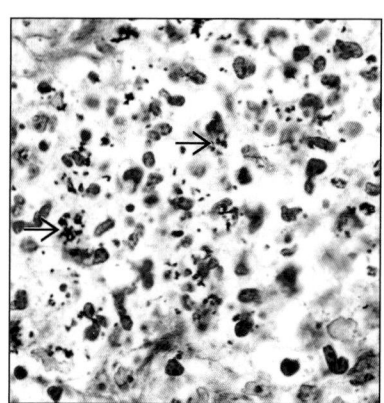

(Left) Intermediate magnification shows a proliferation of small blood vessels arranged in a vaguely lobular configuration with prominent stromal edema, mild fibrosis, and a mixed inflammatory infiltrate. *(Center)* High magnification of bacillary angiomatosis demonstrates a proliferation of small blood vessels with swollen endothelial cells ➡ surrounded by edema and inflammation ➡. *(Right)* Warthin-Starry stain demonstrates positive staining of numerous clusters ➡ and single bacterial organisms.

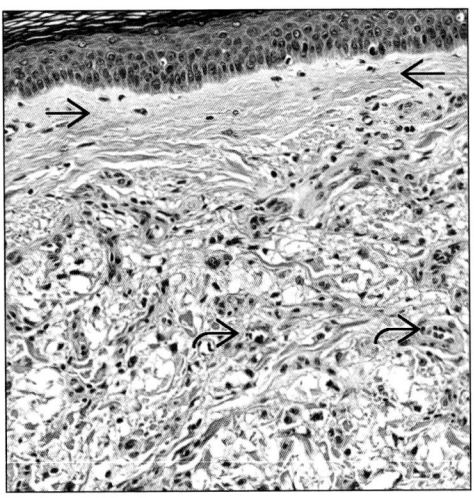

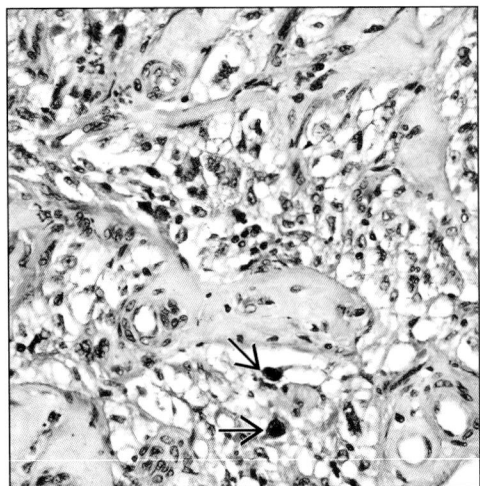

Rare primary cutaneous PEComa shows a dermal-based clear cell neoplasm associated with small blood vessels ➔. There is a grenz zone separating the tumor from the overlying epidermis ➔.

High magnification shows a PEComa with epithelioid cells proliferating around vessels. There are scattered large nuclei ➔ in this field, but no mitoses.

TERMINOLOGY

Abbreviations
- Perivascular epithelioid cell (PEC)
  - Thus, neoplasms are termed "PEComa"

Synonyms
- Perivascular epithelioid cell tumor
- Extrapulmonary sugar tumor
- Monotypic epithelioid angiomyolipoma

Definitions
- Mesenchymal neoplasms composed of distinctive perivascular epithelioid cells; category includes
  - Angiomyolipoma (AML)
  - Clear cell "sugar" tumor of lung (CCST)
  - Lymphangioleiomyomatosis (LAM)
  - Clear cell myomelanocytic tumor of falciform ligament/ligamentum teres (CCMMT)
- In many respects, PEComas are simply angiomyolipomas without fat
- Subset displays overt histologic features of malignancy and malignant clinical behavior

ETIOLOGY/PATHOGENESIS

Association with Tuberous Sclerosis
- Genetic alterations of tuberous sclerosis complex (TSC), losses of *TSC1* (9q34) or *TSC2* (16p13.3) genes
- Autosomal dominant inheritance
- Benign tumors of brain (most common), kidneys, heart, eyes, lungs, and skin
  - Name comes from characteristic tuber or potato-like nodules in brain, which calcify with age and become hard or sclerotic
- AML, CCST, and LAM are associated with tuberous sclerosis but not other types

CLINICAL ISSUES

Epidemiology
- Incidence
  - AML, CCST, LAM are rare
    - Other PEComas extremely rare
- Age
  - CCMMT typically encountered in girls in late childhood
  - Most others seen in adults 50-60 years old
  - AML detected in younger patients in setting of tuberous sclerosis
- Gender
  - Marked overall female predominance

Site
- Reported in multiple sites; rare in skin, but reported
  - Kidney, liver, falciform ligament, deep soft tissues of extremities, uterus, vulva, heart, gallbladder, gastrointestinal tract

Presentation
- CCMMT presents as painful abdominal mass
- Uterine examples manifest as uterine bleeding
- Most other categories of PEComas present as painless masses
- Brain tumors in patients with tuberous sclerosis present with seizures, developmental delay, behavioral problems

Treatment
- Surgical excision

Prognosis
- Most are benign
  - Rare documented examples of malignancy
    - Usually not in AML, LAM, or CCST types
    - Malignant examples behave as aggressive sarcomas

PECOMAS

Key Facts

Terminology

- Mesenchymal neoplasm composed of distinctive perivascular epithelioid cells (PEComa)
  - Includes angiomyolipoma (AML), clear cell "sugar" tumor of lung (CCST), lymphangioleiomyomatosis (LAM), clear cell myomelanocytic tumor of falciform ligament/ligamentum teres (CCMMT)

Etiology/Pathogenesis

- Only AML, CCST, and LAM are associated with tuberous sclerosis, but not other types

Clinical Issues

- Most are benign, but rare malignant cases reported
- Rare tumors overall; very rare in skin

Microscopic Pathology

- PEC cell component consists of epithelioid to spindled cells arranged around vessels extending outward radially
- Clear to granular, lightly eosinophilic cytoplasm and round to oval nuclei with small nucleoli
- Myoid component with densely eosinophilic cytoplasm
- Adipose tissue component present in lesions termed AML

Top Differential Diagnoses

- True smooth muscle tumors
- Renal cell carcinoma
- Clear cell sarcoma
- Melanoma

MICROSCOPIC PATHOLOGY

Histologic Features

- PEC cell component consists of epithelioid to spindled cells arranged around vessels extending outward radially
  - Clear to granular, lightly eosinophilic cytoplasm and round to oval nuclei with small nucleoli
  - Lesions are richly vascular
  - Small arching vessels divide tumor into packets (similar to pattern in renal cell carcinoma)
- Myoid component with densely eosinophilic cytoplasm
  - Nuclei less rounded than those of true smooth muscle
- Adipose tissue component present in lesions termed AML
- CCMMT is almost exclusively spindle cell lesion
  - Uniform moderate-sized cells set in elaborate lace-like vasculature

Rare Malignant Examples

- Criteria for malignancy
  - Infiltrative growth
  - Marked hypercellularity
  - Nuclear enlargement and hyperchromasia
  - Numerous &/or atypical mitotic figures
  - Necrosis

DIFFERENTIAL DIAGNOSIS

True Smooth Muscle Tumors

- Perpendicularly oriented fascicles of spindle cells with brightly eosinophilic cytoplasm and blunt-ended nuclei
  - Criteria for malignancy site specific and related to mitotic activity and nuclear atypia
- Intensely eosinophilic cytoplasm
- Usually lack adipose tissue component (exception is myolipoma)
- Lack PEC differentiation

- Most smooth muscle tumors lack melanocytic antigens and express desmin
- Lack rich vascular pattern (although some leiomyosarcomas arise in association with vessels)
- Some examples are associated with Epstein-Barr virus

Renal Cell Carcinoma

- Clear epithelial cells and rich vascular pattern
  - Sarcomatoid examples overtly high-grade neoplasms
- Usually displays epithelial markers by immunohistochemistry
- Lacks adipose tissue component

Clear Cell Sarcoma

- Usually involves feet and hands of young adults
- Consists of highly uniform cells with clear cytoplasm and uniform nuclei with single large nucleolus
  - Packeted arrangement with groups of cells separated by slender connective tissue septa
- Most examples express S100 protein
- Soft tissue examples express melanocytic markers
  - Subset of visceral examples only express S100 protein but not melanocytic markers
    - This relates to *EWS-CREB1* fusion in visceral examples (in contrast with *EWS-ATF1* fusion in other cases)
- Lack CD117 expression
- No adipose tissue component of myoid component
- Vessels inconspicuous

Melanoma

- Can be spindled to epithelioid
- Marked cytologic atypia with prominent nucleoli is rule
- Some cases display melanin pigment
- Large lesions highly aggressive clinically
- Label with S100 protein
  - Melanocytic markers expressed in most classic examples, negative in spindled lesions
- Vessels inconspicuous

Well-Differentiated Liposarcoma

- Extremely rare in skin

Immunohistochemistry

Antibody	Reactivity	Staining Pattern	Comment
HMB-45	Positive	Cytoplasmic	
Mart-1	Positive	Cytoplasmic	
Tyrosinase	Positive	Cytoplasmic	
MITF	Positive	Nuclear	
α-1-antichymotrypsin	Positive	Cytoplasmic	
HCAD	Positive	Cytoplasmic	
Calponin	Positive	Cytoplasmic	
CD117	Positive	Cell membrane & cytoplasm	
S100	Negative		
CK-PAN	Negative		
Desmin	Equivocal	Cytoplasmic	Often weak and focal

- Shows fat punctuated by atypical nuclei
  - Fibrous septa containing enlarged hyperchromatic nuclei
  - Can have areas of dedifferentiation to high-grade sarcoma
    - Overt high-grade spindle cell sarcoma with numerous mitoses and atypical nuclei
- Most examples not richly vascular
- Show nuclear MDM2 or CDK4 immunolabeling
  - Negative melanocytic markers

Intramuscular Hemangioma

- Capillary or cavernous vascular lesion
- Often has abundant overgrowth of mature adipose tissue
- No spindle cell component
- No immunolabeling with melanocytic markers

Metastatic Gastrointestinal Stromal Tumor

- Epithelioid or spindle cell neoplasms usually involving muscularis propria of gastrointestinal tract
  - Cytoplasmic vacuoles common
  - Cytoplasm eosinophilic
  - Uniform nuclei
  - CD117 immunolabeling and *KIT* mutations in most cases
    - Variable immunolabeling with smooth muscle markers
    - Usually negative for melanocytic markers (some have focal MART-1/Melan-A)
- Lack adipose tissue component and clear cells
- Vessels inconspicuous

Metastatic Hepatocellular Carcinoma

- Large atypical cells with opaque eosinophilic cytoplasm, rich vascularity
- Usually has marked nuclear pleomorphism
- Expresses epithelial markers (CAM5.2), sometimes Hep-Par1
  - Canalicular pattern on immunolabeling with CD10 or polyclonal CEA
- No adipose tissue component
- Some examples have cytoplasmic bile

SELECTED REFERENCES

1. Sukov WR et al: Perivascular epithelioid cell tumor (PEComa) of the urinary bladder: report of 3 cases and review of the literature. Am J Surg Pathol. 33(2):304-8, 2009
2. Hornick JL et al: Sclerosing PEComa: clinicopathologic analysis of a distinctive variant with a predilection for the retroperitoneum. Am J Surg Pathol. 32(4):493-501, 2008
3. Liegl B et al: Primary cutaneous PEComa: distinctive clear cell lesions of skin. Am J Surg Pathol. 32(4):608-14, 2008
4. Martignoni G et al: PEComas: the past, the present and the future. Virchows Arch. 452(2):119-32, 2008
5. Fine SW et al: Angiomyolipoma with epithelial cysts (AMLEC): a distinct cystic variant of angiomyolipoma. Am J Surg Pathol. 30(5):593-9, 2006
6. Folpe AL et al: Perivascular epithelioid cell neoplasms of soft tissue and gynecologic origin: a clinicopathologic study of 26 cases and review of the literature. Am J Surg Pathol. 29(12):1558-75, 2005
7. Harris GC et al: Malignant perivascular epithelioid cell tumour ("PEComa") of soft tissue: a unique case. Am J Surg Pathol. 28(12):1655-8, 2004
8. Vang R et al: Perivascular epithelioid cell tumor ('PEComa') of the uterus: a subset of HMB-45-positive epithelioid mesenchymal neoplasms with an uncertain relationship to pure smooth muscle tumors. Am J Surg Pathol. 26(1):1-13, 2002
9. Folpe AL et al: Clear cell myomelanocytic tumor of the falciform ligament/ligamentum teres: a novel member of the perivascular epithelioid clear cell family of tumors with a predilection for children and young adults. Am J Surg Pathol. 24(9):1239-46, 2000
10. L'Hostis H et al: Renal angiomyolipoma: a clinicopathologic, immunohistochemical, and follow-up study of 46 cases. Am J Surg Pathol. 23(9):1011-20, 1999
11. Tsui WM et al: Hepatic angiomyolipoma: a clinicopathologic study of 30 cases and delineation of unusual morphologic variants. Am J Surg Pathol. 23(1):34-48, 1999
12. Pea M et al: Apparent renal cell carcinomas in tuberous sclerosis are heterogeneous: the identification of malignant epithelioid angiomyolipoma. Am J Surg Pathol. 22(2):180-7, 1998
13. Eble JN et al: Epithelioid angiomyolipoma of the kidney: a report of five cases with a prominent and diagnostically confusing epithelioid smooth muscle component. Am J Surg Pathol. 21(10):1123-30, 1997

Microscopic and Immunohistochemical Features

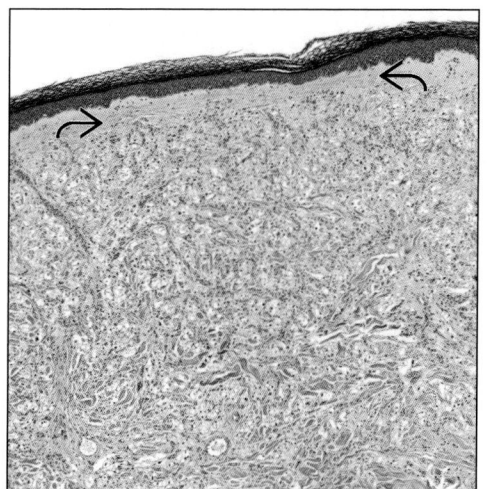

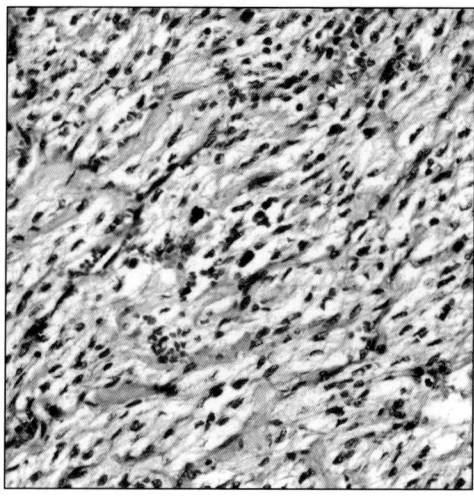

(Left) Primary cutaneous PEComa shows a dermal-based clear cell neoplasm associated with numerous small blood vessels. This tumor diffusely involved the dermis and extended into the subcutaneous adipose tissue. Note the grenz zone separating the tumor from the overlying epidermis ➫. *(Right)* Histologic examination shows a clear cell pattern in PEComa with numerous fibrovascular channels between spindled and epithelioid clear cells.

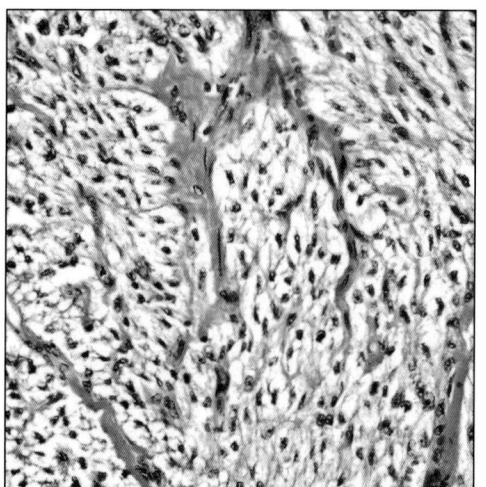

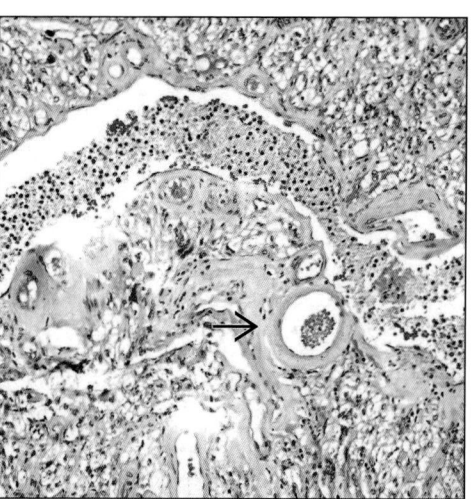

(Left) PEComa often shows a "packeted" appearance formed by fibrovascular separations between bundles of proliferating cells. This pattern is reminiscent of that of renal cell carcinoma or clear cell sarcoma. *(Right)* Higher magnification shows the lesional cells surrounding disorganized, medium-sized vessels ➡.

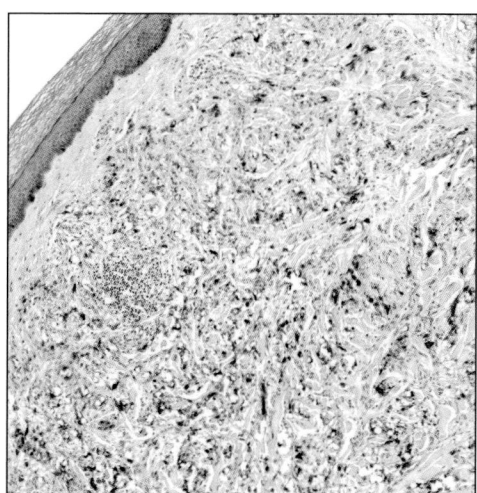

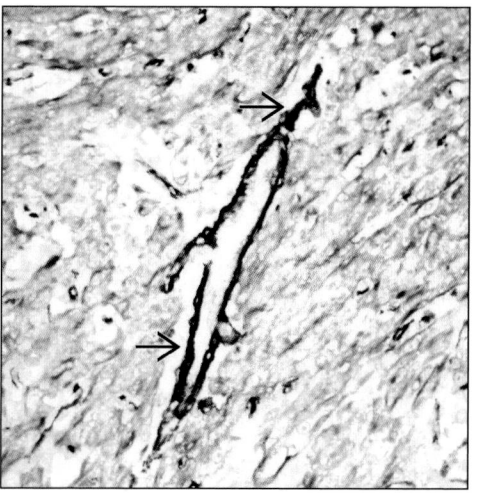

(Left) HMB-45 shows scattered strong cytoplasmic expression in a primary cutaneous PEComa. These lesions also express other markers of melanocytic differentiation, as well as CD117, but typically lack S100 protein and keratin expression. *(Right)* Actin-HHF-35 shows cytoplasmic labeling in a PEComa. Note that the internal control (vessel wall ➡) labels more intensely.

KAPOSI SARCOMA

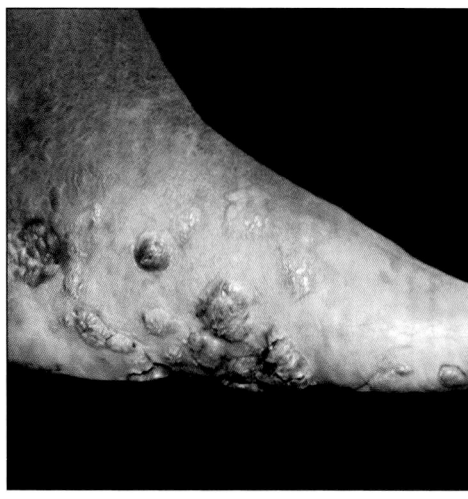

Clinical photograph shows a case of classic Kaposi sarcoma arising in an elderly man who presented with multiple nodular lesions.

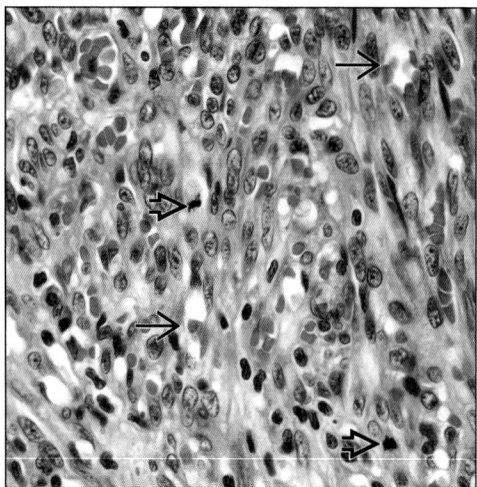

High-power view shows bland tumor cells containing uniform spindled nuclei. Despite the lack of atypia, mitoses are easily found ⊵. Small sieve-like spaces containing erythrocytes are present ⊵.

TERMINOLOGY

Abbreviations
- Kaposi sarcoma (KS)

Definitions
- Locally aggressive endothelial neoplasm associated with human herpes virus 8 (HHV8)

ETIOLOGY/PATHOGENESIS

Infectious Agents
- Associated with HHV8 virus
  - Found in all forms of disease
  - Detected in peripheral blood

CLINICAL ISSUES

Site
- Most typical site of involvement is skin
- Mucosal membranes, lymph nodes, and visceral organs may be affected

Natural History
- 4 main clinical and epidemiologic forms are recognized
  - **Classic indolent form**
    - Occurs predominantly in elderly men of Mediterranean/East European descent
    - Purplish, reddish-blue, dark brown plaques and nodules
    - Usually in distal extremities
  - **Endemic African form**
    - Occurs in middle-aged adults and children in equatorial Africa
    - Patients are not infected by HIV
  - **Iatrogenic form**
    - Occurs in patients treated with immunosuppressive agents
  - **AIDS-associated form**
    - Occurs in patients infected by HIV
    - Most common and most aggressive form
    - Lesions are seen on face, genitals, lower extremities
    - Mucosal membranes, lymph nodes, and visceral organs are frequently involved

Treatment
- Options, risks, complications
  - Chemotherapy &/or radiotherapy
  - Cryotherapy may be useful
- Surgical approaches
  - Surgical treatment of single lesions only

Prognosis
- Classic indolent form
  - Indolent clinical course
  - Lymph node and visceral organ involvement occurs only infrequently
- Endemic African form
  - Protracted clinical course
  - Lymphadenopathic form is progressive and highly lethal
- Iatrogenic form
  - May resolve entirely after withdrawal of immunosuppressive treatment
- AIDS-associated form
  - Most aggressive type of KS
  - May respond to HIV treatment
- Prognosis depends on epidemiological/clinical type of KS
- Prognosis is strongly related to stage of disease and additional infectious diseases

MACROSCOPIC FEATURES

General Features
- Skin lesions range in size from very small to several centimeters

KAPOSI SARCOMA

Key Facts

Terminology

- Locally aggressive endothelial neoplasm associated with human herpes virus 8

Clinical Issues

- Most typical site of involvement is skin
- Mucosal membranes, lymph nodes, and visceral organs may be affected
- 4 main different clinical and epidemiologic forms are recognized
  ○ Classic indolent form
  ○ Endemic African form
  ○ Iatrogenic form
  ○ AIDS-associated form (most common and aggressive)
- Prognosis depends on epidemiological-clinical type

Macroscopic Features

- Skin lesions range in size from very small to several centimeters

Microscopic Pathology

- Histologic features of all forms of KS do not differ
- KS shows different stages of disease
- Patch stage of KS
  ○ Increased vascular spaces in reticular dermis
  ○ Scattered lymphocytes and plasma cells
- Plaque stage of KS
  ○ More extensive vascular proliferation
- Nodular stage of KS
  ○ Well-circumscribed, cellular nodules
  ○ Intersecting fascicles of spindled tumor cells
  ○ Numerous mitoses

- Hemorrhagic nodules of variable size in visceral organs and lymph nodes

MICROSCOPIC PATHOLOGY

Histologic Features

- Histologic features of all forms of KS are similar
- KS shows different stages of disease
- **Patch stage of KS**
  ○ Increased vascular spaces in reticular dermis
    ■ Papillary dermis is not involved in early stages
  ○ Vascular spaces dissect collagen bundles
  ○ Perivascular and periadnexal growth of vascular spaces
  ○ Vascular spaces are lined by flattened, uniform endothelial cells
  ○ Scattered lymphocytes and plasma cells
  ○ Extravasated erythrocytes and hemosiderin deposits
- **Plaque stage of KS**
  ○ More extensive vascular proliferation
  ○ Denser inflammatory infiltrate
  ○ Hyaline globules representing destroyed erythrocytes may be found
- **Nodular stage of KS**
  ○ Well-circumscribed, cellular nodules
  ○ Intersecting cellular fascicles of spindled tumor cells
  ○ Slit- and sieve-like spaces containing erythrocytes
  ○ Mild cytologic atypia
  ○ Numerous mitoses
- Some patients develop lymphangiomatous lesions &/or hemangiomatous lesions

Cytologic Features

- Typically bland-appearing flattened and spindled endothelial tumor cells

DIFFERENTIAL DIAGNOSIS

Hobnail Hemangioma

- Solitary vascular lesions
- Biphasic growth

○ Dilated vessels in superficial parts, narrow vascular spaces in deeper parts of dermis
- Hobnail endothelial cells
- HHV8(-)

Capillary Hemangioma

- Distinctive clinical findings
- Lobular growth of narrow capillaries
- HHV8(-)

Lymphangioma

- Common pediatric lesions
- Rather well-circumscribed lesions
- Dilated vascular spaces
- Usually no inflammatory infiltrate
- HHV8(-)

Progressive Lymphangioma (Benign Lymphangioendothelioma)

- Slowly growing, solitary, plaque-like lesions
- No spindled tumor cells
- No prominent inflammatory infiltrate
- HHV8(-)

Spindle Cell Hemangioma

- Combination of KS-like features with cavernous hemangioma-like features
- No increased mitoses in spindled tumor cells
- Scattered epithelioid tumor cells
- HHV8(-)

Kaposiform Hemangioendothelioma

- Occurs usually in infants and young children
- Often in retroperitoneal and abdominal location
- Only rarely in skin of adult patients
- Infiltrative, cellular lobules
- No increased number of mitoses
- HHV8(-)

Cutaneous Angiosarcoma

- Different clinical findings
- Anastomosing vascular structures
- Prominent nuclear atypia

KAPOSI SARCOMA

Immunohistochemistry

Antibody	Reactivity	Staining Pattern	Comment
CD31	Positive	Cell membrane & cytoplasm	
CD34	Positive	Cell membrane & cytoplasm	
HHV8	Positive	Nuclear	> 90% of cases
FLI-1	Positive	Nuclear	
Actin-sm	Negative		Only around larger, preexisting vessels

- Endothelial multilayering
- HHV8(-)

Microvenular Hemangioma
- Usually solitary vascular lesions
- Narrow vascular structures
- Dermal fibrosis
- Complete rim of actin(+) myopericytes
- HHV8(-)

Lymphangiomatosis (of Limbs)
- Solitary, large, plaque-like lesions
- No increased number of mitoses
- No prominent inflammatory infiltrate
- HHV8(-)

Tufted Hemangioma
- Cannonball distribution of vascular tufts
- CD31(+) endothelial cells are completely surrounded by actin(+) myopericytes
- Crescent-shaped clefts
- HHV8(-)

DIAGNOSTIC CHECKLIST

Clinically Relevant Pathologic Features
- Age, ethnic distribution
- Gross appearance
- Organ distribution

Pathologic Interpretation Pearls
- All clinical forms of KS follow similar morphologic stages
- Dissecting narrow vascular spaces, inflammatory cells, and hemosiderin deposits are useful findings in early stages of KS
- HHV8 immunohistochemical antibodies represent specific and sensitive marker for KS

SELECTED REFERENCES
1. Sharma-Walia N et al: Kaposi's sarcoma associated herpes virus (KSHV) induced COX-2: a key factor in latency, inflammation, angiogenesis, cell survival and invasion. PLoS Pathog. 6(2):e1000777, 2010
2. O'Hara CD et al: Endothelial lesions of soft tissues: a review of reactive and neoplastic entities with emphasis on low-grade malignant ("borderline") vascular tumors. Adv Anat Pathol. 10(2):69-87, 2003
3. Folpe AL et al: Expression of Fli-1, a nuclear transcription factor, distinguishes vascular neoplasms from potential mimics. Am J Surg Pathol. 25(8):1061-6, 2001
4. Goedert JJ: The epidemiology of acquired immunodeficiency syndrome malignancies. Semin Oncol. 27(4):390-401, 2000
5. Guillou L et al: Benign lymphangioendothelioma (acquired progressive lymphangioma): a lesion not to be confused with well-differentiated angiosarcoma and patch stage Kaposi's sarcoma: clinicopathologic analysis of a series. Am J Surg Pathol. 24(8):1047-57, 2000
6. Reed JA et al: Demonstration of Kaposi's sarcoma-associated herpes virus cyclin D homolog in cutaneous Kaposi's sarcoma by colorimetric in situ hybridization using a catalyzed signal amplification system. Blood. 91(10):3825-32, 1998
7. Borroni G et al: Bullous lesions in Kaposi's sarcoma: case report. Am J Dermatopathol. 19(4):379-83, 1997
8. Cossu S et al: Lymphangioma-like variant of Kaposi's sarcoma: clinicopathologic study of seven cases with review of the literature. Am J Dermatopathol. 19(1):16-22, 1997
9. Perniciaro C et al: Familial Kaposi's sarcoma. Cutis. 57(4):220-2, 1996
10. Ioachim HL et al: Kaposi's sarcoma of internal organs. A multiparameter study of 86 cases. Cancer. 75(6):1376-85, 1995
11. Chang Y et al: Identification of herpesvirus-like DNA sequences in AIDS-associated Kaposi's sarcoma. Science. 266(5192):1865-9, 1994
12. Tappero JW et al: Kaposi's sarcoma. Epidemiology, pathogenesis, histology, clinical spectrum, staging criteria and therapy. J Am Acad Dermatol. 28(3):371-95, 1993
13. Nickoloff BJ: The human progenitor cell antigen (CD34) is localized on endothelial cells, dermal dendritic cells, and perifollicular cells in formalin-fixed normal skin, and on proliferating endothelial cells and stromal spindle-shaped cells in Kaposi's sarcoma. Arch Dermatol. 127(4):523-9, 1991
14. Kao GF et al: The nature of hyaline (eosinophilic) globules and vascular slits of Kaposi's sarcoma. Am J Dermatopathol. 12(3):256-67, 1990
15. Dictor M: Kaposi's sarcoma. Origin and significance of lymphaticovenous connections. Virchows Arch A Pathol Anat Histopathol. 409(1):23-35, 1986

KAPOSI SARCOMA

Clinical and Microscopic Features

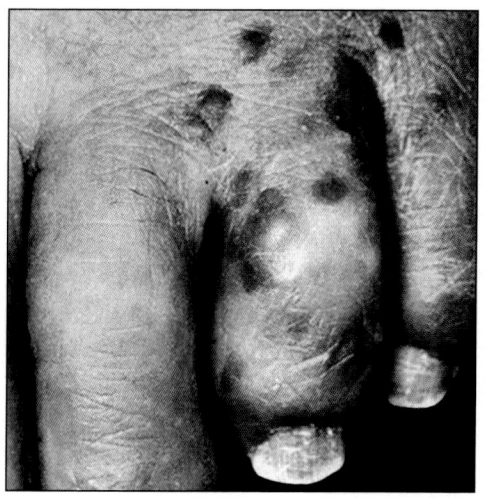

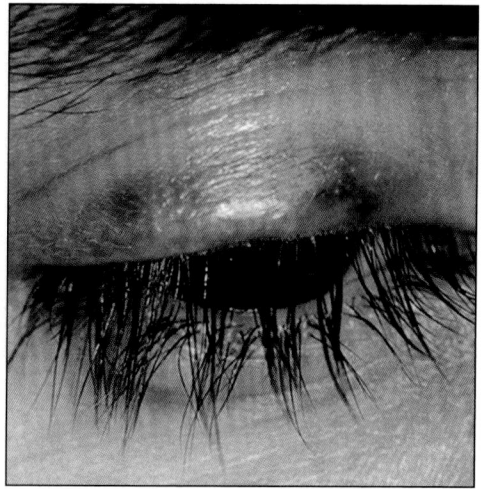

(Left) Early forms of Kaposi sarcoma may cause diagnostic problems. This elderly patient developed multiple small lesions on the toe. Small, slightly elevated, relatively circumscribed brown papules are noted. (Right) Patients with AIDS-related Kaposi sarcoma may present with lesions at unusual anatomic sites, as did this young patient who developed small reddish lesions on his upper eyelid.

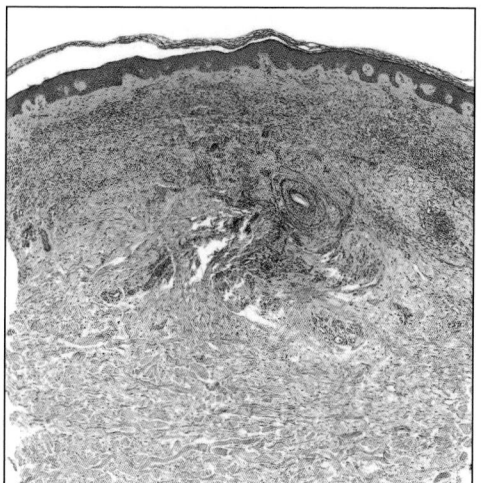

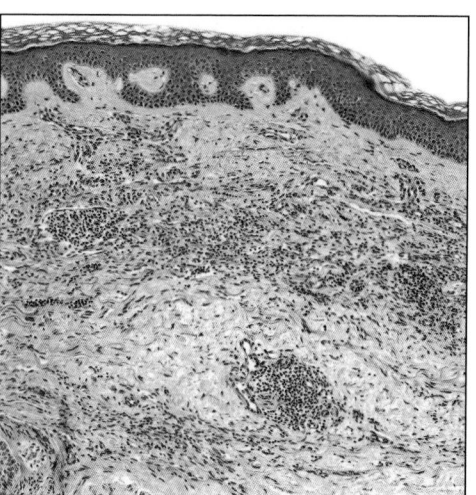

(Left) In early lesions of Kaposi sarcoma, flat, plaque-like lesions are seen. Note that the upper part of the papillary dermis is not involved, which represents an important finding to differentiate from other vascular lesions. (Right) Early lesions of Kaposi sarcoma show a proliferation of thin-walled vessels associated with scattered spindle cells and numerous inflammatory cells.

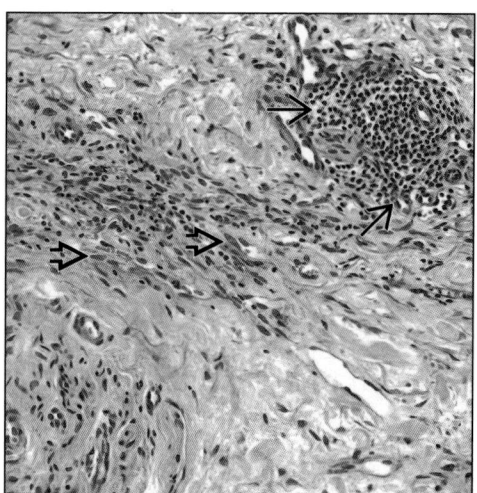

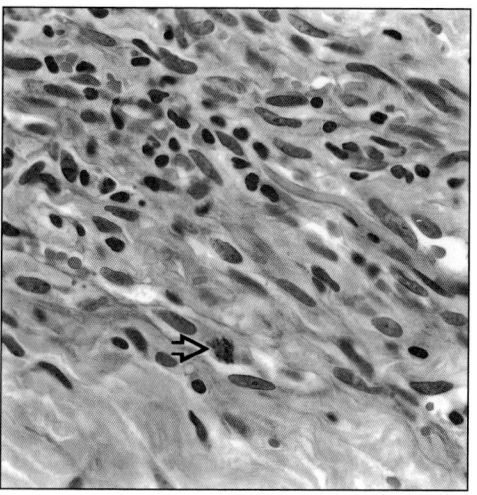

(Left) Dissecting spindle cells ⊃ are associated with numerous inflammatory cells that are arranged in small clusters ⊃ or diffusely between the proliferating spindled cells. (Right) On higher power examination, narrow vascular spaces and cytologically bland spindled cells are seen. Note the presence of inflammatory cells and scattered mitoses ⊃ in the spindled tumor cells.

Microscopic Features and Ancillary Techniques

(Left) The inflammatory infiltrate in Kaposi sarcoma usually contains a number of plasma cells ⮕. In addition, narrow vascular spaces and scattered spindled cells are present. *(Right)* Especially in early lesions of Kaposi sarcoma, the nuclear staining of endothelial cells for HHV8 is very helpful for making the correct diagnosis.

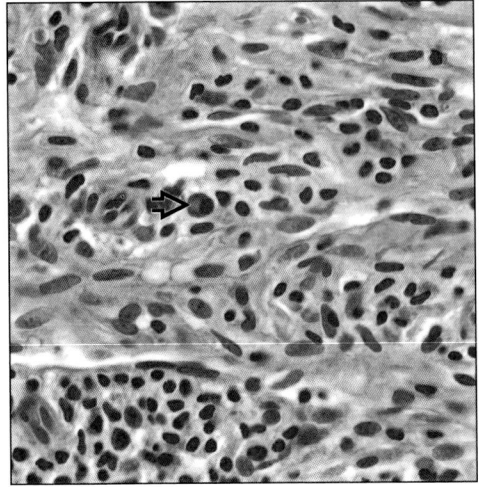
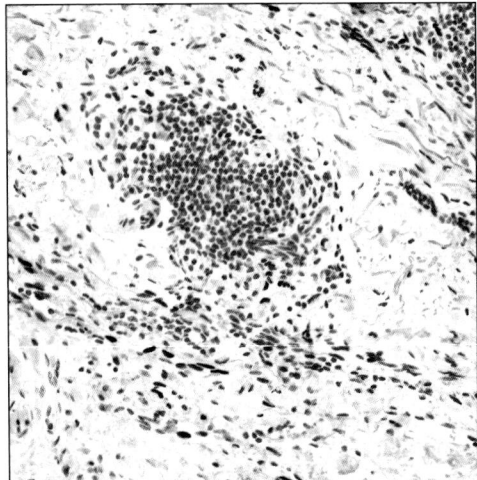

(Left) A very early form of Kaposi sarcoma shows scattered spindled cells, dilated and narrow vascular spaces, as well as a few inflammatory cells set in a slightly fibrosed dermal tissue. *(Right)* Iron staining reveals abundant hemosiderin deposits, which represent an important finding in early forms of Kaposi sarcoma.

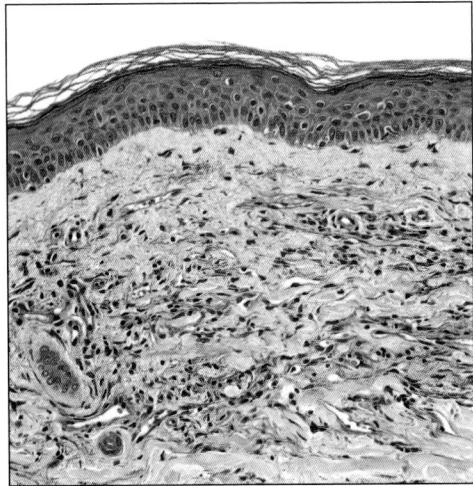
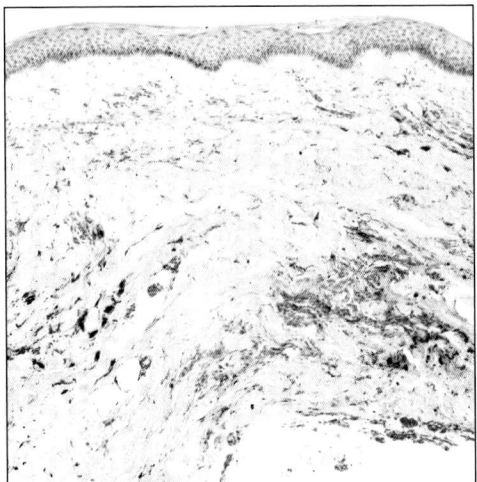

(Left) KS can mimic a pyogenic granuloma in some cases. This example shows an exophytic, ulcerated, and cellular lesion arising on the foot of an elderly male patient with nodular stage Kaposi sarcoma. *(Right)* Higher power view reveals cellular bundles and fascicles of spindle cells, as well as slit-like and sieve-like vascular spaces containing numerous erythrocytes.

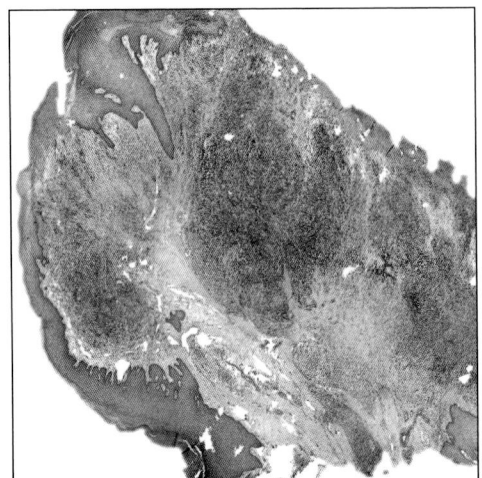
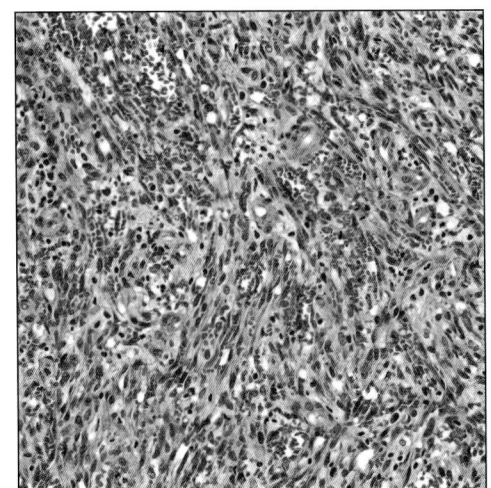

KAPOSI SARCOMA

Microscopic and Immunohistochemical Features

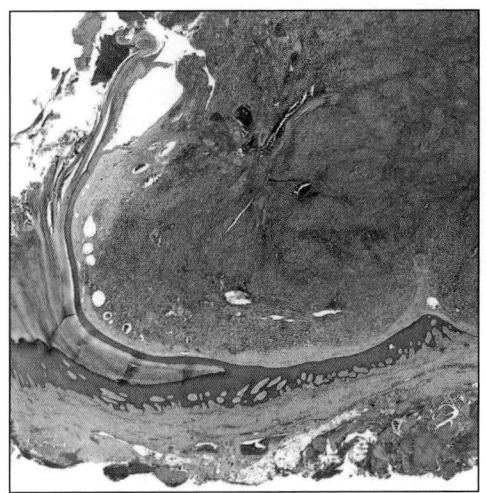
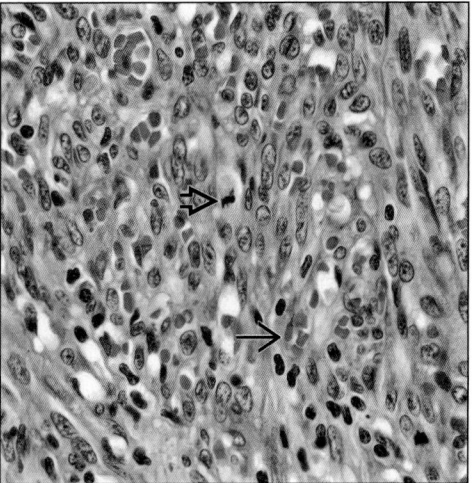

(Left) Low-power view of nodular stage of Kaposi sarcoma shows a well-circumscribed exophytic nodular lesion with ulceration of the epidermis. *(Right)* High-power view shows cytologically bland spindled tumor cells containing uniform spindled nuclei. Despite the lack of atypia, mitoses are easily found ➤. Small, sieve-like spaces that contain erythrocytes ➔ are seen between the spindled cells.

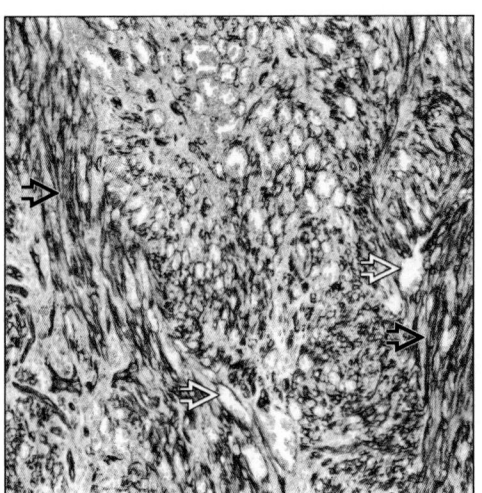
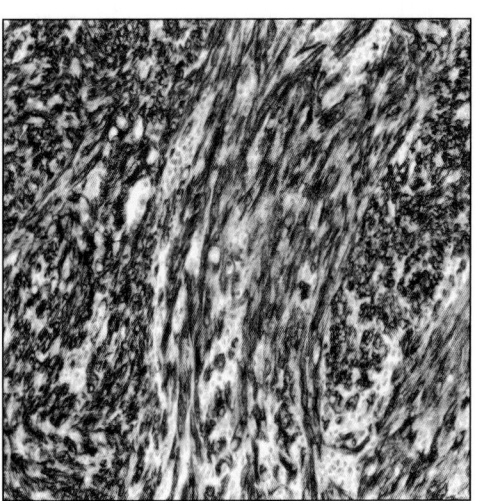

(Left) Tumor cells stain positively for the endothelial marker CD31. In addition to cellular spindle cell fascicles ➤, small vascular spaces lined by CD31(+) endothelial cells are noted ➤. *(Right)* Strong, homogeneous expression of CD34 by neoplastic cells is seen in this example of nodular Kaposi sarcoma.

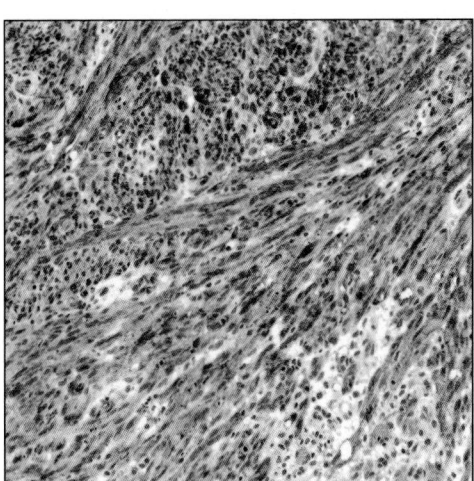
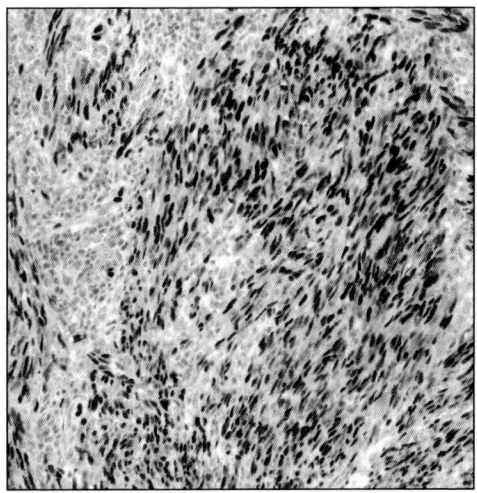

(Left) Expression of podoplanin by neoplastic cells is usually seen in cases of Kaposi sarcoma and can be shown by immunohistochemistry using antibody D2-40. *(Right)* The nuclear staining of tumor cells for HHV8 as shown here is diagnostic for Kaposi sarcoma.

KAPOSIFORM HEMANGIOENDOTHELIOMA

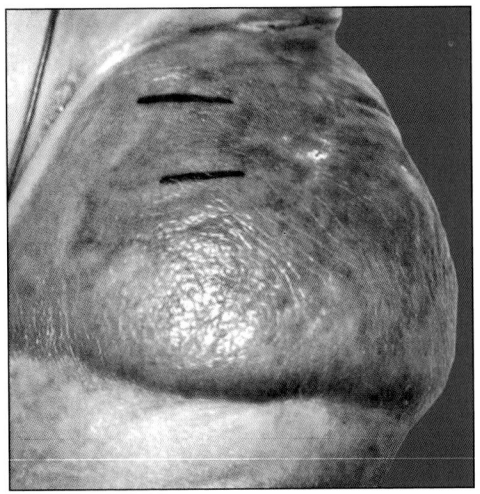

Clinical photograph shows a large inguinal tumor in an infant. More superficial tumors typically present as an erythematous or violaceous mass.

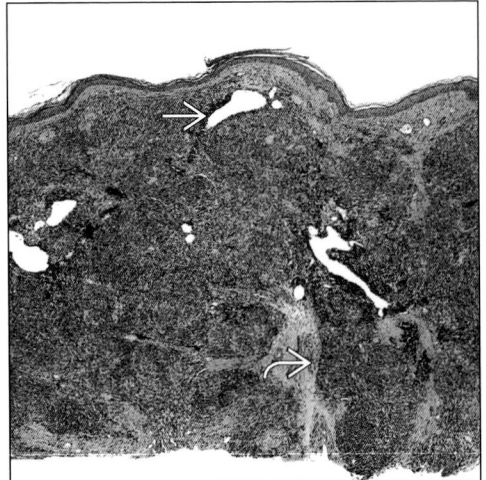

The tumor is composed of irregular nodules ➡ of spindled endothelial cells. At the periphery of the nodules, ectatic vessels ➡ are often present.

ETIOLOGY/PATHOGENESIS

Developmental Anomaly
- Approximately 1/2 of kaposiform hemangioendothelioma cases present in 1st year of life

CLINICAL ISSUES

Epidemiology
- Age
  - Majority present in childhood to teen years

Presentation
- Painful or painless mass
  - Presents as superficial or deep mass
  - Cutaneous lesions present as violaceous plaques
  - Deep tumors, often multiple nodules
- Systemic symptoms
  - Associated with Kasabach-Merritt phenomenon (especially retroperitoneal tumors)
    - Consumptive coagulopathy
    - Thrombocytopenia
    - Majority of all cases of Kasabach-Merritt phenomenon associated with kaposiform hemangioendothelioma

Treatment
- Surgical approaches
  - Wide excision
- Drugs
  - Vincristine, cyclophosphamide, methotrexate, α-interferon

Prognosis
- Rare regional lymph node metastasis
- No distant metastasis
- Mortality approximately 10%, related to local effects of tumor or Kasabach-Merritt phenomenon

MICROSCOPIC PATHOLOGY

Histologic Features
- Multinodular growth pattern
- Spindled areas resembling Kaposi sarcoma
- Capillary hemangioma-like areas with telangiectatic vessels
- Mitoses present, but minimal atypia

Predominant Cell/Compartment Type
- Endothelial

ANCILLARY TESTS

Immunohistochemistry
- Positive for CD31, CD34, FLI-1, and podoplanin (especially in peripheral lymphatic component)
- Negative for GLUT1 (+ in juvenile hemangioma)

DIFFERENTIAL DIAGNOSIS

Tufted Hemangioma (Acquired Tufted Angioma)
- Clinical features
  - Similar demographics as kaposiform hemangioendothelioma
    - Most cases present in children
    - Occasional cases in adults
  - Often associated with Kasabach-Merritt phenomenon
- Microscopic features
  - Nodular proliferation of closely packed capillaries in dermis ("cannonball" pattern)
  - Bland oval to spindled endothelial cells
- May represent part of kaposiform hemangioendothelioma spectrum

KAPOSIFORM HEMANGIOENDOTHELIOMA

Key Facts

Clinical Issues
- Presents in infants and young children
- Deep tumors, often multiple nodules
- Associated with Kasabach-Merritt phenomenon (especially retroperitoneal tumors)
  - Consumptive coagulopathy
  - Thrombocytopenia
- Rare regional lymph node metastases
- No distant metastases reported to date

- Mortality approximately 10%, related to local effects of tumor or Kasabach-Merritt phenomenon

Microscopic Pathology
- Spindled cell areas resembling Kaposi sarcoma
- Zones resembling capillary hemangiomas
- Minimal atypia
- Immunohistochemistry shows positive CD31, CD34, FLI-1, and podoplanin staining
- Negative for HHV8

Kaposi Sarcoma
- Clinical features
  - Immunocompromised and older patients
- Microscopic features
  - Early Kaposi sarcoma shows neoplastic spindle cells and slit-like vessels dissecting through dermal collagen
  - Later lesions show solid spindle cell areas
  - Lacks capillary hemangioma-like areas
  - Positive for HHV8 nuclear antigen

Spindle Cell Hemangioma
- Clinical features
  - Occurs in adults
  - Distal extremities
- Microscopic features
  - Often partially intravascular
  - Ectatic vessels
  - Spindled cells
  - Vacuolated endothelial cells
    - So-called "blister cells"
  - May have areas of thrombosis or phleboliths

DIAGNOSTIC CHECKLIST

Clinically Relevant Pathologic Features
- Age distribution
  - Vast majority occur in children
- Symptom complex
  - Kasabach-Merritt phenomenon

Pathologic Interpretation Pearls
- Vascular tumor in children composed predominantly of spindled endothelial cells

SELECTED REFERENCES

1. Debelenko LV et al: D2-40 immunohistochemical analysis of pediatric vascular tumors reveals positivity in kaposiform hemangioendothelioma. Mod Pathol. 18(11):1454-60, 2005
2. Lyons LL et al: Kaposiform hemangioendothelioma: a study of 33 cases emphasizing its pathologic, immunophenotypic, and biologic uniqueness from juvenile hemangioma. Am J Surg Pathol. 28(5):559-68, 2004
3. Chu CY et al: Transformation between Kaposiform hemangioendothelioma and tufted angioma. Dermatology. 206(4):334-7, 2003
4. Mac-Moune Lai F et al: Kaposiform hemangioendothelioma: five patients with cutaneous lesion and long follow-up. Mod Pathol. 14(11):1087-92, 2001
5. Mentzel T et al: Kaposiform hemangioendothelioma in adults. Clinicopathologic and immunohistochemical analysis of three cases. Am J Clin Pathol. 108(4):450-5, 1997
6. Zukerberg LR et al: Kaposiform hemangioendothelioma of infancy and childhood. An aggressive neoplasm associated with Kasabach-Merritt syndrome and lymphangiomatosis. Am J Surg Pathol. 17(4):321-8, 1993

IMAGE GALLERY

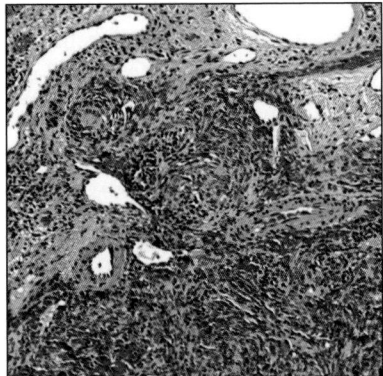 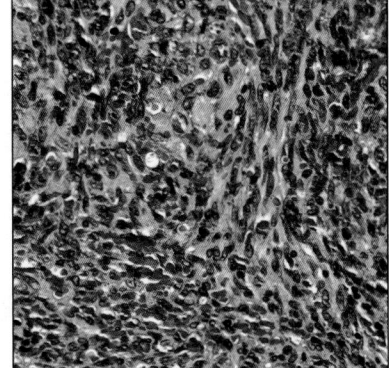 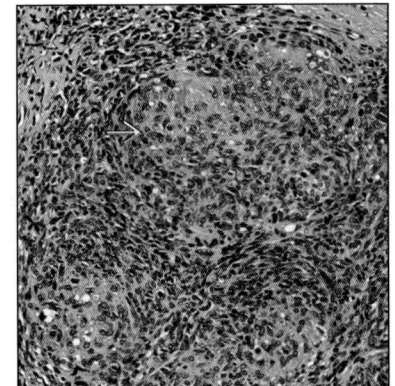

(Left) In the upper left side of the image, the dilated vessels are reminiscent of a capillary hemangioma. The lower portion demonstrates the more solid spindled cell component. (Center) The tumor cells have uniform hyperchromatic spindled nuclei and are arranged in short fascicles with slit-like vascular lumina. (Right) In some areas, the spindled tumor cells can have a somewhat swirling growth pattern, imparting a glomeruloid ➡ appearance.

EPITHELIOID HEMANGIOENDOTHELIOMA

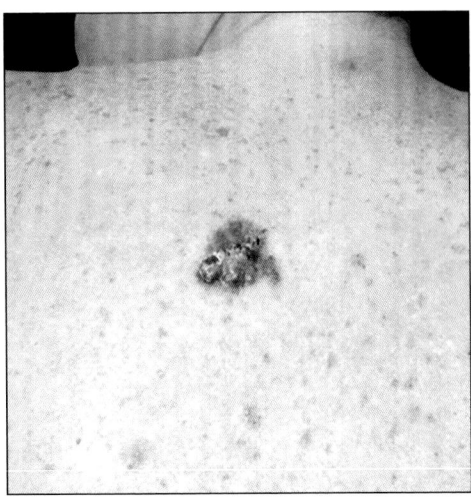

This clinical photograph shows an unusual example of cutaneous epithelioid hemangioendothelioma presenting as a single, discolored, exophytic lesion on the upper back in an adult.

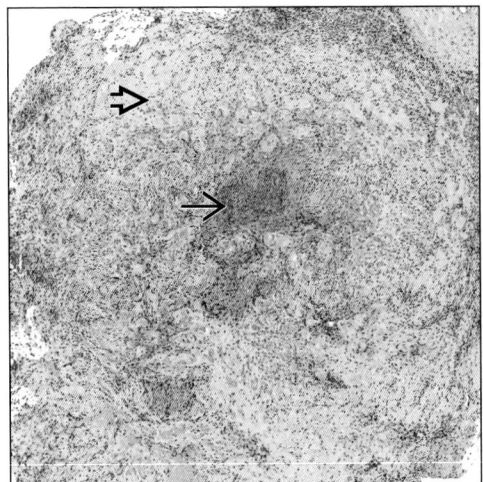

Low-magnification view shows epithelioid hemangioendothelioma with cords of cells ➣ infiltrating the vessel wall and extending into adjacent tissues. The lumen ➣ is filled with thrombotic debris.

TERMINOLOGY

Abbreviations
- Epithelioid hemangioendothelioma (EHE)

Definitions
- Angiocentric vascular neoplasm with metastatic potential, composed of epithelioid endothelial cells

CLINICAL ISSUES

Epidemiology
- Incidence
  - Rare vascular tumor
- Age
  - All age groups, but rare in children
- Gender
  - M = F

Site
- Skin (rare), superficial or deep soft tissue
- Extremities, head and neck, viscera (often multicentric)

Presentation
- Painful mass
- Solitary mass
- Multicentric in a number of cases
- Edema in some cases
- Occlusion of vessels
  - Due to tumor origin in/association with preexisting vessels
  - Can result in ischemic or venous obstructive symptoms

Treatment
- Surgical approaches
  - Wide local excision with clear margins

Prognosis
- Behavior intermediate between hemangioma and angiosarcoma
- Local recurrence rate 10-15%
- Metastatic rate 20-30%, mortality 10-20%
- Superficial cases have better prognosis
- Adverse prognostic factors
  - > 3 mitoses per 50 high-power fields
  - Tumor size > 3 cm

MACROSCOPIC FEATURES

General Features
- Well-circumscribed nodular lesion
- Intravascular mass resembling organizing thrombus

MICROSCOPIC PATHOLOGY

Histologic Features
- Expansion of vessels in angiocentric cases
- Centrifugal extension into soft tissues
- Short strands, cords, solid nests, single cells
- Rare obvious vascular channels
- Bland round to spindled endothelial tumor cells
- Vesicular nuclei, small nucleoli, rare mitoses
- Intracytoplasmic vacuoles, some with red cells
- Myxohyaline or chondroid stroma
- Stromal calcification or ossification in some cases
- Occasionally osteoclast-like giant cells
- Atypical features in ~ 1/3 of cases
  - Increased cellularity with solid nests
  - Marked nuclear atypia, prominent nucleoli
  - Spindling of tumor cells, mitoses, necrosis

ANCILLARY TESTS

Cytogenetics
- t(1;3)(p36.3;q25) in some

EPITHELIOID HEMANGIOENDOTHELIOMA

Key Facts

Terminology

- Vascular neoplasm with metastatic potential composed of epithelioid endothelial cells

Clinical Issues

- Rare vascular tumor
- Superficial or deep soft tissue
  - Rare in skin
- ~ 50% associated with preexisting vessel
- Behavior intermediate between hemangioma and angiosarcoma
  - Metastatic rate (20-30%)
  - Mortality (10-20%)
- Painful mass
- All age groups
- Wide local excision with clear margins
- Adverse prognostic factors
  - > 3 mitoses per 50 high-power fields
  - Tumor size > 3 cm

Macroscopic Features

- Well-circumscribed nodular lesion

Microscopic Pathology

- Rare obvious vascular channels
- Short strands, cords, solid nests, or single cells
- Bland, epithelioid, round, or slightly spindled endothelial cells
- Intracytoplasmic lumina
  - Can contain red blood cells
- Myxohyaline, chondroid-like stroma
- Expression of endothelial markers
  - CD31, CD34, FLI-1
- Some cases are cytokeratin positive

Immunohistochemistry

Antibody	Reactivity	Staining Pattern	Comment
CD31	Positive	Cell membrane & cytoplasm	
CD34	Positive	Cell membrane & cytoplasm	Not specific
FLI-1	Positive	Nuclear	
CK-PAN	Positive	Cytoplasmic	In ~ 20-25% of cases
EMA	Equivocal	Cell membrane & cytoplasm	In ~ 10% of cases

DIFFERENTIAL DIAGNOSIS

Epithelioid Hemangioma

- Lobular architecture, well-formed vascular channels
- Mixed inflammatory infiltrate with eosinophils
- Well-formed vascular channels with SMA positive pericytes

Epithelioid Angiosarcoma

- Sheets of atypical endothelial tumor cells
- Irregular infiltrating vascular channels
- Increased cellularity, atypia and mitoses, necrosis

Myoepithelioma

- Epithelial differentiation with variable CK and EMA expression
- No angiocentric growth
- S100 positivity in most cases

Metastatic Carcinoma

- Clinical findings distinctive
- Higher degree of atypia
- CK, EMA positive, CD34 & CD31 negative

Extraskeletal Myxoid Chondrosarcoma

- Well-demarcated neoplasm, fibrous pseudocapsule
- Gelatinous nodules separated by fibrous septa
- Hypovascular stroma
- Can be focally positive for S100
- t(9;22)(q22;q12) or t(9;17)(q22;q11) in most cases

Myxoid/Round Cell Liposarcoma

- Small undifferentiated mesenchymal tumor cells
- Univacuolated lipoblasts
- Characteristic thin-walled, branching vessels
- S100 protein positive, t(12;16)(q13;p11) in > 90%

DIAGNOSTIC CHECKLIST

Pathologic Interpretation Pearls

- Often arises from preexisting vessel
- Intracytoplasmic vacuoles
- Expression of endothelial markers

SELECTED REFERENCES

1. Clarke LE et al: Cutaneous epithelioid hemangioendothelioma. J Cutan Pathol. 35(2):236-40, 2008
2. Mendlick MR et al: Translocation t(1;3)(p36.3;q25) is a nonrandom aberration in epithelioid hemangioendothelioma. Am J Surg Pathol. 25(5):684-7, 2001
3. Quante M et al: Epithelioid hemangioendothelioma presenting in the skin: a clinicopathologic study of eight cases. Am J Dermatopathol. 20(6):541-6, 1998
4. Mentzel T et al: Epithelioid hemangioendothelioma of skin and soft tissues: clinicopathologic and immunohistochemical study of 30 cases. Am J Surg Pathol. 21(4):363-74, 1997
5. Weiss SW et al: Epithelioid hemangioendothelioma: a vascular tumor often mistaken for a carcinoma. Cancer. 50(5):970-81, 1982

EPITHELIOID HEMANGIOENDOTHELIOMA

Microscopic and Immunohistochemical Features

(Left) Histologic examination shows epithelioid hemangioendothelioma composed of strands, clusters, and single neoplastic epithelioid cells randomly arranged within a myxoid stroma. *(Right)* Higher magnification shows relatively bland epithelioid tumor cells. Note the scattered cells containing intracytoplasmic vacuoles ⊃ possibly representing attempted vascular lumen formation. The cells have moderate amounts of cytoplasm and show minimal nuclear atypia.

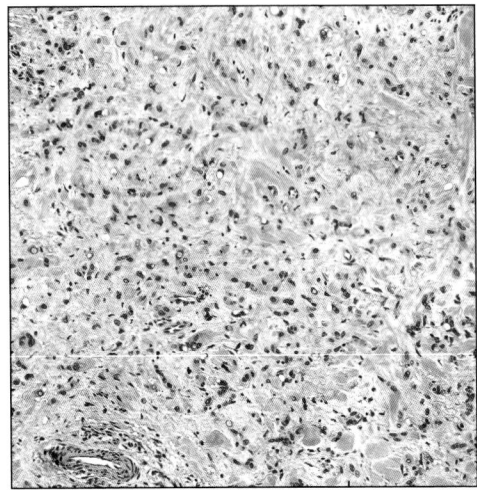
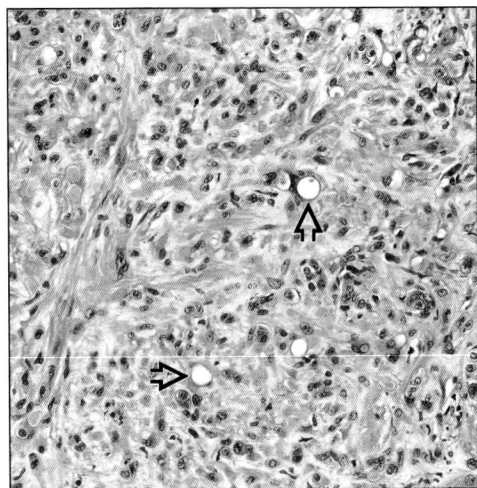

(Left) This tumor is less cellular with epithelioid tumor cells widely dispersed singly and in small clusters within a myxohyaline stroma (sulfated acid mucopolysaccharides). Many cells have intracytoplasmic vacuoles. *(Right)* High magnification shows numerous vacuolated tumor cells mimicking lipoblasts. This can lead to misdiagnosis as myxoid liposarcoma, but this lacks endothelial markers, expresses S100 protein, and has diagnostic chromosomal translocations.

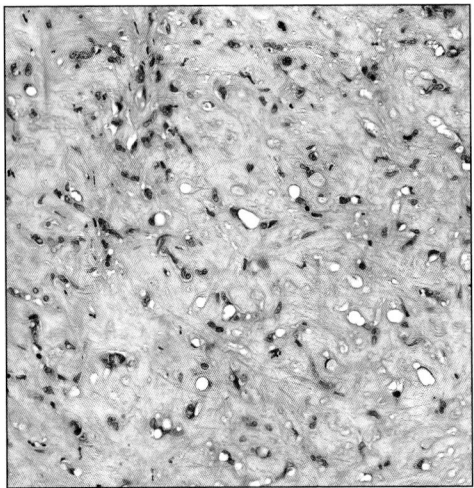
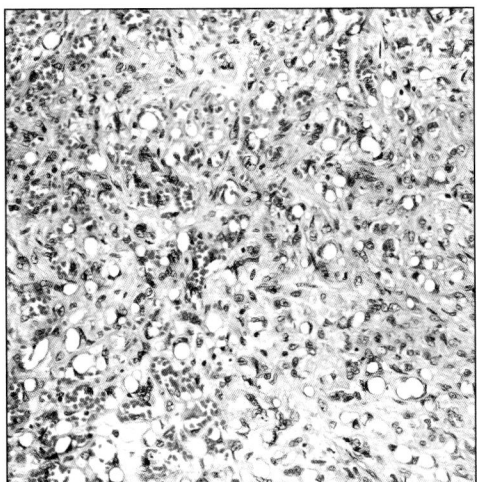

(Left) EHE shows a focus of metaplastic ossification ⊃. Cords of tumor cells → can be seen in the adjacent stroma, which sometimes has a myxohyaline appearance. *(Right)* CD31 shows membranous and cytoplasmic expression. Note scattered vacuolated tumor cells. This marker is highly sensitive for endothelial differentiation, but also is expressed in macrophages and plasma cells. However, carcinoma and melanoma markers are negative.

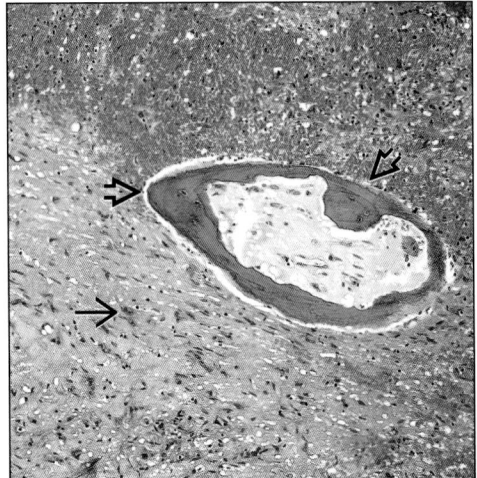
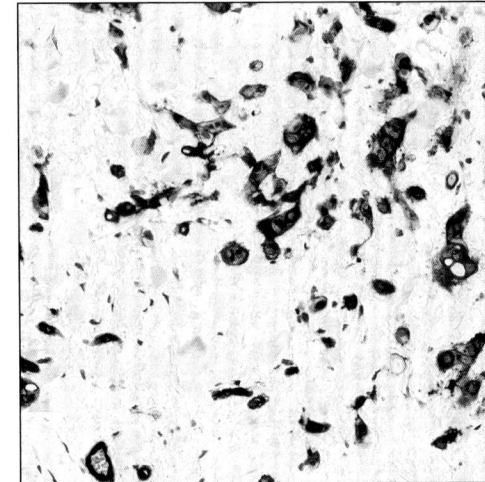

EPITHELIOID HEMANGIOENDOTHELIOMA

Clinical and Microscopic Features

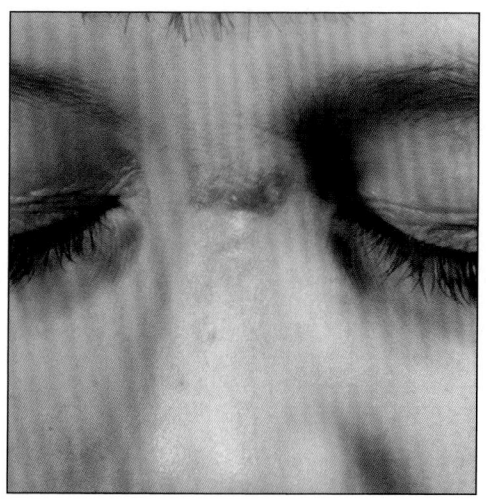

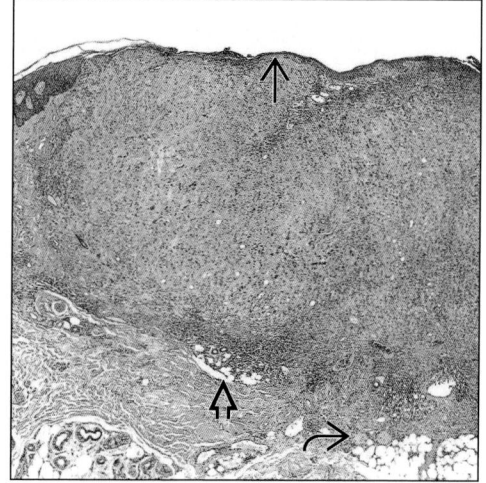

(Left) This clinical photograph shows a poorly circumscribed flat dermal/subcutaneous neoplasm that represents a metastasizing epithelioid hemangioendothelioma arising in a young male. (Right) Low magnification shows an epithelioid hemangioendothelioma in the dermis. Note the ulceration at the surface ➔. There is an inflammatory infiltrate ⮥ at the lower border of the lesion, which is demarcated from adjacent tissue. The tumor extends into the subcutis ➔.

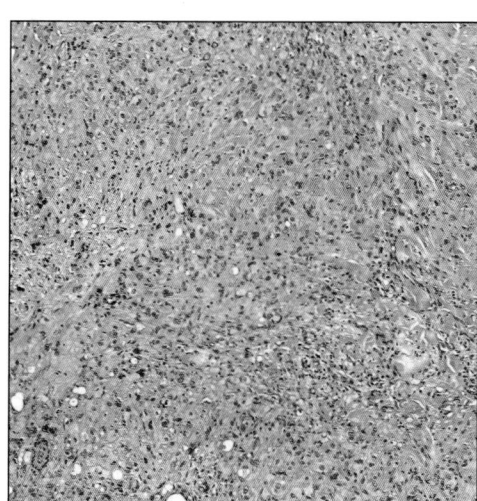

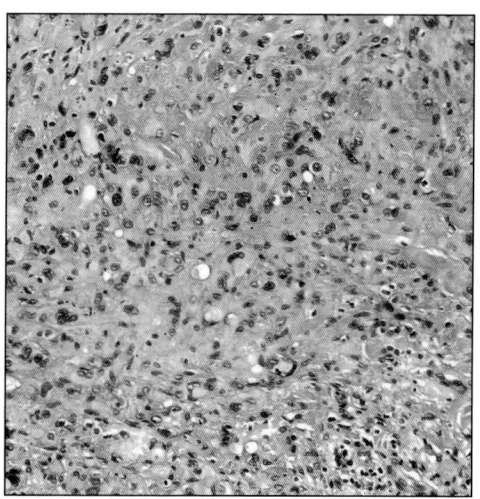

(Left) Higher magnification shows a sheet of epithelioid tumor cells in the dermis. This is less easily recognized as epithelioid hemangioendothelioma, and appearances can overlap with those of epithelioid angiosarcoma. (Right) High magnification shows focal myxohyaline stroma in this dermal lesion. Note the scattered cytoplasmic vacuoles, imparting a characteristic low-power appearance. Immunohistochemistry can, however, be required to exclude carcinoma.

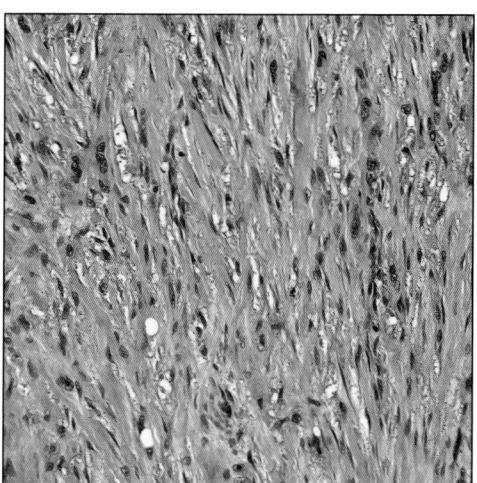

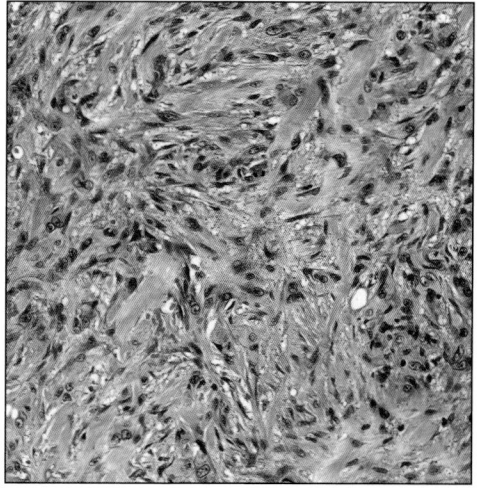

(Left) This is an example of an epithelioid hemangioendothelioma with a prominent spindle cell component. This is an unusual phenomenon that can be focal with more typical areas being found on wide sampling. (Right) Epithelioid hemangioendothelioma can show increased cytologic atypia and scattered mitoses in some cases. Such cases need distinction from angiosarcoma, which is more vasoformative and has more widespread atypia, often with necrosis.

RETIFORM HEMANGIOENDOTHELIOMA

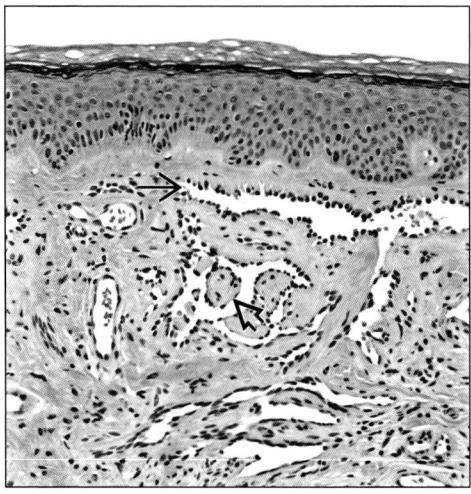

Low-power view of a retiform hemangioendothelioma shows superficial dermal involvement by elongated vascular spaces ⇨. Focal papillary structures are present ⇨.

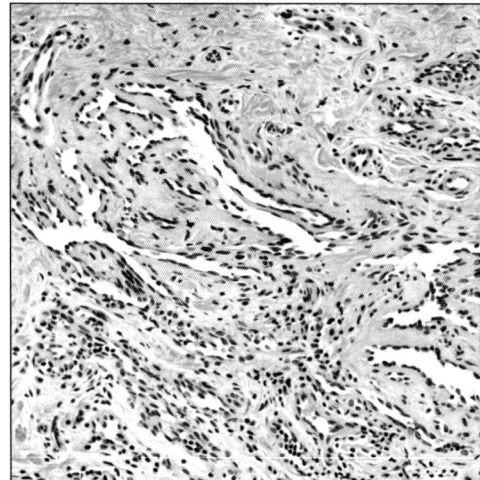

Higher magnification view shows a proliferation of elongated vessels lined by hyperchromatic hobnailed endothelial cells. The surrounding stroma shows fibrosis and scattered lymphocytes.

TERMINOLOGY

Abbreviations
- Retiform hemangioendothelioma (RHE)

Synonyms
- Hobnail hemangioendothelioma

Definitions
- Low-grade malignant vascular tumor composed of elongated vessels resembling rete testis

ETIOLOGY/PATHOGENESIS

Unknown
- Rare cases associated with lymphedema or preceding radiation
- 1 case reported to be positive for HHV8

CLINICAL ISSUES

Epidemiology
- Incidence
  - Rare vascular tumor
- Age
  - Typically middle-aged adults, but may occur in children
- Gender
  - More common in females

Site
- Trunk or extremities

Presentation
- Large nodular to plaque-like lesion

Treatment
- Surgical approaches
  - Complete excision is necessary to prevent recurrence

Prognosis
- Locally aggressive, rarely metastasizing (although lymph node metastases reported in several cases)

MACROSCOPIC FEATURES

General Features
- Typically poorly circumscribed dermal &/or subcutaneous tumor

Size
- May be large tumors (up to 12 cm)

MICROSCOPIC PATHOLOGY

Histologic Features
- Dermal-based infiltrative proliferation of distinctive elongated, arborizing blood vessels resembling rete testis
- Vascular spaces are lined by endothelial cells with characteristic hobnail morphology
  - Endothelial cells show hyperchromasia, but typically do not show prominent cytologic atypia
  - Mitotic figures may be present, but are usually rare
- Very prominent lymphocytic infiltrate in most cases
- May show invasion of subcutaneous tissues
- Some cases show significant overlap with Dabska tumor (both have hobnailed cells), with prominent papillary structures and hyaline cores

Cytologic Features
- Hobnail cells with oval nuclei with mild hyperchromasia

RETIFORM HEMANGIOENDOTHELIOMA

Key Facts

Terminology
- Retiform hemangioendothelioma (RHE)
- Low-grade malignant vascular tumor composed of elongated vessels resembling rete testes

Clinical Issues
- Typically middle-aged adults, but may occur in children
- Locally aggressive, very rarely metastasizing (although lymph node metastases reported)

Microscopic Pathology
- Distinctive elongated, arborizing blood vessels resembling rete testis
- Often show papillary-like intraluminal projections, some of which may have a hyaline core
- Vascular spaces are lined by endothelial cells with characteristic hobnail morphology
- Some cases show significant overlap with Dabska tumor

ANCILLARY TESTS

Immunohistochemistry
- Tumor cells react with vascular endothelial markers CD31, CD34, and FVIIIRAg
- Most cases negative with lymphatic markers D2-40 and VEGFR-3, but rare positive cases

DIFFERENTIAL DIAGNOSIS

Papillary Intralymphatic Angioendothelioma (Dabska Tumor)
- More common in children, but some cases in young adults reported
- Papillary structures more common
- Typically do not show prominent rete-like elongated vessels of RHE
- Some cases show significant overlap with RHE (both have hobnailed cells)
- Most cases (+) for lymphatic markers (D2-40, VEGFR-3)

Composite Hemangioendothelioma (HE)
- By definition, composed of at least 2 distinct HE types
  - Predominant histologic components usually are epithelioid HE and RHE

Kaposi Sarcoma
- Much more common, associated with HIV/AIDS
- Proliferation of small, slit-like vascular spaces lined by spindle cells, lacking rete-like pattern of RHE

- HHV8(+) (only 1 case of RHE reported to be positive)

Angiosarcoma
- Typically occurs in older adults or post-mastectomy
- Proliferation of atypical spindled or epithelioid endothelial cells, often forming anastomosing vascular spaces and showing infiltrative features

DIAGNOSTIC CHECKLIST

Pathologic Interpretation Pearls
- Proliferation of distinctive elongated blood vessels (lined by hobnail cells) resembling rete testis

SELECTED REFERENCES

1. Emberger M et al: Retiform hemangioendothelioma: presentation of a case expressing D2-40. J Cutan Pathol. 36(9):987-90, 2009
2. Parsons A et al: Retiform hemangioendotheliomas usually do not express D2-40 and VEGFR-3. Am J Dermatopathol. 30(1):31-3, 2008
3. Tan D et al: Retiform hemangioendothelioma: a case report and review of the literature. J Cutan Pathol. 32(9):634-7, 2005
4. Schommer M et al: Retiform hemangioendothelioma: another tumor associated with human herpesvirus type 8? J Am Acad Dermatol. 42(2 Pt 1):290-2, 2000
5. Calonje E et al: Retiform hemangioendothelioma. A distinctive form of low-grade angiosarcoma delineated in a series of 15 cases. Am J Surg Pathol. 18(2):115-25, 1994

IMAGE GALLERY

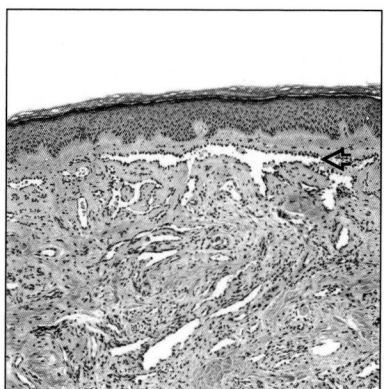 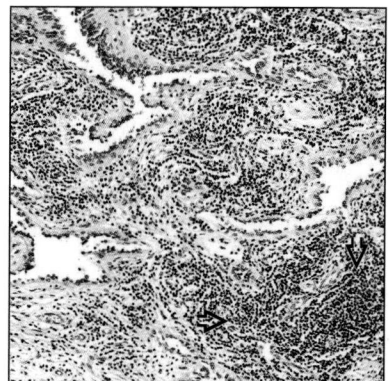 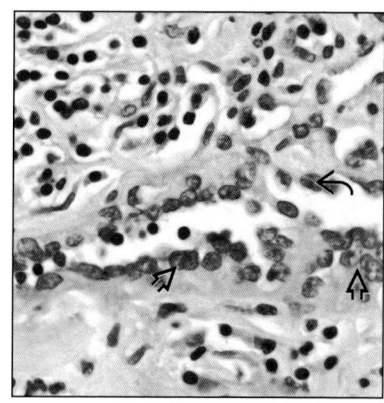

(Left) Low-magnification examination of a RHE shows superficial dermal involvement by irregular, elongated, branching vascular spaces ➡. (Center) Deep area of a retiform HE shows elongated vascular spaces surrounded by prominent lymphoid aggregates ➡. (Right) High-magnification view shows hyperchromatic endothelial cells with hobnail features, nuclear crowding ➡, and focally enlarged nucleoli ➡.

PAPILLARY INTRALYMPHATIC ANGIOENDOTHELIOMA (DABSKA TUMOR)

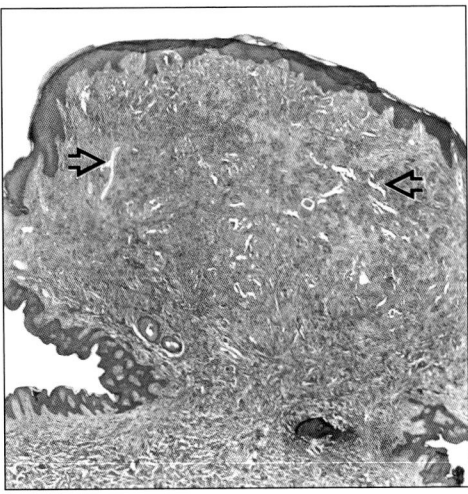

Scanning magnification view of a papillary intralymphatic angioendothelioma (Dabska tumor) shows a polypoid lesion in the skin with irregular dilated vascular spaces ⮞.

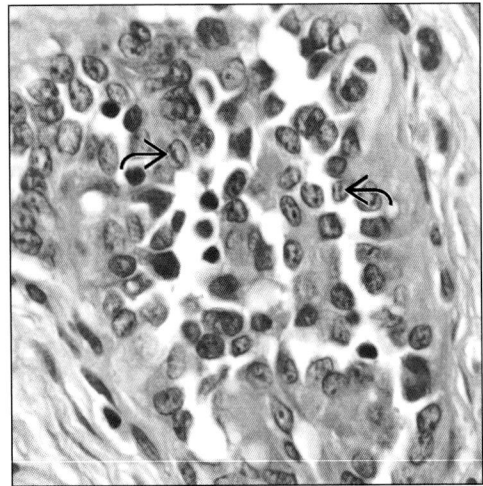

High power shows papillae lined by mildly enlarged hobnailed cells projecting into the vascular lumina. The cells show vesicular chromatin, small nucleoli, and occasional grooves ⮡.

TERMINOLOGY

Abbreviations
- Papillary intralymphatic angioendothelioma (PILA)

Synonyms
- Dabska tumor
- Endovascular papillary angioendothelioma

Definitions
- Low-grade malignant vascular tumor composed of hobnailed endothelial cells

ETIOLOGY/PATHOGENESIS

Unknown
- May be associated with vascular or lymphatic tumor/malformation

CLINICAL ISSUES

Epidemiology
- Incidence
  - Rare tumors
- Age
  - Typically occur in children (minority in adults)
- Gender
  - Slight female predominance

Site
- Distal extremities most common, but may occur in other sites

Presentation
- Plaque-like lesion of dermis & subcutis
  - May show overlying violaceous skin discoloration

Treatment
- Surgical approaches

- Complete surgical excision recommended to prevent metastasis (rare) or recurrence

Prognosis
- High rate of local recurrence, rare metastasis (to lymph nodes)

MACROSCOPIC FEATURES

General Features
- Dermal-based infiltrative tumor with extension into subcutis

Size
- Can be quite large (average: 7 cm)

MICROSCOPIC PATHOLOGY

Histologic Features
- Dermal proliferation of vessels lined by enlarged, cuboidal endothelial cells
  - Intravascular papillary projections with hyaline cores
  - Endothelial cells show prominent hobnail features with plump, rounded profiles protruding into lumina
  - Cytoplasmic vacuolation may be seen
  - Mitotic figures absent or rare
- Typically associated with surrounding lymphoid infiltrate and sclerotic collagen
- Vessels often extend into subcutaneous tissues
- Associated lymphatic or vascular tumor or malformation in some cases

Cytologic Features
- Hobnail cells show high nuclear to cytoplasmic ratio, nuclei may show grooves

PAPILLARY INTRALYMPHATIC ANGIOENDOTHELIOMA (DABSKA TUMOR)

Key Facts

Terminology
- Dabska tumor
- Endovascular papillary angioendothelioma

Clinical Issues
- Typically occur in children (minority in adults)
- Distal extremities most common, but may occur in other sites
- High rate of local recurrence, rare metastasis

Microscopic Pathology
- Dermal proliferation of vessels with papillary projections lined by enlarged, cuboidal endothelial cells
- Endothelial cells show prominent hobnail features with plump, rounded profiles protruding into lumina
- Typically associated with surrounding lymphoid infiltrate and sclerotic collagen

ANCILLARY TESTS

Immunohistochemistry
- Typically positive for vascular markers including FVIIIRAg, CD31, and CD34
- Most cases also positive for lymphatic markers D2-40 and VEGFR-3

DIFFERENTIAL DIAGNOSIS

Retiform Hemangioendothelioma (RHE)
- Most cases occur in adults, but some present in children
- Proliferation of vessels forming distinct elongated rete-like structures lined by hobnail cells
- Some cases of RHE show significant overlap with Dabska tumor, with prominent papillary structures
- Most cases negative with lymphatic markers D2-40 and VEGFR-3, but rare positive cases

Composite Hemangioendothelioma (HE)
- By definition, composed of at least 2 distinct HE types
  - Predominant histologic components usually are epithelioid HE and RHE

Kaposi Sarcoma
- Much more common, associated with HIV infection and AIDS in most cases
- Proliferation of small, slit-like vascular spaces lined by spindle cells, lacking papillary pattern of Dabska

- HHV8(+)

Angiosarcoma
- Typically occurs in older adults or post-mastectomy
- Proliferation of atypical spindled or epithelioid endothelial cells, forming anastomosing vascular spaces and showing infiltrative features

DIAGNOSTIC CHECKLIST

Pathologic Interpretation Pearls
- Dermal proliferation of vessels with papillary projections lined by enlarged, cuboidal endothelial cells

SELECTED REFERENCES

1. Emanuel PO et al: Dabska tumor arising in lymphangioma circumscriptum. J Cutan Pathol. 35(1):65-9, 2008
2. Fukunaga M: Expression of D2-40 in lymphatic endothelium of normal tissues and in vascular tumours. Histopathology. 46(4):396-402, 2005
3. Fanburg-Smith JC et al: Papillary intralymphatic angioendothelioma (PILA): a report of twelve cases of a distinctive vascular tumor with phenotypic features of lymphatic vessels. Am J Surg Pathol. 23(9):1004-10, 1999
4. Dabska M: Malignant endovascular papillary angioendothelioma of the skin in childhood. Clinicopathologic study of 6 cases. Cancer. 24(3):503-10, 1969

IMAGE GALLERY

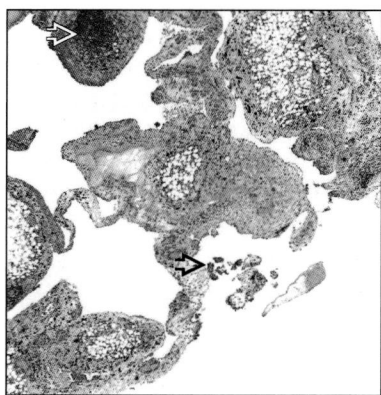 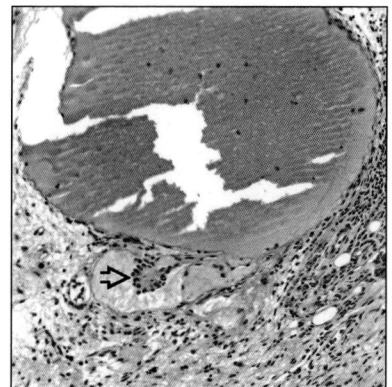 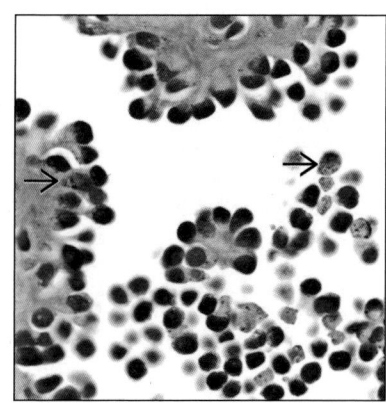

(Left) Low magnification of a PILA shows a background of lymphangioma-like areas with scattered lymphoid aggregates ➡. Note focal intraluminal papillary projections ➡. *(Center)* Dilated vascular space filled with red blood cells overlies a smaller lymphatic space with prominent papillary projection lined by hobnailed cells ➡. *(Right)* Multiple prominent intralymphatic projections of papillary structures with hyaline cores are lined by plump hyperchromatic-staining endothelial cells, some of which contain cytoplasmic hemosiderin pigment ➡.

ATYPICAL VASCULAR LESION

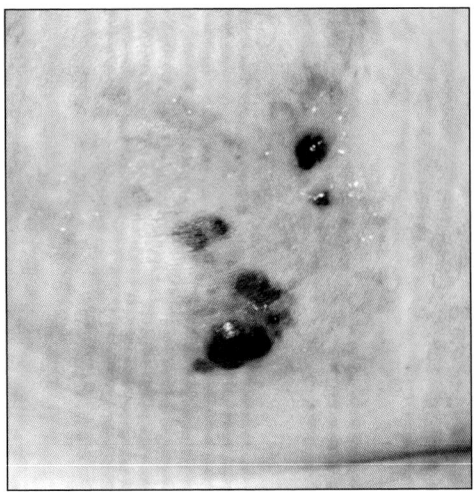

Multiple red papules and nodules on the chest are seen in a patient with an atypical vascular lesion after radiotherapy.

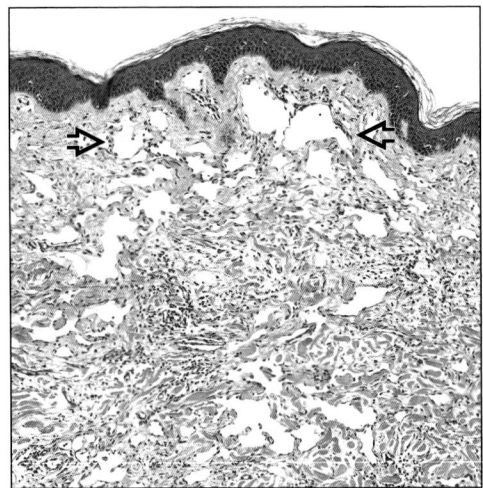

Low-magnification view of an AVL shows a superficially located, lymphangioma-like vascular lesion composed of dilated vascular structures ⊵ lined by cytologically bland endothelial cells.

TERMINOLOGY

Abbreviations
- Atypical vascular lesion (AVL)

Synonyms
- Atypical vascular proliferation (AVP)
- Benign lymphangiomatous papule (BLAP)

Definitions
- Vascular proliferation after radiotherapy excluding obvious angiosarcoma, arising predominantly in breast

ETIOLOGY/PATHOGENESIS

Environmental Exposure
- Occur after radiotherapy (40-60 Gy)
- Develop a median of 3 years after radiotherapy

CLINICAL ISSUES

Epidemiology
- Incidence
  - Exact incidence difficult to establish
  - Relative risk is increased about 10x following radiation therapy
  - Incidence for post-irradiation AVL is equal after mastectomy or breast-conserving therapy
- Age
  - Wide age range; median in late 50s
  - Usually 1 decade earlier than radiation-induced cutaneous angiosarcoma

Site
- Seen in skin of breast &/or chest wall
- Develops less frequently at other sites after radiation for gynecological or other malignancies

Presentation
- Small, red to brown papules (usually < 5 mm)
- Often multifocal lesions
- Presents only rarely as large plaques

Treatment
- Surgical approaches
  - All lesions must be excised completely

Prognosis
- Very difficult to estimate exact prognosis
- Presence of significant cytologic atypia worsens prognosis
- Presence of increased proliferative activity (Ki-67) and p53 expression are worse signs
- Post-irradiation AVL likely represents precursor of cutaneous angiosarcoma in some cases

MICROSCOPIC PATHOLOGY

Histologic Features
- Rather well-circumscribed, superficially located dermal lesions
- Extension into subcutaneous tissue usually not seen
- Small, symmetrical, and often wedge-shaped lesions
- Dilated &/or narrow vascular structures
- Dissection of collagen bundles may be present
- Anastomosing vascular structures may be seen
- Single layer of slightly enlarged endothelial cells
- Neither endothelial multilayering nor prominent cytologic atypia
- No increased endothelial mitoses
- No confluent hemorrhage nor necrosis

Cytologic Features
- Slightly enlarged endothelial cells

ATYPICAL VASCULAR LESION

Key Facts

Terminology

- Vascular proliferation after radiotherapy, excluding obvious angiosarcoma, arising predominantly in breast

Clinical Issues

- Exact incidence is difficult to establish
- Small papules, usually < 5 mm
- Papules are red to brown colored
- All lesions must be excised completely

- Wide age range; median in late 50s

Microscopic Pathology

- Usually well-circumscribed, superficial dermal-based lesions
- Small, symmetrical, and wedge-shaped lesions
- Dilated &/or narrow vascular structures
- Single layer of slightly enlarged endothelial cells
- No endothelial multilayering should be seen
- No prominent cytologic atypia or mitoses

DIFFERENTIAL DIAGNOSIS

Hobnail Hemangioma

- Solitary papules or nodules
- Biphasic growth (superficial dilated vessels, deeper narrow vessels)
- Hobnail endothelial cells
- Stromal fibrosis, hemosiderin deposits

Lymphangioma Circumscriptum

- Represents developmental malformation (infants, adults)
- Clinically, groups of small vesicles containing clear fluid are present
- Small and superficially located lesions

Progressive Lymphangioma

- Presents clinically as large, slowly increasing, pink to reddish brown plaques
- Infiltrating and dissecting lymphatics
- Lymphatics orientated horizontally in dermis

Well-Differentiated Angiosarcoma

- Usually deeper dermis/subcutaneous tumor
- Anastomosing and infiltrating vascular structures
- Endothelial multilayering and endothelial atypia
- Increased number of endothelial mitoses
- Increased Ki-67 and p53 expression
- Evidence of *c-myc* amplification
- Post-irradiation AVLs and angiosarcomas are best regarded as a continuum

DIAGNOSTIC CHECKLIST

Clinically Relevant Pathologic Features

- Symptom time frame
- Gross appearance
- Invasive pattern
- Nuclear features

Pathologic Interpretation Pearls

- AVL and post-irradiation well-differentiated cutaneous angiosarcoma represent morphologic spectrum
- All lesions showing features of AVL have to be excised completely

SELECTED REFERENCES

1. Patton KT et al: Atypical vascular lesions after surgery and radiation of the breast: a clinicopathologic study of 32 cases analyzing histologic heterogeneity and association with angiosarcoma. Am J Surg Pathol. 32(6):943-50, 2008
2. Brenn T et al: Radiation-associated cutaneous atypical vascular lesions and angiosarcoma: clinicopathologic analysis of 42 cases. Am J Surg Pathol. 29(8):983-96, 2005
3. Di Tommaso L et al: The capillary lobule: a deceptively benign feature of post-radiation angiosarcoma of the skin: report of three cases. Am J Dermatopathol. 27(4):301-5, 2005
4. Fineberg S et al: Cutaneous angiosarcoma and atypical vascular lesions of the skin and breast after radiation therapy for breast carcinoma. Am J Clin Pathol. 102(6):757-63, 1994

IMAGE GALLERY

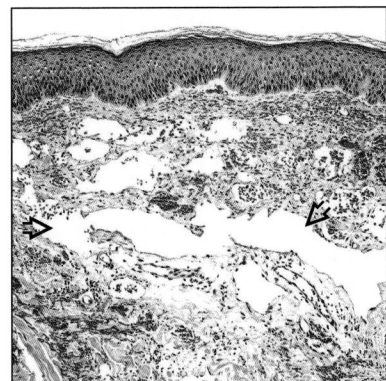 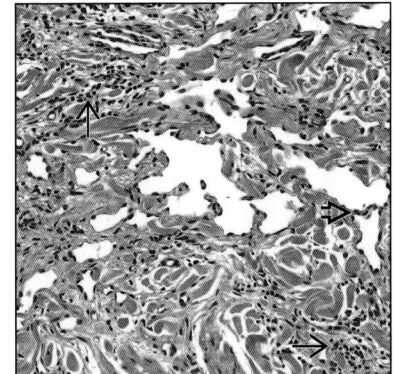 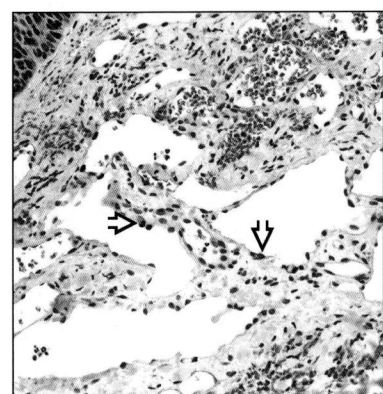

(Left) This AVL is composed of mainly dilated vascular structures ⊵ lined by small to slightly enlarged endothelial cells. *(Center)* The lining endothelial cells are only slightly enlarged and contain uniform nuclei. Note the endothelial bridges ⊵ in the absence of endothelial multilayering. Scattered lymphocytes are present ⊸, a frequent finding in these lesions. *(Right)* The presence of scattered Ki-67(+) endothelial cells ⊵ represents a suspicious finding in cases of AVL after radiotherapy.

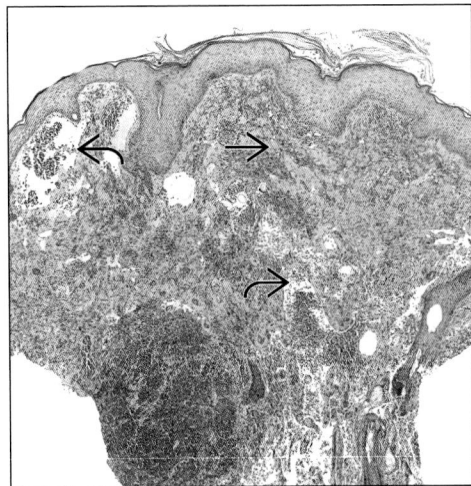

Cutaneous angiosarcoma of the scalp in an elderly man. The dermis contains dilated vascular channels ⊡ lined by plump endothelial cells. There are also spindle cell areas ⊡ and focal hemorrhage.

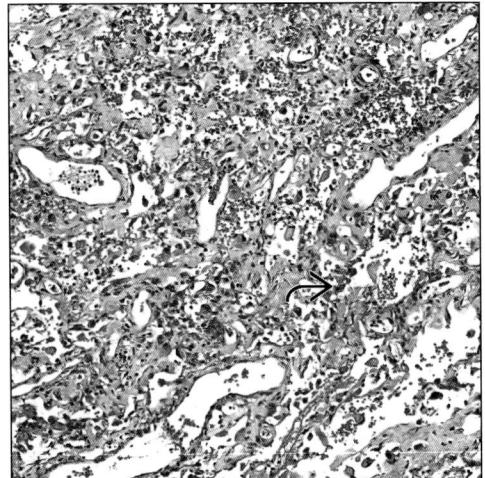

Higher magnification shows well-differentiated angiosarcoma comprising irregularly shaped anastomosing vascular structures with open lumina lined by enlarged, atypical endothelial cells ⊡.

TERMINOLOGY

Synonyms
- Hemangiosarcoma
- Malignant hemangioblastoma
- Malignant hemangioendothelioma

Definitions
- Malignant mesenchymal neoplasm of cells recapitulating variable morphologic and functional features of endothelial cells

ETIOLOGY/PATHOGENESIS

Developmental Anomaly
- Develops rarely in association with genetic syndromes
  - Klippel-Trenaunay syndrome
  - Maffucci syndrome
- In longstanding congenital lymphedema

Environmental Exposure
- Rarely develops adjacent to foreign material or synthetic vascular grafts
- In limbs with longstanding lymphedema
  - After mastectomy: Stewart-Treves syndrome
- Post-therapeutic irradiation

CLINICAL ISSUES

Epidemiology
- Incidence
  - Rare; < 1% of all sarcomas
  - More frequent in superficial locations
    - 1/4 of angiosarcomas arise in deep soft tissues
- Age
  - Occurs at any age, but most common in older adults
  - Rare subset in childhood
- Gender
  - M > F

Site
- Skin of head and neck
- Skin of limbs in longstanding lymphedema
- Skin of breast following therapeutic irradiation for carcinoma
- Deep soft tissue
  - Lower extremities > upper extremities
  - Trunk > head/neck region
  - Significant proportion arises in abdomen and retroperitoneum
  - Rarely multifocal

Presentation
- Slow growing
- Deep mass
  - Usually large mass
  - Hematologic abnormalities
  - Thrombocytopenia may be present
  - Arteriovenous shunting may be present
  - Rarely arises in nonlipogenic component of dedifferentiated liposarcomas
  - Rarely arises in benign or malignant nerve sheath tumors
  - Very rarely arises in preexisting benign hemangioma
- Skin lesions
  - Plaque or nodule with purple discoloration and bruising

Treatment
- Surgical approaches
  - Aggressive surgical resection with wide tumor-free margins
- Adjuvant therapy
  - Response to chemotherapy
  - Inhibition of angiogenesis

Prognosis
- Poor prognosis irrespective of grade of malignancy
  - Local recurrence in 20-30%
  - Distant metastases in 50%

ANGIOSARCOMA

Key Facts

Terminology
- Malignant mesenchymal neoplasm of cells recapitulating variable morphologic and functional features of endothelial cells

Clinical Issues
- Deep soft tissues
  - Lower extremities, followed by upper extremities
  - Trunk > head and neck
  - Significant proportion intraabdominal and retroperitoneal
- Rare (more frequent in superficial locations)
  - < 1% of all sarcomas
- Any age, but most common in older adults
- Poor prognosis irrespective of grade of malignancy
  - 5-year survival 20-30% at best

- Aggressive surgical resection with wide tumor-free margins

Microscopic Pathology
- Irregular, anastomosing vascular spaces
- Variably pleomorphic endothelial tumor cells
- Endothelial multilayering and papillary formation
- Solid areas common
- No complete rim of actin positive myopericytes
- Often intracytoplasmic lumina
- Prominent nuclear atypia
- Numerous mitoses
- Expression of endothelial markers
- Epithelioid angiosarcomas occur relatively frequently in deep soft tissues
  - Solid sheets of large epithelioid cells in epithelioid angiosarcoma

---

- 5-year survival 20-30% at best

MACROSCOPIC FEATURES

General Features
- Infiltrating neoplasm
- Areas of hemorrhage

MICROSCOPIC PATHOLOGY

Histologic Features
- Angiosarcoma
  - Usually no relationship to preexisting vessels
  - Irregular infiltrating and anastomosing vascular spaces
  - Variably pleomorphic endothelial tumor cells
    - Nuclear atypia and prominent nucleoli
  - Endothelial multilayering and papillary formation
  - Solid areas common
  - Neoplastic vascular structures encircled by reticulin fibers
  - No complete rim of SMA positive (myo)pericytes
  - Often intracytoplasmic lumina that may contain erythrocytes
  - Mitoses are usually numerous
  - Areas of hemorrhage and necrosis may be present
  - Clear distinction between lymphatic and vascular differentiation remains problematic
- Epithelioid angiosarcoma
  - In cutaneous or, more commonly, in deep soft tissues
  - Often rapid growth
  - Very aggressive clinical course
  - Solid sheets of large epithelioid cells
  - Tumor cells with abundant eosinophilic cytoplasm and large vesicular nuclei
  - Prominent cytologic atypia and numerous mitoses
  - Often areas of tumor necrosis
- Rare predominantly spindle cell morphology
- Rare granular cell variant
- Rare inflammatory variant

Predominant Pattern/Injury Type
- Diffuse

Predominant Cell/Compartment Type
- Endothelial

DIFFERENTIAL DIAGNOSIS

Hemangioma
- Lobular architecture
- Well-formed vascular structures
- No endothelial multilayering and papillary formation
- Usually complete rim of actin positive myopericytes
- No prominent cytologic atypia
- No/few mitoses in endothelial cells

Malignant Melanoma (Primary or Metastatic)
- Clinical features usually differ
- No vascular spaces
- No intracytoplasmic vacuoles with erythrocytes
- Round tumor cells
- Vesicular nuclei with prominent nucleoli
- Endothelial immunohistochemical markers negative
- Melanocytic markers positive

Poorly Differentiated Carcinoma (Primary or Metastatic)
- Clinical features usually differ
- No vascular spaces (pseudovascular spaces can be seen in acantholytic squamous cell carcinoma)
- Epithelial structures may be present
- Endothelial immunohistochemical markers negative
- Usually strong, diffuse expression of multiple epithelial markers

Proximal-type Epithelioid Sarcoma
- No vascular structures
- Epithelioid and rhabdoid tumor cells
- Endothelial markers negative
- Loss of INI1 expression

Immunohistochemistry

Antibody	Reactivity	Staining Pattern	Comment
CD31	Positive	Cell membrane & cytoplasm	
CD34	Positive	Cell membrane & cytoplasm	Not sensitive, may be negative
FLI-1	Positive	Nuclear	Not specific
Podoplanin	Positive	Cytoplasmic	About 40%, can reflect lymphatic differentiation
CD117	Positive	Cell membrane & cytoplasm	In almost 1/2 of cases; not specific
Actin-sm	Positive	Cytoplasmic	In some cases
CK-PAN	Positive	Cytoplasmic	In some cases (in 50% of epithelioid angiosarcoma)
SNF5	Positive	Nuclear	Consistently expressed
S100P	Negative		
EMA	Equivocal	Cell membrane & cytoplasm	In some cases

Malignant Myoepithelioma
- Epithelial structures usually found at least focally
- Focal myxoid stromal changes often present
- Often show expression of S100 by immunohistochemistry
- Often positive for actins
- Endothelial markers negative

Retiform Hemangioendothelioma
- Distal extremities
- Young patients
- Dermal/subcutaneous location
- Rete testis-like infiltrative pattern
- Hobnail cytomorphology of endothelial cells
- No prominent cytologic atypia
- Usually no endothelial multilayering
- Often focal lymphocytic infiltration

Sclerosing (Pseudovascular) Rhabdomyosarcoma
- Scattered rhabdomyoblasts
- Prominent sclerosis
- No expression of endothelial markers
- Desmin positive
- Scattered cells express myogenin (nuclear)

Large Cell Anaplastic Lymphoma
- No expression of endothelial markers
- Expression of lymphoid markers (CD3, CD30)

Gastrointestinal Stromal Tumor (Metastatic)
- No vascular structures
- CD31 negative
- CD117 positive
- Characteristic molecular findings

DIAGNOSTIC CHECKLIST

Clinically Relevant Pathologic Features
- Gross appearance
- Age distribution
- History of preexisting lesion, associated disease or irradiation

Pathologic Interpretation Pearls
- Irregular anastomosing vascular structures
- Atypical proliferating endothelial tumor cells
- No complete rim of actin positive (myo)pericytes

SELECTED REFERENCES

1. Deyrup AT et al: Pediatric cutaneous angiosarcomas: a clinicopathologic study of 10 cases. Am J Surg Pathol. 35(1):70-5, 2011
2. Suchak R et al: Primary cutaneous epithelioid angiosarcoma: a clinicopathologic study of 13 cases of a rare neoplasm occurring outside the setting of conventional angiosarcomas and with predilection for the limbs. Am J Surg Pathol. 35(1):60-9, 2011
3. Fayette J et al: Angiosarcomas, a heterogeneous group of sarcomas with specific behavior depending on primary site: a retrospective study of 161 cases. Ann Oncol. 18(12):2030-6, 2007
4. Toro JR et al: Incidence patterns of soft tissue sarcomas, regardless of primary site, in the surveillance, epidemiology and end results program, 1978-2001: An analysis of 26,758 cases. Int J Cancer. 119(12):2922-30, 2006
5. Leowardi C et al: Malignant vascular tumors: clinical presentation, surgical therapy, and long-term prognosis. Ann Surg Oncol. 12(12):1090-101, 2005
6. Rossi S et al: Utility of the immunohistochemical detection of FLI-1 expression in round cell and vascular neoplasm using a monoclonal antibody. Mod Pathol. 17(5):547-52, 2004
7. Rossi S et al: Angiosarcoma arising in hemangioma/vascular malformation: report of four cases and review of the literature. Am J Surg Pathol. 26(10):1319-29, 2002
8. Miettinen M et al: Distribution of keratins in normal endothelial cells and a spectrum of vascular tumors: implications in tumor diagnosis. Hum Pathol. 31(9):1062-7, 2000
9. Meis-Kindblom JM et al: Angiosarcoma of soft tissue: a study of 80 cases. Am J Surg Pathol. 22(6):683-97, 1998
10. Schuborg C et al: Cytogenetic analysis of four angiosarcomas from deep and superficial soft tissue. Cancer Genet Cytogenet. 100(1):52-6, 1998
11. Parham DM et al: Angiosarcomas of the breast developing post radiotherapy. Histopathology. 31(2):189-95, 1997
12. Mark RJ et al: Angiosarcoma. A report of 67 patients and a review of the literature. Cancer. 77(11):2400-6, 1996
13. Maddox JC et al: Angiosarcoma of skin and soft tissue: a study of forty-four cases. Cancer. 48(8):1907-21, 1981

Microscopic and Immunohistochemical Features

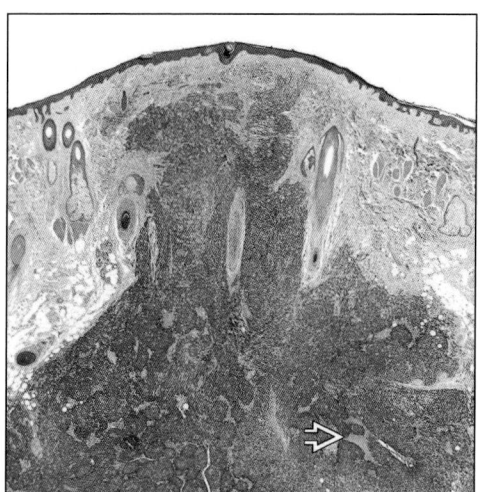

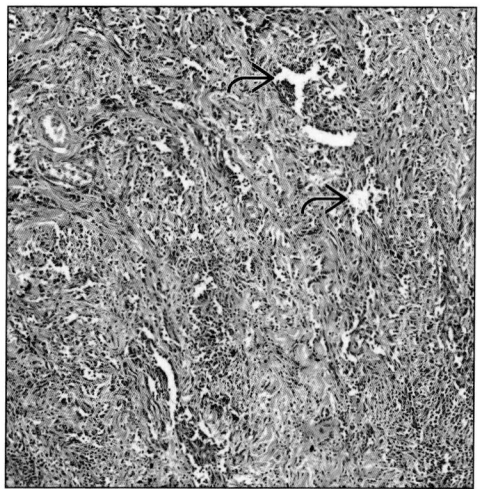

(Left) This is an example of cutaneous epithelioid angiosarcoma arising on the scalp showing a solid cellular infiltrate in the dermis, surrounding adnexa and extending into subcutis. There is focal necrosis ➡. *(Right)* Higher power histologic examination shows narrow to focally dilated vascular structures lined by atypical endothelial cells. Vascular space formation ➡ is often very scanty in epithelioid and spindled cell variants.

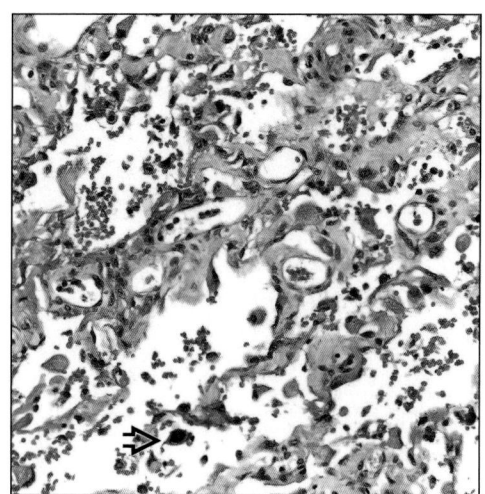

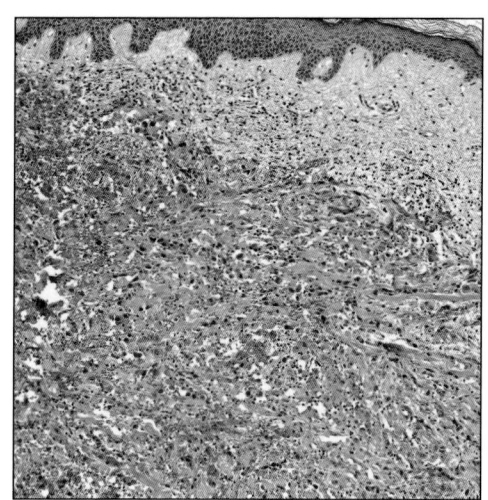

(Left) High magnification of a well-differentiated angiosarcoma shows endothelial cells with enlarged, hyperchromatic and pleomorphic nuclei. Note the free-floating atypical endothelial cells ➡, which are a frequent finding. *(Right)* Epithelioid angiosarcoma shows irregular dermal infiltration by sheets and cords of polygonal cells with hemorrhage. Although often CK positive, unlike carcinoma and epithelioid sarcoma, they express CD31.

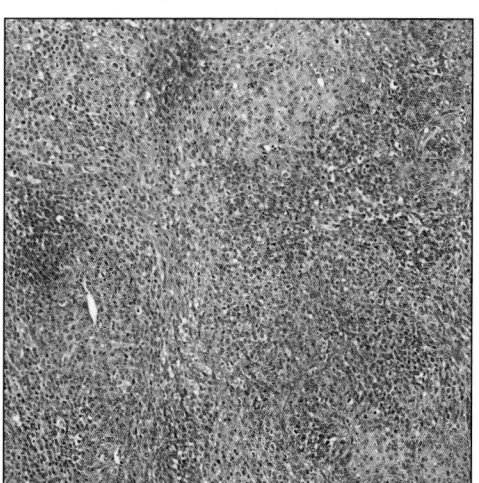

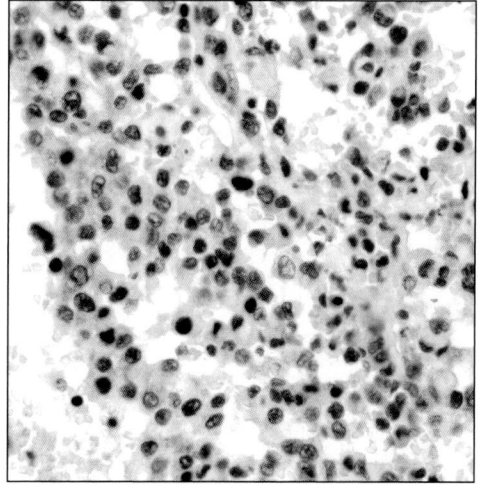

(Left) Intermediate-power examination of this epithelioid angiosarcoma shows variably cellular sheets of atypical epithelioid tumor cells. There is minimal vasoformation or hemorrhage in this example. *(Right)* Immunostaining is positive for INI1 in numerous tumor cell nuclei of this epithelioid angiosarcoma. This helps to distinguish keratin positive epithelioid angiosarcomas from epithelioid sarcoma, which can express CD34, but lacks INI1 in 90% of cases.

Microscopic and Immunohistochemical Features

(Left) Poorly differentiated angiosarcoma shows sheets of atypical epithelioid tumor cells with enlarged vesicular nuclei. This tumor does not have any specific morphological features, and diagnosis essentially requires use of an immunohistochemical panel. *(Right)* The cells of epithelioid angiosarcoma can occasionally show intracytoplasmic lumina ➡, within which a red cell can be seen. The cells have abundant cytoplasm and prominent nucleoli ➡.

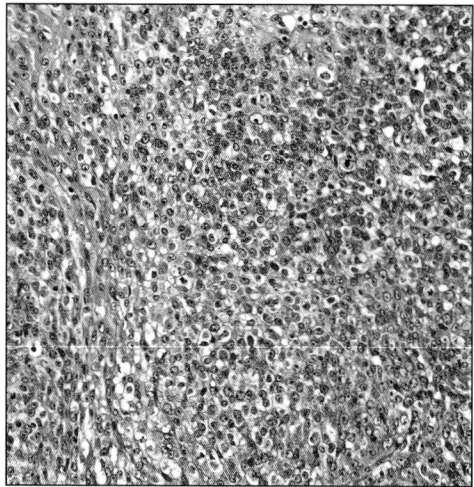

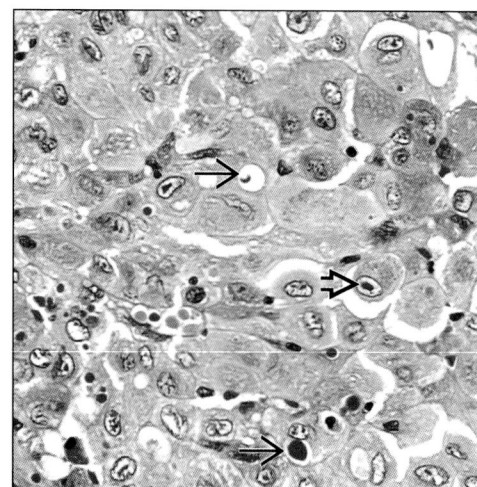

(Left) Rarely, epithelioid angiosarcoma shows rhabdoid cytomorphology. The nucleus is pushed to one side and distorted in shape by a cytoplasmic inclusion ➡. Ultrastructurally, this comprises an aggregate of cytoplasmic intermediate filaments. *(Right)* Immunostaining with antibody to CD31 shows expression of this endothelial marker by epithelioid tumor cells. The antibody shows membranous localization.

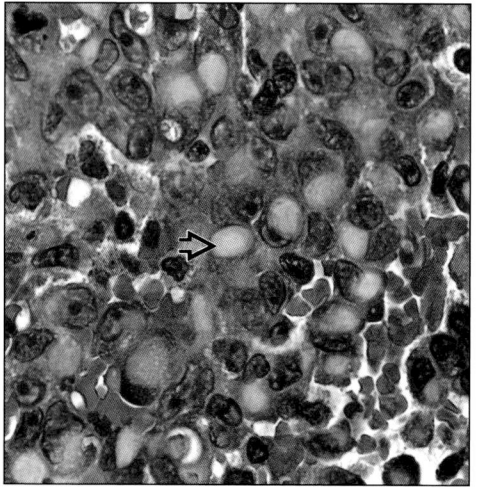

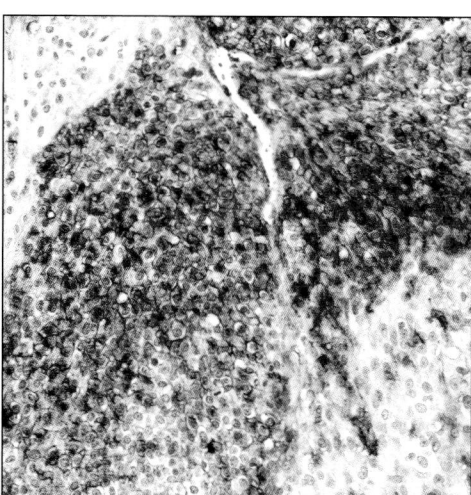

(Left) Histologic examination shows an example of angiosarcoma of soft tissue, which is composed mainly of sheets of atypical spindle-shaped tumor cells. *(Right)* High-power view of spindle cell angiosarcoma. Note the striking cytologic atypia, in contrast to Kaposi sarcoma, which is more uniform. Kaposi sarcoma also expresses markers of endothelial differentiation but can be distinguished from angiosarcoma by its highly specific nuclear positivity for HHV8 on immunostaining.

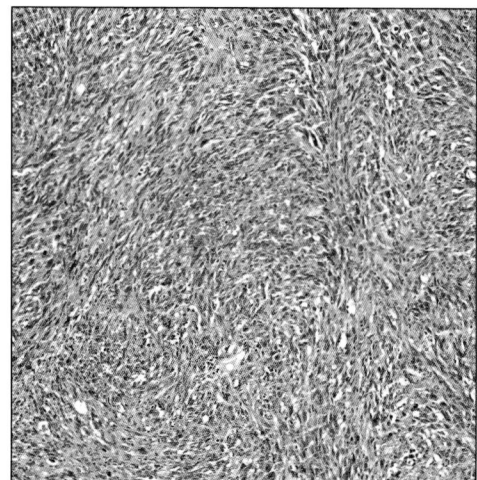

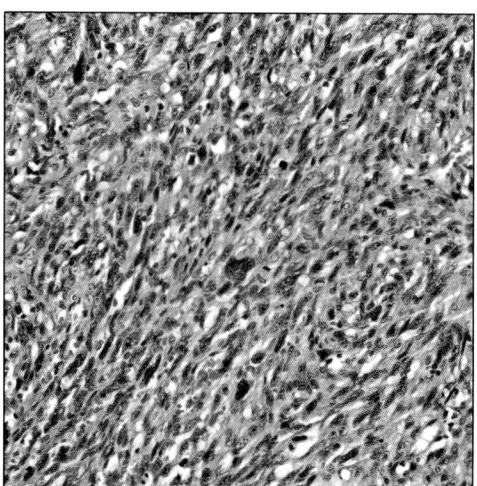

ANGIOSARCOMA

Immunohistochemical and Variant Microscopic Features

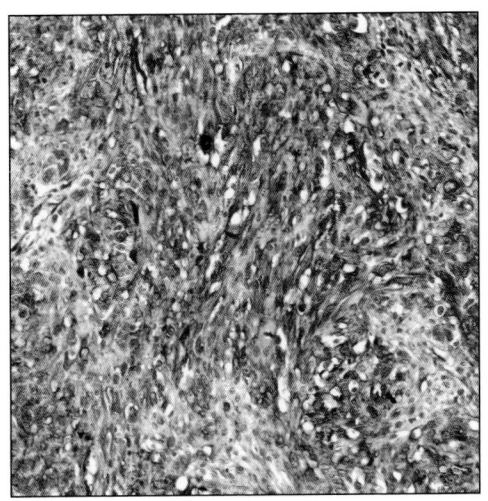

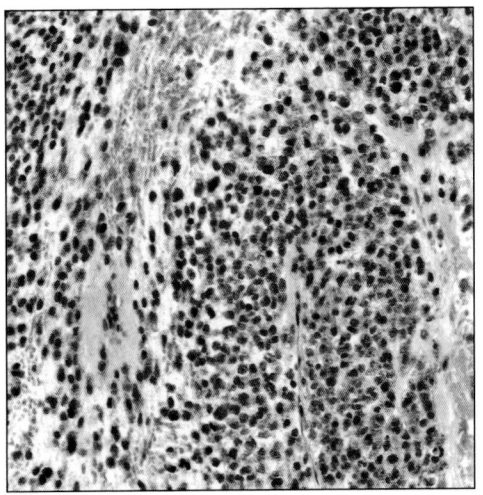

(Left) CD31 immunostaining confirms the endothelial line of differentiation of tumor cells in this spindle cell angiosarcoma. In this context, the marker is specific for endothelial differentiation, but also stains Kaposi sarcoma. (Right) FLI-1 immunostaining shows nuclear expression. This is a marker of endothelial differentiation, but is not specific, as it is expressed in some carcinomas, lymphomas, and Ewing sarcoma. However, epithelioid sarcomas are negative.

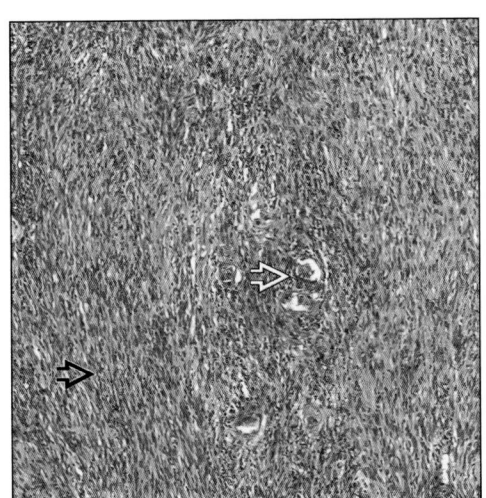

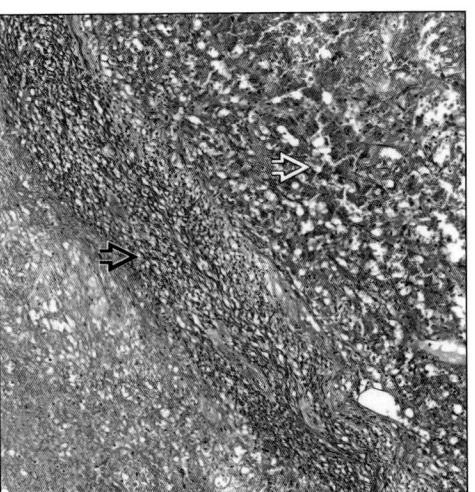

(Left) Angiosarcoma arising in a malignant peripheral nerve sheath tumor. Note the sheets of spindle cells ⊳ and focal atypical epithelioid endothelial tumor cells ⧨. Angiosarcoma has also been described as arising in schwannoma. (Right) This is a rare example of angiosarcoma arising in a low-grade malignant peripheral nerve sheath tumor (MPNST). Note spindle cell areas ⊳ of the nerve sheath tumor, adjacent to anastomosing vascular structures lined by atypical endothelial cells ⧨.

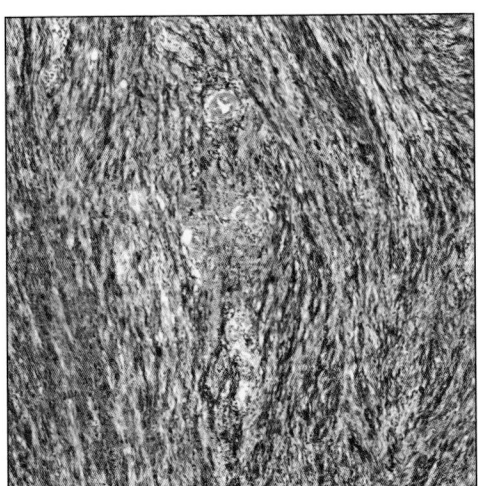

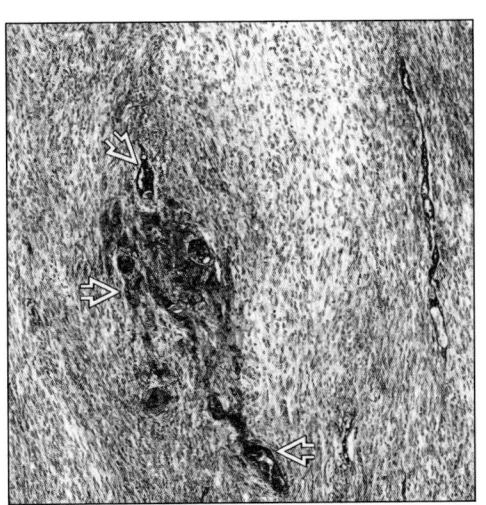

(Left) Immunostaining for S100 protein shows expression by many (but not all) spindle-shaped tumor cells of the low-grade malignant peripheral nerve sheath tumor component. The angiosarcomatous component did not express this antigen. (Right) CD31 immunostaining shows expression by cells of the angiosarcomatous component ⧨, not the areas of MPNST. This marker is more specific than CD34, which can be expressed in nerve sheath tumors as well as endothelial neoplasms.

Tumors and Tumor-like Conditions with Neural, Nerve Sheath, and Neuroendocrine Differentiation

NEUROMAS

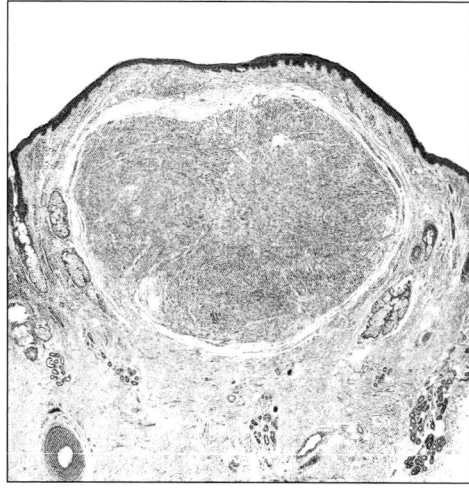

Solitary circumscribed neuroma ("palisaded encapsulated neuroma") represents a well-circumscribed, partially encapsulated, dermal-based neural neoplasm. Note absence of epidermal hyperplasia.

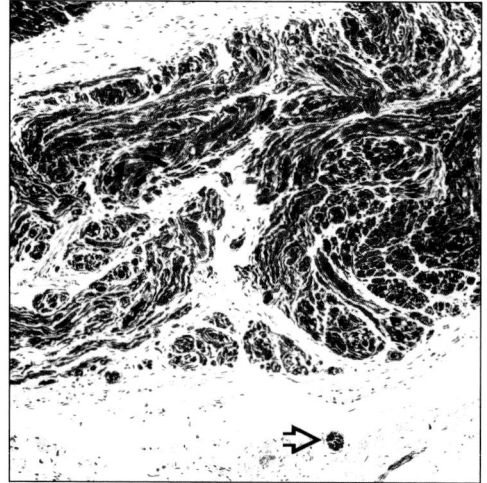

Solitary circumscribed neuroma is composed mainly of S100 protein positive Schwann cells. Preexisting peripheral nerves ➥ can often be seen at the base of these lesions.

TERMINOLOGY

Definitions
- Proliferation of peripheral nerve fibers in which ratio of axons to Schwann cell fascicles approaches 1:1
  - Solitary circumscribed neuroma ("palisaded encapsulated neuroma") represents spontaneous proliferation of peripheral nerve fibers
  - Multiple mucosal neuromas associated with multiple endocrine neoplasia (MEN) syndrome (type 2B) represent rare autosomal dominant condition
  - Traumatic neuroma represents post-traumatic proliferation of peripheral nerve fibers
  - Morton neuroma represents degenerative neural changes with reactive fibrosis on the foot
  - Pacinian neuroma represents painful hyperplasia of pacinian bodies on finger
  - Epithelial sheath neuroma represents proliferation of nerves ensheathed by squamous epithelium

ETIOLOGY/PATHOGENESIS

Developmental Anomaly
- Multiple mucosal neuromas in MEN syndrome
  - Represents rare autosomal dominant condition
  - Also includes medullary carcinoma of thyroid, pheochromocytoma, and somatic abnormalities
  - Mucosal neuromas have been rarely reported without any other systemic features of the syndrome

Environmental Exposure
- Traumatic neuroma
  - Amputation neuroma represents painful, reactive proliferation of nerve fibers after amputation
  - Proliferation of nonencapsulated nerve fibers after intrauterine or perinatal amputation of supernumerary digits
  - Can occur on penis after circumcision
- Morton neuroma

  - Degenerative damage of peripheral nerves

CLINICAL ISSUES

Epidemiology
- Age
  - Solitary circumscribed neuroma most common in 5th and 7th decades
- Gender
  - Solitary circumscribed neuroma occurs in equal ratio in both genders

Site
- Solitary circumscribed neuroma
  - Majority (90%) located on face
  - Rare in other anatomic locations
  - Mucosal involvement has been reported rarely
- Mucosal neuroma
  - Lips, tongue, eyelids
  - Upper GI tract
- Morton neuroma
  - Sole of foot
  - Usually in distal parts of peripheral nerves of 3rd and 4th metatarsals
- Pacinian neuroma
  - Usually on fingers
- Epithelial sheath neuroma
  - Usually on back
  - In superficial dermis

Presentation
- Painful or painless mass
- Slow growing

Treatment
- Surgical approaches
  - Simple excision is curative

Prognosis
- Biologically benign

NEUROMAS

Key Facts

Terminology
- Neuroma represents proliferation of peripheral nerve fibers in which ratio of axons to Schwann cell fascicles approaches 1:1
- Solitary circumscribed neuroma ("palisaded encapsulated neuroma") represents spontaneous proliferation of peripheral nerve fibers
- Multiple mucosal neuromas associated with multiple endocrine neoplasia syndrome (type 2B) represents rare autosomal dominant condition
- Traumatic neuroma represents post-traumatic proliferation of peripheral nerve fibers
- Morton neuroma represents degenerative neural change with reactive fibrosis on foot
- Pacinian neuroma represents painful hyperplasia of Pacinian bodies on finger

- Epithelial sheath neuroma represents proliferation of enlarged dermal nerves ensheathed by squamous epithelium

Clinical Issues
- Solitary circumscribed neuroma occurs predominantly on face
- Morton neuroma arises usually in distal parts of peripheral nerves of 3rd and 4th os metatarsale

Microscopic Pathology
- Proliferation of peripheral nerve fibers
- Proliferation of S100 positive Schwann cells
- Neurofilament positive axons
- No cytologic atypia
- No increased mitotic activity
- Perineural fibrosis in traumatic neuroma

MACROSCOPIC FEATURES

General Features
- Raised dermal, papular or nodular lesions

MICROSCOPIC PATHOLOGY

Histologic Features
- Solitary circumscribed neuroma ("palisaded encapsulated neuroma")
  - Single dermal nodule
  - Multinodular &/or plexiform growth are very uncommon
  - Well-developed fascicles of Schwann cells
  - Numerous associated axons
  - Characteristic clefts
  - Superficial part is rather loosely arranged
  - Capsule-like fibroblasts and perineurial cells are seen in deeper parts
  - Small nerves can grow into lesion from below
  - Epithelioid cytomorphology is seen very rarely
  - Vascular variant has been reported rarely
- Multiple mucosal neuromas associated with MEN syndrome
  - Morphology resembles features of solitary circumscribed neuroma
- Traumatic neuroma
  - Irregular arrangement of proliferating nerve fascicles embedded in fibrous scar tissue
  - Perineural fibrosis
  - Perineurial cells surround each small nerve fascicle
- Morton neuroma
  - Enlargement of plantar digital nerves
  - Edema of the nerve
  - Perineural fibrosis
- Pacinian neuroma
  - Hyperplasia of pacinian bodies
- Epithelial sheath neuroma
  - Large hyperplastic peripheral nerves in upper parts of dermis

- Nerve fibers are surrounded by mature squamous epithelium
- Associated fibroplasia and scattered inflammatory cells

Cytologic Features
- Elongated spindled cells
- Ill-defined, pale eosinophilic cytoplasm
- Bland, elongated fusiform nuclei
- No cytologic atypia

DIFFERENTIAL DIAGNOSIS

Schwannoma
- Encapsulated neoplasms
- Composed of Schwann cells
- Antoni A and Antoni B growth pattern
- Usually no neurofilament positive axons
- Contains blood vessels

Neurofibroma
- Often poorly circumscribed lesions
- Typically shows myxoid stroma
- No proliferation of peripheral nerve fibers

Perineurioma
- Composed of EMA positive perineurial cells
- Spindled tumor cells with elongated nuclei and long, thin cytoplasmic processes
- No S100 positive Schwann cells
- No neurofilament positive axons

Dermal Melanocytic Nevus
- Epithelioid-appearing nevus cells
- At least focal presence of melanin pigment
- Expression of melanocytic antigens HMB-45, MART-1/Melan-A

Dermatofibroma
- Ill-defined dermal lesions
- Composed of "fibrohistiocytic" cells
- S100 negative

9

NEUROMAS

Immunohistochemistry

Antibody	Reactivity	Staining Pattern	Comment
S100	Positive	Nuclear & cytoplasmic	Schwann cells are positive
NFP	Positive	Cytoplasmic	Axons are positive
EMA	Positive	Cell membrane & cytoplasm	Perineurial cells are positive at periphery of lesion
CD56	Positive	Cytoplasmic	In axons
Actin-sm	Negative		
GFAP	Negative		
CK-PAN	Negative		

Dermatomyofibroma
- Plaque-like dermal lesions
- Composed of spindled myofibroblasts
- S100 negative, SMA positive

Pilar Leiomyoma
- Ill-defined dermal neoplasms
- Composed of spindled eosinophilic tumor cells
- S100 negative
- Expression of muscle markers

Ganglioneuroma
- Composed of mature ganglion cells intermixed with fascicles of spindled S100 protein positive cells

Dermatofibrosarcoma Protuberans
- Diffuse infiltrative growth
- Storiform growth pattern
- S100 negative
- CD34 positive spindled cells

Superficial Acral Fibromyxoma
- Fascicles of spindled tumor cells
- Collagenous and myxoid stroma
- S100 negative
- Often focal expression of EMA &/or CD34

Sclerotic Fibroma (Storiform Collagenoma)
- Collagenous stroma with lamellar clefts
- S100 negative, CD34 positive

DIAGNOSTIC CHECKLIST

Clinically Relevant Pathologic Features
- Organ distribution

Pathologic Interpretation Pearls
- Solitary lesions
- Painful or painless lesions
- Biologically benign lesions
- Proliferation of peripheral nerve fascicles
- Proliferation of axons
- Perineural fibrosis

SELECTED REFERENCES

1. Salcedo E et al: Traumatic neuromas of the penis: a clinical, histopathological and immunohistochemical study of 17 cases. J Cutan Pathol. 36(2):229-33, 2009
2. Misago N et al: Unusual benign myxoid nerve sheath lesion: myxoid palisaded encapsulated neuroma (PEN) or nerve sheath myxoma with PEN/PEN-like features? Am J Dermatopathol. 29(2):160-4, 2007
3. Lombardi T et al: [Solitary circumscribed neuroma (palisaded encapsulated neuroma) of the oral mucosa.] Ann Dermatol Venereol. 129(2):229-32, 2002
4. Dubovy SR et al: Palisaded encapsulated neuroma (solitary circumscribed neuroma of skin) of the eyelid: report of two cases and review of the literature. Br J Ophthalmol. 85(8):949-51, 2001
5. Navarro M et al: Palisaded encapsulated neuroma (solitary circumscribed neuroma) of the glans penis. Br J Dermatol. 142(5):1061-2, 2000
6. Requena L et al: Epithelial sheath neuroma: a new entity. Am J Surg Pathol. 24(2):190-6, 2000
7. Magnusson B: Palisaded encapsulated neuroma (solitary circumscribed neuroma) of the oral mucosa. Oral Surg Oral Med Oral Pathol Oral Radiol Endod. 82(3):302-4, 1996
8. Bennett GL et al: Morton's interdigital neuroma: a comprehensive treatment protocol. Foot Ankle Int. 16(12):760-3, 1995
9. Megahed M: Palisaded encapsulated neuroma (solitary circumscribed neuroma). A clinicopathologic and immunohistochemical study. Am J Dermatopathol. 16(2):120-5, 1994
10. Argenyi ZB et al: Plexiform and other unusual variants of palisaded encapsulated neuroma. J Cutan Pathol. 20(1):34-9, 1993
11. Argenyi ZB et al: Vascular variant of palisaded encapsulated neuroma. J Cutan Pathol. 20(1):92-3, 1993
12. Dakin MC et al: The palisaded, encapsulated neuroma (solitary circumscribed neuroma). Histopathology. 20(5):405-10, 1992
13. Tsang WY et al: Epithelioid variant of solitary circumscribed neuroma of the skin. Histopathology. 20(5):439-41, 1992
14. Alexander J et al: An unusual solitary circumscribed neuroma (palisaded encapsulated neuroma) of the skin-- with observations on the nature of pseudo-epitheliomatous hyperplasia. Histopathology. 18(2):175-7, 1991
15. Butterworth DM et al: Solitary circumscribed neuroma of the skin. Histopathology. 19(6):577-9, 1991
16. Albrecht S et al: Palisaded encapsulated neuroma: an immunohistochemical study. Mod Pathol. 2(4):403-6, 1989
17. Dover JS et al: Palisaded encapsulated neuromas. A clinicopathologic study. Arch Dermatol. 125(3):386-9, 1989
18. Fletcher CD et al: Digital pacinian neuroma: a distinctive hyperplastic lesion. Histopathology. 15(3):249-56, 1989
19. Fletcher CD: Solitary circumscribed neuroma of the skin (so-called palisaded, encapsulated neuroma). Am J Surg Pathol. 13(7):574-80, 1989
20. Reed RJ et al: Palisaded, encapsulated neuromas of the skin. Arch Dermatol. 106(6):865-70, 1972

Microscopic Features

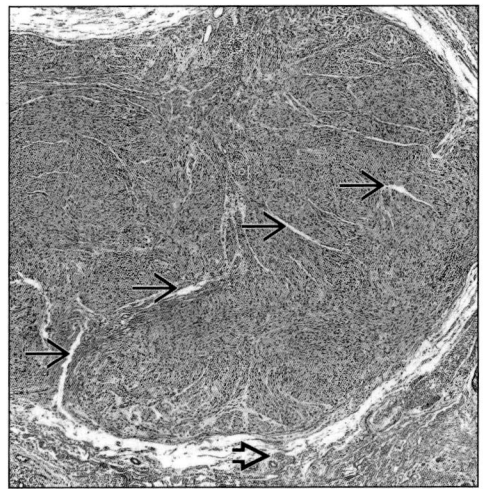

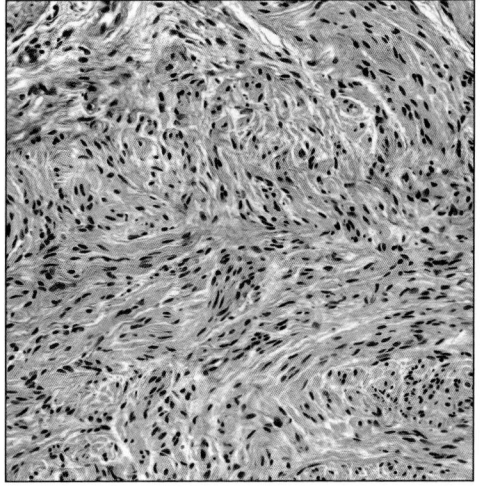

(Left) Solitary circumscribed neuroma is a circumscribed, sometimes partly encapsulated dermal lesion composed of Schwann cells and associated axons. Characteristic clefts ⮕ and a small preexisting nerve at the base of the lesion ⮔ can be seen. (Right) The neoplastic Schwann cells contain ill-defined, pale eosinophilic cytoplasm and cytologically bland spindled nuclei with evenly distributed chromatin. No prominent cytologic atypia and no increased mitoses are present.

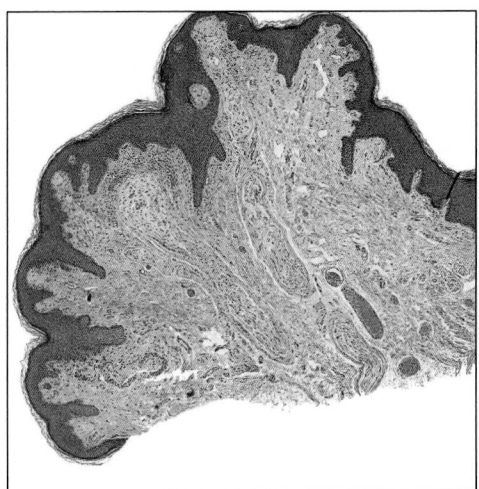

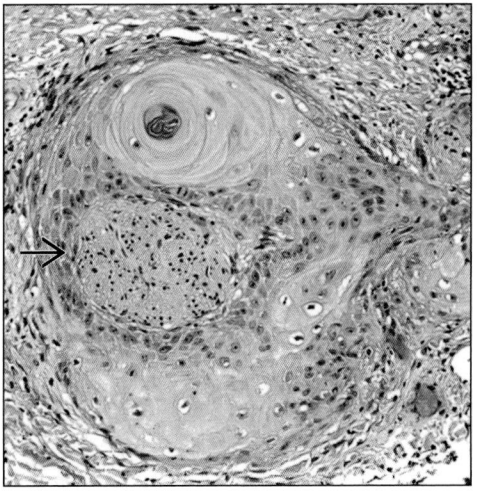

(Left) Traumatic neuroma of the penis after circumcision has hyperplastic nerve fibers with mild perineural fibrosis. This lesion can clinically mimic a condyloma, but attention to the history and the immunohistochemical demonstration of excess nerves lead to the correct diagnosis. (Right) Epithelial sheath neuroma is a rare benign superficial dermal lesion. An enlarged nerve bundle ⮕ is surrounded by keratinizing squamous epithelium. (Courtesy C. Cockerell, MD and C. Etufugh, MD.)

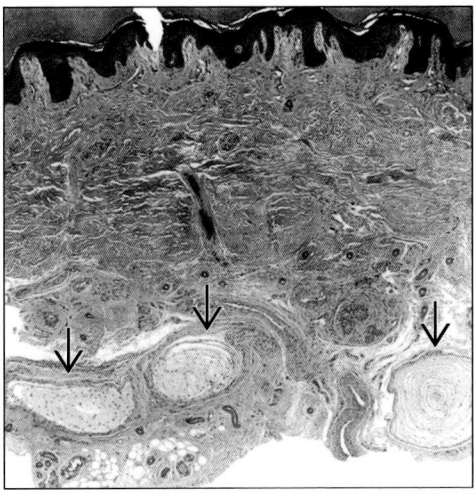

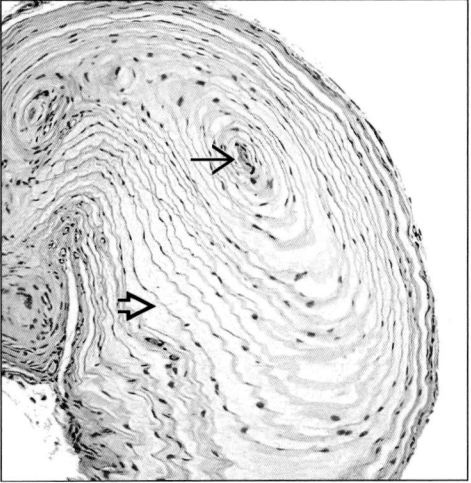

(Left) Pacinian neuroma comprises round or oval nodules with multiple cell layers ⮕, resembling normal Pacinian corpuscles. This occurs mainly in digits in subcutaneous tissue, and can be painful. (Courtesy C. Cockerell, MD and C. Etufugh, MD.) (Right) The corpuscles comprise concentric lamellae ⮔ of perineurial cells with elongated slender processes. These are immunoreactive for epithelial membrane antigen. In the center is an axon ⮕, which is positive for neurofilaments.

9

NEUROFIBROMA

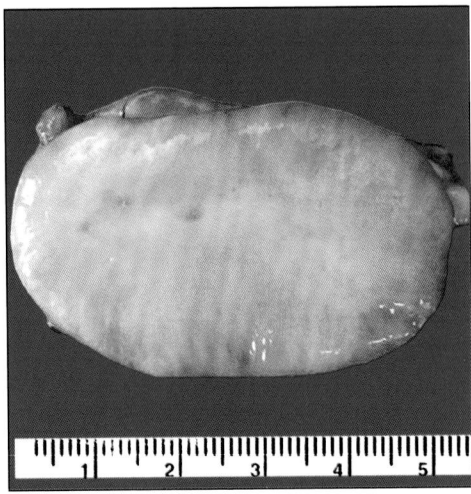

The cut surface of neurofibroma is pale, homogeneous, waxy, and often myxoid in appearance. Degenerative changes typically seen in schwannomas are seldom present in neurofibroma.

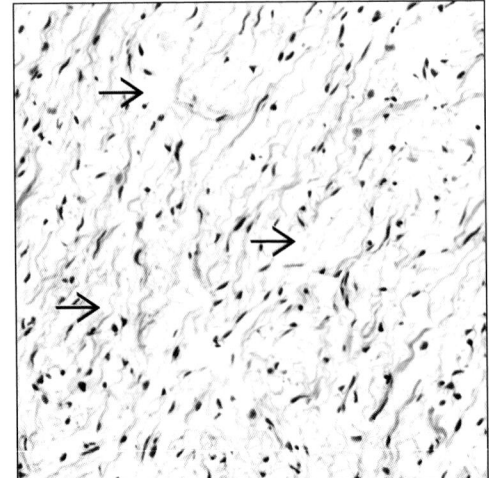

Histologic examination shows the classic hypocellular appearance of spindle and wavy cells with angulated or ovoid nuclei and thin cell processes amid a loose myxoid matrix ➡.

TERMINOLOGY

Abbreviations
- Neurofibroma (NF)

Synonyms
- von Recklinghausen disease = neurofibromatosis type 1 (NF1)

Definitions
- Benign peripheral nerve sheath tumor composed of Schwann cells, fibroblasts, perineurial-like cells, and residual nerves in myxoid/collagen matrix

ETIOLOGY/PATHOGENESIS

Histogenesis
- Neurofibromas are sporadic in about 90% of cases; others are syndromic in association with NF1
  - NF1 results from germline mutation in *NF1* gene on chromosome 17q11.2
    - *NF1* gene encodes for neurofibromin protein, which is a GTPase-activating protein
    - Neurofibromin also acts as a tumor suppressor by downregulating the Ras signal transduction pathway
  - Sporadic tumors arise from somatic mutations in *NF1*
- Evidence supporting neoplastic nature of NF
  - Sporadic tumors are histologically similar to NF1-associated neurofibromas
  - Tumors are monoclonal on X chromosome inactivation studies
  - Lesional cells carry *NF1* gene deletion

CLINICAL ISSUES

Epidemiology
- Incidence

  - Most common tumor of peripheral nerve
  - NF1 incidence: 1 in 2,500-4,000 births
- Age
  - Solitary, sporadic lesions: In patients 20-30 years old
  - Tumors in setting of NF1 present during puberty
  - Plexiform NF may be congenital
- Gender
  - Affects both sexes equally

Presentation
- Most tumors are solitary and sporadic
- Superficial cutaneous or localized intraneural NF present as painless, palpable mass
- Deep intraneural tumors may present with pain or dysesthesia
- Intraspinal (nerve root) NF may show signs of spinal cord compression

Natural History
- Slow-growing tumors in most instances
  - Increased rates of growth may be seen in puberty and pregnancy
- Malignant transformation in NF
  - Rare in sporadic tumors; usually occurs in setting of NF1
  - Very rare in cutaneous NF (0.001%)
  - More common in plexiform NF (2-10%)
  - Clinical suspicion for malignant transformation
    - Rapid enlargement of preexisting NF
    - Pain or change in neurological symptoms

Treatment
- Surgical approaches
  - Complete resection is curative
  - Decompression of spinal cord in symptomatic tumors

Prognosis
- Recurrence rare, even after partial removal

NEUROFIBROMA

Key Facts

Terminology
- Benign peripheral nerve sheath tumor with heterogeneous admixture of axons, Schwann cells, perineurial cells, and fibroblasts
- Most are sporadic; neurofibromatosis type 1 (NF1) associated with multiple, large, or plexiform tumors

Clinical Issues
- Localized cutaneous NF most common subtype
- Diffuse cutaneous NF infiltrate dermis and subcutis
- Localized intraneural NF are deep seated and involve larger nerves
- Plexiform NF involves multiple nerve fascicles or branches ("bag of worms")
- Massive soft tissue NF involves pelvis, shoulder, or extremities ("localized gigantism")

Macroscopic Features
- Variable size and consistency
- Lack degenerative changes seen in schwannomas

Microscopic Pathology
- Bundles of spindle cells with angulated or wavy nuclei
- Loose, myxoid, or thick collagenous matrix
- Coarse collagen bundles resemble "shredded carrots"
- Residual, central, neurofilament-positive axon fibers present
- Atypical NF behave in benign manner

Diagnostic Checklist
- Malignant transformation occurs in about 2-10% of plexiform NF
  - ↑ cellularity, atypia, hyperchromasia, mitoses

Subtypes
- **Localized cutaneous NF**
  - Most common type
  - Nodular or polypoid, usually well-circumscribed
  - Freely movable, soft, round lesions that elevate skin
  - Generally not associated with peripheral nerve
- **Diffuse cutaneous NF**
  - Typically affects children and young adults
  - Large plaque-like tumors that often affect head and neck region
  - 10% associated with NF1
  - Diffuse infiltration of dermis and subcutaneous adipose tissue
  - Entraps dermal vessels, nerves, and adnexa
  - Spreads along subcutaneous connective tissue septa
- **Plexiform NF**
  - Usually presents in early childhood
  - Pathognomonic of NF1 if plexiform architecture is strictly defined
  - Multinodular lesions involving multiple nerves or nerve branches
  - "Bag of worms" appearance is characteristic
  - Generally affects small nerves
  - Entire extremity may be involved ("elephantiasis neuromatosa")
- **Massive soft tissue NF**
  - Tends to be very large, diffuse, or plexiform
  - Widespread infiltration of adipose tissue and muscle
  - Results in large pendulous folds of neurofibromatous tissue ("localized gigantism")

IMAGE FINDINGS

MR Findings
- Irregular or bright on T2WI MR
- Gadolinium enhancing on T1WI
- "Target" sign due to reduced signal in intraneural NF
- "Dumbbell" tumors: Intradural and extradural portions of paraspinal tumor acquire shape of dumbbell

MACROSCOPIC FEATURES

General Features
- Gray to tan cut surface
- Glistening, gelatinous to firm/fibrous consistency
- Relatively well-circumscribed, but not encapsulated
  - Intraneural NF may be covered by epineurium
- Lack degeneration (hemorrhage, cystic change) commonly seen in schwannomas

Size
- Localized cutaneous lesions: Up to 2 cm
- May reach much larger size (e.g., massive soft tissue NF)

MICROSCOPIC PATHOLOGY

Histologic Features
- Irregular interlacing bundles or fascicles of spindle cells
- Ovoid to spindled, wavy, dark nuclei with thin cell processes
- Variable proportions of loose myxoid matrix and coarse collagen bundles
- Collagen bundles impart "shredded carrots" appearance
- Residual axons usually present within tumor
- Mast cells, lymphocytes, and even xanthoma cells may be present
- Some tumors may be more cellular with uniform collagenous matrix ("cellular neurofibroma")
- Nuclear atypia may be present in some cases
  - Atypia in absence of increased cellularity, mitotic activity, and necrosis is not a feature of malignancy in NF
- Rare morphological findings
  - Epithelioid Schwann cells
  - Skeletal muscle
  - Glandular epithelium or rosettes
- NF subtypes
  - **Localized cutaneous NF**

- Dense collagenized stroma is typical; cutaneous NF separated from epidermis by grenz zone
  - **Diffuse cutaneous NF**
    - Uniformly fine fibrillary collagenous matrix
    - Clusters of Meissner body-like structures are often present
  - **Plexiform NF**
    - Tortuous mass of multinodular tumor tissue
    - Early stages of tumor may show only increased endoneurial matrix
    - Large tumors may also have intermixed areas of diffuse NF
    - Nuclear atypia may be present

Cytologic Features
- Bland nuclear features in most cases

Histologic Variants
- Pigmented NF
  - Rare (< 1% of all NF)
  - Melanin pigment present in dendritic or epithelioid tumor cells
  - Pigmented cells cluster in superficial parts of tumor
  - Stain positively with S100 and melanocytic markers, such as HMB-45
  - May recur, but do not metastasize
- Atypical NF
  - Tumors with atypia in which features fall short of diagnosis of low-grade malignant peripheral nerve sheath tumor (MPNST)
  - Nuclear atypia or rare mitotic figures in isolation should not be construed as signs of malignancy
  - Shows variable number of large hyperchromatic nuclei
  - Mitotic activity is low or absent

ANCILLARY TESTS

Immunohistochemistry
- S100 stains subset of tumor cells; may also be positive for GFAP and CD34
- Perineurial cells positive for EMA
- Axons positive for neurofilament protein

Electron Microscopy
- Heterogeneous mixture of cell types, including Schwann cells, small neurites, perineurial cells, and fibroblasts

DIFFERENTIAL DIAGNOSIS

Plexiform Schwannoma
- Biphasic tumor with Antoni A and Antoni B areas
- Verocay bodies, perivascular hyalinization, and hemosiderin deposits present
- Cellular plexiform schwannoma may be mistaken for MPNST arising in plexiform NF
- S100 positivity is more diffuse and uniform

Perineurioma
- Concentric "onion bulb" or whorled proliferations around nerve fibers

- Diffusely and strongly positive for EMA

Ganglioneuroma (GN)
- Large neoplastic ganglion cells interspersed with neurofibroma-like areas
- GN shows abundant unmyelinated axons

Malignant Peripheral Nerve Sheath Tumor (MPNST)
- Cellular NF may be mistaken for MPNST
- Pleomorphism, nuclear enlargement, necrosis, and high mitotic activity (> 4/10 HPF) favor MPNST

Plexiform Fibrohistiocytic Tumors (PFHT)
- PFHT may be mistaken for plexiform NF
- Female predilection; myofibroblastic proliferation with multinucleated histiocytic giant cells in PFHT
- PFHT is actin(+), CD68(+), S100(-)

Dermatofibrosarcoma Protuberans (DFSP)
- Infiltration into subcutaneous adipose tissue in diffuse NF may be mistaken for DFSP
- DFSP is more cellular with uniformly storiform architecture and CD34 positivity

DIAGNOSTIC CHECKLIST

Clinically Relevant Pathologic Features
- Features pathognomonic for NF1
  - Multiple intraneural or cutaneous involvement
  - Plexiform architecture
  - Large (massive) soft tissue lesions
- Cutaneous NF associated with NF1
  - Overlying café au lait spots (pigmented macules)

Pathologic Interpretation Pearls
- Transformation to MPNST evident by increased cellularity, atypia, necrosis, and high mitotic activity

SELECTED REFERENCES
1. Skovronsky DM et al: Pathologic classification of peripheral nerve tumors. Neurosurg Clin N Am. 15(2):157-66, 2004
2. Evans DG et al: Malignant peripheral nerve sheath tumours in neurofibromatosis 1. J Med Genet. 39(5):311-4, 2002
3. Ferner RE et al: Neurofibroma and schwannoma. Curr Opin Neurol. 15(6):679-84, 2002
4. Fetsch JF et al: Pigmented (melanotic) neurofibroma: a clinicopathologic and immunohistochemical analysis of 19 lesions from 17 patients. Am J Surg Pathol. 24(3):331-43, 2000
5. Rasmussen SA et al: NF1 gene and neurofibromatosis 1. Am J Epidemiol. 151(1):33-40, 2000
6. Woodruff JM: Pathology of tumors of the peripheral nerve sheath in type 1 neurofibromatosis. Am J Med Genet. 89(1):23-30, 1999
7. Lin BT et al: Neurofibroma and cellular neurofibroma with atypia: a report of 14 tumors. Am J Surg Pathol. 21(12):1443-9, 1997
8. Lassmann H et al: Different types of benign nerve sheath tumors. Light microscopy, electron microscopy and autoradiography. Virchows Arch A Pathol Anat Histol. 375(3):197-210, 1977

NEUROFIBROMA

Radiographic, Gross, and Microscopic Features

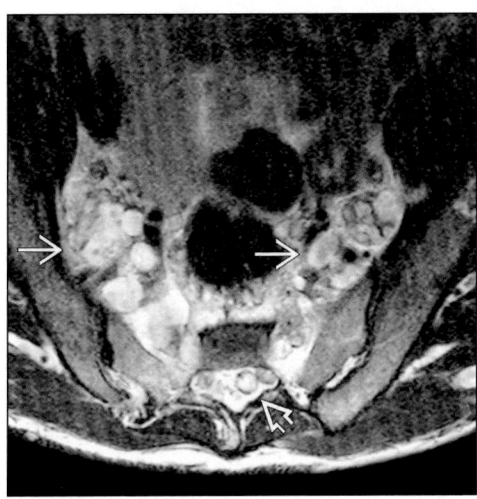

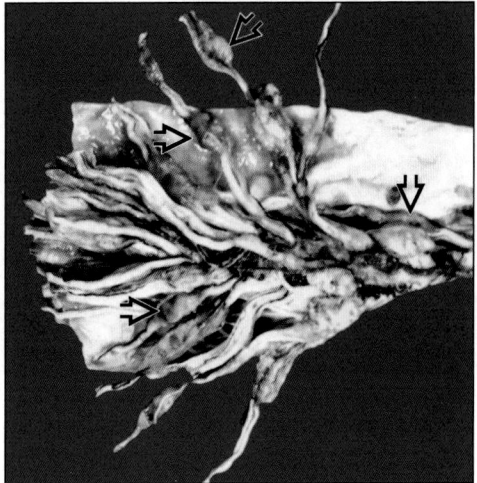

(Left) Axial T2WI MR shows bilateral plexiform neurofibromas ➡ involving the sacral plexus with a characteristic "bag of worms" appearance. There is intraspinal extension ➡. (Right) Gross photograph shows multiple small fusiform tumors ➡ involving spinal nerve roots around the sacral plexus from a patient with NF1.

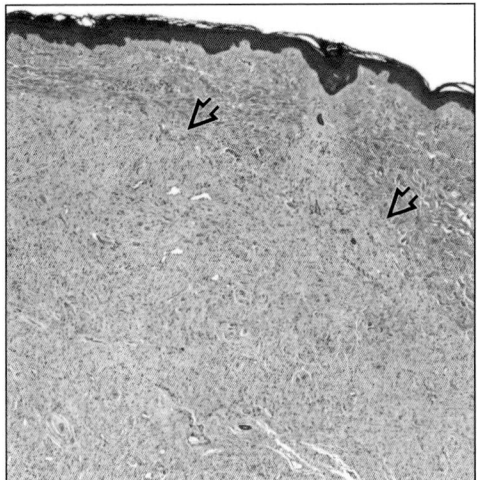

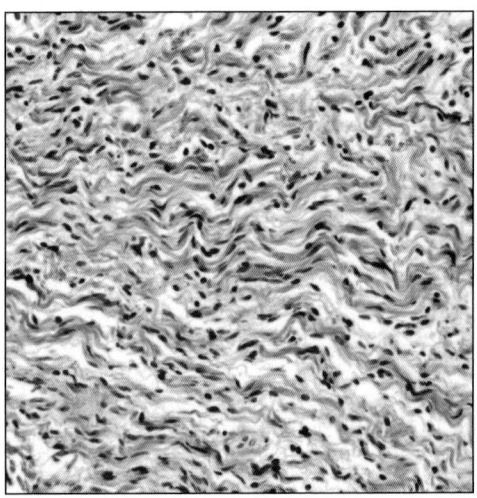

(Left) Localized cutaneous neurofibromas are fairly well-circumscribed ➡ but unencapsulated tumors. Although they may occur in NF1, the majority of localized cutaneous tumors are sporadic in nature. (Right) Neurofibromas are composed of small ovoid to spindled cells with dark wavy nuclei in a variably myxoid or collagenous background.

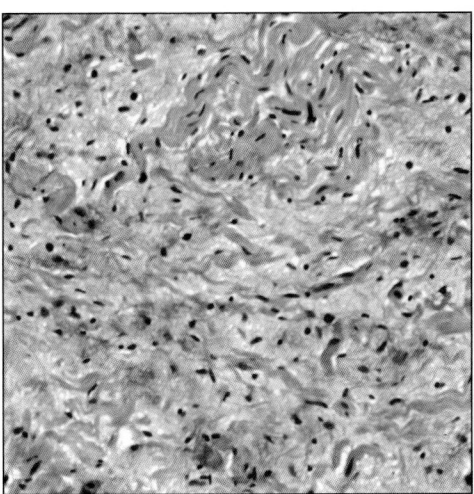

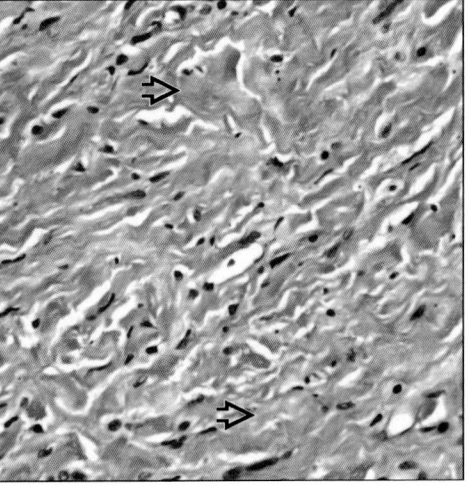

(Left) Some neurofibromas may show prominent myxoid stromal change. When this change is prominent, these tumors may be mistaken for myxoma. (Right) Other neurofibromas may be extremely hypocellular and show a densely collagenized stroma ➡.

SCHWANNOMA (NEURILEMMOMA)

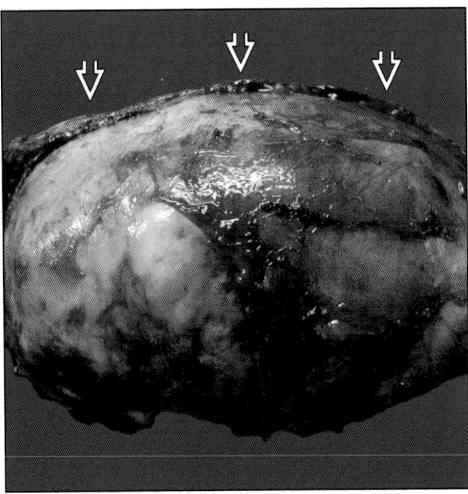

Schwannomas are well-circumscribed, encapsulated tumors and often arise as an eccentric mass loosely attached to an underlying nerve. The underlying nerve ➡ wraps around the tumor in this example.

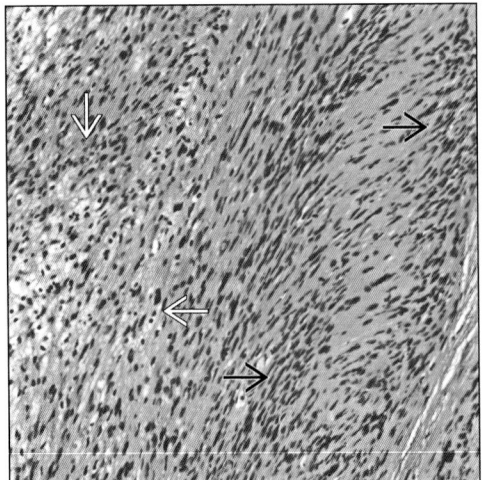

Schwannomas are composed of alternating hypercellular spindle cell areas (Antoni A ➡) and hypocellular round cell areas (Antoni B ➡). Nuclear palisading is often present in Antoni A areas.

TERMINOLOGY

Definitions
- Encapsulated, benign peripheral nerve sheath tumor composed predominantly of Schwann cells

ETIOLOGY/PATHOGENESIS

Molecular Aberrations
- Somatic *NF2* gene mutations present in most tumors
- Bilateral vestibular schwannomas occur in setting of germline *NF2* gene mutations

CLINICAL ISSUES

Epidemiology
- Incidence
  - 90% are sporadic
  - 10% are syndromic
    - About 3% with neurofibromatosis type 2 (NF2)
    - 2% with schwannomatosis
    - 5% with multiple meningiomas
    - Rarely in association with neurofibromatosis type 1 (NF1)
- Age
  - All ages
  - Common between 20-50 years of age
- Gender
  - Affects males and females equally

Site
- Head & neck
- Upper and lower extremities
- Deep-seated tumors occur in mediastinum and retroperitoneum

Presentation
- Slow growing
- Painless mass in most cases

- Large tumors may be painful
- Cystic tumors may show fluctuation in size

Treatment
- Surgical excision is curative

Prognosis
- Excellent

Multiple Schwannoma Syndromes
- **Neurofibromatosis type 2**
  - Autosomal dominant condition
  - Incidence around 1:30,000-40,000
  - Inactivating germline mutations of *NF2* gene on chromosome 22
  - Bilateral vestibular schwannomas are characteristic
  - Schwannomas involving other cranial nerves may be present
  - CNS tumors like meningioma, ependymoma, and gliomas are also part of disease spectrum
  - Schwannomas in NF2 resemble their sporadic counterparts
- **Schwannomatosis**
  - Not associated with germline mutations in *NF1* or *NF2* genes
  - Autosomal dominant inheritance with incomplete penetrance
  - Both sexes affected equally
  - Patients do not develop bilateral vestibular schwannomas or CNS tumors seen in NF2
  - Locus of disease mapped to chromosome 22 proximal to *NF2* gene
  - Morphology similar to sporadic schwannomas

MACROSCOPIC FEATURES

General Features
- Surrounded by true capsule consisting of epineurium
- Eccentric mass loosely attached to underlying nerve

SCHWANNOMA (NEURILEMMOMA)

Key Facts

Terminology
- Encapsulated, benign peripheral nerve sheath tumor composed predominantly of Schwann cells

Clinical Issues
- Common between 20-50 years of age
- Affects males and females equally
- Surgical excision is curative

Macroscopic Features
- Typically presents as eccentric mass loosely attached to underlying nerve

Microscopic Pathology
- Hallmark: Variable amounts of hypercellular Antoni A and hypocellular Antoni B areas
- Spindle cells in short fascicles in Antoni A areas

- Loose matrix with cystic change and inflammatory cells in Antoni B areas
- Bland nuclear features in most instances; degenerative nuclear atypia in "ancient" schwannoma
- Cellular schwannoma may mimic MPNST
- Plexiform schwannoma usually seen in children
- Epithelioid schwannoma may be mistaken for smooth muscle tumor
- Melanotic/psammomatous schwannoma often associated with Carney syndrome
- Schwannomas in NF2 and schwannomatosis similar to sporadic tumors
- Microcystic/reticular schwannoma has predilection for visceral location

Ancillary Tests
- Diffuse, strong S100 positivity is characteristic

- Small tumors may be fusiform in shape and mimic neurofibroma
- Dumbbell-shaped tumors occur in vertebral canal usually in posterior mediastinum
- Cut surface is pink, white-yellow
- Large tumors may show cystic change, hemorrhage, or calcification

Size
- Variable

MICROSCOPIC PATHOLOGY

Histologic Features
- Uninodular mass with fibrous capsule
- Hallmark: Variable amounts of hypercellular Antoni A and hypocellular Antoni B areas
- Antoni A
  - Spindle cells in short fascicles
  - Plump nuclei, indistinct cytoplasmic borders
  - Intranuclear vacuoles in some tumors
  - Nuclear palisading or whorling
  - Verocay bodies
    - Compact rows of palisaded nuclei separated by fibrillary processes
- Antoni B
  - Spindle or oval cells
  - Loose matrix with cystic change and inflammatory cells
  - Large vessels with thick hyalinized walls and luminal thrombi
- Benign epithelial structures and glands may be present in rare instances

Cytologic Features
- Bland nuclear features in most instances

Variants
- "Ancient" schwannoma
  - Marked nuclear atypia of degenerative type
  - Usually seen in deep-seated large tumors of long duration

- Cystic change, hemorrhage, calcification, and hyalinization present
  - Lacks mitotic activity
  - Behavior is similar to ordinary schwannoma
- Cellular schwannoma
  - Composed almost exclusively of hypercellular Antoni A areas, which lack Verocay bodies
  - More common in mediastinum and retroperitoneum
  - Encapsulated tumors; some may be multinodular or plexiform in architecture
  - Long sweeping fascicles of spindle-shaped cells
  - Mitotic activity is low (< 4/10 HPF)
  - Small foci of necrosis may be present
  - Diffuse strong S100 positivity distinguishes cellular schwannoma from malignant peripheral nerve sheath tumors (MPNSTs)
- Plexiform schwannoma
  - Usually involves skin
  - Infrequent in deeper locations
  - Encapsulated tumors with multinodular or plexiform architecture
  - Often more cellular than ordinary schwannoma
  - Association with neurofibromatosis is weak (unlike plexiform neurofibroma, which is almost pathognomonic of NF1)
- Epithelioid schwannoma
  - Small round Schwann cells with eosinophilic cytoplasm and sharp cell borders
  - Arranged in clusters, cords, or as single cells
  - Stroma is collagenous or myxoid
  - Foci of typical schwannoma may be present
  - Degenerative nuclear atypia may be seen
  - Lacks mitotic activity
  - Immunostains for S100 and type IV collagen are positive
- Melanotic/psammomatous schwannoma
  - Distinctive tumor of adults (average age around 33 years) that often arises in spinal or autonomic nerves near midline
  - About 50% of patients have evidence of Carney syndrome (cardiac myxoma, spotty pigmentation,

endocrine overactivity, acromegaly, or sexual precocity)
- o Multiple tumors may be present in 20% of patients
- o Pigmentation may be heavy and mask underlying tumor morphology
- o Syncytial arrangement of spindle to ovoid cells with prominent nucleoli and intranuclear inclusions
- o Psammoma bodies are present in most cases
- o Tumors express not only S100, but also HMB-45
- o Difficult to predict behavior since bland-appearing tumors have also been known to metastasize
- o Overall, metastasis occurs in about 26% of cases
- Neuroblastoma-like schwannoma
  - o Schwann cells are round and small in this variant and cluster around large collagen cores
  - o Mimics rosettes seen in neuroblastoma
- Pseudoglandular schwannoma
  - o Prominent cystic change
  - o Cystic spaces are lined by small round tumor cells
  - o Mimics epithelial neoplasm
- Microcystic/reticular schwannoma
  - o Anastomosing strands of spindle cells in myxoid, fibrillary, or collagenous matrix
  - o Predilection for visceral location
  - o Mimics reticular perineurioma
- Malignant transformation in schwannomas
  - o Extremely rare
  - o Malignant change in schwannomas usually resembles epithelioid MPNST

ANCILLARY TESTS

Immunohistochemistry
- Diffuse, strong S100 positivity is characteristic
- CD57 and GFAP may be positive in some tumors

Electron Microscopy
- Transmission
  - o Almost exclusively composed of Schwann cells
  - o Basal lamina with electron dense material lines surface of Schwann cells
  - o Flat invaginated nucleus and attenuated cell processes
  - o Increased lysosomes in Schwann cells in Antoni B areas

DIFFERENTIAL DIAGNOSIS

Leiomyoma
- Nuclear palisading is also seen in smooth muscle tumors and may mimic schwannoma
- Leiomyomas lack alternating Antoni A and Antoni B areas
- Leiomyomas are positive for desmin and smooth muscle actin, and are negative for S100

Malignant Peripheral Nerve Sheath Tumor (MPNST)
- Cellular schwannomas may be mistaken for MPNST

- Plexiform schwannomas are also cellular and may be mistaken for MPNST arising in plexiform neurofibroma
- MPNSTs show greater nuclear atypia, necrosis, and only focal S100 positivity, unlike benign schwannoma variants, which are diffusely S100 positive

Malignant Melanoma
- Melanotic schwannomas may be mistaken for melanoma due to coexpression of S100 and HMB-45
- Melanotic schwannomas do not have degree of nuclear atypia or mitotic activity seen in melanoma
- Most primary melanomas show overlying junctional component (melanoma in situ)
- Psammoma bodies are present in melanotic schwannoma, but not in melanomas

DIAGNOSTIC CHECKLIST

Pathologic Interpretation Pearls
- Encapsulated tumor with alternating hypercellular and hypocellular areas, and usually diffuse, strong S100 positivity

SELECTED REFERENCES

1. Liegl B et al: Microcystic/reticular schwannoma: a distinct variant with predilection for visceral locations. Am J Surg Pathol. 32(7):1080-7, 2008
2. MacCollin M et al: Diagnostic criteria for schwannomatosis. Neurology. 64(11):1838-45, 2005
3. Woodruff JM et al: Congenital and childhood plexiform (multinodular) cellular schwannoma: a troublesome mimic of malignant peripheral nerve sheath tumor. Am J Surg Pathol. 27(10):1321-9, 2003
4. McMenamin ME et al: Expanding the spectrum of malignant change in schwannomas: epithelioid malignant change, epithelioid malignant peripheral nerve sheath tumor, and epithelioid malignant angiosarcoma: a study of 17 cases. Am J Surg Pathol. 25(1):13-25, 2001
5. Antinheimo J et al: Population-based analysis of sporadic and type 2 neurofibromatosis-associated meningiomas and schwannomas. Neurology. 54(1):71-6, 2000
6. Kindblom LG et al: Benign epithelioid schwannoma. Am J Surg Pathol. 22(6):762-70, 1998
7. Chan JK et al: Pseudoglandular schwannoma. Histopathology. 29(5):481-3, 1996
8. Goldblum JR et al: Neuroblastoma-like neurilemoma. Am J Surg Pathol. 18(3):266-73, 1994
9. Brooks JJ et al: Benign glandular schwannoma. Arch Pathol Lab Med. 116(2):192-5, 1992
10. Carney JA: Psammomatous melanotic schwannoma. A distinctive, heritable tumor with special associations, including cardiac myxoma and the Cushing syndrome. Am J Surg Pathol. 14(3):206-22, 1990
11. Fletcher CD et al: Cellular schwannoma: a distinct pseudosarcomatous entity. Histopathology. 11(1):21-35, 1987
12. Fletcher CD et al: Benign plexiform (multinodular) schwannoma: a rare tumour unassociated with neurofibromatosis. Histopathology. 10(9):971-80, 1986

SCHWANNOMA (NEURILEMMOMA)

Gross and Microscopic Features

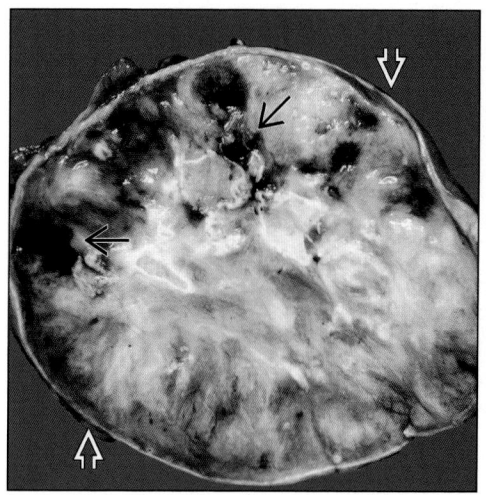

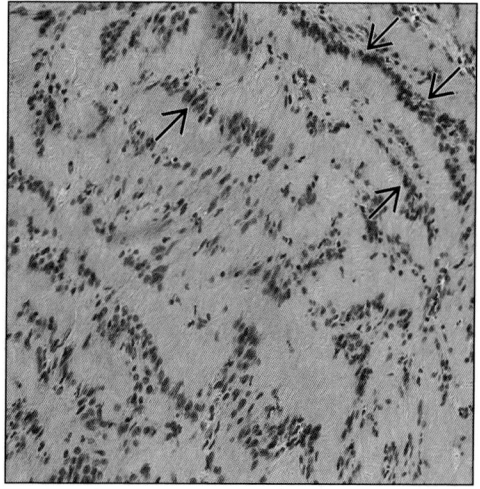

(Left) This tumor shows a thick peripheral capsule ⇨ and a yellow-white cut surface with foci of hemorrhage ➡. (Right) Nuclear palisading in Antoni A areas may be prominent and form nuclear palisades around a collagenous hyalinized core (Verocay bodies) ➡. Verocay bodies can be quite variable in number from case to case.

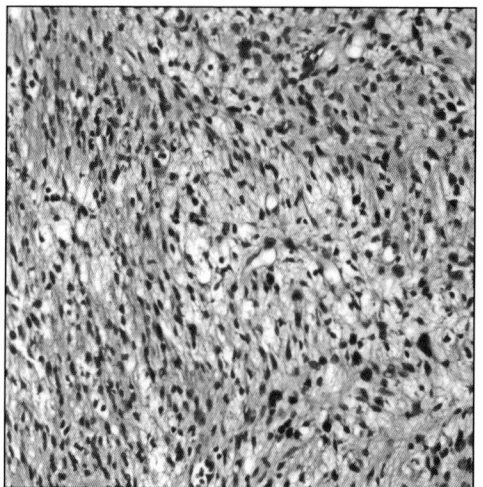

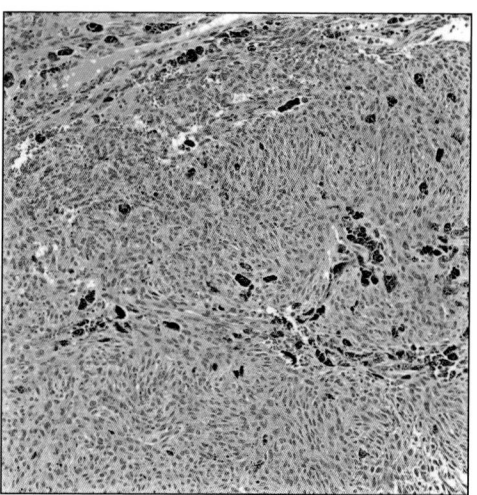

(Left) Antoni B areas are paucicellular with small, round to ovoid tumor cells and may contain foamy macrophages and inflammatory cells. The background stroma is loose and myxoid, in contrast to the more collagenized stroma in Antoni A areas of the tumor. (Right) Melanotic schwannoma occurs sporadically and in association with Carney syndrome. Syncytial arrangement of spindle cells with prominent melanin pigmentation is characteristic of this variant.

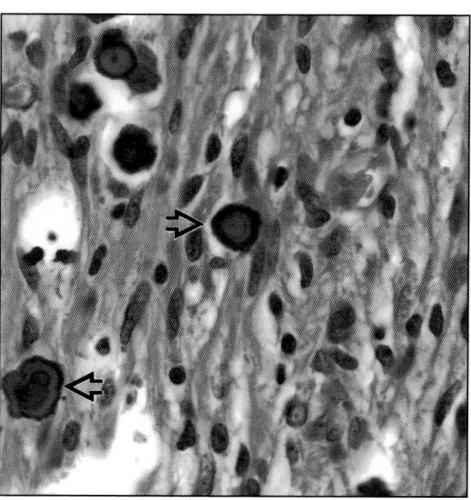

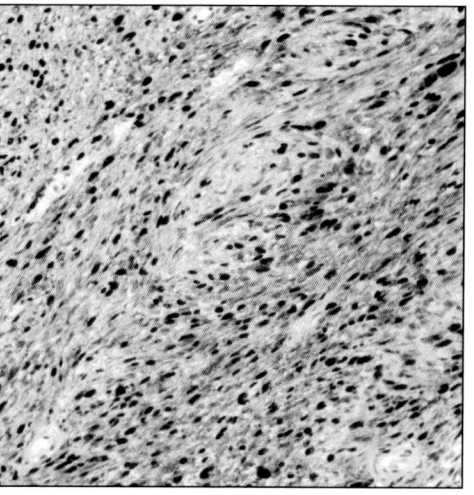

(Left) Psammomatous calcification ⇨ is present in most cases of melanotic schwannoma and is a helpful clue in distinguishing this schwannoma variant from metastatic malignant melanoma. (Right) Schwannomas are characterized by diffuse and strong immunoreactivity for S100 protein. The presence of diffuse positivity is a useful clue to the benign nature of some schwannoma variants that may otherwise be mistaken for a MPNST.

CELLULAR NEUROTHEKEOMA

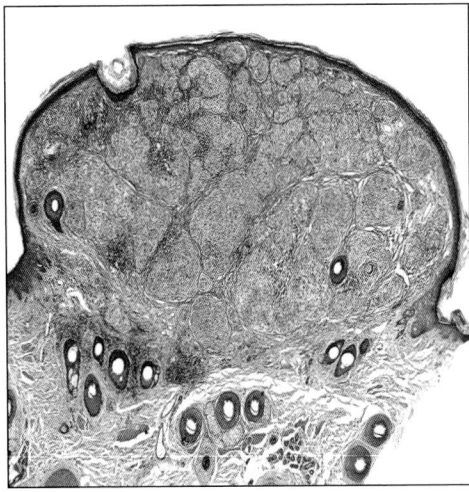

Scanning magnification of a transverse section of whole tumor shows the smooth, dome-shaped outline. The lesion is confined to the dermis. The epidermis is thinned, except at the lateral margins.

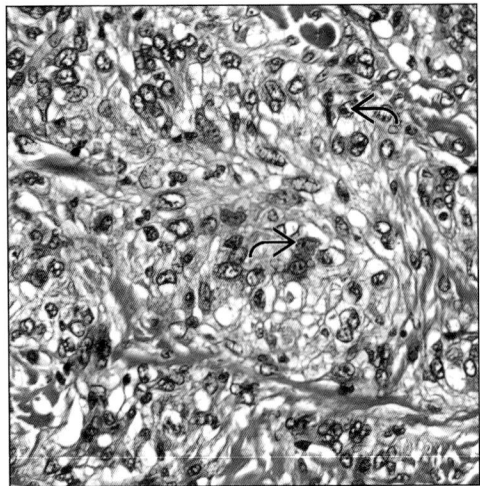

High magnification shows cellular features. The nuclei are uniform, rounded, and vesicular, and some have small nuclei ➔. The cytoplasm is eosinophilic, finely granular, or focally clear.

TERMINOLOGY

Abbreviations
- Neurothekeoma (NTK)

Definitions
- Multinodular dermal tumor composed of nests of rounded cells separated by delicate fibrous septa
- Differs from dermal nerve sheath myxoma (also termed myxoid neurothekeoma)
- Cell type unknown
  o Possibly related to plexiform fibrous histiocytoma
  o Cells may be myofibroblastic or fibrohistiocytic

CLINICAL ISSUES

Epidemiology
- Incidence
  o Rare
- Age
  o Young adults, most 15-25 years
- Gender
  o M = F
- Ethnicity
  o No predilection

Site
- Head and neck and upper extremity most common

Presentation
- Slow growing
  o Elevated dermal nodule
  o Painless

Treatment
- Surgical approaches
  o Simple excision

Prognosis
- Reported cases have behaved in benign fashion

- Occasional recurrence, especially if incompletely excised
- Atypical histologic features have no prognostic significance

MACROSCOPIC FEATURES

General Features
- Rounded or dome-shaped skin lesion
- Pale or tan

Size
- ≤ 2 cm diameter

MICROSCOPIC PATHOLOGY

Histologic Features
- ~ 50% confined to dermis; 48% involve superficial subcutis
- Nests of rounded cells
  o Uniform nuclei, scanty cytoplasm
  o Occasional spindling of cells, especially in myxoid areas
- Nests separated by thin fibrous septa
  o Increased fibrosis in desmoplastic variant
- Myxoid change in 20%
  o 30% are mixed cellular and myxoid lesions
- Nuclear atypia in 25%
- Occasional mitoses, may be up to 3 per 10 HPF
- Multinucleated and osteoclast-like cells in 30-40%
- Occasional plexiform pattern

DIFFERENTIAL DIAGNOSIS

Dermal Nerve Sheath Myxoma (Myxoid Neurothekeoma)
- Well-circumscribed
- Delicate internal septa between myxoid lobules

CELLULAR NEUROTHEKEOMA

Key Facts

Terminology
- Multinodular dermal tumor composed of nests of rounded cells separated by delicate fibrous septa
- Differs from dermal nerve sheath myxoma (also termed myxoid neurothekeoma)

Clinical Issues
- Young adults, most 15-25 years
- Head and neck and upper extremity most common sites
- Elevated dermal nodule
- Reported cases have behaved in benign fashion

Microscopic Pathology
- ~ 50% confined to dermis
- 48% involve superficial subcutis
- Nests of rounded cells

- Occasional spindling of cells, especially in myxoid areas
- Myxoid change in 20%
- Nuclear atypia in 25%
- Mitoses: ≤ 3 per 10 high-power fields
- Osteoclast-like cells in 30%
- Occasional plexiform pattern

Top Differential Diagnoses
- Dermal nerve sheath myxoma
  - Circumscribed, S100 positive
- Plexiform fibrohistiocytic tumor
  - Based at dermal-subcutaneous junction
  - Also has multinucleated cells and fibroblasts
  - Fibroblastic variant has fascicles in subcutis
- Melanocytic nevus
  - S100 protein positive

Immunohistochemistry

Antibody	Reactivity	Staining Pattern	Comment
Actin-sm	Positive	Cytoplasmic	30-60% of cases
CD63	Positive	Cytoplasmic	Same as NKI-C3; in 90%, but not specific
MITF	Positive	Nuclear	80% of cases
CD68	Positive	Cytoplasmic	Nonspecific finding
Podoplanin	Positive	Cell membrane	100%; not in plexiform fibrohistiocytic tumor
S100	Negative		Contrast with dermal nerve sheath myxoma
HMB-45	Negative		Helps to exclude melanoma
melan-A103	Negative		Helps to exclude melanoma

- Schwann cells
  - Sometimes vacuolated
- S100 protein strongly positive
- EMA positive perineurial cells peripherally

Plexiform Fibrohistiocytic Tumor
- More deeply located
  - Based at dermal-subcutaneous junction
  - Extends into dermis and subcutaneous fat
- Fibrohistiocytic nodules composed of histiocyte-like cells, multinucleated cells, fibroblasts
- Fibroblastic pattern in 17%
  - Plexiform bundles of spindle cells within collagen
- Mixed fibroblastic and fibrohistiocytic pattern in 40%

Epithelioid Cutaneous Fibrous Histiocytoma
- Overlying epidermal hyperplasia
- Cells not organized in nests
- NKI/C3 (CD63) and MITF negative

Melanocytic Nevus
- Junctional component is present in most cases
- S100 and other melanocytic markers are positive

Melanoma
- Overlying melanoma in situ usually present
- Nuclear atypia with prominent nucleoli
- Usually multiple mitoses, may be atypical
- S100 positive; HMB-45 and MART-1/Melan-A positive in many cases

SELECTED REFERENCES

1. Jaffer S et al: Neurothekeoma and plexiform fibrohistiocytic tumor: mere histologic resemblance or histogenetic relationship? Am J Surg Pathol. 33(6):905-13, 2009
2. Kaddu S et al: Podoplanin expression in fibrous histiocytomas and cellular neurothekeomas. Am J Dermatopathol. 31(2):137-9, 2009
3. Zedek DC et al: Desmoplastic cellular neurothekeoma: Clinicopathological analysis of twelve cases. J Cutan Pathol. 36(11):1185-90, 2009
4. Alkhalidi H et al: Cellular neurothekeoma with a plexiform morphology: a case report with a discussion of the plexiform lesions of the skin. J Cutan Pathol. 34(3):264-9, 2007
5. Fetsch JF et al: Neurothekeoma: an analysis of 178 tumors with detailed immunohistochemical data and long-term patient follow-up information. Am J Surg Pathol. 31(7):1103-14, 2007
6. Hornick JL et al: Cellular neurothekeoma: detailed characterization in a series of 133 cases. Am J Surg Pathol. 31(3):329-40, 2007
7. Busam KJ et al: Atypical or worrisome features in cellular neurothekeoma: a study of 10 cases. Am J Surg Pathol. 22(9):1067-72, 1998

9

Microscopic Features

(Left) Scanning magnification shows a tumor forming a nodular cluster of cell nests at the dermal-subcutaneous junction ⇨, protruding into fat. Numerous single nests of lesional cells are dispersed throughout the overlying dermis ⇨. *(Right)* Examination of the dermal nests at higher magnification shows small numbers of rounded cells arranged in an ill-defined whorl, with myxoid stroma around the margin. About 20% of cellular neurothekeomas show prominent myxoid change.

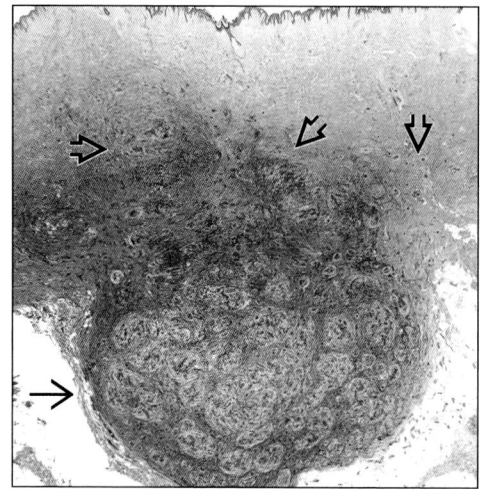
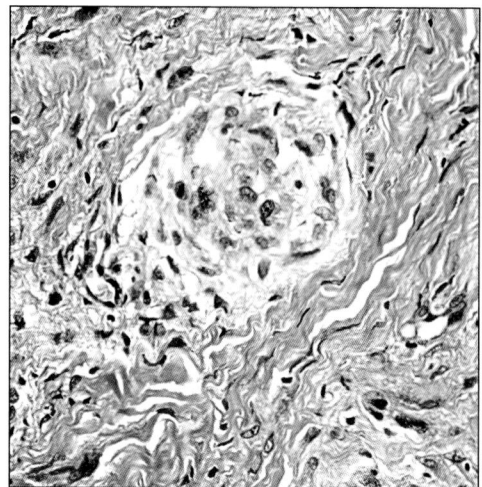

(Left) Intermediate magnification shows a cellular neurothekeoma with confluent dermal nests forming irregularly shaped cellular aggregates. This variant can be misdiagnosed as a nerve sheath tumor or melanocytic lesion. *(Right)* High magnification shows rounded nests of cells separated by thin fibrous septae with some lymphocytes. The cells have uniform nuclei, moderate amounts of cytoplasm, & variably distinct cell borders.

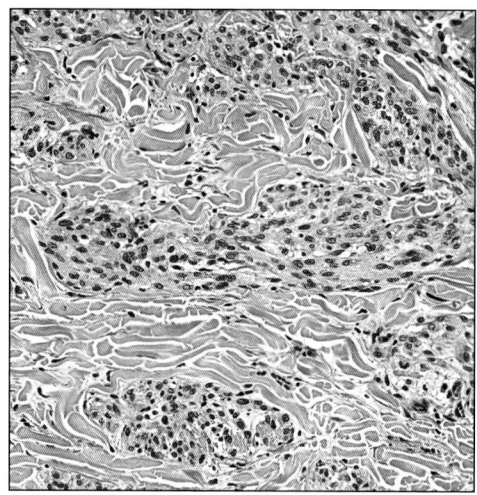
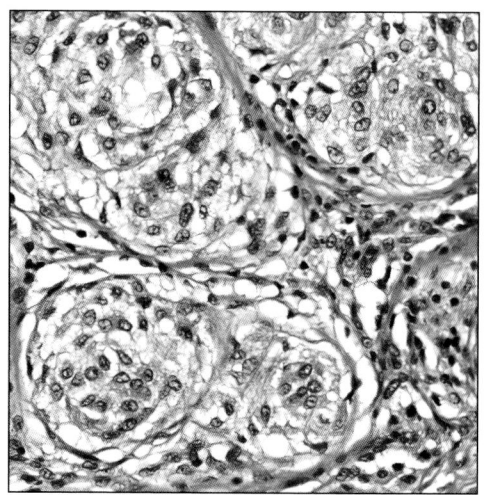

(Left) This is an example of an atypical cellular neurothekeoma. The cell nests are larger and more irregularly shaped than usual. Note the scattered hyperchromatic nuclei ⇨. *(Right)* High magnification shows an atypical cellular neurothekeoma with mild variation in nuclear shape and size, focal hyperchromasia ⇨, and a mitotic figure ⇨. Up to 3 mitoses per 10 high-power fields can be seen, but this does not indicate malignant potential.

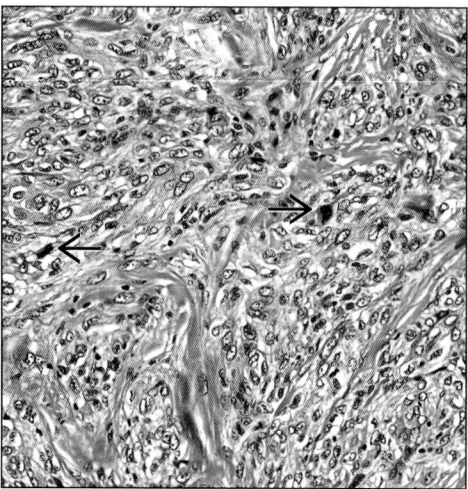
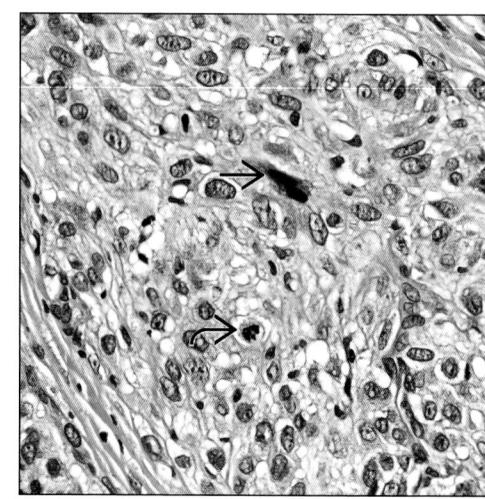

Microscopic Features

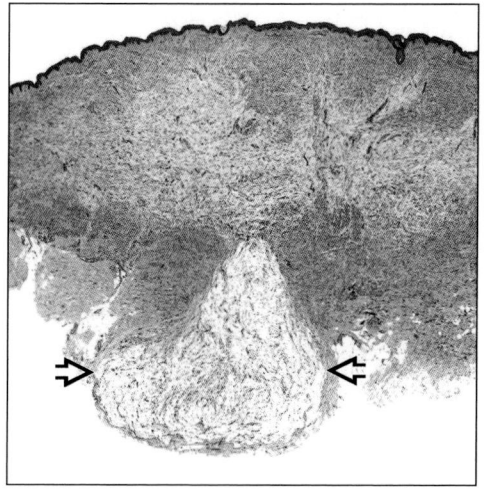
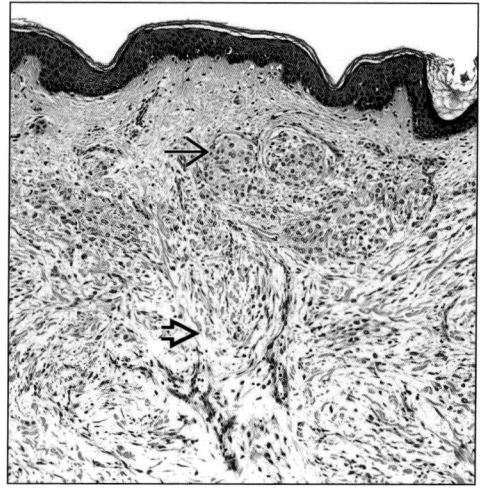

(Left) Low-power view of a cellular NTK shows an example with myxoid change and a nodule ⇨ extending into the subcutis. The cellular composition differs from that of plexiform fibrohistiocytic tumor, which additionally has multinucleated cells and spindle-shaped cells, and rarely shows myxoid change. (Right) This cellular neurothekeoma shows focal myxoid change ⇨ with gradual transition from more typical cellular areas ⇨ in the superficial dermis.

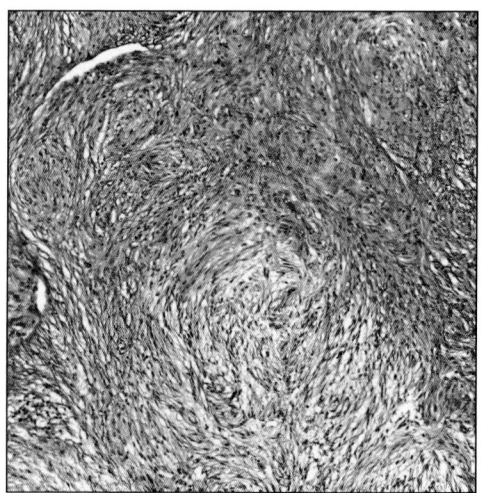
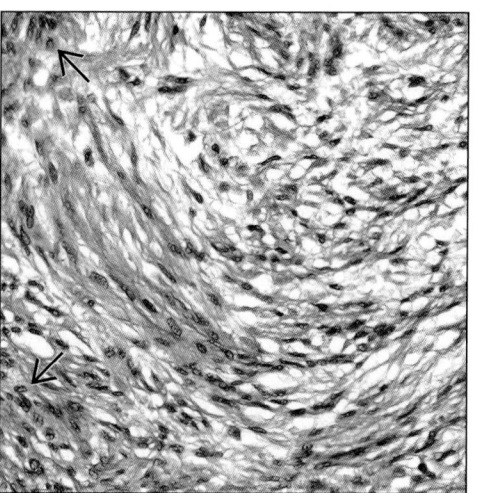

(Left) An example of the myxoid variant of cellular neurothekeoma shows that the myxoid and cellular areas merge. The cells assume a spindled shape in the latter. (Right) High magnification shows a myxoid variant of cellular neurothekeoma. There is a vaguely whorled pattern of spindle cells that retain the typical nuclear and cytoplasmic features. Note the residual foci of the more typical rounded cells at the corners of the field ⇨.

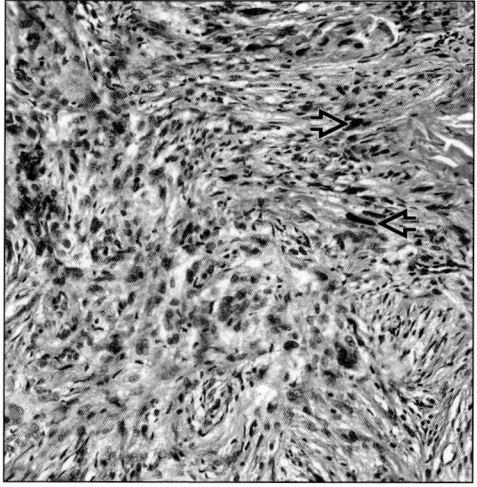
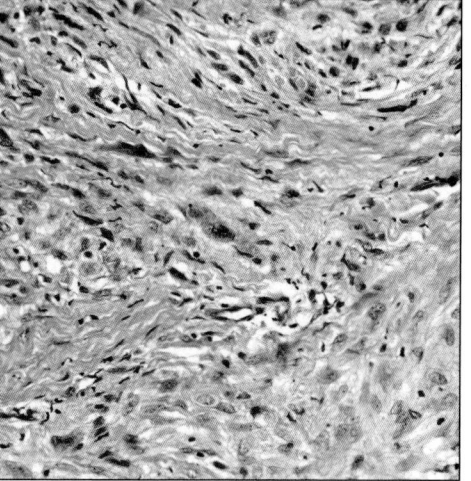

(Left) This cellular neurothekeoma shows the usual pattern of nests of cells with uniform cytologic features in the lower half of the field and transition to spindle cells in the upper half, where there is also focal nuclear atypia ⇨. (Right) Higher magnification shows spindled cells lying within fibrous rather than myxoid stroma. The cell margins are indistinct. This would be difficult to diagnose as a cellular NTK in the absence of more typical areas.

9

DERMAL NERVE SHEATH MYXOMA

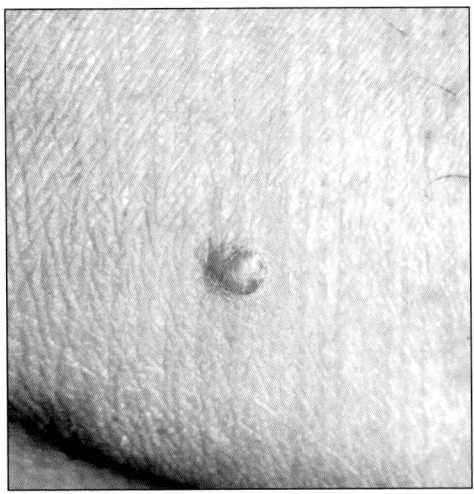

Dermal nerve sheath myxoma presents as a firm papule or nodule that varies from 0.5-4.5 cm in size. It usually occurs in adult patients. Common locations are fingers, hand, and pretibial skin.

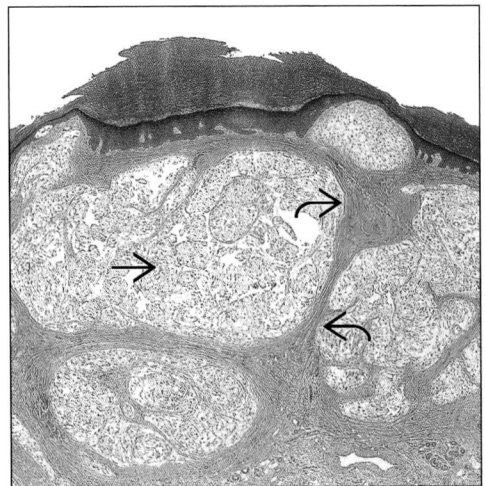

Nerve sheath myxoma is composed of well-defined myxoid lobules ➡ separated by thick fibrous septa ➡. It involves the dermis and often underlying subcutis as well.

TERMINOLOGY

Synonyms
- Cutaneous lobular neuromyxoma, perineurial myxoma, myxoid neurothekeoma

Definitions
- Benign cutaneous nerve sheath tumor with Schwannian differentiation, abundant myxoid matrix, and well-defined lobular architecture

CLINICAL ISSUES

Epidemiology
- Incidence
  o Rare; fewer than 100 cases reported
- Age
  o Mostly adults; median: 34 years

Site
- Extremities
  o Fingers and hand most common
  o Pretibial skin common
- Rare intraoral cases reported
- Uncommon on face

Presentation
- Painless mass
  o Slow growth

Treatment
- Surgical approaches
  o Simple excision

Prognosis
- Benign and nonaggressive, but often excised with positive margins
  o Up to 50% recur

MACROSCOPIC FEATURES

Size
- 0.5-4.5 cm

MICROSCOPIC PATHOLOGY

Histologic Features
- Multiple myxoid lobules
  o Well-defined borders separated by dense fibrous septa
- Usually limited to dermis and subcutis
- Paucicellular proliferation of epithelioid and spindle-shaped Schwann cells
  o Interconnecting cords/networks, syncytial nests, ring-like structures, Verocay-like structures (rare)
  o Stellate and vacuolated cells common
  o No atypia, very low mitotic rate

Predominant Pattern/Injury Type
- Myxoid

Predominant Cell/Compartment Type
- Spindle and epithelioid

ANCILLARY TESTS

Immunohistochemistry
- S100 diffusely positive in 100% of cases
- GFAP positive in most
- Negative for SMA, desmin, CD68, HMB-45, synaptophysin, chromogranin-A, CD31

DIFFERENTIAL DIAGNOSIS

Cellular Neurothekeoma
- Multinodular, but less myxoid matrix and less defined border

Key Facts

Terminology
- Benign myxoid nerve sheath tumor with well-defined lobular architecture and Schwann cell differentiation
- Cutaneous lobular neuromyxoma, perineurial myxoma, myxoid neurothekeoma

Clinical Issues
- Fingers and hand most common
- Pretibial skin common
- Uncommon on face
- Benign, but up to 50% recur (incompletely excised)

Microscopic Pathology
- Multiple myxoid lobules with well-defined borders
- Epithelioid and spindle Schwann cells
- Interconnecting cords/networks, syncytial nests, ring-like structures

- Stellate and vacuolated cells common
- No atypia, very low mitotic rate

Ancillary Tests
- S100 diffusely positive in 100%, GFAP positive in most
- Negative for SMA, desmin, CD68, HMB-45, synaptophysin, chromogranin-A, CD31

Top Differential Diagnoses
- Cellular neurothekeoma
- Superficial angiomyxoma
- Digital mucoid cyst
- Myxoid neurofibroma
- Superficial acral fibromyxoma
- Myxoid dermatofibrosarcoma protuberans
- Low-grade myxofibrosarcoma

- Whorling pattern common
- Spindle and large plump epithelioid cells, ill-defined cytoplasm
- Greater nuclear variability and mitotic activity
- Lacks cords, syncytial aggregates, and vacuolated cells
- S100 negative
- Predilection for face

Superficial Angiomyxoma
- Poorly circumscribed, extends into adjacent tissue
- Fibroblastic cells, often binucleated or multinucleated
- Prominent vascularity; small, thin-walled, curvilinear, congested vessels
- Sparse dispersed inflammation, often neutrophils
- S100 negative
- Predilection for trunk and head and neck region

Cutaneous Myxoma in Carney Complex
- Indistinguishable from superficial angiomyxoma
- Wide anatomic distribution; predilection for ear, eyelid, nipple
- Spotty pigmentation, endocrine overactivity, psammomatous melanotic schwannoma

Digital Mucoid Cyst
- Extruded myxoid material, possibly from underlying joint
- Fibroblastic cells, spindled and stellate-shaped
- Limited to fingers over dorsal aspect of distal interphalangeal joints

Myxoid Neurofibroma
- Small spindle cells with buckled, wavy nuclei, and ill-defined cytoplasm
- Lacks lobular architecture, may be plexiform or diffuse
- Collagen bundles within myxoid stroma

Superficial Acral Fibromyxoma
- Variable amount of fibrous and myxoid stroma
- Lacks well-defined lobules
- CD34 positive, S100 negative
- Acral extremities, often periungual

Myxoid Dermatofibrosarcoma Protuberans
- Storiform or fascicular, lacks lobular architecture
- Infiltrates subcutis, classic "honeycomb" pattern
- Spindle cells with ill-defined cytoplasm, mitotically active
- CD34 positive, S100 negative

Low-Grade Myxofibrosarcoma
- Variable lobular architecture, infiltrative growth into dermis and subcutis
- Pleomorphism and mitotic figures in most cases
- S100 negative

SELECTED REFERENCES

1. Nishioka M et al: Nerve sheath myxoma (neurothekeoma) arising in the oral cavity: histological and immunohistochemical features of 3 cases. Oral Surg Oral Med Oral Pathol Oral Radiol Endod. 107(5):e28-33, 2009
2. Fetsch JF et al: Neurothekeoma: an analysis of 178 tumors with detailed immunohistochemical data and long-term patient follow-up information. Am J Surg Pathol. 31(7):1103-14, 2007
3. Reimann JD et al: Myxoid dermatofibrosarcoma protuberans: a rare variant analyzed in a series of 23 cases. Am J Surg Pathol. 31(9):1371-7, 2007
4. Fetsch JF et al: Nerve sheath myxoma: a clinicopathologic and immunohistochemical analysis of 57 morphologically distinctive, S-100 protein- and GFAP-positive, myxoid peripheral nerve sheath tumors with a predilection for the extremities and a high local recurrence rate. Am J Surg Pathol. 29(12):1615-24, 2005
5. Fetsch JF et al: Superficial acral fibromyxoma: a clinicopathologic and immunohistochemical analysis of 37 cases of a distinctive soft tissue tumor with a predilection for the fingers and toes. Hum Pathol. 32(7):704-14, 2001
6. Calonje E et al: Superficial angiomyxoma: clinicopathologic analysis of a series of distinctive but poorly recognized cutaneous tumors with tendency for recurrence. Am J Surg Pathol. 23(8):910-7, 1999
7. Mentzel T et al: Myxofibrosarcoma. Clinicopathologic analysis of 75 cases with emphasis on the low-grade variant. Am J Surg Pathol. 20(4):391-405, 1996

DERMAL NERVE SHEATH MYXOMA

Microscopic Features

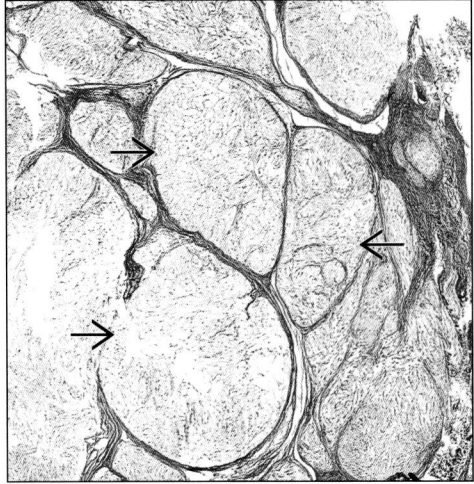

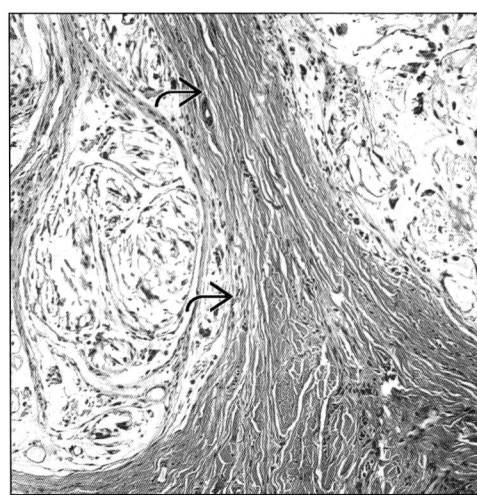

(Left) On low-power examination, nerve sheath myxoma has a very well-defined lobular architecture composed of rounded lobules ⇒ containing copious myxoid matrix. *(Right)* The lobules are typically bordered by thick fibrous septa ⇒. Unlike many other cutaneous myxoid lesions, dermal nerve sheath myxoma has a sharp border and does not tend to infiltrate adjacent structures or entrap dermal collagen.

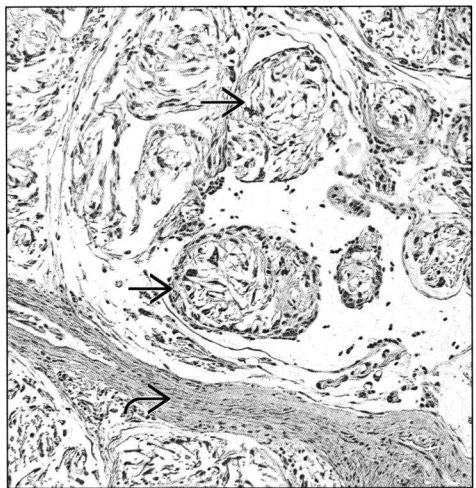

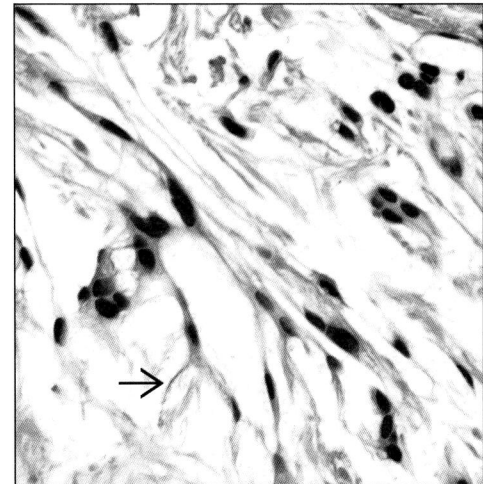

(Left) Nerve sheath myxomas often form cohesive structures/nests ⇒ as well as interconnecting networks of cells. Note the thick fibrous septa at the bottom ⇒, which divides adjacent lobules. *(Right)* The cells are Schwannian cells with uniform nuclei, evenly distributed chromatin, and elongated fibrillary cell processes ⇒ forming bipolar and stellate configurations.

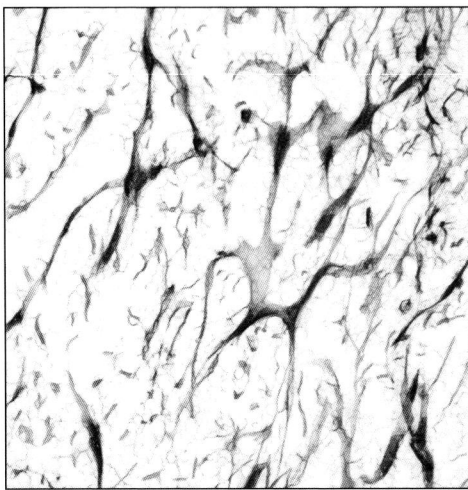

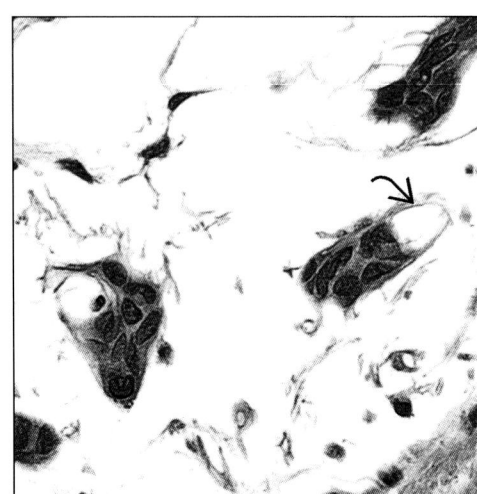

(Left) This micrograph depicts spindled and stellate schwannian cells of a dermal nerve sheath myxoma with abundant eosinophilic cytoplasm and long, interconnecting cell processes, forming a reticulated pattern. *(Right)* The neoplastic cells of nerve sheath myxoma consist of spindled and epithelioid cells with uniform, bland, ovoid nuclei and abundant eosinophilic cytoplasm. They are frequently arranged in syncytial nests and often have intracytoplasmic vacuoles ⇒, as shown.

DERMAL NERVE SHEATH MYXOMA

Microscopic Features and Differential Diagnosis

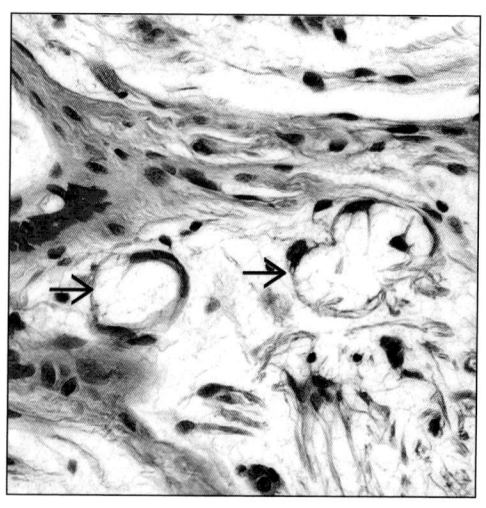
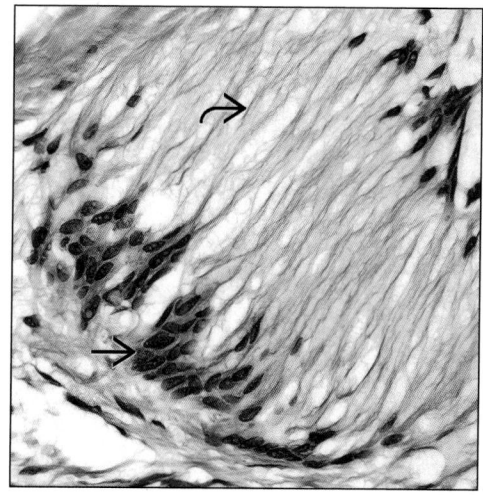

(Left) The neoplastic cells often interconnect to form ring-like structures ➡, as depicted in this micrograph. *(Right)* Verocay-like bodies are rarely seen in nerve sheath myxomas. These provide additional evidence for Schwann cell differentiation. Note the peripheral palisaded nuclei ➡ and fine fibrillary cytoplasmic processes ➡.

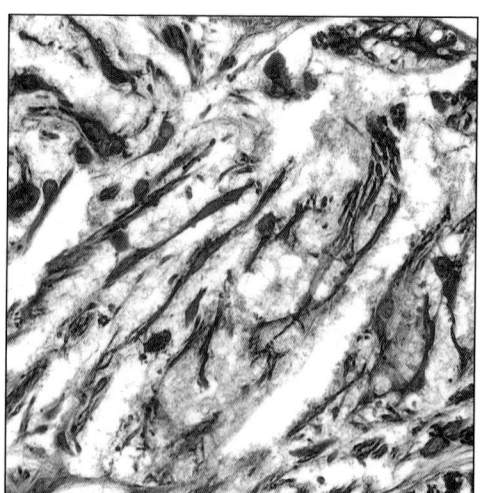
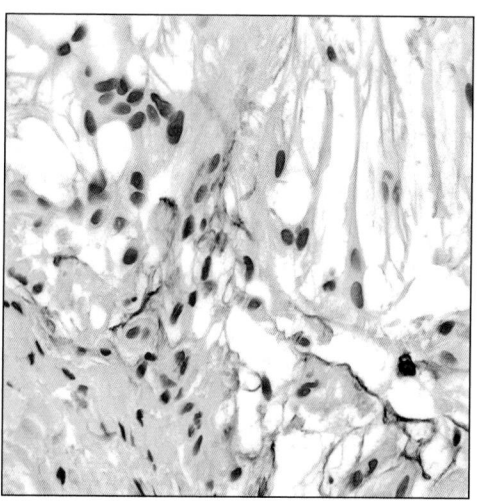

(Left) Nerve sheath myxomas are strongly S100 positive, consonant with Schwannian differentiation. This immunohistochemically stained section depicts diffuse, intense nuclear and cytoplasmic reactivity. *(Right)* This immunohistochemical stain for CD34 highlights long, thin cell processes of intraneural fibroblasts, which are frequently detected in nerve sheath myxoma. In addition, EMA positive perineurial cells (not depicted) are also detected in most tumors.

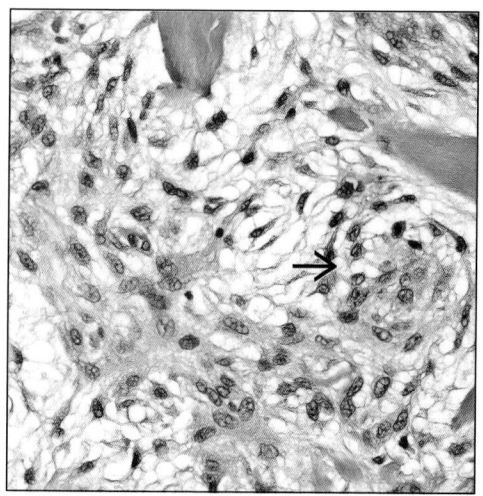
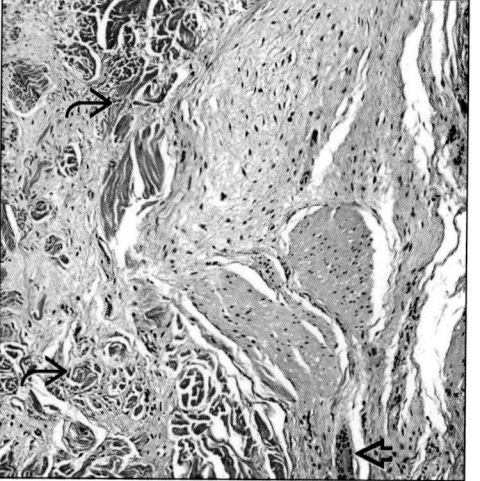

(Left) Like nerve sheath myxoma, neurothekeoma has both spindled and epithelioid cells. However, epithelioid cells are larger and plumper with a tendency to form whorled structures ➡. Neurothekeoma is S100(-). *(Right)* Superficial angiomyxoma differs from nerve sheath myxoma by having a less defined lobular architecture and an infiltrative growth pattern, which includes frequent entrapment of adnexal structures ➡ and dermal collagen ➡.

GRANULAR CELL TUMOR

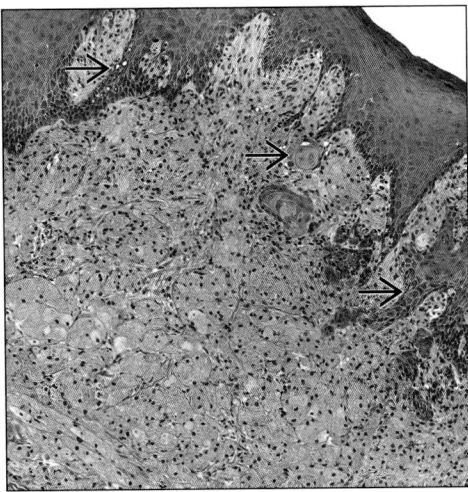

Prominent pseudoepitheliomatous hyperplasia ➡ can be seen overlying granular cell tumors. The tumor is unencapsulated, creating a sheet-like distribution of neoplastic granular cells.

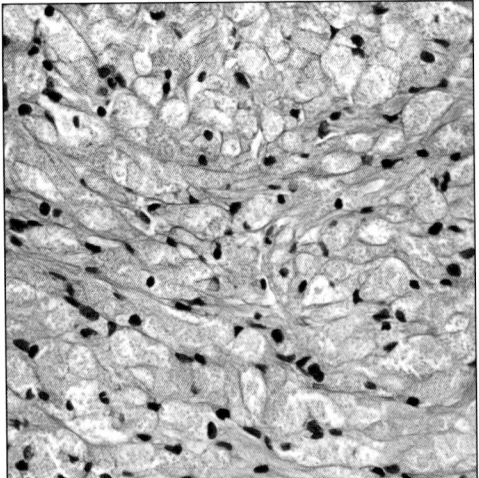

High magnification shows that the cells are polygonal, with a slightly spindled appearance. The cytoplasm contains numerous eosinophilic granules and the nuclei are small, round to oval, and hyperchromatic.

TERMINOLOGY

Abbreviations
- Granular cell tumor (GCT)

Synonyms
- Granular cell myoblastoma
- Abrikossoff tumor

Definitions
- Benign tumor composed of poorly demarcated proliferation of plump granular cells
  ○ Distinct from congenital epulis of newborn (gingival granular cell tumor of infancy)

ETIOLOGY/PATHOGENESIS

Schwannian Derivation
- Thought to arise from Schwann cells
  ○ Positive with neural-associated antibodies
  ○ Granules represent senescent change with accumulation of autophagocytic lysosomes

CLINICAL ISSUES

Epidemiology
- Incidence
  ○ Rare
- Age
  ○ All ages
    ▪ Peak between 40-60 years
- Gender
  ○ Female > male (2:1)
- Ethnicity
  ○ Blacks affected more often than whites

Site
- Over 50% occur in head and neck region
  ○ Up to 70% of these develop in oral cavity (mucosa, tongue, hard palate)
  ○ Tongue is most common site
    ▪ Dorsum more often than lateral margin
- Skin
- Nerve
- Esophagus
- Biliary tract
- Neurohypophysis
- Up to 20% of patients have multiple lesions

Presentation
- Most present as a single painless nodule
  ○ Usually have symptoms for < 12 months
- Rarely, may present with Eagle syndrome
  ○ Elicitation of pain on swallowing, turning head, or extending tongue
    ▪ Syndrome is thought to be caused by irritation of glossopharyngeal nerve

Treatment
- Surgical approaches
  ○ Complete excision with narrow margins
  ○ Laser excision can be performed

Prognosis
- Excellent long-term prognosis
- Recurrence/relapse/persistence is uncommon (~ 10%)
- Malignant GCTs very rare
  ○ Local recurrence in more than 30%
  ○ 50% metastasize, mainly to lymph nodes, lung, bone

MACROSCOPIC FEATURES

General Features
- Smooth-surfaced submucosal or subcutaneous nodule
  ○ Poorly demarcated
- Cut surface firm, pale yellow or cream colored

GRANULAR CELL TUMOR

Key Facts

Terminology

- Benign tumor composed of poorly demarcated accumulation of plump granular cells
- Thought to arise from Schwann cells
- Granular cell myoblastoma

Clinical Issues

- Female > male (2:1)
- Blacks affected more often than whites
- Up to 70% of head and neck lesions develop in oral cavity (tongue most common)
- Up to 20% of patients will have multifocal disease
- Recurrence/relapse/persistence is uncommon (~ 10%)

Macroscopic Features

- Cut surface is firm, pale-cream colored

Microscopic Pathology

- Unencapsulated plump, polygonal to elongated granular cells blending with adjacent soft tissues, especially skeletal muscle
- Cells show indistinct cell membranes, abundant granular, eosinophilic cytoplasm, and small hyperchromatic nuclei
- Overlying pseudoepitheliomatous hyperplasia is common

Ancillary Tests

- Granules are PAS(+), diastase resistant
- Strongly and uniformly positive for S100, NSE

Top Differential Diagnoses

- Squamous cell carcinoma, rhabdomyoma, schwannoma, congenital epulis of newborn

---

- In mouth, concurrent *Candida* infection can form white plaque

Size

- Mean: 1-2 cm

MICROSCOPIC PATHOLOGY

Histologic Features

- Nonencapsulated
  - Blending with adjacent soft tissues, especially skeletal muscle, is common
  - May extend up to epithelium
  - Satellite nodules can develop
    - Rarely plexiform pattern
- Plump, polygonal to elongated eosinophilic cells
- Indistinct cell membranes, creating a syncytium
- Abundant granular eosinophilic cytoplasm
  - Represents lysosomes
- Central small, dark to vesicular round nuclei
- Overlying pseudoepitheliomatous hyperplasia in 30% of cases
  - Usually limited to epithelium immediately overlying tumor
- Marked stromal desmoplasia may be seen
- Malignant GCT has 3 or more of following features
  - Spindling of cells
  - Pleomorphism
  - High nuclear:cytoplasmic ratio
  - Prominent nucleoli
  - Mitoses > 2 per 10 high-power fields
  - Necrosis
- Atypical GCT has 1 or 2 of these features
- Benign GCT has none of these features, or only focal pleomorphism

ANCILLARY TESTS

Frozen Sections

- Pseudoepitheliomatous hyperplasia can mask tumor
- Granular eosinophilic cytoplasm usually evident

Histochemistry

- PAS-diastase
  - Staining pattern
    - Granules are periodic acid-Schiff (PAS) positive, diastase resistant

Immunohistochemistry

- Strongly and uniformly positive for S100 protein (nuclear and cytoplasmic), NSE, and CD68

Electron Microscopy

- Continuous external lamina around cell nests
- Rare rudimentary intercellular junctions
- Pleomorphic secondary lysosomes
  - Autophagosomes
  - Residual bodies
  - Myelin-like figures
  - Angulate lysosomes

DIFFERENTIAL DIAGNOSIS

Squamous Cell Carcinoma

- Pseudoepitheliomatous hyperplasia (PEH) can mimic squamous cell carcinoma (SCC)
  - Especially in oral cavity, tongue
  - Small, superficial surface biopsy specimens can be difficult
  - Must be properly orientated
- SCC usually shows p53 and E-cadherin immunoreactivity, findings not seen in PEH
- Immunohistochemistry does not replace properly orientated H&E sections

Rhabdomyoma

- Sheet-like distribution of polygonal cells with homogeneous, eosinophilic cytoplasm
- Cytoplasmic clearing with "spider web" cells
- PTAH highlights cross-striations in cytoplasm
- Expresses desmin (diffuse, cytoplasmic) and myogenin (in nuclei)

GRANULAR CELL TUMOR

Immunohistochemistry

Antibody	Reactivity	Staining Pattern	Comment
S100	Positive	Nuclear & cytoplasmic	Nearly all tumor cells
CD68	Positive	Cytoplasmic	Schwann cells and histiocytes
NSE	Positive	Cytoplasmic	Weak to strong in most tumor cells
CD57	Positive	Cytoplasmic	Weak reaction but in nearly all tumor cells
PGP9.5	Positive	Cytoplasmic	Most tumor cells
Inhibin-α	Positive	Cytoplasmic	Variably positive in most tumor cells
Calretinin	Positive	Nuclear & cytoplasmic	Variable in most tumor cells
NGFR	Positive	Cell membrane	Same as p75/NGFR
Collagen IV	Positive	Stromal matrix	Basement membrane around tumor cells is positive
Ki-67	Positive	Nuclear	< 2% of nuclei in general
GFAP	Negative		
CK-PAN	Negative		
α-1-antitrypsin	Negative		
Desmin	Negative		

Schwannoma

- Often encapsulated, with well-defined borders
- Has Antoni A and Antoni B areas, with Verocay bodies
- More spindled cellular arrangement
- S100 protein immunoreactivity diffuse, strong
- EMA positive in subcapsular spindle cells
- CD68 usually negative
- Not associated with PEH

Congenital Epulis of Newborn

- Can be histologically indistinguishable from GCT
- Develops in newborns or infants only
- Lacks S100 protein
- Positive for NSE

Smooth Muscle Tumors

- Short to long, sweeping, and interlacing fascicles
- Granular cells rarely seen
- SMA, desmin, and H-caldesmon positive
- S100 protein negative

Nonneural Granular Cell Tumor (Primitive Polypoid Granular Cell Tumor)

- Benign
- Cutaneous lesion, often polypoid
- Mild focal to rare moderate nuclear atypia
- Histologically similar, but lacks S100 staining

Mucosal Lichen Planus

- Significant granular cells can be seen in association with oral lichen planus
  - Also called oral ceroid granuloma
- Characteristic inflammatory infiltrate with Civatte bodies at interface
- Direct immunofluorescence characteristic for lichen planus
- Cells are positive with S100 protein
- Can coexist with granular cell tumor

Granular Cell Change in Other Tumors

- Cutaneous fibrous histiocytoma
  - Typical features present elsewhere in lesion

  - S100 negative
- Dermatofibrosarcoma
  - Mainly long spindle cells in storiform pattern
  - Granular cell change very rare
    - Usually focal, nongranular cell areas elsewhere
  - CD34 positive
  - S100 negative

DIAGNOSTIC CHECKLIST

Pathologic Interpretation Pearls

- Large granular cells
- Coarse cytoplasmic granules
  - PAS positive, diastase resistant
- Diffuse S100 protein positivity

SELECTED REFERENCES

1. Nasser H et al: Malignant granular cell tumor: a look into the diagnostic criteria. Pathol Res Pract. 207(3):164-8, 2011
2. Papalas JA et al: Isolated and synchronous vulvar granular cell tumors: a clinicopathologic study of 17 cases in 13 patients. Int J Gynecol Pathol. 29(2):173-80, 2010
3. Aldabagh B et al: Plexiform pattern in cutaneous granular cell tumors. J Cutan Pathol. 36(11):1174-6, 2009
4. Vered M et al: Granular cell tumor of the oral cavity: updated immunohistochemical profile. J Oral Pathol Med. 38(1):150-9, 2009
5. van der Meij EH et al: Granular cells in oral lichen planus. Oral Dis. 7(2):116-8, 2001
6. Fanburg-Smith JC et al: Malignant granular cell tumor of soft tissue: diagnostic criteria and clinicopathologic correlation. Am J Surg Pathol. 22(7):779-94, 1998
7. Junquera LM et al: Granular-cell tumours: an immunohistochemical study. Br J Oral Maxillofac Surg. 35(3):180-4, 1997
8. Collins BM et al: Multiple granular cell tumors of the oral cavity: report of a case and review of the literature. J Oral Maxillofac Surg. 53(6):707-11, 1995
9. Gordon AB et al: Granular cell tumour of the breast. Eur J Surg Oncol. 11(3):269-73, 1985

Clinical, Microscopic, and Ancillary Features

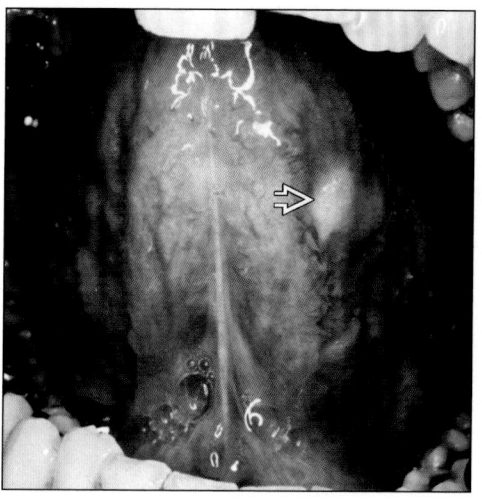

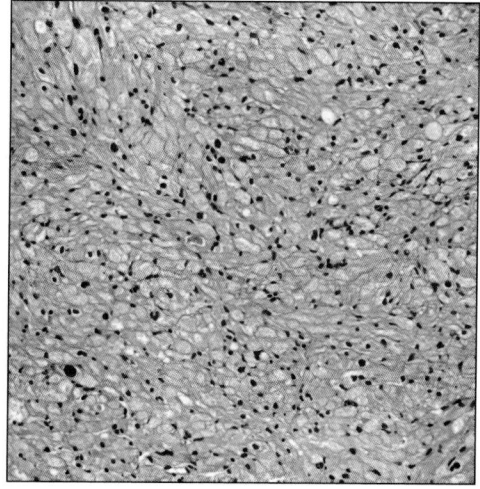

(Left) Granular cell tumors present clinically as either a smooth-surfaced, submucosal swelling or nodule or as a pale to white, discrete, plaque-like lesion ⊵. The overlying epithelium may be pale. Secondary candidiasis can be present. (Right) Granular cell tumor shows a vaguely fascicular arrangement of enlarged, polygonal granular cells. Note the abundant granular cytoplasm. The nuclei are small with a hyperchromatic appearance in this intermediate-power view.

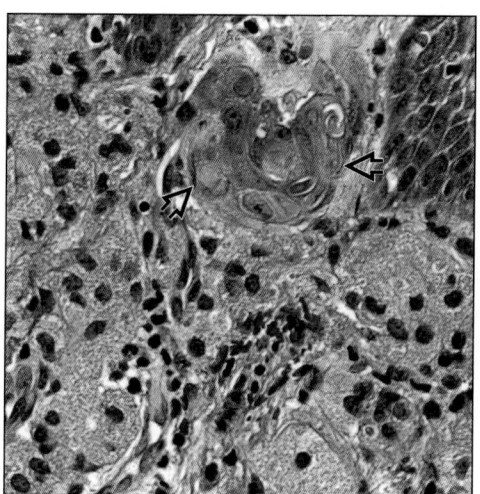

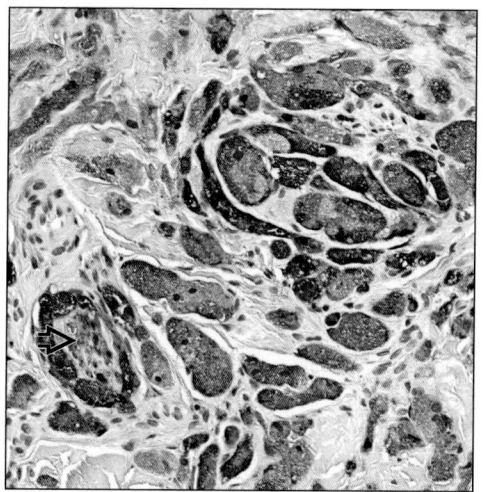

(Left) Pseudoepitheliomatous hyperplasia can mimic squamous cell carcinoma, as seen here ⊵. Note the dyskeratosis and paradoxical maturation. The cells of granular cell tumor have granular cytoplasm with central round nuclei. (Right) S100 protein strongly stains the cytoplasm and the nuclei of the granular cells. Note the entrapped peripheral nerve ⊵. The tumor is derived from Schwann cells, so nerve association is common.

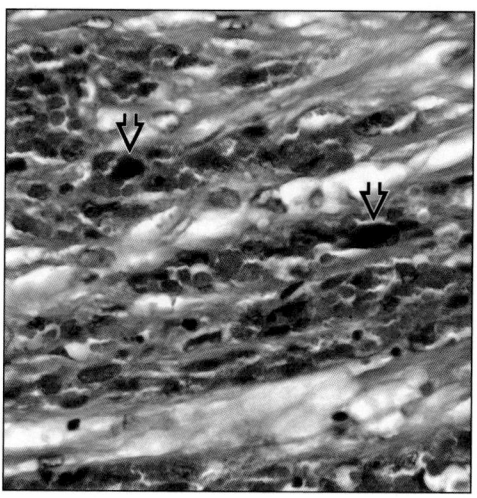

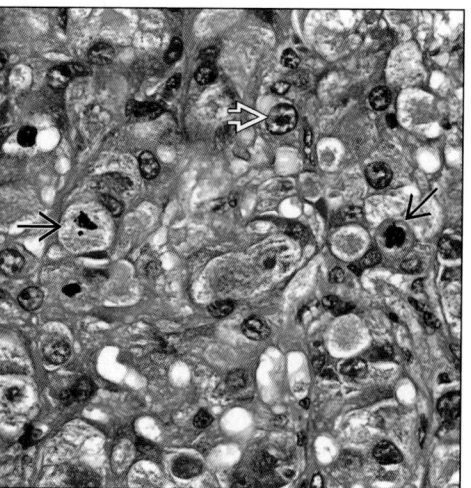

(Left) Atypical granular cell tumor shows focal spindling of cells and enlarged, hyperchromatic nuclei ⊵, but lacks other features of malignancy. (Right) Malignant granular cell tumor shows enlarged nuclei, prominent nucleoli ⊵, and mitotic activity ⊡. Cases with 3 or more of the following features can be regarded as malignant: Pleomorphism, high nuclear:cytoplasmic ratio, prominent nucleoli, mitoses > 2 per 10 high-power fields, spindling, and necrosis.

FIBROLIPOMATOUS HAMARTOMA OF NERVE

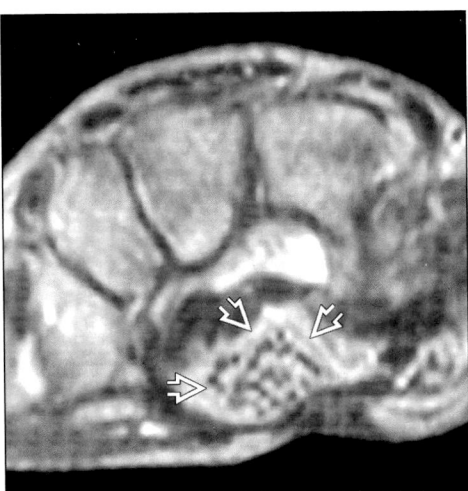

MR of the wrist shows an abnormal fat signal ⇒ in the stroma between the nerve fascicles (black dots) of an enlarged median nerve.

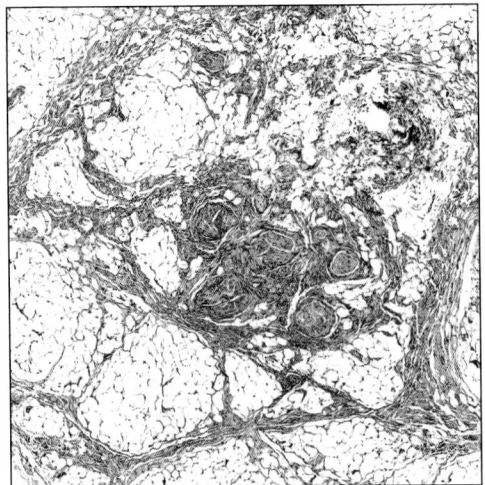

Histologic examination shows an accumulation of mature adipose tissue with hypocellular fibrous septa around and between nerve bundles.

TERMINOLOGY

Synonyms
- Lipofibromatous hamartoma of nerve
- Neural fibrolipoma
- Neurolipomatosis, lipomatosis of nerve

Definitions
- Increased fibrofatty tissue infiltrating and surrounding subcutaneous and, rarely, deep nerves

CLINICAL ISSUES

Epidemiology
- Age
  - Predominantly in children, including congenitally
  - Some cases in young adults up to 30 years of age
  - Rarely in older adults

Site
- Affects palmar surface, wrist, forearm
- Median nerve and branches most commonly affected
- Rarely involves ulnar or radial nerve
- Involves left arm > right arm
- Very rarely involves sciatic, peroneal, or cranial nerve

Presentation
- Subcutaneous mass
  - Slow growing
- Paresthesia
- Macrodactyly (digital gigantism, macrodystrophia lipomatosa)
  - Present in 27% of cases
  - Can be congenital and progressive
  - Increased growth of bone and soft tissue of affected digit

Treatment
- Options, risks, complications

- Complete excision contraindicated because of nerve damage
- Surgical approaches
  - Biopsy confirms diagnosis
  - Debulking or carpal tunnel release for symptomatic control
  - Removal of deformed digit

Prognosis
- Usually stabilizes if incompletely excised

IMAGE FINDINGS

MR Findings
- Fusiform enlargement of affected nerve segment
- "Telephone cable" sign

MACROSCOPIC FEATURES

General Features
- Sausage-shaped mass
- Yellow-white tissue
- Surrounds and expands nerve
- Can extend into adjacent soft tissue of hand and wrist

Size
- Variable, up to 10 cm length of nerve involved

MICROSCOPIC PATHOLOGY

Histologic Features
- Adipose tissue and fibrous tissue
  - Infiltrate around and between nerve branches and along perineurium
- Epineurial and perineurial fibrous thickening
- Perineurium can become hyperplastic
  - Concentric layers
  - "Onion bulb" intraneural hyperplasia
- Nerve bundles become separated

FIBROLIPOMATOUS HAMARTOMA OF NERVE

Key Facts

Terminology
- Increased fibrofatty tissue infiltrating and surrounding nerves

Clinical Issues
- Median nerve most commonly affected
- Predominantly in children, including congenitally
- Macrodactyly
- Complete excision contraindicated because of nerve damage

Macroscopic Features
- Sausage-shaped mass
- Can extend into adjacent soft tissue of hand and wrist

Microscopic Pathology
- Adipose tissue and fibrous tissue
- Perineurium can become hyperplastic
- Nerve bundles become separated

- Nerves can become atrophic in longstanding cases
- Rare metaplastic bone formation

Predominant Pattern/Injury Type
- Diffuse, interstitial
- Fibrosis

Predominant Cell/Compartment Type
- Adipocyte
- Fibroblast

Other Causes of Macrodactyly
- Neurofibromatosis type 1
- Ollier disease
- Maffucci syndrome
- Klippel-Trenaunay syndrome
- Congenital lymphedema
- Proteus syndrome
  - Mutations in *PTEN* tumor suppressor gene
  - Localized gigantism and lipomatous masses

DIFFERENTIAL DIAGNOSIS

Lipoma of Nerve
- Well-circumscribed
- Confined within nerve

Neurofibroma
- Proliferation of neural elements including nerve sheath cells and fibroblasts
- No fatty component

Neuroma
- Increased number of nerve bundles
- No fatty component

Lipomatosis
- Histologically similar
- Usually skin and subcutis
- Spares nerves

SELECTED REFERENCES

1. Woertler K: Tumors and tumor-like lesions of peripheral nerves. Semin Musculoskelet Radiol. 14(5):547-58, 2010
2. Bisceglia M et al: Neural lipofibromatous hamartoma: a report of two cases and review of the literature. Adv Anat Pathol. 14(1):46-52, 2007
3. Razzaghi A et al: Lipofibromatous hamartoma: review of early diagnosis and treatment. Can J Surg. 48(5):394-9, 2005
4. Al-Qattan MM: Lipofibromatous hamartoma of the median nerve and its associated conditions. J Hand Surg [Br]. 26(4):368-72, 2001
5. Marom EM et al: Fibrolipomatous hamartoma: pathognomonic on MR imaging. Skeletal Radiol. 28(5):260-4, 1999
6. Berti E et al: Fibrolipomatous hamartoma of a cranial nerve. Histopathology. 24(4):391-2, 1994
7. Amadio PC et al: Lipofibromatous hamartoma of nerve. J Hand Surg [Am]. 13(1):67-75, 1988
8. Silverman TA et al: Fibrolipomatous hamartoma of nerve. A clinicopathologic analysis of 26 cases. Am J Surg Pathol. 9(1):7-14, 1985

IMAGE GALLERY

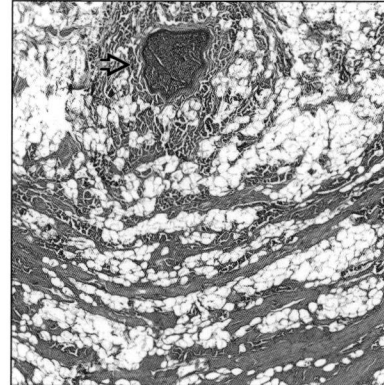
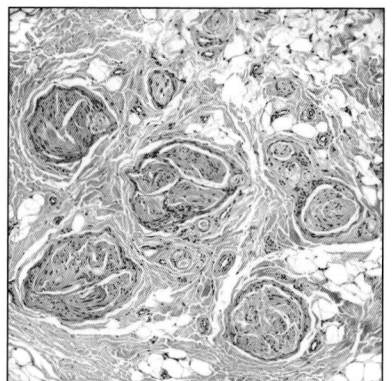
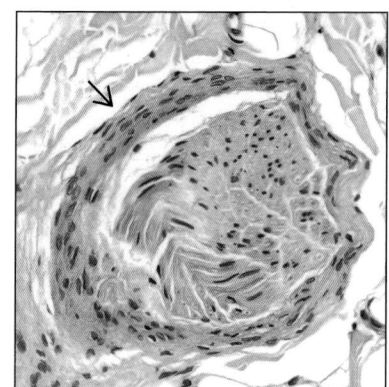

(Left) Low magnification shows fibrous bands and adipose tissue in the subcutis adjacent to a nerve ➡. Note the prominent extension of lesional tissue beyond the nerve. *(Center)* Intermediate magnification shows nerve bundles separated by fibrous tissue within fat. *(Right)* Higher power shows perineurial cell hyperplasia with several layers of elongated spindle cells ➡. These demonstrate immunoreactivity for epithelial membrane antigen (EMA).

PERINEURIOMA

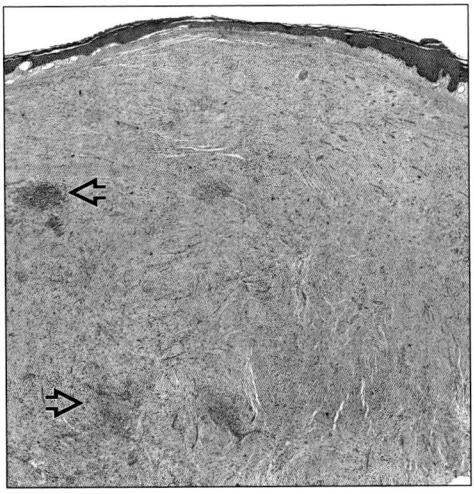

An intact surface epithelium is noted overlying a proliferation of spindled cells arranged in a vaguely storiform pattern with focal small whorls. Collections of inflammatory cells are present ➡.

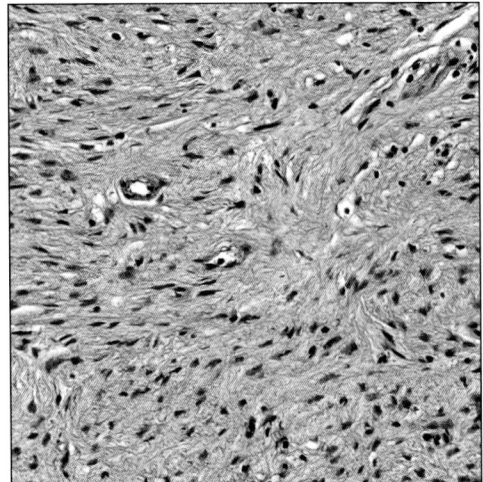

There is a haphazard spindle cell proliferation showing a syncytial appearance. The cells show slightly spindled nuclei with cytoplasmic processes. The background stroma is slightly loose to myxoid.

TERMINOLOGY

Abbreviations
- Soft tissue perineurioma (STP)

Synonyms
- Storiform perineurial fibroma
- Perineurial cell tumor

Definitions
- Benign peripheral nerve sheath tumor, specifically of perineurial cell derivation that surrounds endoneurial connective tissue space of nerve fibers
  - Tumors are traditionally separated into intraneural, sclerosing, and soft tissue perineurioma
  - Perineurial cells can be seen in other tumors, such as neurofibroma and schwannoma

ETIOLOGY/PATHOGENESIS

Pathogenesis
- May be related to Schwann cells, fibroblasts, or arachnoid cap cells

CLINICAL ISSUES

Epidemiology
- Incidence
  - Exceedingly rare
  - Represents < 0.5% of peripheral nerve sheath tumors
- Age
  - Wide age range: 2-85 years
  - Majority: 2nd-5th decades
    - Mean: 45 years
- Gender
  - Slight female preponderance
    - Female > male (1.1-1.2:1)

Site
- Superficial subcutaneous soft tissue
  - Most common in soft tissues of lower and upper extremities
  - 2nd most common in trunk
  - Head and neck sites affected in ~ 15% of all perineuriomas
- Oral cavity is affected ~ 4% of the time

Presentation
- Most patients present with solitary painless mass
- May have syndrome/familial association
  - Neurofibromatosis type 2 (NF2)
  - Nevoid basal cell carcinoma (Gorlin) syndrome
  - Interestingly, both have meningioma in common
    - Perineurium may be derived from arachnoid cap cells

Treatment
- Surgical approaches
  - Excision is treatment of choice
    - Some advocate for wide excision to prevent recurrence

Prognosis
- Local recurrence is uncommon (< 5% of cases)
  - May develop late
  - Only seen if originally incompletely excised
- Metastases are not reported
- Pleomorphic cells and infiltrative margins do not affect clinical outcome

MACROSCOPIC FEATURES

General Features
- Usually discrete, but without easily detected capsule
  - Well-circumscribed

Size
- Wide range: 0.3-20 cm

PERINEURIOMA

Key Facts

Terminology

- Benign peripheral nerve sheath tumor, specifically of perineurial cell derivation that surrounds endoneurial connective tissue space of nerve fibers

Etiology/Pathogenesis

- May be related to Schwann cells, fibroblasts, or arachnoid cap cells

Clinical Issues

- Women affected slightly more often than men
- Presents with solitary, painless mass in superficial subcutaneous soft tissue

Macroscopic Features

- Usually discrete but without easily detected capsule

Microscopic Pathology

- Superficial subcutaneous or dermal site, well circumscribed
- Spindled tumor cells organized in many patterns (fascicles, storiform, pinwheel, whorled, lamellar)
- Bipolar, bland, plump spindled cells with pale, eosinophilic cytoplasm
- Background stroma is collagenous, myxoid or a mixture, without vascular hyalinization

Ancillary Tests

- Variably positive with perineurial markers (EMA, claudin-1, GLUT1, CD34) and collagen IV

Top Differential Diagnoses

- Neurofibroma, schwannoma, solitary fibrous tumor, meningioma

---

- Mean: ~ 3 cm

MICROSCOPIC PATHOLOGY

Histologic Features

- Superficial subcutaneous or dermal site
- Well-circumscribed, focally showing changes suggesting a collagenous capsule
  - "Infiltrating" borders can be seen
  - Significant invasion is rare
- Spindled tumor cells organized in many patterns
  - Fascicles
  - Storiform or pinwheel
  - Whorled to concentrically stratified
  - Lamellar architecture
- Tumors are hypo- or hypercellular
  - Alternating zones can be seen
- Bipolar, bland, plump spindled cells with pale, eosinophilic cytoplasm
  - Indistinct cytoplasmic borders
- Nuclei vary
  - Oval, tapered, elongate, triangular, curved, compressed, twisted, or wavy
  - Intranuclear pseudoinclusions are rare
- Isolated pleomorphic cells ("ancient change") is unusual
- Background stroma is collagenous, myxoid, or a mixture
  - Sclerotic, round to elliptical collagen deposits may be present
  - Pericellular cracking or clefting between collagen and cells
- Mitoses are sparse
  - Most tumors have none
- Degeneration and hemorrhage may be present
- Calcifications (calcospherites or metaplastic bone) are exceptional
- Chronic inflammation is uncommon
- Peripheral nerve association is unique, usually "twigs" of nerves
- Vessel hyalinization is **not** present

- Sclerosing, reticular (retiform), granular and epithelioid subtypes are recognized, although rare
  - Reticular
    - Lace-like growth pattern of anastomosing cords of spindle cells
  - Sclerosing
    - Epithelioid and spindle cells in trabecular or whorled pattern within markedly dense sclerotic stroma

ANCILLARY TESTS

Cytology

- Cellular smears with sheets and clusters of spindle-shaped tumor cells
- Cells are bipolar with cytoplasmic extensions
- May have "signet ring" appearance
- Prominent myxoid background

Immunohistochemistry

- Variably positive with perineurial markers
  - EMA: Strong and diffuse in all cases
  - Claudin-1: Distinctly particulate pattern along cell membrane in nearly all cases
  - GLUT1: Usually membranous to stippled
  - CD34: Up to 65% of tumors may be positive
  - May show smooth muscle actin (~ 20%) and S100 (~ 5%) staining
- Strong membranous staining with type IV collagen

Cytogenetics

- Chromosome 22 abnormalities seen in conventional perineurioma
- Chromosome 10 aberrations seen in sclerosing variants
  - Deletion of 10q
  - t(2;10)(p23;q24)
  - Monosomy 10

PERINEURIOMA

Immunohistochemistry

Antibody	Reactivity	Staining Pattern	Comment
EMA	Positive	Cytoplasmic	Strong and diffuse in all cases
Claudin-1	Positive	Cell membrane	Distinctly particulate pattern along cell membrane in nearly all cases
GLUT1-cytoplasm	Positive	Cell membrane	Usually membranous to stippled
CD34	Positive	Cytoplasmic	Seen in up to 65% of cases
Collagen IV	Positive	Stromal matrix	Strong membranous staining of cells
Actin-sm	Positive	Cytoplasmic	Up to 20% of cases
S100	Positive	Nuclear & cytoplasmic	Only in up to 5% of cases
CK-PAN	Negative		
GFAP	Negative		
NFP	Negative		Axons adjacent to the tumor may be highlighted
Desmin	Negative		

Electron Microscopy

- Long, thin, cytoplasmic processes with incomplete basal lamina (basement membrane) and pinocytotic vesicles
- Tapering nuclei with condensed heterochromatin
- Axons absent

DIFFERENTIAL DIAGNOSIS

Neurofibroma and Schwannoma

- Benign peripheral nerve sheath tumors include neurofibromas, schwannomas, and perineuriomas
  - Hybrid combinations of schwannoma/neurofibroma and perineurioma may occur
  - Show alternating layers of S100 and EMA positive cells layered adjacent to one another
- Have association with a nerve in many cases
- Wavy nuclei with background loose stroma
- Antoni A and Antoni B areas seen in schwannoma
- Perivascular hyalinization and encapsulation are usually found in schwannoma
- Almost always show strong S100 protein immunoreactivity

Solitary Fibrous Tumor

- Cellular tumors with spindled cells in a "patternless pattern"
- Much more heavily collagenized stroma
- Usually shows positive CD34, Bcl-2, and CD99 staining
  - CD34 is of limited utility, as it is positive in many perineuriomas

Ectopic Meningioma

- Central nervous system association is usual
- Whorled architecture with psammoma bodies and intranuclear inclusions
- Lacks collagen IV immunoreactivity
- Will show EMA reactivity
  - Perineurial and arachnoidal cells may be related

SELECTED REFERENCES

1. Fang WS et al: An unusual sinonasal tumor: soft tissue perineurioma. AJNR Am J Neuroradiol. 30(2):437-9, 2009
2. Hornick JL et al: Hybrid schwannoma/perineurioma: clinicopathologic analysis of 42 distinctive benign nerve sheath tumors. Am J Surg Pathol. 33(10):1554-61, 2009
3. Kum YS et al: Intraneural reticular perineurioma of the hypoglossal nerve. Head Neck. 31(6):833-7, 2009
4. Hornick JL et al: Soft tissue perineurioma: clinicopathologic analysis of 81 cases including those with atypical histologic features. Am J Surg Pathol. 29(7):845-58, 2005
5. Ide F et al: Comparative ultrastructural and immunohistochemical study of perineurioma and neurofibroma of the oral mucosa. Oral Oncol. 40(9):948-53, 2004
6. de La Jarte-Thirouard AS et al: Intraneural reticular perineurioma of the neck. Ann Diagn Pathol. 7(2):120-3, 2003
7. Chrysomali E et al: Benign neural tumors of the oral cavity: a comparative immunohistochemical study. Oral Surg Oral Med Oral Pathol Oral Radiol Endod. 84(4):381-90, 1997
8. Li D et al: Intratemporal facial nerve perineurioma. Laryngoscope. 106(3 Pt 1):328-33, 1996
9. Tsang WY et al: Perineurioma: an uncommon soft tissue neoplasm distinct from localized hypertrophic neuropathy and neurofibroma. Am J Surg Pathol. 16(8):756-63, 1992
10. Housini I et al: Fine needle aspiration cytology of perineurioma. Report of a case with histologic, immunohistochemical and ultrastructural studies. Acta Cytol. 34(3):420-4, 1990

Microscopic and Immunohistochemical Features

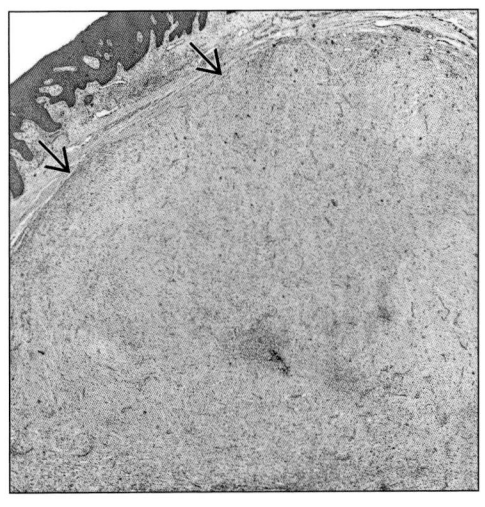

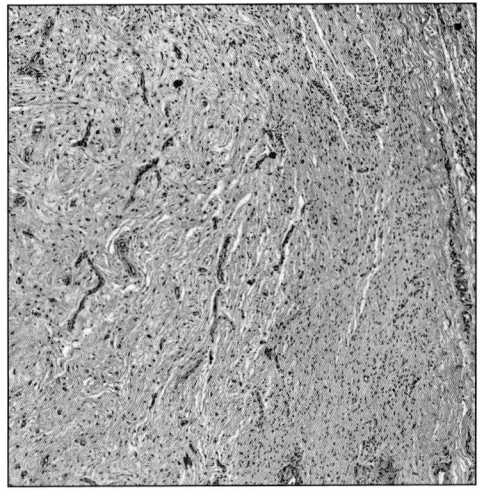

(Left) The periphery of the tumor seems to be well-circumscribed but unencapsulated ➡. The surface epithelium is intact, showing a slightly pseudoepitheliomatous appearance. *(Right)* The tumor blends at the periphery with the densely collagenized stroma. There is a haphazard storiform appearance to the proliferation. The stroma is myxoid to edematous, perhaps having a vaguely tissue culture-like appearance.

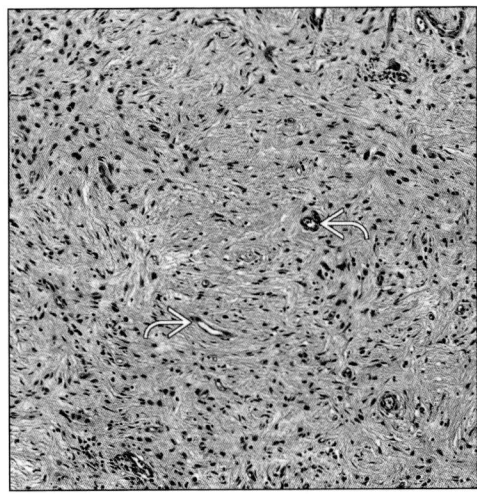

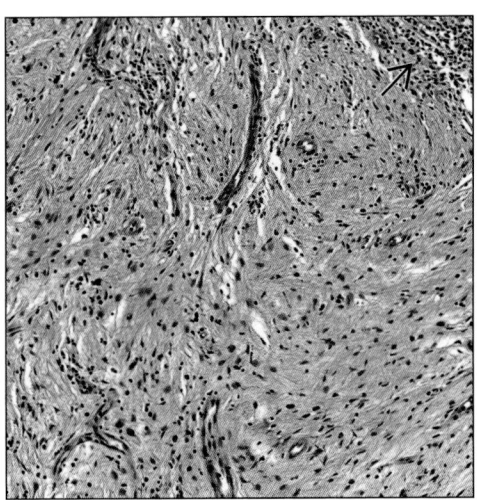

(Left) The cells are arranged in a syncytial pattern, although the spindle cells are easily identified. There are small vessels within the proliferation ➡, but they do not show hyalinized walls. Isolated inflammatory cells are present. *(Right)* The proliferation is less cellular in this field. The vessels are more prominent, but lack perivascular hyalinization. The nuclei of the neoplastic cells are small and spindled. There is a lack of cytologic atypia and mitoses. Inflammatory cells ➡ are seen.

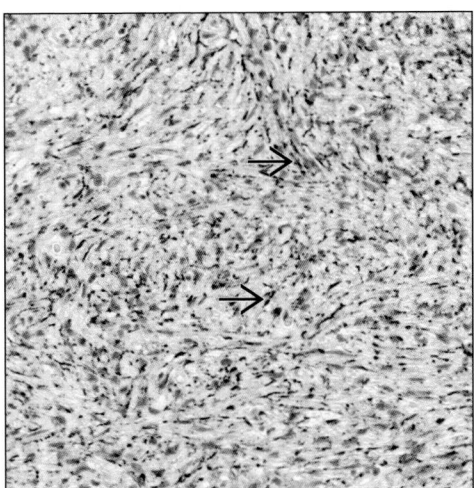

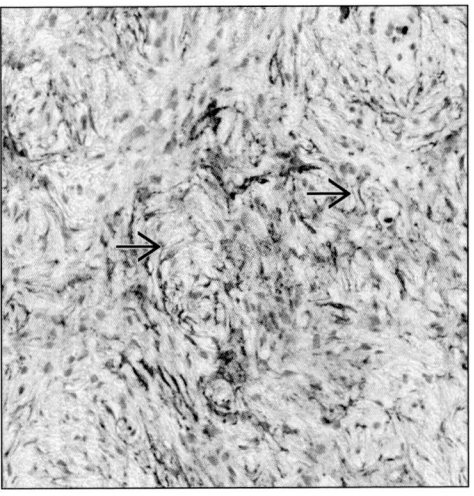

(Left) Claudin-1 will frequently display stippled, beaded, or granular staining ➡, while also highlighting the cell membranes. This staining pattern is quite unique and characteristic of this tumor. *(Right)* The neoplastic spindle cells are highlighted by GLUT1, giving a slightly stippled to granular appearance. The wisps of cytoplasm are stained ➡, creating a feathery appearance to the cells.

NASAL GLIAL HETEROTOPIA

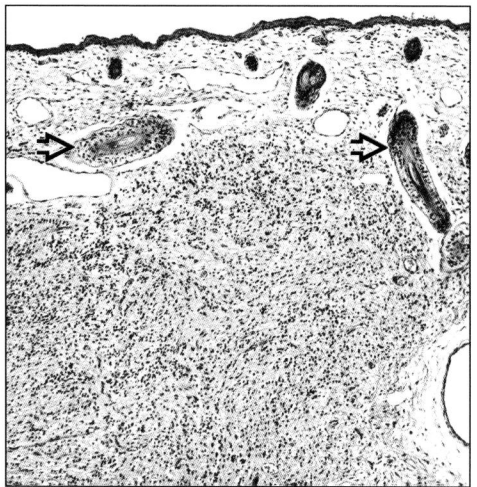

Low magnification shows intact skin with adnexal structures (hair follicles ⊃) surrounding a haphazard collection of neural elements (glial tissue).

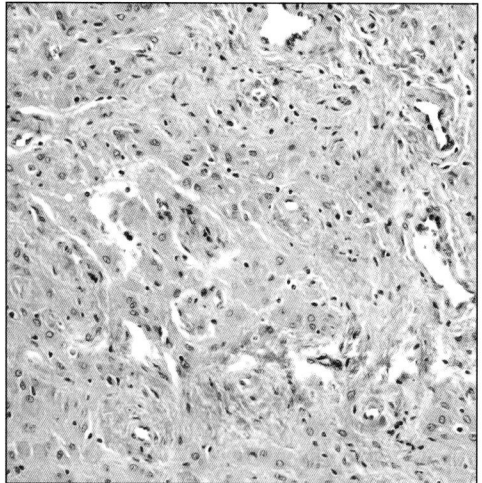

High magnification shows the intermingling of glial elements with fibrosis. This is a very subtle finding, highlighting the reason for performing special studies in many cases.

TERMINOLOGY

Abbreviations
- Nasal glial heterotopia (NGH)

Synonyms
- Glioma (implies tumor, and should be discouraged)

Definitions
- NGH is congenital malformation of displaced normal, mature glial tissue (choristomas)
  - Continuity with intracranial component usually obliterated
- Encephalocele represents herniation of brain tissue and leptomeninges through defect of skull
  - Continuity with cranial cavity is maintained

ETIOLOGY/PATHOGENESIS

Developmental Anomaly
- NGH is congenital malformation of displaced normal and mature glial tissue

Iatrogenic
- Encephalocele is herniation of brain tissue through bony defect
  - Often secondary to infections, trauma, or surgery

CLINICAL ISSUES

Epidemiology
- Incidence
  - NGH is rare
  - Encephalocele is uncommon
- Age
  - NGH usually presents during infancy
  - Encephalocele may present in older children and adults
- Gender

  - Equal sex distribution

Site
- Separated into 2 types, based on location
  - Extranasal (60%): Subcutaneous bridge of nose
  - Intranasal (30%): Superior nasal cavity
  - Mixed (10%)

Presentation
- Firm, subcutaneous nodule at bridge of nose
- Polypoid mass or polyps within superior nasal cavity
- Obstruction
- Chronic rhinosinusitis

Treatment
- Options, risks, complications
  - Radiographs are prerequisite to avoid post-biopsy complications
    - Meningitis and CSF rhinorrhea
- Surgical approaches
  - Excision must be adequate

Prognosis
- Excellent
- Recurrences (up to 30%) if incompletely excised

IMAGE FINDINGS

Radiographic Findings
- Sharply demarcated, expansile mass
- Intracranial extension (tract or cribriform plate defect) must be excluded
  - Especially difficult to document with CT or MR if defect is small

MACROSCOPIC FEATURES

General Features
- Smooth, homogeneous glistening cut surface (similar to brain tissue)

NASAL GLIAL HETEROTOPIA

Key Facts

Etiology/Pathogenesis
- Congenital malformation of displaced normal and mature glial tissue

Clinical Issues
- Separated into extranasal and intranasal types
- NGH usually presents during infancy
- Radiographs are prerequisite to avoid post-biopsy complications
- Recurrences (up to 30%) if incompletely excised

Microscopic Pathology
- Gliosis pattern in glial tissue
- Fibrosis frequently obliterates or obscures glial tissue; special stains required to confirm

Ancillary Tests
- Glial tissue: S100 protein and GFAP positive

Top Differential Diagnoses
- Fibrosed nasal polyp, cutaneous meningioma

- Sometimes fibrous connective tissue dominates, making it firm

Size
- Usually < 2 cm

MICROSCOPIC PATHOLOGY

Histologic Features
- Skin or surface mucosa is intact
- Fibrous connective tissue blended with glial tissue
  - Fibrosis frequently obliterates or obscures glial tissue
  - Special stains required to confirm glial/fibrous tissue
- Nests and sheets of fibrillar neuroglial tissue
- Prominent glial fibrillary network
- Gemistocytes may be noted
- Neurons are uncommon
- Choroid plexus, ependyma, and retinal pigmented cells are exceedingly rare
- Encephalocele shows glial degeneration but requires radiographic/clinical correlation

ANCILLARY TESTS

Histochemistry
- Trichrome will highlight glial tissue and fibrosis
  - Glial tissue: Bright red
  - Fibrosis: Blue

Immunohistochemistry
- Glial tissue is highlighted with S100 protein and GFAP

DIFFERENTIAL DIAGNOSIS

Fibrosed Nasal Polyp
- Lacks glial tissue
- Contains mucoserous glands
- Usually has greater amount of inflammation

Cutaneous Meningioma
- Usually presents as nodule on the scalp or forehead
- Meningothelial (syncytial) lobules and whorls of neoplastic cells
- Psammoma bodies often seen
- EMA positive; S100 weak

SELECTED REFERENCES
1. Penner CR et al: Nasal glial heterotopia. Ear Nose Throat J. 83(2):92-3, 2004
2. Penner CR et al: Nasal glial heterotopia: a clinicopathologic and immunophenotypic analysis of 10 cases with a review of the literature. Ann Diagn Pathol. 7(6):354-9, 2003
3. Kardon DE: Nasal glial heterotopia. Arch Pathol Lab Med. 124(12):1849, 2000

IMAGE GALLERY

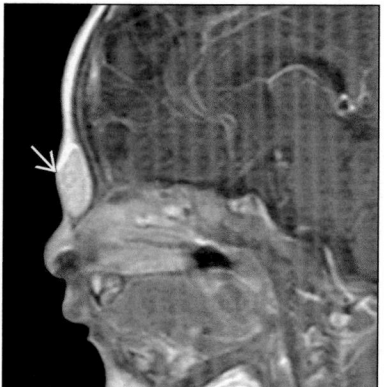
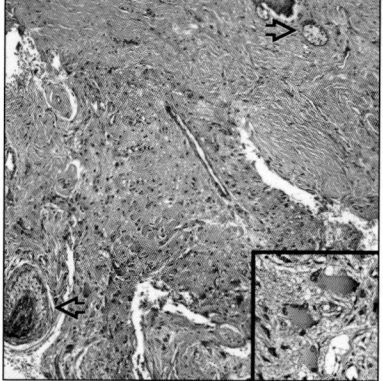
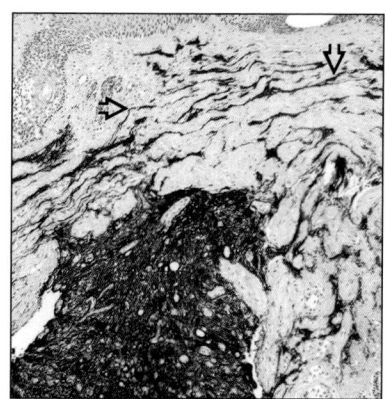

(Left) Sagittal CT scan shows enhancement of an ovoid mass above the nose ➡. There is no intracranial connection. *(Center)* Histologic examination shows pilosebaceous units ➡ surrounded by a gemistocytic-like glial proliferation within the fibrous connective tissue. The inset shows a higher power view of the gemistocytes. *(Right)* GFAP highlights the glial tissue below the intact epithelium. Note the "infiltrative" appearance ➡ of the process as it is separated by reactive fibrosis.

ECTOPIC MENINGIOMA

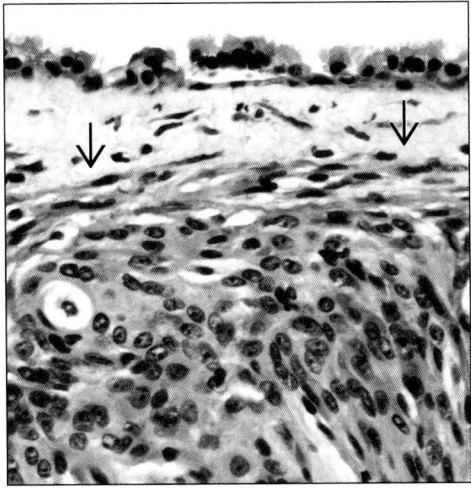

A nasal cavity tumor shows intact mucosa overlying a syncytial-like neoplastic meningothelial cell proliferation ⊟. The nuclei are uniform, and the cells show moderate amounts of cytoplasm.

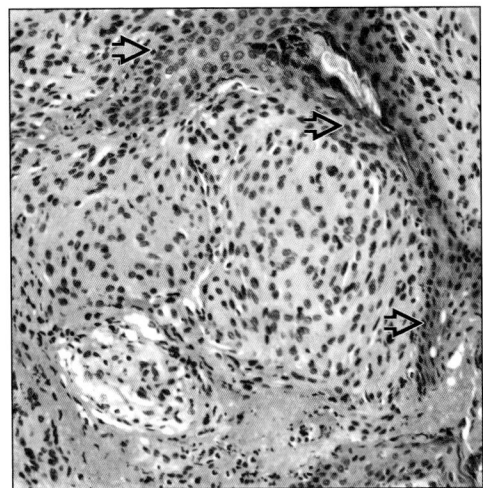

The meningothelial cells are arranged in a distinctive whorled pattern, with uninvolved surface squamous epithelium ⊟. Cell boundaries are indistinct.

TERMINOLOGY

Definitions
- Benign neoplasm of meningothelial cells in scalp, nasal cavity, sinonasal tract, nasopharynx, or lung

ETIOLOGY/PATHOGENESIS

Pathogenesis
- Arachnoid cells from arachnoid granulations or pacchionian bodies lining sheaths of nerves and vessels through skull foramina

CLINICAL ISSUES

Epidemiology
- Incidence
  - Rare tumor of scalp
    - 20% of meningiomas have extracranial extension
  - 0.2% of sinonasal tract and nasopharynx tumors
  - Occasional examples occur outside head and neck
- Age
  - Mean: 40-48 years old
  - Women older than men by more than a decade
- Gender
  - M:F = 1:1.2

Site
- Skin of scalp
- Ear, temporal bone
- Nasal cavity, paranasal sinuses
  - Nasal cavity alone (~ 25%)
  - Frontal sinus most commonly affected in isolation
  - Majority are left sided
- Rare examples in lung, brachial plexus, soft tissue

Presentation
- Subcutaneous nodule
- Sinusitis, obstruction, discharge, and epistaxis
- Exophthalmos, periorbital edema, visual changes, ptosis

Treatment
- Surgical approaches
  - Excision

Prognosis
- About 20% recur, usually < 5 years after primary
- 5-year survival is 78% in scalp tumors
- Young age and complete resection are favorable factors

IMAGE FINDINGS

Radiographic Findings
- Exclude direct CNS extension from en plaque tumor
- Bony sclerosis with focal destruction of bony tissues
- Widening of suture lines and foramina at skull base

MACROSCOPIC FEATURES

General Features
- Intact surface mucosa, but infiltrative into bone
- Multiple fragments of grayish, white-tan, gritty, firm to rubbery masses
- Many in head and neck sites are polypoid

Size
- Range: 1-8 cm, mean: 3.5 cm

MICROSCOPIC PATHOLOGY

Histologic Features
- Infiltrative growth of neoplastic cells, including soft tissue and bone
- Meningothelial (syncytial) lobules of neoplastic cells without distinct borders
- Whorled architecture

ECTOPIC MENINGIOMA

Key Facts

Terminology
- Benign neoplasm of meningothelial cells

Clinical Issues
- Can present in skin of scalp
- Approximately 0.2% of sinonasal tract and nasopharynx tumors
- M:F = 1:1.2
  - Women older by more than a decade
- About 20% recur

- 5-year survival is 78% in scalp tumors

Image Findings
- Must exclude direct CNS extension

Microscopic Pathology
- Infiltrative growth of neoplastic cells, including soft tissue and bone
- Meningothelial (syncytial) lobules of neoplastic cells without distinct borders
- Whorled architecture, psammoma bodies

- Epithelioid cells with round to regular nuclei and even nuclear chromatin
- Intranuclear cytoplasmic inclusions typically seen
- Psammoma bodies or "pre-psammoma" bodies
- Histologic subtypes of meningioma can be seen
  - Transitional, metaplastic, clear cell, atypical

ANCILLARY TESTS

Immunohistochemistry
- Positive: EMA, keratin ("pre-psammoma" body pattern), CAM5.2, claudin-1
- Weak positive: S100 protein
- Negative: Chromogranin, synaptophysin, CD34

DIFFERENTIAL DIAGNOSIS

Perineurioma
- Skin and subcutis
- Perivascular whorls of long thin cells

Cellular Neurothekeoma
- Nodules and nests of ovoid cells in dermis
- Lacks whorled pattern
- EMA and S100 negative

Olfactory Neuroblastoma
- Cribriform plate
- Lobules of small cells with scanty cytoplasm in fibrillary background

- Rosette/pseudorosette formation

Paraganglioma
- Nested architecture
- Chromogranin positive
- Sustentacular cells around cell nests
  - S100 protein positive

Angiofibroma
- Males, in nasopharynx
- Stellate cells in fibrous stroma
  - Nuclei immunoreactive for β-catenin
- "Staghorn" vessels

SELECTED REFERENCES

1. Rushing EJ et al: Primary extracranial meningiomas: an analysis of 146 cases. Head Neck Pathol. 3(2):116-30, 2009
2. Hussein MR et al: Primary cutaneous meningioma of the scalp: a case report and review of literature. J Cutan Pathol. 34 Suppl 1:26-8, 2007
3. Thompson LD et al: Extracranial sinonasal tract meningiomas: a clinicopathologic study of 30 cases with a review of the literature. Am J Surg Pathol. 24(5):640-50, 2000
4. Gabibov GA et al: Meningiomas of the anterior skull base expanding into the orbit, paranasal sinuses, nasopharynx, and oropharynx. J Craniofac Surg. 4(3):124-7; discussion 134, 1993
5. Perzin KH et al: Nonepithelial tumors of the nasal cavity, paranasal sinuses, and nasopharynx. A clinicopathologic study. XIII: Meningiomas. Cancer. 54(9):1860-9, 1984

IMAGE GALLERY

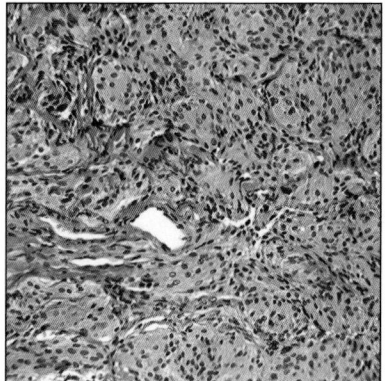 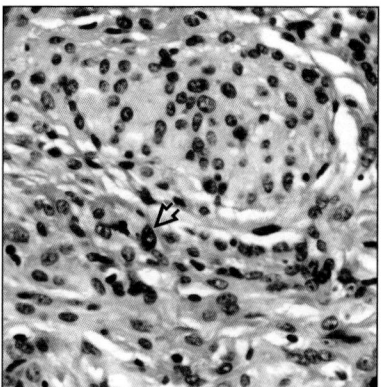 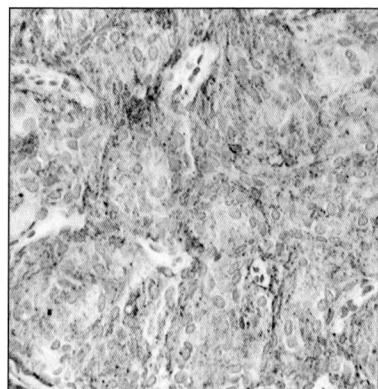

(Left) This example shows multiple small nests of meningothelial cells with a slightly whorled appearance. This appearance resembles paraganglioma, but the latter has sustentacular cells (which can be demonstrated by immunoreactivity for S100 protein). *(Center)* High magnification demonstrates nests of cells without cell borders, showing focal nuclear enlargement ➘. *(Right)* Immunostaining for epithelial membrane antigen is positive on cell membranes or in cytoplasm.

SUPERFICIAL MALIGNANT PERIPHERAL NERVE SHEATH TUMOR

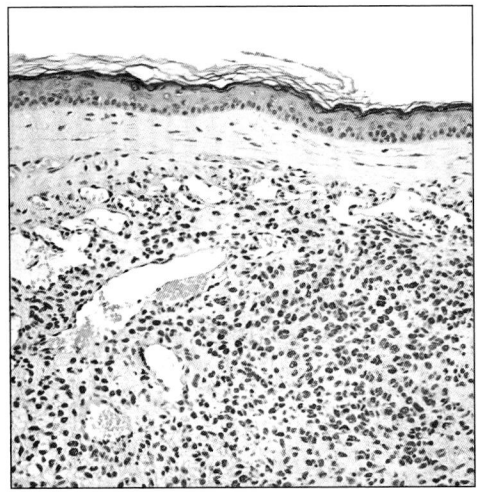

MPNST can rarely present as a primary skin tumor, such as this scalp tumor excised from a 90-year-old woman. Superficial MPNST typically occurs in mid-to-deep dermis or as a subcutaneous primary.

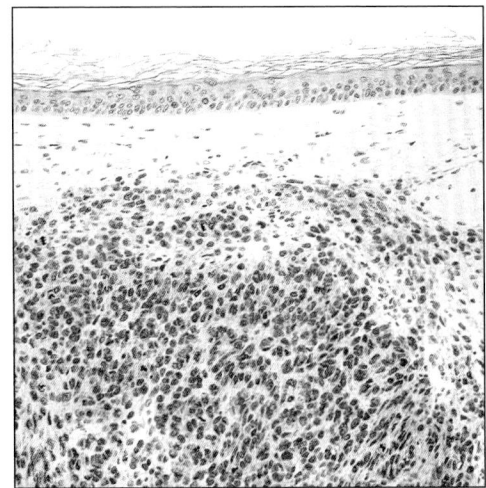

Unless one sees continuity with a cutaneous nerve or adjacent neurofibroma, immunohistochemistry is required for diagnosis. Often negative or patchy, diffuse S100 staining is present in this case.

TERMINOLOGY

Abbreviations
- Malignant peripheral nerve sheath tumor (MPNST)

Synonyms
- Neurofibrosarcoma, "malignant schwannoma" (older terms)

Definitions
- Superficial sarcoma arising from cutaneous nerve or benign nerve sheath tumor, or showing nerve sheath differentiation
  o Diagnostic criteria
    ▪ Arises from nerve or benign nerve sheath tumor
    ▪ Or shows histological evidence of nerve sheath differentiation in a NF1 patient
    ▪ Or shows histological plus immunohistochemical or ultrastructural evidence of nerve sheath differentiation in non-NF1 patient

ETIOLOGY/PATHOGENESIS

Genetic Predisposition
- 40% associated with neurofibromatosis type 1 (NF1)
  o Lifetime incidence: 2-16%

Molecular Pathogenesis
- NF1 caused by germline mutation of *NF1* tumor suppressor gene
  o Somatic loss of 2nd *NF1* allele required for tumorigenesis
- Malignant transformation in both NF1-associated and sporadic MPNST often involves *INK4A* and *P53* and their downstream pathways

CLINICAL ISSUES

Epidemiology
- Incidence
  o MPNST accounts for 5-10% of soft tissue sarcomas
    ▪ Superficial MPNST very rare
- Age
  o Mostly adults (20-50 years)
    ▪ Average: 40 years
    ▪ Wide range: 4-79 years
- Gender
  o Women and men roughly equal

Site
- Head and neck (60%), trunk, upper and lower extremities
- Dermis &/or subcutis
  o Mid- or deep dermis in most cases
  o May invade deeper structures

Presentation
- Painful or painless mass

Treatment
- Surgical approaches
  o Wide excision/resection
- Adjuvant therapy
  o Radiation
- Drugs
  o Generally MPNST shows poor response to chemotherapy

Prognosis
- Local recurrence: 60%
- Metastasis: 25%
  o Lung, lymph node, bone
- 30% die of disease
  o Average survival: 3.3 years

SUPERFICIAL MALIGNANT PERIPHERAL NERVE SHEATH TUMOR

Key Facts

Terminology
- Superficial sarcoma arising from cutaneous nerve or benign nerve sheath tumor, or showing nerve sheath differentiation

Etiology/Pathogenesis
- 40% associated with NF1

Clinical Issues
- Mostly adults, but wide age range (4-79 years)
- Local recurrence: 60%
- Metastasis: 25%

Microscopic Pathology
- Mostly intermediate and high-grade sarcomas
- Spindle cell pattern most common
  - Long fascicles of closely spaced hyperchromatic spindle cells

- Wavy nuclei with tapered ends
- Small round blue cells
- Pleomorphic cells
- Extensive necrosis with perivascular preservation
- Epithelioid MPNST
- Heterologous differentiation

Ancillary Tests
- S100 protein (+) in about 60% of cases (more often in well-differentiated and epithelioid MPNST), usually focal

Top Differential Diagnoses
- Malignant melanoma
- Atypical neurofibroma
- Dermatofibrosarcoma protuberans
- Clear cell sarcoma

IMAGE FINDINGS

General Features
- Morphology
  - Cutaneous nodule
  - Superficial soft tissue mass

MACROSCOPIC FEATURES

General Features
- Epidermal alterations absent
- Coexisting neurofibroma in some cases

Size
- Average: 3 cm (range: 2-16 cm)

MICROSCOPIC PATHOLOGY

Histologic Features
- Wide spectrum of cytoarchitectural patterns
  - Mostly intermediate or high-grade sarcomas
    - High mitotic rate and necrosis
    - Only around 15% are low grade
  - Nerve sheath differentiation
    - Nuclear palisading uncommon, usually focal
    - Tactoid differentiation with whorling or Wagner-Meissner body-like features
  - Intraneural tumors
    - Plexiform architecture
    - Microscopic extension within nerve fascicle
  - Tumors arising from preexisting benign nerve sheath tumor
    - Neurofibroma most common, transitional areas, usually in NF1 patients
  - Diffuse infiltrative sarcomatous proliferation without evidence of nerve or nerve sheath tumor origin
- Spindle cell MPNST (most common pattern)
  - Long fascicles of uniform, closely spaced, hyperchromatic spindle cells

  - Alternating cellular fascicles and hypocellular areas ("tapestry" or "marbled" pattern)
  - Myxoid matrix, focal
  - Storiform arrays
  - Wavy nuclei with tapered ends
  - Small round blue cells
  - Pleomorphic cells
    - Multinucleated giant cells
  - Extensive necrosis with perivascular preservation
- Epithelioid MPNST
  - Multinodular architecture
  - Cords and clusters in some
  - Large epithelioid cells
    - Abundant eosinophilic cytoplasm
    - Large vesicular nuclei with macronucleoli
    - Clear cytoplasm in some
  - Often mixed with spindle cells
- Heterologous differentiation (15% of MPNSTs)
  - Osseous and osteosarcomatous
  - Chondroid and chondrosarcomatous
  - Rhabdomyosarcomatous (Triton tumor)
  - Angiosarcomatous
  - Glandular

Cytologic Features
- Spindle cells
  - Ill-defined cytoplasm
  - Hyperchromatic nucleus with dispersed coarse chromatin
  - Tapered and wavy nuclei in well-differentiated tumors
  - Very brisk mitotic activity in high-grade tumors
- Epithelioid cells
  - Abundant eosinophilic or clear cytoplasm
  - Vesicular nucleus with prominent inclusion-like nucleolus

ANCILLARY TESTS

Immunohistochemistry
- S100 protein (+) in about 60% of cases (more often in well-differentiated and epithelioid MPNST), usually focal

Cytogenetics
- Complex structural and numeric chromosomal abnormalities
  - Frequent loss of *NF1* at 17q11
  - Frequent loss of *P53* at 17q13

DIFFERENTIAL DIAGNOSIS

Malignant Melanoma
- Spindle cell/desmoplastic melanoma
  - Often have overlying melanoma in situ (> 70% of cases), usually lentigo maligna type
  - May have clustered or thèque-like areas
  - Diffusely and strongly S100(+)
    - MPNST often S100(-) or with only weak/focal staining
  - Usually HMB-45, tyrosinase, and MART-1/Melan-A(-)
- Epithelioid melanoma
  - Almost always have overlying melanoma in situ (unless metastatic)
  - Amelanotic melanoma may be indistinguishable from epithelioid MPNST
  - Diffusely S100(+)
    - Epithelioid MPNST often diffusely S100(+) as well
  - Usually HMB-45, tyrosinase, and MART-1/Melan-A(+)
    - MPNST negative for these markers

Atypical Neurofibroma
- Large, hyperchromatic spindle cells
- Degenerated (smudged) chromatin
- Low mitotic rate
- Lacks necrosis
- Usually retains cytoarchitectural features of neurofibroma
  - Edematous fibrillary or myxoid matrix with collagen bundles ("shredded carrots" pattern)

Dermatofibrosarcoma Protuberans (DFSP)
- Dermal-based tumor composed of uniform spindle cells with tapered nuclei and indistinct cytoplasm
- Well-defined storiform architecture usually prominent
- Broadly infiltrates subcutis and entraps adipocytes in a "honeycomb" pattern
- CD34(+), FXIIIA(-), S100(-)
- t(17;22)(q22;q13) by cytogenetics
- *COL1A-PDGFRB* by FISH or RT-PCR

Clear Cell Sarcoma (Malignant Melanoma of Soft Parts)
- Predilection for acral extremities
- Usually deep soft tissue tumor, but can invade skin in some cases
  - Rare cutaneous primary tumors

- Multinodular, packeted or nested architecture
  - Nests often surrounded by fibrous tissue bands
- Uniform epithelioid and spindle cells
- Vesicular chromatin with prominent nucleoli
- Diffuse S100, HMB-45 and MART-1/Melan-A staining in most cases
- t(12:22) by cytogenetics
- *EWSR1* break apart by FISH
- *EWS-ATF1* or *EWS-CREB1* by RT-PCR

SELECTED REFERENCES

1. Salgado R et al: Molecular diagnosis of dermatofibrosarcoma protuberans: A comparison between reverse transcriptase-polymerase chain reaction and fluorescence in situ hybridization methodologies. Genes Chromosomes Cancer. 50(7):510-7, 2011
2. Gottfried ON et al: Neurofibromatosis Type 1 and tumorigenesis: molecular mechanisms and therapeutic implications. Neurosurg Focus. 28(1):E8, 2010
3. Hantschke M et al: Cutaneous clear cell sarcoma: a clinicopathologic, immunohistochemical, and molecular analysis of 12 cases emphasizing its distinction from dermal melanoma. Am J Surg Pathol. 34(2):216-22, 2010
4. Jokinen CH et al: Atypical neurofibroma of the skin and subcutaneous tissue: clinicopathologic analysis of 11 cases. J Cutan Pathol. 37(1):35-42, 2010
5. Tanas MR et al: Utilization of fluorescence in situ hybridization in the diagnosis of 230 mesenchymal neoplasms: an institutional experience. Arch Pathol Lab Med. 134(12):1797-803, 2010
6. Jagdis A et al: Prospective evaluation of TLE1 as a diagnostic immunohistochemical marker in synovial sarcoma. Am J Surg Pathol. 33(12):1743-51, 2009
7. Olsen SH et al: Cluster analysis of immunohistochemical profiles in synovial sarcoma, malignant peripheral nerve sheath tumor, and Ewing sarcoma. Mod Pathol. 19(5):659-68, 2006
8. Allison KH et al: Superficial malignant peripheral nerve sheath tumor: a rare and challenging diagnosis. Am J Clin Pathol. 124(5):685-92, 2005
9. Birindelli S et al: Rb and TP53 pathway alterations in sporadic and NF1-related malignant peripheral nerve sheath tumors. Lab Invest. 81(6):833-44, 2001
10. Lucas DR et al: Clear cell sarcoma of soft tissues. Mayo Clinic experience with 35 cases. Am J Surg Pathol. 16(12):1197-204, 1992
11. Dabski C et al: Neurofibrosarcoma of skin and subcutaneous tissues. Mayo Clin Proc. 65(2):164-72, 1990
12. Hruban RH et al: Malignant peripheral nerve sheath tumors of the buttock and lower extremity. A study of 43 cases. Cancer. 66(6):1253-65, 1990
13. George E et al: Malignant peripheral nerve sheath tumors of the skin. Am J Dermatopathol. 11(3):213-21, 1989
14. Jain S et al: Desmoplastic malignant melanoma and its variants. A study of 45 cases. Am J Surg Pathol. 13(5):358-73, 1989
15. Ducatman BS et al: Malignant peripheral nerve sheath tumors. A clinicopathologic study of 120 cases. Cancer. 57(10):2006-21, 1986
16. Guccion JG et al: Malignant Schwannoma associated with von Recklinghausen's neurofibromatosis. Virchows Arch A Pathol Anat Histol. 383(1):43-57, 1979

SUPERFICIAL MALIGNANT PERIPHERAL NERVE SHEATH TUMOR

Clinical and Microscopic Features

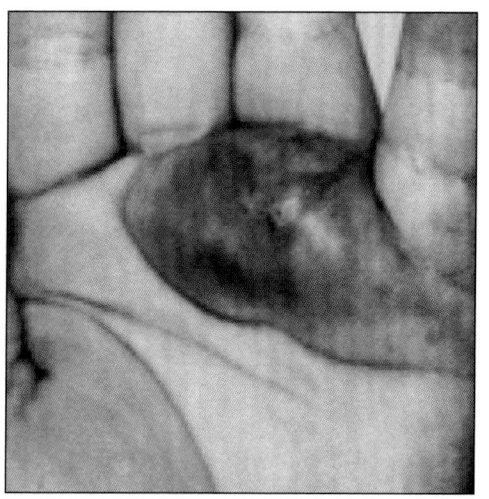

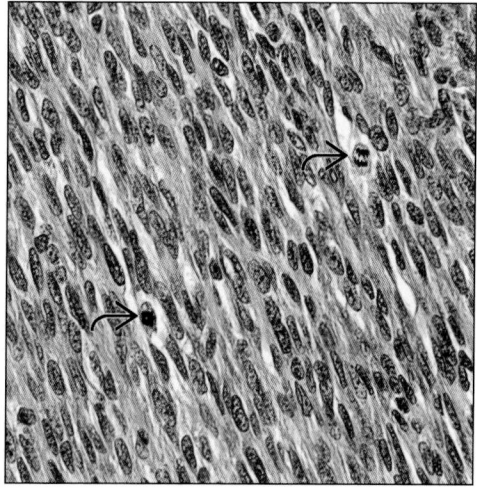

(Left) Superficial MPNST presents as a cutaneous nodule or soft tissue swelling as depicted in this hand tumor. Average size is around 3 cm. However, massive tumors up to 16 cm have been reported. (Right) The most common pattern of MPNST is a high-grade spindle cell sarcoma composed of long fascicles of closely spaced, uniform spindle cells with ill-defined cytoplasmic borders, coarse nuclear hyperchromasia, and very brisk mitotic activity ➔.

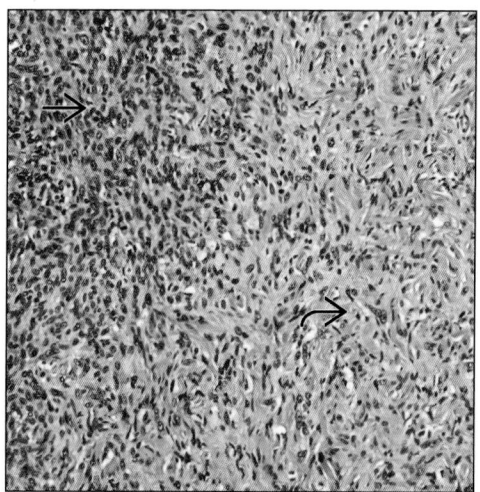

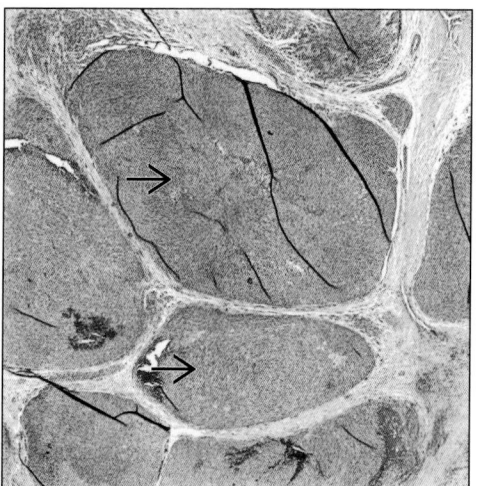

(Left) Superficial MPNSTs may arise from either cutaneous nerves or from benign nerve sheath tumors. This spindle cell MPNST ➔ arose from a neurofibroma ➔ in the neck of a 46-year-old woman with type 1 neurofibromatosis. (Right) MPNSTs that arise within larger nerves frequently have a plexiform architecture, which is formed by very broad nerve fascicles ➔ expanded by the malignant cells.

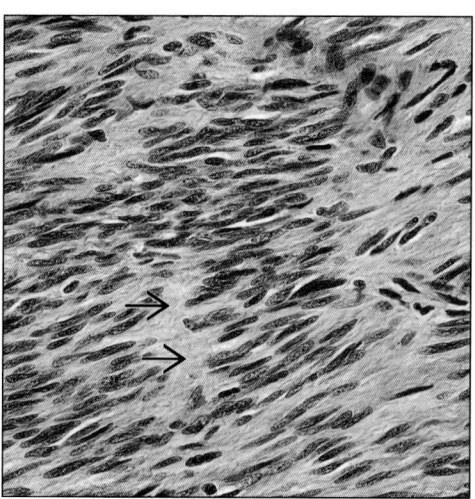

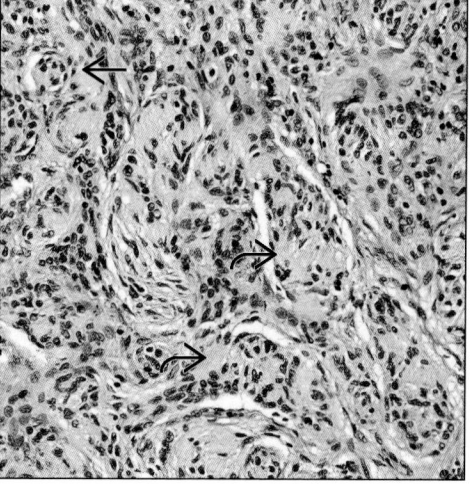

(Left) Microscopic evidence of nerve sheath differentiation is uncommon in MPNST. For example, nuclear palisading with Verocay body formation ➔ is seen in only 15% of MPNSTs, and it is usually a focal finding. (Right) Tactoid differentiation is also seen in MPNSTs. This photomicrograph depicts cell clusters with a vague whorling growth pattern ➔ and hyaline matrix ➔ mimicking tactoid or Wagner-Meissner-like bodies.

I

9

SUPERFICIAL MALIGNANT PERIPHERAL NERVE SHEATH TUMOR

Microscopic Features and Ancillary Techniques

(Left) A distinctive pattern seen in spindle cell MPNST consists of alternating hypercellular fascicles ⇉ and less cellular myxedematous regions ⇉, sometimes referred to as a "tapestry" or "marbled" pattern. *(Right)* Although myxoid matrix ⇉ is common in MPNST, it usually accounts for only a portion of a given tumor with solid areas predominating, but this can occasionally lead to diagnostic difficulty in a core biopsy.

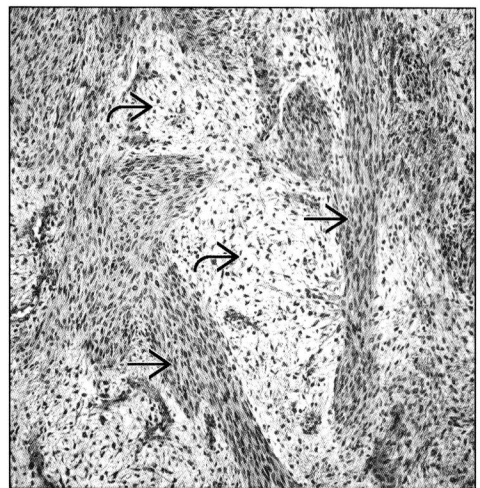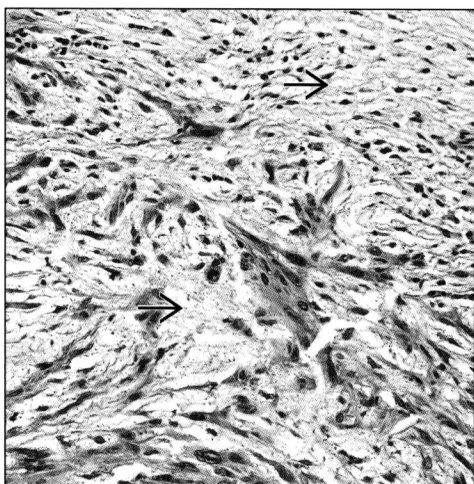

(Left) MPNST can sometimes have a pleomorphic spindle cell pattern with marked nuclear enlargement ⇉ and atypical mitotic figures ⇉, mimicking undifferentiated pleomorphic sarcoma. *(Right)* MPNST can have prominent small round blue cell areas mimicking Ewing sarcoma or poorly differentiated synovial sarcoma. Immunohistochemistry and molecular genetic investigation can resolve these differential diagnoses in most instances.

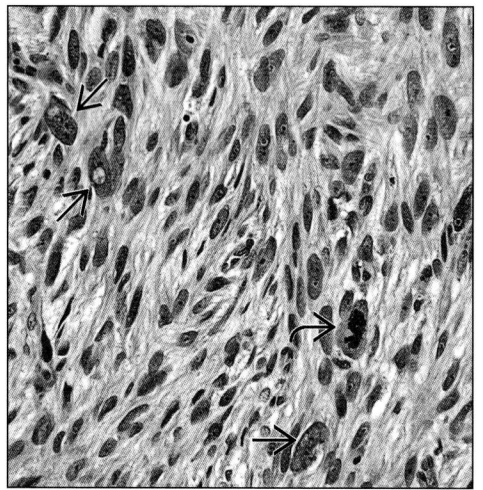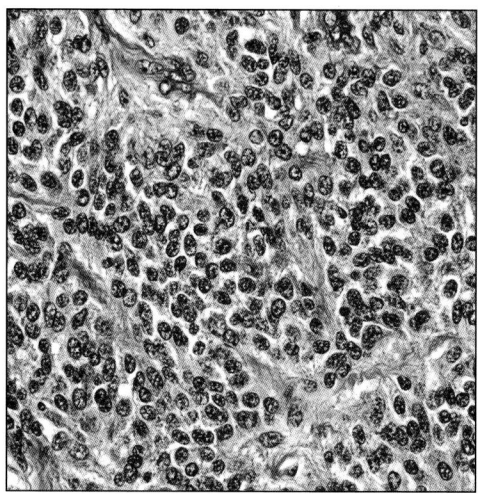

(Left) Large geographic zones of necrosis ⇉ are common in high-grade MPNSTs. In this example, a cuff of viable malignant cells surrounds a blood vessel ⇉ ("perivascular preservation"). *(Right)* Only around 60% of superficial MPNSTs are positive for S100 immunohistochemically, and in most cases the staining reaction is focal as shown. Well-differentiated tumors can show more diffuse staining.

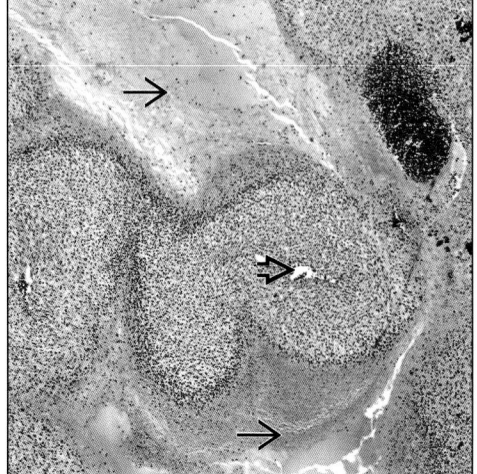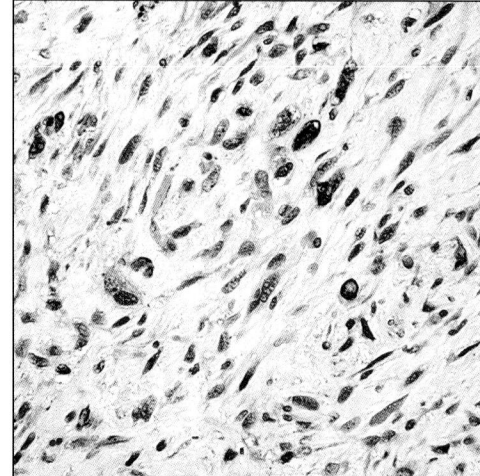

SUPERFICIAL MALIGNANT PERIPHERAL NERVE SHEATH TUMOR

Variant Microscopic Features

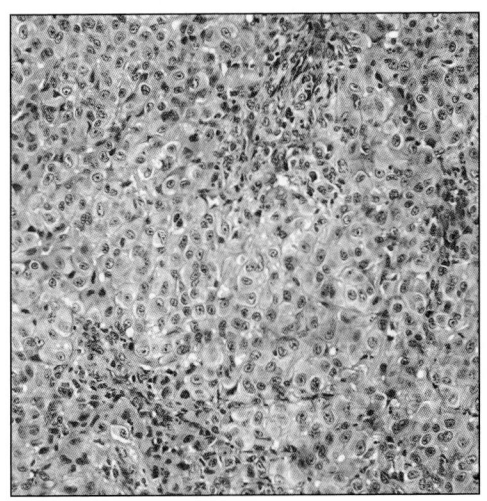
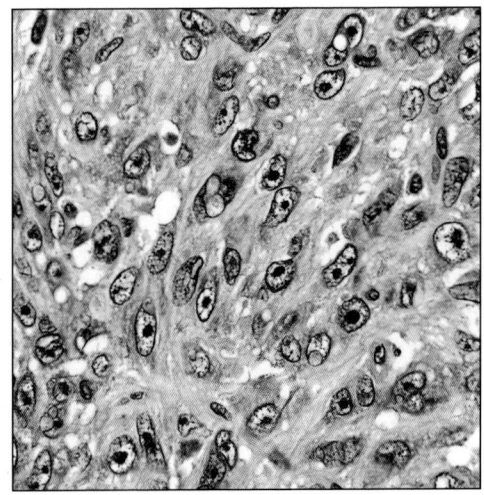

(Left) Epithelioid MPNST may occur as a primary cutaneous tumor. It is characterized by sheets of epithelioid cells with abundant eosinophilic cytoplasm in a vaguely nodular pattern. *(Right)* Epithelioid MPNST is characterized by large polygonal cells with abundant eosinophilic cytoplasm and vesicular nuclei with prominent large nucleoli. It is usually diffusely S100(+), but negative for HMB-45 and MART-1/ Melan-A, which distinguishes it from melanoma.

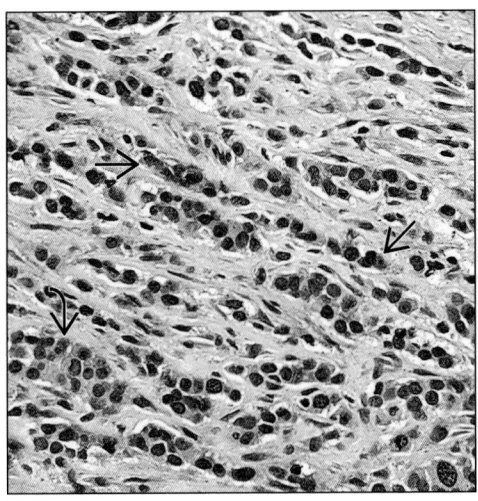
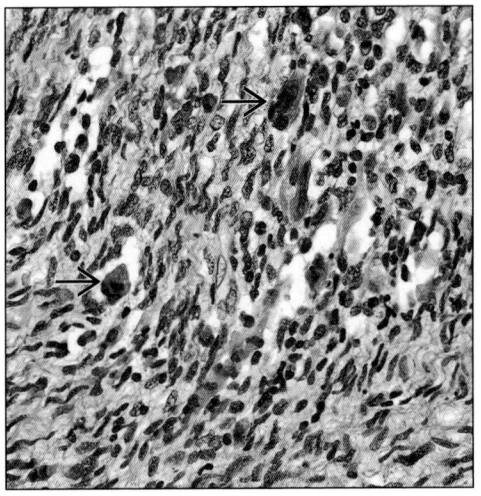

(Left) In some epithelioid MPNSTs, the cells are arranged in single file cords ➡ and small clusters ➡, mimicking carcinoma. However, immunostaining for cytokeratins is negative. *(Right)* Heterologous differentiation is present in around 15% of MPNSTs. Rhabdomyosarcomatous differentiation ("Triton tumor") has been reported in superficial MPNST. Note malignant rhabdomyoblasts with brightly eosinophilic cytoplasm ➡ in a spindle cell MPNST.

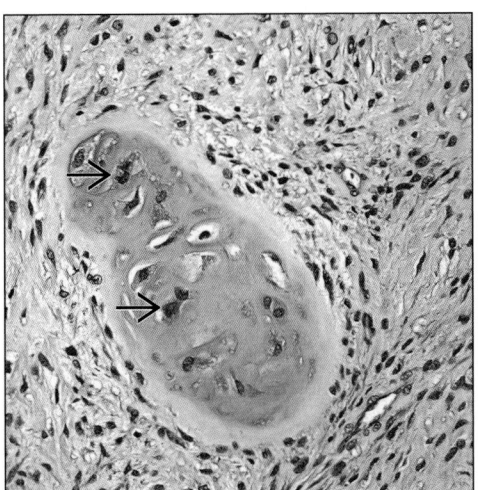
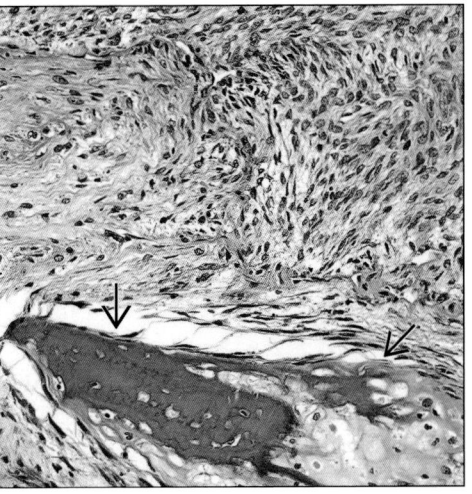

(Left) Cartilaginous differentiation has also been reported in some MPNSTs. It can be benign or malignant (chondrosarcomatous), as indicated in this case by cytological atypia ➡. *(Right)* Heterologous osseous differentiation can occur in some MPNSTs, represented in this example by benign-appearing woven bone ➡. However, osteosarcomatous differentiation as well as other forms of heterologous elements, such as angiosarcoma, have also been described in superficial tumors.

PERIPHERAL NEUROEPITHELIOMA/PRIMITIVE NEUROECTODERMAL TUMOR

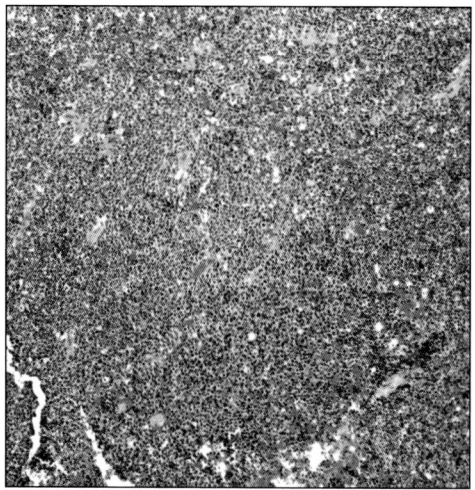

Low-power view shows PNET with the classic appearance of patternless, hypercellular lobules to sheets of undifferentiated, "small round blue" cells.

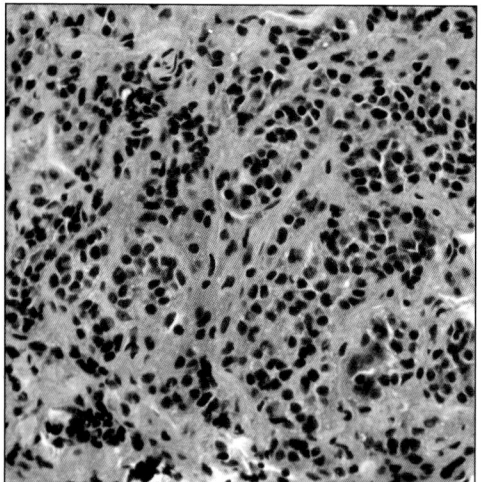

High-power view shows peripheral PNET with the characteristic arrangement of monomorphic cells into nests, lobules, and cords.

TERMINOLOGY

Abbreviations
- Primitive neuroectodermal tumor (PNET)
- Peripheral neuroepithelioma (PNE)

Synonyms
- Primary malignant peripheral PNET
- Peripheral (cutaneous) neuroblastoma
- Extraskeletal Ewing sarcoma

Definitions
- Rare malignant small blue round cell tumor of dermis and superficial subcutis
- Variable evidence of neuroectodermal differentiation (morphologic, ultrastructural, immunohistochemical)

ETIOLOGY/PATHOGENESIS

Histogenesis
- Not entirely clear, regarded as controversial
  - Derived from neural crest cells or neuroepithelium of primitive neuroectodermal tissue
  - Alternatively, from primitive neuroepithelial cell
- Considered PNET of peripheral nervous system
  - Thought to arise from peripheral nerves
  - Not connected to sympathetic nervous system
- Morphologic similarities with other embryonal tumors
  - Assumed to share common histogenetic origins
  - Central nervous system PNET (medulloblastoma)
  - Askin tumor (chest wall/thoracopulmonary PNET)

Genetics
- t(11;22)(q24;q12)
  - Related to Ewing sarcoma (same translocation)
  - Probably phenotypic spectrum of same tumor

CLINICAL ISSUES

Epidemiology
- Incidence
  - Very rare (especially if metastasis excluded)
- Age
  - Children, adolescents, young adults (20s)
  - Occasionally may affect older patients
- Gender
  - No gender predilection reported

Site
- Trunk, extremities, scalp, face, neck, shoulder
- May uncommonly involve vulva, vagina

Presentation
- Mostly painless nodules
  - But may be tender
- May be clinically misdiagnosed as benign tumor or cyst
- Usually do not secrete catecholamines or metabolites

Natural History
- Highly aggressive behavior
  - May grow rapidly
- Distant metastases common
  - Regional lymph nodes, lung, liver, bones, brain

Treatment
- Surgical approaches
  - Goal is complete surgical resection
- Adjuvant therapy
  - Chemotherapy and radiation

Prognosis
- Slightly better than soft tissue counterpart
  - Probably due to earlier detection
- 5-year disease-free survival: ~ 60%
- Improved overall survival correlated with younger age and wide initial surgical excision

PERIPHERAL NEUROEPITHELIOMA/PRIMITIVE NEUROECTODERMAL TUMOR

Key Facts

Terminology
- Rare malignant small round blue cell tumor
- Variable evidence of neuroectodermal differentiation

Etiology/Pathogenesis
- From neural crest cells or primitive neuroepithelium
- t(11;22)(q24;q12) in 90% of cases (*EWS-FLI-1* fusion)
  - Related to Ewing sarcoma (same translocation)
  - Probably phenotypic spectrum of the same entity

Clinical Issues
- Trunk, extremities, scalp, face, neck, shoulder
- Painless nodules, misdiagnosed as benign tumor, cyst
- Highly aggressive behavior, distant metastases
- 5-year disease-free survival: ~ 60%

Macroscopic Features
- Hemorrhagic, ulcerated or polypoid, ill-defined mass

Microscopic Pathology
- In dermis, focal extension into superficial subcutis
- Sheets, nests, lobules, trabeculae and cords of cells
- Delicate reticulin positive fibrovascular stroma
- Monomorphic cells, no nucleoli, scant cytoplasm
- Intercellular vague Homer Wright rosettes
- Mitoses, apoptosis, necrosis (may be confluent)

Ancillary Tests
- Diffusely, strongly positive for membranous CD99
- Positive for 1 or more neural markers (e.g., NSE)
- Membrane-bound dense core neurosecretory granules
- Intracytoplasmic glycogen commonly seen

Diagnostic Checklist
- Primary vs. metastatic, e.g., metastatic neuroblastoma
- Histologically indistinguishable; work-up required

MACROSCOPIC FEATURES

General Features
- Nodular, may be multiple or multinodular
  - May be ulcerated or polypoid
- Mass with ill-defined borders
- Hemorrhagic (red, brown, and purple)
  - Or gray-white and fleshy

Size
- Usually vary between 5-10 cm in largest dimension

MICROSCOPIC PATHOLOGY

Histologic Features
- Usually located in dermis, often with focal extension into superficial subcutis
  - May be entirely subcutaneous
  - Overlying epidermis may be ulcerated
  - Margins pushing or infiltrative
- Sheets, nests, lobules, trabeculae and cords of cells
  - In close approximation to each other
  - Microcystic, pseudoglandular and pseudopapillary formations observed
- Separated by delicate fibrovascular stroma
  - Reticulin-positive fibrils
  - Stromal vessels may form glomeruloid tufts
- Intercellular rosettes may be present, but often vague
  - Homer Wright rosettes with central neuropil
  - Support primitive neural nature of neoplasm
- Spindle cell areas may be present (10-20%)
  - Simulate fibrosarcoma or malignant peripheral nerve sheath tumor
- Areas of confluent necrosis can be seen
- Cartilaginous or osseous metaplasia may be seen

Cytologic Features
- Monomorphic, "small round blue cells"
  - Round to oval, uniform-appearing cells
  - 2-3x size of mature lymphocytes
- Characteristic nuclear details
  - Evenly distributed, dispersed chromatin
  - Small or absent nucleoli
- Little or scant, amphophilic cytoplasm
  - May be vacuolated
- Mitotic activity usually prominent, but may be low
  - Including abnormal mitotic figures
- Individual cell necrosis and cellular apoptosis often present, but may be sparse
- Larger, atypical, and pleomorphic cells may be present
  - Irregular nuclei or binucleated, prominent nucleoli
- Intracytoplasmic glycogen may be seen

Predominant Pattern/Injury Type
- Neoplastic

Predominant Cell/Compartment Type
- Nervous, neural
- Neuroendocrine

ANCILLARY TESTS

Immunohistochemistry
- Diffusely, strongly positive for membranous CD99
  - *MIC2* gene product
- Usually positive for 1 or more neural/neuroendocrine markers
  - Neuron-specific enolase (NSE) may be the most sensitive marker
  - PGP9.5, neurofilament protein (NFP)
  - Synaptophysin, Leu-7 (CD57)
  - Chromogranin usually negative
- FLI-1 positive neoplastic nuclei
- Aberrant cytokeratin, GFAP, S100 expression seen
- Lymphocytic, melanocytic, muscle markers negative

Cytogenetics
- t(11;22)(q24;q12) in 90% of cases
  - *EWS* to *FLI1* gene fusion
  - Maybe detected by cytogenetics, FISH, RT-PCR
  - Also seen in olfactory neuroblastoma, Askin tumor

Electron Microscopy
- Elongated, interdigitating cytoplasmic processes
- Rudimentary intercellular junctions, rarely desmosomes, intermediate filaments, microtubules
- Membrane-bound dense core neurosecretory granules
- Myofilaments or melanosomes are generally absent
- Glycogen usually abundant

DIFFERENTIAL DIAGNOSIS

Extraskeletal Ewing Sarcoma
- Similar entity across phenotypic spectrum
  - Considered same biological entity by most authors
- Usually less differentiated, more primitive-appearing
- Lacks neurosecretory granules, well-developed desmosomes
- Usually negative for NSE, keratin, S100
- Usually contains abundant glycogen

Metastatic Neuroblastoma
- Impossible to distinguish histologically
- Usually multiple nodules
- Usually in young children
- Shows adrenergic expression, metabolic excretion
  - Catecholamines and metabolites
- Neuronal differentiation
  - Neurofilament positive
  - Generally vimentin negative
  - Neurites, granules by EM
- May contain mature neural elements
  - Ganglion cells
  - Neuropil (fibrillary intercellular network)
- Usually negative for CD99
- Chromosome 1, 11, and 17 aberrations

Merkel Cell Carcinoma
- Typically occurs in elderly adults
- Perinuclear whorls of intermediate filaments
- Positive for CK20, EMA, pankeratin
- May have neurosecretory granules
- Typically positive: Synaptophysin, chromogranin, NSE
- Chromosome 1 and 6 abnormalities

Rhabdomyosarcoma (Embryonal and Alveolar)
- Common nuclear pleomorphism and multinucleation
- Hyperchromatic nuclei, eosinophilic cytoplasm (rhabdomyoblasts)
- Positive for actin, desmin, myoglobin by immunohistochemistry
- Ultrastructurally, thick and thin filaments, dense bodies, basal lamina
- 11p allelic loss, t(1;13) or t(2;13)

Lymphoma
- More irregular nuclear contours
- Lacks intercellular attachments, neurosecretory granules
- Positive for CD45 (LCA), CD20 (B cell) or CD3 (T cell)

Malignant Peripheral Nerve Sheath Tumor
- Most cases occur in adults
- Cells are typically spindle-shaped, not round
- S100 usually at least focally positive
- Lacks neurosecretory granules

Small Cell Melanoma
- Very rare in children
- Overlying melanoma in situ usually present
- S100, HMB-45 positive
- Ultrastructurally, premelanosomes, melanosomes

Metastatic Small Cell Carcinoma
- Extremely rare in children
- Cytokeratin, EMA positive
- Synaptophysin, GFAP negative
- Lacks Homer Wright rosettes, neurosecretory granules
- Contains more mature desmosomes, tonofilaments, keratohyalin granules

DIAGNOSTIC CHECKLIST

Clinically Relevant Pathologic Features
- Nuclear features
- Organ distribution
- Metastatic distribution
- Primary vs. metastatic PNET
  - Histologically indistinguishable
  - Extensive clinical examination required
- PNE vs. peripheral neuroblastoma
  - Terms sometimes used interchangeably
  - Association with peripheral nerves not always seen
  - Clinically not different: Both have poor outcomes

Pathologic Interpretation Pearls
- Avoid diagnosis in the absence of
  - CD99 (*MIC2*) immunoreactivity
  - t(11;22)(q24;q12)

SELECTED REFERENCES

1. Banerjee SS: Primary malignant peripheral primitive neuroectodermal tumor (PNET)/Extraskeletal Ewing sarcoma (ES). In LeBoit PE et al: Pathology and Genetics: Skin Tumors. Lyon: IARC Press. 268-9, 2006
2. Sangueza OP et al: Multiple primitive neuroectodermal tumors. J Am Acad Dermatol. 31(2 Pt 2):356-61, 1994
3. Van Nguyen A et al: Cutaneous neuroblastoma. Peripheral neuroblastoma. Am J Dermatopathol. 15(1):7-14, 1993
4. Gorman PA et al: Cytogenetic analysis of primitive neuroectodermal tumors. Absence of the t(11;22) in two of three cases and a review of the literature. Cancer Genet Cytogenet. 51(1):13-22, 1991
5. Jacinto CM et al: Malignant primitive neuroectodermal tumor presenting as a scalp nodule. Am J Dermatopathol. 13(1):63-70, 1991
6. Klapman MH et al: Cutaneous and subcutaneous neuroblastoma in children and adults: case reports and population study. J Am Acad Dermatol. 24(6 Pt 1):1025-7, 1991
7. Argenyi ZB et al: Primitive neuroectodermal tumor in the skin with features of neuroblastoma in an adult patient. J Cutan Pathol. 13(6):420-30, 1986
8. Hashimoto H et al: Malignant neuroepithelioma (peripheral neuroblastoma). A clinicopathologic study of 15 cases. Am J Surg Pathol. 7(4):309-18, 1983

Nonmelanocytic Tumors of the Skin: Tumors and Tumor-like Conditions with Neural, Nerve Sheath, and Neuroendocrine Differentiation

I

9

44

Microscopic Features and Ancillary Techniques

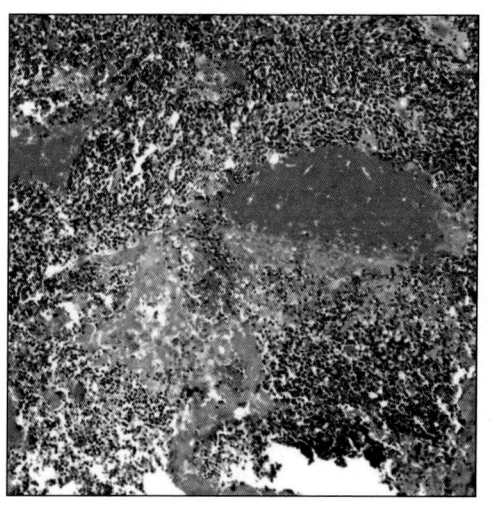
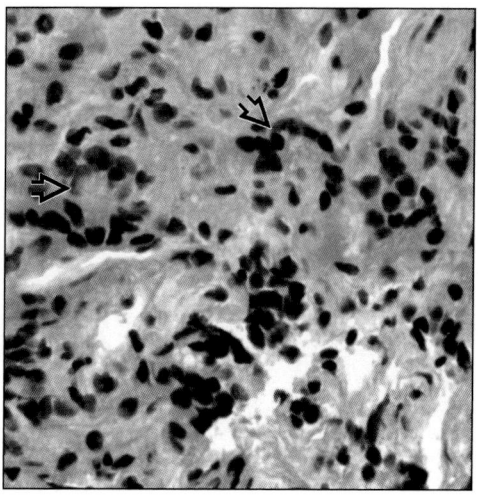

(Left) Deep dermal PNET shows areas of hemorrhage and confluent necrosis, which is usually not geographic or pseudopalisading. (Right) High magnification shows a peripheral PNET with vague arrangement of cells into rosettes ⊡, reminiscent of Homer Wright rosettes with central neuropil.

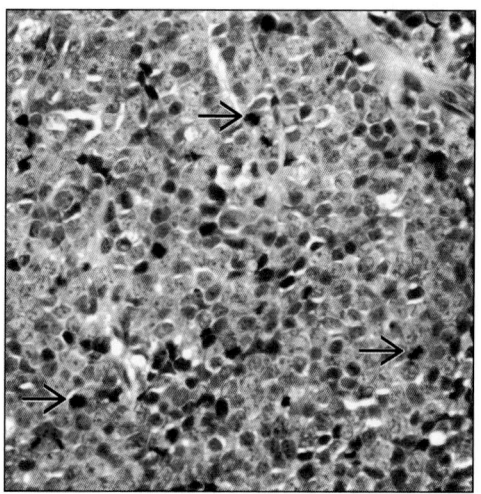
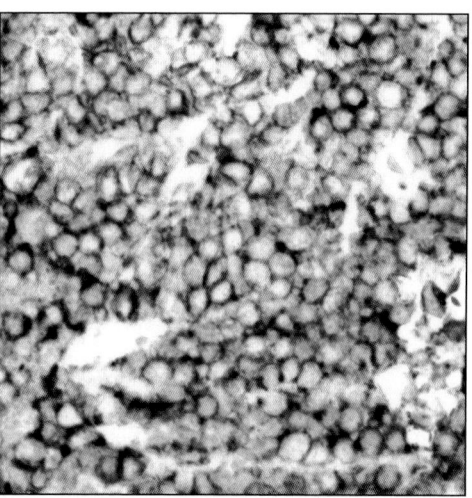

(Left) High-power view shows peripheral PNET with sheet-like areas of dense cellularity composed of monotonous, poorly differentiated tumor cells with little cytoplasm and numerous mitoses ➡. (Right) Immunohistochemical stain for CD99 in peripheral PNET typically shows strong cytoplasmic and membranous immunoreactivity in the tumor cells.

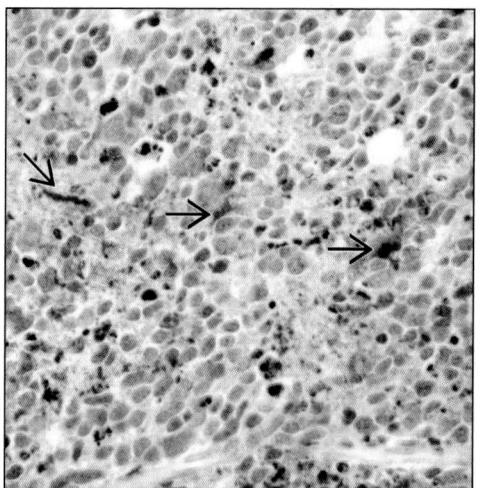
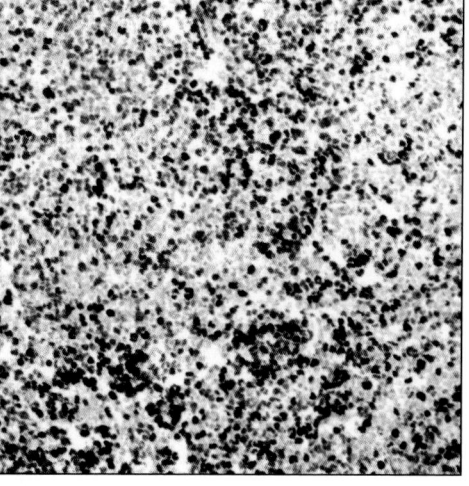

(Left) Immunohistochemical stain for synaptophysin shows a PNET with highlighted areas of neuronal differentiation ➡, characterized by nuclei-free fibrillar zones with tumor cells radially arranged around them, akin to neuroblastic Homer Wright rosettes. (Right) Immunohistochemical stain for Ki-67 (MIB-1) shows a PNET with a very high proliferation index, approaching 80-90%.

PRIMARY NEUROENDOCRINE (MERKEL CELL) CARCINOMA

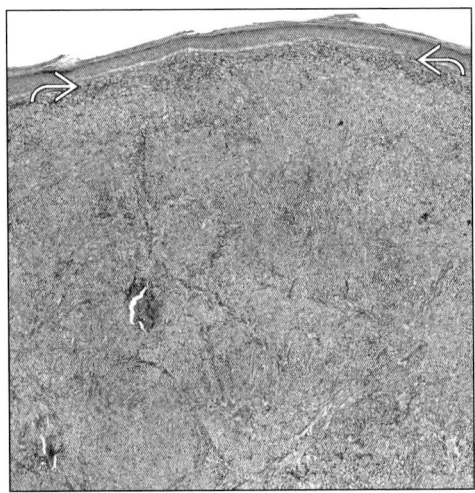

Low magnification of Merkel cell carcinoma shows diffuse dermal involvement by sheets and nodules of atypical basophilic cells. There is a thin grenz zone separating the tumor from the epidermis ➤.

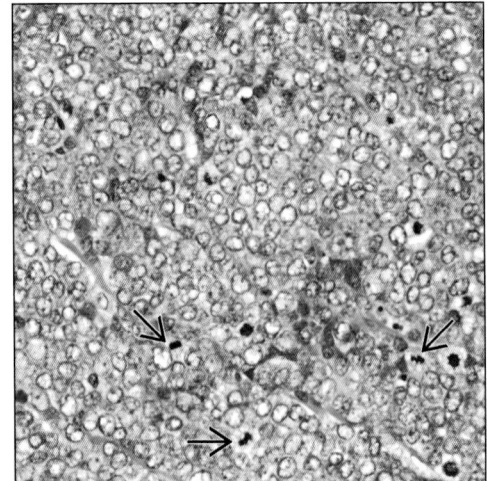

High magnification of MCC shows nuclear molding, hyperchromasia, and vesicular to granular-appearing chromatin. Numerous apoptotic and mitotic figures ➔ are easily identified.

TERMINOLOGY

Abbreviations
- Merkel cell carcinoma (MCC)

Synonyms
- Cutaneous neuroendocrine carcinoma
- Primary small cell carcinoma of skin
- Trabecular carcinoma

Definitions
- Malignant proliferation of cutaneous neuroendocrine cells

ETIOLOGY/PATHOGENESIS

Infectious Agents
- Recent studies have shown strong link to infection with polyomavirus
  - Merkel cell polyoma virus infection is found in up to 90% of cases
- Associated with immunosuppression
  - Organ transplant and HIV(+) patients have much higher incidence

Cell of Origin
- Postulated to represent malignant transformation of cutaneous neuroendocrine (Merkel) cells or pluripotent stem cells, but this remains speculative

CLINICAL ISSUES

Epidemiology
- Incidence
  - Rare
    - Approximately 470 cases/year in USA
- Age
  - Typically in elderly patients (> 65 years old)
- Gender

  - Male > female (2.5:1)
- Ethnicity
  - Caucasians much more commonly affected than other races

Site
- Sun-damaged skin
- Usually head and neck or extremities

Presentation
- Dermal nodular or plaque-like mass lesion
- Rapidly enlarging dermal mass lesion
  - May be ulcerated &/or hemorrhagic

Natural History
- Aggressive tumors with high incidence of local recurrence, lymph node and distant metastasis
- Clinical staging should include imaging studies, especially chest and abdominal CT scans

Treatment
- Surgical approaches
  - Complete and wide excision to ensure complete local removal
  - Consideration may be given to sentinel lymph node (SLN) biopsy
    - However, SLN positivity does not seem to be very sensitive for regional lymph node involvement, as many patients progress to distant metastases
- Adjuvant therapy
  - Radiotherapy is generally used and may lead to remission in some cases
  - Chemotherapy is less effective and does not prolong overall survival

Prognosis
- High incidence of recurrence (up to 30%) and metastasis (up to 75%)
- Overall prognosis is poor
  - Death due to disease is high, even with treatment

PRIMARY NEUROENDOCRINE (MERKEL CELL) CARCINOMA

Key Facts

Terminology
- Cutaneous neuroendocrine carcinoma

Clinical Issues
- Highly aggressive tumors with greater metastatic potential than melanoma
- Rare (approximately 470 cases/year in USA)
- Typically occur in sun-damaged skin of elderly
- More common in males
- Radiotherapy is generally used

Microscopic Pathology
- Highly atypical basaloid neoplasm composed of infiltrative cords, trabeculae, and sheet-like areas
- Typically dermal-based, but may show epidermal (pagetoid) involvement in up to 20% of cases
- Numerous mitoses and apoptotic bodies

- Nuclear crush artifact and streaming may be seen, similar to small cell carcinomas
- Basaloid cells with high N:C ratio, scant cytoplasm, large nuclei, granular to clear chromatin, and indistinct nucleoli

Ancillary Tests
- Immunohistochemistry is important in confirming diagnosis and excluding metastatic carcinoma
- MCC is typically positive for keratins, including CK20, with perinuclear dot-like staining

Top Differential Diagnoses
- Basal cell carcinoma (BCC)
- Metastatic small cell carcinoma (especially pulmonary origin)
- Small cell melanoma

- o Worse prognosis associated with advanced age, head and neck location, large size, and immunosuppression

MACROSCOPIC FEATURES

General Features
- Nodular tumor with blue or red appearance

Size
- Typically < 2 cm

MICROSCOPIC PATHOLOGY

Histologic Features
- Highly atypical invasive basaloid neoplasm
  - o Composed of infiltrative cords, trabeculae, nests, and sheet-like areas
    - Associated dermal desmoplasia may be present
  - o Enlarged, hyperchromatic basaloid tumor cells with scant cytoplasm, large nuclei, granular to clear (vesicular) chromatin, and indistinct nucleoli
  - o Nuclear clearing is a distinctive feature often seen
    - This finding is not present in BCC
  - o Mitotic figures are abundant
  - o Typically, numerous apoptotic bodies
  - o Areas of geographic necrosis often present, especially in larger tumors
  - o Nuclear crush artifact and streaming may be seen, similar to small cell carcinoma
  - o Angiolymphatic invasion identified in significant percentage of cases, often at periphery of tumor
  - o Partial tumor regression may be present
- Typically dermal-based
  - o May show epidermal (pagetoid) involvement in up to 20% of cases
  - o Purely pagetoid (in situ) cases have been reported
- Areas of squamoid or adnexal (including follicular, ductal, or glandular) differentiation may be present in minority of cases
  - o Rarely, melanocytic differentiation may be present

- o These findings suggest that MCC may arise from primitive pluripotential (stem) cell that can differentiate along multiple different lines, rather than specific neuroendocrine cell
- Rarely, spindle cell/sarcomatoid differentiation mimicking atypical fibroxanthoma (AFX), leiomyosarcoma, osteosarcoma, or rhabdomyosarcoma may be seen

Cytologic Features
- Basaloid cells with high N:C ratio, scant cytoplasm, large nuclei, granular to clear chromatin, and indistinct nucleoli

ANCILLARY TESTS

Immunohistochemistry
- Immunohistochemistry (IHC) is important in confirming diagnosis and excluding metastatic neuroendocrine carcinoma
  - o MCC is typically positive for keratins (CK-PAN, CK20, CK8/18/CAM5.2), often with perinuclear dot-like staining
  - o Putative prognostic markers include CD44, p53, and Bcl-2
  - o Negative staining for melanocytic markers and lymphoid markers

Cytogenetics
- Trisomy 6 is identified in many cases of MCC, up to 50% in some studies
- Deletion of short arm of chromosome 1 (1p36) is also commonly identified

DIFFERENTIAL DIAGNOSIS

Basal Cell Carcinoma (BCC)
- Less atypia and mitotic activity
- Most cases show areas of peripheral palisading, mucinous stroma, and tumor-stromal retraction artifact

PRIMARY NEUROENDOCRINE (MERKEL CELL) CARCINOMA

Immunohistochemistry

Antibody	Reactivity	Staining Pattern	Comment
CK-PAN	Positive	Dot positivity	May or may not show dot-like positivity, but will be positive
CK20	Positive	Dot positivity	Rare cases may be negative
CK8/18/CAM5.2	Positive	Dot positivity	Most cases show dot reactivity
NSE	Positive	Cytoplasmic	Most cases are positive (but nonspecific marker)
Chromogranin-A	Positive	Cytoplasmic	Most cases are positive
Synaptophysin	Positive	Cytoplasmic	Most cases are positive
CK7	Negative	Dot positivity	Isolated cases may be CK7 positive when CK20 negative
S100	Negative		
melan-A103	Negative		
HMB-45	Negative		
TTF-1	Negative		
CD45	Negative		
CD99	Negative		

- MCC should always be considered in high-grade/pleomorphic-appearing cases of BCC
- Almost always positive for EpCAM/BER-EP4/CD326, but negative for CK20, chromogranin-A, and synaptophysin

Metastatic Small Cell Carcinoma

- Especially pulmonary origin, which are positive for TTF-1, negative for CK20
- Small cell carcinomas from other sites are TTF-1 negative
- Clinical history and complete examination important to exclude metastasis

Small Cell Melanoma

- Rare variant of melanoma; typically see areas of associated junctional nesting and overlying pagetoid spread
- Cells show more abundant cytoplasm, prominent nucleoli, and may see cytoplasmic pigmentation and intranuclear pseudoinclusions
- S100, HMB-45, MART-1/Melan-A typically positive; negative for cytokeratins, CK20, and neuroendocrine markers

Lymphoma

- Lymphomas are dyscohesive, lacking cord-like and trabecular growth pattern of MCC
- Various lymphoid markers including CD45 will be positive
- CK20 and neuroendocrine markers negative

Small Round Blue Cell Tumors

- These tumors include neuroblastoma, Ewing/primitive neuroectodermal tumor (PNET), rhabdomyosarcoma
- Very rare in skin (typically metastatic from other sites); most cases occur in children
- Immunohistochemistry distinguishes from MCC

DIAGNOSTIC CHECKLIST

Clinically Relevant Pathologic Features

- Mitotic rate
- Angiolymphatic invasion
- Large tumor size
- Small cell size

Pathologic Interpretation Pearls

- High-grade basaloid proliferation with neuroendocrine features
- Composed of infiltrative cords, trabeculae, nests, and sheet-like areas
  ○ Cells are hyperchromatic, with scant cytoplasm, granular-appearing chromatin, and indistinct nucleoli

SELECTED REFERENCES

1. Sastre-Garau X et al: Merkel cell carcinoma of the skin: pathological and molecular evidence for a causative role of MCV in oncogenesis. J Pathol. 218(1):48-56, 2009
2. Feng H et al: Clonal integration of a polyomavirus in human Merkel cell carcinoma. Science. 319(5866):1096-100, 2008
3. Ball NJ et al: Merkel cell carcinoma frequently shows histologic features of basal cell carcinoma: a study of 30 cases. J Cutan Pathol. 34(8):612-9, 2007
4. Calder KB et al: A case series and immunophenotypic analysis of CK20-/CK7+ primary neuroendocrine carcinoma of the skin. J Cutan Pathol. 34(12):918-23, 2007
5. Eng TY et al: A comprehensive review of the treatment of Merkel cell carcinoma. Am J Clin Oncol. 30(6):624-36, 2007
6. Sandel HD 4th et al: Merkel cell carcinoma: does tumor size or depth of invasion correlate with recurrence, metastasis, or patient survival? Laryngoscope. 116(5):791-5, 2006
7. Gancberg D et al: Trisomy 6 in Merkel cell carcinoma: a recurrent chromosomal aberration. Histopathology. 37(5):445-51, 2000
8. Yanguas I et al: Spontaneous regression of Merkel cell carcinoma of the skin. Br J Dermatol. 137(2):296-8, 1997

PRIMARY NEUROENDOCRINE (MERKEL CELL) CARCINOMA

Clinical, Microscopic Features, and Ancillary Techniques

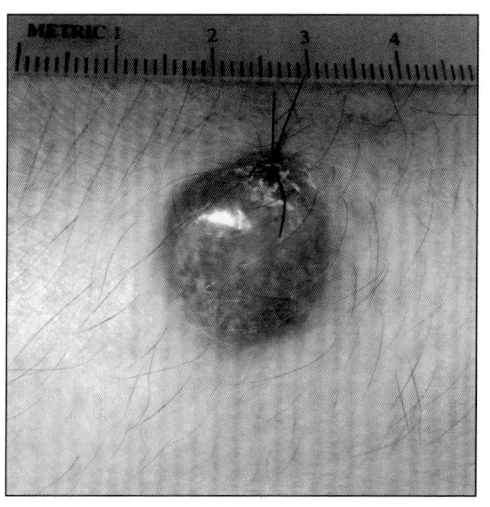

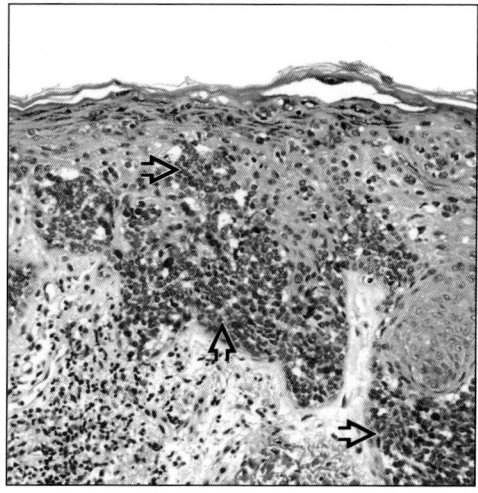

(Left) Clinical photograph of a Merkel cell carcinoma shows a well-circumscribed-appearing erythematous dermal nodule. (Courtesy J. Wu, MD.) (Right) Pagetoid intraepidermal spread of Merkel cell carcinoma ⊡ is seen in a minority of cases (< 20%). No dermal component is present in this image.

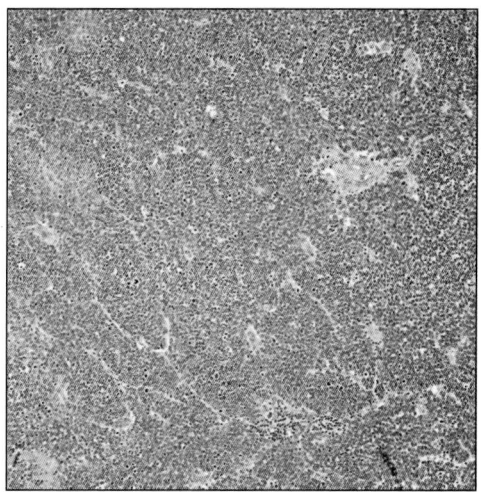

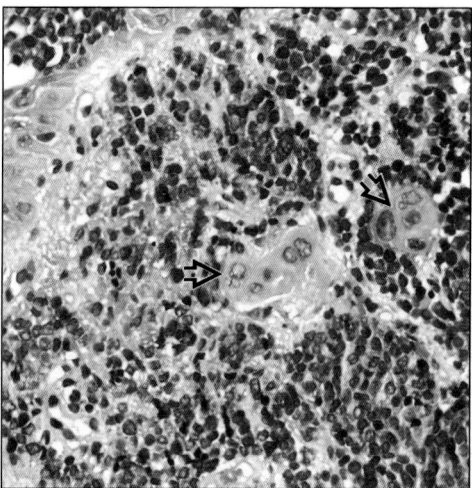

(Left) H&E shows diffuse dermal involvement by Merkel cell carcinoma. The tumor is composed of broad cords and sheet-like collections of highly atypical basaloid cells. There is scant stroma intervening between the neoplastic cells. (Right) Higher magnification of MCC shows that the neoplastic cells are predominantly basophilic with a high nuclear to cytoplasmic ratio. The nuclear chromatin is dense, and nucleoli are not appreciated. Focal squamous differentiation ⊡ is seen in this example.

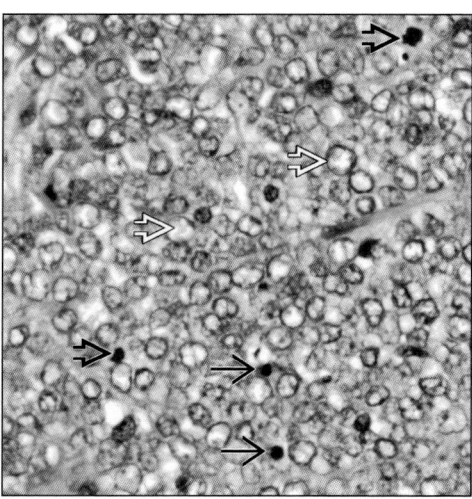

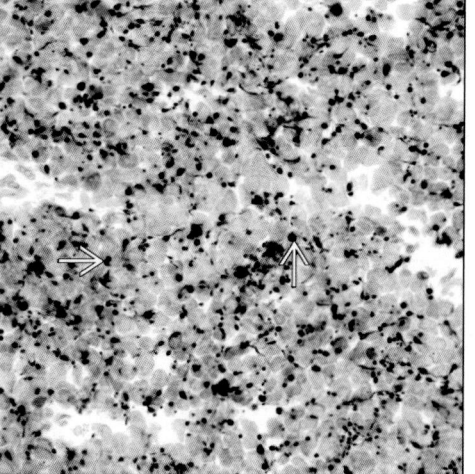

(Left) Nuclear clearing ⊡ is often seen in Merkel cell carcinoma, a feature not seen in basal cell carcinoma or most other small round blue cell tumors. Note the numerous apoptotic bodies ➡ and mitotic figures ⊡. (Right) CK20 immunohistochemistry shows cytoplasmic and perinuclear dot-like ➡ positivity. This pattern is not a feature identified in other basaloid tumor types, helping to confirm the diagnosis.

Merkel Cell Carcinoma of the Skin

Incisional Biopsy, Excision, Reexcision, Lymphadenectomy

Procedure

____ Biopsy, incisional

____ Excision

____ Reexcision

____ Lymphadenectomy, sentinel node(s)

____ Lymphadenectomy, regional nodes (specify): _____

____ Other (specify): _____

____ Not specified

Macroscopic Tumor

____ Present

____ Not identified

Tumor Site

Specify (if known): _____

____ Not specified

Tumor Size

Greatest dimension: _____ cm

*Additional dimensions: _____ x _____ cm

____ Indeterminate

*Tumor Thickness

*Thickness: _____ mm

*Thickness: ≥ _____ mm

Margins

Peripheral margins

____ Cannot be assessed

____ Uninvolved by carcinoma

 Distance of carcinoma from closest margin: _____ mm

 Specify location(s), if possible: _____

____ Involved by carcinoma

 Specify location(s), if possible: _____

Deep margin

____ Cannot be assessed

____ Uninvolved by carcinoma

 Distance of carcinoma from closest margin: _____ mm

 Specify location(s), if possible: _____

____ Involved by carcinoma

 Specify location(s), if possible: _____

Lymph-Vascular Invasion

____ Not identified

____ Present

____ Indeterminate

Invasion of Bone, Muscle, Fascia, or Cartilage

____ Present (specify structures involved): _____

____ Not identified

____ Not applicable (e.g., for superficial biopsy)

*Mitotic Index

*____ < 1/mm²

*____ Specify: _____ /mm²

Nonmelanocytic Tumors of the Skin: Tumors and Tumor-like Conditions with Neural, Nerve Sheath, and Neuroendocrine Differentiation

9

50

PROTOCOL FOR SPECIMENS OF MERKEL CELL CARCINOMA OF THE SKIN

*Tumor-Infiltrating Lymphocytes

*____Not identified

*____Present, nonbrisk

*____Present, brisk

*Tumor Growth Pattern

*____Nodular

*____Infiltrative

*Presence of Second Malignancy

*____Present (specify type): _____

*____Not identified

Lymph Nodes (required only if lymph nodes are present in the specimen)

Number of sentinel nodes examined: _____

Total number of nodes examined (sentinel and nonsentinel): _____

Number of lymph nodes with metastases: _____

Macroscopic tumor

_____ Present

_____ Not identified

_____ Indeterminate

*Size of largest metastatic focus: _____ mm

*Extranodal extension

*_____ Present

*_____ Not identified

Pathologic Staging (pTNM)

TNM descriptors (required only if applicable) (select all that apply)

_____ m (multiple)

_____ r (recurrent)

_____ y (post treatment)

Primary tumor (pT)

_____ pTX: Primary tumor cannot be assessed

_____ pT0: No evidence of primary tumor (e.g., nodal/metastatic presentation without associated primary)

_____ pTis: In situ primary tumor

_____ pT1: ≤ 2 cm maximum tumor dimension

_____ pT2: > 2 cm but ≤ 5 cm maximum tumor dimension

_____ pT3: > 5 cm maximum tumor dimension

_____ pT4: Primary tumor invades bone, muscle, fascia, or cartilage

Regional lymph nodes (pN)

_____ pNX: Nodes not examined pathologically

_____ pN0: Nodes negative by pathologic exam

_____ pN1: Metastasis in regional lymph node(s)

*_____ pN1a: Micrometastasis

*_____ pN1b: Macrometastasis

_____ pN2: In transit metastasis

Distant metastasis (pM)

_____ Not applicable

_____ pM1: Metastasis beyond regional lymph nodes

_____ *pM1a: Metastasis to skin, subcutaneous tissues, or distant lymph nodes

_____ *pM1b: Metastasis to lung

_____ *pM1c: Metastasis to all other visceral sites

*Additional Pathologic Findings

*Specify: _____

*Adapted with permission from College of American Pathologists, "Protocol for the Examination of Specimens from Patients with Merkel Cell Carcinoma of the Skin." Web posting date: February 2011, www.cap.org. Note: Use of checklist is not required for punch or shave biopsies. Protocol applies to Merkel cell carcinoma of cutaneous surfaces only. *Data elements with asterisks are not required. These elements may be clinically important but are not yet validated or regularly used in patient management.*

Tumors of Muscle, Fat, Cartilage, and Bone

CONGENITAL SMOOTH MUSCLE HAMARTOMA

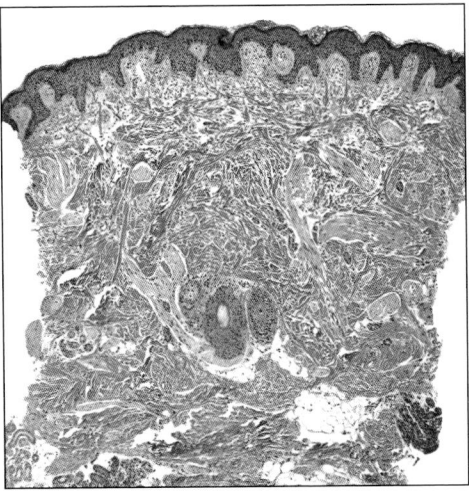

Congenital smooth muscle hamartoma shows a haphazard arrangement of smooth muscle bundles present throughout the dermis.

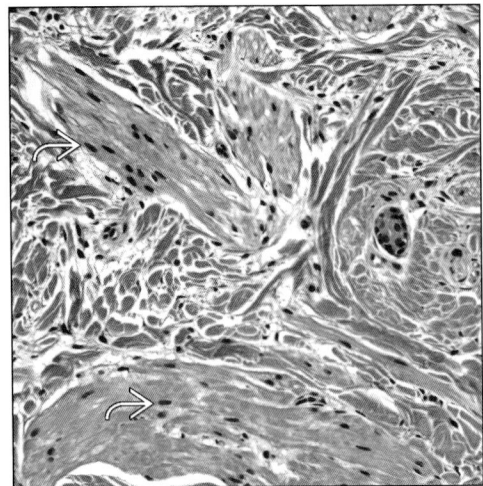

High magnification shows a fascicular arrangement of smooth muscle with characteristic elongated, spindle-shaped to blunt-ended nuclei ➔.

TERMINOLOGY

Synonyms
• Smooth muscle hamartoma

Definitions
• Rare benign smooth muscle tumor presenting in infants
• Characterized by disorganized proliferation of smooth muscle bundles

CLINICAL ISSUES

Epidemiology
• Age
  o Infants

Site
• Lumbosacral area and proximal extremities

Presentation
• Macule or plaque
  o Indurated
  o Often hyperpigmented
  o May have coarse hairs
• Pseudo-Darier sign
  o Piloerection induced by mechanical stimulation
• Occasionally presents as multiple lesions
• Rare familial cases

Treatment
• Surgical approaches
  o Simple excision

Prognosis
• Excellent

MACROSCOPIC FEATURES

General Features
• Ill-defined dermal thickening

Size
• Usually < 2 cm in diameter

MICROSCOPIC PATHOLOGY

Histologic Features
• Haphazard arrangement of benign smooth muscle bundles
  o Resembles arrector pili muscle
  o Spindled cells arranged in fascicles
  o Elongated, spindled to blunt-ended nuclei
  o Eosinophilic cytoplasm
  o No pleomorphism
  o No significant mitotic activity
  o No areas of necrosis

Predominant Pattern/Injury Type
• Fascicular

Predominant Cell/Compartment Type
• Mesenchymal, muscle, smooth

DIFFERENTIAL DIAGNOSIS

Cutaneous Leiomyoma (Pilar Leiomyoma)
• Presents in young adults
• May be multiple
• Solid rather than haphazard fascicles

Leiomyosarcoma
• Diffuse or nodular atypical spindle cell tumor
• Mitotic activity
• Nuclear atypia

CONGENITAL SMOOTH MUSCLE HAMARTOMA

Key Facts

Terminology

- Rare lesion presenting in infants, characterized by disorganized proliferation of benign smooth muscle bundles in dermis, often involving subcutis

Clinical Issues

- Infants
- Most common in lumbosacral area
- Macule or plaque
- Often hyperpigmented, may have coarse hairs

Microscopic Pathology

- Benign smooth muscle bundles
  - Haphazard arrangement
  - Thin fascicles rather than solid growth pattern
  - No atypia
  - No mitoses
  - No necrosis
  - Immunohistochemistry (+) for muscle markers

Immunohistochemistry

Antibody	Reactivity	Staining Pattern	Comment
Actin-sm	Positive	Cytoplasmic	Diffuse
Desmin	Positive	Cytoplasmic	Diffuse
HCAD	Positive	Cytoplasmic	Diffuse
S100P	Negative		
AE1/AE3	Negative		
EMA/MUC1	Negative		
Myogenin	Negative		

Schwannoma

- Circumscribed, deep dermal or subcutaneous lesion
- Often encapsulated
- S100 positive
- EMA/MUC1 positive rim of perineurial cells

Neurofibroma

- Wavy spindle cells
- Meissner bodies in diffuse neurofibroma
- S100 positive

Fetal Rhabdomyoma

- Skeletal muscle differentiation
  - Striations
  - Myogenin, MYOD1 positive

Normal Skin from Special Sites

- Skin from nipple, vulva, or scrotum has high concentration of normal smooth muscle bundles

DIAGNOSTIC CHECKLIST

Pathologic Interpretation Pearls

- Confined to dermis
- No atypical features

SELECTED REFERENCES

1. Gualandri L et al: Multiple familial smooth muscle hamartomas. Pediatr Dermatol. 18(1):17-20, 2001
2. Gagné EJ et al: Congenital smooth muscle hamartoma of the skin. Pediatr Dermatol. 10(2):142-5, 1993
3. Zvulunov A et al: Congenital smooth muscle hamartoma. Prevalence, clinical findings, and follow-up in 15 patients. Am J Dis Child. 144(7):782-4, 1990
4. Johnson MD et al: Congenital smooth muscle hamartoma. A report of six cases and a review of the literature. Arch Dermatol. 125(6):820-2, 1989

IMAGE GALLERY

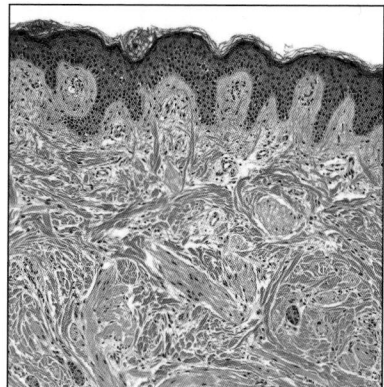 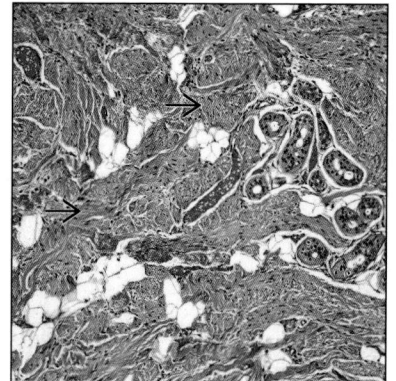 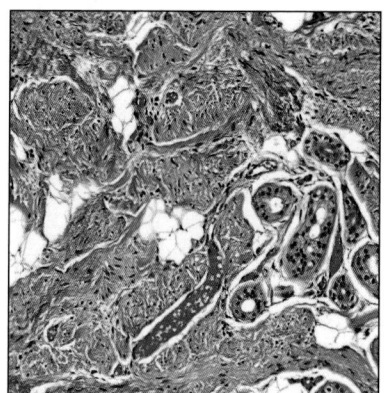

(Left) Low-power view of congenital smooth muscle hamartoma shows a disorganized proliferation of smooth muscle bundles present in the dermis. (Center) This view shows a haphazard pattern of smooth muscle bundles ➡ extending into the deep reticular dermis/subcutis. (Right) Higher magnification shows the numerous bundles of smooth muscle. The smooth muscle resembles arrector pili muscles, but is present in a greater density than normal arrector pili muscles.

LEIOMYOMA (PILAR)

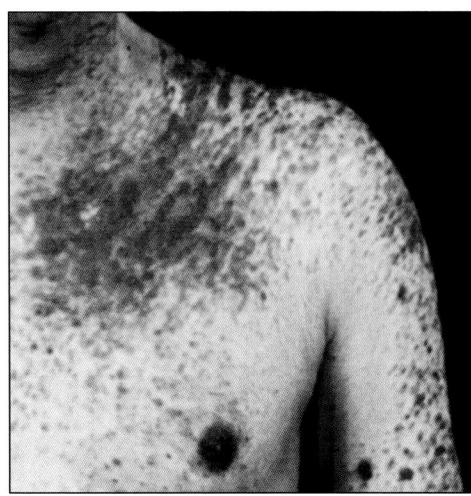

Multiple cutaneous leiomyomas are seen involving the chest, lower neck, shoulder, and upper arm. Typical of superficial leiomyomas, these lesions tend to involve more than 1 body site and extensor surfaces.

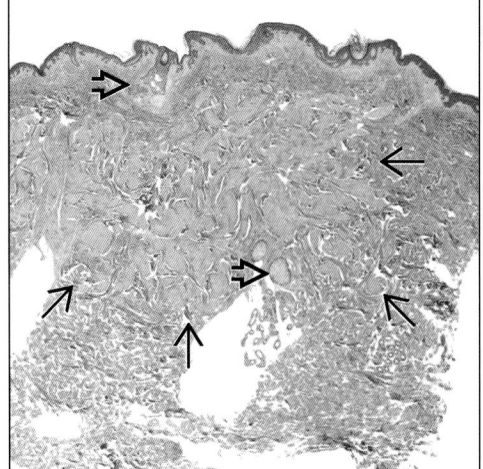

Low-power image shows superficial (pilar) leiomyoma involving most of the dermis. The lesion is unencapsulated and has an irregular border ⇨ with displacement of dermal appendages ⇲.

TERMINOLOGY

Synonyms
- Cutaneous leiomyoma, pilar leiomyoma, piloleiomyoma, leiomyoma cutis

Definitions
- Uncommon benign cutaneous smooth muscle neoplasm originating from arrector pili muscles

ETIOLOGY/PATHOGENESIS

Genetics
- Some cases are familial
  - Autosomal dominant inheritance pattern with incomplete penetrance
- Most patients are shown to have germline fumarate hydratase gene mutations
  - Gene on 1q43 and enzyme involved with tricarboxylic acid (Krebs) cycle
- May be associated with uterine leiomyomas (98%) and renal cell carcinoma (10-15%)
  - Syndrome known as hereditary leiomyomatosis and renal cell cancer, multiple cutaneous and uterine leiomyomatosis syndrome, or Reed syndrome
    - Renal cell carcinomas are usually papillary, tubulopapillary, or collecting duct type

CLINICAL ISSUES

Epidemiology
- Age
  - Most develop in adolescence or early adulthood
  - Some are congenital or develop in childhood

Site
- Predilection for extensor surfaces of extremities, trunk, and head & neck
  - 2 or more body sites are often affected

Presentation
- Most often multiple painful pink or brown papules
  - Papules may coalesce into nodules
  - Lesions tend to follow dermatomal distribution
- Pain can be induced by cold exposure, pressure, or states of emotion
- Rare cases are solitary and painless

Treatment
- Options, risks, complications
  - Depends on number of lesions and symptomatology
  - Medical management with follow-up is option for those with extensive lesions
  - Imaging to rule out renal mass or large atypical uterine lesions is warranted
  - Cryotherapy and laser ablation have been used with mixed results
- Surgical approaches
  - For localized and symptomatic lesions

Prognosis
- Does not undergo malignant change
- Surgically treated lesions often develop recurrence (more likely representing new lesions)

MACROSCOPIC FEATURES

Size
- Most < 2 cm

MICROSCOPIC PATHOLOGY

Histologic Features
- Bundles and fascicles of differentiated smooth muscle cells
  - Cells have abundant fibrillary pink cytoplasm and oval, blunt-ended (cigar-shaped) nuclei
- Unencapsulated, haphazardly arranged, with irregular borders, and confined to dermis

LEIOMYOMA (PILAR)

Key Facts

Terminology
- Benign cutaneous smooth muscle neoplasm arising from arrector pili muscles

Etiology/Pathogenesis
- Many are shown to have germline fumarate hydratase gene mutations
- May be associated with uterine leiomyomas and renal cell carcinoma

Clinical Issues
- Most develop in adolescence or early adulthood
- Predilection for extensor surfaces of extremities as well as trunk
- Most often present with multiple painful pink or brown papules

Microscopic Pathology
- Bundles and fascicles of differentiated smooth muscle cells
- Proliferation is unencapsulated, haphazardly arranged, with irregular borders, and confined to dermis
- Degenerative atypia and occasional mitotic figures (up to 1 per 10 HPF) are acceptable

Top Differential Diagnoses
- Genital leiomyoma
- Angioleiomyoma (vascular leiomyoma)
- Smooth muscle hamartoma
- Dermatomyofibroma
- Myofibroma
- Superficial leiomyosarcoma

  - ○ Often intimately associated with hair follicles
  - ○ Fascicles often dissect between dermal collagen
- Rare cases are circumscribed
- Overlying epidermal hyperplasia is frequently present
- Degenerative atypia and occasional mitotic figures (up to 1 per 10 HPF) are acceptable
  - ○ Higher mitotic activity, diffuse (nondegenerative) atypia, necrosis, and subcutaneous extension suggest leiomyosarcoma

ANCILLARY TESTS

Immunohistochemistry
- Tumor cells are strongly positive for desmin, actin, calponin, and H-caldesmon

DIFFERENTIAL DIAGNOSIS

Genital Leiomyoma
- Usually solitary, painless, & arises from specialized dermal smooth muscle (e.g., dartos in scrotum)
- Common sites include scrotum, penis, nipple, areola, and vulva
- Tend to be more circumscribed, cellular, and histologically heterogeneous than pilar leiomyomas
  - ○ Histologic appearances can include myxoid change and epithelioid cells
  - ○ Can be symplastic
    - ▪ Scattered nuclear atypia but no mitoses

Angioleiomyoma
- Solitary subcutaneous nodule that may be painful
- Most anatomic areas, but most frequent in lower extremities
- Circumscribed, less fascicular
- Intimately associated with evenly distributed, thick-walled to cavernous vascular spaces

Smooth Muscle Hamartoma
- Located in lumbar region
- Usually solitary, larger

- May be associated with increased hair &/or pigment (Becker nevus)
- Smooth muscle bundles tend to be better defined than in leiomyoma, but there is histologic overlap

Myofibroma
- Circumscribed and often nodular with biphasic histology
  - ○ Fascicles and whorls of myofibroblasts
  - ○ Primitive round cell areas
    - ▪ Associated with hemangiopericytomatous pattern
- Necrosis and mitoses can be seen
- Spindle cells are typically negative for desmin

Dermatomyofibroma
- Solitary plaque lesion usually on shoulder or trunk
- Fascicular spindle cell proliferation parallel to epidermis without effacement of adnexa
- Cells appear myofibroblastic
- Typically express SMA, but not desmin or H-caldesmon

Superficial Leiomyosarcoma
- Larger lesions that are usually solitary
- Often extend into subcutis
- More atypia and mitotic activity than in leiomyoma
- Necrosis

SELECTED REFERENCES

1. Badeloe S et al: Clinical and molecular genetic aspects of hereditary multiple cutaneous leiomyomatosis. Eur J Dermatol. 19(6):545-51, 2009
2. Holst VA et al: Cutaneous smooth muscle neoplasms: clinical features, histologic findings, and treatment options. J Am Acad Dermatol. 46(4):477-90; quiz, 491-4, 2002
3. Yokoyama R et al: Superficial leiomyomas. A clinicopathologic study of 34 cases. Acta Pathol Jpn. 37(9):1415-22, 1987
4. Tavassoli FA et al: Smooth muscle tumors of the vulva. Obstet Gynecol. 53(2):213-7, 1979
5. Fox SR Jr: Leiomyomatosis cutis. N Engl J Med. 263:1248-50, 1960

LEIOMYOMA (PILAR)

Clinical and Microscopic Features

(Left) Superficial leiomyomas are usually < 2 cm and appear as multiple pink or brown papules or nodules. Clinically, they tend to elicit pain and are often distributed in a dermatomal fashion. *(Right)* Many superficial leiomyomas have a grenz zone ⇥ and show overlying epidermal hyperplasia with basilar pigmentation (similar to changes seen overlying dermatofibromas), such as this case with elongated, fusing rete ridges →.

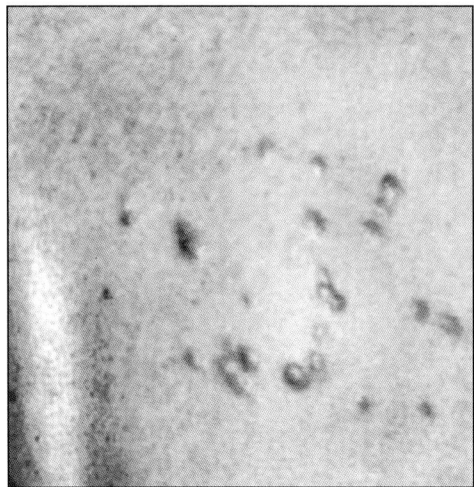 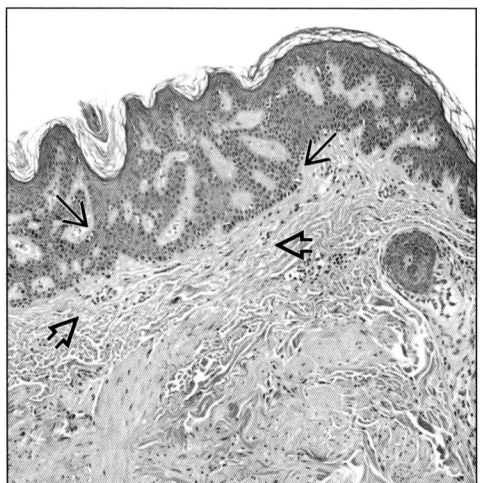

(Left) At higher power, superficial leiomyomas consist of short fascicles or bundles of smooth muscle → that are haphazardly arranged within the dermis and dissect between dermal collagen bundles →. *(Right)* The smooth muscle bundles consist of elongated spindled cells with abundant fibrillary eosinophilic cytoplasm. Nuclei are oval with blunt ends ("cigar-shaped") and show little cytologic atypia or mitotic activity. Note the characteristic dissection between dermal collagen bundles →.

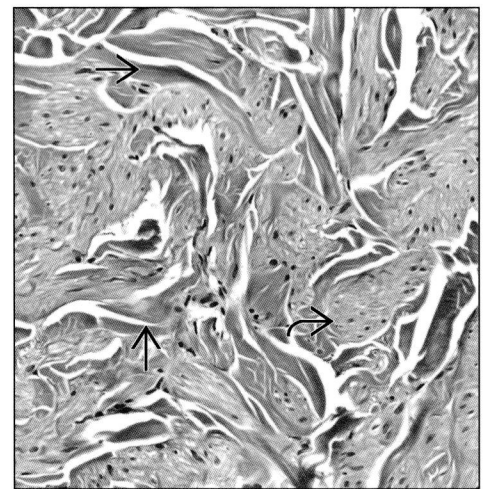 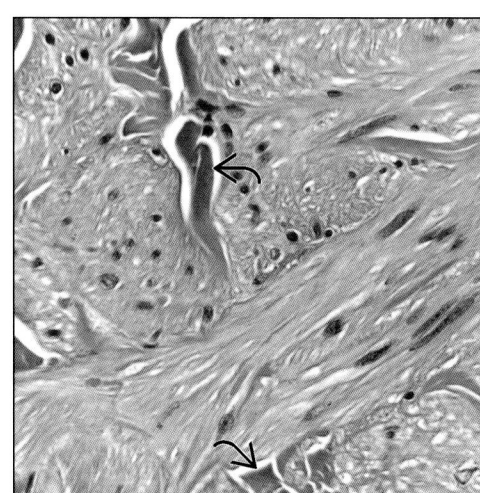

(Left) Surgical specimens often reveal incipient pilar leiomyoma → adjacent to the primary tumor. The main tumor in this example does show areas of circumscription ⇥, but other areas have the more typical infiltrative pattern →. *(Right)* Rare examples of superficial leiomyoma are well-circumscribed, such as this solitary lesion, which shows only focal areas with an irregular border →. Solitary lesions such as this more often present without pain symptoms.

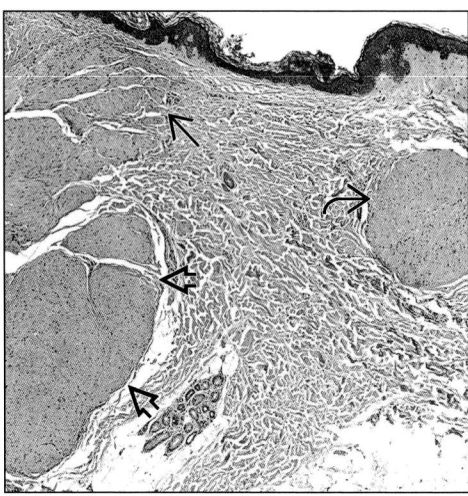 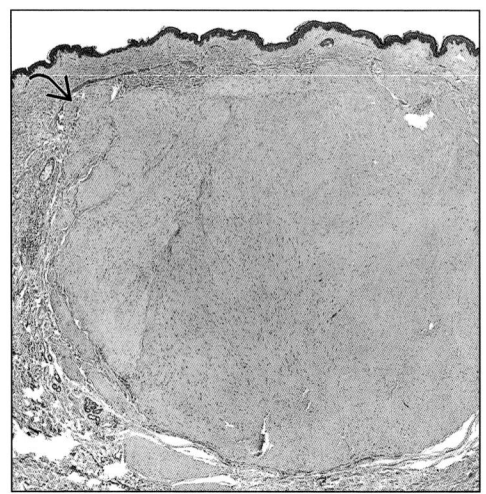

Microscopic Features and Differential Diagnosis

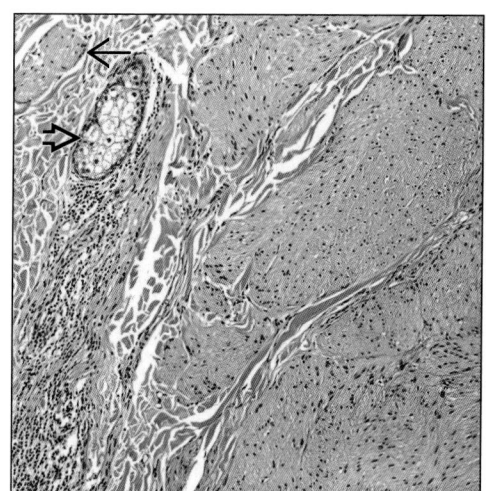

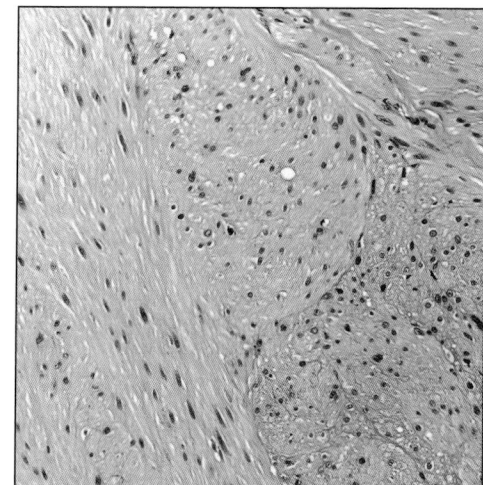

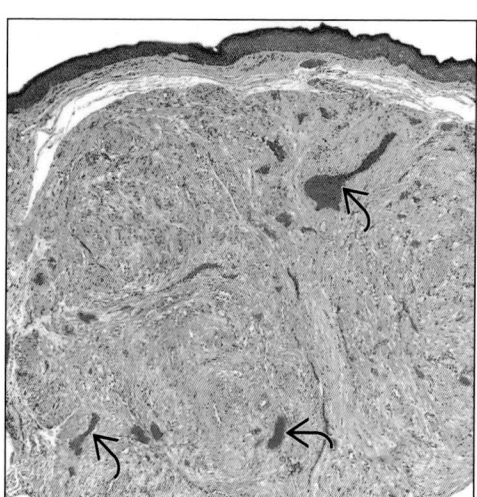

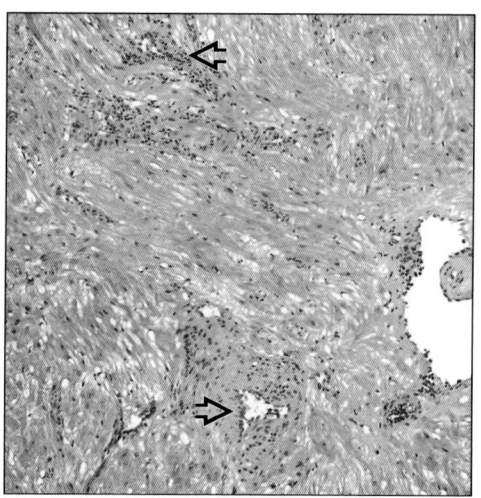

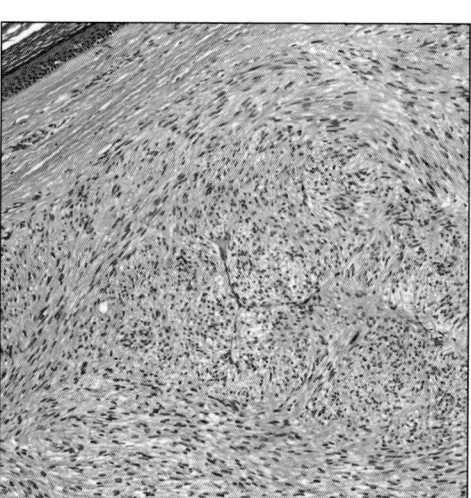

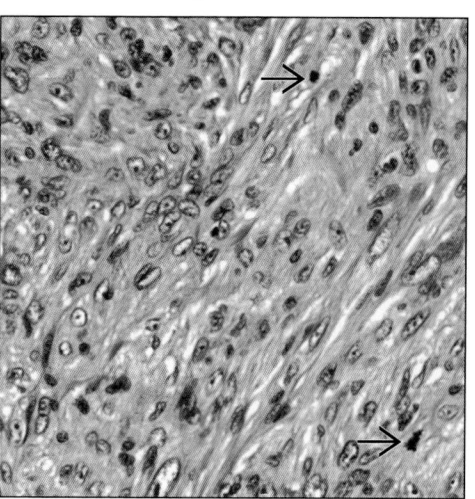

(Left) Similar to typical superficial leiomyomas, solitary and circumscribed cutaneous leiomyomas can arise from the pilar smooth muscle. This solitary and circumscribed tumor was located adjacent to a sebaceous gland ⊵ and pilar smooth muscle bundle ➡, indicating likely origin from this pilosebaceous unit. *(Right)* Solitary superficial leiomyomas are less often characterized by small smooth muscle fascicles intersecting between dermal collagen and are more often solid tumors.

(Left) In contrast to superficial leiomyomas, angioleiomyomas are usually circumscribed and contain numerous variably sized slit-like vascular channels that stand out at low power ➡. In addition, they are usually solitary and located in the lower extremity. *(Right)* Sheets of smooth muscle cells with abundant fibrillary eosinophilic cytoplasm intimately associated with thick-walled ⊵, often slit-like vascular channels characterize angioleiomyomas.

(Left) Superficial leiomyosarcomas also consist of rectilinear fascicles of cells with abundant fibrillary eosinophilic cytoplasm with blunt-ended oval nuclei. However, these are more cellular and show less dissection of dermal collagen. They are usually solitary and larger than superficial leiomyomas. *(Right)* At higher power, superficial leiomyosarcomas will show moderate to marked nuclear atypia with higher nuclear to cytoplasmic ratio and frequent mitotic figures ➡.

ANGIOLEIOMYOMA

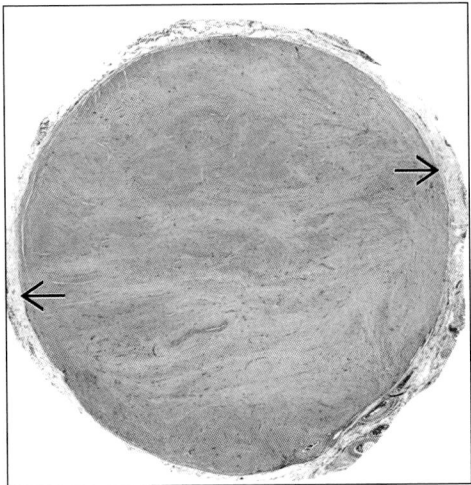

Angioleiomyoma is circumscribed and can be "shelled out." A thin rim of subcutaneous adipose tissue → is seen enclosing the excision specimen. This pattern is sometimes termed the solid variant.

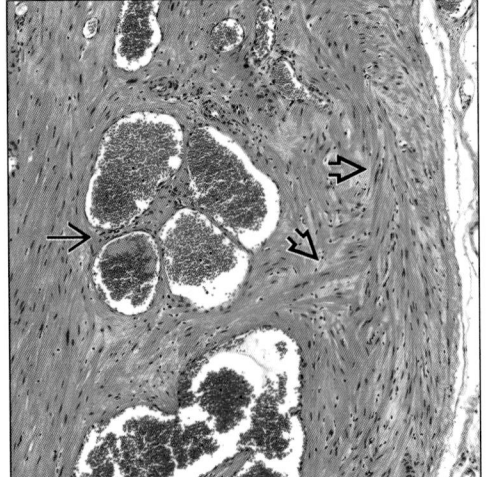

The cavernous type of angioleiomyoma has thin-walled dilated vascular channels arranged in small clusters → within a stroma composed of smooth muscle fibers that form branching fascicles ⇒.

TERMINOLOGY

Synonyms
- Angiomyoma
- Vascular leiomyoma

Definitions
- Benign neoplasm composed of blood vessels and smooth muscle cells in varying proportions

CLINICAL ISSUES

Epidemiology
- Incidence
  - About 25% of superficial leiomyomas
- Age
  - Most common between 40-60 years
- Gender
  - Females > males

Site
- Mostly in subcutis
  - Lower limb, upper limb
  - Trunk and head and neck less common
- Rare similar examples reported in uterus

Presentation
- Painful or painless mass
  - Usually in subcutis
    - Rarely intradermal
  - Pain exacerbated by cold
  - Tenderness worse on pressure

Treatment
- Surgical approaches
  - Local excision is usually curative

Prognosis
- Very occasional recurrence
- Reported examples have not metastasized

MACROSCOPIC FEATURES

General Features
- Well-defined nodule

Size
- Rarely exceeds 2 cm in diameter

MICROSCOPIC PATHOLOGY

Histologic Features
- Circumscribed
- Smooth muscle bundles
  - Arranged around thick-walled vessels
  - Rarely nuclear atypia; no mitoses or necrosis
- Vessels variable
  - Solid variant has vessels with small narrow lumina
  - Venous variant has channels with muscular walls
    - Muscle fibers radiate from vessel wall
  - Cavernous variant is uncommon and has dilated vessels
- Stroma variable
  - Myxoid change
  - Fibrosis or hyalinization
  - Focal calcification
  - Rarely fatty component
  - Nerve fibers can be demonstrated in some cases

DIFFERENTIAL DIAGNOSIS

Leiomyoma
- Cells in sheets or fascicles
  - Lack relationship to blood vessels

Myopericytoma
- Concentric layers of spindle cells without complete smooth muscle differentiation
- Marked hemangiopericytic pattern
- Desmin usually negative

ANGIOLEIOMYOMA

Key Facts

Terminology

- Benign neoplasm composed of blood vessels and smooth muscle cells in varying proportions

Clinical Issues

- Most common between 40-60 years
- Mostly in subcutis; can be painful

Macroscopic Features

- Well-defined nodule

Microscopic Pathology

- Smooth muscle bundles
  - Arranged around thick-walled vessels
  - Fascicles radiate from vessel wall
- Rarely nuclear atypia, no mitoses or necrosis
- Usually have narrow lumina

Top Differential Diagnoses

- Myopericytoma
- Leiomyoma

Immunohistochemistry

Antibody	Reactivity	Staining Pattern	Comment
Actin-sm	Positive	Cytoplasmic	
HCAD	Positive	Cytoplasmic	
Desmin	Positive	Cytoplasmic	In most cases; sometimes absent when myopericytoma-like
CD34	Negative		
S100	Negative		
HMB-45	Negative		
melan-A103	Negative		

- Features can overlap with those of angioleiomyoma

Glomus Tumor

- Solid or angiomatous patterns
- Single or multiple layers of glomus cells outside vessels
- Desmin usually negative

Hemangioma

- Not well-circumscribed
- Lacks smooth muscle component
- Can have capillary, venous, or cavernous vessels

Angiomyolipoma

- Has fatty component
- Can have epithelioid cell morphology
- Myomelanocytic immunophenotype

Leiomyosarcoma

- Often arises in vessel wall
- Cells show atypia, mitotic activity

- Cells not related to blood vessels
- Presence of necrosis

SELECTED REFERENCES

1. Matsuyama A et al: Angioleiomyoma: a clinicopathologic and immunohistochemical reappraisal with special reference to the correlation with myopericytoma. Hum Pathol. 38(4):645-51, 2007
2. McCluggage WG et al: Uterine angioleiomyomas: a report of 3 cases of a distinctive benign leiomyoma variant. Int J Surg Pathol. 15(3):262-5, 2007
3. Hasegawa T et al: Mechanism of pain and cytoskeletal properties in angioleiomyomas: an immunohistochemical study. Pathol Int. 44(1):66-72, 1994
4. Carlà TG et al: Bizarre angiomyomas of superficial soft tissues. Pathologica. 83(1084):237-42, 1991
5. Hachisuga T et al: Angioleiomyoma. A clinicopathologic reappraisal of 562 cases. Cancer. 54(1):126-30, 1984

IMAGE GALLERY

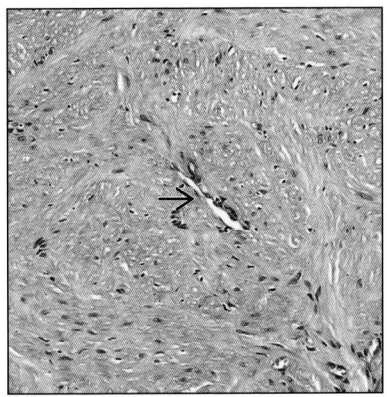 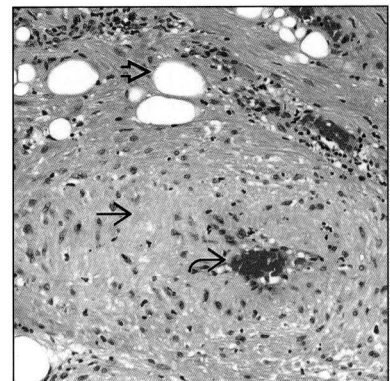 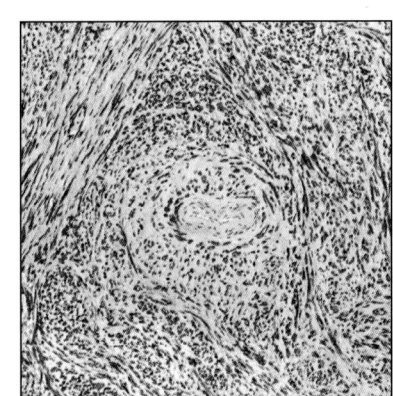

(Left) The vascular lumen is reduced to a narrow slit ➡ by hyalinized stroma between muscle cells. *(Center)* Layers of ill-defined smooth muscle cells ➡ are arranged around the central vascular lumen ➡. This example also contains a small adipose tissue component ➡. *(Right)* Immunohistochemistry shows diffuse positivity for desmin. Other positive markers include SMA and H-caldesmon. Both are also expressed in myopericytoma, but desmin is usually negative.

LEIOMYOSARCOMA

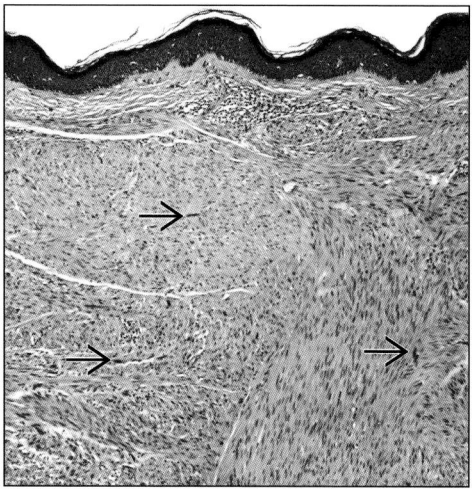
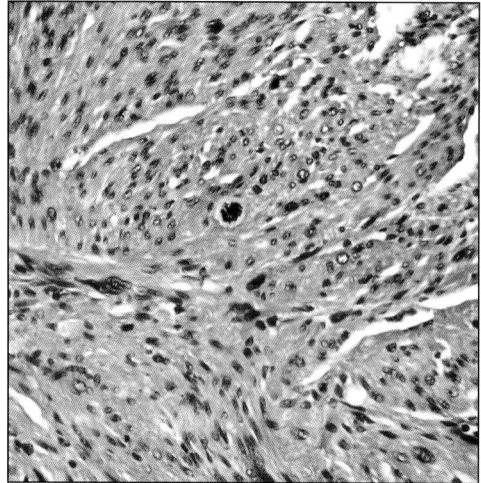

This leiomyosarcoma extended into the subcutis. It is composed of perpendicularly oriented fascicles of brightly eosinophilic cells. At scanning magnification, atypical nuclei stand out ➡.

There is no need to search for numerous mitoses to diagnose leiomyosarcoma, although mitotic counts assist in assigning a sarcoma grade. Note the bright pink color of the cytoplasm.

TERMINOLOGY

Abbreviations
- Leiomyosarcoma (LMS)

Definitions
- Malignant neoplasm composed of cells exhibiting smooth muscle differentiation

ETIOLOGY/PATHOGENESIS

Infectious Agents
- Epstein-Barr virus (EBV) associated in immunosuppressed patients
- Occasional examples are radiation associated

CLINICAL ISSUES

Epidemiology
- Incidence
  - Uncommon: 10-15% of extremity sarcomas
  - Most common overall sarcoma type if uterine and visceral examples are included
- Age
  - Middle-aged adults
- Gender
  - No gender preference overall

Presentation
- Cutaneous LMS presents as a single nodule or plaque-like tumor
  - May be ulcerated or show serum crusting/hemorrhage
- Deep soft tissue tumors present as a mass, often asymptomatic, in extremities
  - Retroperitoneum most common site
  - Vena cava examples often symptomatic
- Uterine examples considered separately with unique diagnostic criteria

Treatment
- Surgical excision
  - Radiation
  - Chemotherapy for metastatic tumors

Prognosis
- Outcome site and stage dependent as with other sarcoma types
  - Lesions restricted to cutis essentially never metastasize
    - Some observers have advocated diagnosing them as "atypical smooth muscle tumors"
  - Subcutaneous lesions
    - Up to 1/3 of tumors metastasize
    - 10-20% of patients with subcutaneous lesion die of disease
  - Retroperitoneum: About 80% of patients die of disease, typically with metastases
  - Bone: Metastases in up to 1/2 of patients
  - Vena cava: 5- and 10-year survival 50% and 30%, respectively
  - Head and neck: Over 1/2 metastasize

MICROSCOPIC PATHOLOGY

Histologic Features
- Perpendicularly oriented fascicles of spindle cells
- Cells show brightly eosinophilic cytoplasm
- Blunt-ended nuclei with nuclear atypia
- Some examples are epithelioid-appearing
- Any number of mitoses sufficient in subcutis, scrotal lesions, or deep soft tissue if nuclear atypia is present
- In vulva, some observers offered > 5 mitosis per 10 HPF as "cutoff," but recurrences reported in lesions with any mitotic activity

Predominant Pattern/Injury Type
- Fascicular

LEIOMYOSARCOMA

Key Facts

Terminology
- Malignant neoplasm composed of cells exhibiting smooth muscle differentiation

Etiology/Pathogenesis
- Epstein-Barr virus associated in immunosuppressed patients

Clinical Issues
- Superficial or deep soft tissue mass, often asymptomatic, in extremities
- Retroperitoneum most common site
- Retroperitoneal and inferior vena cava lesions more common in women
- Uncommon: 10-15% of extremity sarcomas
- Most common sarcoma type if uterine examples are included

- Treatment is complete surgical excision
- Prognosis is site and stage dependent, as with other sarcoma types

Microscopic Pathology
- Perpendicularly oriented fascicles of spindle cells
- Brightly eosinophilic cytoplasm
- Blunt-ended nuclei
- Nuclear atypia

Ancillary Tests
- Labels as per smooth muscle: Desmin, actin, calponin, caldesmon
  - Some cases label with keratins

Top Differential Diagnoses
- Sarcomatoid squamous cell carcinoma
- Atypical fibroxanthoma (AFX)

Predominant Cell/Compartment Type
- Mesenchymal, smooth muscle

Variant and Special Forms
- **Epithelioid leiomyosarcoma**
  - Literature confounded because many epithelioid gastrointestinal stromal tumors (GIST) were termed epithelioid LMS in past
  - Found anywhere in body
  - Distinct epithelioid morphology, but more nuclear atypia than GISTs
  - Older studies reported smooth muscle actin (SMA) and muscle specific actin (MSA) positive, desmin negative immunophenotype, but desmin labels most lesions using modern methods
    - Possible reflection of misdiagnosed GISTs
    - Less sensitive desmin antibodies in past
- **Myxoid leiomyosarcoma**
  - Grossly gelatinous
  - Extensive myxoid change, but zones of typical leiomyosarcoma allow diagnosis
    - Express desmin and actin
    - Subset labels with keratin antibodies
  - Tend to be low grade
  - Clinicopathologic features otherwise same as typical leiomyosarcoma
- **Inflammatory leiomyosarcoma**
  - Characterized by dense inflammation that masks underlying lesion
    - Histiocytes, xanthoma cells, lymphocytes, neutrophils
  - Areas of more typical morphology must be sought
  - Clinicopathologic features otherwise as per typical leiomyosarcoma
- **Pleomorphic leiomyosarcoma**
  - Defined as pleomorphic areas in > 2/3 of tumor
    - Ordinary leiomyosarcomatous fascicular area covers < 1/3
  - More aggressive since higher grade
    - In one series, 65% of patients died of disease
  - Subset features osteoclast-like giant cells
- **Epstein-Barr virus-associated**

- a.k.a. EBV-associated smooth muscle tumors (EBV-SMT)
  - Classified as "leiomyoma" and "leiomyosarcoma," but term EBV-SMT may be more appropriate
  - Appearances are somewhat unique
  - Found in immunosuppressed patients
  - Frequently multifocal
  - No clear-cut metastases reported
- Histologic features
  - Monomorphic, spindled, smooth muscle cells arranged in short intersecting fascicles
  - Subpopulation of more primitive round cells are either admixed with spindled cells or form discrete nodules
  - Variable lymphocytic infiltrate composed primarily of T cells
  - Mitotic activity variable (0-18 per 10 HPF)
  - Necrosis and myxoid change in some cases
  - All are EBV-encoded RNA (EBER) positive
  - All express SMA; desmin in ~ 1/2
- Reducing immunosuppression in transplant patients should be key treatment
  - Rapid tumor reduction following reduced immunosuppression reported, but some lesions persist
  - About 5% die of disease
- Treatment is primarily surgical
- Sirolimus (inhibitor of mTOR-associated protein pathway) effective in some lesions
- **Leiomyosarcoma with osteoclast-like giant cells**
  - Same demographics as conventional LMS
  - Areas with same histology as typical LMS
    - Reactive with smooth muscle markers: Actins and desmin
  - Areas with osteoclast-like giant cells
    - Some giant cells appear bland (like histiocytes), but others cytologically malignant
    - Benign-appearing osteoclast-like giant cells label with CD68, but not muscle markers
    - Cytologically malignant giant cells label with smooth muscle markers
  - No osteoid/matrix formation seen

LEIOMYOSARCOMA

Immunohistochemistry

Antibody	Reactivity	Staining Pattern	Comment
Desmin	Positive	Cytoplasmic	
Actin-sm	Positive	Cytoplasmic	
Calponin	Positive	Cytoplasmic	
Caldesmon	Positive	Cytoplasmic	
CK-PAN	Positive	Cytoplasmic	Reactive in ~ 1/3 of cases; usually focal
ERP	Negative	Not applicable	Occasional gynecologic examples focally reactive
CD34	Negative	Cytoplasmic	Usually negative
S100	Negative	Not applicable	Rare cases focally reactive
HMB-45	Negative	Not applicable	Rare cases focally reactive

ANCILLARY TESTS

Immunohistochemistry
- Label as smooth muscle tumors: (+) for desmin, actin, calponin, caldesmon
  - Some cases label with keratins

Cytogenetics
- Complex variable karyotypes
- No characteristic translocation, mutation, or fusion product known

DIFFERENTIAL DIAGNOSIS

Considered Based on Anatomic Site
- **Skin and subcutaneous fat/fascia**
  - Sarcomatoid squamous cell carcinoma
    - Can have epithelial in situ component
    - Expresses HMWCKs (CK5/6, CK903) and p63, in contrast to LMS
  - Atypical fibroxanthoma (AFX)
    - Occurs in heavily sun-damaged skin of elderly
    - Composed of population of atypical to bizarre and pleomorphic-appearing spindled and epithelioid cells
    - Typically negative for muscle markers including desmin and MSA (although SMA can be positive in some cases); positive for nonspecific markers (CD10, CD68, CD99)
  - Leiomyoma
    - Bland cytology
    - Mitoses infrequent
  - Dermatofibroma/fibrous histiocytoma
    - Uniform, bland-appearing histiocytoid and fibroblastic cells
    - Collagen trapping pattern at periphery
    - Often has secondary inflammatory constituents (lymphoplasmacytic cells, foamy histiocytes, hemosiderin)
    - Typically lacks desmin; is factor XIIIa positive
  - Nodular fasciitis
    - Bland nuclei
    - Loose storiform rather than fascicular pattern
    - Backdrop of lymphocytes and extravasated erythrocytes, often osteoclast-like giant cells

- Immunoreactive for actin or calponin, but not desmin or caldesmon

DIAGNOSTIC CHECKLIST

Pathologic Interpretation Pearls
- Attention to depth of involvement important in evaluating smooth muscle tumors of skin
  - Lesions restricted to cutis essentially never metastasize; subcutaneous tumors have significant metastatic potential

SELECTED REFERENCES

1. Oda Y et al: Pleomorphic leiomyosarcoma: clinicopathologic and immunohistochemical study with special emphasis on its distinction from ordinary leiomyosarcoma and malignant fibrous histiocytoma. Am J Surg Pathol. 25(8):1030-8, 2001
2. Rubin BP et al: Myxoid leiomyosarcoma of soft tissue, an underrecognized variant. Am J Surg Pathol. 24(7):927-36, 2000
3. de Saint Aubain Somerhausen N et al: Leiomyosarcoma of soft tissue in children: clinicopathologic analysis of 20 cases. Am J Surg Pathol. 23(7):755-63, 1999
4. Kaddu S et al: Cutaneous leiomyosarcoma. Am J Surg Pathol. 21(9):979-87, 1997
5. Merchant W et al: Inflammatory leiomyosarcoma: a morphological subgroup within the heterogeneous family of so-called inflammatory malignant fibrous histiocytoma. Histopathology. 27(6):525-32, 1995
6. Mentzel T et al: Leiomyosarcoma with prominent osteoclast-like giant cells. Analysis of eight cases closely mimicking the so-called giant cell variant of malignant fibrous histiocytoma. Am J Surg Pathol. 18(3):258-65, 1994
7. Suster S: Epithelioid leiomyosarcoma of the skin and subcutaneous tissue. Clinicopathologic, immunohistochemical, and ultrastructural study of five cases. Am J Surg Pathol. 18(3):232-40, 1994
8. Miettinen M: Keratin subsets in spindle cell sarcomas. Keratins are widespread but synovial sarcoma contains a distinctive keratin polypeptide pattern and desmoplakins. Am J Pathol. 138(2):505-13, 1991
9. Fields JP et al: Leiomyosarcoma of the skin and subcutaneous tissue. Cancer. 47(1):156-69, 1981

LEIOMYOSARCOMA

Microscopic and Immunohistochemical Features

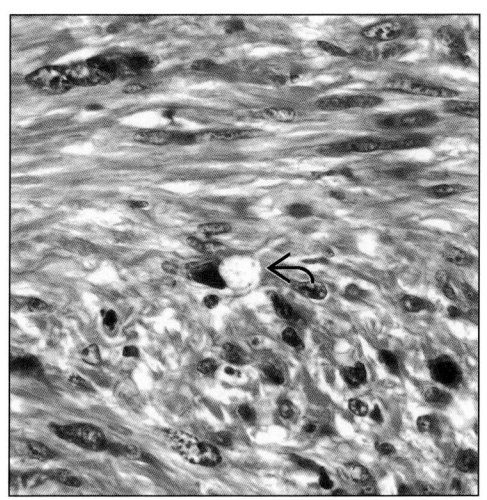
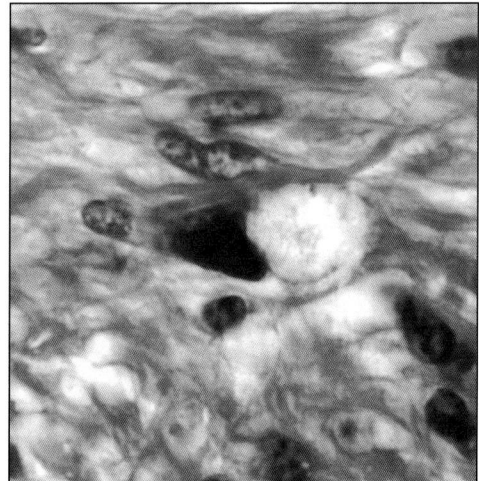

(Left) High magnification shows a classic appearance of a leiomyosarcoma. The proliferating cells contain blunt-ended nuclei and fibrillary eosinophilic cytoplasm. A paranuclear large vacuole is in the center of the field ➡. (Right) High magnification of a paranuclear vacuole is depicted in a leiomyosarcoma. The cells above the vacuolated one have blunt-ended nuclei.

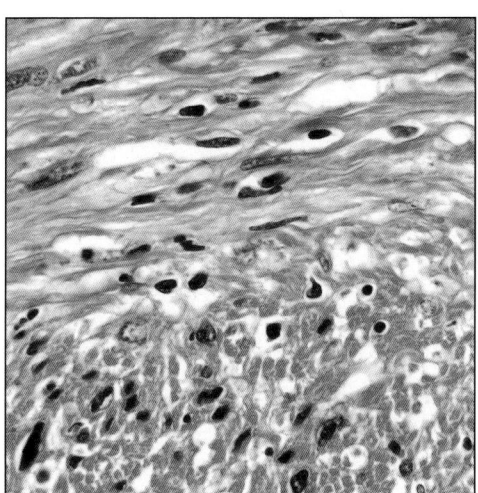
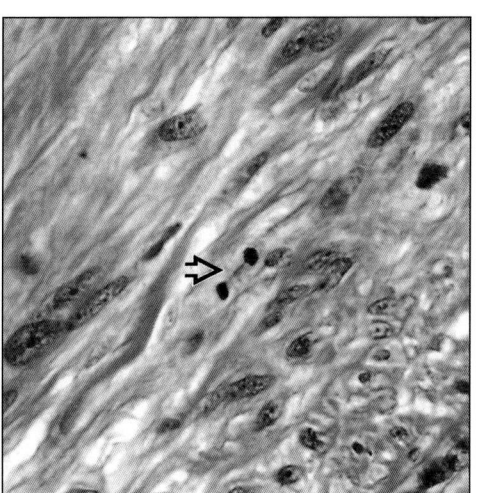

(Left) High magnification shows perpendicularly oriented fascicles. The cells in the upper part of the field are in a fascicular arrangement, whereas the ones at the bottom of the field are mostly aligned en face. (Right) This image shows an anaphase bridge ➡ in the center of the field, an indication that this neoplasm has chromosome instability rather than a characteristic translocation or gene rearrangement.

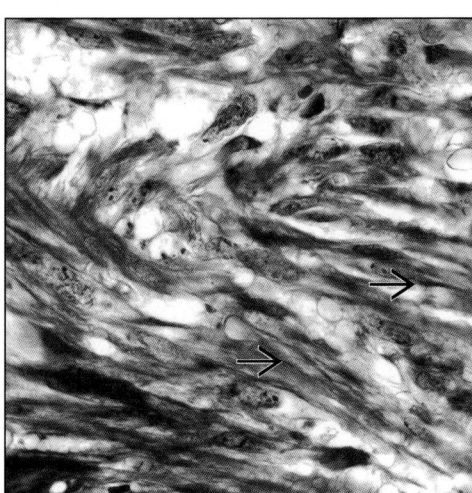
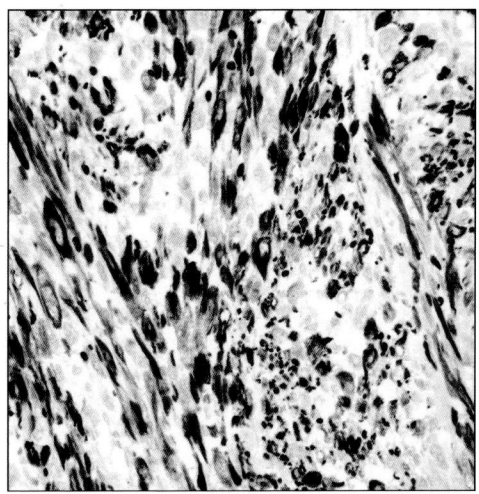

(Left) Masson trichrome stain highlights delicate red cytoplasmic filaments ➡ in this well-differentiated leiomyosarcoma. (Right) Desmin immunostaining shows striking cytoplasmic labeling in this leiomyosarcoma. In contrast to myofibroblastic lesions such as nodular fasciitis (which show smooth muscle actin staining), leiomyosarcomas express desmin and caldesmon, whereas nodular fasciitis usually lacks these markers or shows only focal expression.

LEIOMYOSARCOMA

Variant Microscopic Features

(Left) *The lesional cells in this inflammatory leiomyosarcoma show blunt-ended nuclei and brightly eosinophilic cytoplasm, although obscuring inflammation masks the typical fascicular pattern. This tumor was strongly reactive with desmin and lacked ALK.* *(Right)* *This leiomyosarcoma displays prominent osteoclast-like giant cells* ➡. *In the past, such lesions were sometimes mistaken for undifferentiated pleomorphic sarcomas (or malignant fibrous histiocytomas).*

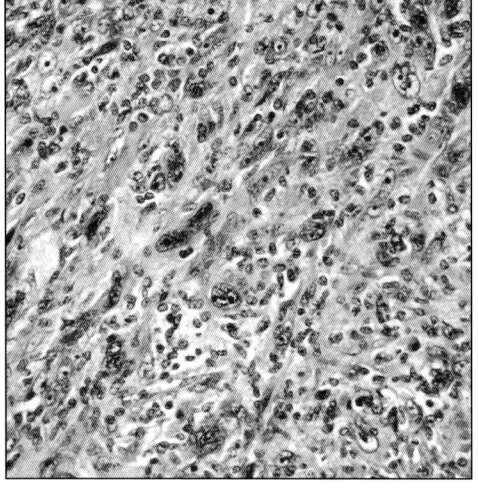
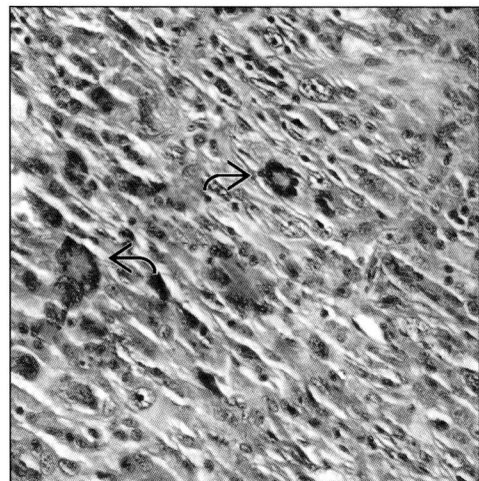

(Left) *Based on the lack of involvement of the subcutaneous adipose tissue, a favorable prognosis would be anticipated for this lesion. In fact, some observers have suggested diagnosing such superficial cutaneous lesions as "atypical smooth muscle tumors." (Right) Note the nuclear palisading in this cutaneous leiomyosarcoma case. Although this pattern could suggest a nerve sheath tumor, the perpendicular arrangement of the fascicles supports the interpretation of leiomyosarcoma.*

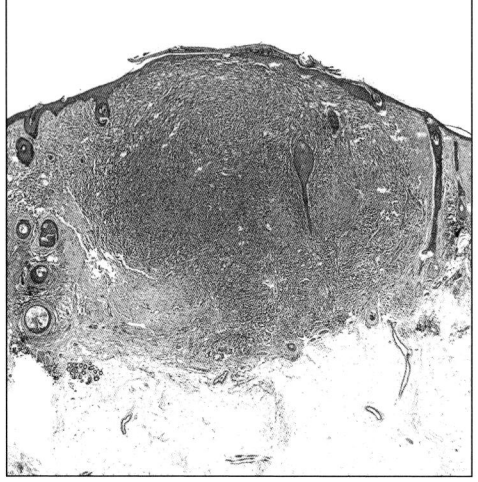
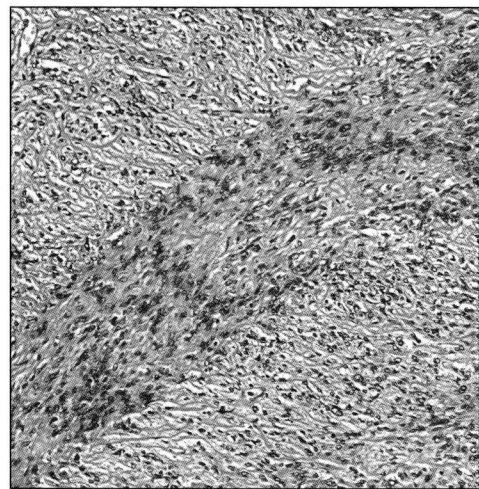

(Left) *Histologic examination of a myxoid leiomyosarcoma is shown. The bottom of the field shows typical leiomyosarcoma features, whereas the top is myxoid with a pleomorphic cell* ➡. *A predominance of pleomorphic zones would qualify a tumor as a "pleomorphic leiomyosarcoma." (Right) This cell, found in the myxoid zone of the myxoid leiomyosarcoma, shows blunt-ended nuclear contours. Note the delicate eosinophilic filaments* ➡ *in the cytoplasm.*

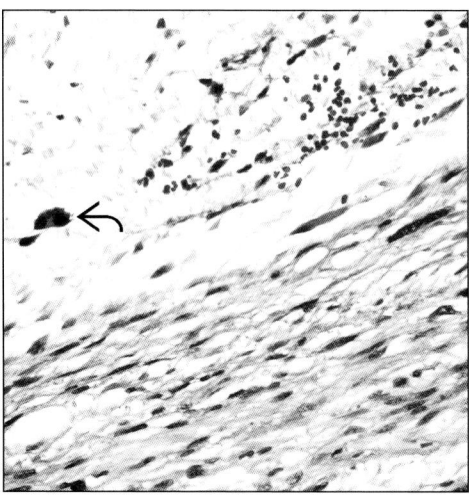
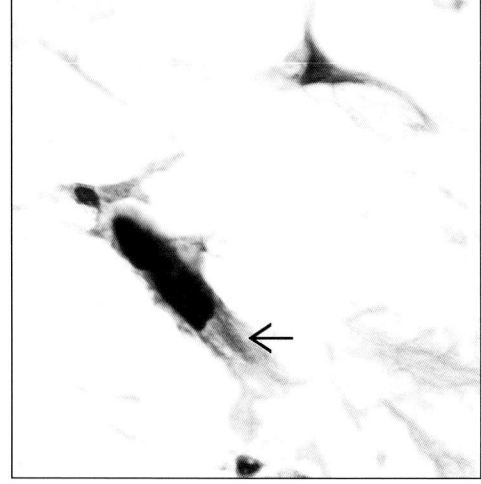

LEIOMYOSARCOMA

Variant Microscopic Features

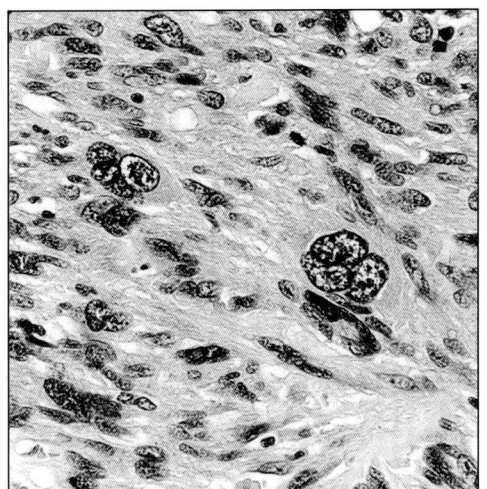

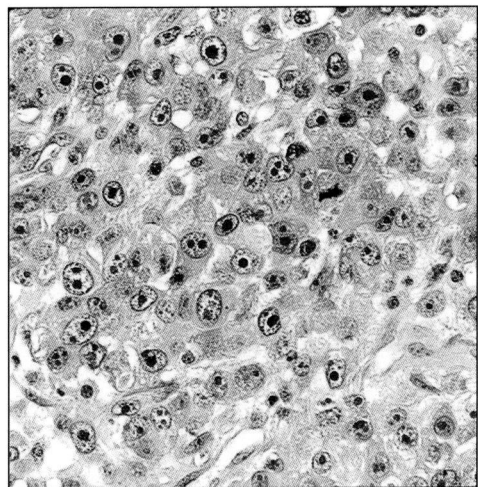

(Left) This leiomyosarcoma displays striking nuclear pleomorphism. When this feature is the overriding one, such tumors have been classified as "pleomorphic leiomyosarcoma," and behave more aggressively. *(Right)* Epithelioid leiomyosarcoma shows abundant eosinophilic cytoplasm and cytologically malignant nuclei. The diagnosis in such cases often requires use of immunohistochemistry to exclude melanoma and poorly differentiated carcinomas.

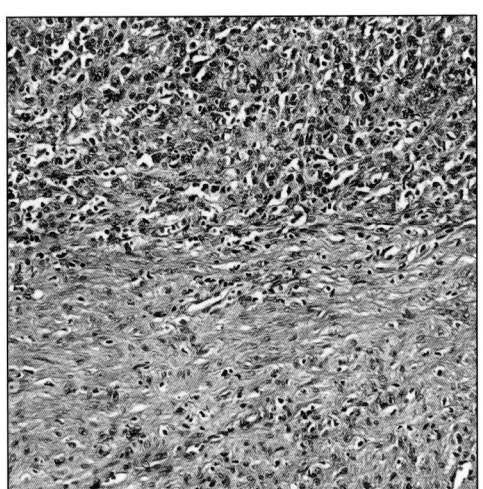

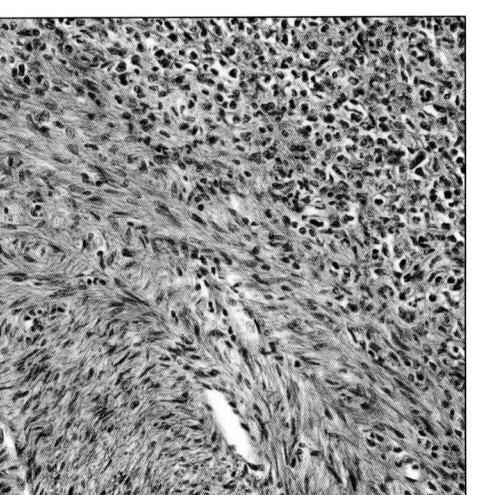

(Left) Epstein-Barr virus-associated smooth muscle tumor manifests a dual population of fascicular eosinophilic cells and smaller darker cells at the top of the field. (Courtesy A. Deyrup, MD.) *(Right)* Higher magnification of an Epstein-Barr virus-associated smooth muscle tumor is shown. These tumors have EBV-encoded RNA (EBER) and express SMA, but only 54% are desmin positive. (Courtesy A. Deyrup, MD.)

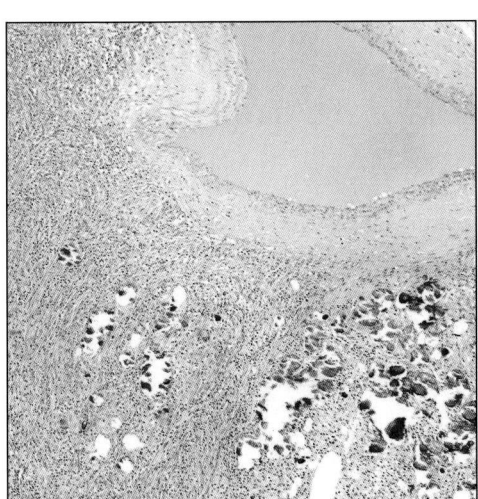

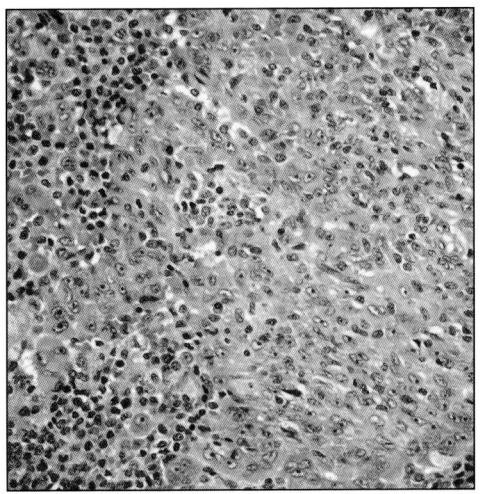

(Left) An inflammatory leiomyosarcoma associated with a large vein and microcalcifications is depicted here. *(Right)* At a higher magnification of an inflammatory leiomyosarcoma, the proliferating cells show epithelioid features. The inflammatory component is primarily lymphoplasmacytic.

RHABDOMYOMA

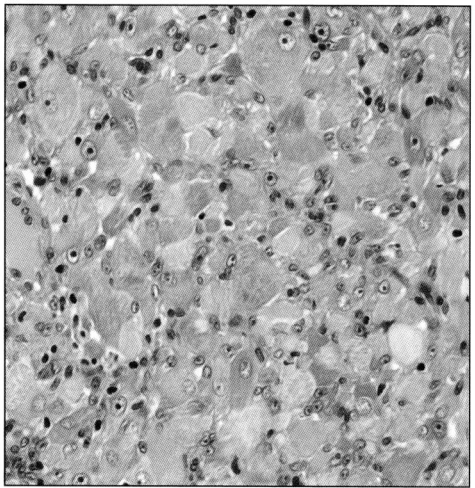

High magnification shows adult rhabdomyoma composed of large polygonal cells with copious eosinophilic cytoplasm (varying in staining intensity) and small round nuclei with uniform nucleoli.

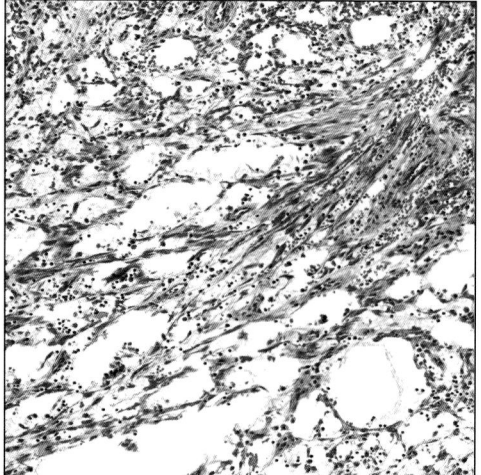

Low magnification shows fetal rhabdomyoma of myxoid (immature) type. Slender spindle cells form loosely organized fascicles in myxoid stroma. Note the absence of pleomorphism and necrosis.

TERMINOLOGY

Definitions
- Benign tumor with skeletal muscle differentiation
- Can arise in heart (cardiac rhabdomyoma) or extracardiac locations
- Extracardiac tumors can be of adult or fetal histologic type

ETIOLOGY/PATHOGENESIS

Developmental Anomaly
- No associations for most extracardiac lesions
- Cardiac rhabdomyoma can be associated with tuberous sclerosis
- Some fetal rhabdomyomas associated with nevoid basal cell carcinoma syndrome
  - *PTCH* mutations
    - Inhibitory receptor in Sonic hedgehog signaling pathway

CLINICAL ISSUES

Epidemiology
- Incidence
  - Rare
- Age
  - Adults; mean: 6th-7th decades
  - Fetal rhabdomyoma mostly in childhood; median: 4 years
    - About 1/2 in 1st year, or congenital
    - Rare examples in adults up to 6th decade
- Gender
  - 75% in males
  - Genital rhabdomyoma mostly in middle-aged women
    - Rare cases in males

Site
- Rarely a cutaneous lesion
- Most often in head and neck region, especially fetal rhabdomyoma
  - Larynx, oropharynx, mouth, neck
- Genital lesions are subepithelial
  - Mostly in vagina, occasionally in vulva or cervix
- Rare examples in males in paratesticular region or epididymis

Presentation
- Incidental finding
- Painless mass
- Difficulty breathing (laryngeal tumors)

Treatment
- Surgical approaches
  - Simple complete excision

Prognosis
- Excellent after complete excision
- Can recur if incompletely excised

MACROSCOPIC FEATURES

General Features
- Usually solitary
- Occasionally multinodular or multicentric

Size
- Most lesions are small (< 10 cm diameter); median: ~ 3 cm

MICROSCOPIC PATHOLOGY

Key Microscopic Features
- Adult rhabdomyoma
  - Circumscribed

RHABDOMYOMA

Key Facts

Terminology
- Benign tumor with skeletal muscle differentiation
- Extracardiac tumors can be of adult or fetal histologic type

Etiology/Pathogenesis
- Some fetal rhabdomyomas associated with nevoid basal cell carcinoma syndrome

Clinical Issues
- Adults; mean: 6th-7th decades; 75% males
- Fetal rhabdomyoma mostly childhood
- Genital rhabdomyoma mostly in middle-aged women
- Most often in head and neck region, especially fetal rhabdomyoma
- Genital lesions mostly in vagina, occasionally vulva or cervix

Microscopic Pathology
- Adult rhabdomyoma
  - Circumscribed
  - Large polygonal cells with abundant eosinophilic cytoplasm
- Fetal rhabdomyoma
  - Immature (myxoid) type has long spindle cells in myxoid stroma
  - Intermediate (juvenile) type has spindled and round cells with variable skeletal muscle differentiation
- No atypia or necrosis; mitoses usually absent

Ancillary Tests
- Lesional cells are immunoreactive for desmin, myogenin, and MYOD1

  - Large polygonal cells with abundant eosinophilic cytoplasm
  - Cross striations and crystalline cytoplasmic inclusions occasionally seen
  - Small bland nuclei, some with prominent nucleoli
  - Some vacuolated ("spider") cells
- Fetal rhabdomyoma, immature (myxoid)
  - Solitary circumscribed lesion, can be polypoid
  - Spindle cells with eosinophilic cytoplasm, occasional cross-striations
  - No atypia or necrosis, mitoses usually absent
  - Myxoid stroma
- Fetal rhabdomyoma, intermediate (juvenile)
  - More mature skeletal muscle: Strap cells, smooth muscle-like cells, and rounded rhabdomyoblasts
- Genital rhabdomyoma
  - Polypoid subepithelial lesion
  - Bundles of strap cells with eosinophilic cytoplasm, scattered rhabdomyoblast-like cells
  - Fibrous stroma

ANCILLARY TESTS

Immunohistochemistry
- Immunoreactive for desmin, myogenin, and MYOD1

Electron Microscopy
- Sarcomeric differentiation: Thick and thin filaments, Z-bands, glycogen deposits associated with filaments

DIFFERENTIAL DIAGNOSIS

DDx of Adult Rhabdomyoma
- Rhabdomyosarcoma
  - Mitoses, pleomorphism, necrosis
- Carcinoma
  - In situ changes in overlying epithelium
  - Mitoses, pleomorphism
  - Epithelial markers positive; desmin absent
- Melanoma
  - Mitoses, pleomorphism

  - S100(+); HMB-45 and MART-1/Melan-A in some cases
  - Desmin usually negative, myogenin(-)
- Hibernoma
  - Lobulated, cells multivacuolated, central nuclei
  - S100(+), desmin(-)
- Granular cell tumor
  - Cytoplasm granular rather than fibrillary
  - S100(+), CEA(+), and inhibin(+); desmin(-)

DDx of Fetal Rhabdomyoma
- Embryonal rhabdomyosarcoma
  - Mitoses, pleomorphism, necrosis

SELECTED REFERENCES

1. Walsh SN et al: Cutaneous fetal rhabdomyoma: a case report and historical review of the literature. Am J Surg Pathol. 32(3):485-91, 2008
2. Davies B et al: Paratesticular rhabdomyoma in a young adult: case study and review of the literature. J Pediatr Surg. 42(4):E5-7, 2007
3. Valdez TA et al: Recurrent fetal rhabdomyoma of the head and neck. Int J Pediatr Otorhinolaryngol. 70(6):1115-8, 2006
4. Kawada H et al: Multiple cutaneous rhabdomyomas in a child. Eur J Dermatol. 14(6):418-20, 2004
5. Watson J et al: Nevoid basal cell carcinoma syndrome and fetal rhabdomyoma: a case study. Ear Nose Throat J. 83(10):716-8, 2004
6. Wehner MS et al: Epididymal rhabdomyoma: report of a case, including histologic and immunohistochemical findings. Arch Pathol Lab Med. 124(10):1518-9, 2000
7. Johansen EC et al: Rhabdomyoma of the larynx: a review of the literature with a summary of previously described cases of rhabdomyoma of the larynx and a report of a new case. J Laryngol Otol. 109(2):147-53, 1995
8. Cleveland DB et al: Adult rhabdomyoma. A light microscopic, ultrastructural, virologic, and immunologic analysis. Oral Surg Oral Med Oral Pathol. 77(2):147-53, 1994
9. Kapadia SB et al: Fetal rhabdomyoma of the head and neck: a clinicopathologic and immunophenotypic study of 24 cases. Hum Pathol. 24(7):754-65, 1993

RHABDOMYOMA

Microscopic and Immunohistochemical Features

(Left) Low magnification shows an adult rhabdomyoma of the larynx. The tumor is separated from the epithelium by a narrow clear zone and forms a solid sheet of cells. Laryngeal rhabdomyomas are most commonly of the adult type, although examples of fetal rhabdomyoma also occur. *(Right)* Intermediate-power examination shows an adult rhabdomyoma. The large, rounded, uniform cells have abundant eosinophilic cytoplasm. They are arranged in confluent sheets with interspersed inflammatory cells.

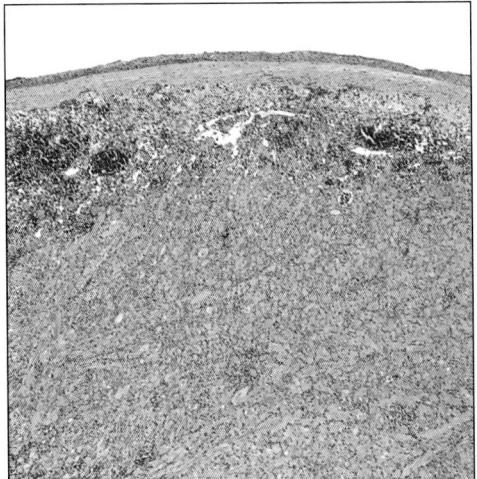
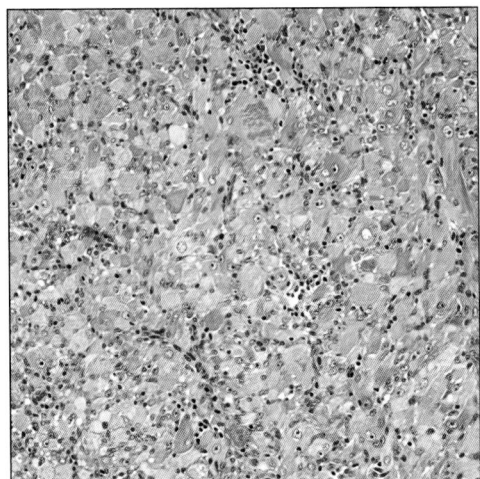

(Left) High magnification shows an adult rhabdomyoma with vacuolated cells, some with strands of cytoplasm extending to the cell's periphery ("spider" cell) ➡️. This appearance is mostly seen in cardiac rhabdomyoma. *(Right)* Adult rhabdomyoma is shown with a large lesional cell containing crystalline rod-shaped intracytoplasmic inclusions ➡️. With electron microscopy, these are seen to be composed of hypertrophic Z-band structures.

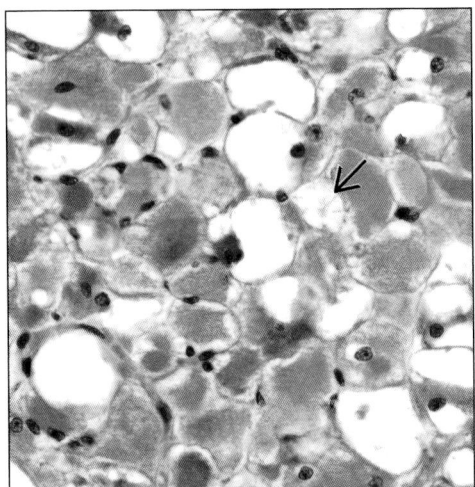
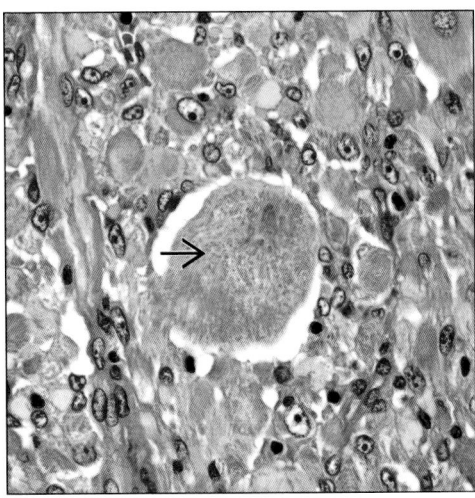

(Left) Desmin stain in an adult rhabdomyoma shows strong, diffuse positivity throughout the lesion. This is a diagnostic finding in rhabdomyoma and can also highlight cross-striations. *(Right)* Positive myogenin in an adult rhabdomyoma shows immunoreactivity in nuclei of many of the lesional cells. This is diagnostic of skeletal muscle differentiation. Cytoplasmic staining is sometimes seen, but it is nonspecific and should be disregarded. MYOD1 is also useful although less sensitive.

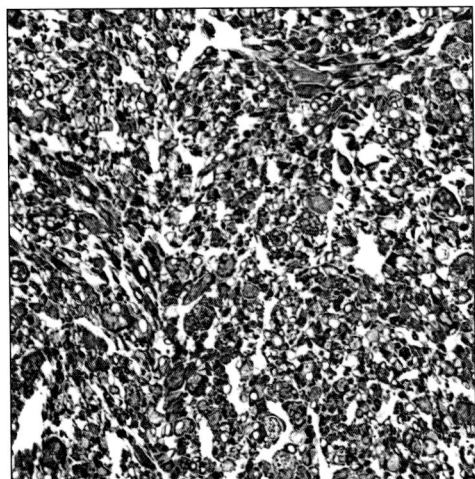
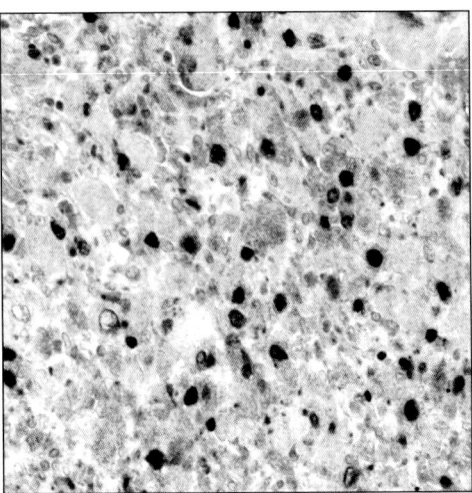

10

RHABDOMYOMA

Microscopic Features

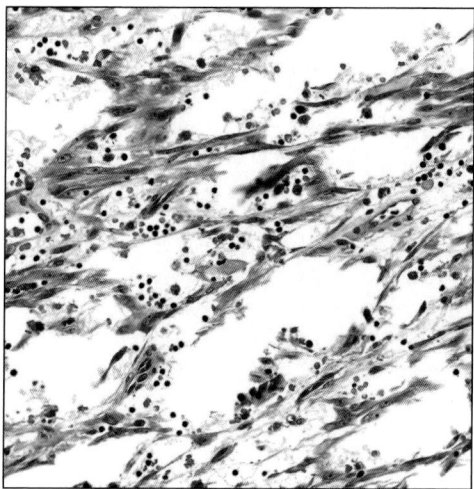

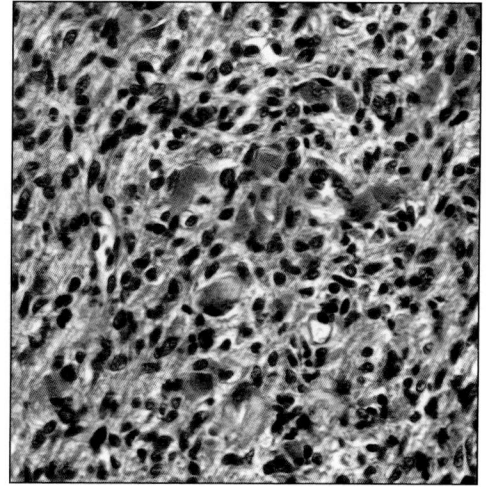

(Left) Fetal rhabdomyoma of myxoid (immature) type, with spindle cells arranged in a vaguely fascicular pattern in a myxoid stroma. Pleomorphism and necrosis are absent. *(Right)* Fetal rhabdomyoma (intermediate type) is shown. Cells show varying stages of skeletal muscle maturation, including rhabdomyoblast-like cells. As in other types of rhabdomyoma, mitotic figures, pleomorphism, and necrosis are absent, which helps to exclude embryonal rhabdomyosarcoma.

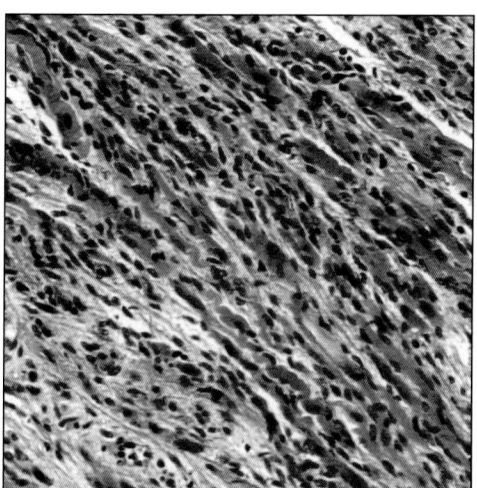

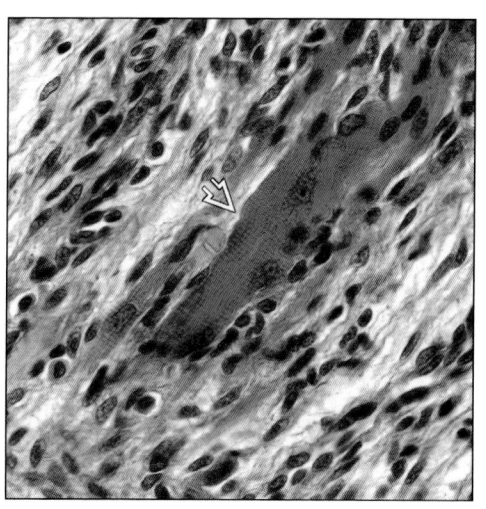

(Left) Intermediate-type fetal rhabdomyoma manifesting relatively uniform spindle cells, with differentiation resembling late-stage embryonic skeletal muscle development. Nuclei are uniform, and no mitotic activity is seen. *(Right)* Intermediate-type fetal rhabdomyoma at higher magnification. Note variation in cell type. Typical cross-striations ➡, characteristic of skeletal muscle differentiation, are apparent in the cytoplasm.

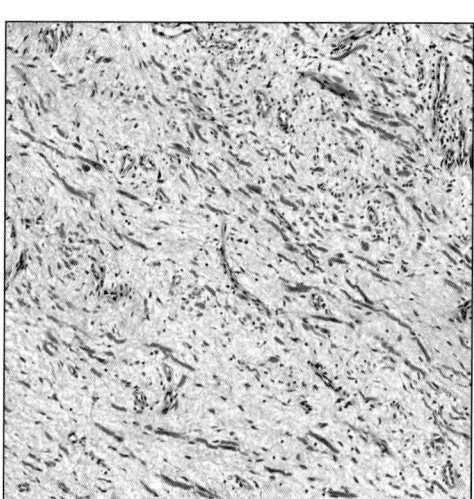

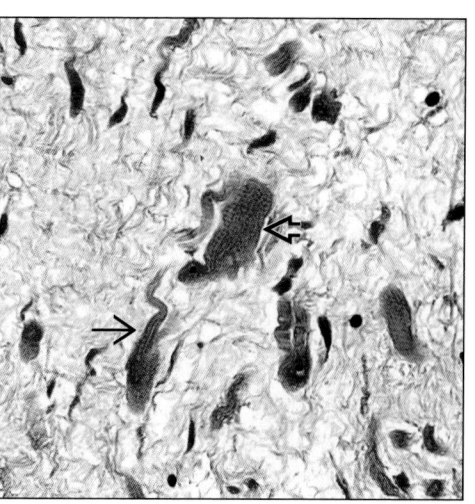

(Left) Genital rhabdomyoma. This is a vaginal tumor with widely separated cords of cells with eosinophilic cytoplasm in a fibrous and myxoid stroma. *(Right)* Higher magnification shows spindle cells that vary in shape and size. Some are slender and wavy, others are tadpole-like ➡, and occasional cells are strap-shaped ➡, with cross-striations evident in this example. As with most rhabdomyomas, no mitoses are seen.

CUTANEOUS RHABDOMYOSARCOMA

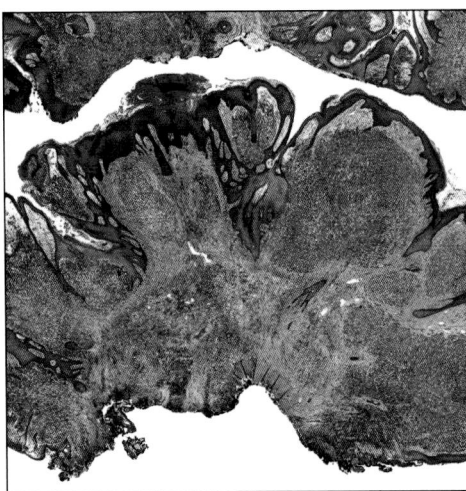

This cutaneous RMS from the ear is a polypoidal tumor with extensive infiltration of the dermis by hypercellular sheets of fairly uniform, small, hyperchromatic, ovoid cells.

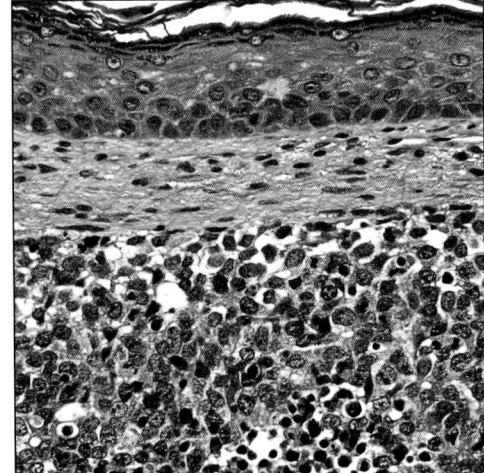

High magnification of a cutaneous RMS shows a nodular dermal proliferation of medium-sized, blue-staining, ovoid cells. A grenz zone separates the tumor from overlying epidermis.

TERMINOLOGY

Abbreviations
- Rhabdomyosarcoma (RMS)
- Embryonal rhabdomyosarcoma (ERMS)
- Alveolar rhabdomyosarcoma (ARMS)

Definitions
- Malignant tumor showing variable differentiation toward skeletal muscle

ETIOLOGY/PATHOGENESIS

Unknown
- Cell of origin still unknown
  - Possible candidate cells include muscle stem cells and multipotent mesenchymal stem cells
- Often occurs in sites lacking skeletal muscle
- May occur in association with inherited syndromes
  - e.g., Beckwith-Wiedemann

CLINICAL ISSUES

Epidemiology
- Incidence
  - Rhabdomyosarcomas are most frequent soft tissue sarcomas in children and young adults
  - Occurrence in skin is rare
    - May occur as metastasis from primary site
    - May very rarely occur as primary cutaneous lesion
    - ARMS, ERMS, and pleomorphic RMS may all occur as primary neoplasms in the skin
  - ERMS is most common RMS subtype
    - Represents 60-70% of RMS
  - Alveolar RMS
    - Approximately 30% of RMS
  - Pleomorphic RMS
    - Rarer amongst pleomorphic sarcomas

- Age
  - RMS occurs most often in children and young adults
  - Cutaneous RMS occurs mostly in children (including congenitally and in infants) and young people
    - However, can occur in all age groups
  - ERMS generally affects youngest population
    - Typically < 10 years
  - ARMS
    - Adolescents and young adults
  - Pleomorphic RMS
    - Older adults
  - Spindle cell RMS
    - Rare variant in children and adolescents; rarely adults
- Gender
  - M = F

Site
- May occur at any cutaneous site
  - Including head and neck, trunk, extremities
- Small numbers arise as heterologous elements of other skin tumors
  - e.g., within congenital melanocytic nevi
  - e.g., in Merkel cell carcinoma
- Embryonal RMS
  - Most common soft tissue sites include head and neck, pelvis (including genitourinary region), and bile duct
  - Trunk and limbs less frequently involved than in ARMS
- Alveolar RMS
  - Extremities, trunk, head and neck
- Spindle cell RMS
  - Paratesticular region, head and neck
- Pleomorphic RMS
  - Extremities

Presentation
- Mass, NOS
  - Often presents as asymptomatic papule or nodule

CUTANEOUS RHABDOMYOSARCOMA

Key Facts

Terminology

- Malignant soft tissue tumor that shows variable differentiation toward skeletal muscle
- 3 main subtypes
  - Alveolar rhabdomyosarcoma (ARMS)
  - Embryonal rhabdomyosarcoma (ERMS)
  - Pleomorphic rhabdomyosarcoma

Clinical Issues

- Rare at cutaneous sites
  - May be primary or secondary
- ERMS: Most common subtype; most in children < 10 years
- ARMS: Adolescents and younger adults; highly aggressive tumor
- Pleomorphic RMS: Older adults; aggressive tumor

Microscopic Pathology

- ERMS
  - Sheets and loose fascicles of spindle and ovoid cells
  - Complex karyotypes by cytogenetics
- ARMS
  - Sheets of small and medium-sized round cells; central dyscohesion resembling pulmonary alveoli
  - Characteristic *PAX-FOXO1* gene fusions in most
- Pleomorphic RMS
  - Malignant fibrous histiocytoma/pleomorphic sarcoma-like morphology with marked anaplasia
- All RMS can have rhabdomyoblasts in variable numbers and stages of differentiation
  - Most frequently seen in ERMS
- All RMS express desmin and at least focal myogenin
  - Expression usually most widespread in ARMS

- May cause pain
  - Nonspecific clinical features
    - Diagnosis may therefore be delayed

Prognosis

- Main prognostic parameters for RMS
  - Histologic type
    - ERMS has significantly better prognosis than ARMS
    - Spindle cell variants (excluding aggressive adult spindle cell variant) have better prognosis
  - Disease stage
  - Site
    - Favorable sites for soft tissue RMS: Head and neck (nonparameningeal), genitourinary (nonbladder, nonprostate), and bile duct
- Number of cases in skin is small for conclusive interpretation of behavior compared to soft tissue RMS
  - However, documented cutaneous cases prone to repeated recurrences and metastases

MACROSCOPIC FEATURES

General Features

- Infiltrative, fleshy mass
- Hemorrhage and necrosis often seen

MICROSCOPIC PATHOLOGY

Histologic Features

- **Embryonal RMS**
  - Loose fascicles and sheets
    - Variable cellularity
  - Spindle, stellate, and ovoid cells
    - Ovoid and elongated, hyperchromatic or vesicular nuclei
    - Varying stages of myogenic differentiation
  - Often have myxoid stroma
  - Mitoses
  - Necrosis
- **Alveolar RMS**
  - Small to medium-sized round cells
  - Nests and sheets, divided by fibrous septa
    - Alveolar-like spaces formed by central loss of cohesion
    - Central cells poorly preserved and necrotic
    - Resemble pulmonary alveoli
  - Solid variant lacks alveolar pattern
  - Tumor giant cells frequent
- **Pleomorphic RMS**
  - Malignant fibrous histiocytoma (MFH)/pleomorphic sarcoma-like morphology
    - Marked cellular pleomorphism and cytological atypia
- **Spindle cell RMS**
  - Spindle cells with elongated nuclei
  - Tumors may have abundant collagenous stroma
  - Adult cases are cellular, fibrosarcoma-like spindle cell sarcomas
- Rhabdomyoblasts
  - Cells with eccentric nuclei and variable amounts of eosinophilic cytoplasm
  - Cytoplasmic cross-striations may be visible
  - Variable numbers and stages of differentiation
  - Can be found in all RMS subtypes
    - Most frequent in ERMS

ANCILLARY TESTS

Immunohistochemistry

- Desmin positivity
  - ARMS has strongest and most widespread expression
  - More focal in ERMS and pleomorphic RMS
- Myogenin and MYOD1 variably positive
  - Myogenic nuclear regulatory proteins
  - Nuclear expression is specific for RMS
  - ARMS usually has most diffuse and strong expression, compared to other subtypes
- SMA variably positive
- CD56(+)
- H-caldesmon, cytokeratin, EMA, and S100 protein (-)

Cytogenetics

- ERMS
  - Complex karyotypes
    - Often gains of chromosomes 2, 8, 12, and 13
    - LOH at 11p15.5 considered hallmark of ERMS
    - Genes located in 11p15.5 region include some that encode proteins involved in growth regulation
- ARMS
  - Characteristic translocations involving *FOXO1* and *PAX3/7* genes
  - t(2;13)(q35;q14) (majority [60%] of ARMS)
  - t(1;13)(p36;q14) (10-15% of ARMS)
    - Generate chimeric fusion oncoproteins that act as aberrant transcription factors
    - *FOXO1* (chromosome 13); member of forkhead transcription factor family
    - *PAX3* or *PAX7* (chromosomes 2 and 1, respectively); members of paired box family of transcription factors with high degree of homology
- Pleomorphic RMS
  - Complex karyotypes

DIFFERENTIAL DIAGNOSIS

Rhabdomyoma

- Head and neck predilection, especially fetal type
- Fetal rhabdomyoma
  - No atypia or necrosis
  - Mitoses usually absent
- Adult rhabdomyoma
  - Middle-aged adults, M > F
  - Circumscribed
  - Large polygonal cells, abundant cytoplasm
- Genital rhabdomyoma
  - Mostly middle-aged women
  - Strap cells, no mitoses

Rhabdomyomatous Mesenchymal Hamartoma

- Congenital or in infants
- Dermal and subcutaneous
  - Rarely in oral cavity
- Mature skeletal muscle, fat, nerves, and adnexa
- No mitoses, necrosis, or atypia

Leiomyosarcoma

- Intersecting fascicular architecture
- Cells may show typical cytological features of smooth muscle, e.g., blunt-ended nuclei
- Strong SMA and H-caldesmon expression
- Lack myogenin and MYOD1 expression

Merkel Cell and Small Cell/Neuroendocrine Carcinoma

- Older adults
- Primary tumor site may be identifiable
- Cells show crush artifact
- Nuclear moulding
- CK-PAN expression

  - Cytoplasmic dot positivity (CK20) in Merkel cell carcinoma
- Desmin negative

Ewing Sarcoma/PNET

- Cells more uniform and smaller
- Many cases CD99 positive
- May rarely express desmin
  - However, negative for myogenic markers
- Expression of neural/neuroectodermal markers in PNET
- Characteristic translocations involving *EWSR1*

Lymphoma/Leukemia

- Often systemic involvement by disease
- Usually sites of lymphadenopathy
- Architecture dispersed and sheet-like, rather than nested (compared with ARMS)
- Expression of broad spectrum hematolymphoid markers
- Desmin negative

Atypical Fibroxanthoma (AFX)

- Elderly adults
- Typically sun-damaged skin
- Should not extend into subcutis
- Can express SMA
  - Desmin typically negative

SELECTED REFERENCES

1. Adhikari LA et al: Merkel cell carcinoma with heterologous rhabdomyoblastic differentiation: the role of immunohistochemistry for Merkel cell polyomavirus large T-antigen in confirmation. J Cutan Pathol. Epub ahead of print, 2011
2. Brecher AR et al: Congenital primary cutaneous rhabdomyosarcoma in a neonate. Pediatr Dermatol. 20(4):335-8, 2003
3. Gong Y et al: Primary cutaneous alveolar rhabdomyosarcoma of the perineum. Arch Pathol Lab Med. 126(8):982-4, 2002
4. Hoang MP et al: Rhabdomyosarcoma arising in a congenital melanocytic nevus. Am J Dermatopathol. 24(1):26-9, 2002
5. Setterfield J et al: Primary cutaneous epidermotropic alveolar rhabdomyosarcoma with t(2;13) in an elderly woman: case report and review of the literature. Am J Surg Pathol. 26(7):938-44, 2002
6. Wong TY et al: Primary cutaneous sarcomas showing rhabdomyoblastic differentiation. Histopathology. 26(1):25-32, 1995
7. de la Luz Orozco-Covarrubias M et al: Malignant cutaneous tumors in children. Twenty years of experience at a large pediatric hospital. J Am Acad Dermatol. 30(2 Pt 1):243-9, 1994
8. Schmidt D et al: Rhabdomyosarcomas with primary presentation in the skin. Pathol Res Pract. 189(4):422-7, 1993
9. Pérez-Guillermo M et al: Infantile cutaneous rhabdomyosarcoma (Li-Fraumeni syndrome): cytological presentation of fine-needle aspirate biopsy, report of a case. Diagn Cytopathol. 8(6):621-6, 1992
10. Wiss K et al: Rhabdomyosarcoma presenting as a cutaneous nodule. Arch Dermatol. 124(11):1687-90, 1988

CUTANEOUS RHABDOMYOSARCOMA

Microscopic and Immunohistochemical Features

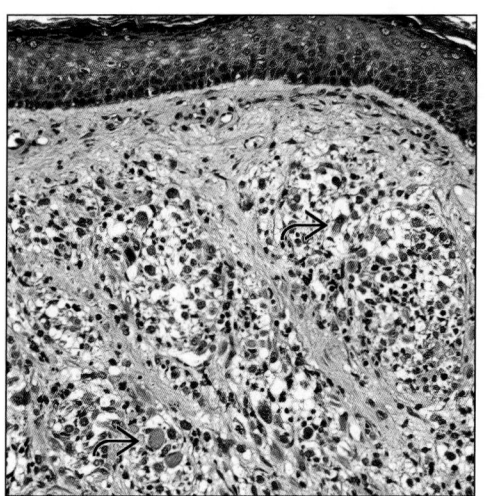
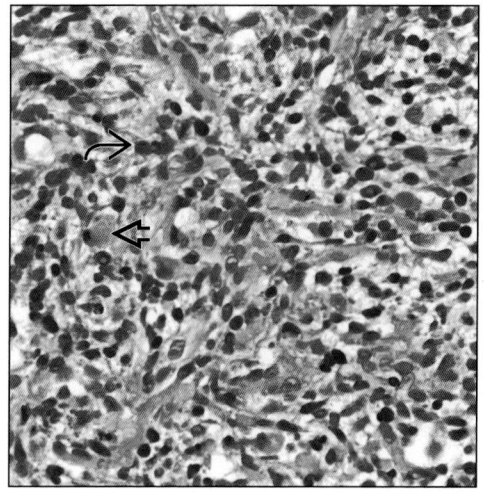

(Left) This embryonal subtype of cutaneous RMS shows extensive dermal invasion by collections of primitive cells with ovoid nuclei within myxoid stroma. Note numerous intermixed rhabdomyoblasts ➡. *(Right)* In this ERMS, the cells show a range of appearances, with relatively undifferentiated ovoid cells with hyperchromatic nuclei ➡ and a few rhabdomyoblasts with large amounts of eosinophilic cytoplasm & eccentric nuclei ➡.

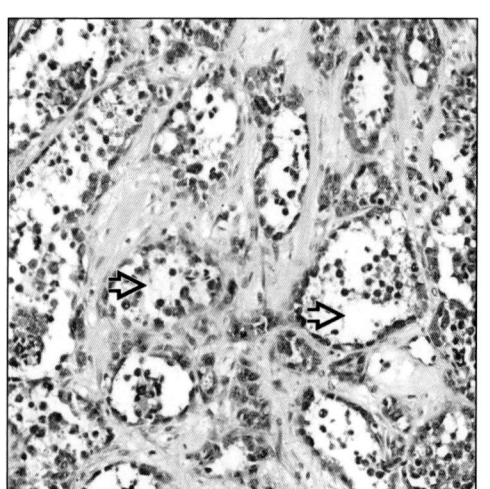
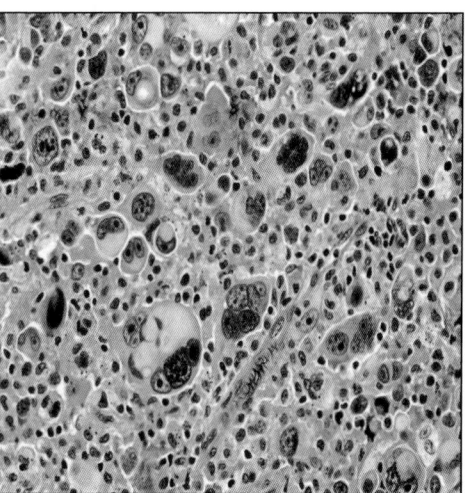

(Left) This example of alveolar rhabdomyosarcoma is composed of nests of round cells separated by fibrous septa. In the nests, there is peripheral cellular preservation but central dyscohesion and necrosis ➡, somewhat resembling the appearance of pulmonary alveoli. *(Right)* This pleomorphic RMS is composed of sheets of large, polygonal, often bizarre-appearing cells with abundant eosinophilic cytoplasm, resembling pleomorphic rhabdomyoblasts.

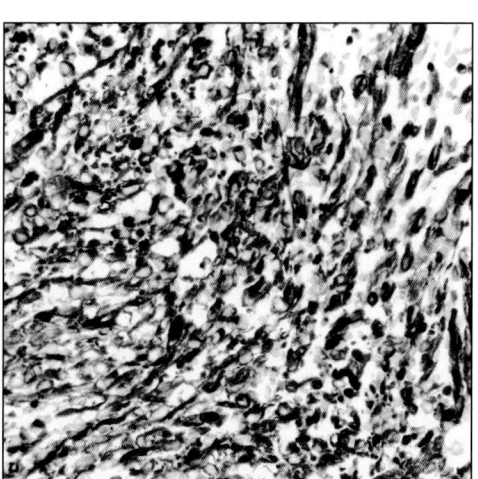
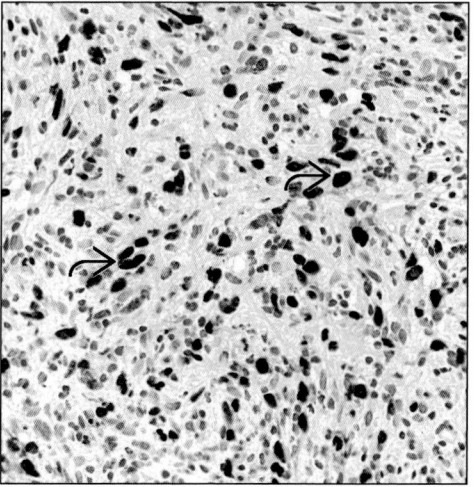

(Left) Desmin expression in rhabdomyosarcoma is typically diffuse and strong in the cytoplasm of the neoplastic cells. Cross-striations may be highlighted. *(Right)* Immunostaining for myogenin shows well-defined nuclear localization ➡. The proportion of nuclei expressing this marker varies. It is most widespread in alveolar rhabdomyosarcoma, with lesser degrees in embryonal and pleomorphic subtypes. Cytoplasmic staining is nonspecific and seen in many tumor types.

LIPOMA

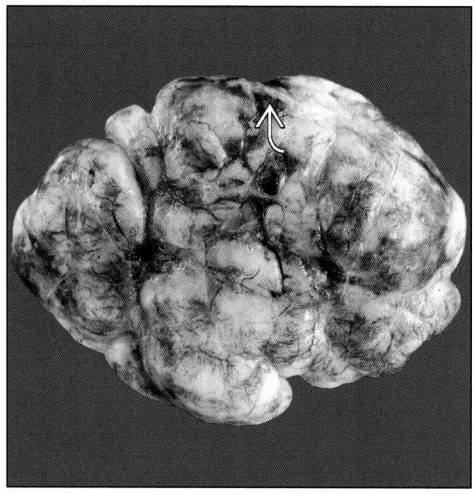

Lipomas are surrounded by a thin, delicate, and transparent capsule ⮒, and often show a lobulated appearance.

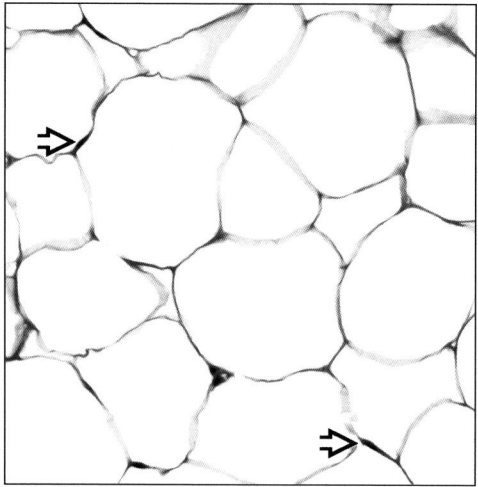

Lipomas are composed of mature white adipocytes, which show minimal size variation. The tumor cells show a peripherally flattened nucleus ⮒ without any atypia.

TERMINOLOGY

Definitions
- Benign tumor of mature white adipocytes

ETIOLOGY/PATHOGENESIS

Unknown
- Although etiology is unknown, lipomas tend to occur more commonly in obese individuals

CLINICAL ISSUES

Presentation
- Painless mass
  - Large lesions may be painful

Treatment
- Surgical excision is curative

Prognosis
- Recurrences in < 5% cases
- Higher recurrence rate in intramuscular lipoma

IMAGE FINDINGS

Radiographic Findings
- Soft tissue mass isodense to subcutaneous tissue
- Delicate fibrous strands may be present, particularly in larger lesions

MACROSCOPIC FEATURES

General Features
- Most common between 40-60 years of age
- Located in subcutaneous or deep soft tissue
- Approximately 5% may be multiple

Gross Features
- Well-circumscribed
- Delicate capsule
- Yellow, greasy cut surface
- Myxoid change, bone, or cartilage may be present in some variants
- Infiltrative margins may be present in intramuscular lipoma
- Nodular and papillary appearance seen in lipoma arborescens involving the synovium

MICROSCOPIC PATHOLOGY

Histologic Features
- Lobules of mature adipocytes
- Minimal variation in adipocytic size
- Foci of fat necrosis or hemorrhage may be present

Cytologic Features
- Adipocytes with peripheral flattened nucleus
- No nuclear atypia

Variants
- Additional mesenchymal component may be present in some lipomas
  - Abundant fibrous tissue: **Fibrolipoma**
    - Sclerotic lipoma is a variant with predilection for scalp and hands in young men
  - Cartilage: **Chondrolipoma**
    - Mature hyaline cartilage admixed with adipose tissue
    - Should be distinguished from chondroid lipoma, which is a distinct entity
  - Bone: **Osteolipoma**
    - Rare
  - Myxoid stromal change: **Myxolipoma**
    - Some myxolipomas may have a prominent vascular component (**angiomyxolipoma**)

LIPOMA

Key Facts

Terminology
- Benign tumor of mature white adipocytes

Clinical Issues
- Surgical excision is curative
- Higher recurrence rate in intramuscular lipoma

Macroscopic Features
- Most common between 40-60 years of age
- Approximately 5% may be multiple

- Well-circumscribed with delicate capsule
- Yellow, greasy cut surface

Microscopic Pathology
- Lobules of mature adipocytes with minimal size variation
- No nuclear atypia

Ancillary Tests
- Lipomas are cytogenetically heterogeneous

- Myxolipomas need to be distinguished from myxomas and myxoid liposarcomas
  - Smooth muscle: **Myoliploma**
    - Considered distinct entity
- Intramuscular lipoma
  - May have infiltrative margins
  - Entrapped skeletal muscle at periphery
  - Also known as "infiltrating lipoma"
  - Mature adipocytes with no atypia
  - Recurrences may occur in about 15% cases

ANCILLARY TESTS

Immunohistochemistry
- Stain like mature adipocytes (S100 and LEP positive)

Cytogenetics
- Lipomas are cytogenetically heterogeneous
- Common anomalies include
  - Aberrations involving 12q13-15
  - Rearrangements involving 6p21-23
  - Deletions involving 13q

DIFFERENTIAL DIAGNOSIS

Angiolipoma
- Lipoma with increased number of vessels, some of which contain fibrinous thrombi

Atypical Lipomatous Tumor (ALT)
- Deep-seated intramuscular lipomas may be mistaken for ALT
- Intramuscular lipomas show no nuclear atypia

Myxoid Liposarcoma (MLS)
- Myxolipomas may be mistaken for MLS
- Myxolipomas lack lipoblasts and plexiform vasculature seen in MLS

DIAGNOSTIC CHECKLIST

Pathologic Interpretation Pearls
- Uniform size of adipocytes, delicate fibrous septa, and lack of nuclear atypia are key to diagnosis

SELECTED REFERENCES

1. Gaskin CM et al: Lipomas, lipoma variants, and well-differentiated liposarcomas (atypical lipomas): results of MRI evaluations of 126 consecutive fatty masses. AJR Am J Roentgenol. 182(3):733-9, 2004
2. Tardío JC et al: Angiomyxolipoma (vascular myxolipoma) of subcutaneous tissue. Am J Dermatopathol. 26(3):222-4, 2004
3. Willén H et al: Comparison of chromosomal patterns with clinical features in 165 lipomas: a report of the CHAMP study group. Cancer Genet Cytogenet. 102(1):46-9, 1998
4. Zelger BG et al: Sclerotic lipoma: lipomas simulating sclerotic fibroma. Histopathology. 31(2):174-81, 1997
5. Fletcher CD et al: Intramuscular and intermuscular lipoma: neglected diagnoses. Histopathology. 12(3):275-87, 1988

IMAGE GALLERY

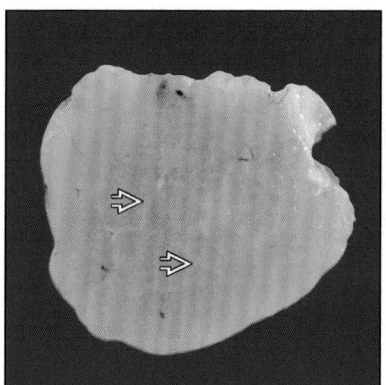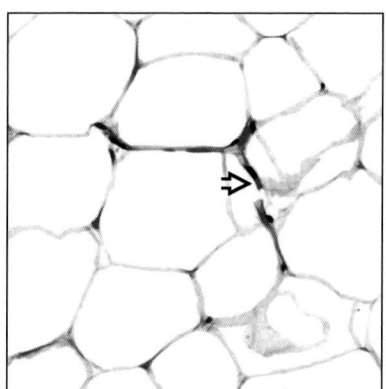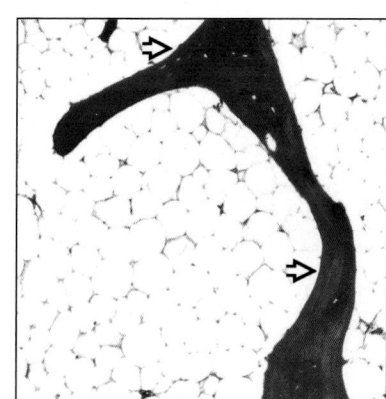

(Left) The cut surface of lipomas is homogeneous, yellow, and greasy. Note the delicate fibrous septa ⧩ in the lesion, which separate it into lobules. *(Center)* The blood vessels in lipomas are delicate and often compressed ⧩ between distended adipocytes, making them inconspicuous. *(Right)* Additional mesenchymal components may be present in some lipomas. Mature lamellar bone ⧩ is seen here in this example of an osteolipoma.

ANGIOLIPOMA

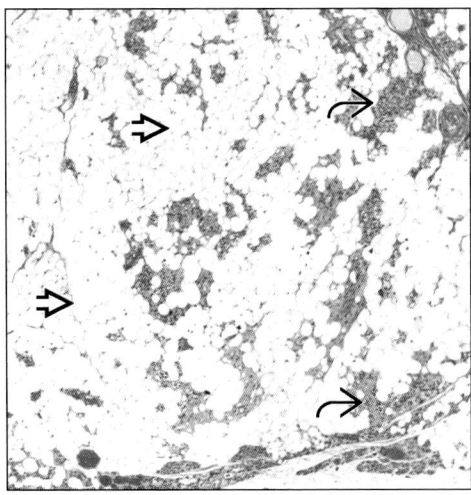

Angiolipomas are biphasic tumors composed of mature adipocytes ⊳ and branching, capillary-sized blood vessels ⇗.

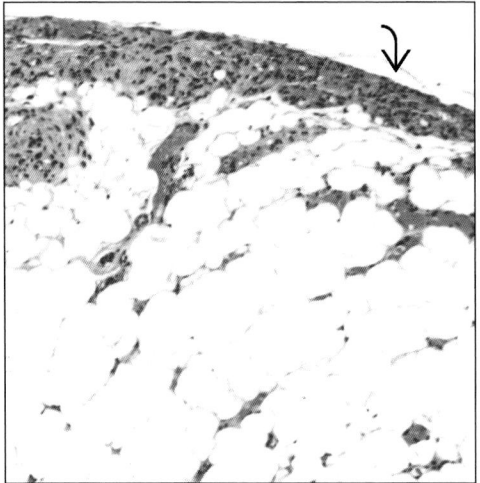

Angiolipomas are surrounded by a delicate capsule ⇗, and the vascular component is often most prominent in the subcapsular region.

TERMINOLOGY

Definitions
- Biphasic tumor consisting of mature adipocytes and thin-walled blood vessels with fibrin thrombi

ETIOLOGY/PATHOGENESIS

Familial Predilection
- In minority of cases (5-10%)

CLINICAL ISSUES

Epidemiology
- Age
  - Common in young adults
- Gender
  - Male predominance

Site
- Forearm, trunk, and upper arm most common sites
- Spinal angiolipomas are considered a distinct entity
  - Infiltrating margins
  - Vascular component mimics arteriovenous malformation or cavernous hemangioma
- Rare instances of visceral involvement (lymph node, duodenum, breast) reported

Presentation
- Painful mass
  - Often present as multiple, subcutaneous nodules
  - No correlation between pain and degree of tumor vascularity

Treatment
- Surgical excision

Prognosis
- Always benign

- Does not recur or undergo malignant transformation

MACROSCOPIC FEATURES

Gross Features
- Encapsulated tumor
- Yellow-red nodules
- Typically < 2 cm in size

MICROSCOPIC PATHOLOGY

Histologic Features
- 2 components are present in these tumors
  - Mature adipocytes
  - Branching, capillary-sized blood vessels with fibrinoid thrombi
    - Vascularity and fibrinoid thrombi often more prominent in subcapsular zone
- Relative proportion of each component is variable
- Variable amount of fibrosis may be present
- Mast cells may be conspicuous in some cases

Cytologic Features
- No significant nuclear atypia is present in adipocytic or vascular component

Variant Subtype
- Cellular angiolipoma
  - Vascular component predominates in this variant
  - May be mistaken for Kaposi sarcoma or angiosarcoma

ANCILLARY TESTS

Cytogenetics
- Karyotypically normal
- t(X;2) has been reported in 1 case

ANGIOLIPOMA

Key Facts

Terminology
- Biphasic tumor consisting of mature adipocytes and thin-walled blood vessels with fibrinoid thrombi

Clinical Issues
- Common in young adults; male predominance
- Painful tender subcutaneous nodule
- May be multiple
- Does not recur or undergo malignant transformation

Macroscopic Features
- Encapsulated, yellow-red nodule
- Typically < 2 cm in size

Microscopic Pathology
- Admixture of mature adipocytes and capillary-sized blood vessels with fibrin thrombi
- Vascular component predominates in cellular angiolipoma

Electron Microscopy
- Transmission
  - Adipocytes and spindle-shaped endothelial cells are seen
  - Fibrin thrombi may be associated with disrupted endothelial cells

DIFFERENTIAL DIAGNOSIS

Lipoma
- Lesions in which adipocytic component predominates may be mistaken for a conventional lipoma
  - Vessels with fibrinoid thrombi are helpful in making diagnosis of angiolipoma

Intramuscular Hemangioma
- Previously known as "**infiltrating angiolipoma**"
- Angiolipomas are small, multiple, and superficial in location, unlike intramuscular hemangioma

Kaposi Sarcoma (KS)
- Cellular angiolipoma may rarely be mistaken for KS
- Endothelial proliferation present in both lesions
- Angiolipomas lack slit-like spaces and PAS positive hyaline globules seen in KS
- Endothelial cells in KS are HHV8 positive

Angiomyolipoma (AML)
- Mixture of mature fat cells, smooth muscle, spindle cells, and vessels

- Spindle cells in AML are HMB-45 positive smooth muscle cells

DIAGNOSTIC CHECKLIST

Pathologic Interpretation Pearls
- Variable admixture of mature adipocytes and branching capillaries with fibrin thrombi

SELECTED REFERENCES

1. Konya D et al: Lumbar spinal angiolipoma: case report and review of the literature. Eur Spine J. 15(6):1025-8, 2006
2. Kazakov DV et al: Primary intranodal cellular angiolipoma. Int J Surg Pathol. 13(1):99-101, 2005
3. Mohl W et al: Duodenal angiolipoma -- endoscopic diagnosis and therapy. Z Gastroenterol. 42(12):1381-3, 2004
4. Sciot R et al: Cytogenetic analysis of subcutaneous angiolipoma: further evidence supporting its difference from ordinary pure lipomas: a report of the CHAMP Study Group. Am J Surg Pathol. 21(4):441-4, 1997
5. Kanik AB et al: Cellular angiolipoma. Am J Dermatopathol. 17(3):312-5, 1995
6. Yu GH et al: Cellular angiolipoma of the breast. Mod Pathol. 6(4):497-9, 1993
7. Dixon AY et al: Angiolipomas: an ultrastructural and clinicopathological study. Hum Pathol. 12(8):739-47, 1981

IMAGE GALLERY

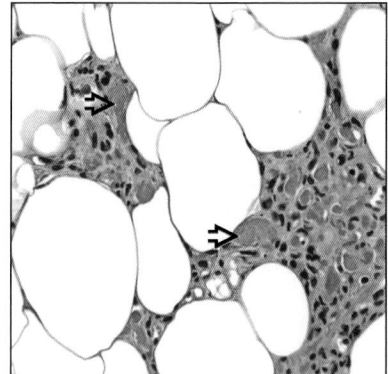
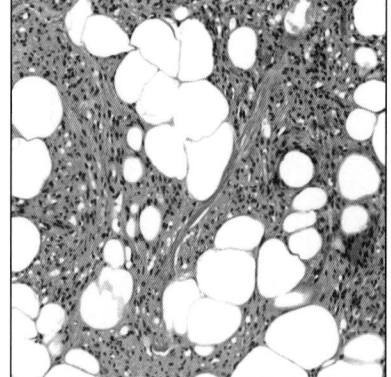
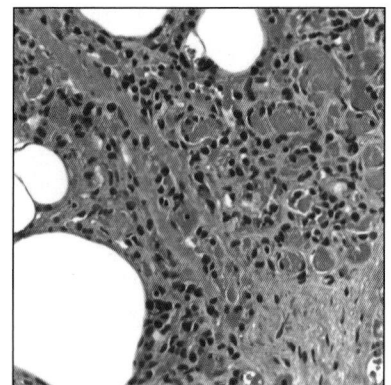

(Left) The vascular component in angiolipomas shows intraluminal fibrin thrombi ⊵. The adipocytic component is benign and shows no nuclear atypia. *(Center)* Cellular angiolipomas show predominance of the vascular component and may be mistaken for Kaposi sarcoma. *(Right)* The presence of intraluminal fibrin thrombi in cellular angiolipoma is helpful in distinguishing it from Kaposi sarcoma or angiosarcoma.

SPINDLE CELL AND PLEOMORPHIC LIPOMA

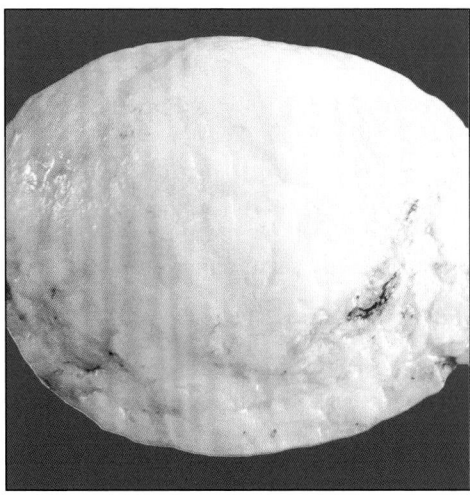

Spindle cell and pleomorphic lipomas are well-circumscribed tumors with a pale yellow, homogeneous appearance that lacks the lobular configuration seen in typical lipomas.

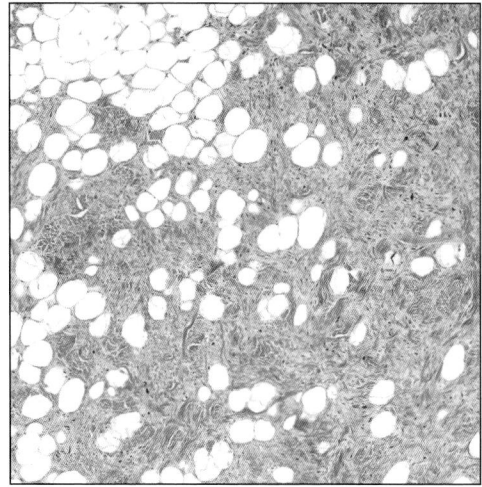

Spindle cell lipomas show mature adipocytes admixed with a bland spindle cell proliferation in a dense collagenous stroma.

TERMINOLOGY

Abbreviations
• Spindle cell lipoma (SCL)/pleomorphic lipoma (PL)

Definitions
• Benign adipocytic tumor with variable admixture of spindle cells, ropey collagen, and multinucleated tumor giant cells

CLINICAL ISSUES

Epidemiology
• Age
  ○ Typically in older age group (> 50 years)
• Gender
  ○ Predominantly in men; < 10% in women

Site
• Shoulder and posterior neck most common sites of involvement
• Other sites
  ○ Upper arm
  ○ Face
  ○ Oral cavity
• Lower extremity involvement is rare

Presentation
• Painless mass
  ○ Dermal or subcutaneous nodule
  ○ Often present for long duration
  ○ Rarely multiple or familial

Treatment
• Conservative surgical excision is adequate

Prognosis
• Benign behavior
• Local recurrence is rare

MACROSCOPIC FEATURES

Gross Appearance
• Well-circumscribed tumor
• Yellow-gray white appearance
• Firm consistency
• Some cases may show myxoid appearance

MICROSCOPIC PATHOLOGY

Histologic Features
• Spindle cell lipoma is composed of variable admixture of 3 components
  ○ Mature adipocytes
  ○ Bland spindle cell proliferation
  ○ Myxoid stroma with ropey collagen and mast cells
• Pleomorphic lipoma is part of same spectrum
  ○ In addition to above features, also shows multinucleated tumor giant cells with peripherally arranged nuclei ("floret cells")
  ○ Lipoblasts may be present in pleomorphic lipoma

Cytologic Features
• Bland nuclei in spindle cell lipoma
• Hyperchromatic nuclei in multinucleated tumor giant cells in pleomorphic lipoma

Variants
• Pseudoangiomatoid variants
  ○ Prominent slit-like spaces resembling vascular channels
  ○ May be mistaken for vascular neoplasm, since SCL is also CD34 positive
  ○ SCL is CD31 negative, unlike tumors with true endothelial differentiation
• Fat-free and fat-poor variant
  ○ Spindle cell proliferation dominates the picture
  ○ Adipocytes may be scarce or completely absent
  ○ Similar site predilection as typical SCL/PL

SPINDLE CELL AND PLEOMORPHIC LIPOMA

Key Facts

Terminology
- Benign adipocytic tumors with variable admixture of spindle cells, mucinous stroma, ropey collagen, and multinucleate giant cells

Clinical Issues
- Typically in older men (> 50 years)
- Shoulder and posterior neck most common sites
- Benign behavior

Macroscopic Features
- Well-circumscribed subcutaneous lesions
- Yellow-gray white, firm with myxoid areas

Microscopic Pathology
- Spindle cells with ropey collagen, mature adipose tissue, and myxoid stroma with mast cells
- Spindle cells are diffusely/strongly positive for CD34

- Pleomorphic lipoma shows multinucleated tumor giant cells with peripheral nuclei ("floret" cells)
- Lipoblasts may be present in some PL
- Variants
  - Pseudoangiomatoid variant of SCL shows prominent slit-like spaces resembling vascular channels
  - Spindle cell proliferation dominates the picture in fat-free and fat-poor variant of SCL

Ancillary Tests
- Deletions of 16q and 13q occur in SCL/PL

Top Differential Diagnoses
- Dermatofibrosarcoma protuberans (DFSP)
- Peripheral nerve sheath tumors
- Solitary fibrous tumor (SFT)

ANCILLARY TESTS

Immunohistochemistry
- SCL/PL are diffusely and strongly positive for CD34
- Rare cases may stain focally for S100

Cytogenetics
- More complex karyotype than typical lipoma
- Deletions of 16q, usually involving the 16q13 region
- Deletions of 13q have also been reported

DIFFERENTIAL DIAGNOSIS

Dermatofibrosarcoma Protuberans (DFSP)
- Typically occurs in young individuals
- Spindle cells arranged in storiform pattern and infiltrate into subcutaneous tissue
- Shares CD34 positivity with SCL/PL

Peripheral Nerve Sheath Tumors
- Some SCL/PL may show nuclear palisading and mimic peripheral nerve sheath tumors
- S100 and CD34 immunostains useful in making this distinction

Solitary Fibrous Tumor (SFT)
- Also diffusely CD34 positive
- Ectatic branching "staghorn" vascular pattern present in SFT

Sclerosing Well-Differentiated Liposarcoma (WDLPS)
- Unlike WDLPS, SCL/PL are well-circumscribed subcutaneous tumors with diffuse CD34 positivity
- Giant ring chromosomes and MDM2 and CDK4 positivity present in well-differentiated liposarcoma

Spindle Cell Liposarcoma
- Spindle cells arranged in fascicles in spindle cell liposarcoma and lack ropey collagen of SCL/PL
- CD34 positivity present in SCL/PL

Myxoid Liposarcoma
- SCL/PL with prominent vascular proliferation may be mistaken for myxoid liposarcoma

DIAGNOSTIC CHECKLIST

Clinically Relevant Pathologic Features
- Gross appearance
  - Well-circumscribed subcutaneous tumors
- Age distribution
  - Typically occur in older men
- Site of involvement
  - Posterior neck and shoulder

Pathologic Interpretation Pearls
- Spindle cell lipoma
  - Mature adipocytes admixed with bland spindle cells, ropey collagen, and myxoid stroma with mast cells
- Pleomorphic lipoma
  - Hyperchromatic, round or spindle-shaped nuclei
  - Multinucleated floret cells with peripheral arrangement of nuclei

SELECTED REFERENCES

1. Billings SD et al: Diagnostically challenging spindle cell lipomas: a report of 34 "low-fat" and "fat-free" variants. Am J Dermatopathol. 29(5):437-42, 2007
2. Fanburg-Smith JC et al: Multiple spindle cell lipomas: a report of 7 familial and 11 nonfamilial cases. Am J Surg Pathol. 22(1):40-8, 1998
3. Dal Cin P et al: Lesions of 13q may occur independently of deletion of 16q in spindle cell/pleomorphic lipomas. Histopathology. 31(3):222-5, 1997
4. Hawley IC et al: Spindle cell lipoma--a pseudoangiomatous variant. Histopathology. 24(6):565-9, 1994
5. Shmookler BM et al: Pleomorphic lipoma: a benign tumor simulating liposarcoma. A clinicopathologic analysis of 48 cases. Cancer. 47(1):126-33, 1981
6. Enzinger FM et al: Spindle cell lipoma. Cancer. 36(5):1852-9, 1975

Gross and Microscopic Features

(Left) Both spindle cell and pleomorphic lipomas may show gray-white foci ⊵ that are firm in consistency and correlate histologically with spindle cell areas with ropey collagenous matrix. *(Right)* The spindle cells in the tumor show no nuclear atypia and are present in a background of a ropey collagenous matrix ⊵.

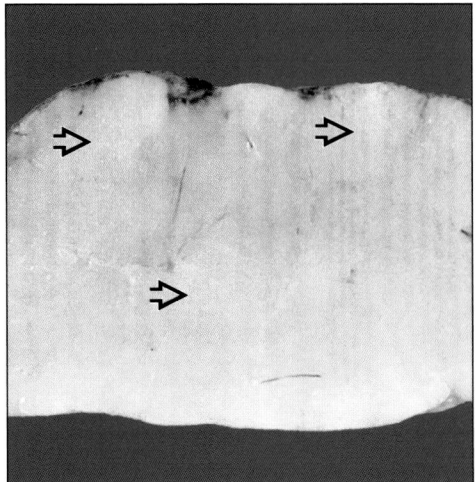
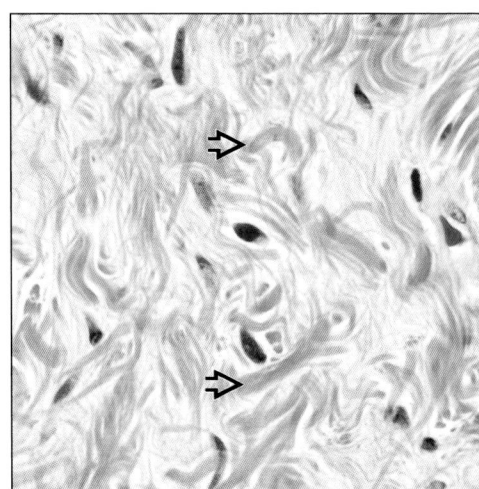

(Left) Myxoid stromal change can be prominent ⊵ in some examples of SCL. These cases may be mistaken for myxolipomas or myxoid liposarcomas. SCL are diffusely and strongly CD34 positive. *(Right)* Myxoid zones in spindle cell lipoma are also devoid of any nuclear atypia. The background of thick collagen bundles ⊵ points toward the correct diagnosis of spindle cell lipoma in these cases.

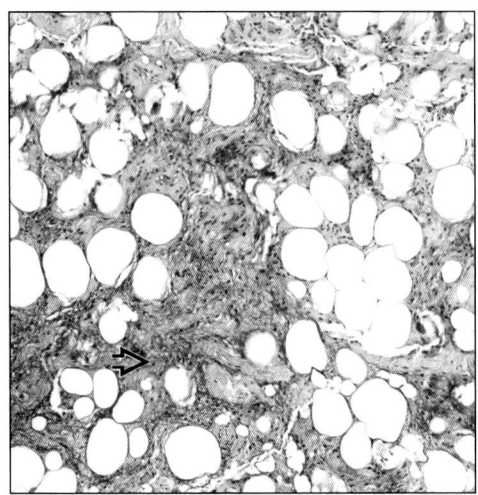
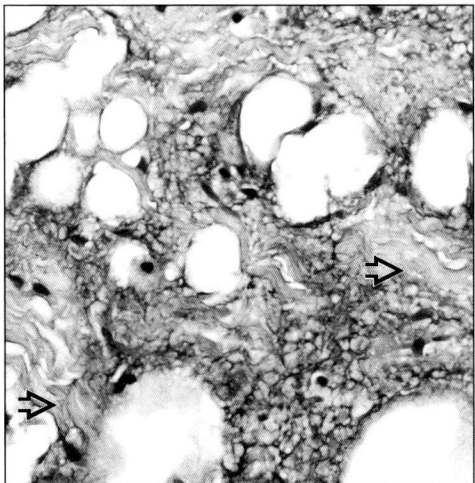

(Left) In some cases, the spindle cell proliferation with ropey collagen ⊵ may dominate the overall picture, with only a few adipocytes present. These tumors are recognized as fat-poor or (fat-free if lacking adipocytes) variants of spindle cell lipoma. *(Right)* Both spindle cell and pleomorphic lipoma share diffuse and strong positivity for CD34.

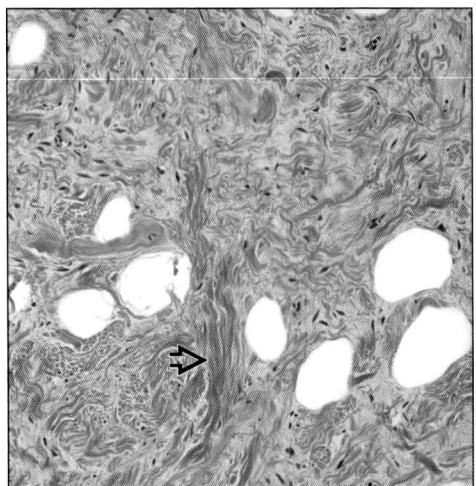
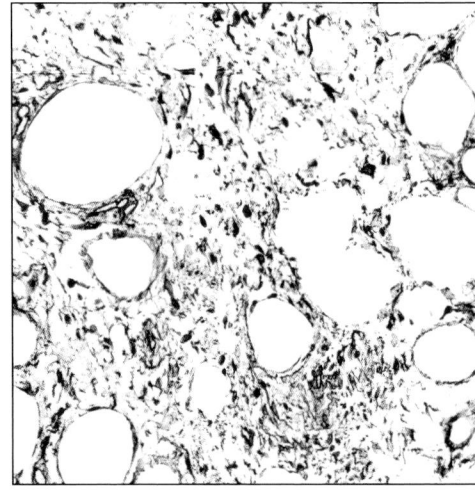

SPINDLE CELL AND PLEOMORPHIC LIPOMA

Microscopic and Immunohistochemical Features

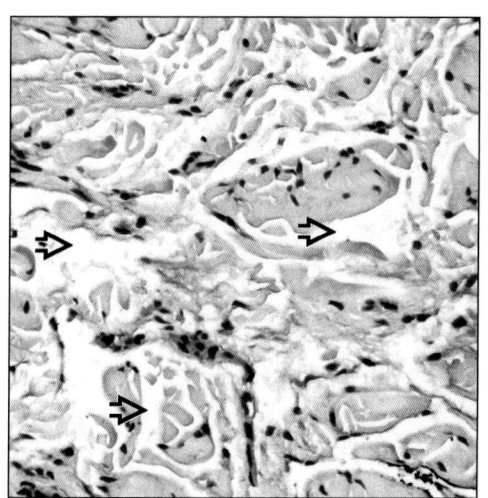

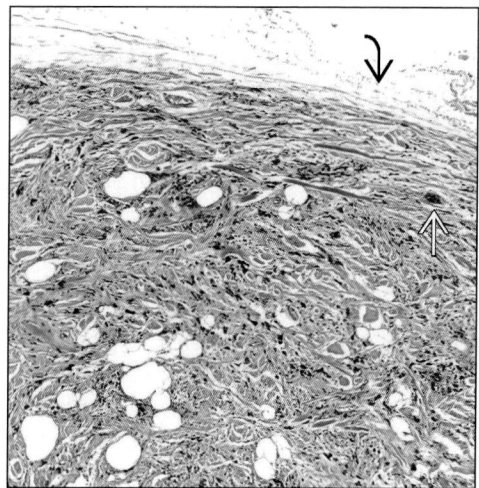

(Left) Exaggerated slit-like spaces ⊅ are present in the pseudoangiomatous variant of SCL, which may be mistaken for a vascular neoplasm. *(Right)* Pleomorphic lipomas are well-circumscribed tumors ⇗ with hyperchromatic spindled and round nuclei and a variable number of multinucleated tumor giant cells ➡.

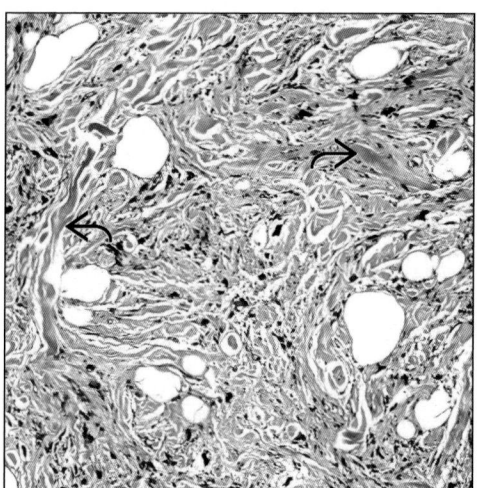

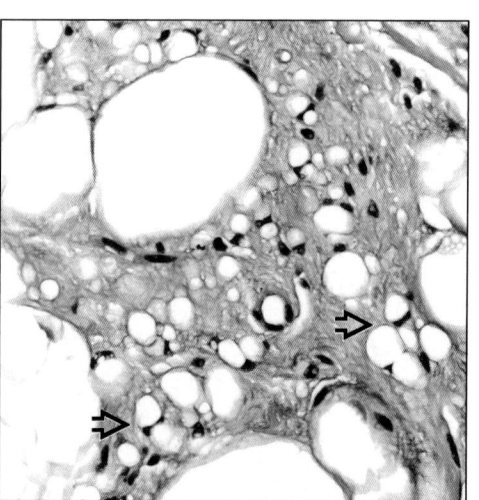

(Left) The ropey collagen ⇗ that is characteristic of SCL is also present in pleomorphic lipomas, suggesting that the 2 lesions are part of the same spectrum. *(Right)* Scattered lipoblasts ⊅ may be present in pleomorphic lipoma. The presence of lipoblasts or mitotic activity does not affect prognosis in pleomorphic lipoma.

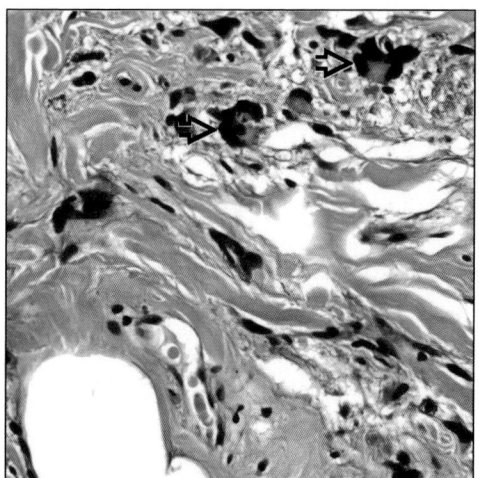

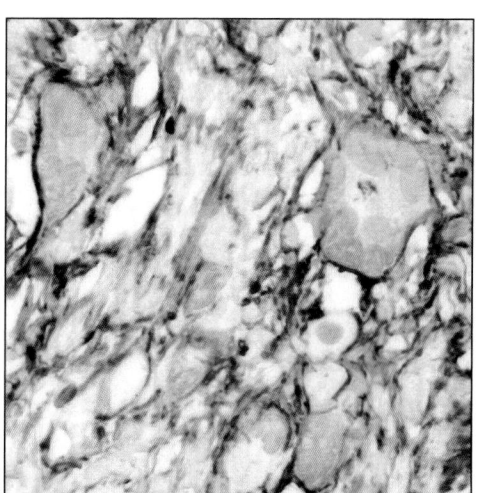

(Left) The multinucleated tumor giant cells in pleomorphic lipoma have peripherally arranged nuclei ⊅ and are described as "floret cells." *(Right)* CD34 immunostain is strongly positive in spindle cells and multinucleated floret cells in pleomorphic lipoma.

CHONDROID LIPOMA

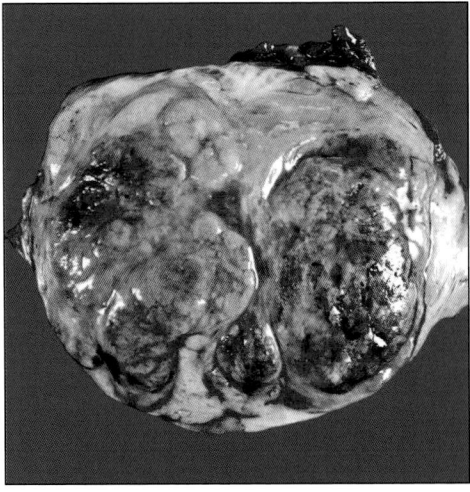

Gross photograph of chondroid lipoma shows a circumscribed lesion with a multilobulated, yellow to tan cut surface and prominent hemorrhage.

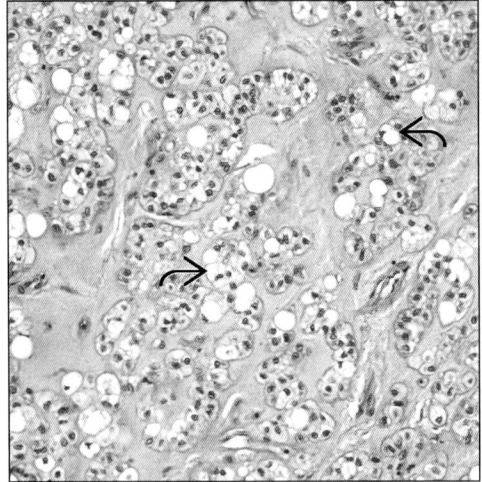

Chondroid lipoma shows islands of rounded cells in a hypocellular chondroid-like stroma. The cells are lipoblastic-like, with multivacuolated, lipid-containing cytoplasm ⇗. Mature adipocytes are present.

TERMINOLOGY

Definitions
- Uncommon benign neoplasm with features of embryonal fat and embryonal cartilage
  - Most frequently affects proximal limbs and limb girdles of adult women
- Often mistaken for sarcomas

ETIOLOGY/PATHOGENESIS

Developmental Anomaly
- Etiology unknown

CLINICAL ISSUES

Epidemiology
- Age
  - Adults, peak incidence in 3rd and 4th decades
- Gender
  - M:F = 1:4

Site
- Predominantly proximal limbs and limb girdles
- Trunk, head and neck (especially oral cavity)
- Both superficial (subcutaneous) and deep locations

Presentation
- Painless mass
  - Recent enlargement in 1/2 of cases

Treatment
- Surgical approaches
  - Simple complete excision

Prognosis
- Excision is curative
- Does not recur locally or metastasize

MACROSCOPIC FEATURES

General Features
- Frequently encapsulated with yellow to tan, sometimes hemorrhagic cut surface

Size
- 1.5-11 cm (median: 4 cm)

MICROSCOPIC PATHOLOGY

Histologic Features
- Lobulated
- Nests and cords of rounded cells
- Cytoplasm is eosinophilic and granular with intracytoplasmic glycogen or with lipid vacuoles, consistent with lipoblastic differentiation
- No significant atypia or mitotic activity
- Variable mature adipose tissue component
- Prominent myxoid to hyalinized chondroid matrix, containing Alcian blue(+), hyaluronidase-resistant chondroitin sulphate
- Interspersed thick- and thin-walled vessels
- Variable hemorrhage, hemosiderin deposition, fibrosis, and calcification

Margins
- Circumscribed

Predominant Pattern/Injury Type
- Adipocytic

ANCILLARY TESTS

Immunohistochemistry
- Variable positivity for S100 in lipoblasts
- Occasional focal cytokeratin positivity, but EMA(-)
- Focal CD68 positivity in vacuolated cells
- High expression of cyclin-D1 in all 4 cases in 1 study

CHONDROID LIPOMA

Key Facts

Terminology

- Uncommon benign neoplasm with features of embryonal fat and embryonal cartilage
- Balanced translocation t(11;16)(q13; p12-13) in some cases; thought to be specific for lesion

Clinical Issues

- Peak incidence in 3rd and 4th decades
- Female preponderance
- Occurs in superficial and deep locations

- Most frequently affects proximal limbs and limb girdles

Microscopic Pathology

- Nests and cords of rounded cells with granular eosinophilic cytoplasm or multivacuolated cytoplasm containing lipid
- Prominent myxohyaline stroma
- Variable amount of mature adipose tissue
- S100 protein and CD68 positive

Cytogenetics

- t(11;16)(q13;p12-13) in a few cases
  - Appears characteristic for this lesion
- Novel *C11orf95-MKL2* identified as resulting fusion oncogene in 3 cases

Electron Microscopy

- Spectrum of cellular differentiation
  - Primitive cells sharing features of prelipoblasts and chondroblasts
  - Lipoblasts and mature adipocytes
- Abundant intracytoplasmic lipid and glycogen
- Characteristic knob-like cytoplasmic protrusions

DIFFERENTIAL DIAGNOSIS

Soft Tissue Chondroma

- Hands and feet
- True hyaline cartilage matrix
- No adipocytic component

Myoepithelial Tumor

- Ductal/epithelial structures often present
- More pronounced and uniform cytokeratin positivity
- SMA, EMA, calponin positive

Myxoid Liposarcoma

- Deep location; can reach large size
- Spindle cell component
- Plexiform vascular pattern
- Round cell liposarcoma has larger cells, few vacuoles

- Characteristic translocations: t(12;16), t(12;22)

Extraskeletal Myxoid Chondrosarcoma

- Deep, slow-growing infiltrative tumor
- Can reach large size
- Multilobulated with fibrous septa
- Cells form anastomosing cords
- Cytoplasmic vacuoles usually absent
- No fatty component
- Characteristic translocations: t(9;17), t(9:22)

SELECTED REFERENCES

1. de Vreeze RS et al: Delineation of chondroid lipoma: an immunohistochemical and molecular biological analysis. Sarcoma. 2011:638403, 2011
2. Huang D et al: C11orf95-MKL2 is the resulting fusion oncogene of t(11;16)(q13;p13) in chondroid lipoma. Genes Chromosomes Cancer. 49(9):810-8, 2010
3. Ballaux F et al: Chondroid lipoma is characterized by t(11;16)(q13;p12-13). Virchows Arch. 444(2):208-10, 2004
4. Thomson TA et al: Cytogenetic and cytologic features of chondroid lipoma of soft tissue. Mod Pathol. 12(1):88-91, 1999
5. Kindblom LG et al: Chondroid lipoma: an ultrastructural and immunohistochemical analysis with further observations regarding its differentiation. Hum Pathol. 26(7):706-15, 1995
6. Meis JM et al: Chondroid lipoma. A unique tumor simulating liposarcoma and myxoid chondrosarcoma. Am J Surg Pathol. 17(11):1103-12, 1993

IMAGE GALLERY

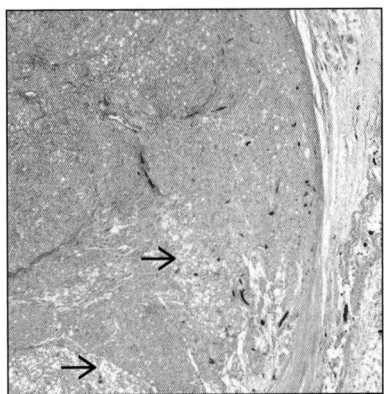 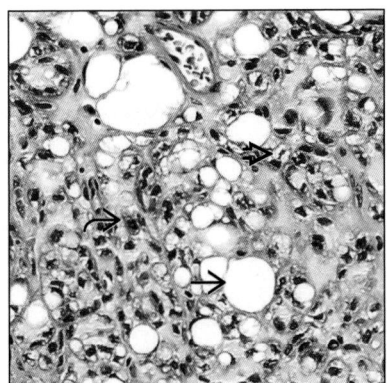 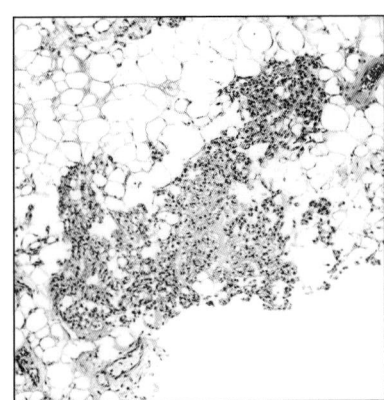

(Left) Low magnification shows a well-demarcated, encapsulated lesion within the subcutis. Cells with eosinophilic granular cytoplasm are admixed with mature adipocytes ➡. *(Center)* The cells have eosinophilic granular cytoplasm ➡ admixed with lipoblast-like cells ⇒ and mature adipocytes ➡. *(Right)* Core biopsy of chondroid lipoma shows a cellular proliferation of rounded cells within myxoid stroma, which can lead to an erroneous diagnosis of myxoid liposarcoma.

NEVUS LIPOMATOSUS

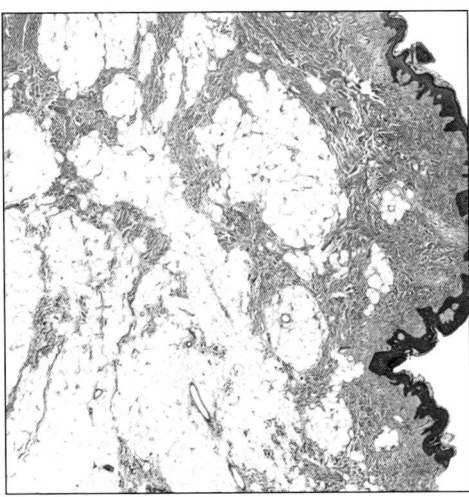

Nevus lipomatosus often appears polypoid and consists of mature fat within the dermis.

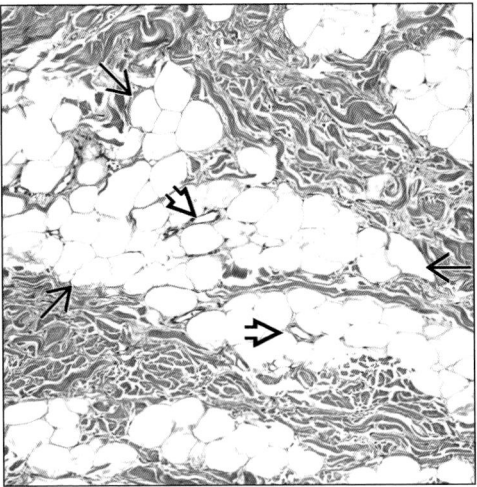

The aggregates of mature adipose tissue ➡ are often found around dermal blood vessels ⊅.

TERMINOLOGY

Synonyms
- Nevus lipomatosus superficialis
- Pedunculated lipofibroma

Definitions
- Connective tissue nevus/hamartoma characterized by mature adipose tissue in reticular dermis

ETIOLOGY/PATHOGENESIS

Unknown
- Most cases are idiopathic

Genetic
- Single case described with 2p24 deletion
  - Importance in pathogenesis remains unclear

CLINICAL ISSUES

Epidemiology
- Incidence
  - Uncommon
- Age
  - Classic form: Children and young adults
  - Solitary form: Adults
- Gender
  - Equal incidence in males and females

Site
- Posterior surfaces
  - Buttocks
  - Upper thigh
  - Lower back

Presentation
- Classic form
  - Multiple, grouped papules, polypoid lesions, or plaques
  - Rarely diffuse
  - Rarely associated with
    - Lipedematous scalp
    - Dermoid cysts
    - Folliculosebaceous cystic hamartoma
    - Angiokeratoma
- Solitary form
  - Locations similar to classic form
  - May also occur in areas where acrochordons present

Treatment
- Surgical approaches
  - Simple excision is curative
  - Laser removal also reported

Prognosis
- Excellent: Benign lesions
  - Primarily a cosmetic issue

MACROSCOPIC FEATURES

General Features
- Papule, plaque, or nodule with smooth or wrinkled surface
- Skin-colored to yellow appearance

MICROSCOPIC PATHOLOGY

Histologic Features
- Polypoid silhouette at low magnification
- Mature adipose tissue in upper dermis
  - Often clustered around dermal blood vessels
  - A few small, immature-appearing lipocytes may be present
- Increased numbers of small blood vessels
- Absence of adnexal structures
- No increased cellularity or cytologic atypia

NEVUS LIPOMATOSUS

Key Facts

Terminology
- Connective tissue nevus characterized by mature adipose tissue in reticular dermis

Clinical Issues
- Solitary or multiple grouped papules or polypoid lesions

Microscopic Pathology
- Mature adipose tissue in upper dermis

- Absence of adnexal structures

Top Differential Diagnoses
- Acrochordon (skin tag)
  ○ Lacks mature adipose tissue
- Lipoma
- Fibrolipoma
- Spindle cell lipoma
- Focal dermal hypoplasia
  ○ Clinically different

DIFFERENTIAL DIAGNOSIS

Acrochordon/Fibroepithelial Polyp (Skin Tag)
- Similar clinical/gross appearance
  ○ However, acrochordons typically show a thin stalk
- Acrochordons usually lack mature adipose tissue

Lipoma
- Presents deep to the dermis
- Well-circumscribed nodule of mature adipose tissue
- Lacks admixed reticular dermal collagen

Fibrolipoma
- Typically presents deep to the dermis
- Collagen bands represent fibrotic areas within lipoma, not reticular dermal collagen
- Term is also commonly used for acrochordons with adipose tissue

Spindle Cell Lipoma
- Presents on upper back, head and neck
- Usually tumor of subcutis
- Short fascicles of bland spindled cells
- Ropey collagen and myxoid stroma
- Frequent mast cells

Focal Dermal Hypoplasia (Goltz Syndrome)
- Histologically appears similar
  ○ But reticular dermis diminished
- Clinically different
  ○ Widespread, depressed, atrophic lesions

○ May have polypoid lesions from herniation of fat through atrophic dermis
○ Associated with skeletal abnormalities

SELECTED REFERENCES

1. Fatah S et al: Successful CO2 laser treatment of naevus lipomatosus cutaneous superficialis. Clin Exp Dermatol. 35(5):559-60, 2010
2. Cardot-Leccia N et al: Naevus lipomatosus superficialis: a case report with a 2p24 deletion. Br J Dermatol. 156(2):380-1, 2007
3. Kang H et al: Nevus lipomatosus cutaneous superficialis with folliculosebaceous cystic hamartoma. J Am Acad Dermatol. 56(2 Suppl):S55-7, 2007
4. Mansur AT et al: Colocalization of lipedematous scalp and nevus lipomatosus superficialis: a case report. J Cutan Pathol. 34(4):342-5, 2007
5. Orteu CH et al: Naevus lipomatosus cutaneous superficialis: overlap with connective tissue naevi. Acta Derm Venereol. 76(3):243-5, 1996
6. Eyre SP et al: Rubbery zosteriform nodules on the back. Nevus lipomatosus cutaneous superficialis (Hoffmann-Zurhelle). Arch Dermatol. 128(10):1395, 1398, 1992
7. Dotz W et al: Nevus lipomatosus cutaneus superficialis. A light and electron microscopic study. Arch Dermatol. 120(3):376-9, 1984
8. Lynch FW et al: Nevus lipomatosus cutaneus superficialis (Hoffmann-Zurhelle); presentation of a case and review of the literature. AMA Arch Derm. 78(4):479-82, 1958

IMAGE GALLERY

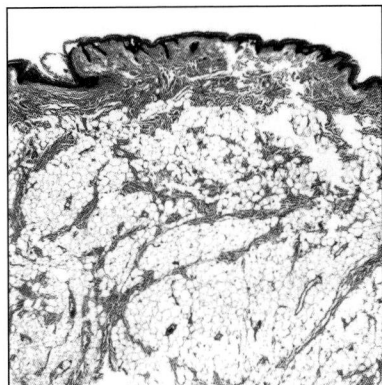 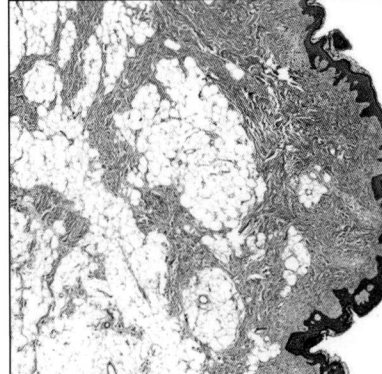 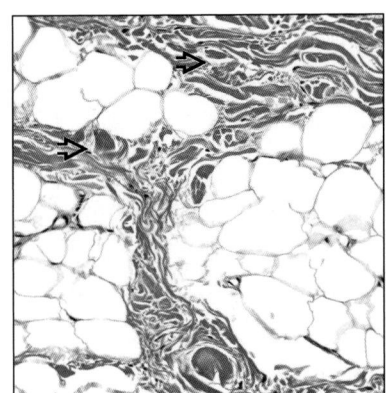

(Left) In this case of nevus lipomatosus superficialis, the mature adipose tissue is quite prominent and diffusely present throughout the dermis. *(Center)* There are lobular aggregates of mature adipose tissue in the dermis. Note the absence of normal adnexal structures. *(Right)* Note that the collagen otherwise resembles normal reticular dermis ⮞, with the characteristic spaces between the bands of eosinophilic-staining collagen.

HIBERNOMA

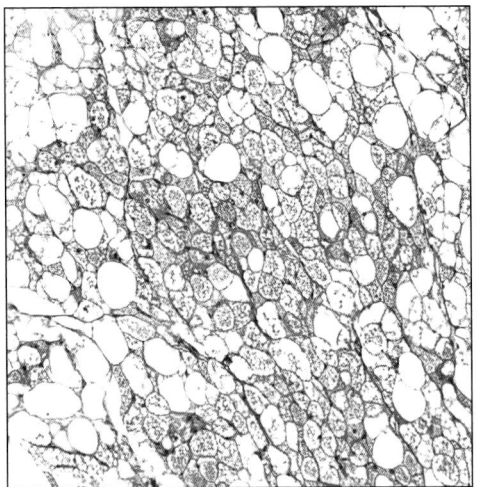

Low-power histologic view shows hibernoma, which is composed of well-defined lobules of polygonal cells. Bland cells with the appearance of brown fat are mixed with mature adipocytes. No atypia is present.

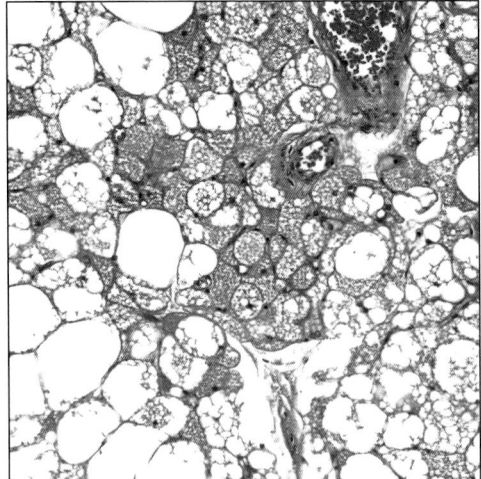

Hibernoma is shown at higher magnification, comprising an admixture of polygonal cells with granular eosinophilic or multivacuolated cytoplasm. Univacuolated adipocytes are also seen.

TERMINOLOGY

Synonyms
- Fetal lipoma, lipoma of embryonic fat

Definitions
- Benign tumor most frequently occurring in younger adults, with differentiation toward brown fat
  o Tumor has characteristic cytogenetic aberrations, mainly involving 11q13-21

ETIOLOGY/PATHOGENESIS

Developmental Anomaly
- Etiology unknown
  o Many occur at sites of normal brown fat in fetuses and newborns
  o Genetic changes in some

CLINICAL ISSUES

Epidemiology
- Incidence
  o Rare; approximately 1% of all adipocytic tumors
- Age
  o Peak incidence: 3rd decade
  o Rare in children
- Gender
  o M = F

Site
- Most tumors subcutaneous; approximately 10% intramuscular
- Thigh is most common site
- Shoulder, back, trunk, abdomen, retroperitoneum

Presentation
- Painless mass
- Slow enlargement

Treatment
- Surgical approaches
  o Simple complete excision

Prognosis
- Excellent; excision is curative
- Does not recur or metastasize

MACROSCOPIC FEATURES

General Features
- Circumscribed, lobulated lesions
- Tan to brown, greasy, sometimes mucoid cut surface

Size
- Range: 1-24 cm (mean: 9.3 cm)

MICROSCOPIC PATHOLOGY

Histologic Features
- Lobulated tumor composed of sheets of cells of varying types
  o Polygonal cells with granular eosinophilic cytoplasm
  o Multivacuolated cells with lipid droplets
  o Univacuolated adipocytes
- Small, bland, central nuclei
- Mitotic figures exceptional
- Myxoid variant
  o Predominantly occurs in males, head and neck region
  o Constituent cells separated by acellular myxoid stroma
- Lipoma-like variant
  o Most common in thigh
  o Mostly univacuolated adipocytes, few hibernoma cells
- Spindle cell variant
  o Rare; found in posterior neck or scalp

HIBERNOMA

Key Facts

Terminology
- Benign tumor with differentiation toward brown fat, most frequently seen in younger adults

Clinical Issues
- Peak incidence in 3rd decade
- Most tumors subcutaneous
- Thigh is most common site
- Can occur in abdomen and retroperitoneum

Microscopic Pathology
- Variable differentiation toward brown fat
- Cells are granular, multivacuolated, or univacuolated adipocytes
- Myxoid, lipoma-like, and spindle cell variants
- Cellular atypia unusual; mitoses exceptional

Ancillary Tests
- Variable, sometimes strong positivity for S100
- Rearrangements of 11q13-21 in several cases

  - ○ Hibernoma cells, thick collagen bundles, mast cells, mature fat

Predominant Cell/Compartment Type
- Adipose

ANCILLARY TESTS

Immunohistochemistry
- Variable, sometimes strong positivity for S100 protein
- Spindle cell variant may show CD34 positivity

Cytogenetics
- Rearrangements of 11q13-21 in several cases
  - ○ t(9;11)(q34;q13) in 1 case

Electron Microscopy
- Transmission
  - ○ Numerous mitochondria, lipid droplets

DIFFERENTIAL DIAGNOSIS

Residual Brown Fat
- Upper chest and neck, no mass lesion
- Associated with reactive lymph nodes

Lipoblastoma
- Usually in 1st 3 years of life
- Spindle cells, myxoid stroma, vascular pattern

Adult Rhabdomyoma
- Most common in head and neck
- Large polygonal cells, abundant cytoplasm
- Cross striations
- Immunoreactive for desmin and myogenin (nuclear)

Chondroid Lipoma
- Clusters of vacuolated cells
- Chondromyxoid stroma

Atypical Lipomatous Tumor/Well-Differentiated Liposarcoma
- Atypical cells in fibrous septa
- Lipoblasts with hyperchromatic scalloped nuclei
- Immunoreactivity for MDM2 and CDK4

Myxoid Liposarcoma
- Deep location
- Plexiform vascular pattern, lipoblasts
- Round cell component
- Characteristic translocations t(12;16), t(12;22)

SELECTED REFERENCES

1. Chirieac LR et al: Characterization of the myxoid variant of hibernoma. Ann Diagn Pathol. 10(2):104-6, 2006
2. Furlong MA et al: The morphologic spectrum of hibernoma: a clinicopathologic study of 170 cases. Am J Surg Pathol. 25(6):809-14, 2001
3. Mertens F et al: Hibernomas are characterized by rearrangements of chromosome bands 11q13-21. Int J Cancer. 58(4):503-5, 1994

IMAGE GALLERY

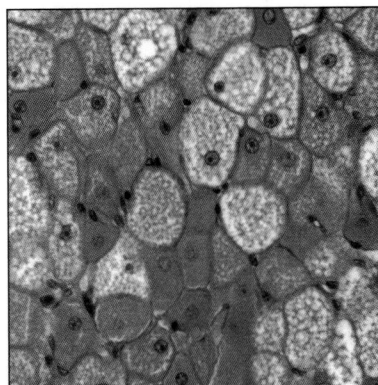 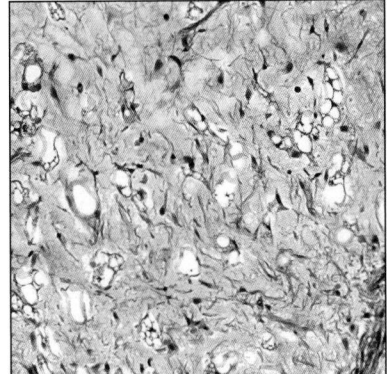 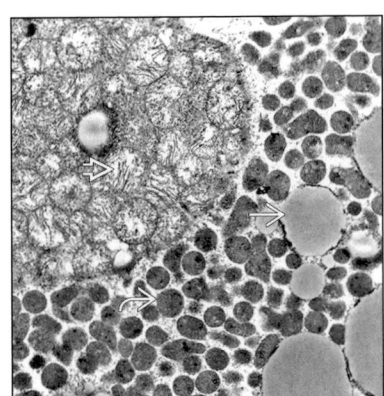

(Left) High-power view of hibernoma shows polygonal cells with well-defined cell borders and abundant finely granular eosinophilic cytoplasm or numerous cytoplasmic lipid vacuoles. *(Center)* Myxoid variant of hibernoma. Small foci of brown fat cells and mature adipocytes are dispersed in a myxoid stroma. *(Right)* EM of hibernoma shows numerous tightly packed mitochondria displaying transverse cristae ➡. There are also small electron-dense lysosomes ➡ and lipid droplets ➡.

ATYPICAL LIPOMATOUS TUMOR AND LIPOSARCOMA

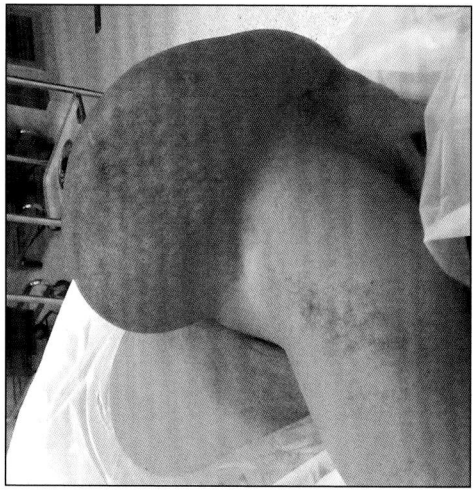

A large lipomatous tumor on the shoulder of a male patient is shown. This image was taken at the time of an operation to remove the lesion.

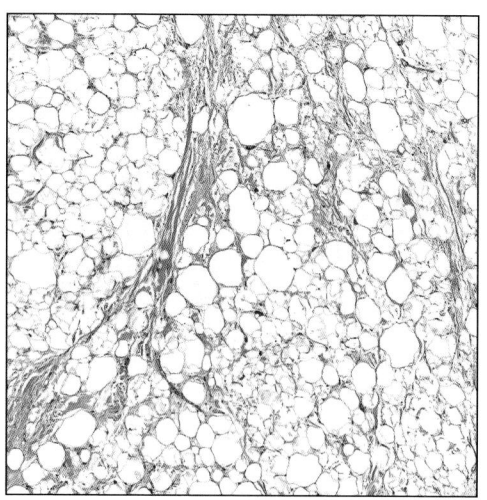

Histologic examination of ALT shows striking variations in size and shape of lipogenic cells, as well as scattered enlarged cells with enlarged hyperchromatic nuclei.

TERMINOLOGY

Abbreviations
- Atypical lipomatous tumor (ALT)

Synonyms
- Well-differentiated liposarcoma (WDLS)

Definitions
- Intermediate (locally aggressive, nonmetastasizing) lipogenic neoplasm composed of atypical adipocytes

CLINICAL ISSUES

Epidemiology
- Incidence
  - Accounts for 40-45% of all liposarcomas
  - Most frequently in deep soft tissues
    - Retroperitoneum, abdominal cavity, paratesticular region, mediastinum
    - Limbs
  - May also arise in subcutaneous tissue and very rarely in skin
- Age
  - Middle-aged to elderly adults
  - Extremely rare in childhood
- Gender
  - M = F

Presentation
- Deep-seated, painless, slowly enlarging tumor mass

Treatment
- Complete surgical excision

Prognosis
- In surgically amenable sites
  - Recur only rarely after complete excision
- Intraabdominal, retroperitoneal, mediastinal, or paratesticular lesions
  - Often recur locally and may be fatal
- Variable risk of dedifferentiation in extremities (< 2%) and in retroperitoneum (> 20%)

IMAGE FINDINGS

General Features
- Best diagnostic clue
  - Circumscribed, lobular mass
- Location
  - Deep soft tissues
- Size
  - Variable
  - Usually > 5 cm
- Morphology
  - Circumscribed, lipomatous lesion

MACROSCOPIC FEATURES

General Features
- Well-circumscribed lobular neoplasms
- Color varies from yellow to white
- Fat necrosis may be seen in large lesions

Sections to Be Submitted
- Sample margins and representative sections of tumor
- Look for indurated, firm areas

Size
- May attain very large size

MICROSCOPIC PATHOLOGY

Histologic Features
- **Lipoma-like subtype**
  - Adipocytes show significant variation in size and shape
  - Enlarged hyperchromatic nuclei
  - Hyperchromatic and multinucleated stromal cells

ATYPICAL LIPOMATOUS TUMOR AND LIPOSARCOMA

Key Facts

Terminology

- Intermediate (locally aggressive, nonmetastasizing) lipogenic neoplasm composed of atypical adipocytes

Clinical Issues

- Accounts for 40-45% of all liposarcomas
- Occurs most frequently in deep soft tissues of limbs followed by retroperitoneum, abdominal cavity, paratesticular region, and mediastinum
- Usually presents as deep-seated, painless, and slowly enlarging tumor mass
- Lesions located in surgically amenable soft tissues recur only rarely after complete excision
- Neoplasms arising in intraabdominal, retroperitoneum, mediastinum, or spermatic cord often recur repeatedly and may cause death

- Variable risk of dedifferentiation in extremities (< 2%) and retroperitoneum (> 25%)
- May also arise in subcutaneous tissue and very rarely in skin
- Middle-aged to elderly adults
- Intermediate (locally aggressive but nonmetastasizing) malignant mesenchymal tumor

Microscopic Pathology

- Atypical adipocytes, atypical stromal cells, lipoblasts
  ○ Adipocytes show striking variations in size and shape
  ○ Enlarged hyperchromatic nuclei
- Lipoma-like subtype
- Sclerosing subtype
- Inflammatory subtype
- Spindle cell subtype

○ Lipoblasts may be seen, but are not essential for diagnosis
○ Involvement of large vessel walls by atypical tumor cells
○ Prominent myxoid stromal changes may be present
○ Rare chondroid stromal changes
- **Sclerosing subtype**
  ○ Scattered bizarre stromal cells with hyperchromatic nuclei
  ○ Rare atypical lipogenic cells and multivacuolated lipoblasts
  ○ Fibrillary, collagenous stroma
- **Inflammatory subtype**
  ○ Prominent inflammatory infiltrate (lymphocytes, plasma cells)
  ○ Scattered atypical lipogenic cells/lipoblasts
  ○ Often edematous stroma
- **Spindle cell subtype**
  ○ Atypical lipogenic cells
  ○ Slightly atypical neuroid spindle cells
  ○ Fibrous, fibromyxoid stroma
- **Heterologous differentiation rarely seen**
  ○ Smooth or striated muscle
  ○ Cartilage, bone

Predominant Pattern/Injury Type

- Circumscribed

Predominant Cell/Compartment Type

- Adipose
  ○ Atypical adipocytes, atypical stromal cells, lipoblasts

Grade

- Intermediate (locally aggressive but nonmetastasizing) malignant mesenchymal tumor

ANCILLARY TESTS

Cytogenetics

- Supernumerary ring and giant marker chromosomes
  ○ Contain amplified sequences originating from 12q14-15 region

○ *MDM2, CDK4, SAS, HMGIC* are amplified

In Situ Hybridization

- *MDM2* and *CDK4* amplification can be identified by FISH-technique

DIFFERENTIAL DIAGNOSIS

Lipoma

- Lobular growth pattern
- No or only slight atypia of adipocytes
- Lack increased number of enlarged and hyperchromatic nuclei
- No lipoblasts should be identifiable
- No amplification of *MDM2* &/or *CDK4*

Spindle Cell and Pleomorphic Lipoma

- Usually occurs in elderly male patients
- Arises usually in subcutaneous tissues of neck, shoulder, or upper back
- No or only slight atypia of adipocytes
- Bland CD34 positive spindled &/or multinucleated giant cells ("floret-like giant cells")
- Rope-like collagen bundles
- Often myxoid stromal changes
- Scattered mast cells
- No amplification of *MDM2* &/or *CDK4*

Pseudolipoblastic Granulomatous Foreign Body Reaction

- Multivacuolated, CD68 positive histiocytes
- No atypical lipogenic cells

Angiomyolipoma

- Myogenic tumor cells expressing myogenic and melanocytic markers (currently considered type of PEComa)
- Often associated with tuberous sclerosis
- Thick-walled blood vessels
- Predominantly renal/perirenal tissues

ATYPICAL LIPOMATOUS TUMOR AND LIPOSARCOMA

Immunohistochemistry

Antibody	Reactivity	Staining Pattern	Comment
CDK4	Positive	Nuclear	Focal expression; may be negative; reactive histiocytes may be positive as well
MDM2	Positive	Nuclear	Focal expression; may be negative; reactive histiocytes may be positive as well

Inflammatory Myofibroblastic Tumor

- Fascicles of myofibroblastic spindled cells in mixed inflammatory cell background
- No atypical lipogenic tumor component
- Expression of ALK in a number of cases (especially in children and adolescents)

Sclerosing Lipoma

- Dermal-based neoplasms
- Typically present on scalp or hands of young adult males
- No atypical lipogenic tumor cells

Dedifferentiated Liposarcoma

- Abrupt or gradual transition from atypical lipomatous tissue to nonlipogenic component
- Atypical nonlipogenic tumor component with variable morphologic features, but typically high-grade spindle cell tumor
- Strong expression of MDM2 and CDK4

Angiolipoma

- Subcutaneous nodules in young adults
- Often multiple lesions
- Often tender to painful clinically
- Forearm represents most common site
- Mature fat separated by small blood vessels
- Vascular channels typically contain fibrin thrombi

DIAGNOSTIC CHECKLIST

Clinically Relevant Pathologic Features

- Gross appearance
- Organ distribution
- Age distribution

Pathologic Interpretation Pearls

- Atypical lipogenic cells
- Atypical stromal cells
- Often focal nuclear expression of MDM2 &/or CDK4
- Amplification of MDM2 and CDK4 detected by FISH-analysis

SELECTED REFERENCES

1. Evans HL: Atypical lipomatous tumor, its variants, and its combined forms: a study of 61 cases, with a minimum follow-up of 10 years. Am J Surg Pathol. 31(1):1-14, 2007
2. Sirvent N et al: Detection of MDM2-CDK4 amplification by fluorescence in situ hybridization in 200 paraffin-embedded tumor samples: utility in diagnosing adipocytic lesions and comparison with immunohistochemistry and real-time PCR. Am J Surg Pathol. 31(10):1476-89, 2007
3. Binh MB et al: MDM2 and CDK4 immunostainings are useful adjuncts in diagnosing well-differentiated and dedifferentiated liposarcoma subtypes: a comparative analysis of 559 soft tissue neoplasms with genetic data. Am J Surg Pathol. 29(10):1340-7, 2005
4. Folpe AL et al: Lipoleiomyosarcoma (well-differentiated liposarcoma with leiomyosarcomatous differentiation): a clinicopathologic study of nine cases including one with dedifferentiation. Am J Surg Pathol. 26(6):742-9, 2002
5. Micci F et al: Characterization of supernumerary rings and giant marker chromosomes in well-differentiated lipomatous tumors by a combination of G-banding, CGH, M-FISH, and chromosome- and locus-specific FISH. Cytogenet Genome Res. 97(1-2):13-9, 2002
6. Dei Tos AP et al: Coordinated expression and amplification of the MDM2, CDK4, and HMGI-C genes in atypical lipomatous tumours. J Pathol. 190(5):531-6, 2000
7. Pedeutour F et al: Structure of the supernumerary ring and giant rod chromosomes in adipose tissue tumors. Genes Chromosomes Cancer. 24(1):30-41, 1999
8. Dei Tos AP et al: Primary liposarcoma of the skin: a rare neoplasm with unusual high grade features. Am J Dermatopathol. 20(4):332-8, 1998
9. Kraus MD et al: Well-differentiated inflammatory liposarcoma: an uncommon and easily overlooked variant of a common sarcoma. Am J Surg Pathol. 21(5):518-27, 1997
10. Fletcher CD et al: Correlation between clinicopathological features and karyotype in lipomatous tumors. A report of 178 cases from the Chromosomes and Morphology (CHAMP) Collaborative Study Group. Am J Pathol. 148(2):623-30, 1996
11. Mentzel T et al: Lipomatous tumours of soft tissues: an update. Virchows Arch. 427(4):353-63, 1995
12. Nilbert M et al: Characterization of the 12q13-15 amplicon in soft tissue tumors. Cancer Genet Cytogenet. 83(1):32-6, 1995
13. Dal Cin P et al: Cytogenetic and fluorescence in situ hybridization investigation of ring chromosomes characterizing a specific pathologic subgroup of adipose tissue tumors. Cancer Genet Cytogenet. 68(2):85-90, 1993
14. Weiss SW et al: Well-differentiated liposarcoma (atypical lipoma) of deep soft tissue of the extremities, retroperitoneum, and miscellaneous sites. A follow-up study of 92 cases with analysis of the incidence of "dedifferentiation". Am J Surg Pathol. 16(11):1051-8, 1992
15. Azumi N et al: Atypical and malignant neoplasms showing lipomatous differentiation. A study of 111 cases. Am J Surg Pathol. 11(3):161-83, 1987
16. Bolen JW et al: Liposarcomas. A histogenetic approach to the classification of adipose tissue neoplasms. Am J Surg Pathol. 8(1):3-17, 1984
17. Kindblom LG et al: Atypical lipoma. Acta Pathol Microbiol Immunol Scand [A]. 90(1):27-36, 1982
18. Evans HL et al: Atypical lipoma, atypical intramuscular lipoma, and well differentiated retroperitoneal liposarcoma: a reappraisal of 30 cases formerly classified as well differentiated liposarcoma. Cancer. 43(2):574-84, 1979

ATYPICAL LIPOMATOUS TUMOR AND LIPOSARCOMA

Gross and Microscopic Features

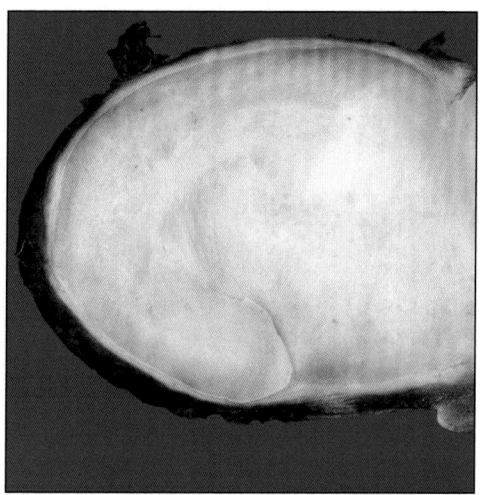

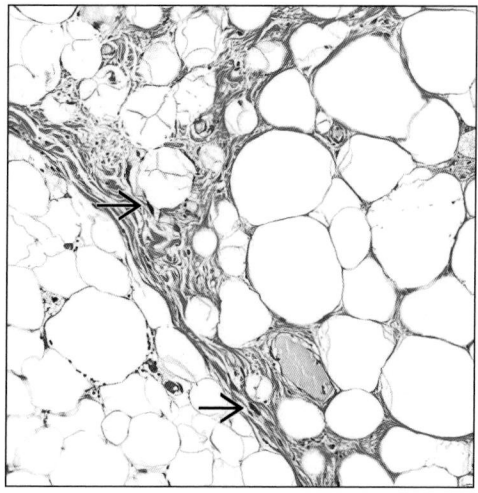

(Left) *Gross pathology photograph shows indurated, gray-white cut surface in this example of an atypical lipomatous tumor, in contrast to nonneoplastic fatty tissue.* **(Right)** *Histologic examination shows the lipoma-like subtype of an atypical lipomatous tumor with variation in size and shape of lipogenic tumor cells and scattered cells with enlarged, hyperchromatic-staining nuclei* ➡.

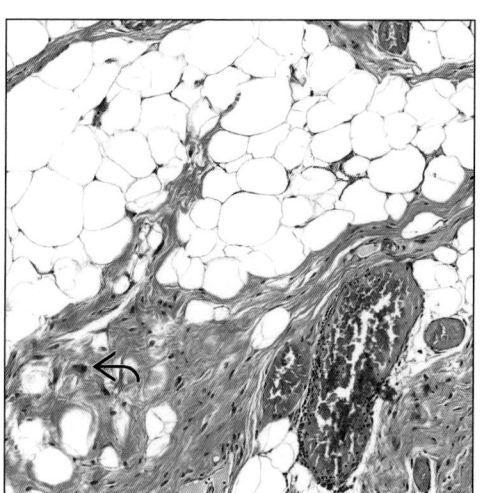

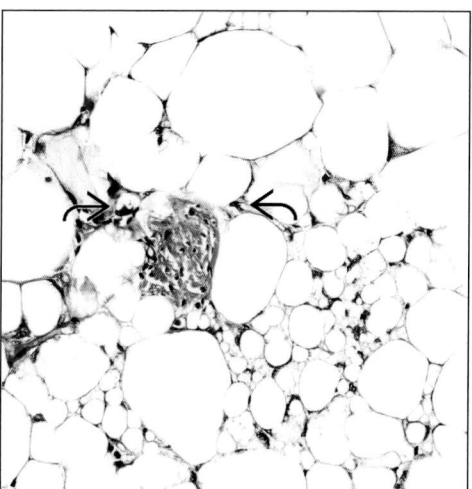

(Left) *Low magnification of ALT shows fibrous septa with enlarged cells containing irregularly shaped, hyperchromatic nuclei* ➡. **(Right)** *Examination of another example of ALT shows scattered lipoblasts* ➡ *in a perivascular location.*

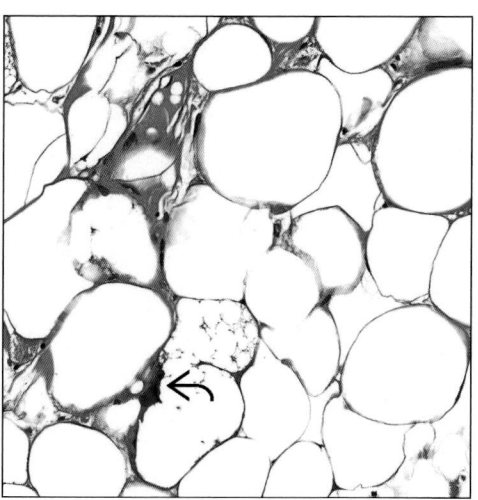

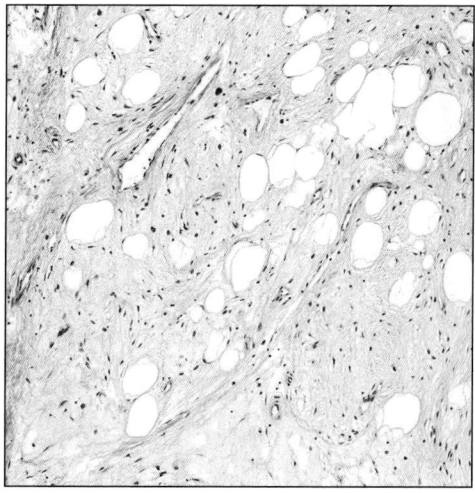

(Left) *Higher magnification shows multivacuolated lipoblasts containing hyperchromatic nuclei* ➡. *Note the indentation of the hyperchromatic nuclei.* **(Right)** *Low magnification shows the lipoma-like subtype of an atypical lipomatous tumor with myxoid stromal changes.*

Microscopic and Immunohistochemical Features

(Left) Low magnification shows the lipoma-like subtype of an atypical lipomatous tumor with a focus of chondroid metaplasia. The cartilaginous tissue appears histologically benign. *(Right)* S100 immunostaining shows lipogenic cells of variable size and shape and multivacuolated lipoblasts.

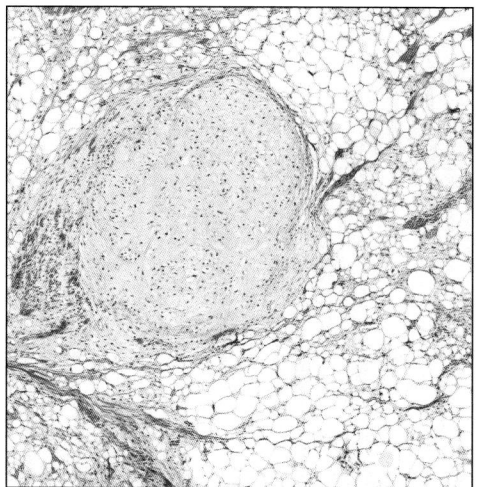
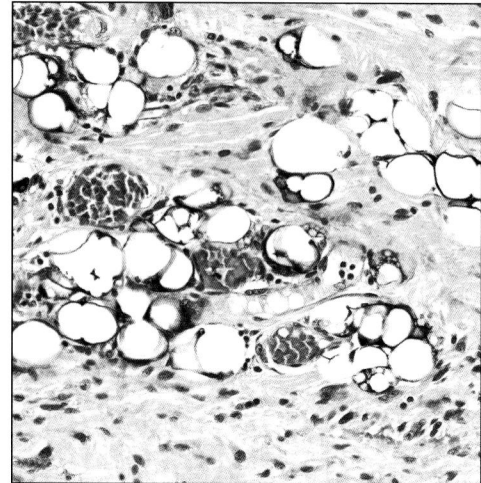

(Left) MDM2 immunostaining shows focal nuclear expression ➡. *(Right)* CDK4 immunostaining shows focal nuclear expression in this atypical lipomatous tumor.

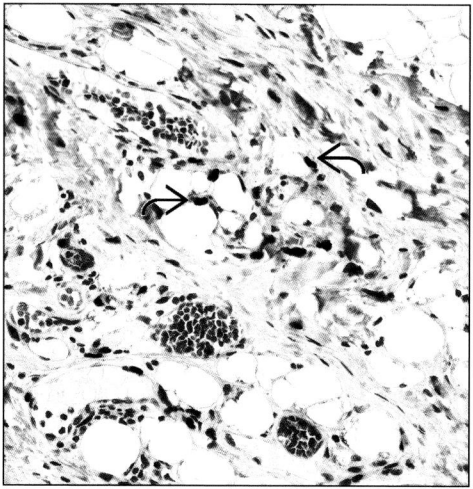
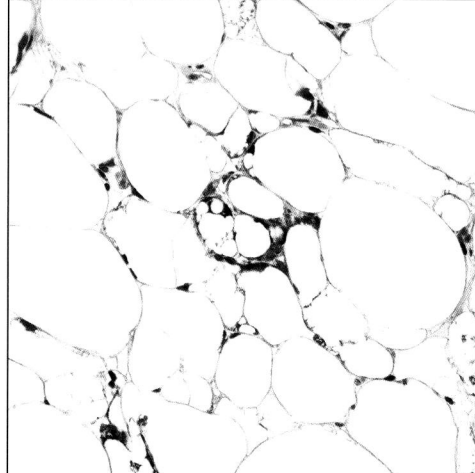

(Left) Histologic examination shows scattered lipogenic cells including bivacuolated lipoblasts ➡ set in a prominent collagenous stroma in this example of the sclerosing subtype of an atypical lipomatous tumor. *(Right)* Low magnification shows an example of the inflammatory subtype of an atypical lipomatous tumor with a prominent inflammatory infiltrate, edematous stroma, and only scattered atypical lipogenic tumor cells ➡.

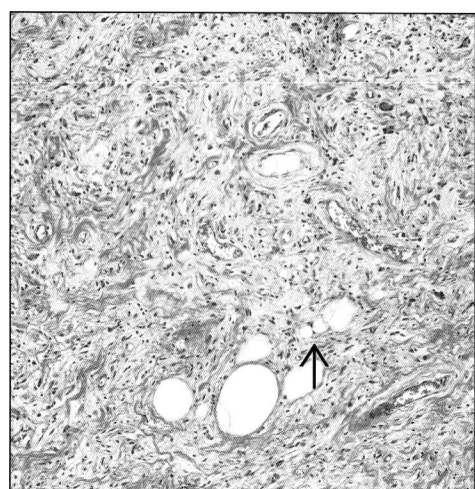
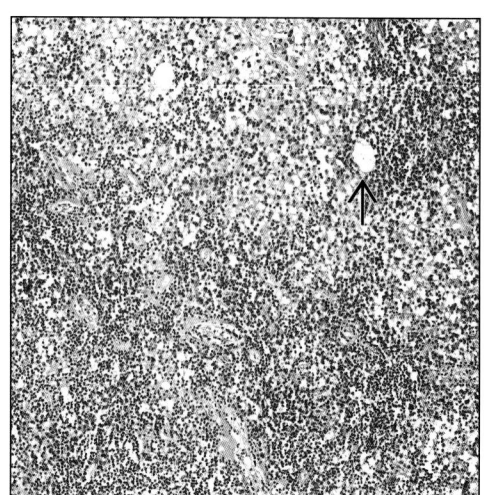

ATYPICAL LIPOMATOUS TUMOR AND LIPOSARCOMA

Microscopic Features and FISH-Analysis

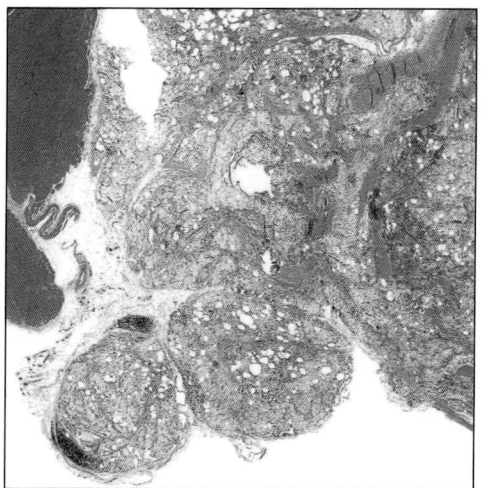

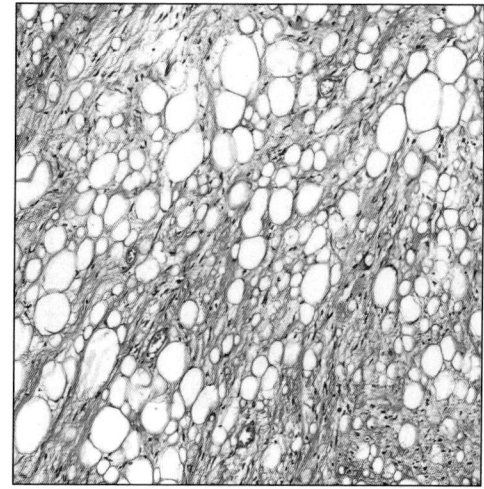

(Left) Low-magnification examination of this spindle cell subtype of an atypical lipomatous tumor shows a deep-seated lobular neoplasm. *(Right)* Higher magnification shows an atypical lipomatous tumor of the spindle cell subtype with atypical lipogenic cells admixed with slightly enlarged spindled tumor cells.

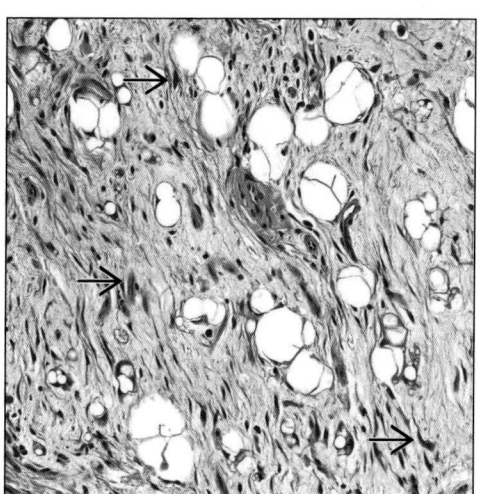

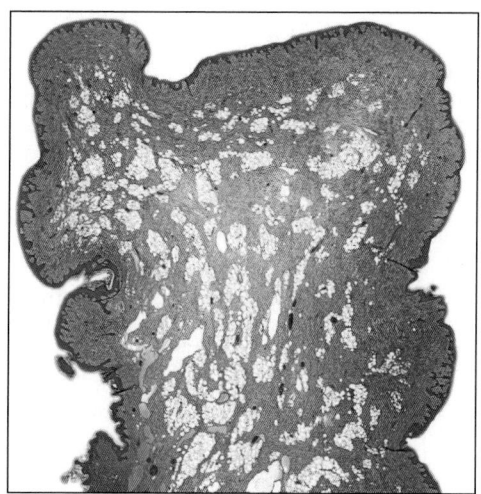

(Left) High-power examination shows a neoplasm composed of atypical lipogenic and spindled tumor cells ➡ with enlarged and hyperchromatic nuclei. *(Right)* Histologic examination shows a low-power view of a rare cutaneous atypical lipomatous tumor with a polypoid configuration.

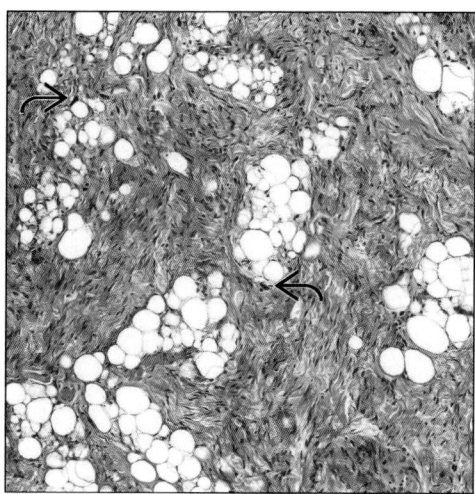

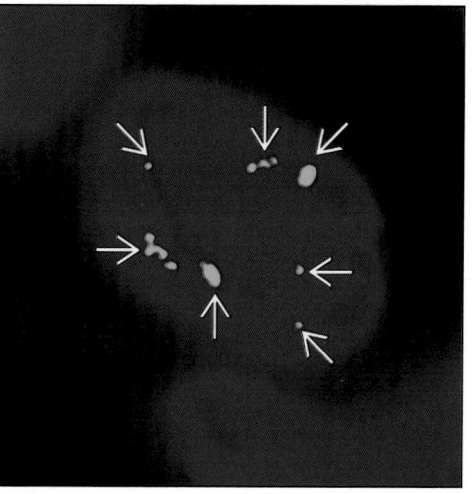

(Left) Higher power examination shows a cutaneous atypical lipomatous tumor as an ill-defined dermal neoplasm composed of atypical lipogenic cells with enlarged and hyperchromatic-staining nuclei ➡. *(Right)* In situ hybridization FISH-analysis shows MDM2 amplification. Note numerous signals ➡ in an analyzed tumor cell nucleus.

CHONDROMA

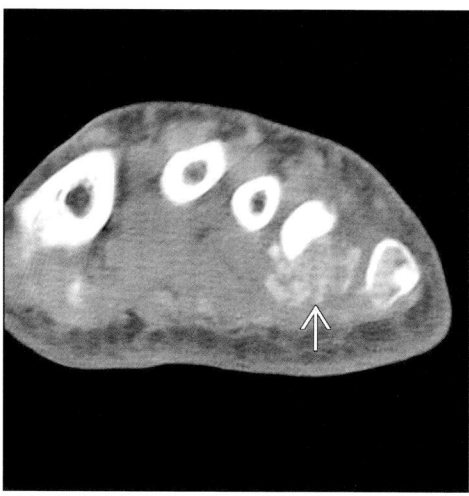

CT depicts a mineralized soft tissue chondroma ➡️ adjacent to the 4th metatarsal. Soft tissue chondroma has a predilection for the hands and feet, often near a joint or tendon.

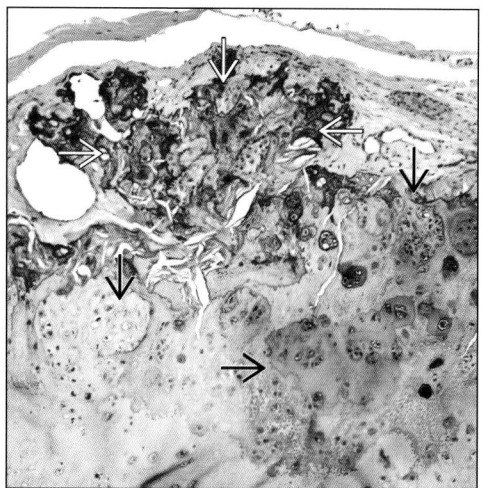

Soft tissue chondroma typically appears as a well-circumscribed tumor composed of hyaline cartilage lobules ➡️ with extensive calcification ➡️ and sharp demarcation from adjacent soft tissue (top).

TERMINOLOGY

Synonyms
- Extraskeletal chondroma, chondroma of soft parts, fibrochondroma, osteochondroma, myxochondroma, chondroblastoma-like chondroma of soft tissue

Definitions
- Benign hyaline cartilage neoplasm of soft tissue with predilection for hands and feet
- Only rare reports of primary cutaneous tumors (chondroma cutis)

CLINICAL ISSUES

Epidemiology
- Incidence
  - Uncommon; exact incidence unknown
  - Exceedingly rare as cutaneous primary
- Age
  - Median: 4th decade; range: Infancy to 9th decade
- Gender
  - Women and men equally affected

Presentation
- Painless mass
- Most common in hands and feet (60-95%), especially fingers (40-50%)
  - Rare reports in proximal extremities, trunk, head and neck, upper aerodigestive tract, dura, skin, fallopian tube

Treatment
- Surgical approaches
  - Simple excision

Prognosis
- Low recurrence rate (15-20%)
  - Recurrences controlled by reexcision
- No reports of malignant degeneration

IMAGE FINDINGS

General Features
- Best diagnostic clue
  - Small, well-demarcated, mineralized soft tissue mass in acral extremity
- Location
  - Hands and feet
  - Often in vicinity of joint or tendon
  - No intraarticular or subperiosteal localization by definition
- Morphology
  - Most are calcified or ossified
  - Sometimes erode and deform underlying bone

MACROSCOPIC FEATURES

General Features
- Well demarcated, spherical or ovoid
- Rubbery or hard
- Sometimes soft, friable, gelatinous, or cystic

Size
- Median: 1.6 cm; range: 0.3-6.5 cm

MICROSCOPIC PATHOLOGY

Histologic Features
- Well-circumscribed and lobulated deep dermal &/or subcutaneous tumor
- Mostly composed of mature hyaline cartilage
- Chondrocytes located in lacunae
  - Arranged diffusely or in small clusters
  - Some have enlarged nuclei and moderate pleomorphism
  - Very low mitotic rate
- Variable amounts of calcification

CHONDROMA

Key Facts

Terminology

- Benign hyaline cartilage neoplasm of soft tissue with predilection for hands and feet
- Synonyms: Extraskeletal chondroma, chondroma of soft parts, osteochondroma, myxochondroma

Clinical Issues

- Low recurrence rate (15-20%)
- Recurrences controlled by reexcision
- No reports of malignant degeneration

Image Findings

- Small, well-demarcated, mineralized soft tissue mass in acral extremity

Macroscopic Features

- Median size: 1.6 cm; range: 0.3-6.5 cm

Microscopic Pathology

- Well-circumscribed and lobulated
- Mostly composed of mature hyaline cartilage
- Variable amounts of calcification
- Ossification common
- Granulomatous inflammation in 15% of cases
- Rare tumors with extensive xanthogranulomatous inflammation
- Chondroblastoma-like chondroma

Top Differential Diagnoses

- Tumoral calcinosis
- Tophaceous pseudogout
- Synovial chondromatosis
- Extraskeletal myxoid chondrosarcoma
- Calcifying aponeurotic fibroma

- o Granular stippled calcification that surrounds chondrocytes in lace-like pattern
- o Some have extensive calcification with deep basophilia of matrix
- Ossification common
- Granulomatous inflammation in 15% of cases
  - o Epithelioid macrophages and osteoclastic giant cells
  - o Most pronounced in heavily calcified tumors
- Rare tumors with extensive xanthogranulomatous inflammation mimicking fibrous histiocytoma or giant cell tumor of tendon sheath
- Rare tumors with extensive stromal fibrosis (fibrochondroma)
- **Chondroblastoma-like chondroma**
  - o Abundant myxoid matrix
  - o Immature chondrocytes
    - Polygonal or elongated cells
    - Abundant eosinophilic or vacuolated cytoplasm
    - Eccentrically located nuclei, often grooved or reniform, resembling cells of chondroblastoma

DIFFERENTIAL DIAGNOSIS

Tumoral Calcinosis

- Predilection for large joints
- Calcium hydroxyapatite crystals (psammomatous)
- Histiocytic giant cells with intracytoplasmic calcifications

Tophaceous Pseudogout

- Wide distribution, including acral extremities, but predilection for temporomandibular joint
- Heavily calcified lesions with metaplastic cartilage formation
- Rhomboid-shaped CPPD crystals with positive birefringence under polarized light

Synovial Chondromatosis

- Larger tumors
- Most often in synovium of large joints, especially knee, but also tenosynovium of acral extremities

- More discrete lobular architecture and chondrocyte clusters

Calcifying Aponeurotic Fibroma

- Hands and feet, especially palm of children
- Geographic areas of calcification surrounded by chondrocytic cells
- Extensive fibromatous areas

Extraskeletal Myxoid Chondrosarcoma

- Large, lobulated soft tissue mass
- Myxoid matrix, thick fibrous septa, and cords of neoplastic cells

DIAGNOSTIC CHECKLIST

Clinically Relevant Pathologic Features

- Tissue distribution

Pathologic Interpretation Pearls

- Features that can lead to misdiagnosis
  - o Chondrocyte atypia
  - o Increased cellularity
  - o Extensive calcification and ossification
  - o Granulomatous or xanthogranulomatous reaction
  - o Fibrous, myxoid, and chondroblastoma-like features

SELECTED REFERENCES

1. Fetsch JF et al: Tenosynovial (extraarticular) chondromatosis: an analysis of 37 cases of an underrecognized clinicopathologic entity with a strong predilection for the hands and feet and a high local recurrence rate. Am J Surg Pathol. 27(9):1260-8, 2003
2. Cates JM et al: Chondroblastoma-like chondroma of soft tissue: an underrecognized variant and its differential diagnosis. Am J Surg Pathol. 25(5):661-6, 2001
3. Ando K et al: Cutaneous cartilaginous tumor. Dermatol Surg. 21(4):339-41, 1995
4. Hsueh S et al: Cartilaginous lesions of the skin and superficial soft tissue. J Cutan Pathol. 9(6):405-16, 1982
5. Dahlin DC et al: Cartilaginous tumors of the soft tissues of the hands and feet. Mayo Clin Proc. 49(10):721-6, 1974

CHONDROMA

Microscopic Features

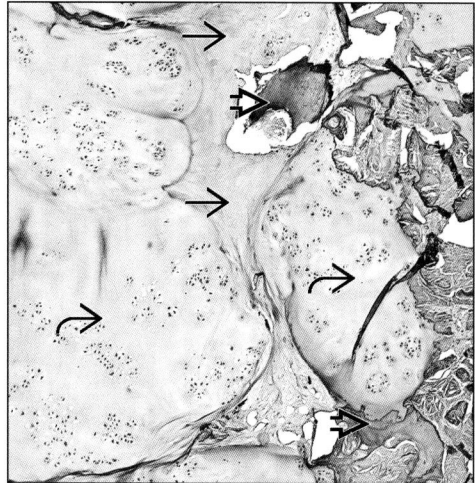

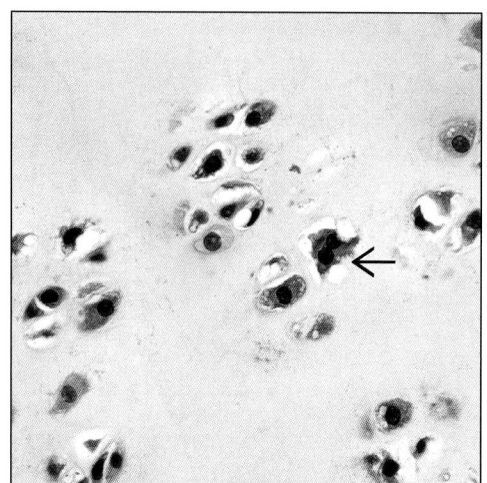

(Left) Soft tissue chondroma typically has a lobular architecture with islands of hyaline cartilage ⇗ separated by fibrous bands ⇥. Ossification ⇲ is common. (Right) High-power micrograph illustrates typical cytological features. The chondrocytes are often arranged in clusters, situated in lacunar spaces within pale blue hyaline matrix, and have uniform round nuclei and abundant eosinophilic cytoplasm. Rare binucleated cells can be seen ⇥. Mitoses are rare.

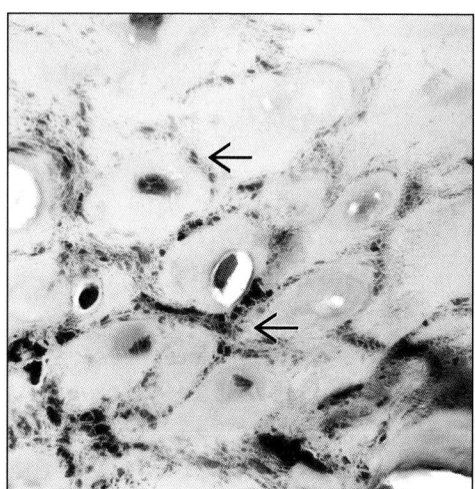

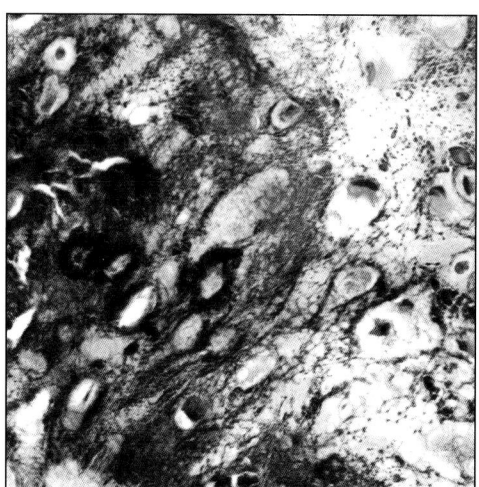

(Left) Calcification is very common in soft tissue chondroma. It appears as granular basophilic stippling of the matrix, which often surrounds individual chondrocytes to form a lace-like pattern ⇥. (Right) Areas of very dense calcification are also common, illustrated by heavy basophilic staining of the cartilage matrix.

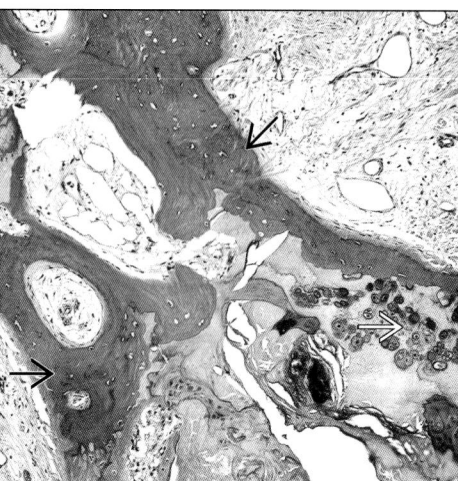

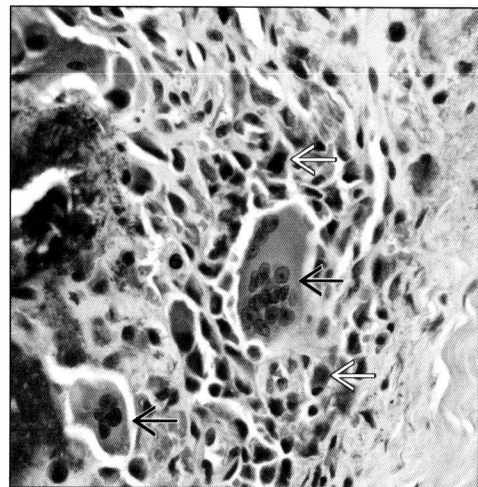

(Left) Ossification ⇥ is also common and can sometimes be extensive, as illustrated here. It can be located either at the center or periphery of the tumor and is formed via endochondral ossification of calcified cartilage matrix ➡. (Right) Granulomatous inflammation is common, especially in calcified tumors. This micrograph illustrates epithelioid macrophages ➡ and osteoclastic giant cells ⇥ in a calcified tumor. When extensive, this mimics giant cell tumor of tendon sheath.

CHONDROMA

Microscopic Features

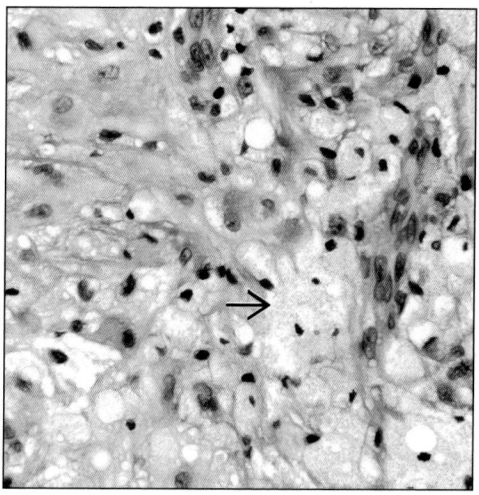

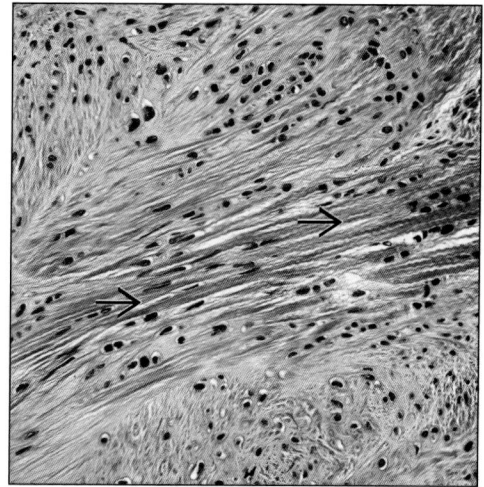

(Left) Xanthogranulomatous inflammation can be present in soft tissue chondroma, consisting of sheets or clusters of foamy histiocytes ➡. When extensive, such a tumor can be mistaken for fibrous histiocytoma or giant cell tumor of tendon sheath. (Right) Soft tissue chondroma can have extensive fibrosis exemplified by numerous collagen bundles traversing this tumor ➡. Tumors with extensive fibrosis are sometimes referred to as fibrochondromas.

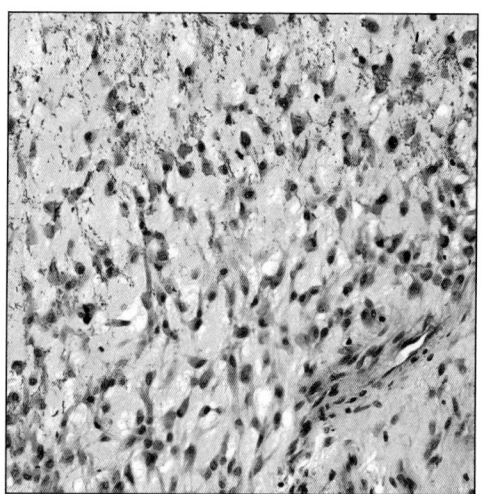

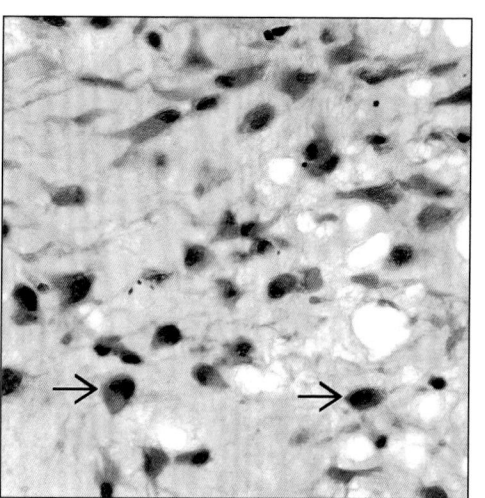

(Left) Soft tissue chondroma can have extensive myxoid matrix where chondrocytes assume elongated & stellate configurations, sometimes interconnecting with each other to form a fine network, mimicking extraskeletal myxoid chondrosarcoma. Tumors with extensive myxoid matrix are sometimes called myxochondromas. (Right) Chondrocytes can resemble chondroblasts consisting of rounded cells with abundant eosinophilic cytoplasm & eccentric grooved or reniform nuclei ➡.

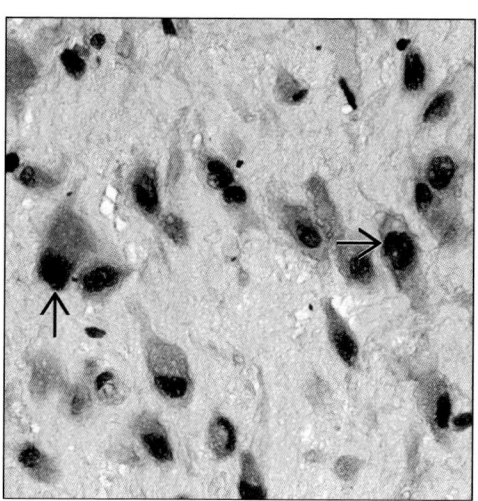

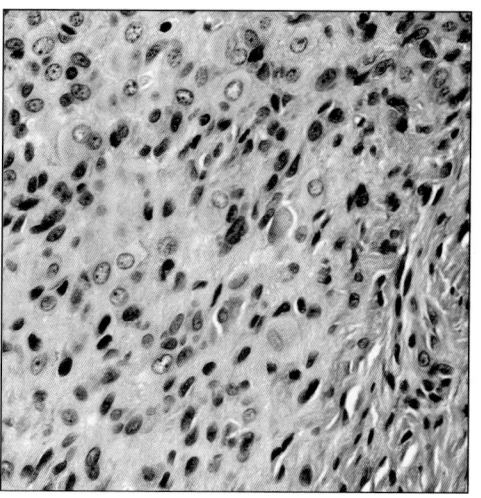

(Left) Degenerative cytologic atypia is not uncommon in soft tissue chondroma. This high-power micrograph illustrates chondrocytes with nuclear enlargement ➡ and pleomorphism, which, out of context, would be suspicious for chondrosarcoma. (Right) Focal areas of increased cellularity can also be present in soft tissue chondroma, as exemplified by this tumor, and should not be regarded as worrisome for malignancy.

OSTEOMA CUTIS

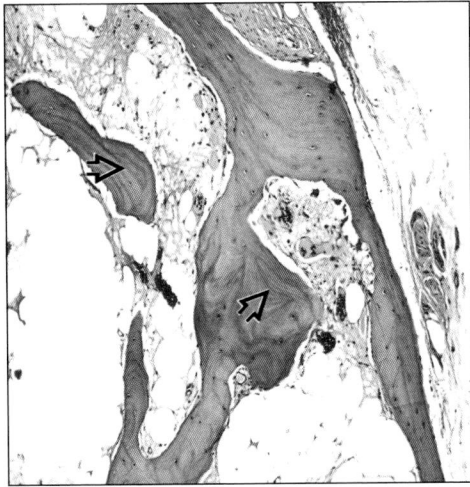

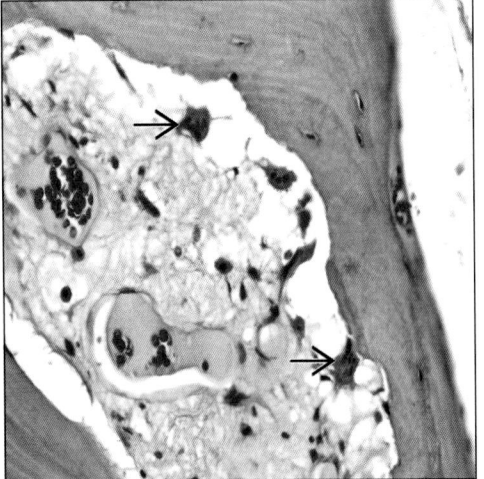

Low-magnification image of an osteoma cutis shows mature bone-forming trabeculae, with cement lines ⮑ surrounding adipocytes and small blood vessels.

Higher power view shows mature trabeculae composed of lamellar-type bone lined by scattered osteoclasts ➔.

TERMINOLOGY

Synonyms
- Primary cutaneous osteoma cutis
- Metaplastic (secondary) ossification
- Cutaneous ossification

Definitions
- Primary or secondary cutaneous mature bone formation

ETIOLOGY/PATHOGENESIS

Primary (Rare)
- Often genetic or developmental in origin; presents at early age
- May be part of Albright hereditary osteodystrophy or other genetic syndromes
  - Albright: X-linked dominant condition associated with characteristic facies, mental retardation, basal ganglia calcification, and cataracts
  - Other rare syndromes include congenital plaque-like osteomatosis, progressive osseous heteroplasia, and fibrodysplasia ossificans progressiva

Secondary (Common)
- Associated with preexisting lesions, such as nevi, benign tumors (including adnexal tumors, especially pilomatrixomas), basal cell carcinoma, scars, acne, and ruptured cysts

CLINICAL ISSUES

Epidemiology
- Age
  - Primary cases often present at birth or in early childhood
  - Secondary cases typically present in adulthood

Site
- Variable, but often involve extremities or face

Presentation
- Dermal papule, plaque, or nodule
  - Multiple lesions more common in primary types

Treatment
- Surgical approaches
  - Complete conservative excision is not necessary but curative

Prognosis
- Excellent in vast majority of cases; no malignant potential
- Genetic cases may develop numerous debilitating lesions

MACROSCOPIC FEATURES

General Features
- Nodular, dermal-based solid bony lesion

MICROSCOPIC PATHOLOGY

Histologic Features
- Appearance varies from small spicules to large masses of bone
  - Typically located in deep dermis &/or subcutis
  - Mature-appearing bone, often with Haversian systems and cement lines
  - Cartilaginous precursor usually absent
  - Osteoblastic activity may be present (especially in Albright syndrome); osteoclasts are less common
  - Stromal fat may be present
  - Hematopoietic cells occasionally present
- Transepidermal elimination may be seen, particularly in plaque-like osteomas

OSTEOMA CUTIS

Key Facts

Etiology/Pathogenesis

- Primary: May be part of Albright hereditary osteodystrophy or other genetic syndromes
- Secondary: Associated with preexisting lesions, such as nevi, tumors, scars, and ruptured cysts

Clinical Issues

- Primary cases often present at birth or in early childhood; secondary cases in adults

Microscopic Pathology

- Appearance varies from small spicules to large masses of bone
- Mature-appearing bone, often with Haversian systems and cement lines
- Osteoblastic activity may be present (especially in Albright syndrome), osteoclasts are less common
- Typically located in deep dermis &/or subcutaneous tissue

- Associated/precursor lesions often present in secondary ossification, including
  - Nevi (especially on face)
  - Pilomatrixomas (often ruptured lesions)
  - Basal cell carcinomas
  - Other tumors, including trichoepitheliomas, hemangiomas, schwannomas, lipomas, and dermatofibromas
  - Cysts, including epidermoid and pilar (tricholemmal) cysts, especially ruptured
  - Sites of trauma, scars, injections, and previous infection
- Pigmentation has been reported in patients treated with minocycline or tetracycline

Cytologic Features

- Osteocytes, osteoblasts, and osteoclasts show bland cytologic features without atypia

DIFFERENTIAL DIAGNOSIS

Calcinosis Cutis

- Nodules of dense basophilic material typically lacking well-formed bone
- Peripheral rim of secondary ossification may form

Chondroma

- Very rare dermal or subcutaneous tumor
- Cartilaginous tumor, which often lacks mature bone formation

Myositis Ossificans

- Subcutaneous tumor showing shell of reactive bone
- Central proliferation of fibroblastic cells with "tissue-culture" appearance (similar to nodular fasciitis)

Osteosarcoma

- Exceptionally rare in skin, most cases likely metastatic or from underlying bone tumor invading dermis
- Proliferation of highly atypical epithelioid, spindled, and multinucleated tumor giant cells

SELECTED REFERENCES

1. Haro R et al: Plaque-like osteoma cutis with transepidermal elimination. J Cutan Pathol. 36(5):591-3, 2009
2. Burford C: Pigmented osteoma cutis secondary to long-term tetracyclines. Australas J Dermatol. 48(2):134-6, 2007
3. Thielen AM et al: Multiple cutaneous osteomas of the face associated with chronic inflammatory acne. J Eur Acad Dermatol Venereol. 20(3):321-6, 2006
4. Bergonse FN et al: Miliary osteoma of the face: a report of 4 cases and review of the literature. Cutis. 69(5):383-6, 2002
5. Shoji T et al: Basal cell carcinoma with massive ossification. Am J Dermatopathol. 21(1):34-6, 1999
6. Cottoni F et al: Primary osteoma cutis. Clinical, morphological, and ultrastructural study. Am J Dermatopathol. 15(1):77-81, 1993
7. Prendiville JS et al: Osteoma cutis as a presenting sign of pseudohypoparathyroidism. Pediatr Dermatol. 9(1):11-8, 1992

IMAGE GALLERY

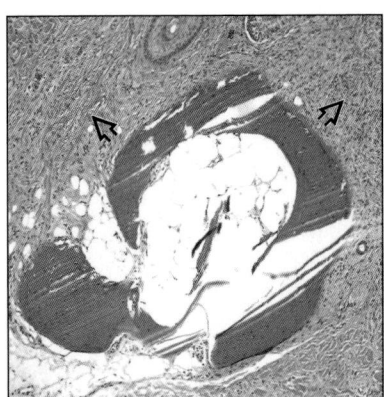 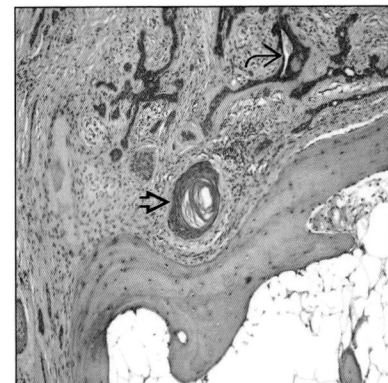 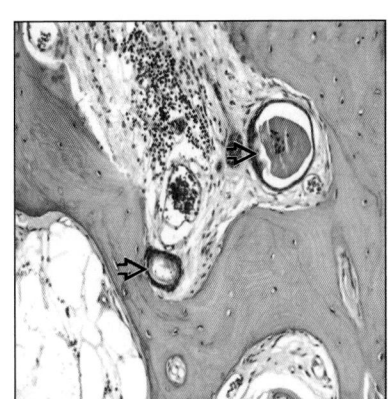

(Left) Low-power view of an osteoma cutis arising in association with a dermatofibroma ⊵ shows a proliferation of mature osteoid surrounding large bland fat cells. *(Center)* Low magnification of an osteoma cutis associated with a chondroid syringoma (cutaneous mixed tumor) shows a proliferation of bland ductal ⊿ and folliculocystic structures ⊵ surrounding the bone. *(Right)* Higher power examination of the same osteoma cutis shows a few bland adnexal ducts ⊵ trapped between the mature bony trabeculae.

Histiocytic Proliferations

JUVENILE AND ADULT-TYPE XANTHOGRANULOMA

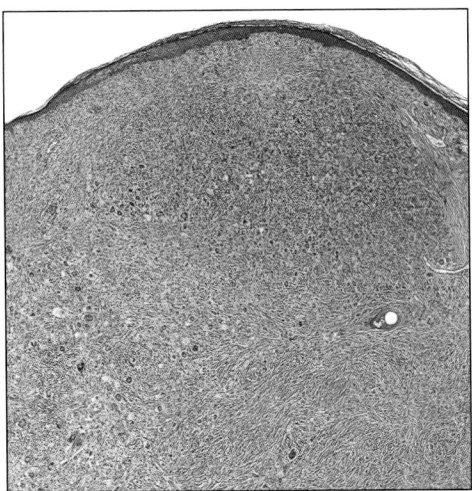

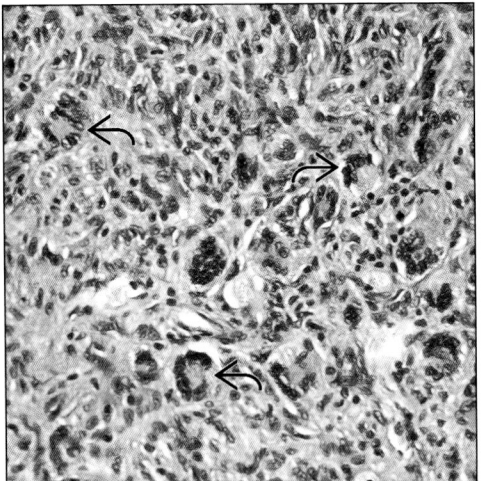

This is a typical appearance of a juvenile xanthogranuloma removed from the face of a small boy. The lesion is uniform and cellular and proliferates in the dermis with no grenz zone.

Many Touton giant cells ➔ can be seen in this juvenile xanthogranuloma. The background cells are spindled to ovoid with eosinophilic cytoplasm, which shows only minimal lipid in this case.

TERMINOLOGY

Abbreviations
- Juvenile xanthogranuloma (JXG)

Synonyms
- Nevoxanthoendothelioma

Definitions
- Stable or regressing histiocytic lesion that usually occurs in childhood
  - Form of non-Langerhans histiocytosis

CLINICAL ISSUES

Epidemiology
- Incidence
  - Rare
- Age
  - Majority in individuals under 3 years
    - Visceral examples almost exclusively in infants and children
  - 13-30% in older children and adults
- Gender
  - Slight male predominance

Presentation
- Solitary cutaneous lesion in majority of cases
  - Head and neck > trunk > extremities
- Up to 10% of patients with multiple cutaneous lesions
- Up to 5% of patients with visceral-systemic disease

Treatment
- Simple excision
- Chemotherapy administered to rare patients with systemic disease

Prognosis
- Usually excellent

- Most lesions regress or stabilize (including large visceral ones)
- Rare deaths associated with multiorgan disease

MICROSCOPIC PATHOLOGY

Histologic Features
- Mononuclear cells
- Multinucleated cells ± Touton features
- Spindle cells
  - Variable finely vacuolated cytoplasm
  - Often lightly eosinophilic
- Variable lipid and foamy histiocytes
  - Minimal lipid in early lesions
- Inflammatory cell background
  - Acute and chronic inflammatory cells
    - Eosinophils are a consistent finding
    - Neutrophils uncommon
- Negligible nuclear atypia
- Minimal mitotic activity

DIFFERENTIAL DIAGNOSIS

Langerhans Cell Histiocytosis
- Usually presents as skeletal disease
- Atypical histiocytic cells
- Background eosinophils
- S100(+), CD1a(+)

Xanthoma
- Foamy histiocytes
- No Touton giant cells
- No background inflammation
- Can be associated with hyperlipidemia
  - Usually lesions of adults
- Benign

Fibrous Histiocytoma/Dermatofibroma
- Usually in adults

JUVENILE AND ADULT-TYPE XANTHOGRANULOMA

Key Facts

Terminology
- Stable or regressing histiocytic lesion that usually occurs in childhood
- Form of non-Langerhans histiocytosis

Clinical Issues
- Majority in individuals under 3 years
- Visceral examples almost exclusively in infants and children
- Solitary cutaneous lesion in majority of cases

- Head and neck > trunk > extremities

Microscopic Pathology
- Mononuclear cells
- Multinucleated cells ± Touton features
- Variable lipid and foamy histiocytes
- Spindle cells
- Inflammatory cell background
- Eosinophils are a frequent finding

Immunohistochemistry

Antibody	Reactivity	Staining Pattern	Comment
CD68	Positive	Cytoplasmic	Essentially all cases reactive
FXIIIA	Positive	Nuclear	Essentially all cases reactive
CD1a	Negative		
S100	Equivocal	Nuclear & cytoplasmic	Most cases are negative; if positive, staining is weak

- Prominent storiform pattern
- Eosinophils usually inconspicuous
- Peripheral collagen trapping in cutaneous examples
- Overlying epidermal hyperplasia
- Intralesional hemorrhage, hemosiderin
- Benign
  - Rare metastases, but no deaths associated with superficial lesions

Rosai-Dorfman Disease
- Also known as sinus histiocytosis with massive lymphadenopathy
- Usually involves lymph nodes but may present in skin and soft tissues
- Form of non-Langerhans histiocytosis
- Histiocytes and lymphoid aggregates
- Emperipolesis is key diagnostic feature
- Histiocytes are S100(+), CD1a(-)
- Most patients have good outcome

Reticulohistiocytoma
- Benign histiocytic proliferation, which typically occurs in adults

- Brown-yellow papules at any site
- Nodules composed of brightly eosinophilic histiocytes, some multinucleated
- Nuclear atypia
- CD68(+), S100(-), CD1a(-)

SELECTED REFERENCES

1. Janssen D et al: Clonality in juvenile xanthogranuloma. Am J Surg Pathol. 31(5):812-3, 2007
2. Janssen D et al: Juvenile xanthogranuloma in childhood and adolescence: a clinicopathologic study of 129 patients from the kiel pediatric tumor registry. Am J Surg Pathol. 29(1):21-8, 2005
3. Dehner LP: Juvenile xanthogranulomas in the first two decades of life: a clinicopathologic study of 174 cases with cutaneous and extracutaneous manifestations. Am J Surg Pathol. 27(5):579-93, 2003
4. Zelger B et al: Juvenile and adult xanthogranuloma. A histological and immunohistochemical comparison. Am J Surg Pathol. 18(2):126-35, 1994

IMAGE GALLERY

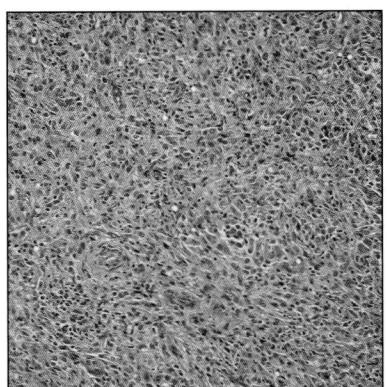 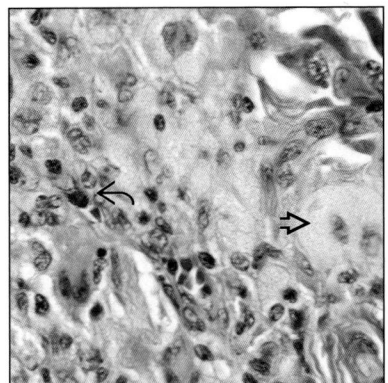 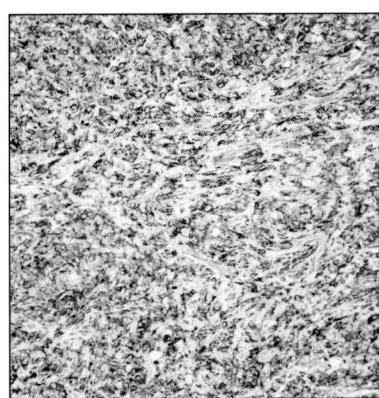

(Left) A cellular example shows juvenile xanthogranuloma featuring an inflammatory background composed mostly of mononuclear cells. *(Center)* Eosinophils ➡ and foamy histiocytes ⮞ are commonly encountered in juvenile xanthogranuloma. *(Right)* Essentially all examples of juvenile xanthogranuloma are reactive with CD68 (shown) and factor XIIIa antibodies on immunohistochemistry, but are negative for S100 and CD1a.

RETICULOHISTIOCYTOMA

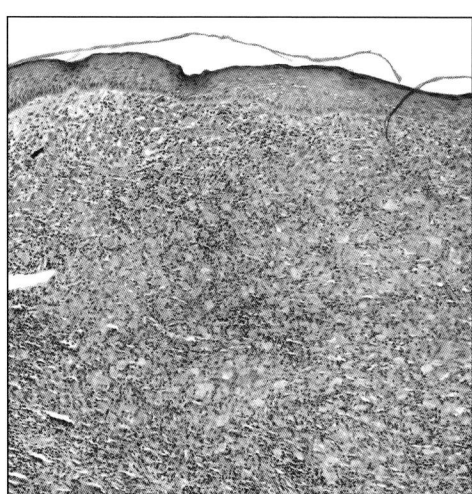

Low-power examination shows a dense nodular to sheet-like collection of large histiocytic cells in the dermis.

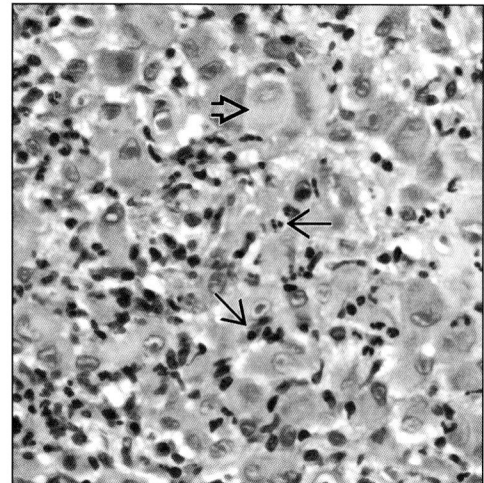

High-power view shows large histiocytic cells with abundant dense, glassy-appearing cytoplasm ⇨ and a background inflammatory infiltrate containing neutrophils and eosinophils ➡.

TERMINOLOGY

Synonyms
- Solitary cutaneous reticulohistiocytoma (SCR)
- Reticulohistiocytic granuloma
- Giant cell reticulohistiocytoma

Definitions
- Proliferation of histiocytes with abundant dense, glassy-appearing eosinophilic cytoplasm

ETIOLOGY/PATHOGENESIS

Environmental Exposure
- May be related to stimuli, such as insect bites, infection, trauma, or ruptured folliculitis or cyst in some cases

CLINICAL ISSUES

Epidemiology
- Incidence
  - Rare tumor
- Age
  - Usually occurs in adults > 40 years old
    - However, some cases have been reported in adolescents
- Gender
  - Equal male and female incidence
- Ethnicity
  - Most cases occur in Caucasians

Site
- Usually head and neck region, including mucosal sites
  - However, may present at almost any cutaneous site

Presentation
- Skin papule or nodule
  - Usually single lesion, but several may be present in some cases
- Firm, rapidly growing lesion
- Usually appear as red-brown or yellow-brown
- May be preceded by trauma in some cases
- Lack of systemic symptoms, including fever, weight loss, or weakness (which may be seen in multicentric reticulohistiocytosis)

Treatment
- Surgical approaches
  - Complete conservative excision is curative
    - Usually not required unless lesion is very large or fails to resolve

Prognosis
- Excellent; lesions often involute spontaneously
- No definite relationship with more aggressive multicentric reticulohistiocytosis
  - However, multiple skin lesions should suggest possibility of generalized cutaneous reticulohistiocytosis

MACROSCOPIC FEATURES

General Features
- Dermal-based nodular, well-circumscribed but unencapsulated lesion

Size
- Lesions typically range in size from 0.5-2 cm

MICROSCOPIC PATHOLOGY

Histologic Features
- Dermal-based nodular proliferation of large mononuclear and multinucleated histiocytes
  - Cells show characteristic abundant glassy/hyalinized-appearing eosinophilic cytoplasm

RETICULOHISTIOCYTOMA

Key Facts

Terminology
- Proliferation of histiocytes with abundant dense, glassy-appearing eosinophilic cytoplasm

Clinical Issues
- Usually occurs in adults > 40 years old, but cases have been reported in adolescents
- Usually head and neck region, including mucosal sites, but may present at any cutaneous site
- Usually red-brown or yellow-brown appearing

Microscopic Pathology
- Dermal-based nodular proliferation of large mononuclear and multinucleated histiocytes
- Cells show characteristic abundant glassy/hyalinized-appearing eosinophilic cytoplasm

- Occasional Touton-type giant cells containing lipid may be present
- Early lesions characterized by more mononuclear cells with lymphocytes

Ancillary Tests
- Cells are typically positive for CD68 (KP1), CD163, and lysozyme

Top Differential Diagnoses
- Multicentric reticulohistiocytosis and generalized cutaneous reticulohistiocytosis
- Juvenile xanthogranuloma (JXG)
- Langerhans cell histiocytosis (LCH)
- Rosai-Dorfman disease (sinus histiocytosis with massive lymphadenopathy)

- o Some cells may show finely granular cytoplasm
- o Occasional Touton-type giant cells containing lipid may be present, but not prominent
- o Cytologic atypia is usually minimal, and mitoses are few and nonatypical
- o No infiltrative features are present
- Overlying epidermis may show atrophy/thinning
  - o Often grenz zone separating infiltrate from epidermis
- Early lesions characterized by background inflammatory infiltrate with many small mononuclear cells and lymphocytes
- Later lesions show greater numbers of large mononuclear and multinucleated cells, with background infiltrate including neutrophils and eosinophils
- Phagocytosis of inflammatory cells and collagen may be present
- Occasional bizarre-appearing cells may be present, but do not indicate malignancy
- Rare cases may show deep subcutaneous, and even lymph node, involvement

Cytologic Features
- Large but cytologically bland-appearing cells that show characteristic abundant glassy/hyalinized-appearing eosinophilic cytoplasm

Predominant Pattern/Injury Type
- Inflammatory, granulomatous

Predominant Cell/Compartment Type
- Histiocyte

ANCILLARY TESTS

Histochemistry
- Periodic acid-Schiff with diastase digestion and Sudan black
  - o Reactivity: Positive
  - o Staining pattern
    - Cytoplasmic; highlights granules

Immunohistochemistry
- Cells are typically positive for CD68 (KP1), CD163, and lysozyme
- Variable positivity reported for FXIIIA, CD64, and α-1-antitrypsin
- S100 negative in most cases, but has been reported to be rarely positive (usually weak/focal)
- Cells negative for CD1a, CD3, CD20, CD34, actin, desmin, HMB-45, MART-1/Melan-A

Electron Microscopy
- Large cells showing abundant granular cytoplasm containing numerous mitochondria, phagolysosomes, dense bodies, and myelin figures
- Also contain so-called "pleomorphic cytoplasmic inclusions"
  - o Highly complex structures consisting mainly of unit membranes, which may surround vesicles
- Birbeck granules are absent

DIFFERENTIAL DIAGNOSIS

Multicentric and Generalized Cutaneous Reticulohistiocytosis
- These entities show different clinical features
  - o Multicentric cutaneous reticulohistiocytosis (MCR) presents with multiple lesions involving skin, mucosal sites, joints, and occasionally internal organs
    - MCR may show aggressive course with destructive arthropathy and constitutional symptoms
  - o Generalized cutaneous reticulohistiocytosis (GCR) is characterized by eruption of multiple small cutaneous lesions
    - Some cases may progress to MCR
- Histologically, there is considerable overlap with solitary reticulohistiocytoma, but some differences have been described
  - o Solitary lesions may be better circumscribed and show more multinucleated giants cells

o Neutrophils and xanthomatized cells have been reported to be more common in solitary reticulohistiocytoma
o FXIIIA expression may be lower in systemic cases

Juvenile Xanthogranuloma (JXG)
- Typically occurs in children, but some cases occur in adults ("adult type xanthogranuloma")
- Multiple papules are common, and dozens of lesions have been reported in some cases
- Histologically, JXG typically shows more foamy histiocytes and Touton-type giant cells with peripheral wreath-like arrangement of nuclei
  o Cells lack dense glassy eosinophilic cytoplasm of reticulohistiocytoma
- Cells positive by immunohistochemistry for CD68 and CD163, but negative for S100 and CD1a

Langerhans Cell Histocytosis (LCH)
- LCH includes Letterer-Siwe, Hand-Schüller Christian, eosinophilic granuloma, and congenital self-healing reticulohistiocytosis variants
- Predominantly occur in children
  o Also a 2nd peak in elderly adults (usually eosinophilic granuloma variant)
- Typically characterized by multiple skin lesions and systemic involvement (especially bone)
- Histologic examination shows proliferation of mononuclear cells in dermis and occasionally in epidermis
  o Cells show large, folded or reniform vesicular nuclei, and abundant eosinophilic cytoplasm
  o Cells lack dense eosinophilic cytoplasm of reticulohistiocytoma
  o Background infiltrate often contains numerous eosinophils and variable numbers of lymphocytes
- CD1a and S100 should be positive in vast majority of cases (both are typically negative in reticulohistiocytoma)

Rosai-Dorfman Disease
- Also known as sinus histiocytosis with massive lymphadenopathy (SHML)
- Often show concomitant lymphadenopathy and constitutional symptoms
- Lesions may be solitary or multiple
- Histologic examination shows proliferation of large, pale-staining histiocytes with emperipolesis of lymphocytes, plasma cells, and erythrocytes
  o Cells lack dense, glassy cytoplasm of reticulohistiocytoma
- S100(+) (typically negative in reticulohistiocytoma), CD68(+), lysozyme(+), CD1a(-)

DIAGNOSTIC CHECKLIST

Pathologic Interpretation Pearls
- Nodular proliferation of large mononuclear and multinucleated histiocytes
  o Cells show characteristic abundant glassy/ hyalinized-appearing eosinophilic cytoplasm

o Occasional Touton-type giant cells containing lipid may be present, but not prominent (as in JXG)
- Cells positive for CD68, CD163, and lysozyme
- Cells typically negative for S100, CD1a, CD3, CD20, and CD34

SELECTED REFERENCES

1. Caputo R et al: Unusual variants of non-Langerhans cell histiocytoses. J Am Acad Dermatol. 57(6):1031-45, 2007
2. Chen CH et al: Multicentric reticulohistiocytosis presenting with destructive polyarthritis, laryngopharyngeal dysfunction, and a huge reticulohistiocytoma. J Clin Rheumatol. 12(5):252-4, 2006
3. Miettinen M et al: Reticulohistiocytoma (solitary epithelioid histiocytoma): a clinicopathologic and immunohistochemical study of 44 cases. Am J Surg Pathol. 30(4):521-8, 2006
4. Wang KH et al: Cutaneous Rosai-Dorfman disease: clinicopathological profiles, spectrum and evolution of 21 lesions in six patients. Br J Dermatol. 154(2):277-86, 2006
5. Nguyen TT et al: Expression of CD163 (hemoglobin scavenger receptor) in normal tissues, lymphomas, carcinomas, and sarcomas is largely restricted to the monocyte/macrophage lineage. Am J Surg Pathol. 29(5):617-24, 2005
6. Bakri SJ et al: Recurrent solitary reticulohistiocytoma of the eyelid. Ophthal Plast Reconstr Surg. 19(2):162-4, 2003
7. Ka MM et al: [Multicentric reticulohistiocytosis with a 20-year follow-up .] Rev Med Interne. 23(9):779-83, 2002
8. Busam KJ et al: Immunohistochemical distinction of epithelioid histiocytic proliferations from epithelioid melanocytic nevi. Am J Dermatopathol. 22(3):237-41, 2000
9. Burgdorf WH et al: The non-Langerhans' cell histiocytoses in childhood. Cutis. 58(3):201-7, 1996
10. Shy SW et al: A solitary congenital self-healing histiocytosis. Report of a case and review of the literature. Pathol Res Pract. 192(8):869-74; discussion 875-6, 1996
11. Suwabe H et al: Reticulohistiocytoma involving the skin, subcutaneous tissue and a regional lymph node. Pathol Int. 46(7):531-7, 1996
12. Hunt SJ et al: Solitary reticulohistiocytoma in pregnancy: immunohistochemical and ultrastructural study of a case with unusual immunophenotype. J Cutan Pathol. 22(2):177-81, 1995
13. Zelger B et al: Reticulohistiocytoma and multicentric reticulohistiocytosis. Histopathologic and immunophenotypic distinct entities. Am J Dermatopathol. 16(6):577-84, 1994
14. Caputo R et al: Solitary reticulohistiocytosis (reticulohistiocytoma) of the skin in children: report of two cases. Arch Dermatol. 128(5):698-9, 1992
15. Chun SI et al: Congenital self-healing reticulohistiocytosis--report of a case of the solitary type and review of the literature. Yonsei Med J. 33(2):194-8, 1992
16. Anaguchi S et al: [Solitary reticulohistiocytic granuloma--a report of three cases and a review of literature.] Nippon Hifuka Gakkai Zasshi. 101(7):735-42, 1991
17. Coode PE et al: Multicentric reticulohistiocytosis: report of two cases with ultrastructure, tissue culture and immunology studies. Clin Exp Dermatol. 5(3):281-93, 1980
18. Davies BT et al: The so-called reticulohistiocytoma of the skin; a comparison of two distinct types. Br J Dermatol. 67(6):205-11, 1955

I
11

Microscopic and Immunohistochemical Features

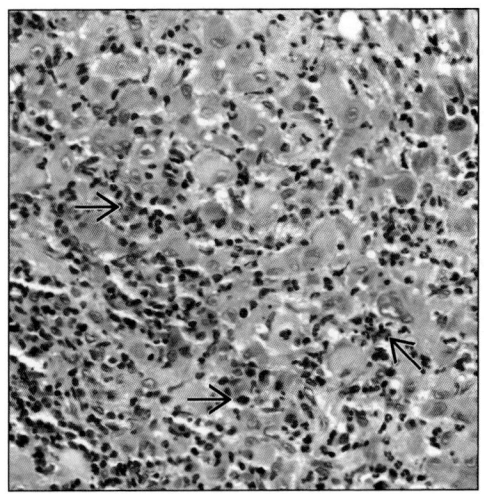 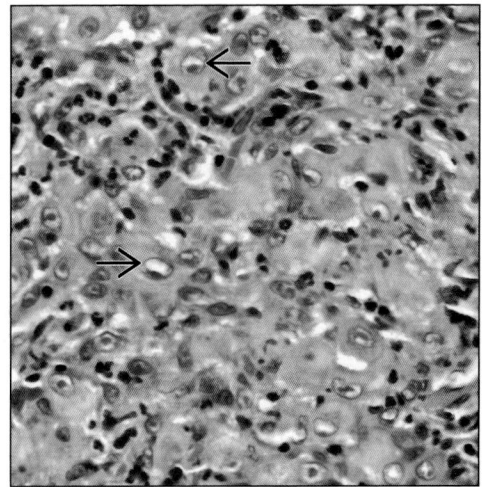

(Left) Intermediate-power view shows sheets of eosinophilic cells associated with an inflammatory infiltrate containing lymphocytes, neutrophils, and numerous eosinophils ➔. (Right) Higher power examination shows the cytologic features of the cells, with abundant dense eosinophilic to glassy-appearing cytoplasm and vesicular nuclei ➔ with prominent nucleoli.

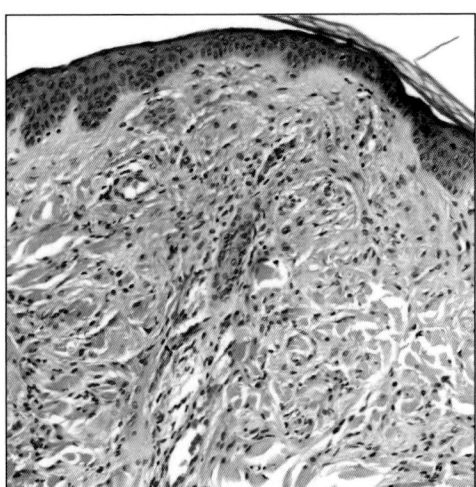 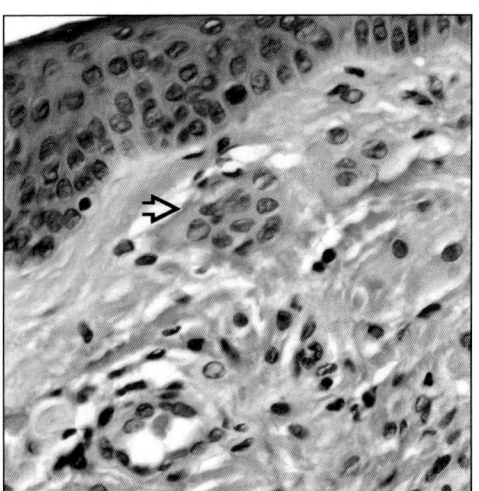

(Left) Low-power view of a hypocellular (possibly regressing) lesion shows only scattered large histiocytes in the superficial dermis. (Right) Higher power examination of the cells shows typical histologic features of reticulohistiocytoma, with enlarged mononuclear and multinucleated ➔ cells with abundant eosinophilic cytoplasm.

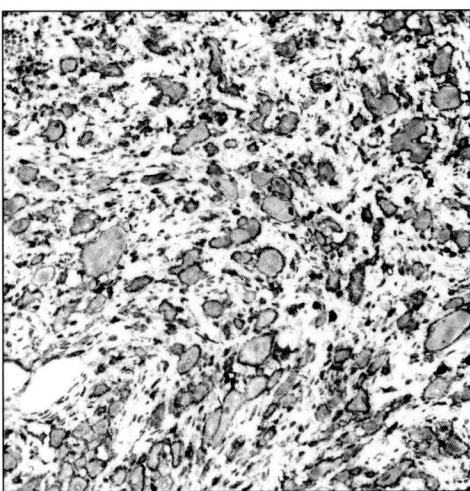 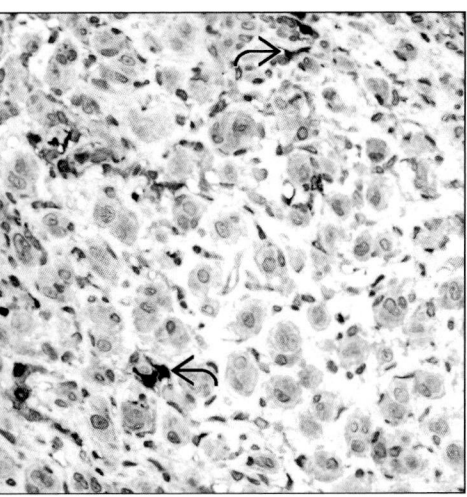

(Left) CD163 immunohistochemical stain is strongly and diffusely positive, highlighting the tumoral cell cytoplasm and membranes. (Right) S100 is essentially negative, with only very weak cytoplasmic, and no nuclear, staining. A few background dendritic cells are strongly positive ➔.

11

MULTICENTRIC RETICULOHISTIOCYTOSIS

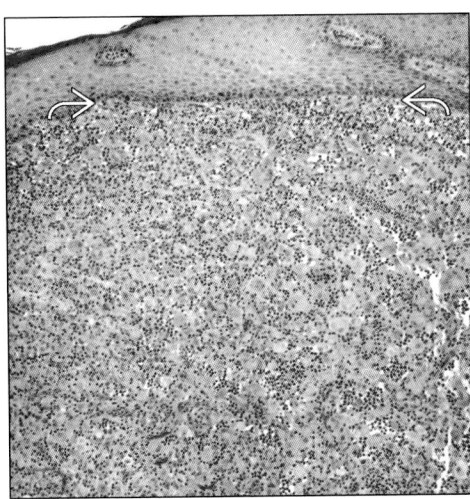

Low magnification of MCR shows a nodular proliferation of enlarged histiocytic cells in the dermis. There is a very thin grenz zone ➡, and the epidermis shows flattening of the rete ridges.

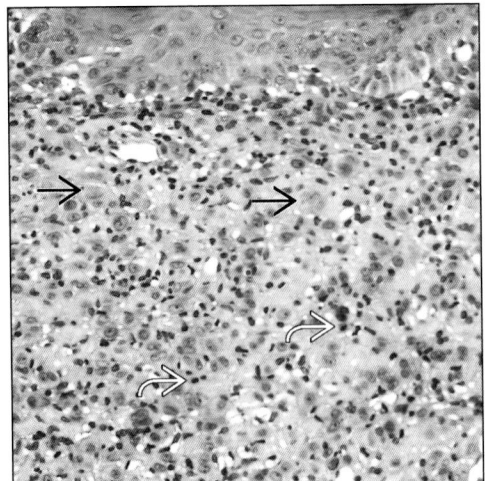

Higher magnification of MCR shows a proliferation of numerous enlarged histiocytic-appearing cells ➡ associated with a background mixed inflammatory infiltrate containing scattered eosinophils ➡.

TERMINOLOGY

Abbreviations
- Multicentric reticulohistiocytosis (MCR)

Synonyms
- Giant cell reticulohistiocytosis
- Reticulohistiocytosis of skin and synovia

Definitions
- Proliferation of large histiocytes with dense eosinophilic cytoplasm involving multiple organs

ETIOLOGY/PATHOGENESIS

Associated Conditions
- Autoimmune disorders and internal malignancies

CLINICAL ISSUES

Epidemiology
- Age
  - Most cases occur in adults > 40 years old

Site
- Can affect multiple sites, including hands, face, juxtaarticular regions, oral, nasal/pharyngeal mucosa

Presentation
- Multiple nodules and arthropathy
  - Most cases present with multiple cutaneous/mucocutaneous papulonodules and severe arthropathy, other visceral symptoms

Treatment
- Drugs
  - Immunosuppressive medications typically used
  - Underlying autoimmune disease or malignancy should be treated

Prognosis
- Variable; some cutaneous lesions may regress
- Osteoarticular involvement shows progressive course in approximately 50% of cases

MACROSCOPIC FEATURES

General Features
- Dermal-based nodular, nonencapsulated lesion

Size
- Typically range from 2 mm to 2 cm in diameter

MICROSCOPIC PATHOLOGY

Histologic Features
- Dermal-based nodular proliferation of large mononuclear and multinucleated histiocytes
  - Cells show characteristic abundant glassy/hyalinized-appearing eosinophilic cytoplasm
  - Some cells may show finely granular cytoplasm
  - Cytologic atypia is minimal; only few mitoses should be present
  - Less well-circumscribed than solitary reticulohistiocytoma, but no infiltrative features
- Overlying epidermis may show atrophy/thinning
- Early lesions characterized by background inflammatory infiltrate with many small mononuclear cells and lymphocytes
- Later lesions show greater numbers of large cells, neutrophils, and eosinophils

ANCILLARY TESTS

Immunohistochemistry
- Typically positive for histiocytic markers, including CD68, lysozyme, and CD45

MULTICENTRIC RETICULOHISTIOCYTOSIS

Key Facts

Terminology
- Giant cell reticulohistiocytosis

Clinical Issues
- Most cases occur in adults > 40 years old
- Multiple nodules and arthropathy
- Prognosis is variable; some cutaneous lesions may regress
- Osteoarticular involvement shows progressive course in 1/2 of cases

Microscopic Pathology
- Dermal-based nodular proliferation of large mononuclear and multinucleated histiocytes
- Often overlying epidermal atrophy
- Cells show characteristic abundant glassy/hyalinized-appearing eosinophilic cytoplasm
- Occasional Touton-type giant cells containing lipid may be present, but not prominent
- Background of neutrophils and eosinophils

○ Variable reactivity reported for FXIIIA; may be greater than in solitary reticulohistiocytoma
- Cells are typically negative for S100 (may be focally positive in some cases), CD1a, and MAC387

- Characterized by multiple skin lesions and systemic involvement (especially bone)
- Cells show folded or reniform vesicular nuclei and abundant eosinophilic cytoplasm
- CD1a and S100 are strongly positive in vast majority

DIFFERENTIAL DIAGNOSIS

Solitary Cutaneous Reticulohistiocytoma (SCR) and Generalized Cutaneous Reticulohistiocytosis (GCR)
- SCR presents as single papular or nodular cutaneous lesion
  ○ Histologically, there is considerable overlap with MCR, but some differences may be seen
    ▪ May be better circumscribed and show more multinucleated giant cells and neutrophils
- GCR is characterized by eruption of multiple small cutaneous lesions
  ○ Some cases may progress to MCR

Juvenile Xanthogranuloma (JXG)
- Typically single lesion occurring in children, but can be multiple, and some cases occur in adults
- Histologically, shows more foamy histiocytes and Touton-type giant cells with peripheral wreath-like rim of nuclei and foamy cytoplasm

Langerhans Cell Histocytosis (LCH)
- Predominantly occurs in children, but 2nd peak in elderly adults (usually eosinophilic granuloma variant)

DIAGNOSTIC CHECKLIST

Pathologic Interpretation Pearls
- Nodular proliferation of large mononuclear and multinucleated histiocytes
  ○ Cells show characteristic abundant glassy/hyalinized-appearing eosinophilic cytoplasm

SELECTED REFERENCES

1. Luz FB et al: Multicentric reticulohistiocytosis: a proliferation of macrophages with tropism for skin and joints, part I. Skinmed. 6(4):172-8, 2007
2. Baghestani S et al: Multicentric reticulohistiocytosis presenting with papulonodular skin eruption and polyarthritis. Eur J Dermatol. 15(3):196-200, 2005
3. Snow JL et al: Malignancy-associated multicentric reticulohistiocytosis: a clinical, histological and immunophenotypic study. Br J Dermatol. 133(1):71-6, 1995
4. Coode PE et al: Multicentric reticulohistiocytosis: report of two cases with ultrastructure, tissue culture and immunology studies. Clin Exp Dermatol. 5(3):281-93, 1980

IMAGE GALLERY

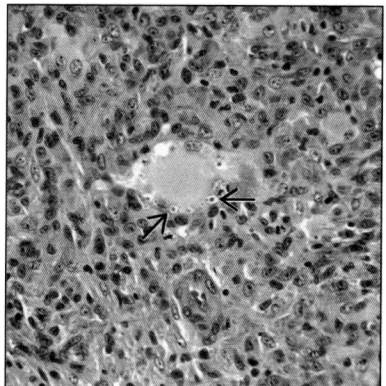 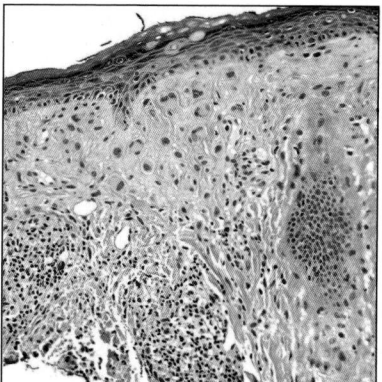 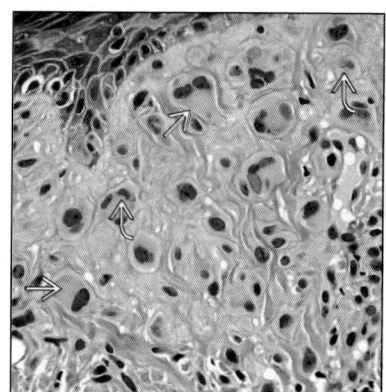

(Left) High magnification of a cellular MCR shows a very large, central multinucleated cell containing fragments of phagocytosed erythrocytes ➡. *(Center)* A hypocellular example of MCR shows a superficial dermal-based proliferation of large epithelioid histiocytes and a mild associated lymphocytic infiltrate. *(Right)* Higher magnification shows a population of enlarged histiocytic cells with abundant dense eosinophilic cytoplasm ➡ and 1 to several oval to reniform nuclei ➡.

NON-LANGERHANS CELL HISTIOCYTOSES

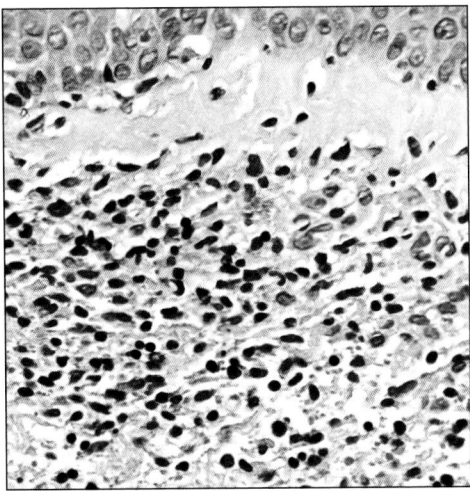

Indeterminate cell histiocytosis is a very rare histiocytosis composed of cells with histologic and immunohistochemical similarities to Langerhans cells, but lacking Birbeck granules by electron microscopy.

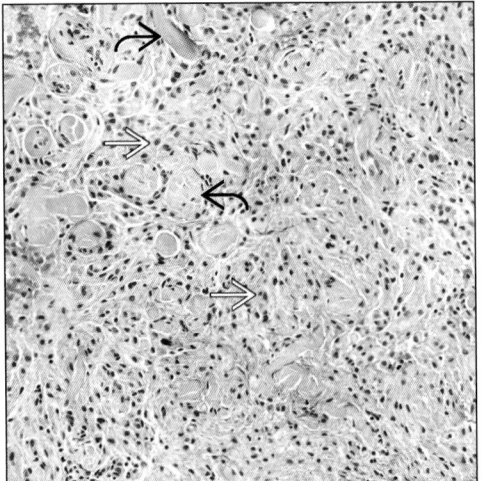

Hereditary progressive mucinous histiocytosis shows a dermal proliferation composed of epithelioid histiocytes ➤ and mucin separating broad bundles of collagen ⬈.

TERMINOLOGY

Synonyms
- Non-X histiocytoses

Definitions
- Wide range of histiocytic disorders that are not derived from Langerhans cells
  - Sometimes difficult to categorize because of overlapping morphologic and clinical findings
  - Includes juvenile xanthogranuloma, reticulohistiocytoma, and Rosai-Dorfman disease
- Histiocyte = bone marrow-derived cell belonging to monocytes/macrophage &/or dendritic cell lineage and functional variants
  - Includes macrophages, Langerhans cells, interstitial dendritic cells, interdigitating dendritic cells, plasmacytoid dendritic cells, microglia, Kupffer cells, and alveolar macrophages

CLINICAL ISSUES

Epidemiology
- Age
  - Depends on type of histiocytosis

Treatment
- Benign tumors that do not require treatment in most cases

Prognosis
- Depends on type of histiocytosis

MICROSCOPIC PATHOLOGY

Histologic Features
- Macrophages are large (15-25 μm in diameter) phagocytic cells with irregular shapes and pseudopodia

- Nucleus is round, but may be indented or reniform
- Nuclear membrane is indistinct, and chromatin is fine
- Cytoplasm is abundant and can be granulated
- Cytoplasmic vacuoles may be seen, and phagocytosed material may be present
- Other features depend on the type of histiocytosis

ANCILLARY TESTS

Immunohistochemistry
- Depends on type of histiocytosis
  - Macrophages are typically positive for CD14, CD68, and CD163
  - Dermal/interstitial dendritic cells are positive for FXIIIA, CD14, CD163, and fascin
  - Indeterminate cells are S100(+), CD1a(+), FXIIIA(+)

Electron Microscopy
- Non-Langerhans cell histiocytoses do not have Birbeck granules by ultrastructural studies, unlike Langerhans cell histiocytosis (LCH)

DIFFERENTIAL DIAGNOSIS

Benign Cephalic Histiocytosis
- Rare histiocytosis characterized by asymptomatic, self-healing reddish to brownish macules and papules on the head, which spread later to trunk and arms
  - Begins in children ≤ 3 years old
- Morphology
  - Dermal histiocytes, fairly small with round nuclei
    - ± vacuolated cytoplasm
    - Positive for CD68, CD11a, and CD11c; negative for S100 and CD1a
  - Patterns include papillary dermal, lichenoid, and diffuse
    - Usually no epidermotropism

NON-LANGERHANS CELL HISTIOCYTOSES

Key Facts

Terminology

- Wide range of histiocytic disorders that are not derived from Langerhans cells
  - Sometimes difficult to categorize because of overlapping morphologic and clinical findings

Microscopic Pathology

- Macrophages are large (15-80 μm in diameter) phagocytic cells with irregular shapes and pseudopodia
- Indented nuclei, fine chromatin, abundant cytoplasm

Ancillary Tests

- Macrophages are positive for CD14, CD68, CD163
- Dermal/interstitial dendritic cells are positive for CD14, CD163, FXIIIA, fascin

Top Differential Diagnoses

- Benign cephalic histiocytosis
  - Rare cutaneous condition in children characterized by skin lesions that initially present on the head and consist of histiocytes
- Indeterminate cell histiocytosis
  - Features of macrophages, dendritic cells, and Langerhans cells, and is S100(+), CD68(+), CD1a(+)
- Progressive nodular histiocytosis
  - Part of xanthogranuloma family of disease, but more clinically aggressive and disfiguring than others
- Atypical granuloma annulare
  - May be either clinically atypical (associated with malignancies) or histologically atypical (more cellular, pleomorphic, and mitoses)

- Electron microscopy shows comma-shaped bodies, coated vesicles, and desmosome-like structures with absence of Birbeck granules

Generalized Eruptive Histiocytoma

- Rare benign histiocytosis characterized by crops of hundreds of blue-red papules, affecting mainly adults, and self-healing
  - Symmetrically distributed on trunk and extremities
    - May become hyperpigmented macules when they regress
- Clinical course
  - Usually self-limiting; may last from 1 month to over 12 years
    - May persist, may resolve, or may relapse
  - Sometimes associated with underlying tumors
    - Macules/papules may regress when underlying malignancy is treated
- Morphology
  - Histiocytes in upper dermis
    - Sometimes small and vacuolated cytoplasm
    - ± perivascular distribution
  - Usually no multinucleated giant cells
  - Older lesions may show fibrosis or giant cells
  - CD68(+), S100(-), CD1a(-)
- Electron microscopy shows dense bodies with myelin, but no Birbeck granules

Indeterminate Cell Histiocytosis (ICH)

- Dendritic cells in dermis with features of histiocytes and Langerhans cells but no Birbeck granules
  - Only few cases reported
- Presentation
  - Numerous red/brown papules
    - May coalesce
- Morphology
  - Monomorphous infiltrate of mononuclear histiocytes intermixed with clusters of lymphocytes
    - Rarely multinucleated cells
    - Often increased numbers of reactive T cells interspersed among histiocytic cells
    - Usually ample pale cytoplasm and clefted nuclei

- Rare spindle cell variant has been described
- Stroma can be myxoid
  - Immunohistochemistry
    - S100(+), CD68(+), CD1a(+), FXIIIA(±)
- Sometimes look like Langerhans cells with ample cytoplasm and grooves
  - But lack some Langerhans markers such as Langerin and Birbeck granules

Progressive Nodular Histiocytosis

- Normolipemic non-Langerhans cells histiocytosis with multiple yellow-brown papules and nodules on skin and mucous membranes; part of xanthomatous family of lesions
  - Nodules mostly on trunk
  - Rarely systemic lesions
  - Disfiguring, much more aggressive than other xanthogranulomas
- Positive for CD68, CD163, and FXIIIA, but negative for CD1a and S100
- Young adults present with numerous lesions

Erdheim-Chester Disease

- Rare infiltrative histiocytic disorder characterized by symmetrical bone sclerosis involving long bones and systemic manifestations, mostly in lung, kidney, retroperitoneal, and heart with aggressive biology
  - ~ 30% involve skin
- Epidemiology
  - Mean age: 43 (range: 7-84 years)
  - Slight male predominance
- Symptoms include fever, weight loss, dyspnea, diabetes insipidus, exophthalmos, periorbital xanthomas
  - Diaphyses of long bones show symmetrical osteosclerosis
- Morphology
  - Part of xanthogranuloma family of lesions
  - Collections of foamy histiocytes
    - Histiocytes have round to oval nuclei and moderate to abundant cytoplasm
    - May be multinucleated

- Cytoplasm is usually eosinophilic and foamy
  - Varying degrees of fibrosis
  - Other inflammatory cells (lymphocytes, plasma cells, and eosinophils) may be present
  - Immunohistochemistry
    - Histiocytes positive for CD68, factor XIIIa, ± S100
    - Histiocytes negative for PAS, CD1a, CD45RB
  - Ultrastructural studies show histiocytic cells with phagolysosomes containing lipid but no Birbeck granules
- Treatment and prognosis
  - Systemic adult form, fatal in ~ 50% of patients after 5 years
  - Attempted treatments include corticosteroids, chemotherapy, radiotherapy, surgery, and immunotherapy
- Differentiated from Langerhans cell histiocytosis because it lacks grooved nuclei and is CD1a negative
- Lacks the emperipolesis of Rosai-Dorfman disease

Atypical Granuloma Annulare

- Very rare histiocytic proliferation, whereas granuloma annulare (GA) is common
  - Usually affects older age than typical GA
- Can either be clinically atypical or histologically atypical
  - Clinically atypical
    - Often associated with underlying malignancies including lymphoma
    - Can be painful lesions on palms and soles
  - Histologically atypical
    - Often more cellular as compared to typical granuloma annulare
    - Histiocytes can have increased pleomorphism, including enlarged size, nuclear irregularity, and prominent nucleoli
    - Still areas of palisading, necrobiosis, and mucin
    - Can have increased mitotic figures as well as atypical mitoses, ≥ 1 mitoses per HPF
- Immunohistochemistry
  - Ki-67 shows fairly high proliferation rate
    - Up to 29% of the histiocytes can be positive
- Need to exclude
  - Infections, which usually have true necrosis
  - Other histiocytic tumors, lymphomas, and epithelioid sarcoma
    - Recognition of atypical granuloma annulare is important to not overdiagnose as a malignant condition

Hereditary Progressive Mucinous Histiocytosis (HPMH)

- Rare, often hereditary histiocytosis characterized by multiple persistent papules with prominent mucinosis
  - Reported primarily in female patients
  - Multiple small papules all over the skin appearing in 1st decades of life and increasing gradually in number with age
- Histology
  - Unencapsulated dermal nodules composed of epithelioid histiocytes and abundant Alcian blue-positive mucin separating broad bundles of collagen

- Histiocytes are positive for CD68 and factor XIIIa, but negative for S100, CD1a, and CD34
- Ultrastructural studies show histiocytes with cytoplasmic inclusions similar to zebra bodies and myelin bodies
- Genetic pattern remains unclear
  - Similar to autosomal dominant transmission, but much more likely in women

SELECTED REFERENCES

1. Kim MS et al: Erdheim-chester disease. Ann Dermatol. 22(4):439-43, 2010
2. Kunimoto K et al: Progressive nodular histiocytosis. J Dermatol. 37(12):1071-3, 2010
3. Schlegel C et al: Hereditary progressive mucinous histiocytosis: first report in a male patient. Acta Derm Venereol. 90(1):65-7, 2010
4. Hasegawa S et al: Japanese case of benign cephalic histiocytosis. J Dermatol. 36(1):69-71, 2009
5. Watanabe T et al: Progressive nodular histiocytosis - A five-year follow up. Eur J Dermatol. 18(2):200-2, 2008
6. Stefanaki K et al: Histological and immunohistochemical study of granuloma annulare and subcutaneous granuloma annulare in children. J Cutan Pathol. 34(5):392-6, 2007
7. Kiliç A et al: Generalized eruptive histiocytoma: a pediatric case. Eur J Dermatol. 16(6):694-5, 2006
8. Shimizu S et al: Atypical generalized granuloma annulare associated with two visceral cancers. J Am Acad Dermatol. 54(5 Suppl):S236-8, 2006
9. Jih DM et al: Benign cephalic histiocytosis: a case report and review. J Am Acad Dermatol. 47(6):908-13, 2002
10. Rosenberg AS et al: Cutaneous indeterminate cell histiocytosis: a new spindle cell variant resembling dendritic cell sarcoma. J Cutan Pathol. 28(10):531-7, 2001
11. Gonzalez Ruíz A et al: Progressive nodular histiocytosis accompanied by systemic disorders. Br J Dermatol. 143(3):628-31, 2000
12. Sass U et al: A sporadic case of progressive mucinous histiocytosis. Br J Dermatol. 142(1):133-7, 2000
13. Matsushima Y et al: Generalized eruptive histiocytoma of childhood associated with rheumatic fever. Eur J Dermatol. 9(7):548-50, 1999
14. Manente L et al: Indeterminate cell histiocytosis: a rare histiocytic disorder. Am J Dermatopathol. 19(3):276-83, 1997
15. Trotter MJ et al: Mitotic granuloma annulare: a clinicopathologic study of 20 cases. J Cutan Pathol. 23(6):537-45, 1996

Indeterminate Cell Histiocytosis

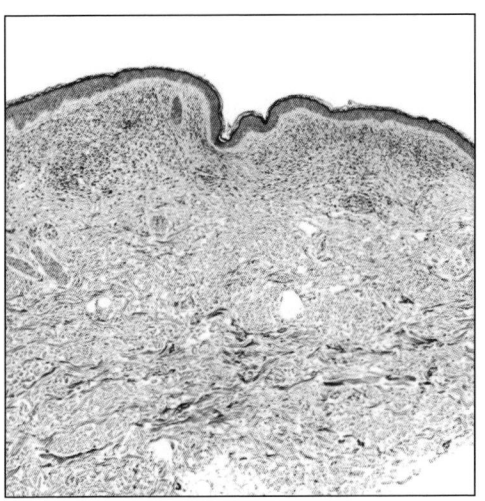

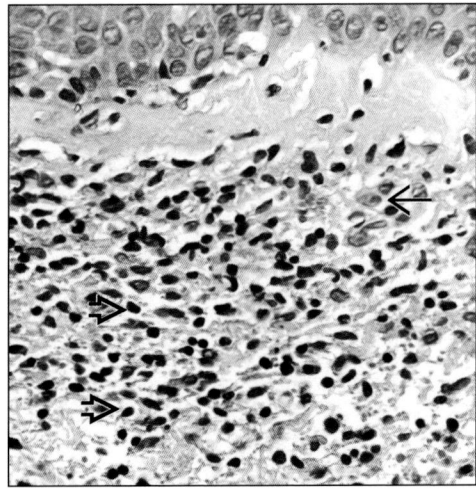

(Left) In this case of indeterminate cell histiocytosis, the superficial dermis contains a histiocytic lesion intermixed with scattered lymphocytes. No epidermotropism is seen. The patient presented with numerous red/brown papules that were coalescing on his face. (Right) At higher power, 2 populations of cells are seen. The histiocyte-like cells appear with fine chromatin and clefted nuclei ➡. There are also scattered small T cells with more coarse chromatin ➡.

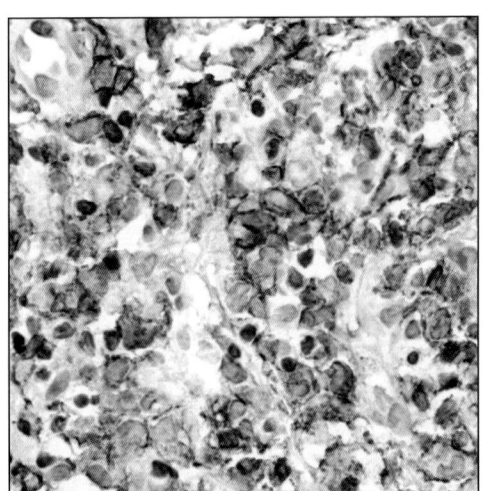

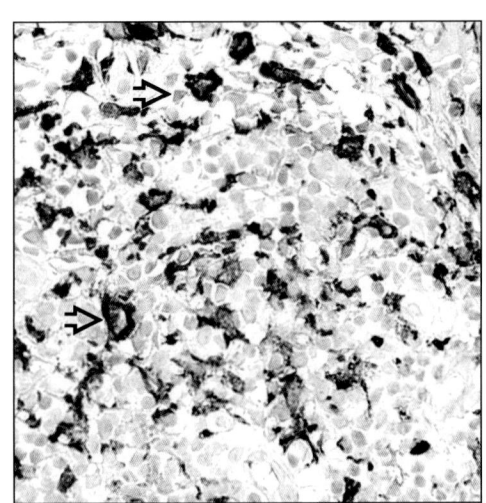

(Left) Indeterminate cell histiocytosis shows features of histiocytes and Langerhans cells. This is an image showing strong, diffuse positive CD1a in the cells of ICH. CD1a is often a marker of Langerhans cells. (Right) ICH shares phenotypic similarities with histiocytes, as the ICH cells are highlighted by CD163 ➡, a macrophage marker. CD68 was also positive (not shown).

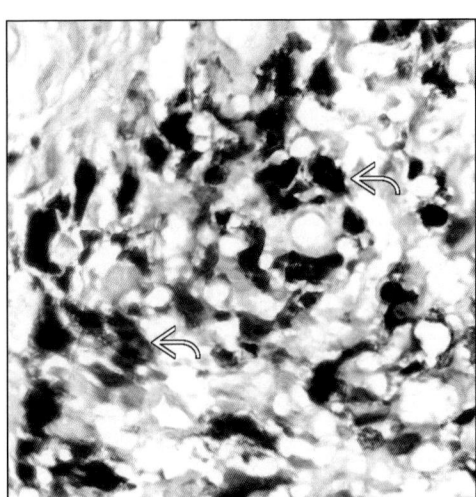

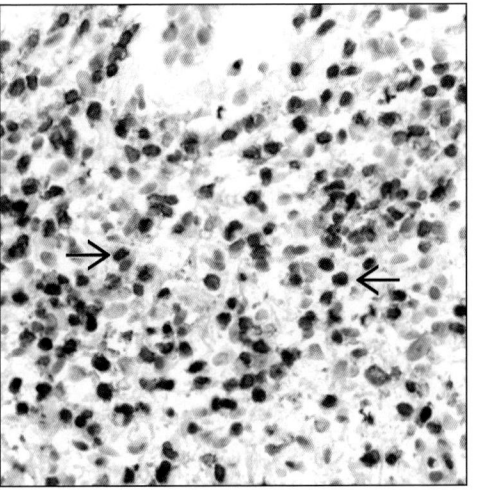

(Left) In this case of ICH, the cells are immunoreactive for S100 ➡. The immunophenotype of histiocyte-like cells that are positive for CD1a, CD163, and S100 is unusual and points to the diagnosis of ICH instead of LCH. Langerin was negative, and no Birbeck granules were seen ultrastructurally, arguing against LCH. (Right) This CD3 immunostain shows increased numbers of small T cells ➡ among the histiocyte-like cells.

NON-LANGERHANS CELL HISTIOCYTOSES

HPMH and Atypical Granuloma Annulare

(**Left**) This is a biopsy specimen from a 40-year-old woman with hereditary progressive mucinous histiocytosis (HPMH). She had multiple papules on her face, similar to those of her mother and daughter. HPMH has an autosomal dominant-like transmission mostly involving women. The dermal lesions consist of histiocytes and mucin. (**Right**) The dermal nodule is composed of epithelioid histiocytes ➡ and mucin separating broad bundles of collagen ➘.

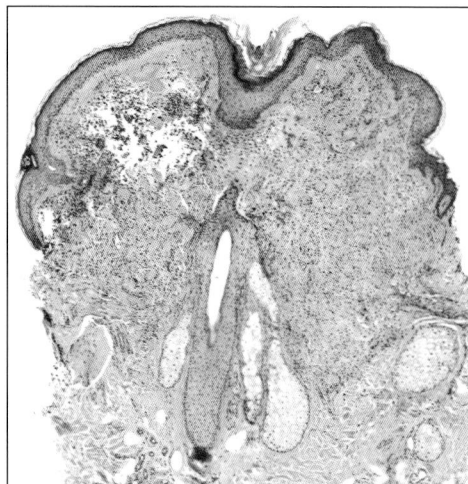
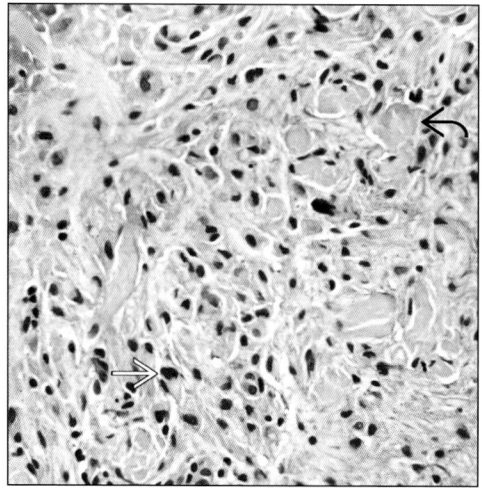

(**Left**) In this case of HPMH, CD68 shows moderate to strong cytoplasmic staining. (**Right**) CD163, another macrophage marker, is also strongly positive ➡ in the histiocytes of HPMH. S100 and CD1a were negative (not shown). Ultrastructural studies showed myelin and zebra bodies.

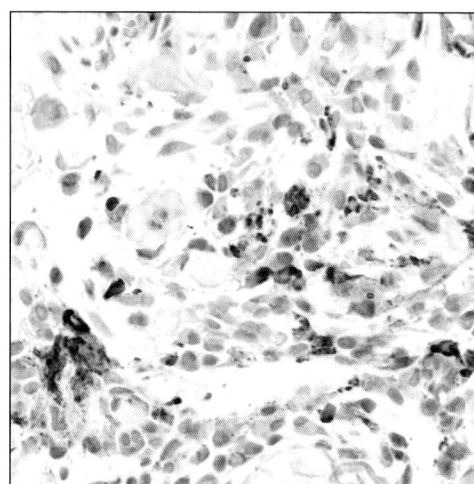
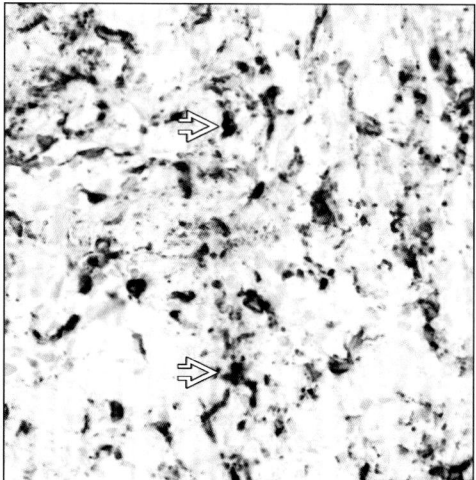

(**Left**) Low-power magnification of a case of atypical granuloma annulare (AGA) shows that there are vaguely formed granulomas ➡ with palisading though the collagen in the superficial and deep dermis. There is more cellularity than would be seen in a typical granuloma annulare. (**Right**) High-power magnification of a case of AGA shows that there are more mitotic figures ➡ than in a typical granuloma annulare. AGA usually has ≥ 1 mitotic figures per HPF.

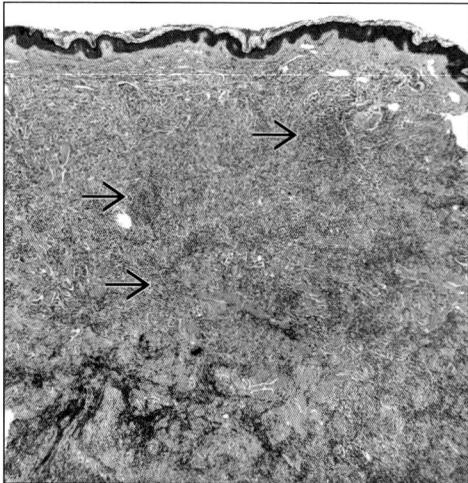
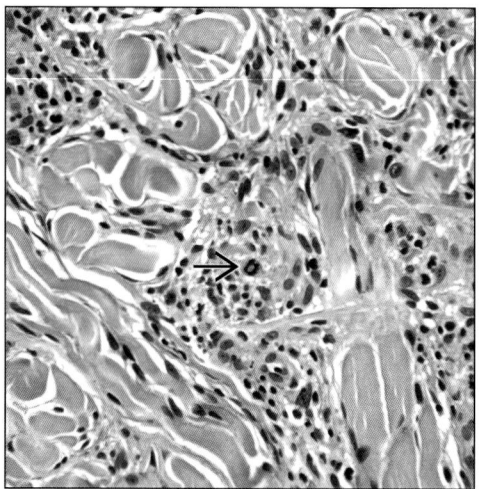

Differential Diagnosis

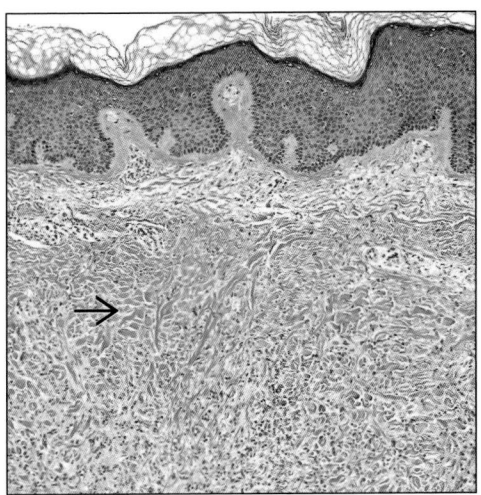

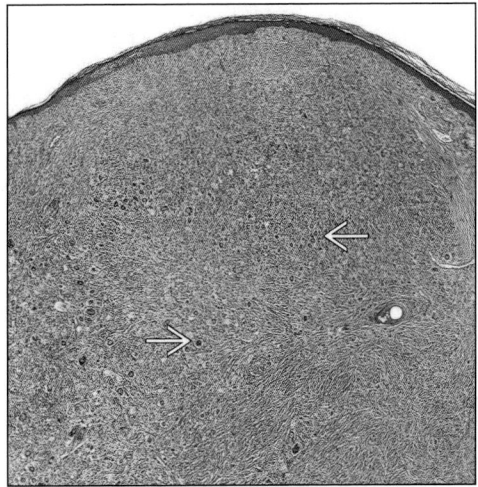

(Left) This dermatofibroma shows bland spindled to histiocytoid-appearing cells in the dermis with overlying epidermal hyperplasia and basilar pigmentation. The spindled cells are entrapping numerous hyalinized balls of collagen ➡. *(Right)* This juvenile xanthogranuloma shows a uniform cellular lesion in the dermis with no grenz zone and scattered Touton giant cells ➡ with peripheral wreath-like arrangement of nuclei.

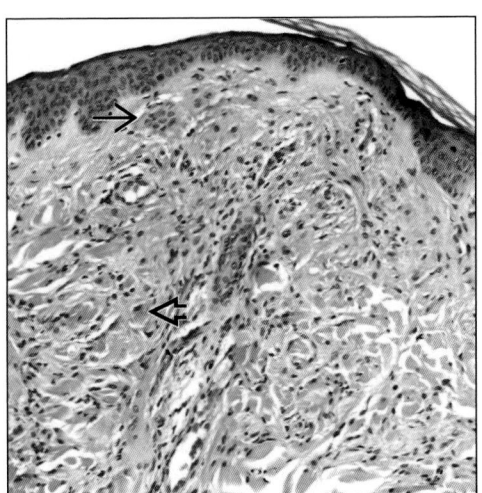

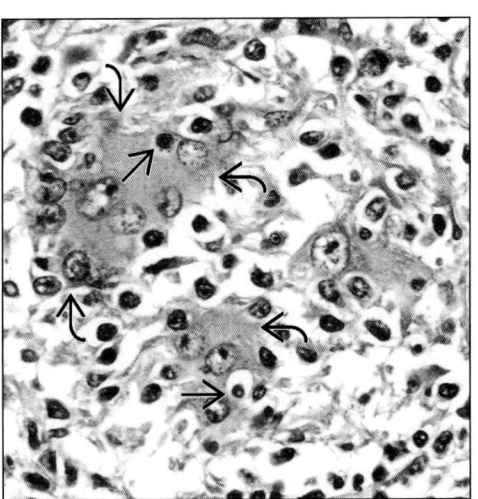

(Left) This reticulohistiocytoma is seen as a hypocellular dermal lesion consisting of scattered large histiocytes with characteristic glassy cytoplasm ➡ and rare multinucleated giant cells ➡. *(Right)* This example of Rosai-Dorfman disease shows striking emperipolesis by the proliferating histiocytes. Lymphocytes ➡ are seen within the cytoplasm of histiocytes ➡.

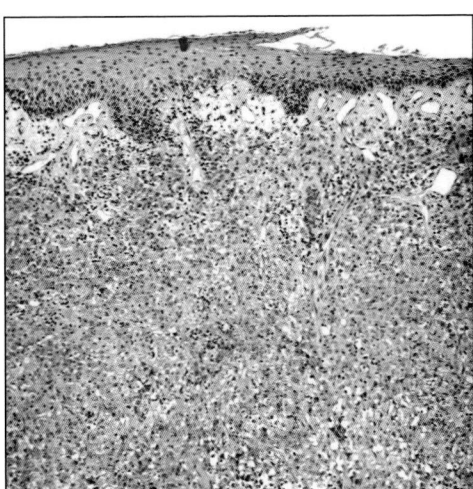

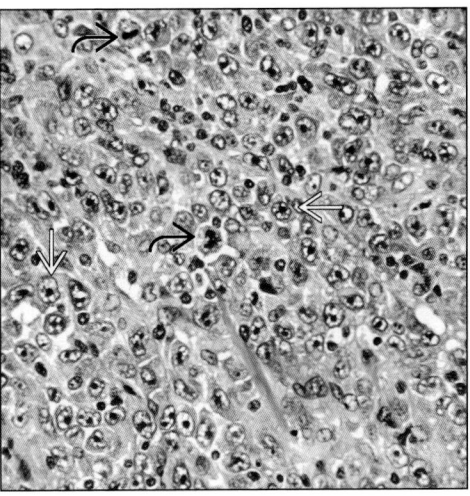

(Left) This histiocytic sarcoma shows a diffuse, dermal-based, sheet-like proliferation of enlarged, undifferentiated-appearing cells at low-power magnification. *(Right)* High magnification of histiocytic sarcoma shows sheets of markedly enlarged and atypical cells ➡ with abundant cytoplasm, enlarged nuclei with prominent nucleoli, and scattered mitotic figures ➡.

LANGERHANS CELL HISTIOCYTOSIS

This example of Langerhans cell histiocytosis of the skin presented as a seborrheic-like erythematous rash with petechiae on the abdomen of a 23-month-old child. (Courtesy S. Vanderhooft, MD.)

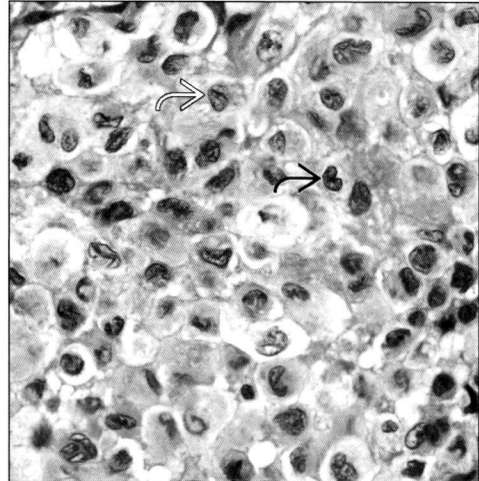

This high-power view shows the characteristic features of Langerhans cells: Folded ⇗ or grooved ↗ nuclei, and abundant pink cytoplasm.

TERMINOLOGY

Abbreviations
- Langerhans cell histiocytosis (LCH)

Synonyms
- Histiocytosis X
- Eosinophilic granuloma

Definitions
- Clonal proliferation of Langerhans cells

CLINICAL ISSUES

Epidemiology
- Age
  - 1st 3 decades of life, but rarely may also occur in older adults
- Gender
  - Male to female ratio = 2:1

Site
- Skin
  - Erythematous, crusted, vesiculopustular rash, or salmon-colored macular-papular rash
- Bone and bone marrow
  - Skull, pelvis, long bones, vertebrae
- CNS
  - Primary in dura, leptomeninges, or parenchyma
  - May be secondary to skull or vertebral involvement
- Other organs that may be affected include lung, lymph nodes, liver, thymus, and GI tract

Presentation
- Newborns and infants usually present with limited skin or bone lesions
- Generalized disease is more common in young children
- Rash may precede systemic findings by several months
- **Eosinophilic granuloma**
  - Single or multiple lesions restricted to bone
- **Hand-Schüller-Christian disease**
  - Multiple organ involvement
  - Diabetes insipidus and exophthalmos
- **Letterer-Siwe disease**
  - Disseminated disease with skin, lymph node, visceral, and marrow involvement
  - Aggressive; many die within 1 year due to extensive lung involvement

Natural History
- May spontaneously resolve or progress

Treatment
- Surgical approaches
  - Local excision for limited disease
- Drugs
  - Chemotherapy for disseminated disease
- Radiation
  - Low-dose radiation for difficult-to-resect lesions

Prognosis
- Poor prognosis associated with
  - Hepatosplenomegaly
  - Thrombocytopenia
  - Young age at diagnosis

IMAGE FINDINGS

Radiographic Findings
- Bone lesions generally well-defined and lytic

MICROSCOPIC PATHOLOGY

Histologic Features
- Langerhans cells infiltrate dermis and subcutis and often extend throughout epidermis to stratum corneum
- Langerhans cells show

LANGERHANS CELL HISTIOCYTOSIS

Key Facts

Terminology
- LCH is also known as
  - Histiocytosis X
  - Eosinophilic granuloma
- Defined as clonal proliferation of Langerhans cells

Clinical Issues
- Newborns and infants usually present with limited skin or bone lesions
- Erythematous, crusted, vesiculopustular rash
- Common sites include skin, bone and bone marrow, and lung
- Male to female ratio = 2:1
- **Eosinophilic granuloma** is restricted to bone
- **Hand-Schüller-Christian disease** has multiple organ involvement and diabetes insipidus

- **Letterer-Siwe disease** is aggressive with multisystem involvement

Microscopic Pathology
- Langerhans cells infiltrate dermis and subcutis and often extend throughout epidermis to stratum corneum
- Langerhans cells show
  - Abundant eosinophilic show cytoplasm
  - Coffee bean-shaped nucleus
- Large numbers of eosinophils and other inflammatory cells typically present
- Mitoses common, but usually not atypical

Ancillary Tests
- CD1a and S100 immunostaining
- Birbeck granules seen on EM

  - Abundant eosinophilic cytoplasm
  - Coffee bean-shaped nuclei or lobulated nucleus with central groove
  - Small nucleolus
- Large numbers of eosinophils frequently present
  - Other inflammatory cells also seen, including multinucleated giant cells
- Necrosis is common
- Mitoses common, but usually not atypical
- Bone marrow aspirates
  - Langerhans cells may be single or in small groups intermixed with hematopoietic precursors
- Lymph nodes
  - Architecture generally preserved
  - Sinuses are distended by Langerhans cells
- Liver
  - Portal or parenchymal nodules, or diffusely infiltrates sinusoids
  - May result in sclerosing cholangitis
    - 15% of all sclerosing cholangitis in children caused by LCH
- Disease passes through various stages
  - Necrosis and increasing fibrosis seen in older lesions

ANCILLARY TESTS

Immunohistochemistry
- CD1a is very specific for Langerhans cells
- Langerin is also specific for Langerhans cells
- S100 is not specific but stains Langerhans cells

Electron Microscopy
- Birbeck granules
  - Tubular pentilaminar membrane-bound cytoplasmic bodies, often with terminal oval protrusion
  - Tennis racket shaped

DIFFERENTIAL DIAGNOSIS

Granulomatous Infiltrates
- Multinucleated, foreign body giant cells typically present
- Histiocytic cells are CD68 positive, CD1a negative

Rosai-Dorfman Disease
- LCH does not display emperipolesis
- Histiocytes are S100(+) but CD1a(-)

Indeterminate Cell Histiocytosis
- Histologic and immunohistochemical features essentially identical to LCH
- Lack Birbeck granules by ultrastructural examination

Hodgkin and Non-Hodgkin Lymphoma
- Cells lack characteristic nuclear features of LCH
- Neoplastic cells are usually CD15 and CD30(+), CD1a(-)

SELECTED REFERENCES

1. Ezra N et al: CD30 positive anaplastic large-cell lymphoma mimicking Langerhans cell histiocytosis. J Cutan Pathol. 37(7):787-92, 2010
2. Degar BA et al: Langerhans cell histiocytosis: malignancy or inflammatory disorder doing a great job of imitating one? Dis Model Mech. 2(9-10):436-9, 2009
3. Gavhed D et al: Biomarkers in the cerebrospinal fluid and neurodegeneration in Langerhans cell histiocytosis. Pediatr Blood Cancer. 53(7):1264-70, 2009
4. Imashuku S et al: Langerhans cell histiocytosis with multifocal bone lesions: comparative clinical features between single and multi-systems. Int J Hematol. 90(4):506-12, 2009
5. Jaffe R: Is there a role for histopathology in predicting the clinical outcome in congenital and infant Langerhans cell disease? Pediatr Blood Cancer. 53(6):924-5, 2009

LANGERHANS CELL HISTIOCYTOSIS

Microscopic and Immunohistochemical Features

(Left) Cutaneous involvement by Langerhans cell histiocytosis can often resemble a melanocytic proliferation at low-power examination. The correct diagnosis is easily made by looking for the characteristic nuclear features and using confirmatory immunohistochemical stains. *(Right)* Higher power view of Langerhans cell histiocytosis in the skin shows numerous Langerhans cells infiltrating into the epidermis ➡. Usually they are present as nests or small aggregates, as seen here.

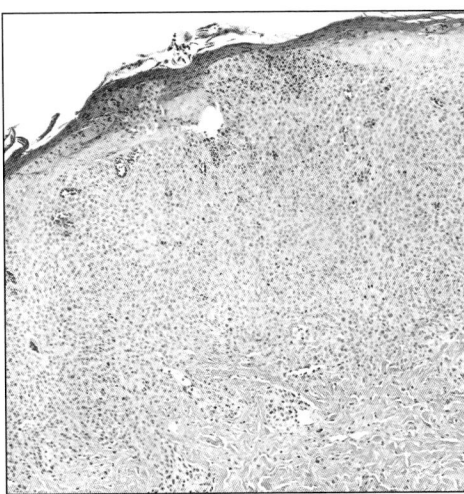
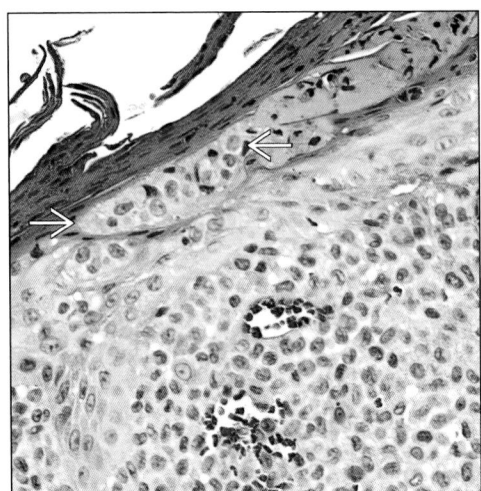

(Left) High-power view highlights the typical nuclear features of Langerhans cells. The nuclei are folded, show long grooves ➡, and often resemble coffee beans. An eosinophil is seen ➡. *(Right)* Low-power view of Langerhans cell histiocytosis shows a collection of eosinophils ➡ representing an eosinophilic granuloma. Eosinophilic granuloma is another term for Langerhans cell histiocytosis, which is used to describe nodules restricted to bone.

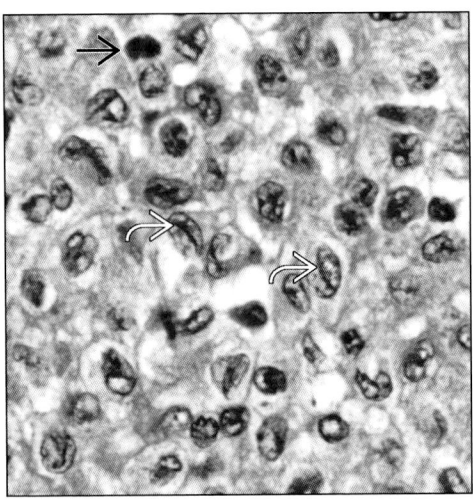
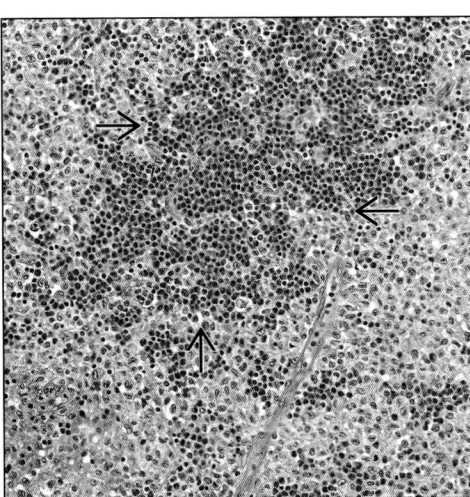

(Left) Langerhans cells show positive membranous and cytoplasmic immunoreactivity for CD1a. Grooved nuclei ➡ can be seen within the positive staining cells. CD1a is very specific for Langerhans cells and is very useful in cases where the cellularity is low. *(Right)* Langerhans cells show positive nuclear and cytoplasmic immunoreactivity for S100. While S100 is not as specific as CD1a for Langerhans cells, it still can be quite useful as a confirmatory marker.

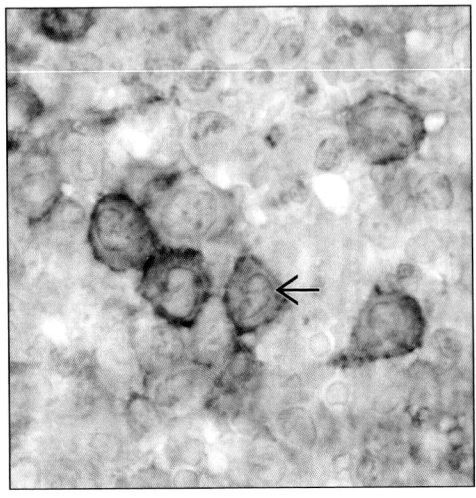
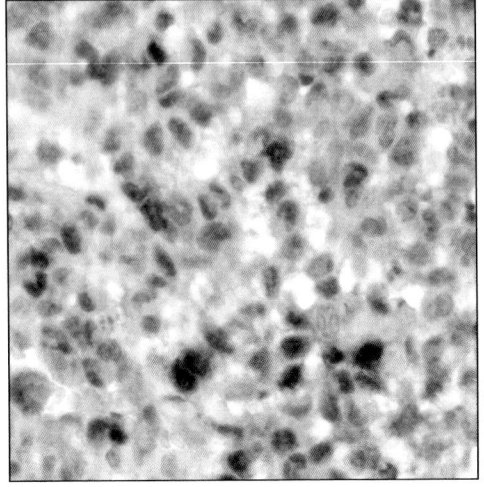

LANGERHANS CELL HISTIOCYTOSIS

Imaging and Microscopic Features

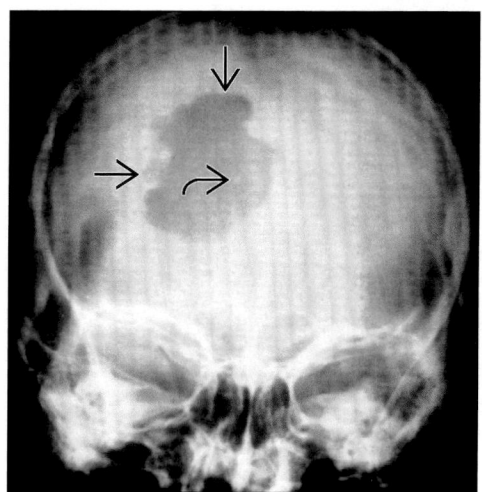
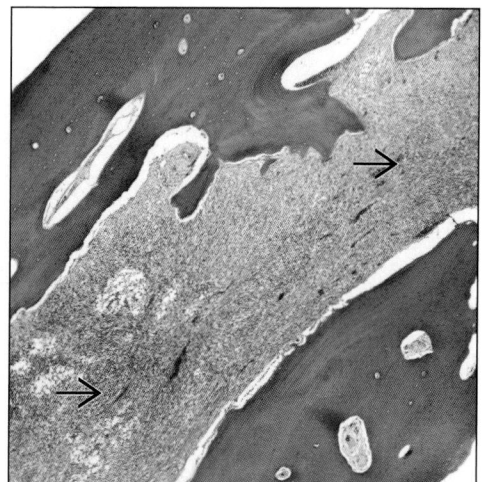

(Left) This radiograph of the skull shows the typical appearance of Langerhans cell histiocytosis in bone ➡. The lesion is lytic with scalloped edges and sharp borders, with a radiodense focus ➡ that is commonly seen in skull lesions. *(Right)* This low-power view of the skull shows Langerhans cell histiocytosis infiltrating through and replacing the marrow space ➡. The skull is a common location for LCH to occur.

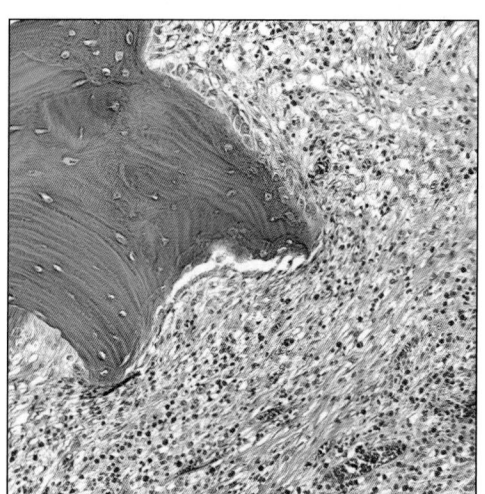
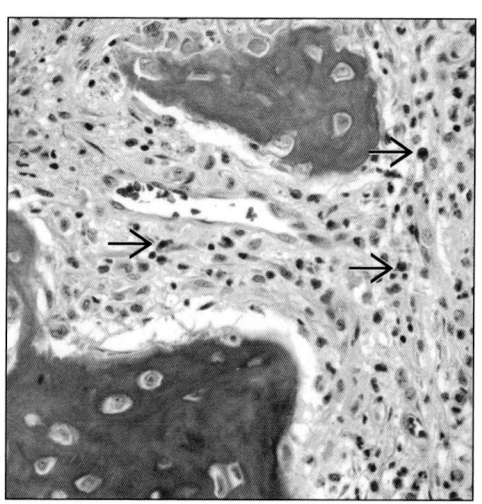

(Left) The histology of Langerhans cell histiocytosis in bone can vary widely. In this example, there is fibrosis and less cellularity; Langerhans cells can be hard to find without the aid of immunostains. *(Right)* High-power view of this Langerhans cell histiocytosis in bone shows less cellularity and a fibrous stroma, with scattered eosinophils ➡. Langerhans cells can be difficult to identify, making immunostains, especially CD1a, very helpful.

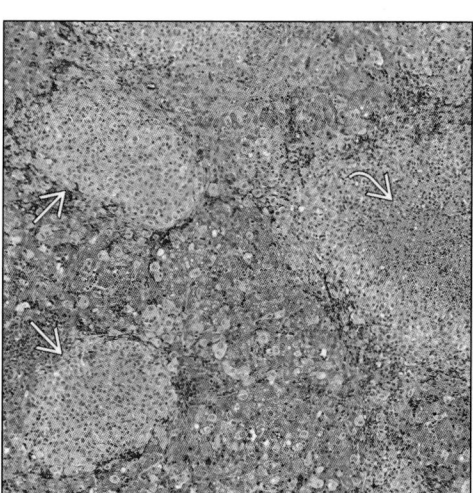
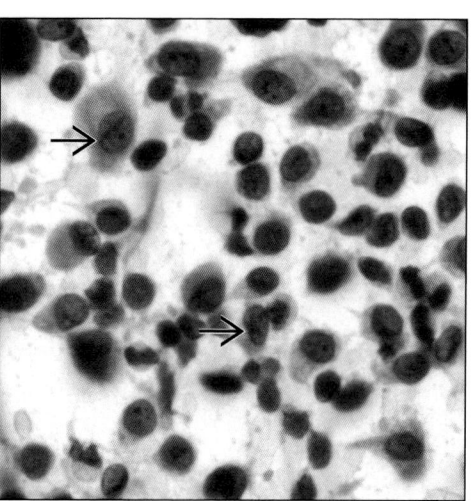

(Left) This low-power example of Langerhans cell histiocytosis in the liver shows multiple scattered nodules ➡. The large nodule on the right ➡ has a necrotic center; necrosis is common in Langerhans cell histiocytosis. *(Right)* Touch preps made at the time of frozen section can be very helpful. The characteristic Langerhans cell features are easily identified, with grooved nuclei ➡ and abundant pink cytoplasm.

ROSAI-DORFMAN DISEASE

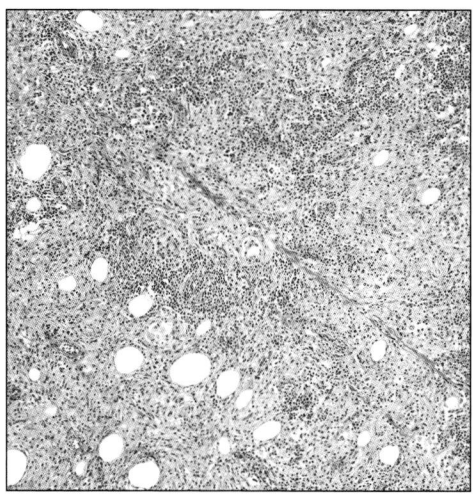

Histologic examination shows a low-power image of extranodal (soft tissue) Rosai-Dorfman disease. The proliferating histiocytes are spindled, infiltrating fat. Small lymphoid aggregates are present.

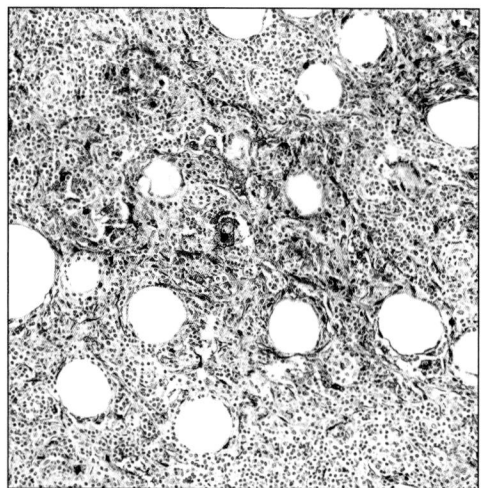

S100 protein shows labeling of the proliferating histiocytes. The staining pattern is not diffuse and must be correlated with the morphology. Some labeled cells are dendritic cells.

TERMINOLOGY

Abbreviations
- Rosai-Dorfman disease (RDD)

Synonyms
- Sinus histiocytosis with massive lymphadenopathy (SHML)
  - Applies to disease involving lymph nodes

Definitions
- Rare, acquired, nonmalignant proliferation of distinctive histiocytes that presents with lymphadenopathy or extranodal disease
  - Lesional histiocytes contain variable numbers of intact lymphocytes within cytoplasm
    - Phenomenon referred to as lymphophagocytosis or emperipolesis
  - Primarily in children and young adults

ETIOLOGY/PATHOGENESIS

Exuberant Hematopoietic Response to Undetermined Immunologic Trigger
- Association with autoimmune lymphoproliferative syndrome has been described
  - Inherited disorder of lymphocyte-programmed cell death with mutations in death receptor genes that specifically eliminate apoptosis in lymphocyte subsets
  - Occurs primarily in early childhood
  - May represent acquired disorder of deregulation of apoptotic signaling pathways
- Various infections associated with cases of RDD/SHML, but none proven as etiologic infectious agent
  - Parvovirus
  - Epstein-Barr virus
  - HHV6
  - Polyoma virus

CLINICAL ISSUES

Presentation
- Varies with site
  - Painless lymphadenopathy is most frequent presenting symptom
    - Involves cervical region in up to 90% of patients
  - 30-45% of patients have at least 1 site of extranodal involvement as well as lymph node involvement
    - Hepatosplenomegaly uncommon
  - ~ 25% of patients have extranodal disease only
  - Skin and soft tissue most common extranodal sites
    - Approximate frequency of extranodal sites
    - Skin and soft tissue (16%)
    - Nasal cavity and paranasal sinuses (16%)
    - Eye, orbit, and ocular adnexa (11%)
    - Bone (11%)
    - Salivary gland (7%)
    - Central nervous system (7%)
    - Oral cavity (4%)
    - Kidney and genitourinary tract (3%)
    - Respiratory tract (3%)
    - Liver (1%)
    - Tonsil (1%)
    - Breast (< 1%)
    - Gastrointestinal tract (< 1%)
    - Heart (< 1%)
  - Simultaneous involvement of multiple extranodal sites not unusual
  - Involvement of kidney, lower respiratory tract, and liver associated with worse clinical outcome (as is number of extranodal sites)

Treatment
- Most patients require little intervention

Prognosis
- Most patients have complete and spontaneous remission

ROSAI-DORFMAN DISEASE

Key Facts

Terminology
- Lesional histiocytes contain variable numbers of intact lymphocytes within their cytoplasm
  - Referred to as lymphophagocytosis or emperipolesis
- Sinus histiocytosis with massive lymphadenopathy (term for disease involving lymph nodes)

Clinical Issues
- Painless lymphadenopathy most frequent presenting symptom
- Skin and soft tissue most common extranodal site
- Poor prognosis correlates with widespread dissemination
  - Involves kidneys, lower respiratory tract, liver, and immunologic abnormalities or anemia
- Most patients have complete & spontaneous remission

- Some may experience recurrent or persistent but stable lymphadenopathy

Microscopic Pathology
- Skin and soft tissue cases have more subtle histologic features than lymph node counterparts
- Emperipolesis less conspicuous
- Proliferating histiocytes frequently spindled
- Majority of lesions label with S100
- Vague storiform pattern
- Scattered lymphoplasmacytic aggregates

Top Differential Diagnoses
- Langerhans cell histiocytosis (LCH)
- Juvenile xanthogranuloma
- Disorders featuring granulomatous inflammation
- Histiocytic sarcoma (histiocytic lymphoma)

- Some may experience recurrent or persistent but stable lymphadenopathy
- In very few cases, disease follows aggressive course and may be fatal
  - Poor prognosis correlates with widespread dissemination, involvement of kidneys, lower respiratory tract, and liver, and immunologic abnormalities or anemia

MACROSCOPIC FEATURES

General Features
- In soft tissues and other extranodal sites
  - Firm, poorly marginated lesion
- In lymph nodes
  - Firm massively enlarged lymph nodes

MICROSCOPIC PATHOLOGY

Histologic Features
- RDD of skin and soft tissue has more subtle histologic features than its lymph node counterpart
  - Emperipolesis less conspicuous
  - Proliferating histiocytes frequently spindled
  - Abundant associated collagen deposition
  - Vague storiform pattern
  - Scattered lymphoplasmacytic aggregates
  - Mild cytologic atypia
- In lymph nodes ("sinus histiocytosis with massive lymphadenopathy")
  - Expanded sinuses contain histiocytic cells with abundant cytoplasm, sometimes multinucleated
  - Emperipolesis a striking feature
  - Lesional cells S100 protein reactive
- Majority of lesions label with S100 protein

Predominant Cell/Compartment Type
- Hematopoietic, histiocytic

DIFFERENTIAL DIAGNOSIS

Langerhans Cell Histiocytosis (LCH)
- Cells with nuclear grooves ("coffee-bean"-shaped), backdrop of eosinophils
- Expresses both S100 and CD1a

Juvenile Xanthogranuloma (JXG)
- Non-Langerhans cell histiocytosis
- Cutaneous form most common
  - Nodules often develop shortly after birth
  - Most common site head and neck, followed by trunk and extremities
  - Many nodules regress spontaneously
- Rare deep cases
  - Skeletal muscle, parenchymal organs
- No association with lipid metabolism disorders
- Histiocytic cells with variable giant cells, lipid
- Background inflammatory cells, often many eosinophils
- CD68(+), CD31(+), S100 protein (-), CD1a(-)

Various Disorders Featuring Granulomatous Inflammation
- Mycobacterial infection
  - Granulomas composed of S100 negative histiocytes
  - No emperipolesis
  - Organisms can be detected by culture/special stains
- Chronic granulomatous disease (CGD)
  - Rare primary inherited immunodeficiency (incidence 1:200,000 in USA)
  - Affects phagocytes (neutrophils & macrophages) that contain nicotinamide adenine dinucleotide phosphate (reduced NADPH) oxidase enzyme
    - Generates superoxide required for killing microorganisms
  - Dysfunction of NADPH oxidase in CGD results in ineffective respiratory burst in phagocytes
    - Unable to kill and digest certain bacteria and fungi, predisposing patients to infections
  - Functional diagnosis of CGD

ROSAI-DORFMAN DISEASE

Immunohistochemistry

Antibody	Reactivity	Staining Pattern	Comment
S100	Positive	Nuclear & cytoplasmic	Intracytoplasmic hematopoietic cells negative
CD68	Positive	Cytoplasmic	
CD1a	Negative		RDD is a non-Langerhans cell histiocytosis

- ■ Demonstrates absence or marked reduction in phagocytic respiratory burst to form superoxides, using tests such as nitroblue tetrazolium (NBT) reduction
- ■ Neutrophils stimulated with phorbol myristate acetate and incubated with yellow dye NBT
- ■ Normal phagocytes reduce this to dark pigment formazan, with mixed NBT-positive and NBT-negative cells, denoting carrier status
  - ○ Features loose collections of pigmented histiocytes typically in lung and GI tract with variable granuloma formation
  - ○ S100 protein stain negative
- • Malakoplakia
  - ○ Acquired granulomatous disorder (1st described by Michaelis & Gutmann)
  - ○ Believed to result from acquired bacteriocidal defect in macrophages
    - ■ Occurring mostly in immunosuppressed patients or in setting of autoimmune disease
  - ○ Usually in bladder or GI tract
  - ○ Collections of histiocytes
    - ■ S100 negative
  - ○ Contain targetoid inclusions that stain with von Kossa stain
    - ■ Believed to reflect concretions of phagocytosed bacteria

Sarcoidosis

- • Well-formed granulomas with mild background infiltrate
- • Histiocytes lack S100 labeling
- • Emperipolesis not a typical feature

Histiocytic Sarcoma (Histiocytic Lymphoma)

- • Marked cytologic atypia
- • Expresses host of histiocytic markers, but not S100 protein
- • Aggressive clinical course

Malignant Fibrous Histiocytoma (High-Grade Pleomorphic Undifferentiated Sarcoma)

- • Composed of highly pleomorphic spindle cells
- • Negative S100 protein
- • Emperipolesis not a typical feature

Follicular Dendritic Cell Tumor/Sarcoma

- • Oval to spindle-shaped cells with eosinophilic cytoplasm in sheets & fascicles, focal storiform pattern & whorls (similar to those seen in meningioma)
- • Oval or elongated nuclei with thin nuclear membranes, inconspicuous or small eosinophilic nucleoli, and clear or dispersed chromatin

- • Tumor cells are intimately admixed with small lymphocytes, with prominent perivascular cuffing
- • Multinucleate cells common
- • Necrosis, marked cellular atypia, high mitotic rate, &/ or abnormal mitoses common
- • Express CD21, CD35, podoplanin (D2-40), S100 protein

SELECTED REFERENCES

1. Al-Daraji W et al: Soft tissue Rosai-Dorfman disease: 29 new lesions in 18 patients, with detection of polyomavirus antigen in 3 abdominal cases. Ann Diagn Pathol. 14(5):309-16, 2010
2. Gaitonde S: Multifocal, extranodal sinus histiocytosis with massive lymphadenopathy: an overview. Arch Pathol Lab Med. 131(7):1117-21, 2007
3. Mehraein Y et al: Parvovirus B19 detected in Rosai-Dorfman disease in nodal and extranodal manifestations. J Clin Pathol. 59(12):1320-6, 2006
4. Wang KH et al: Cutaneous Rosai-Dorfman disease: clinicopathological profiles, spectrum and evolution of 21 lesions in six patients. Br J Dermatol. 154(2):277-86, 2006
5. Maric I et al: Histologic features of sinus histiocytosis with massive lymphadenopathy in patients with autoimmune lymphoproliferative syndrome. Am J Surg Pathol. 29(7):903-11, 2005
6. Rodriguez-Galindo C et al: Extranodal Rosai-Dorfman disease in children. J Pediatr Hematol Oncol. 26(1):19-24, 2004
7. Anders RA et al: Rosai-Dorfman disease presenting in the gastrointestinal tract. Arch Pathol Lab Med. 127(2):E74-5, 2003
8. Andriko JA et al: Rosai-Dorfman disease isolated to the central nervous system: a report of 11 cases. Mod Pathol. 14(3):172-8, 2001
9. Lauwers GY et al: The digestive system manifestations of Rosai-Dorfman disease (sinus histiocytosis with massive lymphadenopathy): review of 11 cases. Hum Pathol. 31(3):380-5, 2000
10. Levine PH et al: Detection of human herpesvirus 6 in tissues involved by sinus histiocytosis with massive lymphadenopathy (Rosai-Dorfman disease). J Infect Dis. 166(2):291-5, 1992
11. Montgomery EA et al: Rosai-Dorfman disease of soft tissue. Am J Surg Pathol. 16(2):122-9, 1992
12. Eisen RN et al: Immunophenotypic characterization of sinus histiocytosis with massive lymphadenopathy (Rosai-Dorfman disease). Semin Diagn Pathol. 7(1):74-82, 1990
13. Foucar E et al: Sinus histiocytosis with massive lymphadenopathy (Rosai-Dorfman disease): review of the entity. Semin Diagn Pathol. 7(1):19-73, 1990
14. Foucar E et al: Sinus histiocytosis with massive lymphadenopathy. An analysis of 14 deaths occurring in a patient registry. Cancer. 54(9):1834-40, 1984
15. Rosai J et al: Sinus histiocytosis with massive lymphadenopathy. A newly recognized benign clinicopathological entity. Arch Pathol. 87(1):63-70, 1969

ROSAI-DORFMAN DISEASE

Microscopic Features and Differential Diagnosis

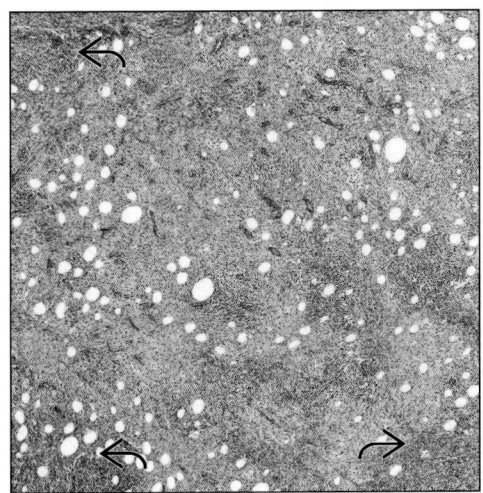

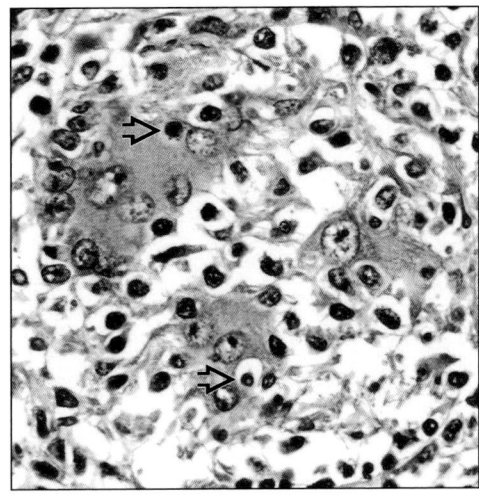

(Left) Histologic examination at low magnification shows a case of soft tissue Rosai-Dorfman disease. Note the scattered lymphoid aggregates ➘ arranged throughout the lesion in a random distribution. *(Right)* High magnification shows the key microscopic feature of Rosai-Dorfman disease, namely striking emperipolesis by the proliferating histiocytes. The cytoplasmic lymphocytes are fully intact ➘.

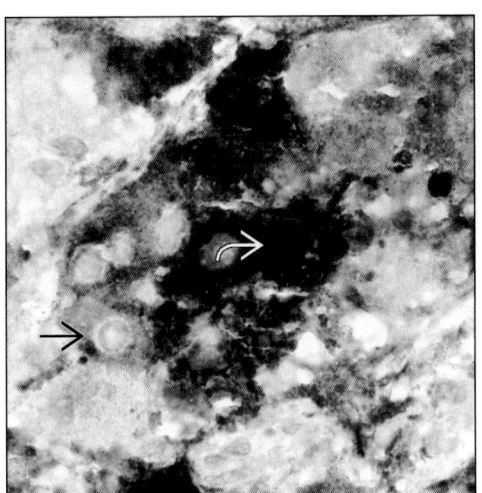

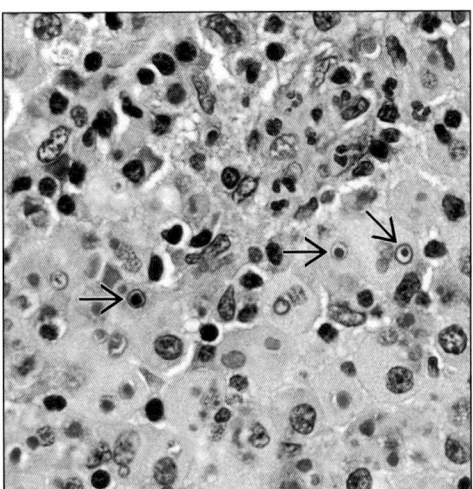

(Left) S100 shows nuclear ➘ and cytoplasmic labeling in the histiocytes. Note that the engulfed lymphocytes in the field do not express S100 protein. They are undamaged and surrounded by a "halo" ➘. The S100 stain sometimes accentuates this emperipolesis. *(Right)* Histologic examination shows an example of malakoplakia. There are several Michaelis-Gutmann bodies indicated ➘. These consist of incompletely eradicated engulfed bacteria.

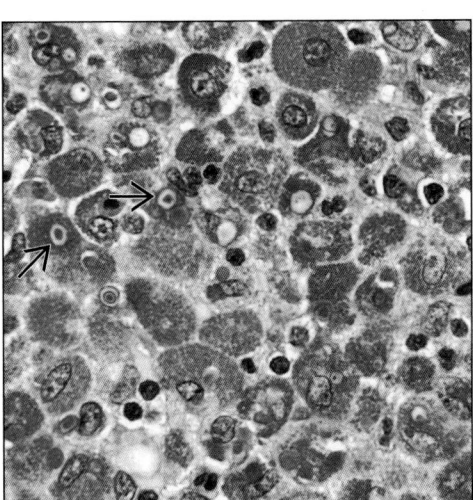

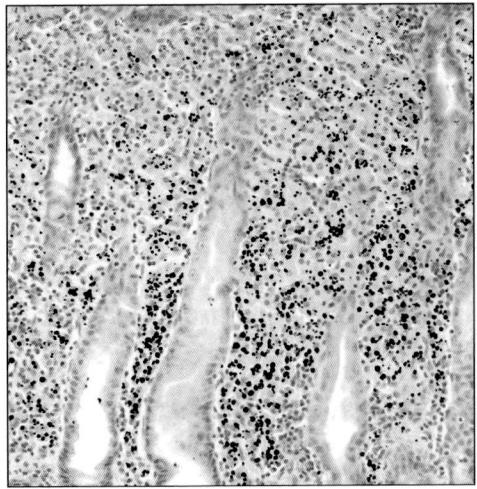

(Left) Periodic acid-Schiff with diastase digestion in malakoplakia shows Michaelis-Gutmann bodies that are PAS negative ➘, despite strong staining in the histiocytes' cytoplasm. *(Right)* von Kossa stain highlights many Michaelis-Gutmann bodies in malakoplakia. In this dramatic example, the bodies are numerous, but most cases display fewer Michaelis-Gutmann bodies.

HISTIOCYTIC SARCOMA

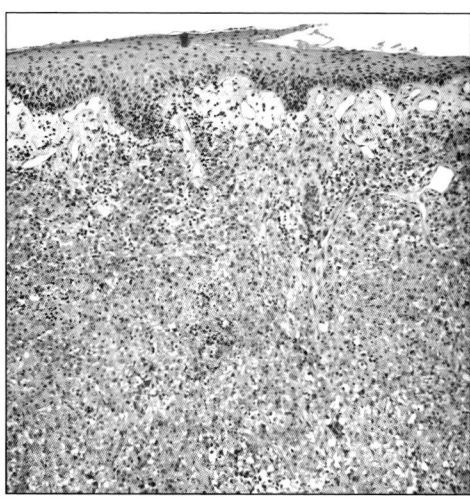

Histiocytic sarcoma at low magnification shows a diffuse, dermal-based sheet-like proliferation of enlarged, undifferentiated-appearing cells at this power.

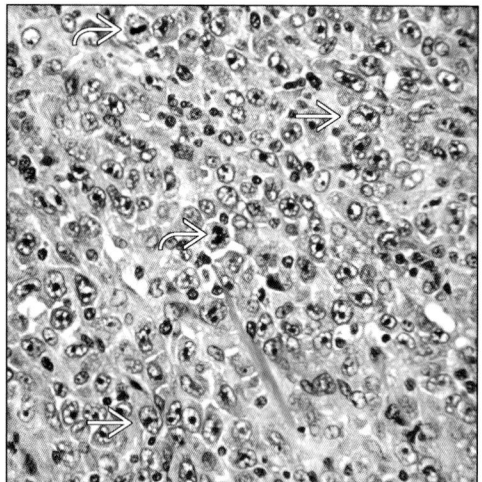

High magnification of histiocytic sarcoma shows sheets of markedly enlarged and atypical cells ➡ with abundant cytoplasm, enlarged nuclei with prominent nucleoli, and scattered mitotic figures ➡.

TERMINOLOGY

Abbreviations
- Histiocytic sarcoma (HS)

Synonyms
- Extramedullary monocytic tumor
- Malignant histiocytosis
- True histiocytic lymphoma

Definitions
- Malignant tumor of mature histiocytes
  - Neoplasms associated with acute monocytic leukemia are excluded
    - Are now classified as monocytic sarcoma

ETIOLOGY/PATHOGENESIS

Etiology
- Idiopathic
  - Sometimes associated with germ cell tumors
  - Also can be associated with lymphoma, leukemia, or myelodysplastic syndrome

Postulated Normal Counterpart
- Mature histiocyte

CLINICAL ISSUES

Epidemiology
- Incidence
  - Extremely rare tumor
- Age
  - Mostly in adults
    - Median age = 52 years old
    - Rare in children
- Gender
  - Approximately equal male:female ratio
- Ethnicity

- No known ethnic predilection

Site
- Most cases are extranodal
  - Skin, gastrointestinal tract, and soft tissue most common
- Lymph node less common

Presentation
- Often a single painless mass
  - B symptoms common
- Skin
  - Variable presentation
    - Can be seen as a rash, a single lesion, or multiple lesions (disseminated)
- Gastrointestinal tract
  - Abdominal pain
  - Intestinal obstruction
- Bone marrow
  - Focal/patchy bone marrow involvement is considered HS
    - Diffuse bone marrow involvement is currently classified as acute monocytic leukemia

Laboratory Tests
- Cytopenias in some patients
  - Thrombocytopenia is most common

Natural History
- Some patients develop both histiocytic tumors and lymphoid tumors
  - Lineage promiscuity (a.k.a. transdifferentiation)
  - Both tumors share molecular findings
    - HS can have t(14;18)(q32;q21)
    - HS can have clonal *IgH* gene rearrangements
    - Identical *IgH* rearrangements or *BCL2* gene breakpoints in same patients with HS and B-cell lymphoma

Treatment
- Surgical approaches

HISTIOCYTIC SARCOMA

Key Facts

Terminology
- Histiocytic sarcoma (HS)
- Malignant histiocytosis
- Extramedullary monocytic tumor

Clinical Issues
- Extremely rare tumor
- Mostly seen in adults
- Usually rash or single lesion on skin
- Some patients develop both histiocytic tumors and lymphoid tumors (transdifferentiation)

Microscopic Pathology
- Dermal and subcutaneous infiltrate sparing epidermis
- Composed of large, noncohesive, atypical epithelioid tumor cells with abundant cytoplasm

Immunohistochemistry: CD163(+), CD68(+), lysozyme(+), CD4 (+/-), S100(-)/focal(+)
- B-cell markers, melanoma markers, carcinoma markers, and myeloid markers negative

Ancillary Tests
- B- and T-cell gene rearrangements usually negative

Top Differential Diagnoses
- Myeloid sarcoma
- Langerhans cell histiocytosis and Langerhans cell sarcoma
- Anaplastic large cell lymphoma (ALCL)
- Diffuse large B-cell lymphoma
- Classic Hodgkin lymphoma
- Melanoma
- Carcinoma

- o Surgical excision with wide margins
- Adjuvant therapy
  - o Chemotherapy and radiation therapy
    - Non-Hodgkin lymphoma protocols (i.e., CHOP)
    - Acute leukemia protocols

Prognosis
- Low-stage (localized) lesions may be less clinically aggressive
- High-stage lesions (multiple lesions, systemic disease, recurrences) resistant to adjuvant therapy
  - o 80% of patients die of disease

MACROSCOPIC FEATURES

General Features
- Skin with rash or tumor nodule
  - o 1 or more firm lesions

MICROSCOPIC PATHOLOGY

Histologic Features
- Skin
  - o Dermal and subcutaneous infiltrate with infiltrative borders
  - o Spares epidermis, separated by grenz zone
- Lymph node
  - o Usually diffuse effacement of lymph node architecture
  - o Focal involvement is often in paracortex
  - o Rare tumor is seen in sinuses
- Hemophagocytosis, sometimes
  - o Emperipolesis in some cases
- Mitotic figures
- Inflammatory background
  - o Often prominent
    - Reactive T cells, plasma cells, eosinophils
    - Especially in HS of central nervous system

Cytologic Features
- Neoplastic cells, large and noncohesive

- o Nuclei
  - Usually epithelioid
  - Rarely spindle-shaped
  - Often highly pleomorphic cells, sometimes monomorphic
  - Vesicular chromatin
  - Nucleoli, prominent sometimes
  - Multinucleated cells can be seen
- o Cytoplasm is abundant
  - Eosinophilic
  - Cytoplasmic vacuoles sometimes
  - Xanthomatous appearance sometimes

ANCILLARY TESTS

Immunohistochemistry
- Histiocyte markers positive
  - o CD163, CD68 (KP1), CD68 (PGM1), lysozyme, CD4 (+/-)
- Other positive markers
  - o LCA(+), HLA-DR(+), CD15 (+/-, weak), S100 (+/-, partial and weak)
- B- and T-cell markers negative
  - o CD2, CD3, CD20, CD79, pax-5
- Melanoma markers negative
  - o MART-1/Melan-A, HMB-45, tyrosinase
- Carcinoma markers negative
  - o Cytokeratin AE1/3, EMA
- Myeloid cell markers negative
  - o MPO, CD13, CD33
- Langerhans cell markers negative
  - o CD1a, langerin, S100(+/-)
- Follicular dendritic cell markers negative
  - o CD21, CD23, CD35

Cytogenetics
- No specific chromosomal abnormalities
- Isochromosome 12p in cases with germ cell tumors

PCR
- HS can show clonal *IgH* gene rearrangement

HISTIOCYTIC SARCOMA

Phenotype of Histiocytic Sarcoma

CD163	CD68	Lysozyme	CD4	MPO	CD1a	CK7	CD21
+	+	+	+/-	-	-	-	-

- HS can have molecular abnormalities seen in other lymphoma/leukemia, i.e., t(14;18)

Electron Microscopy
- Tumor cells with ↑ cytoplasm and lysosomes

DIFFERENTIAL DIAGNOSIS

Myeloid Sarcoma
- Often has monocytic, myelomonocytic, or monoblastic component
- Morphology and phenotype overlap with HS
- Differences from HS
  - Usually less atypia than HS
  - MPO (+/-) in myeloid sarcoma but negative in HS
- Bone marrow with patchy involvement (< 25% cellularity) classified as HS
- Bone marrow with extensive involvement (> 25% cellularity) classified as acute monocytic leukemia

Langerhans Cell Histiocytosis and Langerhans Cell Sarcoma
- Similarities to HS
  - Histiocytic lineage
  - Often eosinophils in background
- Differences from HS
  - Tumor cells have less atypia than HS
    - Grooved nuclei and twisted nuclei
  - Clusters of tumor cells often in epidermis, unlike HS
  - S100(+), CD1a(+), langerin(+)
  - Birbeck granules by electron microscopy

Diffuse Large B-cell Lymphoma
- Large cell proliferation that is often indistinguishable from HS by histology
- Different immunophenotype
  - B-cell markers expressed (CD20[+], CD79[+], pax-5[+])
- Clonal *IgH* gene rearrangement
- Sometimes t(14;18)

Anaplastic Large Cell Lymphoma (ALCL)
- Similarities to HS
  - Large atypical dyscohesive cells
  - Sometimes sinusoidal infiltration pattern
  - CD68 may be dimly (+)
- Differences from HS
  - Hallmark cells with multiple nuclei in a wreath-like or kidney-shaped pattern
  - Immunohistochemistry
    - T-cell antigens (+), CD30(+), ALK(+/-)
    - Histiocyte markers (CD163[-]), cytotoxic markers (+)
  - Molecular translocations involving *ALK* gene
    - More often in systemic ALK(+) cases, usually not in primary cutaneous ALCL cases

Classic Hodgkin Lymphoma
- HS with ↑ background inflammatory cells can be mistaken for classic Hodgkin lymphoma
- Reed-Sternberg cells, binucleate with prominent nucleoli, favor classic Hodgkin lymphoma
- Immunohistochemistry
  - CD30(+), CD15(+/-), LCA(-), pax-5(+/-)
  - Histiocyte markers (-)
- Epstein-Barr encoded receptor (EBER) in 50% of cases

Rosai-Dorfman Disease
- Similarities to HS
  - Large histiocytes with abundant cytoplasm, bland cytologic features
  - Often plasma cells in the background
- Differences from HS
  - Emperipolesis
  - Strongly S100(+)

Juvenile Xanthogranuloma (JXG)
- Also expresses CD14, CD68, and CD163
  - But factor XIIIa(+), fascin(+), and LCA(-), contrary to HS
- Scattered Touton giant cells

Melanoma
- Nodular and metastatic melanomas often highly pleomorphic and may appear similar to HS
  - CD68 may be positive in melanoma
  - Other histiocyte markers are usually negative
- Melanoma markers are needed to diagnose melanoma
  - S100, HMB-45, tyrosinase, MART-1/Melan-A, and KBA-62
- Look for past medical history of melanoma

Carcinoma
- Poorly differentiated carcinoma has overlapping morphology with HS
  - Immunophenotyping necessary to differentiate from HS
    - Cytokeratins, HMWCK, p63, and EMA (+) in most carcinomas
    - Histiocyte markers (-)

SELECTED REFERENCES

1. Wang E et al: Histiocytic sarcoma arising in indolent small B-cell lymphoma: report of two cases with molecular/genetic evidence suggestive of a 'transdifferentiation' during the clonal evolution. Leuk Lymphoma. 51(5):802-12, 2010
2. Feldman AL et al: Clonally related follicular lymphomas and histiocytic/dendritic cell sarcomas: evidence for transdifferentiation of the follicular lymphoma clone. Blood. 111(12):5433-9, 2008
3. Vos JA et al: Histiocytic sarcoma: a study of five cases including the histiocyte marker CD163. Mod Pathol. 18(5):693-704, 2005

HISTIOCYTIC SARCOMA

Microscopic and Immunohistochemical Features

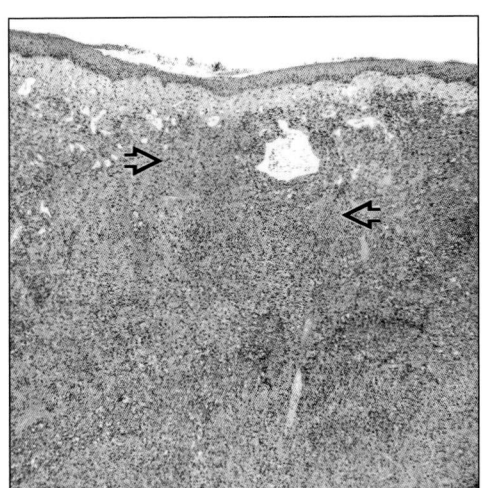

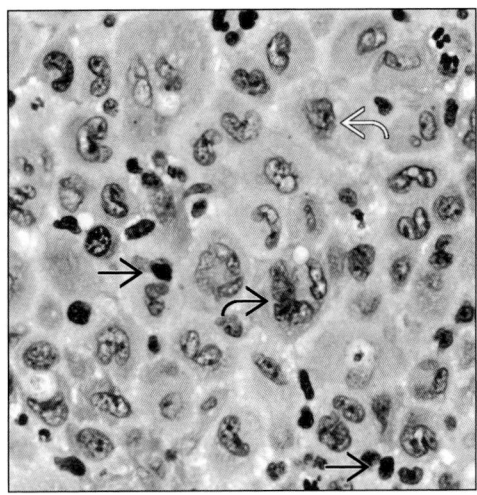

(Left) Histiocytic sarcoma at scanning magnification shows a diffuse, dermal-based sheet-like proliferation of enlarged, undifferentiated-appearing cells with large areas of tumor necrosis ⟹. (Right) Histiocytic sarcoma at high magnification shows large histiocytes ⟹ with abundant eosinophilic-staining cytoplasm and atypical nuclei ⟹ with pleomorphic shapes. There are also scattered small reactive lymphocytes ⟹. (Courtesy R. Miranda, MD.)

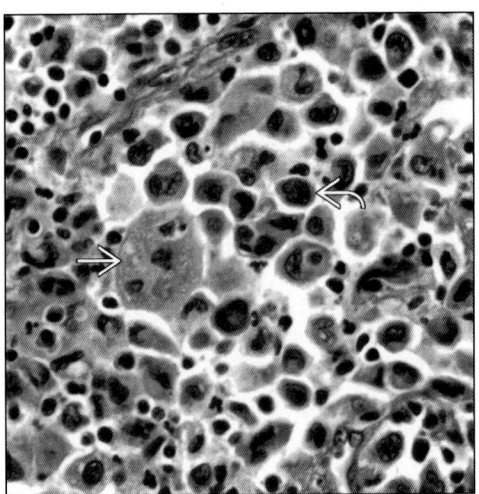

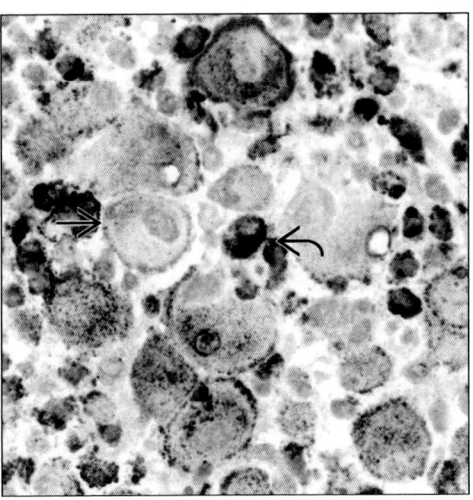

(Left) Another high magnification of histiocytic sarcoma shows pleomorphic neoplastic cells ⟹ as well as reactive histiocytes ⟹ with hemophagocytosis. (Courtesy R. Miranda, MD.) (Right) CD68(+) histiocytic sarcoma. CD68 immunohistochemistry highlights dim reactivity in large neoplastic cells ⟹ and strong reactivity in small nonneoplastic histiocytes ⟹. (Courtesy R. Miranda, MD.)

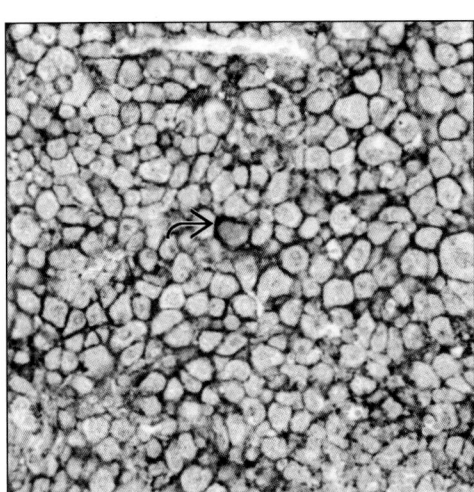

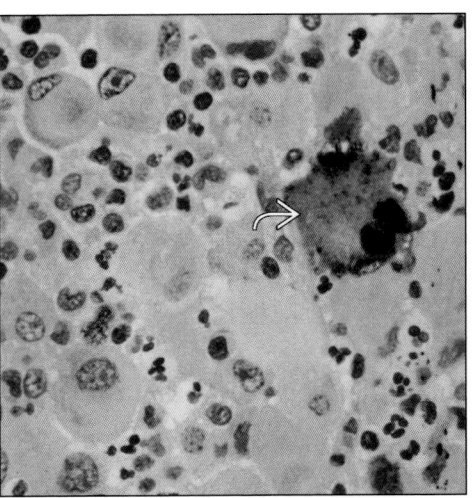

(Left) CD4(+) histiocytic sarcoma. CD4 immunohistochemistry highlights membrane reactivity in the large neoplastic cells ⟹. (Courtesy R. Miranda, MD.) (Right) Histiocytic sarcoma. A neoplastic cell is positive for S100 protein ⟹ by immunohistochemistry. Reactivity occurs in the nucleus and in the cytoplasm. In certain cases of histiocytic sarcoma, a subset (< 25%) of neoplastic cells may express S100 protein. (Courtesy R. Miranda, MD.)

Differential Diagnosis

(Left) Histiocytic sarcoma vs. acute monocytic leukemia (AMoL) in bone marrow aspirate shows a large cell ➡ with irregular nucleus and abundant cytoplasm. The WHO recommends classifying this case as AMoL, but a diagnosis of HS can be suggested if these cells are few or < 25% of cellularity. *(Courtesy R. Miranda, MD.)* *(Right)* This is an acute monocytic leukemia in bone marrow. The neoplastic cells ➡ are similar to histiocytic sarcoma cells and represent ≥ 25% of BM cellularity.

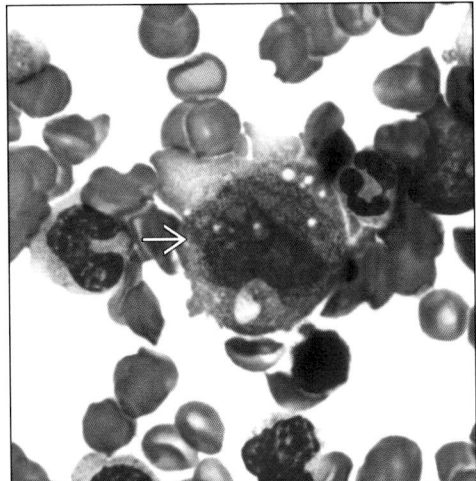
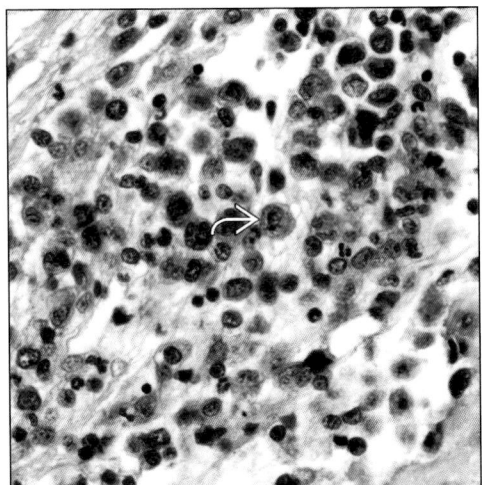

(Left) In this case of myeloid sarcoma, the neoplastic cells are immature but show evidence of myeloid differentiation, seen by cells with granular cytoplasm ➡. Myelocytes and a few neutrophils are present. *(Right)* Myeloid sarcoma involving cervical lymph node. The neoplastic cells are strongly positive for MPO ➡ shown by immunohistochemistry. Uninvolved lymphoid tissue ➡ is negative. *(Courtesy C. Bueso-Ramos, MD.)*

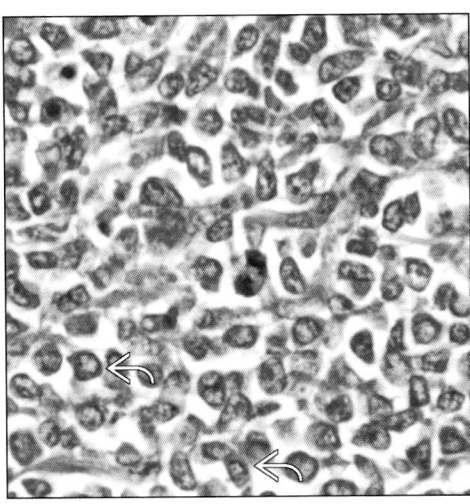
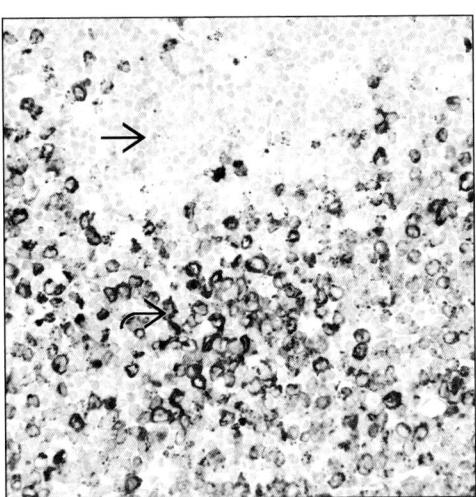

(Left) This case of diffuse large B-cell lymphoma, leg type (DLBCL-L) may be indistinguishable from HS by histology, showing a large cell proliferation with nuclear hyperchromasia. However, DLBCL-L will express B-cell markers such as CD20 and lack histiocyte markers. *(Right)* Strong and diffuse CD20 staining in DLBCL-L. DLBCL-L will typically express B-cell markers such as CD20, CD79a, and pax-5 and lack histiocyte markers such as CD68 and CD163.

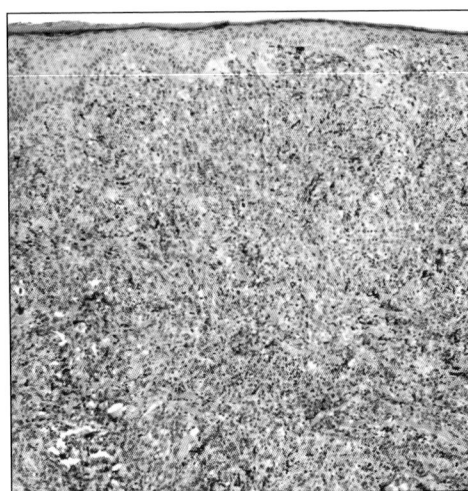
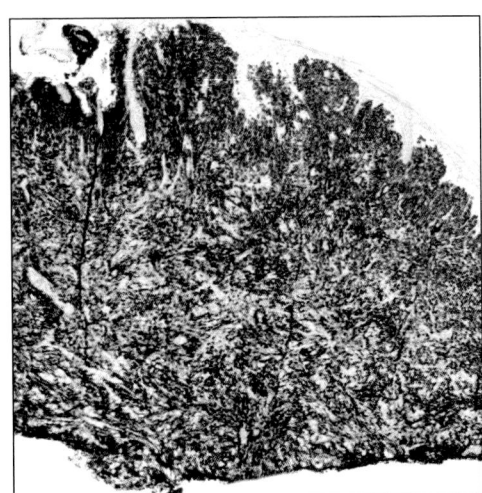

HISTIOCYTIC SARCOMA

Differential Diagnosis

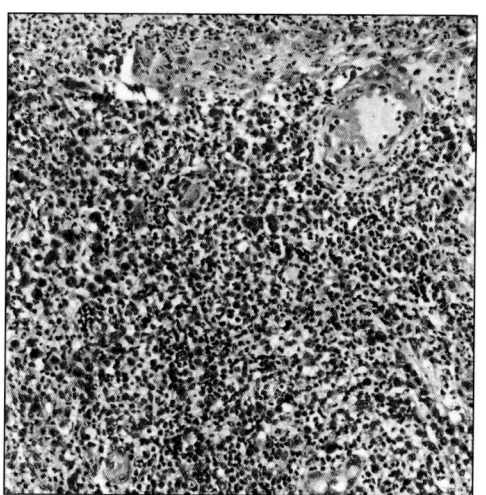

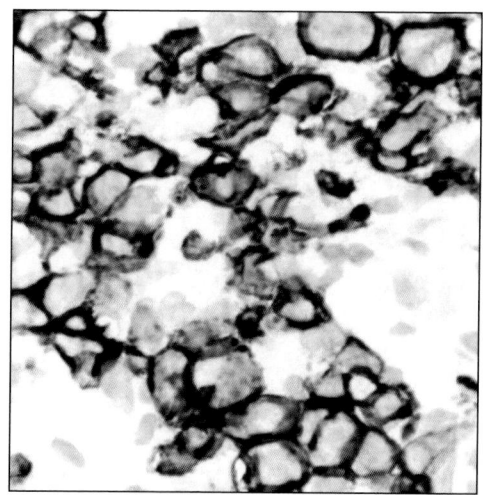

(Left) Anaplastic large cell lymphoma (ALCL) can be mistaken for HS. There is epidermal ulceration over a diffuse dermal collection of large cells with irregular nuclei and abundant cytoplasm, similar to HS, with a background of mixed infiltrate including neutrophils and eosinophils. *(Right)* The large malignant cells in ALCL show strong immunoexpression of CD30. The malignant cells of histiocytic sarcoma do not typically mark with CD30, but should be positive for markers such as CD163.

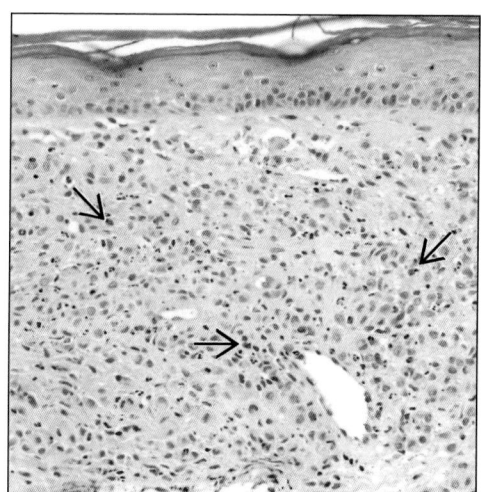

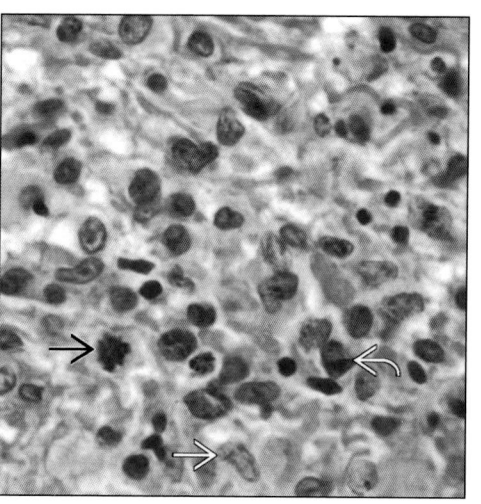

(Left) Langerhans cell histiocytosis (LCH) is in the differential diagnosis of HS. The skin shows a diffuse dermal infiltrate ➡ of ovoid cells with relatively uniform reniform-appearing nuclei and numerous eosinophils. *(Right)* At higher magnification, note that the histiocytes of LCH have grooved ➡ &/or twisted ➡ nuclei. They also show relatively bland fine chromatin. Only a few eosinophils are identified (not shown). A mitotic figure ➡ is also seen.

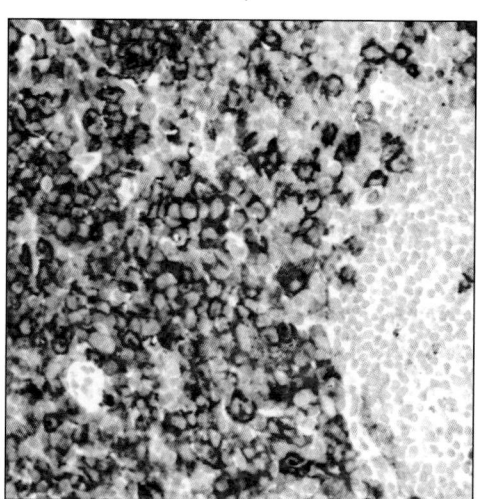

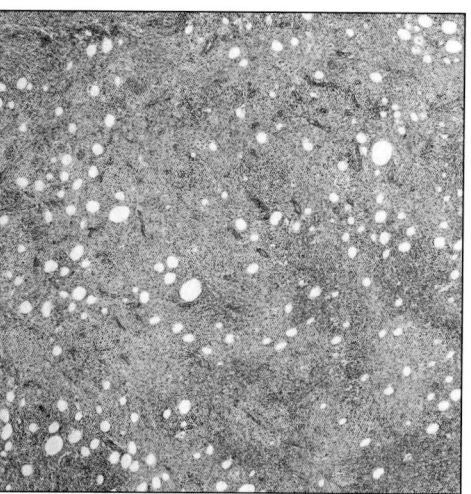

(Left) This CD1a marker stains LCH. The Langerhans cells are strongly CD1a(+), with cytoplasmic staining, as well as S100(+) and langerin(+) (not shown). *(Right)* Also in the differential is Rosai-Dorfman disease. The proliferating histiocytes are epithelioid-shaped and have abundant foamy cytoplasm. Lymphoid aggregates are present. The histiocytes show emperipolesis at high power.

POLYVINYLPYRROLIDONE STORAGE DISEASE

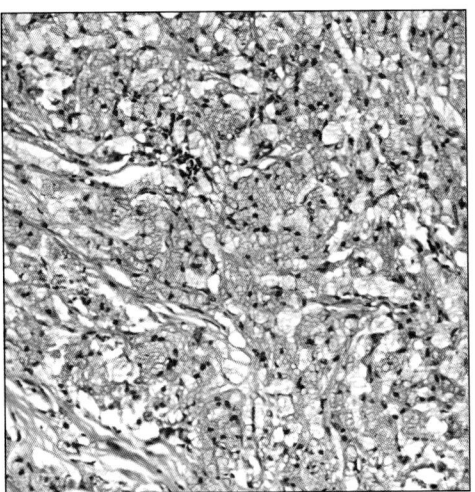

Low-magnification image of PVP storage disease shows soft tissue infiltrated by sheets and nests of uniform macrophages containing basophilic material in their cytoplasm.

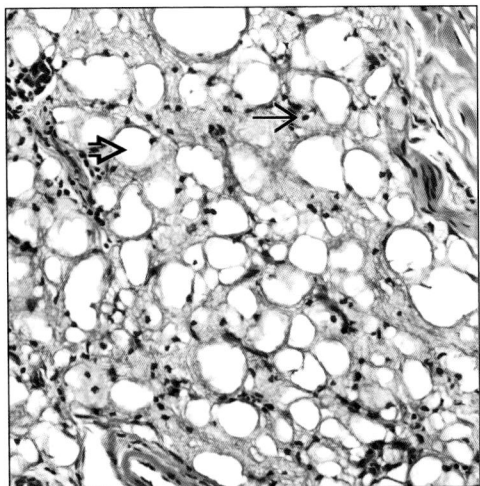

Higher magnification shows histiocytic infiltrate with "bubbly" basophilic cytoplasm containing PVP and circular spaces ⊳. The nuclei ⇉ are small and lack atypia and mitotic activity.

TERMINOLOGY

Abbreviations
- Polyvinylpyrrolidone (PVP) storage disease

Synonyms
- Mucicarminophilic histiocytosis
- Polyvinylpyrrolidone granuloma

Definitions
- Phagocytic foreign body-type reactive condition in which PVP is deposited and retained in tissue

ETIOLOGY/PATHOGENESIS

Causes
- Synthesized during World War II, used intravenously as plasma expander
- PVP found in aerosol hair sprays, adhesives, and lithographic solutions, and in cosmetics, including shaving products, plastics, and inks
- Used to improve clarity and stability of wine and fruit juice
- Used as component in oral medications and Betadine

CLINICAL ISSUES

Epidemiology
- Incidence
  - Associated with IV drug use

Site
- Skin, bone marrow, lung

Presentation
- Skin rash
  - Localized reactions may present as induration at injection site
  - Plaques, erythematous nodules, and purpuric to brown macules
  - Found during work-up for gastrointestinal bleeding in Munchausen syndrome
- Anemia
  - Due to marrow involvement, bony destruction

Treatment
- Prevent additional administration of high molecular weight PVP
- No effective treatment for removal of high molecular weight PVP

Prognosis
- Depending on amount of PVP accumulation, PVP storage disease may be incidental finding
- Can lead to severe irreversible anemia when there is bone marrow involvement
- Pulmonary angiothrombotic granulomatosis involving PVP (crospovidone) may lead to cor pulmonale and death

MICROSCOPIC PATHOLOGY

Histologic Features
- Microscopic
  - Blue-gray bubbly histiocyte with bubbly cytoplasmic contents, no pleomorphism
  - Multinucleated giant cells, foam cells, and granulomas present
  - Blue-gray material in extracellular pools, as well as within histiocyte cytoplasm
- Histochemistry
  - Mucicarmine red, Congo red, Sirius red, and colloidal iron positive
  - PAS, Alcian blue, and Giemsa negative
- Immunohistochemistry
  - CK, S100, and CD1a negative
  - CD68 and CD163 positive

POLYVINYLPYRROLIDONE STORAGE DISEASE

Key Facts

Etiology/Pathogenesis

- Phagocytic foreign body-type reactive condition
- Found in aerosol hair sprays, adhesives, lithographic solutions, shaving products, plastics
- Used to improve clarity and stability of wine and fruit juice; used in oral medications and Betadine
- Presents as skin rash with nodules and macules, untreatable anemia due to bone marrow involvement

Microscopic Pathology

- Histiocytes with blue-gray, bubbly cytoplasm, in small groups or large sheets
- No nuclear atypia or mitotic activity
- Giant cells may be present
- PAS, Alcian blue, and Giemsa negative
- Mucicarmine, Congo red, Sirius red, and colloidal iron positive
- Immunoreactive for CD68 and CD163

Predominant Pattern/Injury Type

- Inflammatory

Predominant Cell/Compartment Type

- Mesenchymal, histiocytic

DIFFERENTIAL DIAGNOSIS

Sea-Blue Histiocytosis

- Histiocytic proliferation
- Primary or secondary in hematologic/systemic disorders
- Blue with Giemsa; PAS positive

Signet Ring Cell Adenocarcinoma

- Signet ring cells appear similar to PVP-containing histiocytes
- Positive for mucicarmine and cytokeratin
- Negative for PAS

Myxofibrosarcoma

- Atypical spindle cells with presence of mitotic activity, cytologic activity, and prominent vasculature
- Positive for Alcian blue

DIAGNOSTIC CHECKLIST

Clinically Relevant Pathologic Features

- May present as subcutaneous masses
- Material may be present at injection site

- Tissue distribution
  - Skin, bone marrow
  - Can be extensive

Pathologic Interpretation Pearls

- Histiocytes with blue-gray, bubbly cytoplasm, in small groups or large sheets, giant cells
- Nuclear pleomorphism, mitoses, necrosis are absent
- CD68 positive, cytokeratin negative

SELECTED REFERENCES

1. Groisman GM et al: Mucicarminophilic histiocytosis (benign signet-ring cells) and hyperplastic mesothelial cells: two mimics of metastatic carcinoma within a single lymph node. Arch Pathol Lab Med. 122(3):282-4, 1998
2. Kuo TT et al: Cutaneous involvement in polyvinylpyrrolidone storage disease: a clinicopathologic study of five patients, including two patients with severe anemia. Am J Surg Pathol. 21(11):1361-7, 1997
3. Hizawa K et al: Subcutaneous pseudosarcomatous polyvinylpyrrolidone granuloma. Am J Surg Pathol. 8(5):393-8, 1984
4. Kuo TT et al: Mucicarminophilic histiocytosis. A polyvinylpyrrolidone (PVP) storage disease simulating signet-ring cell carcinoma. Am J Surg Pathol. 8(6):419-28, 1984
5. Bubis JJ et al: Storage of polyvinylpyrrolidone mimicking a congenital mucolipid storage disease in a patient with Munchausen's syndrome. Isr J Med Sci. 11(10):999-1004, 1975

IMAGE GALLERY

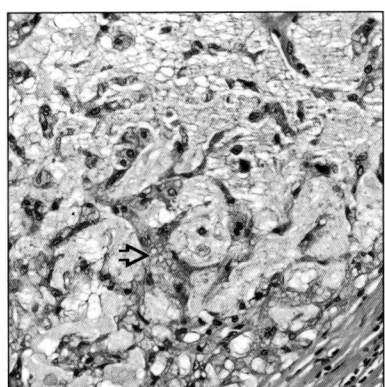 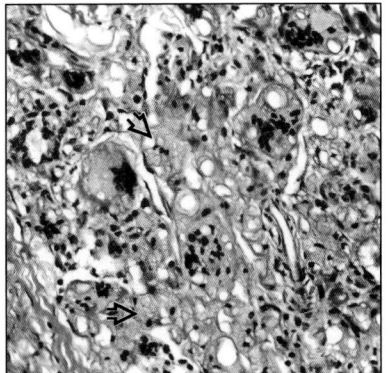 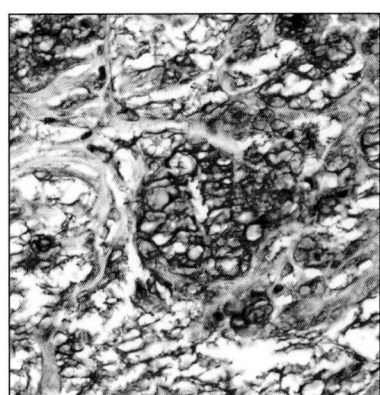

(Left) Histologic examination shows basophilic bubbly material (PVP), largely extracellular but also within histiocytes ➤, mimicking extraskeletal myxoid chondrosarcoma or myoepithelioma. *(Center)* High magnification shows multinucleated histiocytes with abundant blue cytoplasm ➤. *(Right)* Mucicarmine shows positivity in PVP. The term "mucicarminophilic histiocytosis" has been applied to this condition, which resembles adenocarcinoma but lacks epithelial markers.

Lymphomas and Hematopoietic Proliferations

CUTANEOUS PLASMACYTOMA

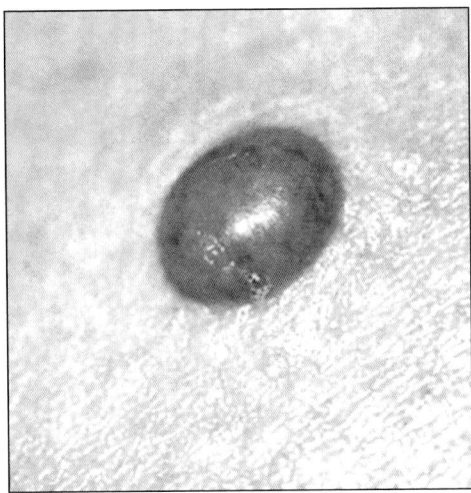

A single red solitary plaque on the forearm is shown, which microscopically is a cutaneous plasmacytoma.

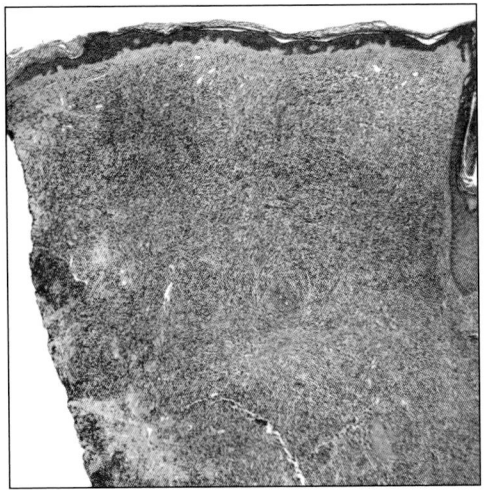

Low-magnification examination of a cutaneous plasmacytoma shows a diffuse dermal-based lymphoid infiltrate with deep extension.

TERMINOLOGY

Abbreviations
- Cutaneous plasmacytoma (CP)

Synonyms
- Extraosseous plasmacytoma of skin

Definitions
- Neoplasm of monoclonal plasma cells in the skin
  - Must 1st exclude cutaneous involvement in multiple myeloma and plasmacytoid B-cell lymphoma such as primary cutaneous extranodal marginal zone lymphoma

CLINICAL ISSUES

Epidemiology
- Incidence
  - Extremely rare
    - Only 3-5% of all plasma cell neoplasms
    - Many cases previously reported as primary cutaneous plasmacytomas would now be reclassified as extranodal marginal zone lymphomas
  - Rarely involve skin, more common in respiratory tract (80% of extraosseous plasmacytomas in oropharynx, nasopharynx, and nasal sinuses)
  - Rarely, may be seen as post-transplant lymphoproliferative disorder (PTLD)
    - Morphologically identical to other plasmacytomas, but PTLD plasmacytoma-like tumors are often EBV(+)
- Age
  - Median age: 55 years
- Gender
  - Mostly in men; male:female = 2:1

Presentation
- Usually single or multiple skin masses

  - Upper airway presents with rhinorrhea, nasal obstruction, epistaxis
- 20% monoclonal gammopathy (small M-protein)

Treatment
- Usually local radiation or surgery

Prognosis
- Local recurrence can occur
- Rare metastases
- Better prognosis if single lesion

MICROSCOPIC PATHOLOGY

Histologic Features
- Diffuse or nodular collections of plasma cells, usually in deep dermis/subcutis
- Usually well differentiated; rarely dysplastic with higher nuclear to cytoplasmic ratio and visible nucleoli
- Rarely, plasma cells may contain eosinophilic, homogeneous cytoplasmic inclusions, known as Russell bodies
- Sometimes binucleate plasma cells are present

Cytologic Features
- Oval-shaped plasma cells with eccentric nucleus, "clock face" or "spoke wheel" chromatin without prominent nucleoli
- Moderate to abundant pink cytoplasm with perinuclear hof (Golgi apparatus)

ANCILLARY TESTS

Immunohistochemistry
- Usually CD38(+), CD138 (syndecan)(+), pax-5(-), CD79a(+)
- CD56(+) in malignant plasma cells; usually CD56(-) in reactive plasma cells

CUTANEOUS PLASMACYTOMA

Key Facts

Terminology
- Neoplasm of monoclonal plasma cells
  - Must 1st rule out plasmacytoid B-cell lymphoma

Clinical Issues
- Skin is rare site for plasmacytomas; most occur in respiratory tract

Microscopic Pathology
- Diffuse or nodular collections of dermal plasma cells

- Oval-shaped plasma cells with eccentric nucleus, "clock face" or "spoke wheel" chromatin without prominent nucleoli
- Increased pink cytoplasm with perinuclear hof

Ancillary Tests
- Usually CD38(+), CD138(+), pax-5(-), CD79a(+)
- Flow cytometry underestimates number of plasma cells
- Molecular shows clonal *IgH* rearrangement

- κ and λ monoclonality by immunohistochemistry or in situ hybridization
- CD20 usually negative, but rarely can aberrantly express CD20; also can express CD117 and CD10
- Sometimes cyclin D1(+)

Flow Cytometry
- Underestimates number of plasma cells because of mechanical fragility; defer to morphology and immunohistochemistry to evaluate plasma cells

Molecular Genetics
- Can show Ig heavy chain (*IgH*) gene rearrangement

DIFFERENTIAL DIAGNOSIS

Benign Plasma Cell Infiltrates
- Also well-differentiated plasma cells without dysplasia, often no mass lesion, polyclonal by κ/λ, CD56(-); look for infectious organisms such as spirochetes (i.e., syphilis)

Extranodal Marginal Zone Lymphoma (ENMZL) with Plasmacytic Differentiation
- Can be difficult to exclude, but usually express B-cell antigens (CD20, pax-5, CD79), contain reactive germinal centers
- Often have admixed mature B cells and show disrupted follicular dendritic cells on CD21

Cutaneous Involvement by Multiple Myeloma
- Increased plasma cells in bone marrow or peripheral blood, unlike plasmacytoma, which by definition spares bone marrow
- Clinical findings: Lytic bone lesions, monoclonal gammopathy, anemia, hypercalcemia

Plasmablastic Lymphoma
- Rare tumors characterized by larger plasmacytoid cells with more atypia, usually EBER or HHV8(+), unlike plasmacytoma; often HIV(+) patients

SELECTED REFERENCES

1. Wang E et al: Primary cutaneous giant cell plasmacytoma in an organ transplant recipient: a rare presentation of a posttransplant lymphoproliferative disorder. Am J Dermatopathol. 32(5):479-85, 2010
2. Bayer-Garner IB et al: Detection of clonality with kappa and lambda immunohistochemical analysis in cutaneous plasmacytomas. Arch Pathol Lab Med. 128(6):645-8, 2004
3. Alexiou C et al: Extramedullary plasmacytoma: tumor occurrence and therapeutic concepts. Cancer. 85(11):2305-14, 1999
4. Hussong JW et al: Extramedullary plasmacytoma. A form of marginal zone cell lymphoma? Am J Clin Pathol. 111(1):111-6, 1999

IMAGE GALLERY

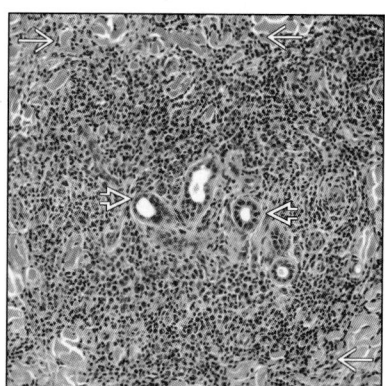 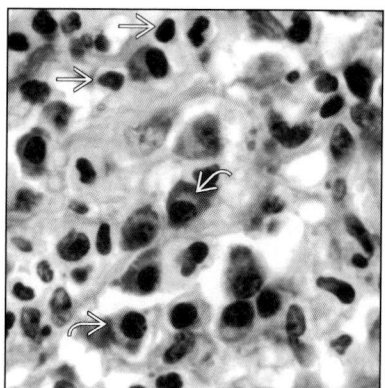 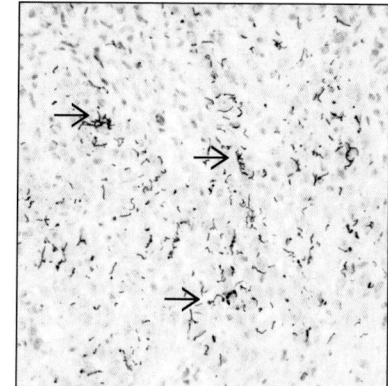

(Left) This cutaneous plasmacytoma shows a prominent plasmacytoid infiltrate surrounding multiple adnexal ducts ➡ and infiltrating between collagen bundles ➡. *(Center)* This cutaneous plasmacytoma shows multiple mature-appearing plasma cells with prominent perinuclear hofs ➡ as well as scattered small lymphocytes ➡. *(Right)* Infectious diseases, including spirochetal infections, are in the differential diagnosis in cases with prominent plasma cell infiltrates. This is an example of syphilis, with numerous coiled organisms ➡ (by spirochetal histochemistry).

CUTANEOUS MARGINAL ZONE B-CELL LYMPHOMA

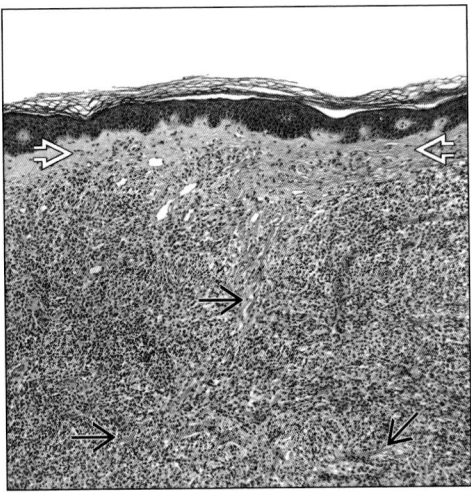

Low magnification of a primary cutaneous MZL shows a prominent, diffuse dermal lymphoid infiltrate, which infiltrates between collagen bundles ⇒ and is separated from the epidermis by a grenz zone ⊞.

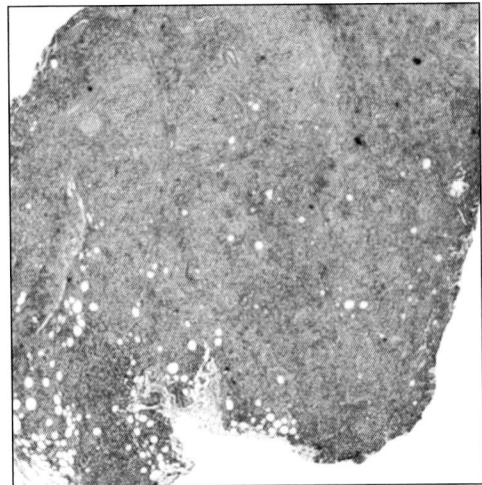

This is another case of cutaneous marginal zone B-cell lymphoma that is extending into the subcutaneous tissue with a nodular and diffuse growth pattern.

TERMINOLOGY

Abbreviations
- Primary cutaneous marginal zone lymphoma (PCMZL)

Synonyms
- Primary cutaneous immunocytoma

Definitions
- Non-Hodgkin small B-cell lymphoma of centrocyte-like marginal zone cells
  - Recapitulates architecture of Peyer patches
    - Usually in sites without significant lymphoid tissue
  - Malignant B cells expanding marginal zones surrounding reactive follicles and colonizing them
- May be difficult to diagnose because of nonspecificity of many of the morphologic features, absence of 1 or more classic features, and nature of the small biopsies

ETIOLOGY/PATHOGENESIS

Infectious Agents
- *Borrelia burgdorferi* DNA found in skin in some European cases, but not in other populations
  - Other infectious diseases noted in tissue other than skin
    - *Helicobacter pylori* implicated in gastric marginal zone lymphoma
    - *Campylobacter jejuni* implicated in small intestine marginal zone lymphoma
    - *Chlamydia psittaci* implicated in ocular marginal zone lymphoma

Autoimmune Diseases
- Marginal zone lymphoma has been associated with patients who have autoimmune diseases
  - Sjögren syndrome and parotid gland marginal zone lymphoma
  - Hashimoto thyroiditis and thyroid marginal zone lymphoma

CLINICAL ISSUES

Epidemiology
- Age
  - Usually adults > 40 years old
- Gender
  - No gender predominance
- Ethnicity
  - No ethnic propensity

Site
- Mostly upper extremity
  - Also head and neck and torso

Presentation
- 1 or more plaques or nodules
  - Rarely ulcerates
  - Multiple nodules often seen in systemic marginal zone lymphoma with secondary spread to dermis

Treatment
- Excision or radiation therapy
  - If solitary or only a few lesions
    - Chemotherapy only considered for widespread disease, metastasis
- Antibiotics
  - Sometimes therapy for *Borrelia burgdorferi* infection

Prognosis
- Excellent
  - 5-year survival: 90-100%
  - But tendency to recur
    - Rarely transforms to large B-cell lymphoma
    - So look for sheets of large B cells for diagnosis of large B-cell lymphoma
    - Scattered large B cells are often seen in PCMZL

CUTANEOUS MARGINAL ZONE B-CELL LYMPHOMA

Key Facts

Terminology
- Non-Hodgkin small B-cell lymphoma of centrocyte-like marginal zone cells
- Malignant B cells expanding marginal zones surrounding reactive follicles and colonizing them

Etiology/Pathogenesis
- *Borrelia burgdorferi* in some cases
- Associated with autoimmune disease

Clinical Issues
- Excellent prognosis; 5-year survival: 90-100%
- Usually treated with excision or radiation

Microscopic Pathology
- Small B cells, monocytoid, plasmacytoid
- Colonized germinal centers
- Lymphoepithelial lesions rare

- ± Dutcher bodies

Ancillary Tests
- B cells positive for CD20, may coexpress CD43 and Bcl-2
- Germinal centers Bcl-6(+), CD10(+), Bcl-2(-)
- CD21(+) loose follicular dendric cell meshworks
- Usually light chain restriction and clonally rearranged immunoglobulin genes
- t(11;18) negative

Top Differential Diagnoses
- Follicular hyperplasia
- Primary cutaneous follicle center lymphoma
- Plasmacytoma
- Secondary involvement by systemic marginal zone lymphoma

MACROSCOPIC FEATURES

General Features
- 1 or more firm red nodules on skin

MICROSCOPIC PATHOLOGY

Histologic Features
- Nodular to diffuse dermal infiltrate
  - Spares epidermis with grenz zone
  - Sometimes involves subcutis
  - Malignant B cells expanding marginal zones surrounding reactive follicles and colonizing them
- Lymphoepithelial lesions (very rare in skin)
- Neoplastic cells
  - Sometimes monocytoid with ample pale/clear cytoplasm
  - Sometimes plasmacytoid with eccentric nucleus and pink cytoplasm
  - Variable numbers of plasma cells, neutrophils, and eosinophils
  - Mostly small in size with coarse chromatin and mild atypia
- Dutcher bodies (intranuclear inclusions)
  - Sometimes seen
  - More often in marginal zone lymphoma than plasmacytoma
  - Russell bodies are cytoplasmic inclusions that may also be seen, but are less specific
- Reactive germinal centers
  - Colonized by neoplastic marginal zone B cells
  - Still contain tingible body macrophages
  - Retain mantle zones
    - If tissue is small, may not see follicles
- Follicular dendric cell meshworks
  - Often disrupted/loosened in colonized germinal centers
- Lymphoepithelial lesions
  - 3 or more lymphocytes entering epithelial structure (usually a gland) and destroying it
  - Very rarely seen in skin

Cytologic Features
- Small to medium-sized B cells with mild atypia, 1 or more inconspicuous nucleoli, and scant pale cytoplasm

ANCILLARY TESTS

Immunohistochemistry
- Neoplastic B cells
  - Express B-cell markers
    - Positive for CD19, CD20, CD22, CD79a
    - Shows predominance of B cells
    - Sheets of B cells with few T cells are concerning for B-cell lymphoma
    - If there is a mix of B and T cells, then look for other features (IHC, clonality) to diagnose lymphoma
  - Coexpression of T-cell markers is a feature of malignancy
    - B cells may coexpress CD43
    - B cells may coexpress Bcl-2
    - Bcl-2 is normally expressed on reactive mantle zone cells
  - Neoplastic B cells do not express
    - CD5, CD10, Bcl-6, CD21, or CD23
  - Light chain restriction
    - Usually in plasma cells &/or lymphoplasmacytic cells
- Germinal centers
  - Positive markers
    - Bcl-6(+), CD10(+)
  - Negative markers
    - Bcl-2(-)
- Follicular dendritic cell meshworks
  - Highlighted by CD21 and CD23
  - Show an expanded or loose pattern
- Lymphoepithelial lesions
  - CD20 or other B-cell markers positive in B cells in the gland
  - Cytokeratin stains can highlight disrupted glands

CUTANEOUS MARGINAL ZONE B-CELL LYMPHOMA

Differential Diagnosis of Cutaneous Marginal Zone Lymphoma

	Primary Cutaneous Marginal Zone Lymphoma	Primary Cutaneous Follicle Center Lymphoma	Systemic Small B-cell Lymphoma Involving Skin	Primary Cutaneous Large B-cell Lymphoma, Leg Type	Follicular Hyperplasia
Gross	Plaques or nodules	Plaques/nodules/tumor	Often nodules	Often multiple nodules	Papules/nodules
Clinical stage	Stage I	Stage I	High stage, disease in lymph node or BM	Stage I with rapid progression to ↑ stages	No staging
Growth pattern	Follicular or diffuse	Follicular or diffuse	Follicular or diffuse	Diffuse	Follicular
Follicles	Colonized	Malignant	Malignant	None	Reactive
Cell type	Marginal zone, monocytoid, plasmacytoid	Centrocytes and centroblasts	Centrocytes and centroblasts	Large cells	Centrocytes and centroblasts
Molecular studies	Monoclonal; no t(11;18)	Monoclonal; rarely t(14;18)	Monoclonal; t(14;18)(+) (in follicular lymphoma); t(11;18) in some MZL	Monoclonal; no t(14;18), translocations of *MYC*, *IgH*, or *BCL6*	Polyclonal
Treatment	No chemotherapy	Usually no chemotherapy	Chemotherapy	Chemotherapy	No treatment

In Situ Hybridization

- Cutaneous marginal zone lymphoma negative for t(11;18) *API2/MLT*
  - t(11;18) in 25-50% gastric marginal zone lymphoma
    - t(11;18)(+) cases are often more aggressive tumors
- t(14;18)(q32;q21) almost always negative
  - Rarely positive; present in 1 series

Molecular Genetics

- Clonal *IgH* gene rearrangement
- *Fas* gene mutations
  - Rare

DIFFERENTIAL DIAGNOSIS

Follicular Hyperplasia (FH)

- Contains reactive germinal centers like PCMZL
  - But germinal centers are not colonized in FH
- Lacks expanded/confluent neoplastic marginal zones
- Lacks light chain restriction
- Polyclonal *IgH* gene rearrangement

Primary Cutaneous Follicle Center Lymphoma (PCFCL)

- Follicles are neoplastic, not reactive like PCMZL
  - Monomorphic
  - Lack tingible body macrophages
  - Attenuated mantle zones
- Nodular or diffuse growth pattern
- Immunohistochemistry
  - Bcl-6(+)
  - CD10(+/-)
    - Often negative in diffuse areas
  - No coexpression of CD43
  - Bcl-2(-/+)
    - Often negative in diffuse areas
    - More common in nodal follicular lymphoma

Plasmacytoma

- Sheets of frank plasma cells

- Not plasmacytoid B cells
- Must exclude cutaneous marginal zone lymphoma
  - Marginal zone lymphoma should have at least a small population of malignant small B cells
- Must exclude plasmacytoid variants of other small B-cell lymphomas
- Must exclude multiple myeloma that is involving skin

Secondary Involvement by Systemic Marginal Zone Lymphoma

- Immunohistochemistry and morphology identical to PCMZL
  - Secondary involvement favors head and neck regions and is limited to older patients
  - t(11;18) may be positive

SELECTED REFERENCES

1. Gerami P et al: Cutaneous involvement with marginal zone lymphoma. J Am Acad Dermatol. 63(1):142-5, 2010
2. Takino H et al: Primary cutaneous marginal zone B-cell lymphoma: a molecular and clinicopathological study of cases from Asia, Germany, and the United States. Mod Pathol. 21(12):1517-26, 2008
3. Mandekou-Lefaki I et al: Primary cutaneous MALT-type lymphoma and Helicobacter pylori: a possible relationship. J Eur Acad Dermatol Venereol. 20(5):606-8, 2006
4. Hoefnagel JJ et al: Primary cutaneous marginal zone B-cell lymphoma: clinical and therapeutic features in 50 cases. Arch Dermatol. 141(9):1139-45, 2005
5. Li C et al: Primary cutaneous marginal zone B-cell lymphoma: a molecular and clinicopathologic study of 24 asian cases. Am J Surg Pathol. 27(8):1061-9, 2003
6. Baldassano MF et al: Cutaneous lymphoid hyperplasia and cutaneous marginal zone lymphoma: comparison of morphologic and immunophenotypic features. Am J Surg Pathol. 23(1):88-96, 1999

Microscopic Features

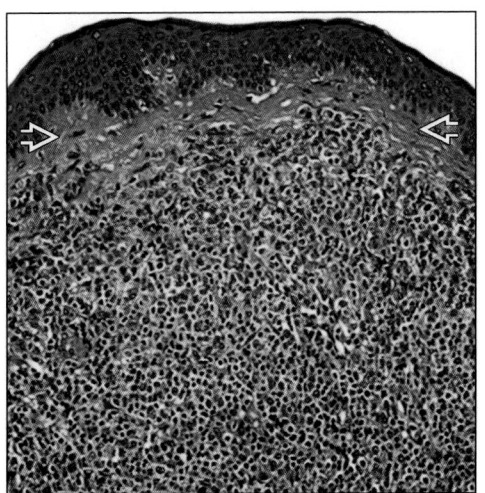

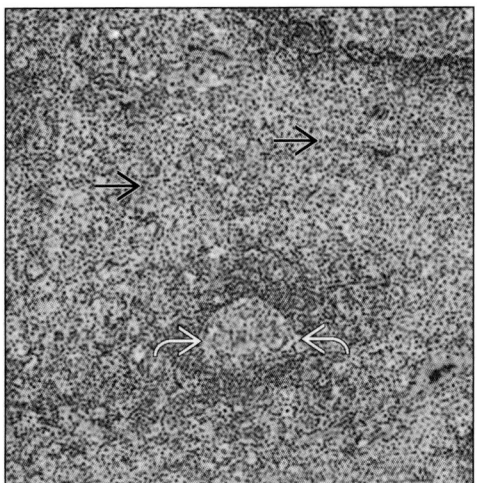

(Left) Low magnification of a primary cutaneous MZL shows a dense, diffuse dermal lymphoplasmacytoid infiltrate, which infiltrates between collagen bundles. Note that it is separated from the epidermis by a grenz zone ⊟. (Right) The marginal zones ⊟ are expanded around a reactive germinal center ⊟. The cells in the marginal zone are more pale than the darker mantle zone cells surrounding the germinal center.

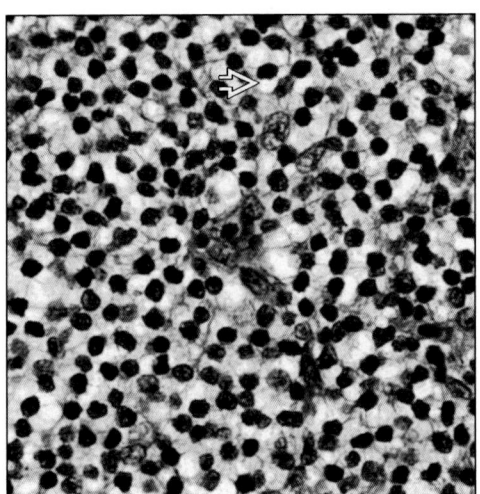

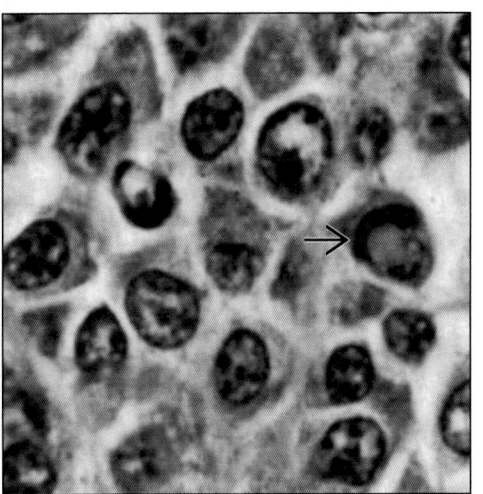

(Left) In many cases of primary cutaneous marginal zone lymphoma, the tumor cells have a monocytoid appearance. In this image, the monocytoid cells have increased amounts of clear cytoplasm ⊟. (Right) There is a Dutcher body ⊟ in this case of primary cutaneous marginal zone lymphoma. Dutcher bodies are intranuclear inclusions that have a round pink appearance.

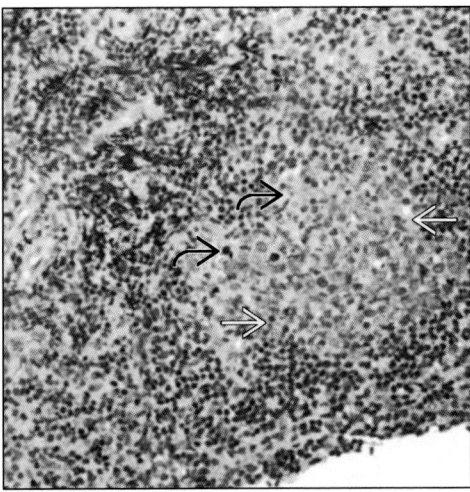

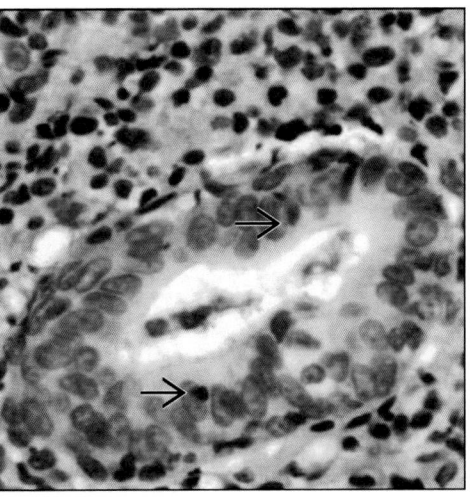

(Left) As in this image, most cases of PCMZL have reactive germinal centers ⊟. However, the germinal centers are colonized or infiltrated by lymphoma. There are small cleaved neoplastic B cells ⊟ penetrating this reactive germinal center. (Right) Lymphoepithelial lesions are common in systemic MZL, although rarely seen in cutaneous marginal zone lymphoma. This gland has a few lymphocytes ⊟ penetrating it.

CUTANEOUS MARGINAL ZONE B-CELL LYMPHOMA

Immunohistochemical Features

(Left) This is a CD20(+) marginal zone lymphoma. CD20 is strongly positive in the neoplastic B cells. Other B-cell markers, such as CD79a and pax-5, are also positive. **(Right)** CD3 is negative in the neoplastic B cells ⇨, but there are numerous reactive-appearing T cells ⇗ that are positive for CD3. Compared to CD20 staining, there is much less CD3 staining.

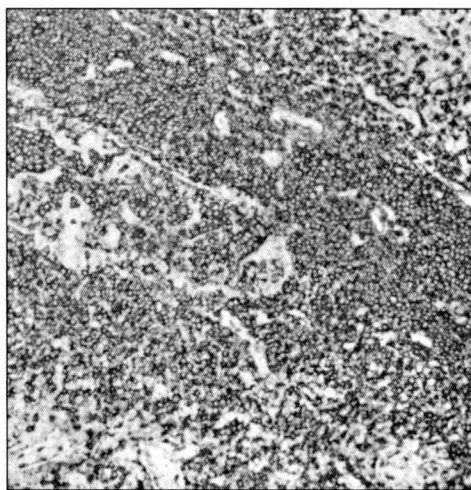 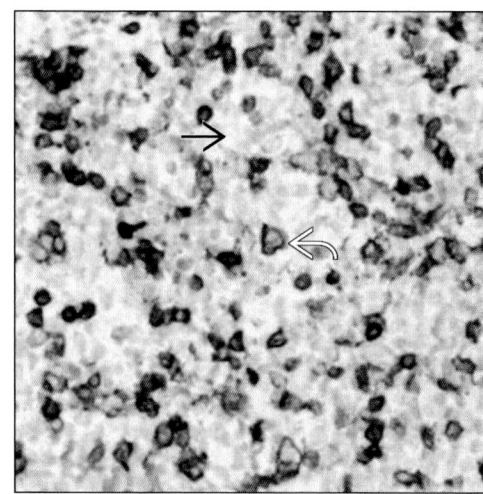

(Left) Bcl-2 immunostain is expressed on the B cells in most cases of PCMZL. Bcl-2 normally marks reactive T cells. However, if compared to CD20 and CD3 staining results, the staining pattern resembles that of CD20, indicating that the B cells coexpress Bcl-2. **(Right)** This is an image showing coexpression of CD43 in PCMZL. This CD43 immunostain is also expressed on the B cells and has a staining pattern similar to CD20.

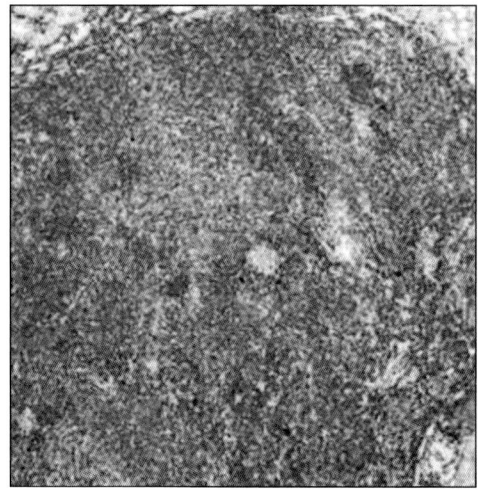 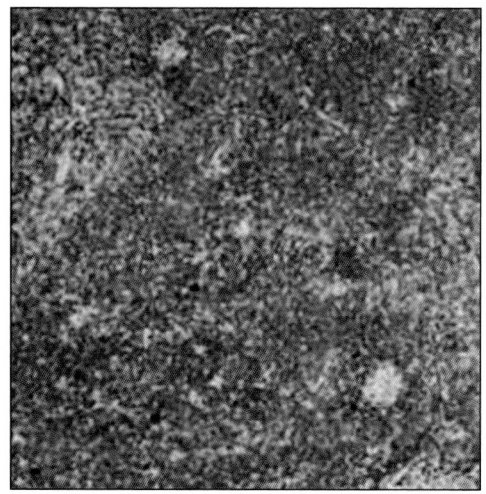

(Left) This image shows CD21 expressed on follicular dendritic cells (FDCs) ⇗, but it is negative in the neoplastic cells in PCMZL. Because the germinal centers are colonized by malignant B cells, the FDCs show a loose/disrupted pattern as seen here. **(Right)** CD20 can be used to highlight the neoplastic B cells in lymphoepithelial lesions. In this case, there are large numbers of small B cells ⇨ in a glandular structure ⇨.

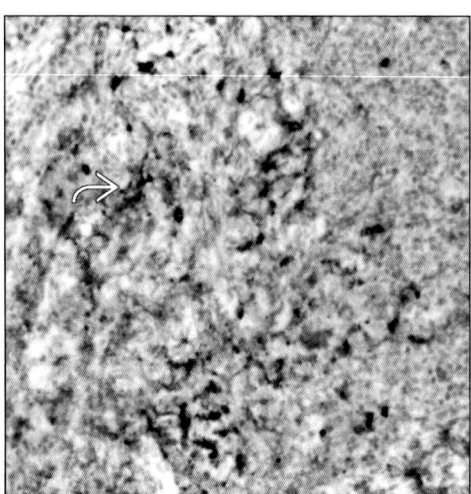 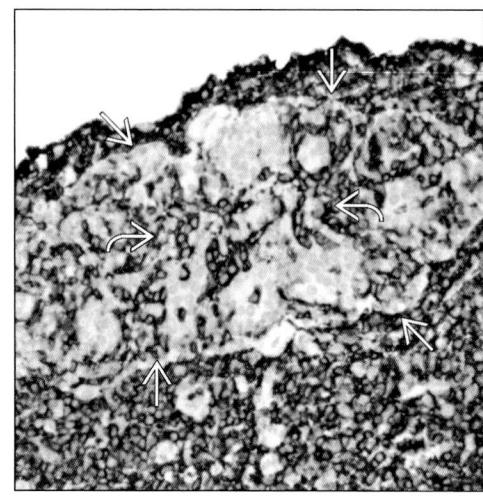

Differential Diagnosis

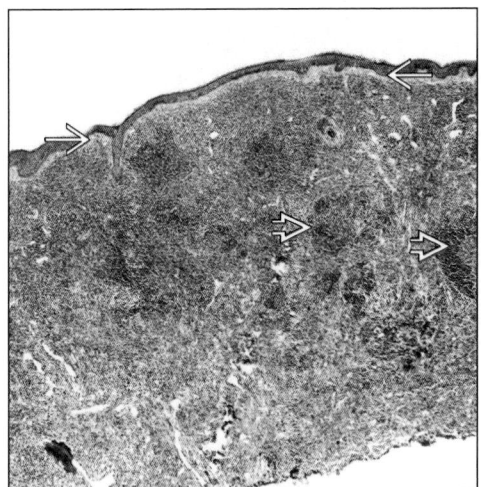

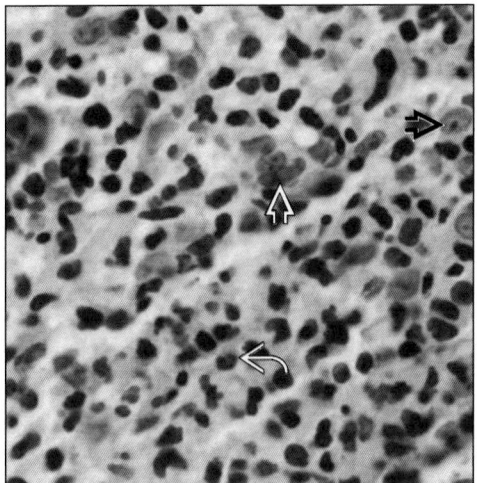

(Left) Primary cutaneous follicle center lymphoma (PCFCL) displays a dense lymphocytic infiltrate in the dermis, sparing the subepidermal layer (grenz zone ➡). The neoplasm contains ill-defined follicles ➡. *(Courtesy R. Miranda, MD.)* *(Right)* PCFCL shows a mix of centrocytes ➡ and centroblasts ➡ and rare follicular dendritic cells ➡. Monocytoid change, plasmacytoid change, and Dutcher bodies typical to PCMZL are not usually seen in PCFCL.

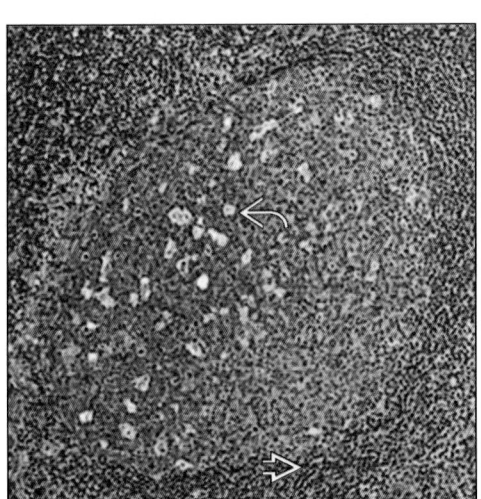

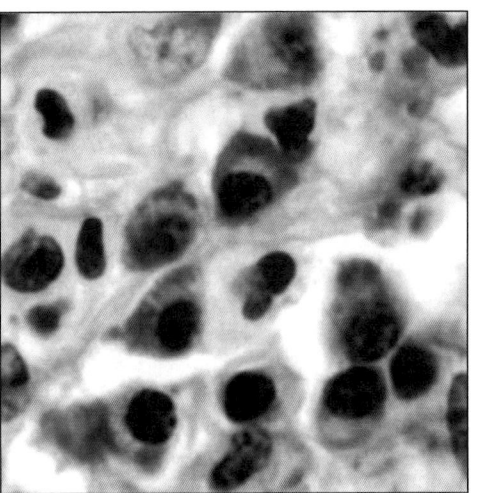

(Left) Follicular hyperplasia (FH) is seen in many pseudolymphomas. FH shows polarized follicles, tingible body macrophages ➡, and well-formed mantle zones ➡. However, germinal centers are not colonized with malignant B cells as in PCMZL. *(Right)* Cutaneous plasmacytoma (CP) is very rare, and most are reclassified as PCMZL today. These are collections of plasma cells, not plasmacytoid B cells, as in PCMZL.

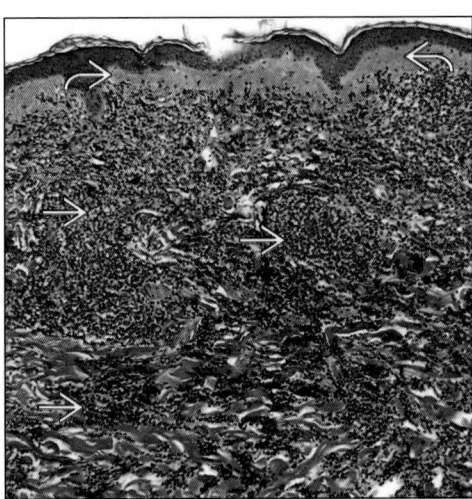

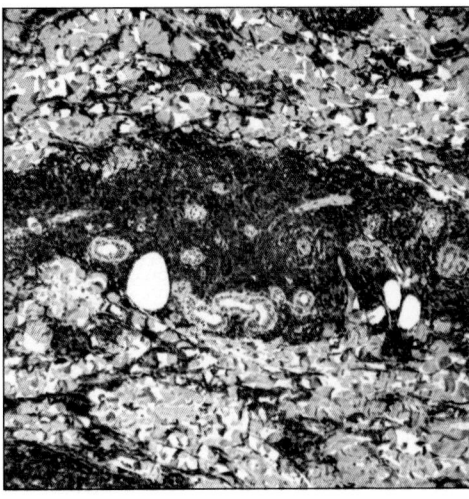

(Left) This image is of chronic lymphocytic leukemia (CLL) of the skin. Atypical lymphocytes ➡ are seen in superficial and deep dermis with an infiltrative growth pattern. Epidermis is uninvolved and separated from proliferation by a grenz zone ➡. *(Right)* A CD5 immunohistochemical stain in CLL shows that the cells are strongly CD5(+). CLL is typically CD5 and CD23(+). With PCMZL, CD5 is expressed by reactive T cells, and not by the tumor B cells.

PRIMARY CUTANEOUS FOLLICLE CENTER LYMPHOMA

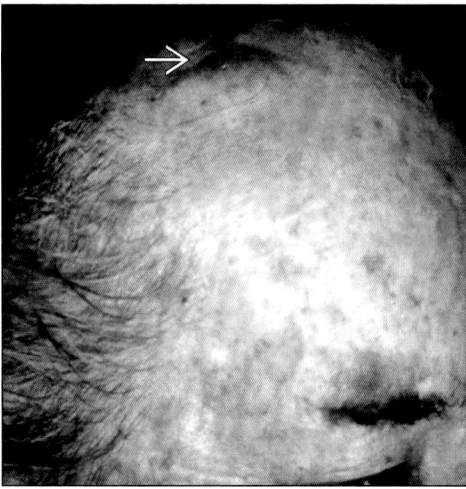

There is a single large raised red nodule ➡ on the scalp, 5 cm in largest dimension. Microscopically, the nodule was diagnosed as PCFCL. (Courtesy M. Tomaszewski, MD.)

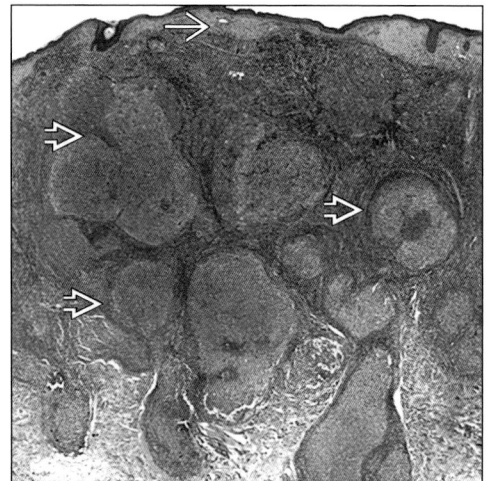

Low-power magnification shows PCFCL with a multinodular ➡ dermal infiltrate that is separated from the epidermis by a grenz zone ➡. (Courtesy M. Tomaszewski, MD.)

TERMINOLOGY

Abbreviations
- Primary cutaneous follicle center lymphoma (PCFCL)

Synonyms
- Follicular lymphoma of skin
- Crosti disease (reticulohistiocytoma of dorsum)
  - Plaques/tumors surrounded by erythematous macules/papules

Definitions
- Mature B-cell lymphoma of follicle center cells, primary in skin
  - Disease limited to skin for 6 months after diagnosis
- Distinct disease from systemic follicular lymphoma
  - Better prognosis
  - Fewer *BCL2* rearrangements than systemic follicular lymphoma

CLINICAL ISSUES

Epidemiology
- Incidence
  - 0.1-0.2 cases per 100,000 people per year
  - Most common primary cutaneous B-cell lymphoma
    - ~ 20% of all skin lymphomas
    - ~ 60% of all B-cell skin lymphomas
- Age
  - Usually adults
    - Median age: 60 years
    - But can also be seen in childhood
- Gender
  - Male:female = 1.5:1

Site
- Usually head and neck, especially scalp
  - Less commonly trunk

Presentation
- Usually single lesion
  - ~ 15% multifocal
- Plaques, nodules, or tumors of differing sizes
  - From < 1 cm to > 40 cm in greatest dimension
- Rarely ulcerates

Treatment
- Observation, surgical removal or local radiation
- Chemotherapy only if extensive disease or extracutaneous disease

Prognosis
- Good
  - Much better than systemic follicular lymphoma
  - Usually complete remission with treatment
  - ~ 95% 5-year survival
- Not affected by
  - Grade or growth pattern
  - Bcl-2 expression or t(14;18) status
- ~ 35% recurrence (often proximal to original lesion); extracutaneous spread ~ 10%
- ~ 10% disseminate to extracutaneous sites

MICROSCOPIC PATHOLOGY

Histologic Features
- Dermal B-cell infiltrate, often extends into subcutis (~ 75%)
  - No overlying epidermotropism
- Growth pattern
  - Nodular, diffuse, or nodular and diffuse
  - May be classified as follicular (> 75% follicular architecture), follicular and diffuse (25-75% follicular architecture), or diffuse (< 25% follicular architecture) growth pattern
- Follicles
  - Often not well-defined
  - Usually seen in small lesions

PRIMARY CUTANEOUS FOLLICLE CENTER LYMPHOMA

Key Facts

Terminology
- PCFCL
- Mature B-cell lymphoma of follicle center cells, primary to skin and not originating in another anatomic site

Clinical Issues
- Mostly single lesion on scalp; trunk 2nd most common site
- > 95% 5-year survival with local recurrences

Microscopic Pathology
- Nodular, diffuse, and nodular/diffuse growth patterns
- Lack of mantle zones, lack tingible body macrophages

Ancillary Tests
- CD20(+), Bcl-6(+), CD10(+/-) (often negative in diffuse variant)

- Bcl-2(-/+) and MUM1(-)
- CD23, CD21, and CD35 positive in FDC meshworks
- Usually CD43(-), unlike other B-cell lymphomas
- CD5(-), Bcl-1(-)
- Clonal Ig heavy chain (*IgH*) gene rearrangement
- t(14;18), often not detected
- Gene expression profiling findings akin to germinal center-like large B-cell lymphoma

Top Differential Diagnoses
- Reactive follicular hyperplasia
- Primary cutaneous marginal zone lymphoma
- Secondary skin involvement of follicular lymphoma
- Primary cutaneous diffuse large B-cell lymphoma, leg type
- Primary cutaneous diffuse large B-cell lymphoma, NOS

- ○ Lack mantle zones
- ○ Lack tingible body macrophages
- ○ Contain follicular dendritic cells
- Tumor cells
  - ○ Mostly centrocytes (small to medium-sized, cleaved)
  - ○ Variable numbers of centroblasts (larger in size)
- Cases with ↑ numbers of centroblasts
  - ○ Diagnose as PCFCL if nodular or nodular and diffuse growth pattern
  - ○ Diagnose as diffuse pattern PCFCL if large cells and only diffuse growth pattern
- Grading of follicular lymphoma
  - ○ Not necessary or of prognostic value for PCFCL
  - ○ Is necessary for systemic follicular lymphoma
    - Grade 1: < 5 centroblasts per high-power field; grade 2: 6-15 centroblasts per high-power field; grade 3: > 15 centroblasts per high-power field
    - Grades 1 and 2 show minimal differences in long-term outcome
    - Thus, 2008 WHO classification lumps cases with few centroblasts as "follicular lymphoma grade 1-2 (low grade)" in systemic follicular lymphoma, and does not advise grading of PCFCL

Cytologic Features
- Small cleaved cells with coarse chromatin and 1 or more indistinct nucleoli on peripheral smear

ANCILLARY TESTS

Immunohistochemistry
- B-cell markers positive
  - ○ CD20, CD19, CD79a, pax-5
  - ○ Mostly MUM1 negative, unlike primary cutaneous diffuse large B-cell lymphoma, leg type
- Follicle center markers positive
  - ○ Bcl-6(+); CD10(+/-) (usually negative in diffuse areas)
  - ○ HGAL (human germinal center-associated lymphoma), E2A, and AID can be positive in PCFCL
- Bcl-2(+/-)
  - ○ Often weak if positive (~ 40% of cases)

- Usually CD43(-), unlike other B-cell lymphomas
- CD23, CD21, and CD35(+) in follicular dendritic cell meshwork
- Express surface immunoglobulins IgM, IgD, IgG, and rarely IgA
- Kappa and lambda can show restriction ~ 1-20% of cases

In Situ Hybridization
- t(14;18) only seen in ~ 30% of cases
  - ○ More common in systemic (lymph node) follicular lymphoma

Molecular Genetics
- Clonal Ig heavy chain gene rearrangement in ~ 45% by PCR
- 10% p15 inactivation and 30% p16 inactivation by promotor hypermethylation

Gene Expression Profiling
- Findings akin to germinal center-like large B-cell lymphoma
  - ○ Often *REL* gene amplification

DIFFERENTIAL DIAGNOSIS

Secondary Skin Involvement by Follicular Lymphoma
- Similar morphology and phenotype to PCFCL
- Follicular lymphoma present in other anatomic site such as lymph node or bone marrow
- CD10(+), Bcl-2(+), unlike many PCFCL cases
- t(14;18)(q32;q21) more common in secondary follicular lymphoma
  - ○ Present in ~ 80-90% of secondary follicular lymphoma cases
- More commonly treated with chemotherapy than PCFCL
- Worse overall prognosis as compared to PCFCL

Nonmelanocytic Tumors of the Skin: Lymphomas and Hematopoietic Proliferations

Primary Cutaneous Marginal Zone Lymphoma

- Malignancy of marginal zone cells (post germinal center cells), and not malignant follicles
- Clinical differences
  - More often multifocal than PCFCL
  - Associated with *Borrelia burgdorferi* in some (European) studies
- Often monocytoid cells ± plasmacytoid cells
- Germinal centers often small/reactive and not larger/irregular as in PCFCL
  - Colonization of germinal centers by marginal zone lymphoma
- Immunohistochemistry
  - CD21 shows expanded follicular dendritic cell meshwork, contrary to tight follicular dendritic cell meshwork in PCFCL
  - More often Bcl-2(+) than PCFCL
  - Clusters of CD123(+) plasmacytoid cells
  - CD10(+)/Bcl-6(+) residual germinal centers

Primary Cutaneous Diffuse Large B-cell Lymphoma, Leg Type (PCDLBCL-LT)

- Clinical differences
  - Older median age, worse prognosis with only 50% 5-year survival
  - More commonly treated with chemotherapy than PCFCL
  - Usually on leg
    - Cases of PCFCL on leg have worse prognosis than patients with PCFCL at other anatomic sites
    - Cases of PCFCL on leg have a similar prognosis to PCDLBCL-LT
- Morphology
  - Diffuse growth pattern, unlike PCFCL, which usually has follicular pattern
  - Large malignant B cells, unlike PCFCL, which has mix of large centroblasts and smaller centrocytes
- Immunohistochemistry
  - IRF-4/MUM1(+), FOXP1(+) in PCDLBCL-LT and IRF-4/MUM1(-), FOXP1(-) in PCFCL
  - More often expresses cytoplasmic staining for IgM, which may be an additional tool for differentiating this lymphoma from PCFCL in clinical practice

Primary Cutaneous Diffuse Large B-cell Lymphoma, NOS (PCDLBCL)

- Needs to be differentiated from PCFCL with diffuse growth pattern and large cells
  - Diagnose as PCFCL if there is at least partial nodular architecture, or if there are fewer centroblasts
  - Diagnose as PCDLBCL if there are all large cells and only a diffuse growth pattern
- Bcl-2(-/+), Bcl-6(+/-)
- Need to exclude PCDLBCL-LT
- Need to exclude systemic DLBCL

Reactive Follicular Hyperplasia, Cutaneous "Pseudolymphoma"

- Can be caused by infection or folliculitis, but often idiopathic

- Reactive follicles
  - Well-defined with polarization
  - Tingible body macrophages present
  - Well-formed mantle zones
  - Often in superficial dermis and not in deeper tissue
- Germinal centers CD10(+), Bcl-6(+), Bcl-2(-)
- Polyclonal plasma cells, and no clonal *IgH* gene rearrangement
- Negative for t(14;18)

Small Lymphocytic Lymphoma/Chronic Lymphocytic Leukemia (CLL)

- Common peripheral blood involvement, unlike follicular lymphoma
- Mostly diffuse architecture
- Different immunophenotype: CD23(+), CD5(+), CD10(-), Bcl-6(-)
- t(11;14) negative

B-cell Lymphoblastic Lymphoma

- Lymphoblasts with sparse cytoplasm, finely stippled chromatin, and inconspicuous nucleoli
- TdT(+), variably CD34(+), CD19(+), CD10(+), variable CD20

Mantle Cell Lymphoma

- Only rarely involves skin
- Bcl-1/cyclin-D1(+) (nuclear), CD5(+), CD10(-), Bcl-6(-)
- t(11;14)(+)

DIAGNOSTIC CHECKLIST

Pathologic Interpretation Pearls

- Nodules to sheet-like collections of B cells, back-to-back, lacking tingible body macrophages, showing attenuated mantle zones
- Similar features as in systemic follicle center lymphoma, but often lacks Bcl-2 and t(14;18)
- Must exclude primary cutaneous diffuse large B-cell lymphoma, leg type, which has worse prognosis and expresses MUM1 and Bcl-2

SELECTED REFERENCES

1. Senff NJ et al: Reclassification of 300 primary cutaneous B-Cell lymphomas according to the new WHO-EORTC classification for cutaneous lymphomas: comparison with previous classifications and identification of prognostic markers. J Clin Oncol. 25(12):1581-7, 2007
2. Zinzani PL et al: Prognostic factors in primary cutaneous B-cell lymphoma: the Italian Study Group for Cutaneous Lymphomas. J Clin Oncol. 24(9):1376-82, 2006
3. Hoefnagel JJ et al: Distinct types of primary cutaneous large B-cell lymphoma identified by gene expression profiling. Blood. 105(9):3671-8, 2005
4. Kim BK et al: Clinicopathologic, immunophenotypic, and molecular cytogenetic fluorescence in situ hybridization analysis of primary and secondary cutaneous follicular lymphomas. Am J Surg Pathol. 29(1):69-82, 2005
5. Willemze R et al: WHO-EORTC classification for cutaneous lymphomas. Blood. 105(10):3768-85, 2005

Microscopic Features

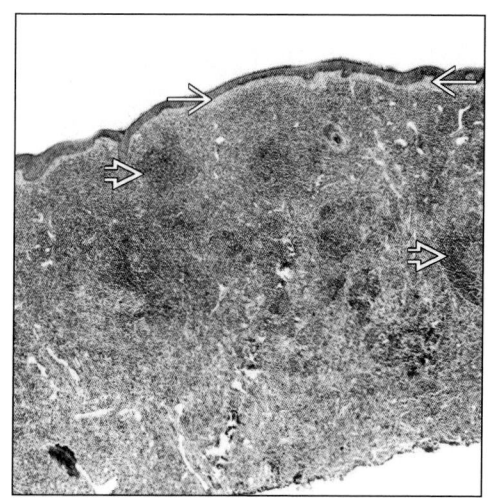
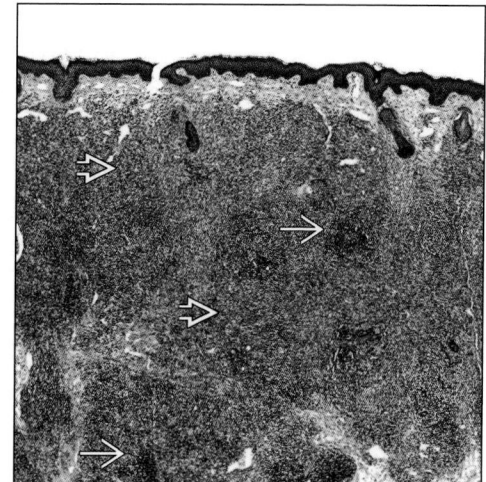

(Left) PCFCL displays a dense, multinodular-appearing lymphocytic infiltrate in the dermis, sparing the subepidermal layer (grenz zone ➡). The neoplasm contains ill-defined follicles ⮕. (Courtesy R. Miranda, MD.) (Right) This example of PCFCL shows a mostly diffuse growth pattern ⮕ with only vaguely follicular-appearing areas ➡.

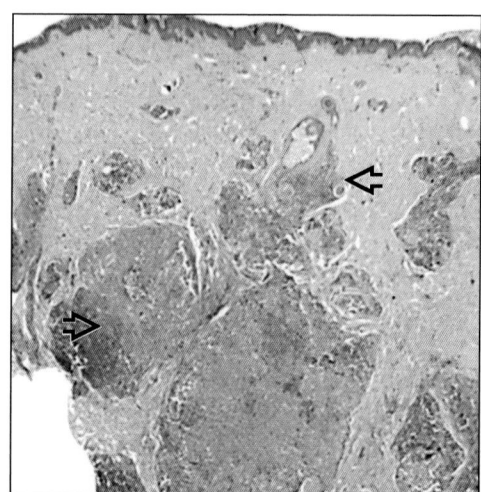
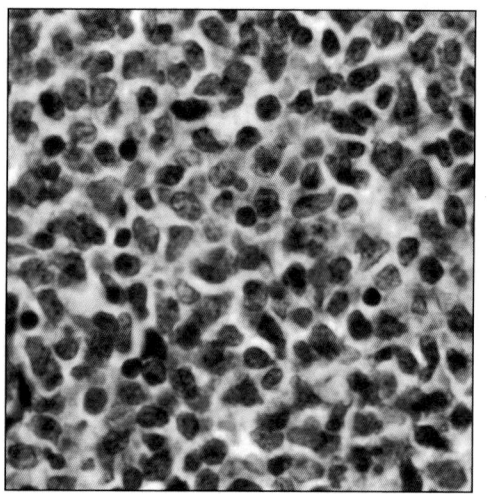

(Left) In this case of PCFCL, the follicles are irregularly shaped and not well-defined ➡. Also, there is loss of the mantle zones surrounding these follicles. (Courtesy M. Tomaszewski, MD.) (Right) Within the follicles of a PCFCL, there is loss of the normal tingible body macrophages that are typically seen in reactive follicles.

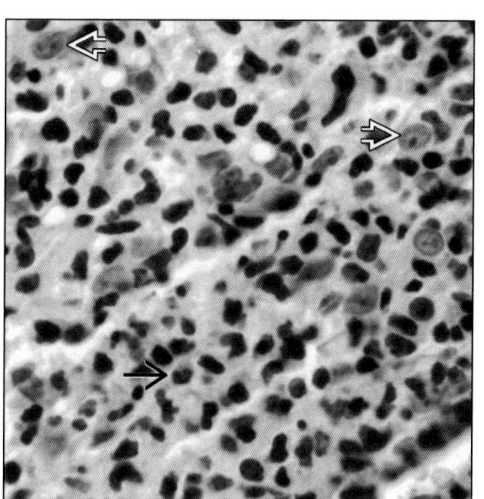
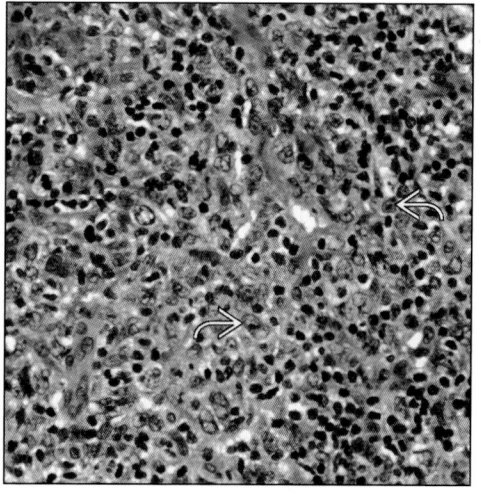

(Left) In most cases of PCFCL, there is a mixture of small cleaved centrocytes ➡ and larger centroblasts. Centroblasts ⮕ are bigger cells and usually have 1 or more nucleoli near the edge of the nuclear membrane. (Right) This is a PCFCL with a diffuse pattern, composed of sheets of markedly enlarged and atypical-appearing cells, many of which have large nucleoli ⮕.

Immunohistochemical Features

(Left) CD20 is strongly expressed in the B cells throughout the dermal infiltrate. Note that the epidermis is uninvolved, with a grenz zone separating the infiltrate from the epidermis ⮕. Other B-cell markers such as CD79a and pax-5 (not shown) are also immunoreactive in the malignant cells. **(Right)** Higher magnification shows that CD20 is very strongly expressed in the B cells throughout the dermal infiltrate.

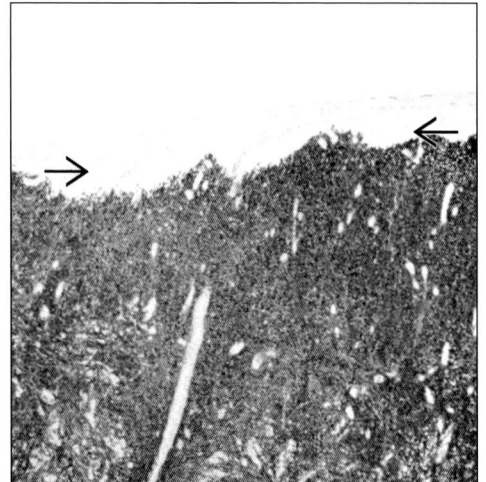
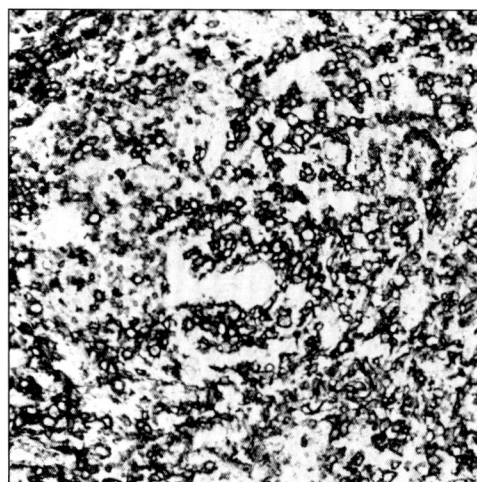

(Left) Bcl-6 is positive in the vast majority of cases of PCFCL. The neoplastic lymphocytes express Bcl-6 even in diffuse areas, as is shown here, with strong and diffuse nuclear staining ⮕. **(Right)** Bcl-2 can be positive or negative in the neoplastic cells in PCFCL. In this case, there is weak to moderate Bcl-2 staining in the tumor cells ⮕, with stronger staining of background T cells ⮕. Bcl-2 tends to be positive in follicular areas, but negative in diffuse areas. *(Courtesy R. Miranda, MD.)*

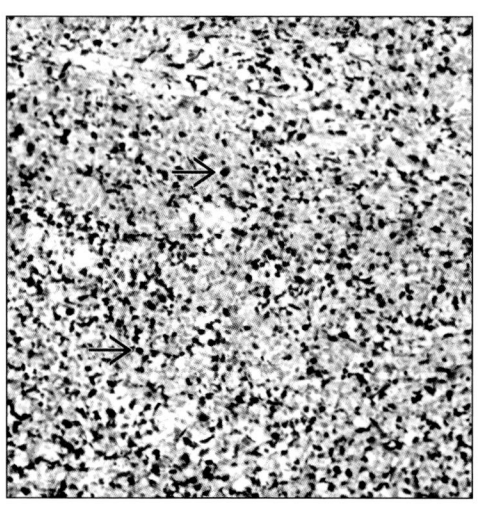
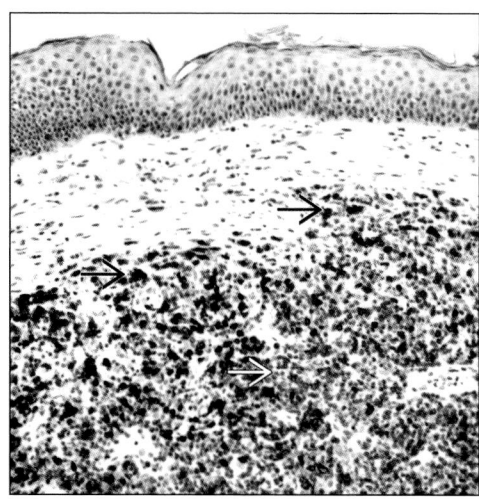

(Left) This is a CD10 immunostain. This case of PCFCL is negative for CD10 in the neoplastic cells. CD10 is often negative in the diffuse areas of PCFCL, whereas it is more commonly positive in the follicular/nodular areas. **(Right)** Anti-CD10 strongly highlights the follicular pattern in this nodular PCFCL case. CD10 is usually reactive in PCFCL with a follicular pattern and tends to be negative in diffuse areas. *(Courtesy R. Miranda, MD.)*

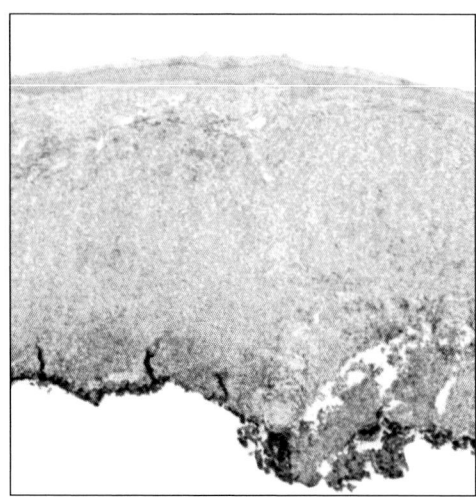
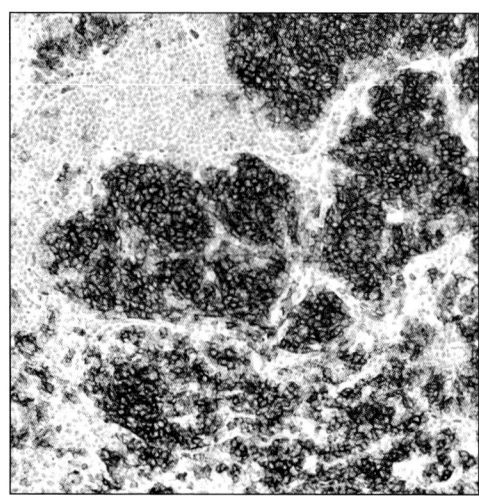

Differential Diagnosis

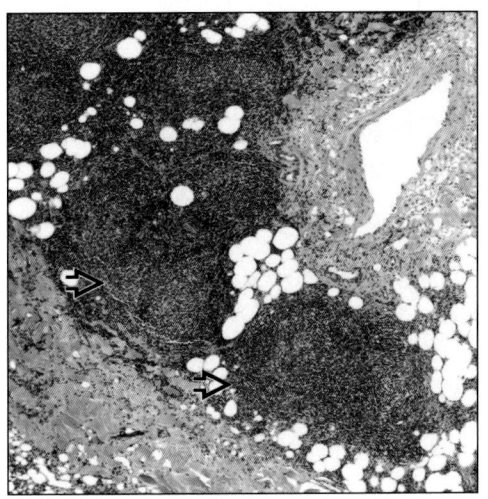

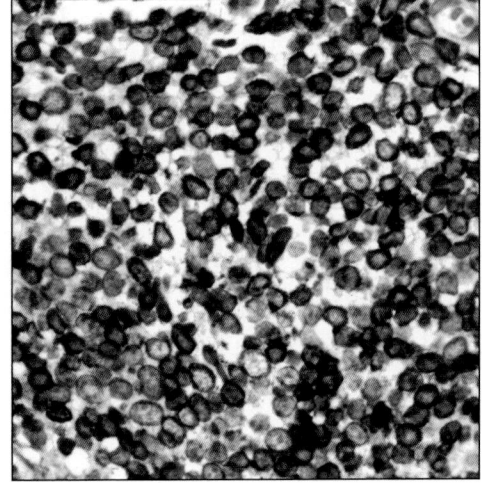

(Left) Secondary follicular lymphoma (FL) of the skin has a similar morphology and phenotype to PCFCL. There are neoplastic follicles ⇗ in the subcutis. (Courtesy R. Miranda, MD.) **(Right)** This is a Bcl-2(+) stain. This case of secondary FL of skin is Bcl-2(+), which is often negative in PCFCL. It is crucial to differentiate secondary FL from PCFCL since it is treated with chemotherapy and has a worse prognosis. (Courtesy R. Miranda, MD.)

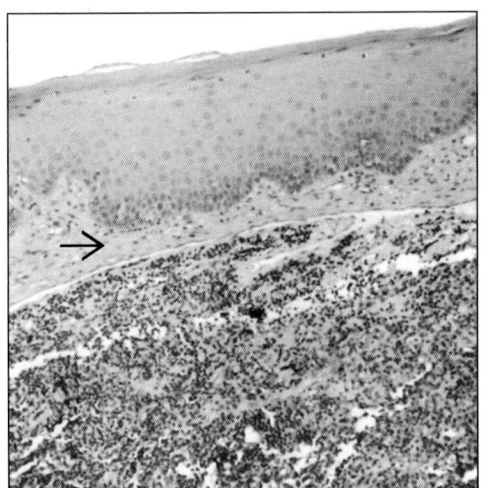

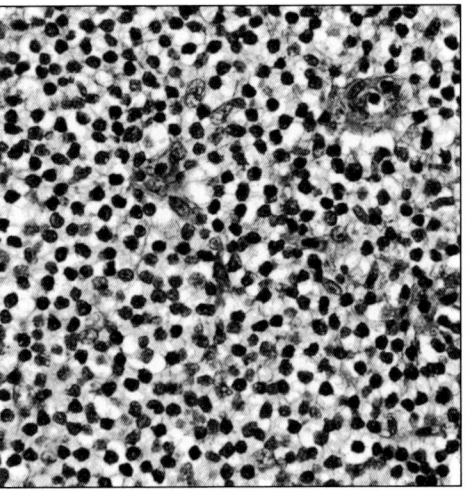

(Left) This case of primary cutaneous marginal zone B-cell lymphoma (PCMZL) shows a dermal infiltrate, and a grenz zone ⇗ separates the tumor from the epidermis. **(Right)** This primary cutaneous marginal zone lymphoma is composed of monocytoid small lymphocytes that have little nuclear irregularity and are surrounded by pale/ clear cytoplasm. There were also colonized germinal centers and an expanded FDC meshwork on CD21 (not shown).

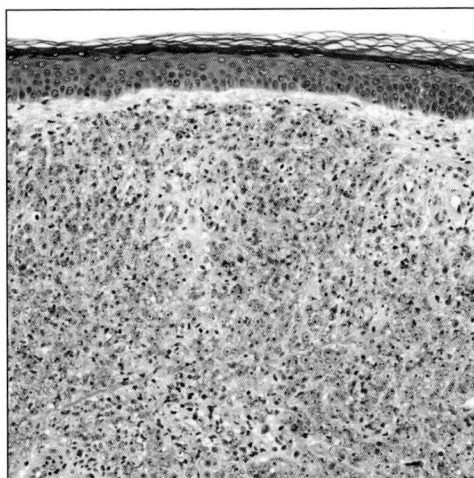

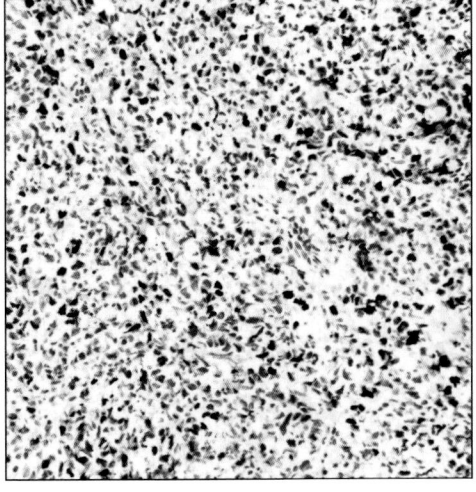

(Left) This image of primary cutaneous diffuse large B-cell lymphoma, leg type shows a diffuse infiltrate of markedly enlarged and atypical-appearing cells. PCDLBCL-LT has a diffuse growth pattern, unlike PCFCL, which usually has, at least in part, follicular areas. PCFCL also differs by containing smaller centrocytes. **(Right)** This is MUM-1, a nuclear marker strongly and diffusely positive in this case of PCDLBCL-LT. MUM-1 is typically negative in PCFCL.

DIFFUSE LARGE B-CELL LYMPHOMA, LEG TYPE

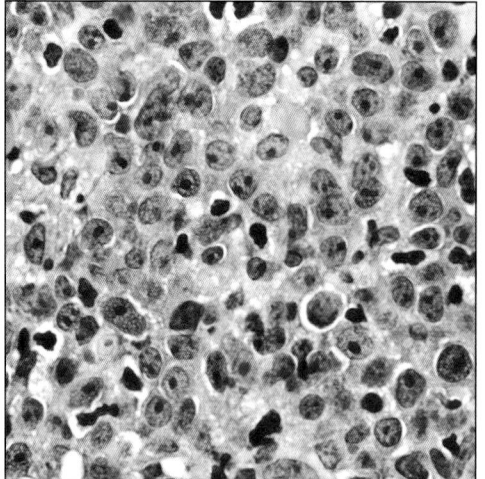

Primary cutaneous diffuse large B-cell lymphoma, leg type (PCDLBCL-LT) shows a diffuse infiltrate replacing the dermis with sparing of the epidermis ➡.

The lymphoma cells in PCDLBCL-LT are large and strikingly round with centrally located nucleoli (immunoblasts).

TERMINOLOGY

Abbreviations
- Primary cutaneous diffuse large B-cell lymphoma, leg type (PCDLBCL-LT)

Synonyms
- Primary cutaneous large B-cell lymphoma, leg type
- Primary cutaneous diffuse large B-cell lymphoma

Definitions
- Primary cutaneous diffuse large B-cell lymphoma composed exclusively of large transformed B cells
  - Often occurs in lower leg(s), but can arise at other sites

ETIOLOGY/PATHOGENESIS

Cell of Origin
- Peripheral B cell of post-germinal center cell origin
  - Immunophenotype: IRF-4/MUM1(+), FOXP1(+)
  - High frequency of somatic mutations of *IgH* variable (V)-region genes

Possible Role of Antigen Selection
- Preferential use of certain *IgHV* gene segments
  - Suggests that antigen stimulation may be involved in pathogenesis

Role of Molecular Abnormalities
- Number of genetic rearrangements and deletions reported
- No abnormality consistently present

CLINICAL ISSUES

Epidemiology
- Incidence
  - Rare

- 4% of all cutaneous lymphomas
- 20% of primary cutaneous B-cell lymphomas
- Age
  - Elderly patients; median age: 7th decade
- Gender
  - More common in women
    - Male to female ratio: 1:1.6; as high as 1:4 in some studies

Site
- Most cases arise in skin of lower leg(s): 1 or both legs may be involved
  - ~ 85% of all cases
- Subset of cases arise in skin of other sites (trunk, arms, head and neck)
  - ~ 15% of cases
  - Similar morphologic and immunophenotypic characteristics
- Single or multiple lesions at time of presentation
  - Some patients have dissemination at initial diagnosis

Presentation
- Red or blue-red cutaneous lesions
  - Plaque, verrucous plaques, or deep plaques
  - Nodular, tumoral lesions
  - Often associated with ulcer
  - Multiple lesions are common
- B symptoms in 10-20% of patients

Treatment
- Anthracycline-containing systemic chemotherapy plus rituximab (R-CHOP)
- Radiotherapy has role for localized lesions in elderly patients

Prognosis
- Relapse is common
- 40-50% 5-year survival rate
  - Factors adversely correlated with prognosis
    - Older age

DIFFUSE LARGE B-CELL LYMPHOMA, LEG TYPE

Key Facts

Terminology
- Primary cutaneous DLBCL composed exclusively of large transformed cells

Clinical Issues
- 20% of primary cutaneous B-cell lymphomas
- Most cases arise in skin of lower leg(s)
  - ~ 85% of all cases
- Subset of cases arise in skin of other sites (trunk, arms, head and neck)
  - ~ 15% of cases
- Single or multiple lesions at time of presentation
- Relapse is common; 50% 5-year survival
- Treated with systemic R-CHOP

Microscopic Pathology
- Diffuse pattern of involvement in dermis

- Monotonous sheets of large immunoblasts or centroblasts
- Few small reactive T cells in background
- No centrocytes (or small B cells) present
- No epidermotropism

Ancillary Tests
- Pan-B-cell antigens (+), Bcl-2(+), Bcl-6(+)
- MUM1(+), FOXP1(+), IgM(+), CD10(-)

Top Differential Diagnoses
- Primary cutaneous follicle center lymphoma
- Systemic DLBCL involving skin
- Plasmablastic lymphoma involving skin
- EBV(+) DLBCL of elderly
- Monomorphic post-transplant lymphoproliferative disorder

- Multiple lesions at presentation
- Inactivation of *CDKN2A*
- Factors not correlated with prognosis
  - Duration of lesions before diagnosis
  - Gender, B symptoms, performance status, or serum lactate dehydrogenase level
  - Bcl-2 or IRF-4/MUM1 expression

MICROSCOPIC PATHOLOGY

Histologic Features
- Diffuse pattern of involvement of dermis
  - Infiltrate can be deep, often extending into superficial subcutaneous adipose tissue
- Cohesive, monotonous sheets of atypical-appearing large cells
  - Centroblasts or immunoblasts
  - Often very round nuclei
- Mitotic figures numerous
- Few small reactive T cells in background
- No centrocytes (or small B cells) present
- No epidermotropism

ANCILLARY TESTS

Immunohistochemistry
- Pan-B-cell antigens (+)
- Cytoplasmic IgM(+), IgD(+/-)
- Bcl-2(+), IRF-4/MUM1(+), FOXP1(+)
- Bcl-6(+), CD10(-)
- No follicular dendritic cell (FDC) meshworks
  - CD21(-), CD23(-), CD35(-)
- T-cell antigens (-), LMP1(-), HHV8(-)

In Situ Hybridization
- FISH often shows rearrangements of *MYC*, *BCL6*, or *IgH* genes
  - No evidence of *IgH-BCL2*/t(14;18) or *BCL2* rearrangements
- EBER(-)

Array CGH
- Amplification of 18q21.31-33 involving *BCL2* and *MALT1* genes

Molecular Genetics
- Monoclonal *IgH* gene rearrangements
- No evidence of *IgH-BCL2*/t(14;18)

Gene Expression Profiling
- Profile is consistent with activated B-cell phenotype

DIFFERENTIAL DIAGNOSIS

Primary Cutaneous Follicle Center Cell Lymphoma (PCFCL)
- Most PCFCL have follicular pattern and can therefore be distinguished from PCDLBCL-LT
- PCFCL cases with diffuse pattern and predominance of large centrocytes or centroblasts are challenging
  - Used to be designated as diffuse large B-cell lymphoma (DLBCL)
    - However, clinically they are confined to skin, and prognosis is good
    - Could lead to over-treatment with multiagent chemotherapy
- Sites of skin involvement
  - Mostly in head and neck, trunk, back, arms
  - Some cases of PCFCL can present on leg
    - Patients with PCFCL on leg often have worse prognosis than patients with PCFCL at other sites
    - Prognosis of PCFCL of leg is similar to, or slightly better than, PCDLBCL-LT
- Histologic features of PCFCL
  - Areas of follicular pattern can be predominant, focal, or absent
  - Often, perivascular &/or periadnexal pattern in dermis is present
  - Mixture of centrocytes and centroblasts
    - Cells can be polylobated or spindle-shaped
  - Stromal reaction with fibrosis and sclerosis is common

DIFFUSE LARGE B-CELL LYMPHOMA, LEG TYPE

- Immunophenotype
  - CD10(+), Bcl-6(+); Bcl-2 often negative; if positive, often weak and focal
  - FDC meshwork is present
    - CD21, CD23, CD35, or other markers
  - IRF-4/MUM1(-), FOXP1(-)
  - Small B cells/centrocytes positive (absent in PCDLBCL-LT)
  - CD3(+) reactive T cells relatively numerous (compared with PCDLBCL-LT)
  - Cases of PCFCL with diffuse pattern
    - CD10 often negative in areas of diffuse pattern
    - Residual FDC meshwork usually can be identified

Systemic DLBCL Involving Skin
- Can be difficult to distinguish from PCDLBCL-LT based on morphology and immunophenotype
- Clinical history of systemic disease is key for differential diagnosis
- If patient has systemic and skin involvement at time of initial presentation
  - Can be difficult to distinguish systemic DLBCL from PCDLBCL-LT
  - Large tumors on lower leg(s) support PCDLBCL-LT

Plasmablastic Lymphoma Involving Skin
- Most patients have high-stage disease at time of presentation
  - Mucosal involvement is common
- Any skin site can be involved; leg uncommon
- Histologic features
  - Cohesive sheets of monomorphic plasmablasts can closely mimic PCDLBCL-LT
  - Some cases may show plasmacytic differentiation
- Immunophenotype
  - CD138(+), CD38(+)
  - Cytoplasmic monotypic Ig light chain (+)
  - EBER(+)

EBV(+) DLBCL of Elderly
- Cutaneous involvement can be initial presentation
- Histologic features
  - Tumor cells are often more polymorphic than PCDLBCL-LT
    - Plasmacytoid or plasmacytic differentiation positive
    - Large transformed cells, Reed-Sternberg-like cells
    - Background often has small lymphocytes, neutrophils, plasma cells, and histiocytes
  - Necrosis is common
- Immunophenotype is similar to PCDLBCL-LT; EBER(+)

Monomorphic Post-Transplant Lymphoproliferative Disorder (PTLD)
- Monomorphic PTLD can involve skin
- Histologic features
  - Tumor cells are often more polymorphic than PCDLBCL-LT
    - Plasmacytoid or plasmacytic differentiation positive
    - Large transformed cells, Reed-Sternberg-like cells
  - Necrosis is common, often with geographic pattern
- Immunophenotype is similar to PCDLBCL-LT; EBER(+)

- Clinical history of organ transplantation

DIAGNOSTIC CHECKLIST

Clinically Relevant Pathologic Features
- PCDLBCL-LT usually involves lower leg(s), but can present at other sites
  - Leg location is adverse prognostic factor

Pathologic Interpretation Pearls
- Diffuse involvement of dermis by sheets of round immunoblasts or centroblasts
  - Very few or absent small B cells
  - Relatively few reactive T cells (compared with PCFCL)
- Immunophenotype
  - Bcl-2(+), Bcl-6(+), MUM1(+), FOXP1(+), IgM(+)

SELECTED REFERENCES
1. Demirkesen C et al: The expression of IgM is helpful in the differentiation of primary cutaneous diffuse large B cell lymphoma and follicle center lymphoma. Leuk Res. 35(9):1269-72, 2011
2. Gokdemir G et al: Primary cutaneous diffuse large B-cell lymphoma of the leg, with an atypical clinical picture of verrucous plaques associated with stasis dermatitis. Clin Exp Dermatol. 35(3):e87-9, 2010
3. Guyot A et al: Combined treatment with rituximab and anthracycline-containing chemotherapy for primary cutaneous large B-cell lymphomas, leg type, in elderly patients. Arch Dermatol. 146(1):89-91, 2010
4. Koens L et al: IgM expression on paraffin sections distinguishes primary cutaneous large B-cell lymphoma, leg type from primary cutaneous follicle center lymphoma. Am J Surg Pathol. 34(7):1043-8, 2010
5. Perez M et al: Primary cutaneous B-cell lymphoma is associated with somatically hypermutated immunoglobulin variable genes and frequent use of VH1-69 and VH4-59 segments. Br J Dermatol. 162(3):611-8, 2010
6. Pham-Ledard A et al: IRF4 expression without IRF4 rearrangement is a general feature of primary cutaneous diffuse large B-cell lymphoma, leg type. J Invest Dermatol. 130(5):1470-2, 2010
7. Grange F et al: Primary cutaneous diffuse large B-cell lymphoma, leg type: clinicopathologic features and prognostic analysis in 60 cases. Arch Dermatol. 143(9):1144-50, 2007
8. Senff NJ et al: Reclassification of 300 primary cutaneous B-Cell lymphomas according to the new WHO-EORTC classification for cutaneous lymphomas: comparison with previous classifications and identification of prognostic markers. J Clin Oncol. 25(12):1581-7, 2007
9. Zinzani PL et al: Prognostic factors in primary cutaneous B-cell lymphoma: the Italian Study Group for Cutaneous Lymphomas. J Clin Oncol. 24(9):1376-82, 2006
10. Kodama K et al: Primary cutaneous large B-cell lymphomas: clinicopathologic features, classification, and prognostic factors in a large series of patients. Blood. 106(7):2491-7, 2005
11. Wiesner T et al: Genetic aberrations in primary cutaneous large B-cell lymphoma: a fluorescence in situ hybridization study of 25 cases. Am J Surg Pathol. 29(5):666-73, 2005
12. Grange F et al: Prognostic factors in primary cutaneous large B-cell lymphomas: a European multicenter study. J Clin Oncol. 19(16):3602-10, 2001

DIFFUSE LARGE B-CELL LYMPHOMA, LEG TYPE

Comparison of PCDLBCL-LT with PCFCL with Diffuse Pattern and Increased Large Cells

Parameter	PCDLBCL-LT	PCFCL with Diffuse Pattern and Increased Large Cells
Demographic Information		
Age	Older, 7th decade	6th decade
Gender	Female preponderance	Slight male preponderance
Sites of Involvement		
Location	Leg, 1 or both	Head and neck most frequent, followed by trunk or arms
	15% involving other sites, e.g., trunk, arm, head and neck	Rarely on leg, which has worse prognosis than PCFCL on other sites
	Multiple lesions common, some with deep plaques	Multiple sites of involvement are common
Risk for developing extracutaneous disease	~ 50%	~ 10%
Disseminated	~ 30%	~ 10%
Morphologic Features		
	Cohesive sheets of centroblasts or immunoblasts	Diffuse growth pattern with predominance of large centrocytes or centroblasts
	Cells often have strikingly round nuclei with many mitoses	Often cleaved, polylobated, irregular, or spindle-shaped
	No centrocytes (or small B cells) present	Often have admixed small centrocytes
Small reactive T cells	Very few, often in perivascular areas	Less pronounced, but more than PCDLBCL-LT
Epidermotropism	Not present	Not present
Perivascular/periadnexal	Not present	Often
Follicular dendritic cell (FDC) meshwork	Not present	Small broken clusters of FDC may be present
Immunohistochemistry		
Bcl-6	Mostly positive	Positive
Bcl-2	Positive ~ 90%	Often negative; if positive, often weak or focal
CD10	Negative	Often negative in diffuse areas; often positive in follicular areas
MUM1	(+, 50-80%)	Negative
FOXP1	Positive	Negative
IgM &/or IgD	Positive	Negative
Molecular Genetics		
	Similar to systemic DLBCL	Different from nodal follicular lymphoma
MYC, *BCL6*, and *IgH* rearrangement by FISH	Can be present	Often absent
Amplification of *BCL2* and *MALT1* genes	Can be present	Absent
Deletions of chromosome 9p21.3 (containing *CDKN2a* and *CDKN2b)*	Reported in 67% of cases	Absent
t(14;18)(q32;q21)	Absent	Reported in 10-40% of cases
Treatment		
	Anthracycline-containing chemotherapy plus rituximab	If single lesion, radiation therapy or surgical excision
	Radiation therapy for localized lesion in elderly	If multiple lesions, systemic chemotherapy may be used
Prognosis		
Relapse	Yes, frequent	Yes, ~ 30% of patients
5-year survival rate	50%	85-100%

PCDLBCL-LT = primary cutaneous diffuse large B-cell lymphoma, leg type; PCFCL = primary cutaneous follicle center cell lymphoma; DLBCL = diffuse large B-cell lymphoma.

DIFFUSE LARGE B-CELL LYMPHOMA, LEG TYPE

Microscopic and Immunohistochemical Features

(Left) This case of PCDLBCL-LT almost completely fills the dermis. The neoplasm has a diffuse pattern with a grenz zone ⇨ between the neoplasm and the uninvolved epidermis. *(Right)* PCDLBCL-LT often appears confluent at low-power magnification. Small reactive T cells can be seen in 1 corner ⇲ of the field, but relatively few are admixed with the lymphoma cells.

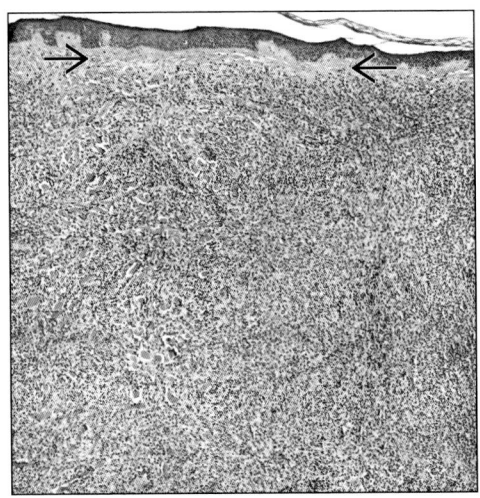 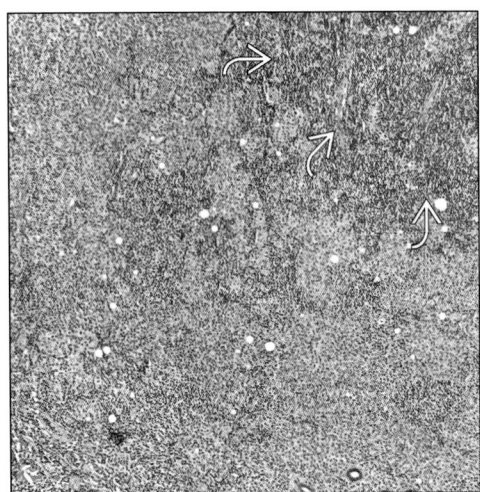

(Left) In PCDLBCL-LT, the lymphoma cells often have a striking round cell morphology and grow in sheets that appear cohesive, and surround a central vessel in this field. *(Right)* In this case of PCDLBCL-LT, the lymphoma cells are centroblasts that appear very similar to each other, imparting a monotonous appearance.

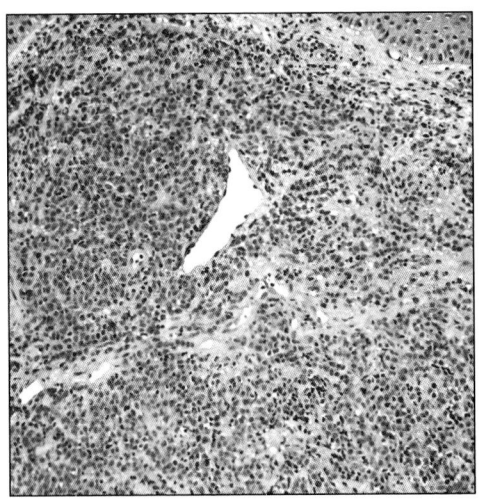 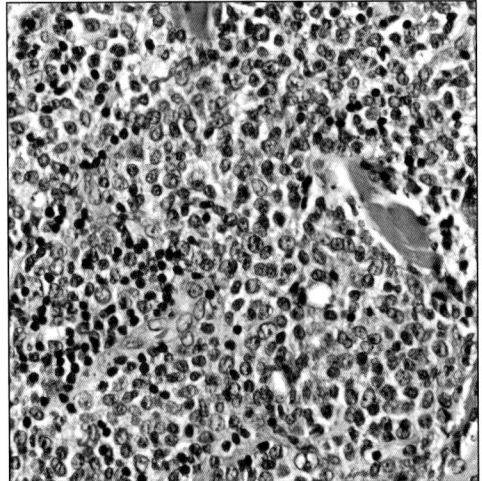

(Left) In this case of PCDLBCL-LT, the lymphoma cells are strongly CD20(+) and form cohesive-appearing sheets. The epidermis ⇨ is not involved, and a thin grenz zone is present ⇲. *(Right)* Most cases of PCDLBCL-LT are strongly and diffusely Bcl-2(+), as shown in this case.

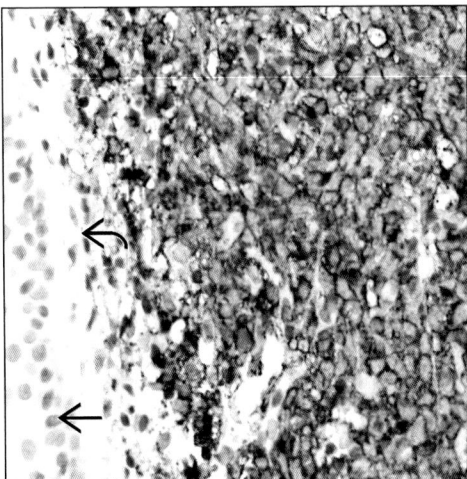 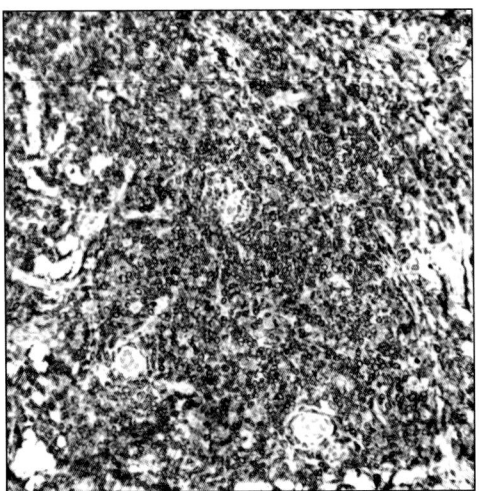

DIFFUSE LARGE B-CELL LYMPHOMA, LEG TYPE

Immunohistochemical Features

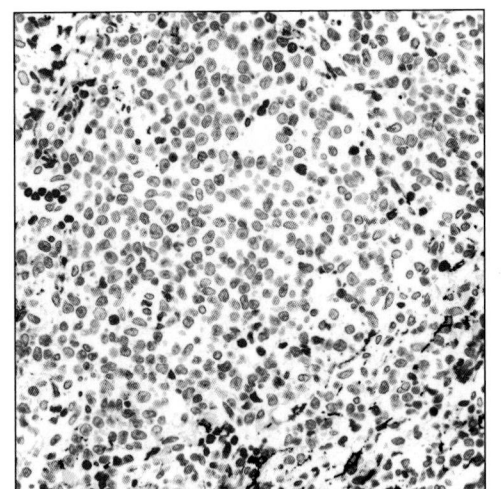
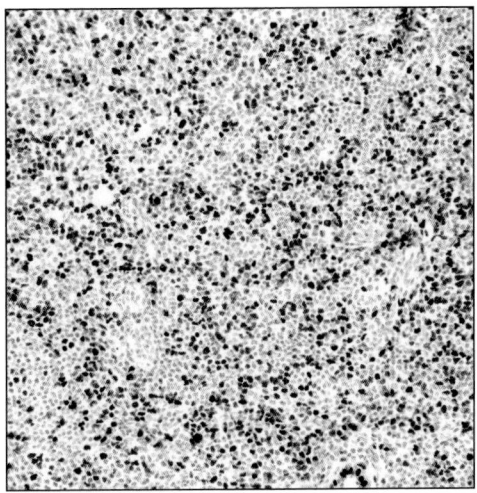

(Left) In PCDLBCL-LT, the lymphoma cells are usually CD10(-), consistent with a post-germinal center origin of lymphoma cells. *(Right)* In PCDLBCL-LT, the lymphoma cells are often at least partially Bcl-6(+).

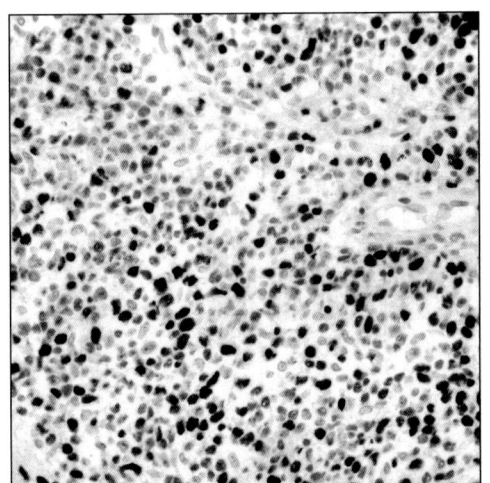
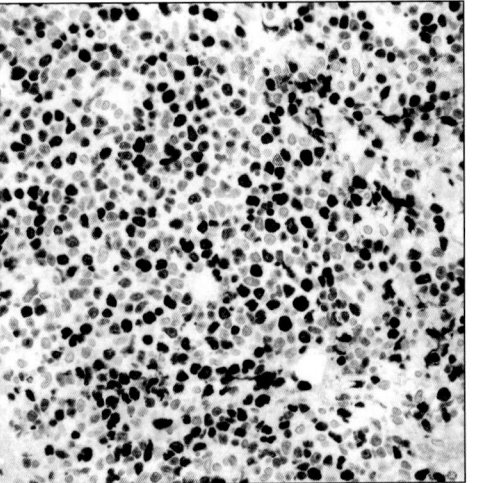

(Left) Approximately 50-80% of cases of PCDLBCL-LT are IRF-4/MUM1(+), a marker associated with more aggressive lymphomas, and indicating a post-germinal center origin. *(Right)* In PCDLBCL-LT, Ki-67 shows a high proliferation fraction in the lymphoid cells.

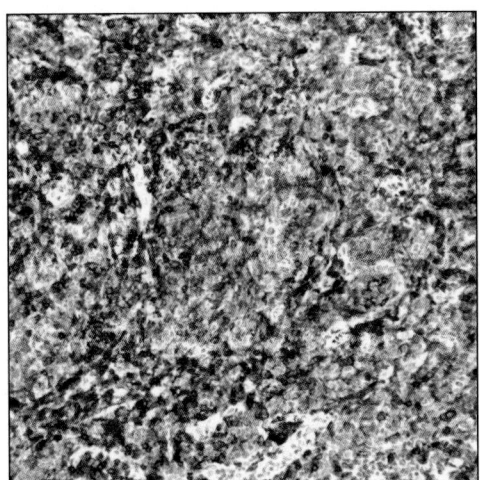
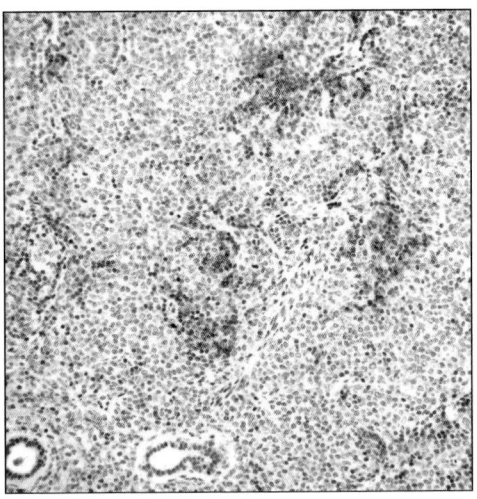

(Left) This case of PCDLBCL-LT is strongly CD23(+). A subset of these tumors are CD23(+), unlike primary cutaneous follicle center lymphoma. Also note that no CD23(+) follicular dendritic cells are present, confirming the presence of a diffuse growth pattern. *(Right)* In this case of PCDLBCL-LT, a CD21 immunostain does not highlight any follicular dendritic cells, supporting a diffuse growth pattern. A small subset of lymphoma cells are CD21(+) in this field.

Differential Diagnosis

(Left) Primary cutaneous follicular center lymphoma (PCFCL) with a diffuse pattern is shown. As with PCDLBCL-LT, the lymphoma cells spare the epidermis, leaving a grenz zone ➡. **(Right)** This case of PCFCL also shows a predominance of large cells. In contrast with PCDLBCL-LT, the tumor cells are cleaved, polylobated, irregular, spindle-shaped (large centrocytes and centroblasts), and admixed with many small lymphocytes.

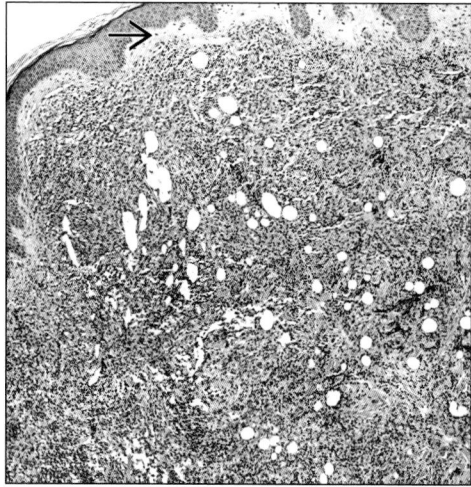
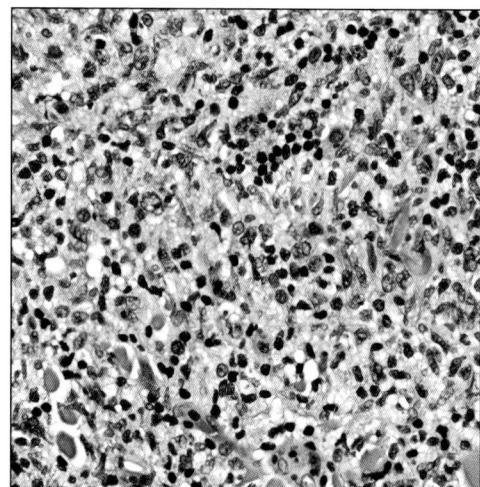

(Left) PCFCL with a predominance of large cells is shown. The infiltrate appears to be noncohesive and is associated with a fibrotic stromal reaction, unlike cases of PCDLBCL-LT. **(Right)** PCFCL often shows vascular invasion or has a perivascular pattern of infiltration. These features are uncommon in PCDLBCL-LT.

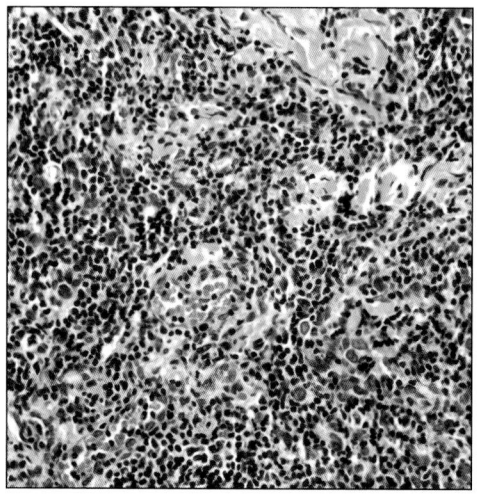
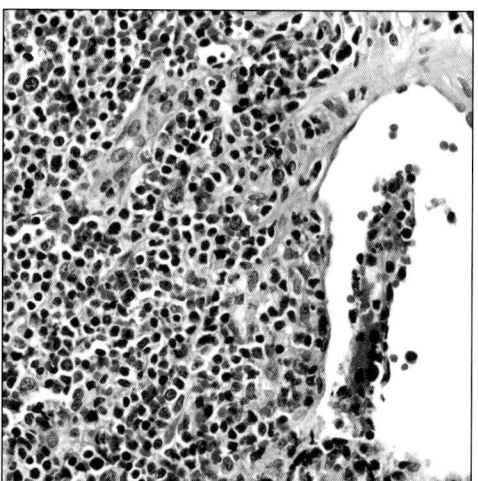

(Left) This case of PCFCL with a diffuse pattern was CD10(-). It should be remembered that CD10 is commonly expressed in follicular areas, but is often negative in diffuse areas of PCFCL. **(Right)** Many cases of PCFCL are negative for Bcl-2. In some cases of PCFCL, the lymphoma cells can be Bcl-2(+), but expression is often weak or present in only a subset of cells ➡, as shown in this field. Small reactive T cells are strongly Bcl-2(+).

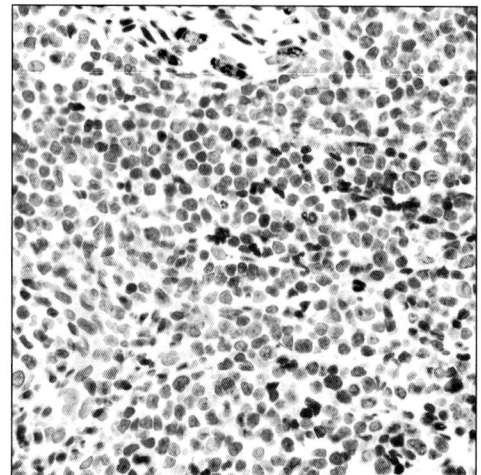
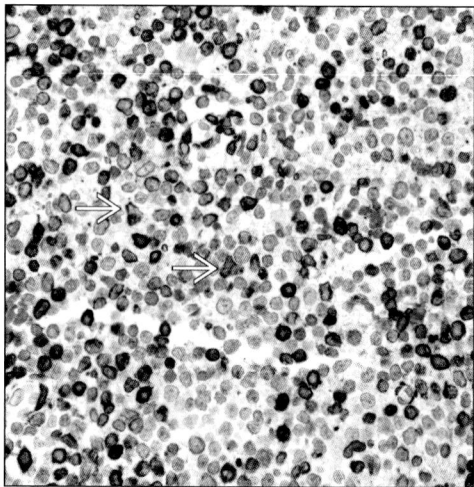

DIFFUSE LARGE B-CELL LYMPHOMA, LEG TYPE

Differential Diagnosis

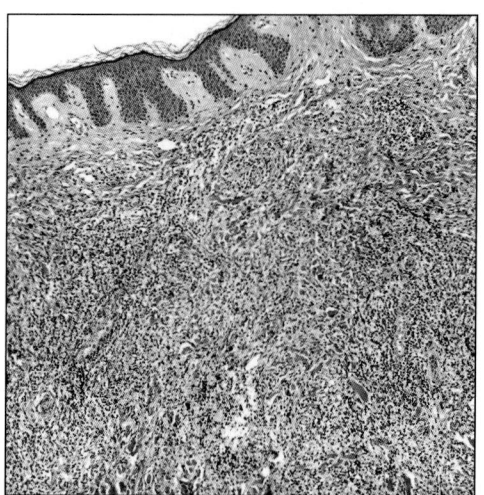

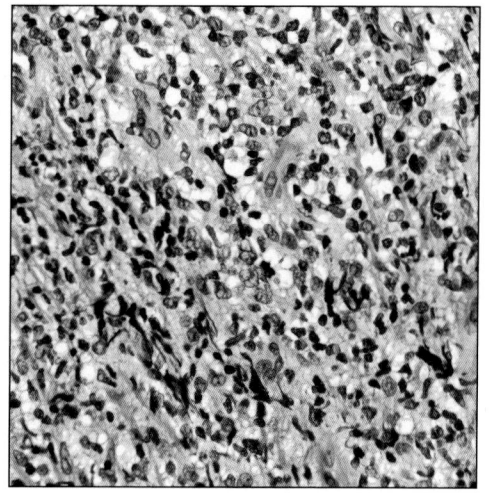

(Left) A case of primary mediastinal (thymic) large B-cell lymphoma disseminated to skin. The pattern of infiltration mimics primary cutaneous lymphoma at low-power magnification. *(Right)* High magnification of a primary mediastinal (thymic) large B-cell lymphoma disseminated to skin. The lymphoma cells are polylobated and spindle-shaped.

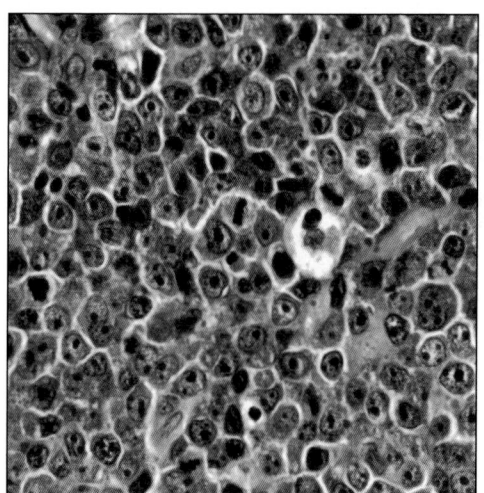

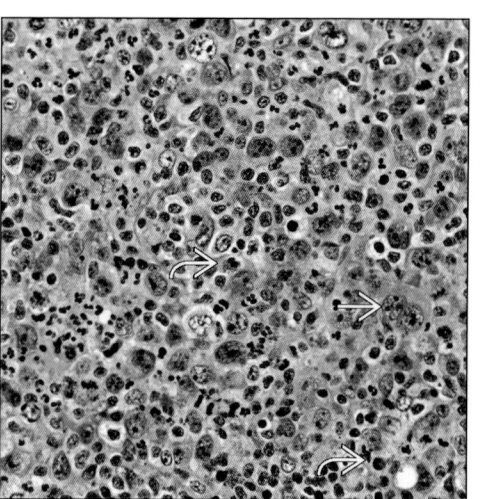

(Left) A case of systemic diffuse large B-cell lymphoma, immunoblastic variant, involving the skin is shown. The lymphoma cells resemble the immunoblasts observed in some cases of PCDLBCL-LT. *(Right)* EBV(+) diffuse large B-cell lymphoma of the elderly involving skin is shown. The lymphoma cells are large and polymorphous, with Reed-Sternberg-like cells ➡ and plasmacytoid cells present. Many neutrophils as well as eosinophils ➡ are also present in the background.

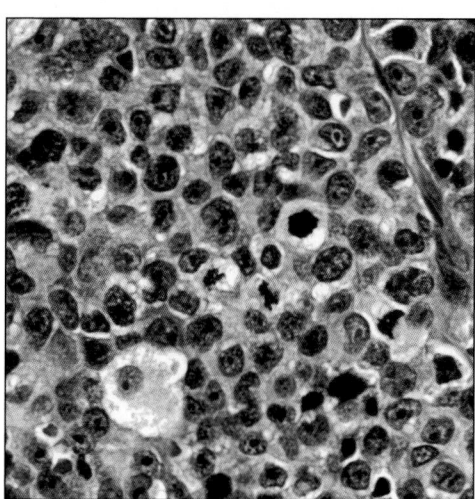

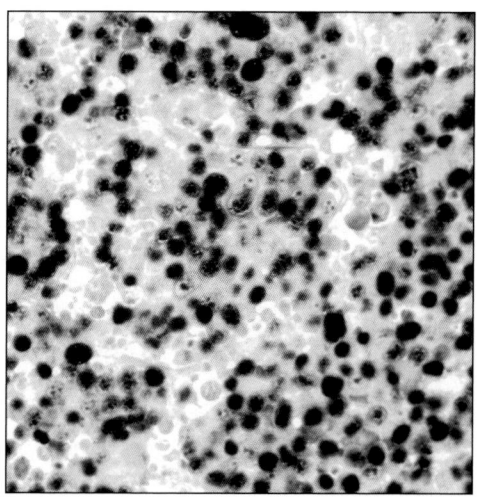

(Left) Plasmablastic lymphoma involving the skin is shown. Plasmablastic lymphoma usually shows a cohesive proliferation of plasmablasts or immunoblasts, and these features overlap with PCDLBCL-LT. *(Right)* Plasmablastic lymphoma involving the skin is shown. In situ hybridization for Epstein-Barr virus small-encoded RNA (EBER) is usually positive in plasmablastic lymphoma, unlike in PCDLBCL-LT.

LYMPHOMATOID GRANULOMATOSIS

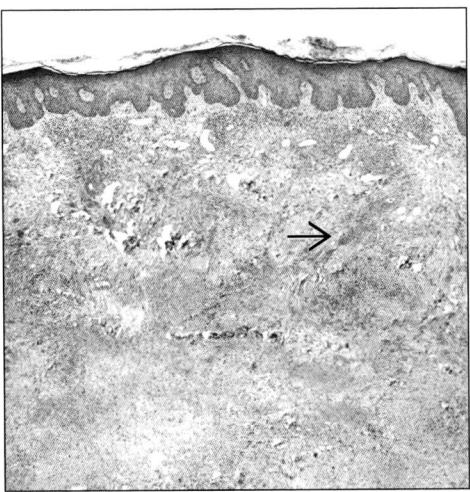

Low-power view of LYG shows an extensive B-cell infiltrate with a perivascular angiodestructive distribution ➡. The epidermis is not involved. (Courtesy M. Royer, MD.)

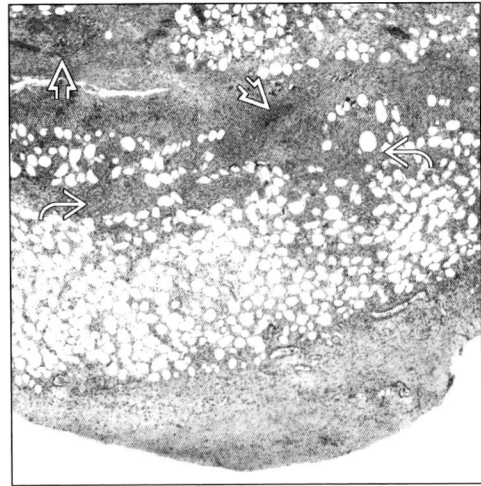

LYG diffusely infiltrating into the fat ➡ can mimic a reactive panniculitis. There is angiocentric involvement with tumor cells surrounding and infiltrating blood vessels ➡.

TERMINOLOGY

Abbreviations
- Lymphomatoid granulomatosis (LYG)

Synonyms
- Angiocentric immunoproliferative lesion, angiocentric lymphoma

Definitions
- Extranodal angiocentric mature B-cell lymphoma that expresses Epstein-Barr virus (EBV) antigens

ETIOLOGY/PATHOGENESIS

Immunodeficiency
- Associated with immunodeficiency, ↑ involvement with allogeneic organ transplant, human immunodeficiency virus infection, X-linked lymphoproliferative disorder, and Wiskott-Aldrich syndrome

Cytokines
- IP10 and Mig are implicated in pathogenesis of blood vessel damage

CLINICAL ISSUES

Epidemiology
- Age
  - Mostly adults, commonly in 50s, also in children with immunodeficiency syndromes
- Gender
  - M:F > 2.0:1.0

Site
- Most common site is lung (usually multiple nodules); skin is most frequent extrapulmonary site

- For skin lesions, often trunk or limbs, cutaneous nodules often develop after pulmonary disease
- Also involve kidney, liver, and brain; usually not found in lymph nodes or spleen

Presentation
- Variable cutaneous lesions can be papules or nodules, often multiple and sometimes with ulceration; plaques are less common
- Pulmonary symptoms (cough and dyspnea)

Prognosis
- Variable, but often related to grading
  - Most patients have aggressive disease, survival < 2 years
  - Cases with increased numbers of small lymphocytes and histiocytes have more favorable prognosis
  - Cases with larger number of atypical B cells expressing EBV have worse prognosis
  - Grading based on number of EBV(+) B cells compared to background reactive T cells
    - Grade 1: < 5 EBER(+) cells per high-power field, large atypical B cells are rare, polymorphous background infiltrate, focal or no necrosis
    - Grade 2: 5-20 EBER(+) cells per high-power field, small clusters of B cells, more necrosis
    - Grade 3: > 20 EBER(+) cells per high-power field, large atypical B cells, larger B-cell aggregates, often Reed-Sternberg-like cells, more necrosis
  - Grade 3 lesions show some response to aggressive chemotherapy + rituximab

MICROSCOPIC PATHOLOGY

Histologic Features
- Dense, atypical lymphoid infiltrate usually in subcutis and sometimes in dermis
  - B cells scattered and do not form sheets
  - B cells may be immunoblasts, multinucleated, and Reed-Sternberg cell-like

LYMPHOMATOID GRANULOMATOSIS

Key Facts

Terminology
- Extranodal angiocentric mature B-cell lymphoma that expresses Epstein-Barr virus (EBV) antigens

Etiology/Pathogenesis
- Associated with immunodeficiency, ↑ involvement with allogeneic organ transplant, human immunodeficiency virus infection, X-linked lymphoproliferative disorder, and Wiskott-Aldrich syndrome

Clinical Issues
- Most common site is lung (usually multiple nodules); skin is most common extrapulmonary site
- Cases with larger number of atypical B cells expressing EBV have worse prognosis

Microscopic Pathology
- B cells in subcutis and sometimes dermis are scattered and often do not form sheets; B cells may be immunoblasts, multinucleated, and Reed-Sternberg cell-like
- Tumor cells angiocentric, angiodestructive with lymphocytic vasculitis and fibrinoid necrosis of injured blood vessels

Ancillary Tests
- CD20(+), pax-5(+), EBV(+) (less in skin than lung), CD30(+/-), CD15(-)
- Clonal Ig heavy chain (IgH) gene rearrangement more often in higher grades lesions
- Mixed population of T cells, but most express CD4

- ○ Cells are small to medium in size, without coarse chromatin
- ○ Often numerous reactive T cells, ↑ plasma cells and histiocytes, usually normal neutrophils and eosinophils, sometimes granulomatous inflammation in subcutis
- Tumor cells angiocentric, angiodestructive with lymphocytic vasculitis and fibrinoid necrosis of injured blood vessels
- Sometimes shows panniculitis

Cytologic Features
- Medium to large atypical lymphocytes, sometimes with 1 or more prominent nucleoli

ANCILLARY TESTS

Immunohistochemistry
- Malignant cells are positive for B-cell markers (CD20[+], CD19[+], pax-5[+]), EBV(+) (less in skin than lung), CD30(+/-), CD15(-)
- Mixed population of T cells, but most express CD4

Molecular Genetics
- Clonal Ig heavy chain (IgH) gene rearrangement more often detected in higher grades lesions
- Polyclonal for T-cell receptor gene rearrangement studies

DIFFERENTIAL DIAGNOSIS

NK/T-cell Lymphoma
- Also angiocentric with necrosis and EBV(+), but tumor cells are NK or T cells (CD56[+] &/or CD3[+] and CD4[+])

Diffuse Large B-cell Lymphoma
- Usually presents with sheets or aggregates of large pleomorphic B cells, whereas LYG may only show scattered B cells not forming sheets

- Most cases do not involve blood vessels, except for intravascular diffuse large B-cell lymphoma, a rare variant
- Less frequently EBV positive, although the subtype diffuse large B-cell lymphoma of the elderly expresses EBV
- Often lacks mixed background infiltrate seen in LYG
- Rare cases may be due to transformation from preexisting LYG

Vasculitis
- Can show similar histologic features to LYG with inflammation of blood vessels and involvement of multiple organ systems
- Usually not EBV(+), vasculitis has nonmonoclonal B cells

SELECTED REFERENCES

1. Wu SM et al: Lymphomatoid granulomatosis: a rare mimicker of vasculitis. J Rheumatol. 32(11):2242-5, 2005
2. Culhaci N et al: Pulmonary lymphomatoid granulomatosis evolving to large cell lymphoma in the skin. Pathol Oncol Res. 8(4):280-2, 2002
3. Beaty MW et al: Cutaneous lymphomatoid granulomatosis: correlation of clinical and biologic features. Am J Surg Pathol. 25(9):1111-20, 2001
4. Jaffe ES et al: Lymphomatoid granulomatosis: pathogenesis, pathology and clinical implications. Cancer Surv. 30:233-48, 1997
5. Angel CA et al: Epstein-Barr virus in cutaneous lymphomatoid granulomatosis. Histopathology. 25(6):545-8, 1994
6. Carlson KC et al: Cutaneous signs of lymphomatoid granulomatosis. Arch Dermatol. 127(11):1693-8, 1991
7. James WD et al: Cutaneous manifestations of lymphomatoid granulomatosis. Report of 44 cases and a review of the literature. Arch Dermatol. 117(4):196-202, 1981
8. Katzenstein AL et al: Lymphomatoid granulomatosis: a clinicopathologic study of 152 cases. Cancer. 43(1):360-73, 1979

Microscopic and Immunohistochemical Features

(Left) High-power magnification of LYG shows that some of the malignant B-cells have considerable atypia including irregular nuclear shapes, enlarged nuclei ➡, and vesicular chromatin ➡. There were also rare multinucleated cells and Reed-Sternberg-like cells. Note that the malignant cells are scattered and not forming large aggregates. *(Right)* Lymphocytes cuff blood vessels ➡ and penetrate the vessel walls, causing prominent fibrinoid necrosis of injured vessels ➡.

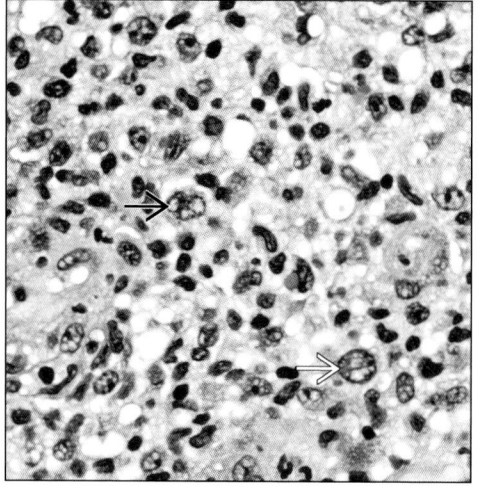
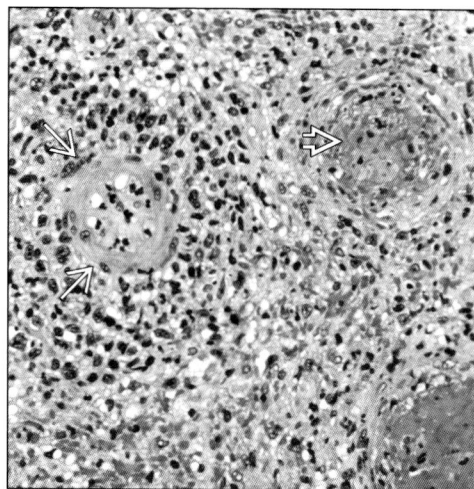

(Left) In a high-power field, mononuclear cells ➡ penetrate the wall of the blood vessel, and many lymphocytes are seen surrounding the blood vessel ➡. Mononuclear cells continue to invade the blood vessel until the vessel is destroyed. *(Right)* This CD20 immunohistochemical stain reveals that the mononuclear cells in the blood vessel ➡ in the center of the slide are B cells. CD20 also highlights increased numbers of lymphocytes outside of the vessel ➡.

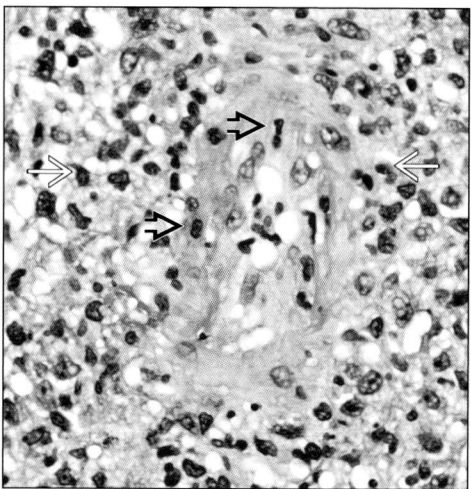
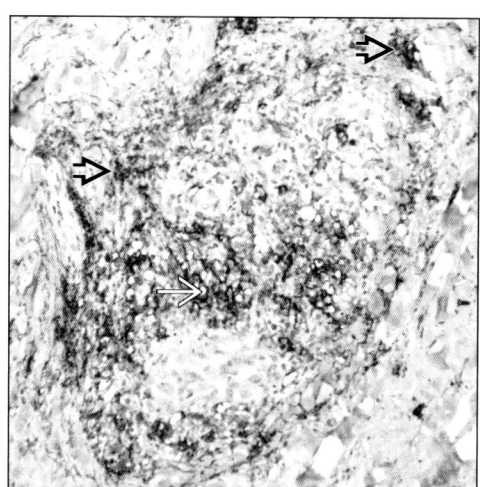

(Left) A CD3 immunostain is not reactive in the larger, malignant B cells ➡ within and surrounding the blood vessel in the center. The CD3 immunostain marks increased numbers of scattered, reactive T cells ➡, which are commonly seen in LYG. *(Right)* A CD7 immunostain is mostly negative in the lymphocytes penetrating the blood vessel in the center of the image ➡. Reactive T cells are seen surrounding the fat cells at the top of the image ➡. *(Courtesy M. Royer, MD.)*

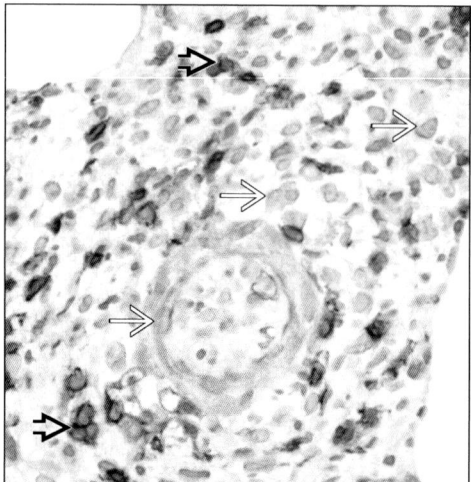
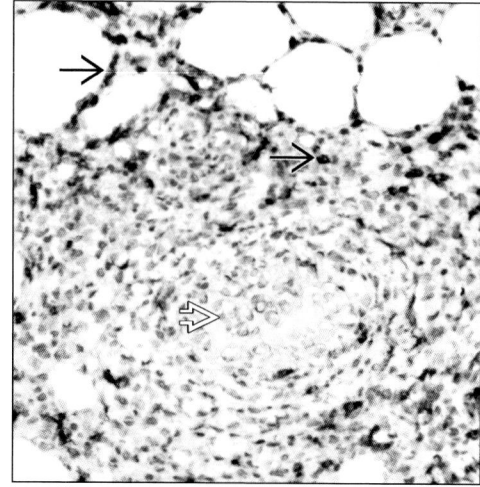

Ancillary Techniques and Differential Diagnosis

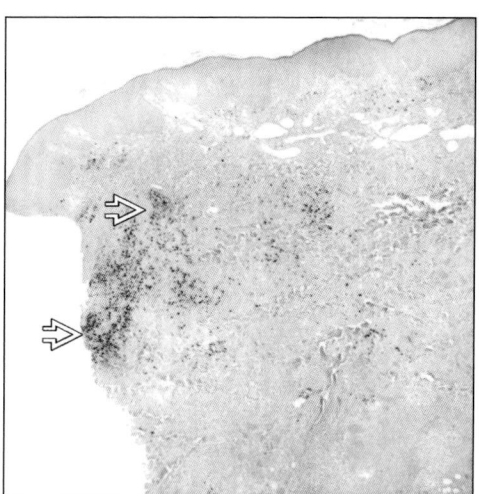

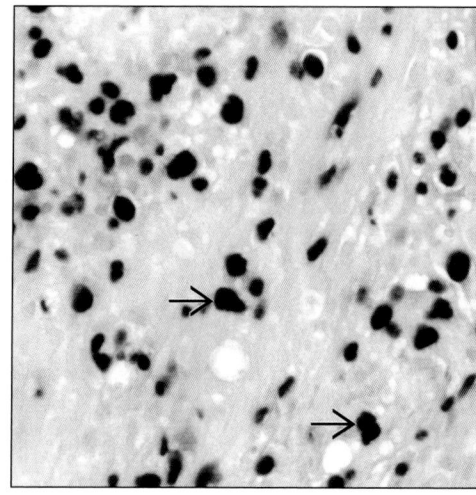

(Left) Low-power image of in situ hybridization for Epstein-Barr encoded receptor (EBER) in a case of cutaneous LYG shows clusters of EBER-positive cells (blue) within the dermis in a perivascular distribution ⮞. There are no EBER-positive cells in the epidermis. (Right) A higher power magnification of the same lesion shows that many of the EBER-positive cells are large in size ➾ and show some nuclear irregularity. The smaller reactive T cells are EBER negative.

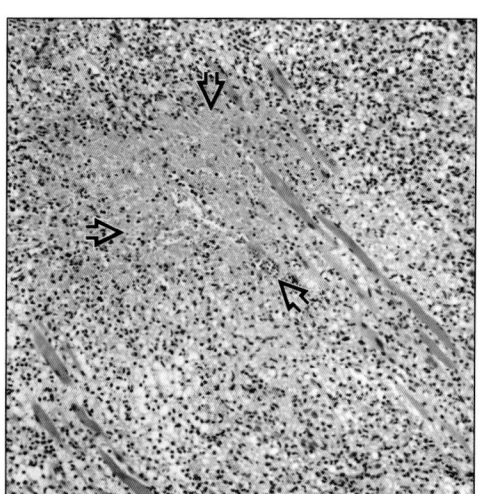

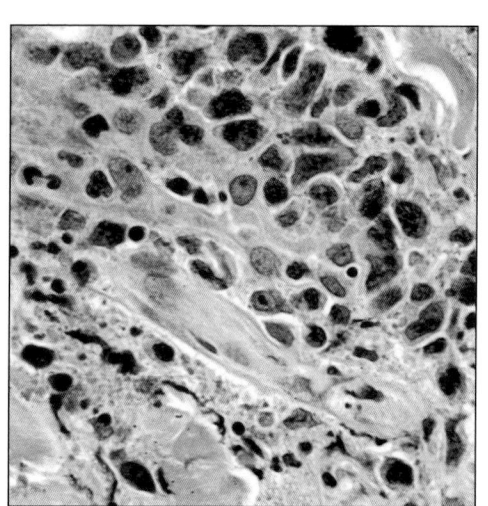

(Left) The differential diagnosis includes extranodal NK/T-cell lymphoma, nasal type, a case of which is shown here involving the deep soft tissue of the cheek. Necrosis is present ⮞ surrounding a vessel. (Courtesy L. J. Medeiros, MD.) (Right) H&E shows high magnification of a nasal-type extranodal NK/T-cell lymphoma of NK cell lineage. The neoplastic cells are large and atypical and were positive for CD3, CD56, cytotoxic proteins, & EBER. (Courtesy L. J. Medeiros, MD.)

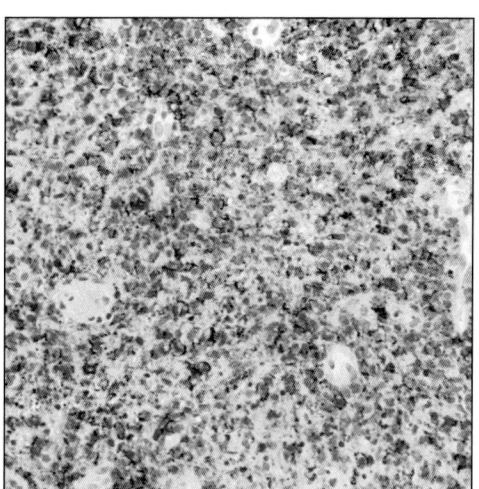

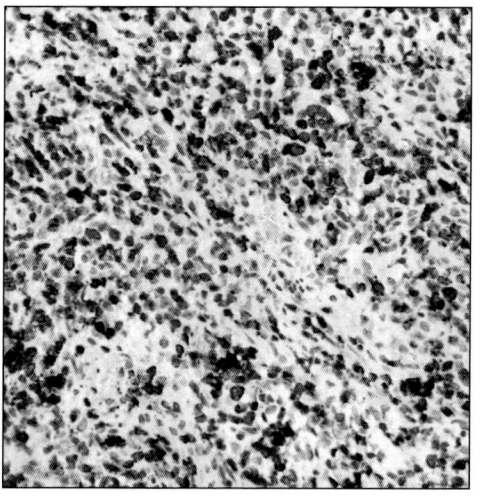

(Left) CD56 immunohistochemical stain shows many positive neoplastic cells in extranodal NK/T-cell lymphoma, nasal type, and is highly suggestive of, but not specific for, NK-cell lineage. (Courtesy L. J. Medeiros, MD.) (Right) CD3 IHC stain shows that the neoplastic cells are positive in NK/T-cell lymphoma. This antibody detects the epsilon chain of CD3 within the cell cytoplasm. Expression of CD3 epsilon chain is seen in both T cells & NK cells. (Courtesy L. J. Medeiros, MD.)

INTRAVASCULAR LARGE B-CELL LYMPHOMA

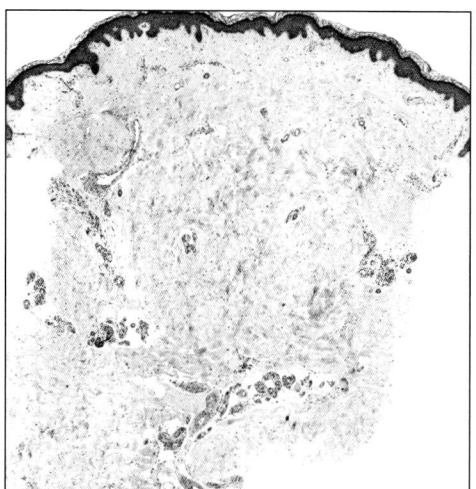

Intravascular large B-cell lymphoma (IVLBCL) involving skin is shown. Note that the infiltration by neoplastic cells is difficult to recognize at this low magnification.

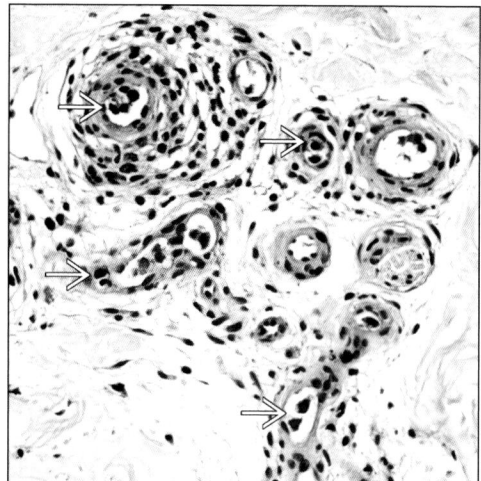

IVLBCL involving the skin is shown. At high power, atypical lymphoid cells are seen inside of small dermal vessels ➡.

TERMINOLOGY

Abbreviations
- Intravascular large B-cell lymphoma (IVLBCL)

Synonyms
- Angiotropic large cell lymphoma
- Angioendotheliotropic (intravascular) lymphoma
- Intravascular lymphomatosis

Definitions
- Large B-cell lymphoma characterized by selective intravascular growth
- Preferential intravascular growth is a condition sine qua non for diagnosing IVLBCL
  - Concomitant and minimal extravascular location of neoplastic cells, usually surrounding involved vessels, can be seen

CLINICAL ISSUES

Site
- Selective tumor growth within lumina of small blood vessels, particularly capillaries
- Widely disseminated
- Any organ can be involved
- Absence of marked lymphadenopathy
- Mechanisms responsible for selective growth of neoplastic cells within blood vessel lumina are unknown; possible explanations include
  - Chemokine-chemokine receptor interactions
    - e.g., CXCL9 (expressed in endothelium) and CXCR3 (expressed in IVLBCL)
  - Decreased expression of adhesion molecules on surface of IVLBCL cells
    - e.g., CD29 and CD54

Presentation
- Middle-aged or elderly patients; median: 67 years
- M:F ratio = 1.3:1

- IVLBCL can involve any organ with heterogeneous, often nonspecific symptoms
  - Fever of unknown origin
  - General fatigue
  - Deterioration in performance status
- Diagnosis can be clinically difficult and some cases are diagnosed postmortem
- 2 major patterns of clinical presentation
  - Western IVLBCL
    - Predominant neurologic and dermatologic manifestations
    - Central nervous system is involved in most patients
  - Asian IVLBCL
    - Hemophagocytic syndrome
    - Fever and B symptoms
    - Pancytopenia and bone marrow infiltration
    - Skin and central nervous system involvement are uncommon
- Skin
  - Heterogeneous clinical presentation: Nodules/plaques (49%), macules (22.5%), telangiectatic patches (20%), cellulitis, ulcerated nodules
  - Waxing and waning lesions (16%)
  - Lower and upper extremities, trunk and lower abdomen
  - Skin involvement is sometimes detected by random skin biopsy of grossly unremarkable skin
  - Cutaneous variant
    - Most frequent in females
    - Younger than other IVLBCL patients
    - Usually not associated with leucopenia or thrombocytopenia
    - Better prognosis (3-year survival rate of 56%, systemic variant: 22%)
- Kidney
  - Increased creatinine
  - Proteinuria
  - Renal insufficiency
- Liver

INTRAVASCULAR LARGE B-CELL LYMPHOMA

Key Facts

Terminology
- Rare large B-cell lymphoma characterized by selective intravascular growth

Clinical Issues
- Heterogeneous clinical signs: Nodules/plaques (49%), macules (23%), telangiectatic patches (20%)
- Absence of marked lymphadenopathy
- Middle-aged or elderly patients
- Neurologic and dermatologic manifestations common
- Patients from Asia often show hemophagocytic syndrome
- Cutaneous variant
  - Most frequent in females, usually younger patients
  - Better prognosis (3-year survival rate of 56%, systemic variant: 22%)

Microscopic Pathology
- IVLBCL cells are large, with vesicular nuclear chromatin, distinct nucleoli, and frequent mitoses
- Lymphoma cells are mainly located in lumina of small vessels

Ancillary Tests
- Pan-B-cell markers (+), Bcl-2(+), MUM1(+)
- CD5(+) (30%); other T-cell markers (-)
- Ki-67 high

Top Differential Diagnoses
- Peripheral T- or NK-cell lymphomas with intravascular pattern
- Hepatosplenic T-cell lymphoma
- T-cell large granular lymphocytic leukemia
- Diffuse large B-cell lymphoma, NOS

- Hepatomegaly
- Increased bilirubin and liver enzymes
- Central nervous system
  - Alteration of consciousness
  - Motor and sensory deficits
  - Seizures
- Lungs
  - Dyspnea and hypoxia
- Hematopoietic system
  - Splenomegaly
  - Hemophagocytosis
  - Anemia, thrombocytopenia, and leukopenia
- Other
  - Increased LDH
  - Endocrine dysfunction (hypopituitarism)
  - Multiorgan failure

Treatment
- Rituximab-containing chemotherapy plus central nervous system-oriented therapy
  - R-CHOP plus high-dose methotrexate

Prognosis
- Aggressive behavior and often fatal course
- Predictive factors that are useful for risk stratification are not established

MICROSCOPIC PATHOLOGY

Histologic Features
- Large, atypical cells mainly located in lumina of small vessels in reticular dermis and subcutis
- Minimal extravascular location of tumor cells can be seen
  - Usually surrounding involved vessels
- Fibrin thrombi, hemorrhage, and necrosis
- Overlying telangiectases can be prominent
- Mitoses are frequent
- No criteria enable distinction between lesions restricted to the skin and skin lesions concurrent with IVLBCL in other organs

- Sinusoidal involvement of liver, spleen, and bone marrow
- Spleen: Red pulp involvement
- Kidney: Neoplastic cells within glomerular capillaries and peritubular capillaries
- Circulating lymphoma cells can be occasionally seen in peripheral blood

Cytologic Features
- Usually tumor cells are large, with vesicular nuclear chromatin with prominent nucleoli
- In some cases, tumor cells have coarse nuclear chromatin and irregular or indented nuclei
- IVLBCL cell size may be smaller than usual in some cases

ANCILLARY TESTS

Immunohistochemistry
- Pan-B-cell markers typically positive
  - CD19, CD20, CD22, CD79a, and pax-5
- Bcl-2(+) (90%), MUM1(+) (95%)
- Less frequently: CD5(+) (30%), CD10(+) (10%), Bcl-6(+) (25%)
- Ki-67: High proliferative activity
- T-cell markers negative
  - CD2(-), CD3(-), CD4(-), CD8(-)

Cytogenetics
- Pathognomonic cytogenetic abnormalities have not been reported

Molecular Genetics
- Monoclonal rearrangements of the *IgH* gene can be detected by PCR
- *TCR* genes in germline configuration

INTRAVASCULAR LARGE B-CELL LYMPHOMA

Lymphomas with Intravascular Pattern of Growth

Lymphoma/Leukemia Type	Immunophenotype
Intravascular large B-cell lymphoma	CD19(+), CD20(+), CD22(+), CD79(+), CD5(-/+), CD10(-/+), MUM1(+/-), CD3(-)
Peripheral T- or NK-cell lymphomas with intravascular pattern	Positive for T-cell (CD2, CD3, CD43, CD5, CD7) &/or NK markers (CD16, CD56, CD57)
Hepatosplenic T-cell lymphoma	CD2(+), CD3(+), TIA(+), GZM-M(+), GZM-B(-), perforin(-), CD4(-), CD5(-), CD16(+/-), CD56(+), CD20(-)
T-cell large granular lymphocytic leukemia	CD3(-), CD8(+), CD4(-), CD56(+), CD57(-), TIA(+), GZM-B(+), GZM-M(+), perforin(+), CD20(-)
Aggressive NK-cell leukemia/lymphoma	CD2(+), surface CD3(-), CD3-ε(+), CD4(-), CD8(-), CD16(+), CD56(+), TIA(+), GZM-B(+), CD57(-), EBV(+/-)
Splenic marginal zone B-cell lymphoma	Pax-5(+), CD19(+), CD20(+), CD22(+), CD43(-), CD5(-), CD10(-), CD23(-), annexin-A1(-)
Diffuse large B-cell lymphoma	Similar immunophenotype to IVLBCL

DIFFERENTIAL DIAGNOSIS

Peripheral T- or NK-cell Lymphomas with Intravascular Pattern

- Rare cases of T-cell lymphoma or NK-cell lymphoma can be purely intravascular
- Positive for T-cell or NK-cell markers
- These rare lymphomas do not have a diagnostic category in 2008 WHO classification

Hepatosplenic T-cell Lymphoma

- Some reported cases of intravascular T-cell lymphomas are probably γ-δ T-cell lymphoma or hepatosplenic T-cell lymphoma
- More frequent in young men
- Splenomegaly and hepatomegaly
- Bone marrow biopsy
  - Early stage disease: Small to intermediate in size lymphoma cells; intrasinusoidal pattern
  - Late stage disease: Large blastic lymphoma cells; interstitial or diffuse pattern
- T-cell markers: CD2(+), CD3(+), and cytotoxic markers TIA(+), GZM-B(+)
- Isochromosome 7q is consistent abnormality

T-cell Large Granular Lymphocytic Leukemia (T-LGL)

- Indolent clinical course with long survival
- Peripheral blood: Increased large granular lymphocytes
- Bone marrow, usually interstitial pattern, but sinusoidal pattern can be seen
- CD8(+), GZM-B(+), perforin(+), CD16(+), CD57(+), CD5(+) (dim)

Aggressive NK-cell Leukemia/Lymphoma

- Leukemic cells can have cytoplasmic azurophilic granules
- NK-cell markers (+), GZM-B(+), perforin(+), EBV(+/-)
- Surface CD3(-), CD5(-)
- No *TCR* gene rearrangements

Splenic B-cell Marginal Zone Lymphoma

- Patients often present with cytopenias
- Small neoplastic cells with abundant pale cytoplasm
- Pan-B-cell markers (+), CD3(-), CD10(-)
- Allelic loss of chromosome 7q22-36 (40%)

Diffuse Large B-cell Lymphoma (DLBCL), NOS

- Tumor cells are cytologically (and can be immunophenotypically) identical
  - IVLBCL does not present with lymphadenopathy or mass, unlike most cases of systemic DLBCL
- Cases of nodal DLBCL can relapse with the appearance of IVLBCL
- Rare cases of IVLBCL may have derived from low-grade B-cell lymphomas
  - Identical *IgH* gene rearrangements in low-grade B-cell lymphoma and IVLBCL (in some cases)

DIAGNOSTIC CHECKLIST

Pathologic Interpretation Pearls

- Large lymphoid cells in intravascular spaces
  - B-cell immunophenotype (CD19, CD20, CD22, CD79a, and pax-5)

SELECTED REFERENCES

1. Kong YY et al: Intravascular large B-cell lymphoma with cutaneous manifestations: a clinicopathologic, immunophenotypic and molecular study of three cases. J Cutan Pathol. 36(8):865-70, 2009
2. Gleason BC et al: Intravascular cytotoxic T-cell lymphoma: A case report and review of the literature. J Am Acad Dermatol. 58(2):290-4, 2008
3. Ponzoni M et al: Definition, diagnosis, and management of intravascular large B-cell lymphoma: proposals and perspectives from an international consensus meeting. J Clin Oncol. 25(21):3168-73, 2007
4. Röglin J et al: Skin manifestations of intravascular lymphoma mimic inflammatory diseases of the skin. Br J Dermatol. 157(1):16-25, 2007
5. Shimizu I et al: Asian variant of intravascular lymphoma: aspects of diagnosis and the role of rituximab. Intern Med. 46(17):1381-6, 2007
6. Ferreri AJ et al: Intravascular lymphoma: clinical presentation, natural history, management and prognostic factors in a series of 38 cases, with special emphasis on the 'cutaneous variant'. Br J Haematol. 127(2):173-83, 2004

INTRAVASCULAR LARGE B-CELL LYMPHOMA

Microscopic and Immunohistochemical Features

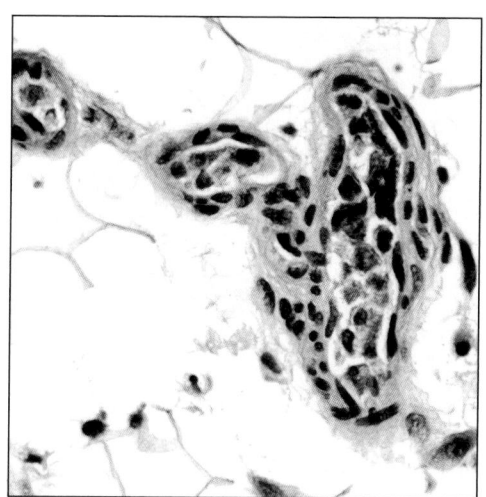

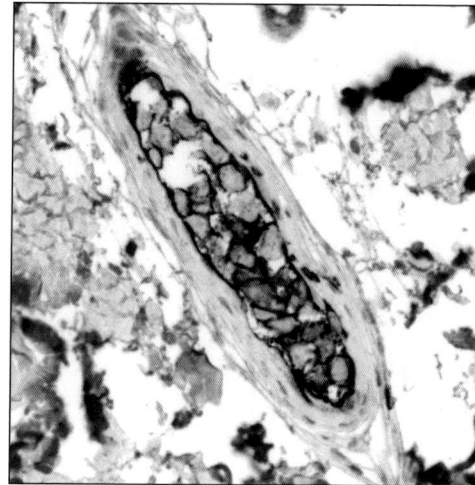

(Left) Subcutaneous adipose tissue shows involvement by IVLBCL. Small blood vessels are filled with large atypical neoplastic cells. (Right) CD20 highlights the intravascular large neoplastic cells, supporting B-cell lineage and the diagnosis of IVLBCL involving subcutaneous adipose tissue.

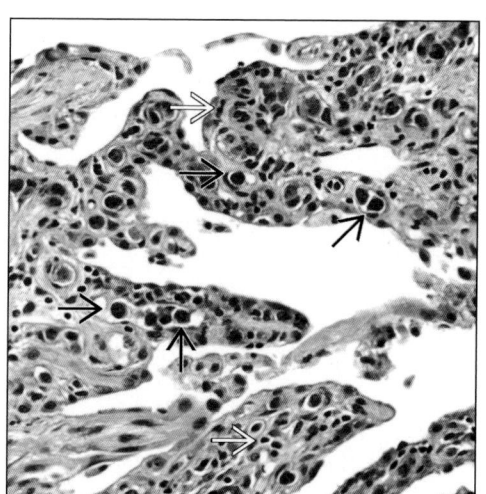

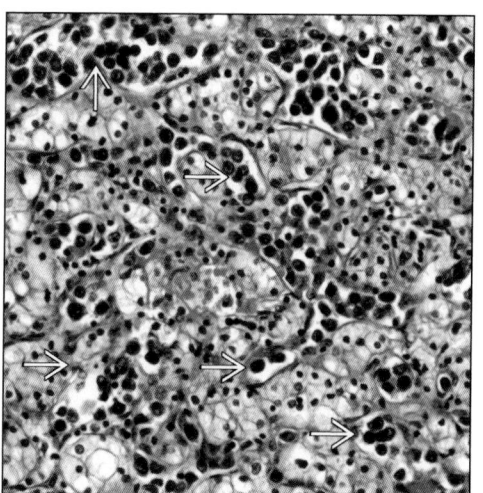

(Left) IVLBCL involving a lung biopsy specimen is shown. The tumor cells are large and located within the alveolar capillaries. Some of the tumor cells are highlighted ➡. Note the size of the neoplastic cells compared with that of small reactive lymphocytes ➡. (Right) IVLBCL in nephrectomy specimen of a patient with renal clear cell carcinoma. Large atypical lymphoid cells are seen inside of small sinusoid-like vessels ➡.

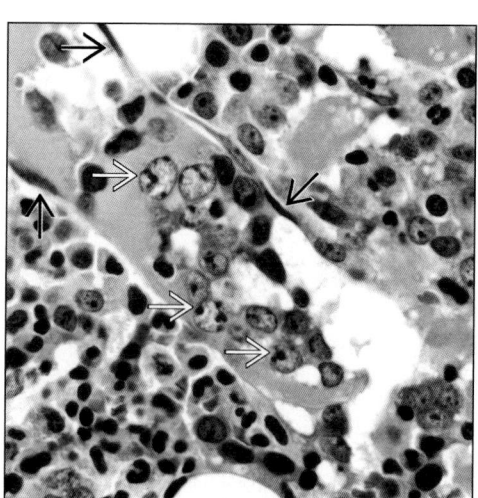

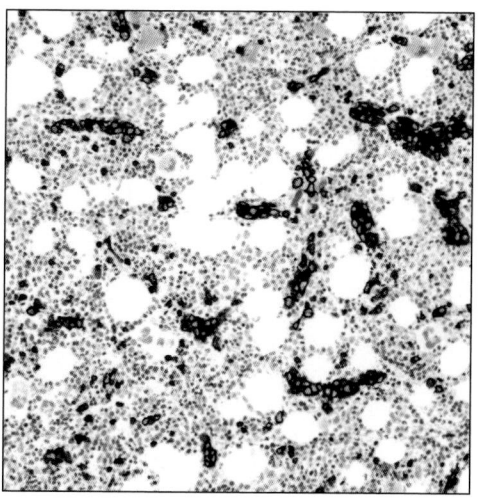

(Left) IVLBCL involving bone marrow is shown. Note the presence of large atypical lymphoid cells inside this small blood vessel. The neoplastic cells characteristically have open nuclear chromatin, distinct nucleoli ➡, and are larger than adjacent endothelial cells ➡. (Right) CD20(+) IVLBCL involving bone marrow is shown. The intrasinusoidal infiltrate is easily recognized using immunostains specific for B-cell markers, such as CD20.

SYSTEMIC B-CELL LYMPHOMAS INVOLVING THE SKIN

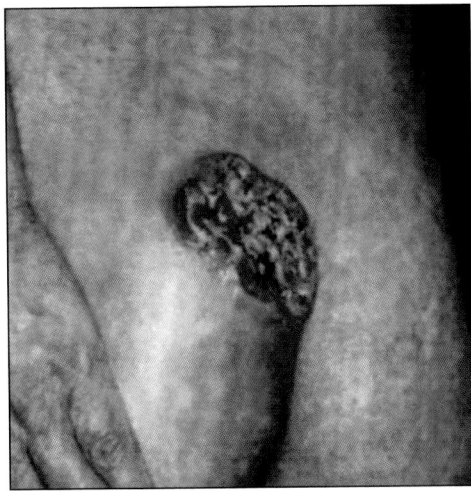

This clinical photograph of cutaneous Hodgkin lymphoma shows a solitary ulcerating skin lesion. The lesion in the left gluteal area enlarged from 2-10 cm over several months. (Courtesy C. Hsai, MD.)

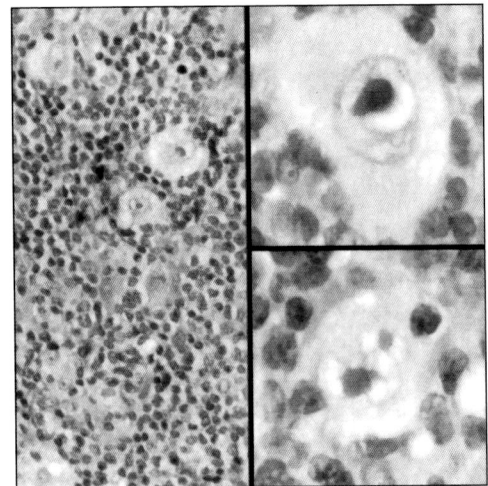

Examination of the gluteal lesion shows Reed-Sternberg cells in the deep dermis, which expressed CD30 and CD15. Note the mixed inflammatory background with many eosinophils. (Courtesy C. Hsai, MD.)

TERMINOLOGY

Synonyms
- Secondary cutaneous B-cell lymphoma

Definitions
- B-cell lymphoma that has spread to skin as a secondary site of disease

ETIOLOGY/PATHOGENESIS

Infectious Agents
- EBV infection in some lymphomas

Radiation
- Can be therapy related

CLINICAL ISSUES

Epidemiology
- Incidence
  - Systemic B-cell lymphoma more often involves skin, compared to systemic T-cell lymphoma
  - 25% of systemic peripheral T-cell lymphomas also have skin lesions
- Age
  - Any age, but mostly adults
- Gender
  - Occurs in both males and females

Presentation
- Single or multiple lesions, usually tumors or nodules
  - Any cutaneous site; no site of predilection
- Skin involvement may present at diagnosis or develop later

Treatment
- Adjuvant therapy

- Frequently aggressive chemotherapy, unlike most primary cutaneous B-cell lymphomas

Prognosis
- Higher stage than primary cutaneous lymphoma
- Usually much worse prognosis than primary cutaneous lymphoma

MICROSCOPIC PATHOLOGY

Histologic Features
- Depend on type of lymphoma
- Morphology and immunophenotype often identical to systemic disease

DIFFERENTIAL DIAGNOSIS

Hodgkin Lymphoma
- Rare skin involvement, unlike non-Hodgkin B-cell lymphoma
  - Skin lesion in < 5% of cases and < 1% at presentation, more common in immunosuppressed
  - Extremely poor prognosis
- Microscopic features
  - Scattered Reed-Sternberg cells with multinucleated giant cells, enlarged nuclei, and > 1 nucleoli sitting within lacunae
  - Many small lymphocytes, eosinophils, and plasma cells
  - Sometimes collagen bands
  - Most common subtype is nodular sclerosing Hodgkin lymphoma
    - Lymphocyte predominant Hodgkin lymphoma not reported in skin
- Immunohistochemistry
  - Reed-Sternberg cells positive for CD15, CD30, pax-5, LMP, CD20 (weak), and EBER
  - Rarely (+) for T-cell antigens and show T-cell receptor gene rearrangement

SYSTEMIC B-CELL LYMPHOMAS INVOLVING THE SKIN

Key Facts

Terminology
- B-cell lymphoma that has spread to skin as a secondary site of disease

Clinical Issues
- Systemic B-cell lymphoma more often involves skin, compared to systemic T-cell lymphoma
- Single or multiple lesions, usually tumors or nodules
- May present at diagnosis or develop during disease progression
- Often requires aggressive chemotherapy
- Higher stage than primary cutaneous lymphomas
- Generally, much worse prognosis than primary cutaneous lymphoma

Top Differential Diagnoses
- Hodgkin lymphoma

- Direct extension to chest by tumor cells in patients with mediastinal disease
  ○ Reed-Sternberg cells CD30(+), CD15(+), pax-5(+), EBER(+)
- Mantle cell lymphoma
  ○ CD5(+), cyclin-D1(+), CD43(+), Bcl-2(+), t(11;14)(+)
- Burkitt lymphoma
  ○ CD10(+), Bcl-6(+), Bcl-2(-), t(8;14)(+)
- SLL/CLL
  ○ CD5(+), CD23(+), cyclin-D1(-)
- Follicular lymphoma
  ○ CD10(+), Bcl-6(+)
  ○ Often Bcl-2(+), unlike primary cutaneous follicle center lymphoma
  ○ Often t(14;18)(+), unlike primary cutaneous follicle center lymphoma

---

  ○ Must differentiate from anaplastic large cell lymphoma, which is CD30(+), CD15(-), pax-5(-), LMP(-), EBER(-)
- Presentation
  ○ Single or multiple dermal or subcutaneous nodules
  ○ Usually direct extension to skin (chest) by tumor cells in patients with mediastinal disease
    ▪ Rare primary skin cases
  ○ Sometimes pruritus, hyperpigmentation, or urticaria, may be due to paraneoplastic syndrome, and not tumor

Non-Hodgkin B-cell Lymphoma
- **Mantle cell lymphoma**
  ○ Involves skin ≤ 2% of cases
    ▪ Primary to skin, extremely rare
  ○ Presentation
    ▪ Often multiple macules, papules, plaques, or nodules on trunk or extremities
  ○ Microscopic features
    ▪ Nodular, diffuse, mantle zone or follicular growth pattern
    ▪ B cells in dermis with grenz zone, often perivascular, sometimes surrounds reactive germinal center
    ▪ Irregular nuclear contours, inconspicuous nucleoli
    ▪ Scattered single epithelioid histiocytes
    ▪ Blastoid variant may be more common in skin; has cells with dispersed chromatin, resembling lymphoblasts, or more atypia, similar to diffuse large B-cell lymphoma
  ○ Immunohistochemistry
    ▪ B-cell marker positive CD5(+), cyclin-D1(+), CD23(-), CD43(+), Bcl-2(+)
- **Burkitt lymphoma**
  ○ 12% of Burkitt lymphoma at autopsy have skin lesions
    ▪ Sometimes direct invasion from underlying lesion
    ▪ Can relapse with cutaneous lesions
  ○ Presentation
    ▪ Often in Africa (jaw tumors), in immunosuppressed, and in gastrointestinal tract

    ▪ Often infection with Epstein-Barr virus
  ○ Microscopic features
    ▪ Patchy dermal and subcutaneous infiltrate with grenz zone
    ▪ Medium to large size B cells with squared-off borders (i.e., cobblestone or jigsaw puzzle)
    ▪ Dispersed chromatin with multiple medium-sized nucleoli
    ▪ Can have basophilic cytoplasm, especially on touch preparation
    ▪ ↑ mitosis and apoptosis
    ▪ Tingible body macrophages creates "starry sky" appearance
  ○ Immunohistochemistry
    ▪ B-cell markers including CD20(+), CD10(+), Bcl-6(+), Bcl-2(-) (usually)
- **Small lymphocytic lymphoma/chronic lymphocytic leukemia (SLL/CLL)**
  ○ 2% show skin lesions, usually already peripheral blood involvement
    ▪ No apparent worse prognosis with skin involvement
  ○ Presentation
    ▪ Cutaneous lesion frequently follows initial diagnostic lesion
    ▪ May develop at previous sites of viral infection
    ▪ May occur at same site as other tumors
    ▪ Cases with plasmacytoid differentiation are usually a single nodule on trunk or extremity
  ○ Microscopic features
    ▪ Nodular or diffuse dermal B-cell infiltrate with small lymphocytes and minimal atypia
    ▪ Sometimes patchy, sometimes perivascular
    ▪ Small B cells with indistinct nucleoli and coarse chromatin
    ▪ Rarely see proliferation centers in skin
    ▪ Rare cases contain large cells (i.e., Richter syndrome) and may have worse prognosis
  ○ Immunohistochemistry
    ▪ B-cell markers positive
    ▪ Usually CD5(+), CD23(+) and cyclin-D1(-) (unlike mantle cell lymphoma)

SYSTEMIC B-CELL LYMPHOMAS INVOLVING THE SKIN

Immunohistochemistry of Secondary Cutaneous B-cell Lymphomas

Neoplasm	CD5	CD10	CD23	CD43	Bcl-1	Bcl-6	MUM1
Burkitt lymphoma	Negative	Positive	Negative	+/-	Negative	Positive	-/+
CLL/SLL	Positive	Negative	Positive	Positive	Negative	Negative	+ proliferation centers
Diffuse large B-cell lymphoma	-/+	+/-	-/+	-/+	Negative	+/-	+ activated B cell type
Follicular lymphoma	Negative	+/-	-/+	Negative	Negative	+	-/+
Mantle cell lymphoma	Positive	Negative	Negative	Positive	Positive	Negative	Negative
Marginal zone lymphoma	Negative	Negative	-/+	-/+	Negative	Negative	Positive
Plasma cell myeloma	Negative	-/+	Negative	-/+	-/+	Negative	+

Positive, > 90% of cases; +/- > 50% of cases; -/+ 10-50% of cases; negative, < 10% of cases.

Genetics of Lymphomas

Neoplasm	Molecular Changes	Genes
Small lymphocytic lymphoma/chronic lymphocytic leukemia	del(6q); del(11q); +12; del(13q); del(17p)	Many
Follicular lymphoma	t(14;18)(q32;q21)	BCL2, IgH
Lymphoplasmacytic lymphoma	del(6q21)	
Mantle cell lymphoma	t(11;14)(q13;q32)	CCND1, IgH
Marginal zone lymphoma extranodal	t(11;18)(q21;q32)	API2, MLT1
	t(14;18)(q32;q21)	IgH, MLT1
	t(1;14)(p22;q32)	BCL10, IgH
	+3, +8, +18	
Burkitt lymphoma	t(8;14)(q24;q32)	IgH, C-MYC
	t(2;8)	C-MYC, kappa
	t(8;22)	lambda, C-MYC

- **Follicular lymphoma**
  - Secondary skin involvement is uncommon
  - Microscopic features
    - Nodular or diffuse dermal infiltrate, usually with grenz zone
    - Germinal centers with decreased tingible body macrophages
    - Attenuated mantle zones
  - Immunohistochemistry/molecular testing
    - B-cell antigens(+), CD10(+), Bcl-6(+)
    - Often Bcl-2(+), unlike primary cutaneous follicle center lymphoma
    - Often t(14;18)(+), unlike primary cutaneous follicle center lymphoma
- **Plasmablastic lymphoma**
  - Diffuse neoplasm with immunoblastic or plasmablastic features and plasma cell immunophenotype
  - Aggressive course and associated with HIV infection
  - Often arises in mucosa of oral cavity
  - "Starry sky" pattern frequent and high mitotic rates
  - Pan-B-cell antigens (CD20, pax-5) are weak or absent
  - Plasma cell markers such as CD138(+)
    - EBER(+), HHV8(-)

SELECTED REFERENCES

1. Pettey AA et al: Cutaneous involvement with Burkitt-like lymphoma. Am J Dermatopathol. 29(2):184-6, 2007
2. Jacobson MA et al: Cutaneous involvement by Burkitt lymphoma. J Am Acad Dermatol. 54(6):1111-3, 2006
3. Fullen DR et al: Granuloma annulare-like infiltrates with concomitant cutaneous involvement by B-cell non-Hodgkin's lymphoma: report of a case. Am J Dermatopathol. 25(1):57-61, 2003
4. Kim BK et al: Primary and secondary cutaneous diffuse large B-cell lymphomas: a multiparameter analysis of 25 cases including fluorescence in situ hybridization for t(14;18) translocation. Am J Surg Pathol. 27(3):356-64, 2003
5. Cerroni L et al: Specific cutaneous infiltrates of B-cell chronic lymphocytic leukemia (B-CLL) at sites typical for Borrelia burgdorferi infection. J Cutan Pathol. 29(3):142-7, 2002
6. Dubus P et al: Value of interphase FISH for the diagnosis of t(11;14)(q13;q32) on skin lesions of mantle cell lymphoma. Am J Clin Pathol. 118(6):832-41, 2002
7. Starz H et al: Secondary lymph node involvement from primary cutaneous large B-cell lymphoma of the leg: sentinel lymph nodectomy as a new strategy for staging circumscribed cutaneous lymphomas. Cancer. 85(1):199-207, 1999

SYSTEMIC B-CELL LYMPHOMAS INVOLVING THE SKIN

Differential Diagnosis

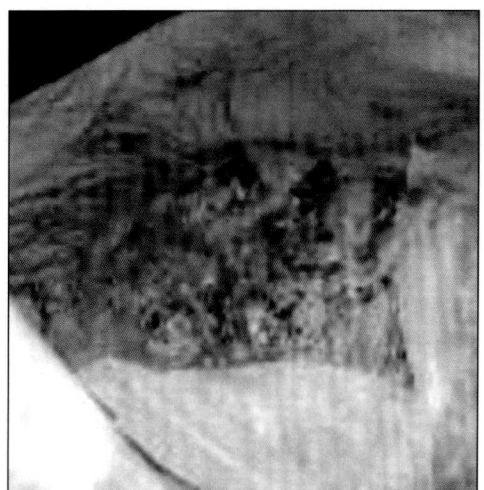

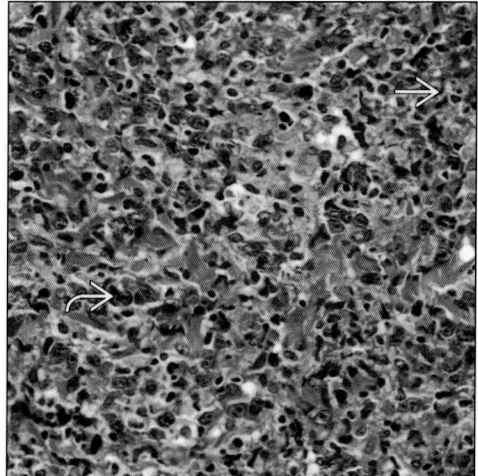

(Left) This clinical photograph of Burkitt lymphoma involving the skin shows a large erythematous, slightly indurated verrucous plaque along the left chest and abdomen with erosions and bullae. (Courtesy D. Berke, MD.) (Right) This is a cutaneous Burkitt lymphoma with atypical B cells ➡ (CD10[+], Bcl-2[-], t(8;14)[+] by FISH) in the dermis and rare tingible body macrophages ➡. Patient was also diagnosed with cecal Burkitt lymphoma.

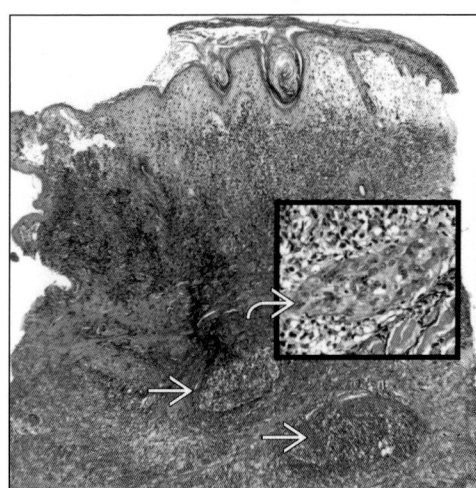

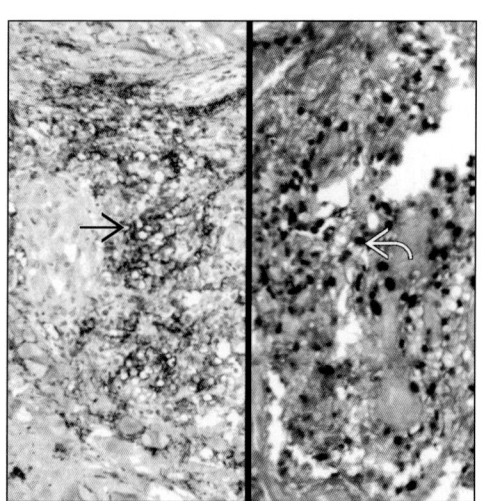

(Left) This is lymphomatoid granulomatosis, and the patient had documented pulmonary LYG. The skin shows an angiocentric lymphoid infiltrate ➡. In the inset, there are medium-sized atypical lymphocytes in the wall of the blood vessel ➡. (Right) Ancillary testing on the same skin biopsy with LYG shows CD20(+) ➡ on the left and EBER(+) ➡ on the right, a phenotype consistent with LYG.

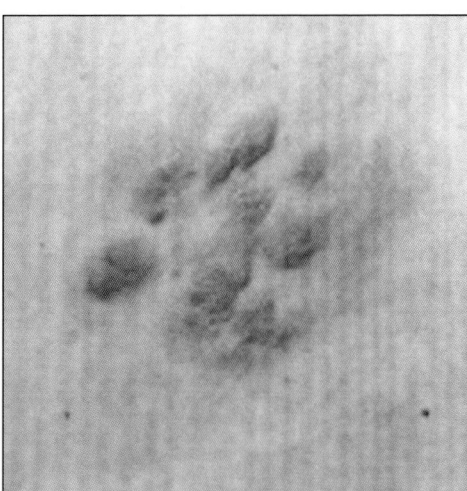

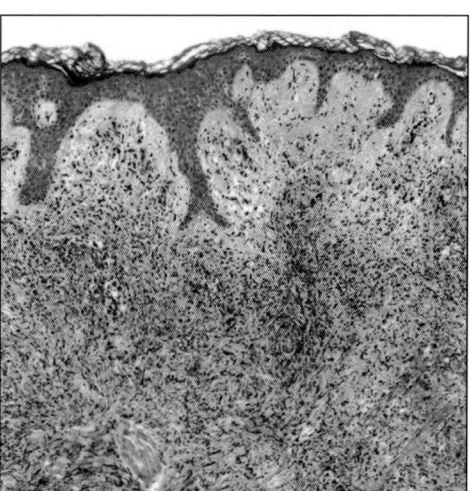

(Left) This is a clinical photograph of systemic follicular lymphoma presenting in the skin, which shows nodules on the lower back in a grouped/zosteriform pattern. The patient was diagnosed with follicular lymphoma in the left axilla 10 months earlier. (Courtesy E. Moreira, MD.) (Right) Skin with follicular lymphoma. The patient also has follicular lymphoma in lymph nodes. The malignant B cells have a mostly diffuse and vaguely nodular pattern (and were CD10[+], Bcl-6[+], Bcl-2[+]).

SYSTEMIC B-CELL LYMPHOMAS INVOLVING THE SKIN

Differential Diagnosis

(Left) This is skin with small lymphocytic lymphoma/chronic lymphocytic leukemia, and the B cells ⇒ are in the superficial and deep dermis with a sheet-like growth pattern. The epidermis is uninvolved and separated from the malignant B cells by a thin grenz zone ⇗. No germinal centers are present. *(Right)* A CD20 immunohistochemical stain shows that the chronic lymphocytic leukemia consists of aggregates of B cells. Pax-5 (not shown) marked the same population of B cells.

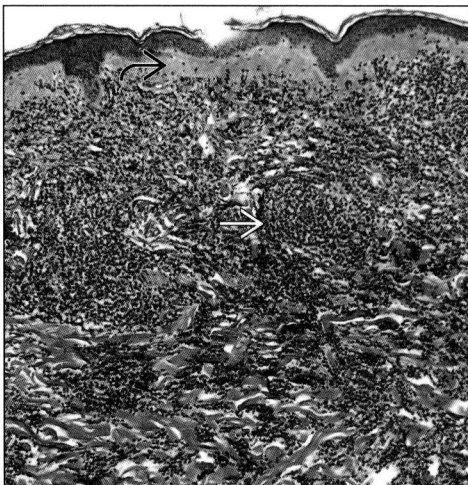
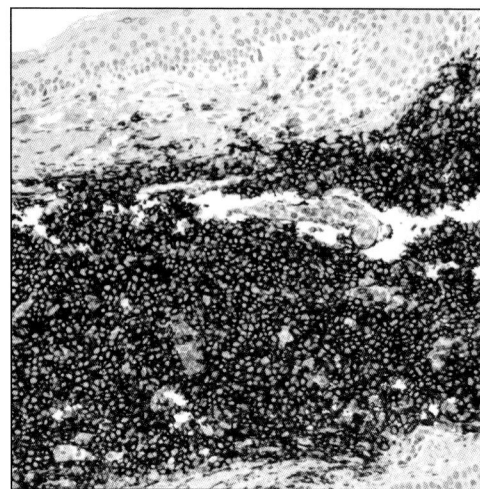

(Left) CD5 immunohistochemical stain shows that the CLL is CD5(+). With reactive lymphocytes, CD5 is expressed in T cells and not B cells, but in CLL, CD5 is usually immunoreactive in the malignant B cells. *(Right)* CD23 immunohistochemical stain shows that the CD20(+), CD5(+) B cells also are positive for CD23. CLL is typically CD20(+), CD5(+), and CD23(+), although a subset of cases do not express CD5 or CD23.

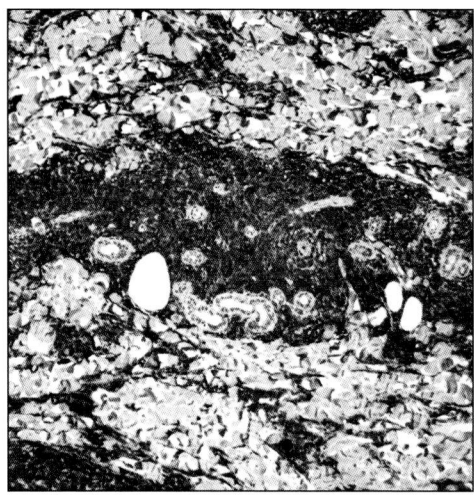
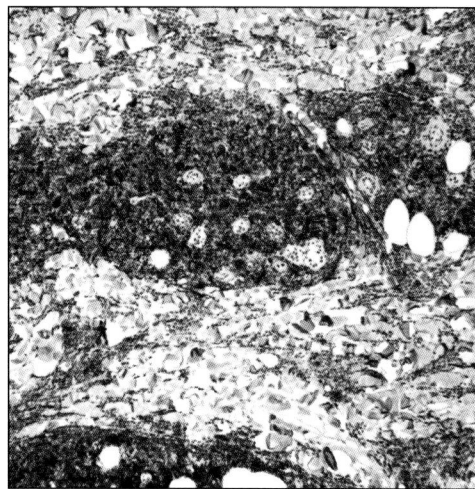

(Left) This peripheral blood with CLL shows B cells ⇗ that are small and round with minimal atypia and coarse chromatin. Numerous smudge cells ⇘ are usually identified. *(Right)* Flow cytometry shows a population of cells with coexpression CD19 and CD5, typical of CLL. These cells also expressed CD23, CD43, and Bcl-2 (not shown).

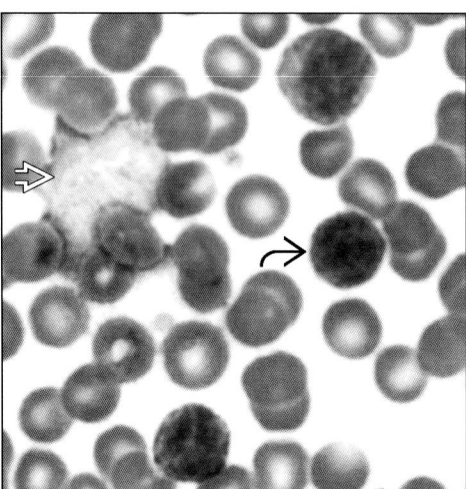
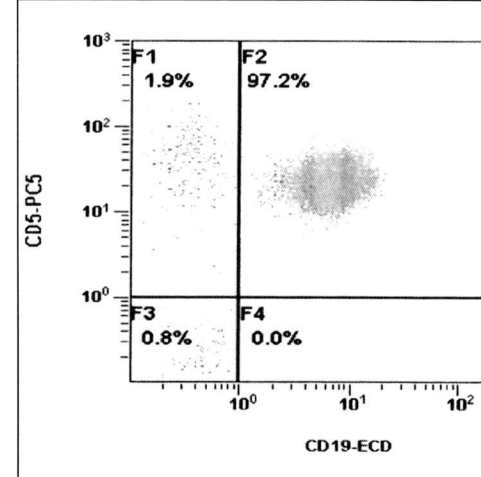

Differential Diagnosis

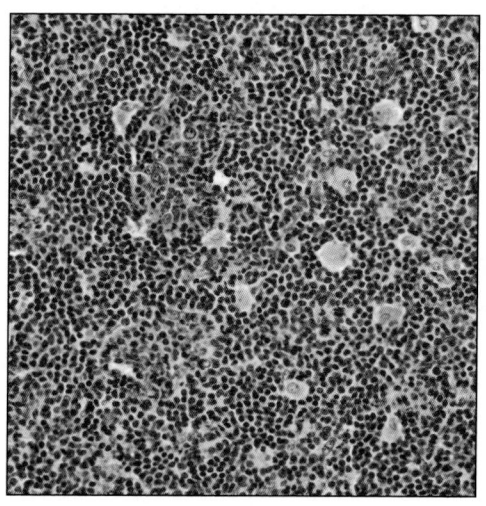

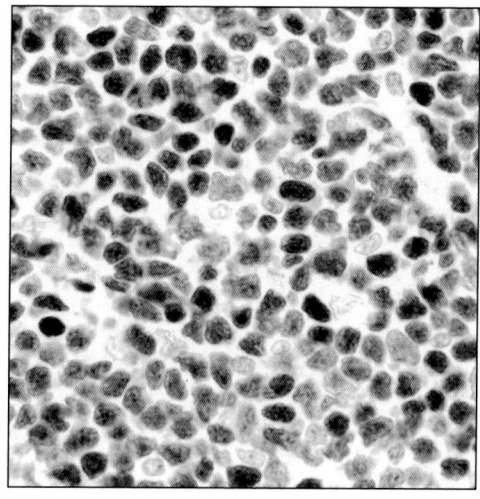

(Left) A case of mantle cell lymphoma shows small lymphocytes and many benign histiocytes with eosinophilic cytoplasm (so-called pink histiocytes). Pink histiocytes are a helpful clue for the diagnosis of MCL, but are not specific. Mantle cell lymphoma is uncommon in the skin. (Courtesy C. Yin, MD.) **(Right)** Cyclin-D1 immunostain shows nuclear expression in the cells of mantle cell lymphoma. PRAD1 and Bcl-1 are different names for cyclin-D1. (Courtesy C. Yin, MD.)

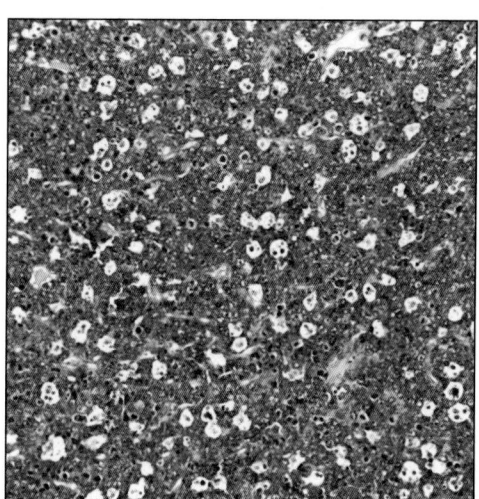

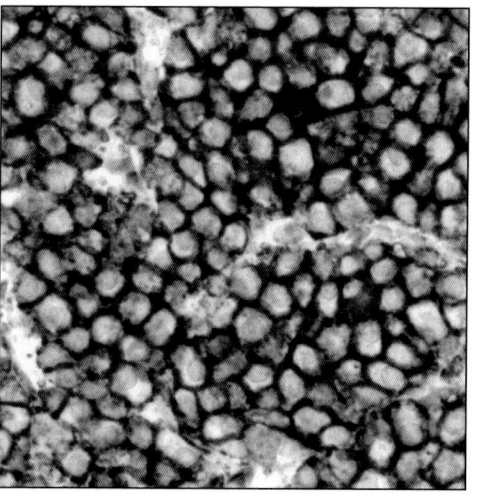

(Left) This case of plasmablastic lymphoma (PBL) is characterized by diffuse infiltrate of large atypical lymphoid cells with a "starry sky" pattern. (Courtesy F. Vega, MD.) **(Right)** In plasmablastic lymphoma, the neoplastic cells show strong expression of CD138/syndecan (shown). Other plasma cell-associated antigens that are usually strongly expressed in PBL cases include IRF-4/MUM1, Vs38/p63, and CD38.

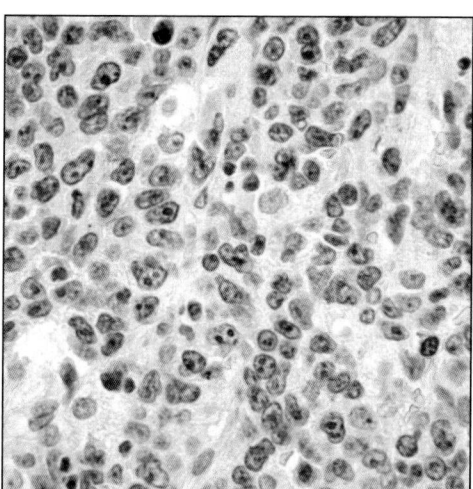

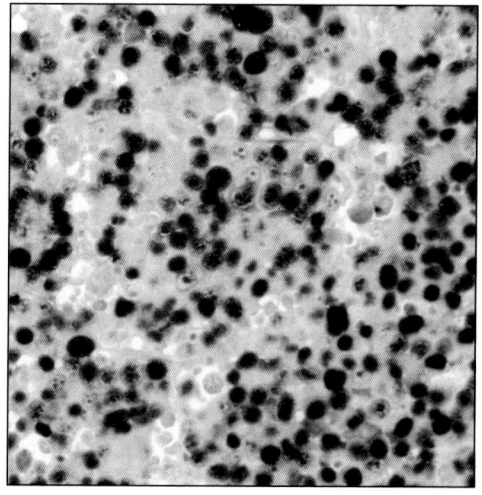

(Left) The tumor cells in plasmablastic lymphoma are negative for pax-5. Strong expression of B-cell markers supports the diagnosis of diffuse large B-cell lymphoma over PBL. (Courtesy F. Vega, MD.) **(Right)** In situ hybridization for Epstein-Barr virus small-encoded RNA (EBER) is usually positive in plasmablastic lymphoma. (Courtesy F. Vega, MD.)

MYCOSIS FUNGOIDES (AND SUBTYPES)

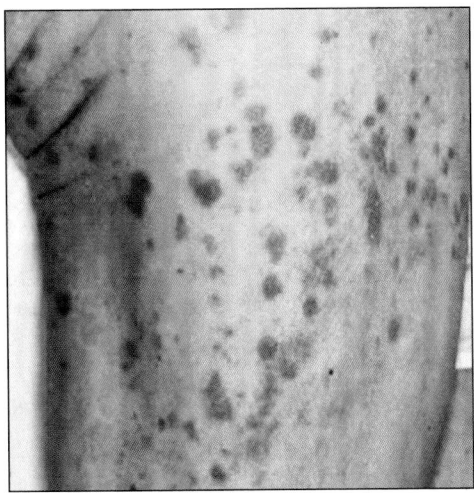

The plaque stage of mycosis fungoides shows the presence of multiple red plaques on much of the body surface of this patient.

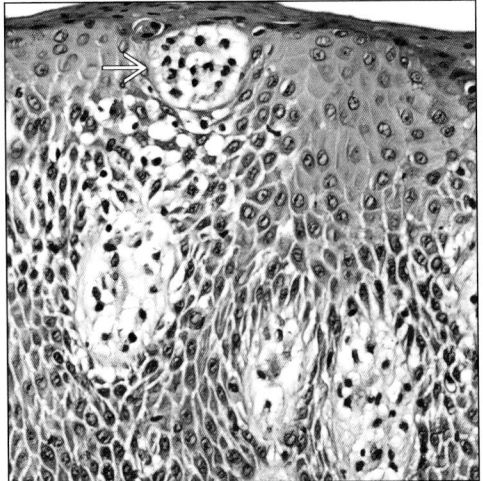

The plaque stage of mycosis fungoides shows the presence of a Pautrier microabscess ➡ containing small atypical tumor cells.

TERMINOLOGY

Abbreviations
- Mycosis fungoides (MF)

Definitions
- Primary cutaneous T-cell lymphoma characterized by
  - Epidermotropism
  - Clinical course showing stepwise evolution of patches, plaques, and tumors

ETIOLOGY/PATHOGENESIS

Unknown
- Chronic antigenic stimulation, possibly due to infectious agent, may play a role
- Genetic abnormalities are likely to be involved

CLINICAL ISSUES

Epidemiology
- Incidence
  - 0.6/100,000 people per year
  - 50% of all cases of primary cutaneous lymphoma
- Age
  - Adults, 5th-6th decade
  - Can be seen in patients < 35 years
- Gender
  - M:F = 2:1
- Ethnicity
  - Incidence is 1.7x higher in African-Americans than in whites

Presentation
- Premycotic period
  - Nonspecific skin lesions; often slight scaling, pruritus
    - Lesions can wax and wane for years; may never progress to MF

- Skin biopsy findings are nondiagnostic
- Stepwise evolution of disease with appearance of patches, plaques, and tumors
  - Patches
    - Mostly on trunk, but can arise anywhere on body, including palms and toes
    - Can be associated with alopecia
  - Plaques
    - Palpable lesions rise above skin surface
    - Can be associated with patch lesions
  - Tumors
    - Usually manifest as skin nodule(s)
    - Can coexist with patches and plaques
- MF variants
  - **Pagetoid reticulosis (localized)**
    - Also referred to as Woringer-Kolopp disease
    - Solitary, slow-growing, psoriasiform, crusty or hyperkeratotic patch or plaque
    - Often arises on distal limb
  - **Folliculotropic (pilotropic) MF**
    - Often involves head and neck area
    - Follicular papules (often grouped), alopecia, and acneiform lesions
    - Clinically more aggressive than other MF types; responds less well to skin-directed therapy
  - **Syringotropic MF**
    - Solitary, well-circumscribed, red-brown plaque, often associated with alopecia
    - Skin-directed therapy may be inadequate (similar to folliculotropic MF)
  - **Granulomatous slack skin**
    - Circumscribed areas of pendulous folds of lax skin in intertriginous areas (axillae, groin)
    - May coexist with classical MF lesions or classical Hodgkin lymphoma

Laboratory Tests
- Morphologic assessment of peripheral blood for Sézary cells
  - Insensitive

MYCOSIS FUNGOIDES (AND SUBTYPES)

Key Facts

Terminology
- Primary cutaneous T-cell lymphoma characterized by
  - Epidermotropism
  - Clinical course showing stepwise evolution of patches, plaques, and tumors

Clinical Issues
- Overall indolent clinical course
- Clinical stage is most important predictor of prognosis

Microscopic Pathology
- Skin biopsy findings may be nondiagnostic in premycotic and some early patch stage lesions
- Superficial band-like or lichenoid infiltrate in patch and thin plaque stage
- Dense, band-like infiltrate in thick plaque stage

- Nodular dermal infiltrate in tumor stage
- Neoplastic lymphocytes are small, slightly cerebriform, and some have halos
- Large cell transformation: Large cells are ≥ 25%

Ancillary Tests
- Immunophenotype
  - CD3(+), TCR-αβ/βF1(+)
  - CD4(+), CD8(-), CD5(+/-), CD7(-), CD26(-)

Top Differential Diagnoses
- Drug reactions, inflammatory dermatoses
- Primary cutaneous CD30(+) T-cell lymphoproliferative disorders (LyP and ALCL)
- Primary cutaneous γ/δ T-cell lymphoma
- Primary cutaneous aggressive epidermotropic CD8(+) cytotoxic T-cell lymphoma

---

- Flow cytometry immunophenotypic analysis
  - Aberrant T-cell immunophenotypes support involvement by MF
- Assessment of T-cell clonality by PCR
- Serum lactate dehydrogenase &/or β-2-microglobulin
  - High levels associated with poorer prognosis

Natural History
- Evolution from patches to plaques to tumors over time
- Some patients develop visceral involvement by MF
  - Most common sites: Lungs, liver, spleen

Treatment
- Early-stage disease (stages I and IIA): Direct skin therapy
  - Topical chemotherapy with nitrogen mustard or carmustine
  - Topical corticosteroids and retinoids
  - Phototherapy; local radiation (radiograph or electron beam)
- Advanced-stage disease (stages IIB-IV)
  - Extracorporeal photopheresis
  - Single-agent chemotherapy
    - Methotrexate, pegylated liposomal doxorubicin (Doxil), purine analogs (fludarabine, 2-deoxycoformycin), others
  - Combination chemotherapy: Many regimens have been used
    - Cyclophosphamide, doxorubicin, vincristine, and prednisone (CHOP)
    - Cyclophosphamide, vincristine, and prednisone (CVP)
    - CVP with methotrexate (COMP)
  - Hematopoietic stem cell transplantation

Prognosis
- Indolent clinical course overall
- Disease prognosis depends on clinical stage
- Clinical significance of T-cell receptor (TCR) gene rearrangements in MF staging is controversial
  - Monoclonal TCR gene rearrangement in blood is extremely common in early-stage disease

- Not synonymous with blood involvement by MF in absence of morphologic or immunophenotypic evidence of disease
  - Monoclonal TCR gene rearrangement in lymph nodes is a common finding
    - Not prognostically significant in multivariate analysis

MACROSCOPIC FEATURES

General Features
- Patches
  - Circumscribed lesions with discoloration of variable size, color, and shape
  - Little scaling, not palpable
- Plaques
  - Palpable infiltrate of variable stage (thin and thick)
- Tumors
  - Often exophytic and ulcerated (hence, term "fungoides")

MICROSCOPIC PATHOLOGY

Histologic Features of Skin
- Premycotic stage
  - Biopsy findings are typically nondiagnostic
  - Lymphocytic infiltrate
    - Mainly in upper dermis, not in subepidermal zone
    - Lacks obvious epidermotropism
- Patch and early (thin) plaque stage
  - Superficial band-like or lichenoid infiltrate of lymphocytes and histiocytes
    - Atypical lymphocytes often line up along the basilar layer, especially at tips of rete ridges
    - Epidermotropism by single cells
    - Neoplastic lymphocytes are small, slightly cerebriform, some with halos
  - Other changes
    - Mild acanthosis, hyperkeratosis; basal layer damage

MYCOSIS FUNGOIDES (AND SUBTYPES)

- Edema and fibrosis, increased postcapillary venules
  - In some early lesions, biopsy findings may be nondiagnostic
- Thick plaque stage
  - Dense, subepidermal, band-like infiltrate with many cerebriform lymphocytes
  - Epidermotropism is more prominent with
    - Intraepidermal clusters and Pautrier microabscesses
    - Confluent Pautrier microabscesses that can result in subcorneal and subepidermal bullae
- Tumor stage
  - Dermal infiltrate becomes more diffuse and prominent
    - Tumor cells range in size from small to large
  - Epidermotropism may be lost
  - Large cell transformation
    - Often occurs in tumor stage
    - Large cells comprise ≥ 25% of tumor
    - CD30 can be (+); high proliferation rate (Ki-67)
- MF variants
  - **Pagetoid reticulosis**
    - Marked intraepidermal proliferation of T cells
    - Sponge-like disaggregation of epidermis
    - Atypical cells have medium or large-sized, sometimes hyperchromatic and cerebriform nuclei
    - CD4(+), CD8(-), or CD4(-), CD8(+)
    - Often CD30(+); Ki-67 > 30%
  - **Folliculotropic MF (pilotropic MF)**
    - Atypical lymphocyte infiltrating epithelium of hair follicles
    - Infiltrate often spares epidermis
    - Often associated with mucinosis (mucinous degeneration)
  - **Syringotropic MF**
    - Hyperplastic eccrine ducts and glands infiltrated by atypical lymphocytes
    - Often abundant eosinophils present
  - **Granulomatous slack skin**
    - Dense granulomatous dermal infiltrate containing atypical T cells, macrophages, and often many multinucleated giant cells
    - Infiltrate often shows destruction of elastic tissue; ± epidermotropism
    - CD4(+), CD8(-)

Histologic Features of Lymph Nodes
- Best to biopsy lymph nodes draining area of involved skin or node with highest standardized uptake value on FDG PET scan
- Early involvement by MF (N1 and N2)
  - LN architecture is well-maintained
  - Dermatopathic changes common
  - Cerebriform lymphocytes are either absent, singly scattered, or in small clusters or aggregates
    - Often difficult to identify morphologically
- Ancillary testing is important to demonstrate involvement by MF
  - Flow cytometric immunophenotyping
  - Assessment for *TCR* gene rearrangement
- Extensive involvement by MF (N3)

- Overt involvement or complete effacement of architecture
- May show large cell transformation

Cytologic Features
- Small- to medium-sized lymphocytes (unless large cell transformation)
- Cerebriform nuclear contours and hyperchromatic nuclei

ANCILLARY TESTS

Immunohistochemistry
- CD4(+), CD8(-)
  - Rare cases can be CD4(-), CD8(+) or CD4(+), CD8(+)
- CD2(+), CD3(+), CD5(+), βF1(+)
- Often shows CD7 loss (all disease stages)
- CD45/LCA(+), CLA(+), CD52(+), CD25(-/+)
- CD30(+/-), usually expressed by large cells
- Ig(-), B-cell antigens(-)

Flow Cytometry
- Can be performed on skin, peripheral blood, lymph nodes, and other tissue specimens
- Flow panel should include
  - CD2, CD3, CD4, CD5, CD7
  - CD8, CD25, CD26, TCR-αβ, TCR-γδ
- CD4:CD8 ratio is often increased
- Typical immunophenotype: CD3(+), CD4(+), CD8(-), CD5(+), TCR-αβ(+)
- Frequent immunophenotypic aberrancies
  - CD26(-), loss of CD7
  - Dim expression of CD2, CD3, CD4, or CD5
- Clonality assessment by Vβ analysis
  - Can be used to follow treatment response

Molecular Genetics
- Monoclonal *TCR* gene rearrangements
- Inactivation of *P16/CDKN2A* or *PTEN* in subsets of cases

Gene Expression Profiling
- Deregulation of genes involved in tumor necrosis factor (TNF) signaling pathway

DIFFERENTIAL DIAGNOSIS

Drug Reactions, Inflammatory Dermatoses
- Exocytosis of lymphocytes can simulate MF, but there is often a background of spongiosis &/or interface changes
- Perivascular lymphocytic infiltrate
- Often increased numbers of eosinophils in dermis
- Dyskeratotic keratinocytes and parakeratosis may or may not be present

Lymphomatoid Papulosis, Type B
- Recurrent, self-healing, waxing and waning lesions
  - Papular, papulonecrotic, &/or nodular skin lesions at different stages of development
- Morphological features
  - Often wedge-shaped infiltrate in the dermis

- o Epidermotropic infiltrate of small atypical cells with cerebriform nuclei similar to MF
- Immunophenotype: T-cell antigens(+), TCR-αβ(+), TCL1(+); CD30 often (-)
- Differential diagnosis in some cases can only be made by obtaining complete clinical information

Cutaneous Anaplastic Large Cell Lymphoma (C-ALCL)

- Cases of MF with large cell transformation can be uniformly CD30(+), similar to C-ALCL
- Clinical findings are different: Usually single nodule in C-ALCL, patches/plaques in MF

Primary Cutaneous γ/δ T-cell Lymphoma

- Clinical presentation
  - o Patients often present with generalized skin lesions, preferentially affecting extremities
  - o Disease may be predominantly epidermotropic and present with patches/plaques that simulate MF
  - o Patients can present with deep dermal or subcutaneous tumor, ± epidermal necrosis and ulceration
  - o B symptoms are common
- Morphologic features
  - o Can be epidermotropic, dermal, or subcutaneous infiltrate
  - o Medium to large lymphoid cells with coarse chromatin
  - o Apoptosis and necrosis are common
- Immunophenotype
  - o CD2(+), CD3(+), CD7(+/-), CD56(+), TCR-γδ(+)
  - o Cytotoxic proteins (+), CD30(-/+)
  - o CD4(-), CD5(-), CD8(-), TCR-αβ/βF1(-)

Primary Cutaneous Aggressive Epidermotropic CD8(+) Cytotoxic T-cell Lymphoma

- Clinical presentation
  - o Generalized skin lesions
  - o Eruptive papules, nodules, and tumors with central ulceration and necrosis
  - o May disseminate to other visceral sites, but often spares lymph nodes
  - o Aggressive clinical course; median survival 32 months
- Morphological features
  - o Variable, ranging from lichenoid pattern to marked, pagetoid epidermotropism and subepidermal to deeper nodular infiltrates
  - o Epidermis may show necrosis, ulceration, and blister formation
  - o Tumor cells are small to medium in size
  - o Angiocentricity and angioinvasion may be present, and tissue destruction is often present
- Immunophenotype
  - o CD3(+), CD8(+), βF1(+)
  - o Cytotoxic proteins (+), CD45RA(+/-), CD2(-/+), CD7(+/-)
  - o CD4(-), CD5(-), CD45RO(-)

Primary Cutaneous Small/Medium Pleomorphic T-cell Lymphoma

- Clinically indolent
  - o Most cases present with a solitary skin lesion; no evidence of patches and plaques typical of MF
    - ▪ Commonly on face, neck, or upper trunk
- Morphological features
  - o Dense, diffuse, or nodular infiltrates within dermis with tendency to infiltrate subcutis
  - o Epidermotropism may be present focally, but if conspicuous, consideration should be given to diagnosis of MF
  - o Small/medium-sized pleomorphic T cells
- Immunophenotype
  - o CD3(+), CD4(+), CD8(-), βF1(+)

T-cell Prolymphocytic Leukemia (T-PLL) Involving Skin

- T-PLL can involve skin, usually with dermal involvement, but epidermotropism can be seen
- Clinical history is helpful, as patients usually have history of T-PLL with
  - o High peripheral blood leukocyte count; bone marrow involvement
- Immunophenotype: T-cell antigens(+), TCR-αβ(+), TCL1(+)

STAGING

Advanced Stage Predicts Poor Prognosis

- Erythematous skin (T4)
- Blood involvement with high tumor volume (blood stage B2)
- Histologic evidence of lymph node involvement (N3)
- Visceral organ involvement (M1)

SELECTED REFERENCES

1. Feng B et al: Flow cytometric detection of peripheral blood involvement by mycosis fungoides and Sézary syndrome using T-cell receptor Vbeta chain antibodies and its application in blood staging. Mod Pathol. 23(2):284-95, 2010
2. Nikolaou VA et al: Clinical characteristics and course of CD8+ cytotoxic variant of mycosis fungoides: a case series of seven patients. Br J Dermatol. 161(4):826-30, 2009
3. Olsen E et al: Revisions to the staging and classification of mycosis fungoides and Sezary syndrome: a proposal of the International Society for Cutaneous Lymphomas (ISCL) and the Cutaneous Lymphoma Task Force of the European Organization of Research and Treatment of Cancer (EORTC). Blood. 2007 Sep 15;110(6):1713-22. Epub 2007 May 31. Review. Erratum in: Blood. 111(9):4830, 2008
4. Gerami P et al: The spectrum of histopathologic and immunohistochemical findings in folliculotropic mycosis fungoides. Am J Surg Pathol. 31(9):1430-8, 2007
5. Agnarsson BA et al: Cutaneous T cell lymphoma with suppressor/cytotoxic (CD8) phenotype: identification of rapidly progressive and chronic subtypes. J Am Acad Dermatol. 22(4):569-77, 1990

MYCOSIS FUNGOIDES (AND SUBTYPES)

TNMB Staging of Mycosis Fungoides

Tumor Stage (T)

T1	Limited patches, papules, &/or plaques covering < 10% of skin surface; may further stratify into T1a (patch only) vs. T1b (plaque ± patch)
T2	Patches, papules, or plaques covering ≥ 10% of skin surface; may further stratify into T2a (patch only) vs. T2b (plaque ± patch)
T3	1 or more tumors (1 cm diameter)
T4	Confluence of erythema covering 80% of body surface area

Lymph Node Stage* (lymph nodes > 1.5 cm in greatest dimension) (N)

N0	No clinically abnormal peripheral lymph nodes; biopsy not required
N1	Dermatopathic lymphadenopathy; no or a few scattered atypical cerebriform mononuclear cells with nuclei > 7.5 μm
N2	Dermatopathic lymphadenopathy; aggregates or clusters of atypical cerebriform mononuclear cells with nuclei > 7.5 μm; architecture is preserved
N3	Partial or complete effacement of architecture with many atypical lymphocytes

Extracutaneous Disease (visceral involvement) (M)

M0	No visceral organ involvement
M1	Visceral involvement (must have pathologic confirmation)
	Splenomegaly as visceral disease, even without biopsy confirmation
	Bone marrow involvement has not been considered as visceral involvement by ISCL/EORTC

Blood Stage** (B)

B0	Absence of significant blood involvement: 5% of peripheral blood lymphocytes are atypical (Sézary) cells
B1	Low blood tumor burden: > 5% of peripheral blood lymphocytes are atypical (Sézary) cells, but < 1,000/μL, or > 1,000/μL atypical cells with no clonality
B2	High blood tumor burden: ≥ 1,000/μL Sézary cells with positive clonality studies

*Central adenopathy may be secondary to a 2nd malignancy (especially a 2nd lymphoma), infection, or a reactive process. The ISCL/EORTC recommends that central enlarged nodes be excluded from the determination of "N" status, except in cases where an excisional biopsy of a central node has proven lymphomatous (N3) involvement with MF. **Morphological assessment of Sézary cells is insensitive to identify tumor cells. Flow cytometry immunophenotyping with proven clonality either by TCR gene rearrangement or Vβ flow cytometric analysis can better assess tumor cell burden.

Clinical Staging of Patients with Mycosis Fungoides (ISCL/EORTC)*

Stage	T	N	M	B	Clinical Presentation
Stage I					
IA	T1	N0	M0	B0 or B1	Disease confined to skin with patches/papules/plaques < 10% of skin surface; no clinically abnormal lymph nodes
IB	T2	N0	M0	B0 or B1	Disease confined to skin with patches/papules/plaques > 10% of skin surface; no clinically abnormal lymph nodes
Stage II					
IIA	T1 or T2	N1 or N2	M0	B0 or B1	Skin involvement with patches/papules/plaques associated with no or early lymph node involvement
IIB	T3	N0 to N2	M0	B0 or B1	Skin involvement with patches/papules/plaques and with 1 or more tumors (> 1 cm) associated with no or early lymph node involvement
Stage III					
IIIA	T4	N0 to N2	M0	B0	Skin involvement with erythroderma, no or early lymph node involvement, and absent blood tumor burden (< 5% Sézary cells)
IIIB	T4	N0 to N2	M0	B0	Skin involvement with erythroderma, no or early (N1-N2) lymph node involvement, and low blood tumor burden (> 5% but < 1,000/μL circulating Sézary cells)
Stage IV					
IVA1	T1 to T4	N0 to N2	M0	B2	High blood tumor burden (> 1,000/μL circulating Sézary cells) with no or early lymph node involvement and no visceral involvement
IVA2	T1 to T4	N3	M0	B0 to B2	High blood tumor burden (> 1,000/μL circulating Sézary cells) with extensive lymph node involvement and no visceral involvement
IVB	T1 to T4	N0 to N3	M1	B0 to B2	High blood tumor burden (> 1,000/μL circulating Sézary cells) with or without extensive lymph node involvement and positive for visceral involvement

*International Society for Cutaneous Lymphomas (ISCL) and the Cutaneous Lymphoma Task Force of the European Organization of Research and Treatment of Cancer (EORTC).

MYCOSIS FUNGOIDES (AND SUBTYPES)

Stages of Disease

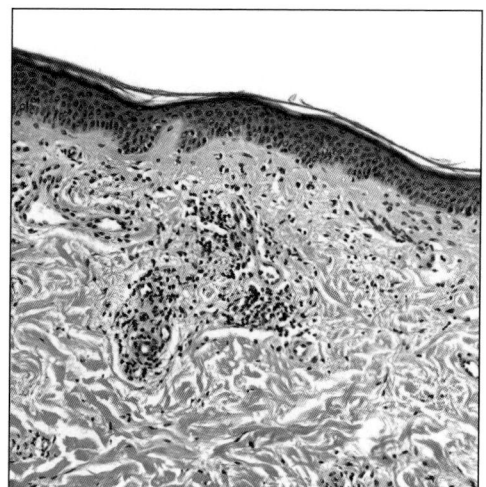

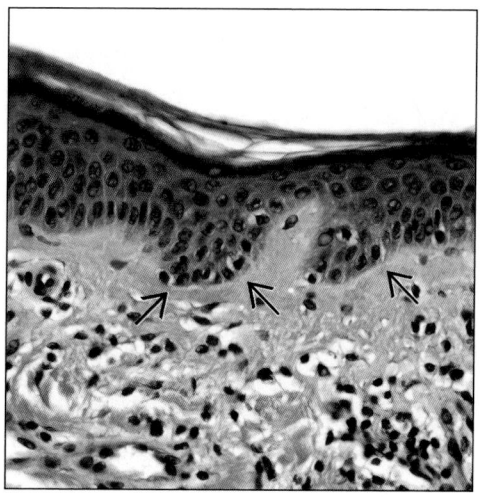

(Left) This biopsy shows the patch stage of mycosis fungoides of the skin. Changes in the early patch stage are often very subtle. This specimen shows a perivascular lymphocytic infiltrate consisting of small lymphocytes and minimal epidermal infiltrate. (Right) This higher power view of patch stage of mycosis fungoides of the skin reveals an epidermal basal layer infiltrate ⮕. The tumor cells are small but have irregular nuclear contours.

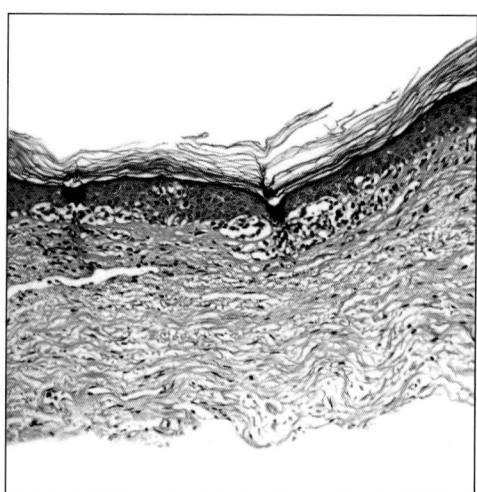

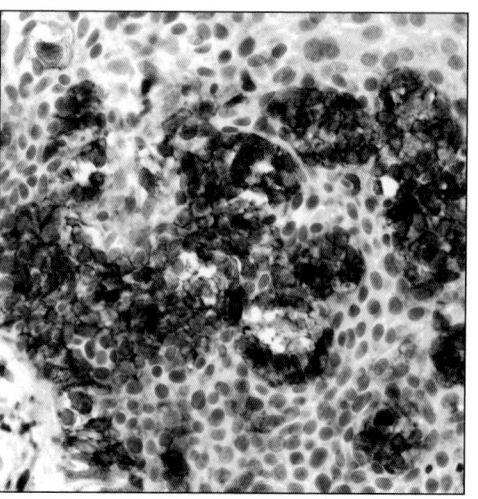

(Left) Later patch stage and early plaque stage of mycosis fungoides shows intraepidermal clusters of atypical lymphocytes. There is minimal subepidermal infiltrate. (Right) Immunohistochemistry in the plaque stage of mycosis fungoides shows that the intraepidermal atypical cerebriform lymphocytes within Pautrier microabscesses are CD4(+).

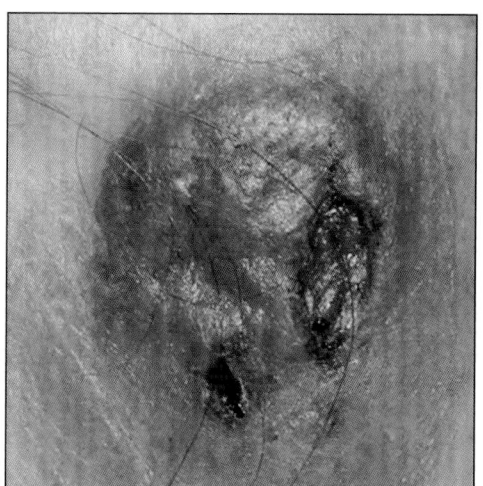

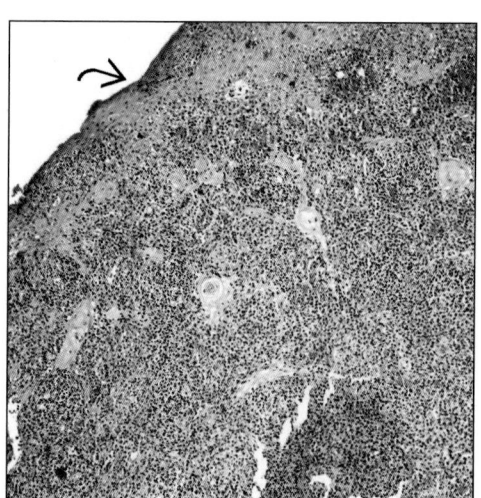

(Left) Clinical photograph of the tumor stage is shown in a patient with mycosis fungoides. (Right) The tumor stage of mycosis fungoides shows a diffuse and prominent dermal infiltrate. Also present is dermal hemorrhage and focal overlying erosion ⮕.

Large Cell Transformation

(Left) Higher power view of the tumor stage of mycosis fungoides shows no significant epidermotropism and large tumor cells growing in sheets in the dermis. *(Right)* Another case of mycosis fungoides with large cell transformation shows a diffuse dermal infiltrate with increased large cells. There is no significant epidermotropism.

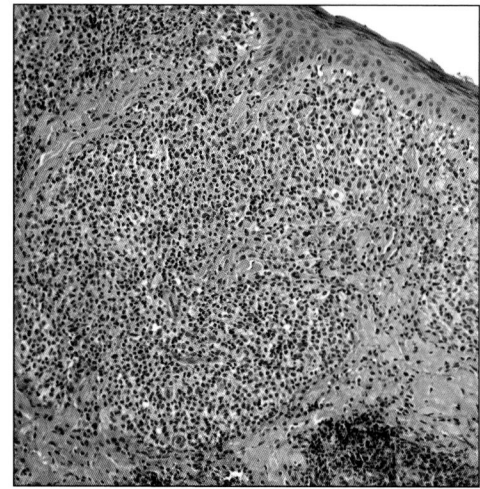
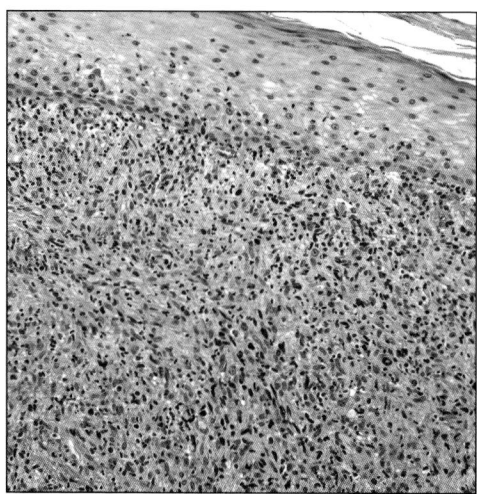

(Left) Mycosis fungoides with large cell transformation involves skin. The tumor cells are large and pleomorphic with angulated nuclei and nuclear hyperchromasia ➡. *(Right)* Immunohistochemistry in mycosis fungoides with large cell transformation shows that the large tumor cells are strongly CD3(+).

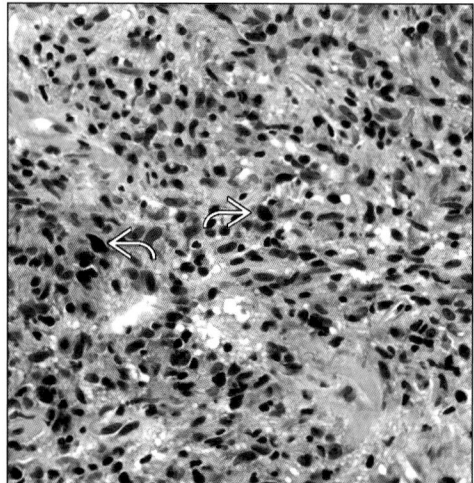
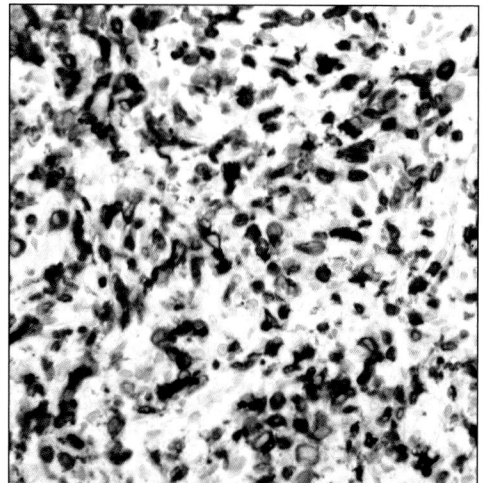

(Left) In mycosis fungoides with large cell transformation, the large tumor cells are CD7(-), with only small reactive T cells staining. *(Right)* The large tumor cells are strongly CD30(+) in MF with large cell transformation; MF with large cell transformation often, but not always, shows CD30 expression.

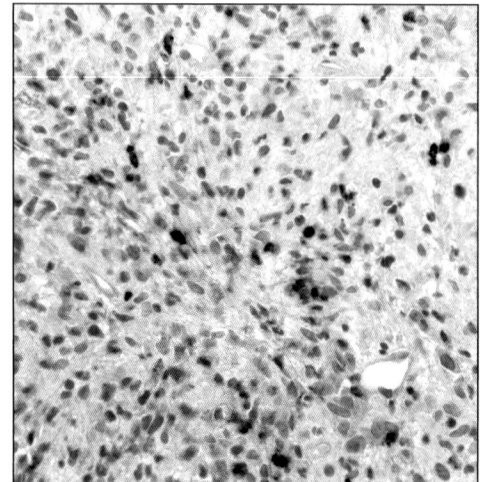
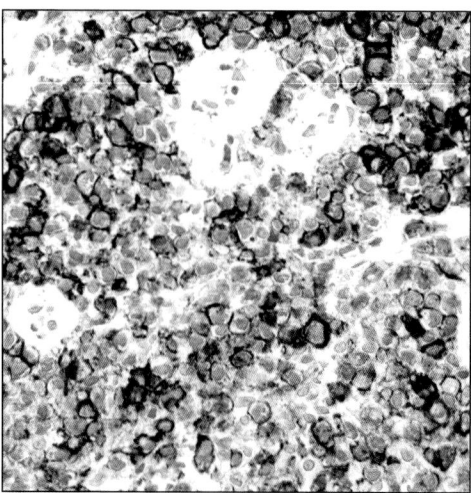

MYCOSIS FUNGOIDES (AND SUBTYPES)

Variant Microscopic Features

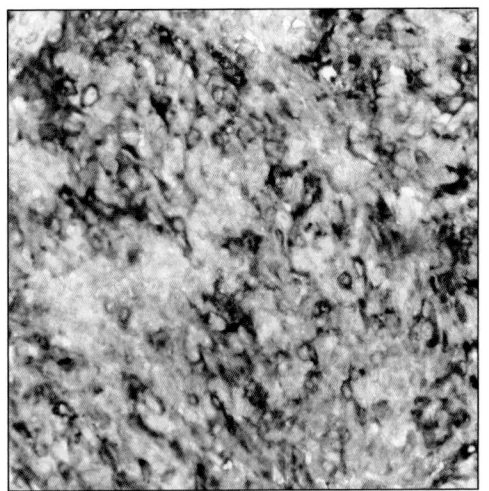

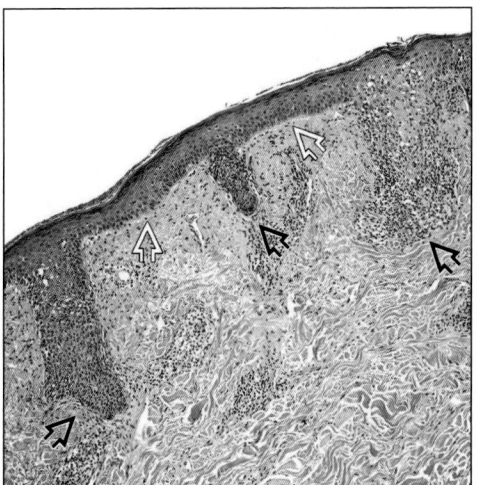

(Left) In mycosis fungoides with large cell transformation, the large tumor cells are often CD25(+). (Right) A case of folliculotropic variant mycosis fungoides (pilotropic mycosis fungoides) shows a lymphocytic infiltrate in and around the hair follicles ⊳ with relative sparing of the interfollicular skin ⊳.

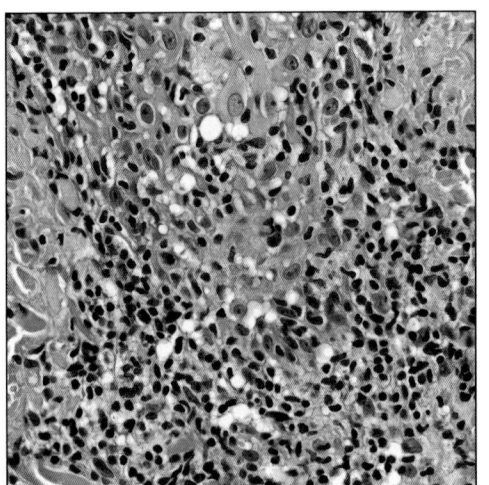

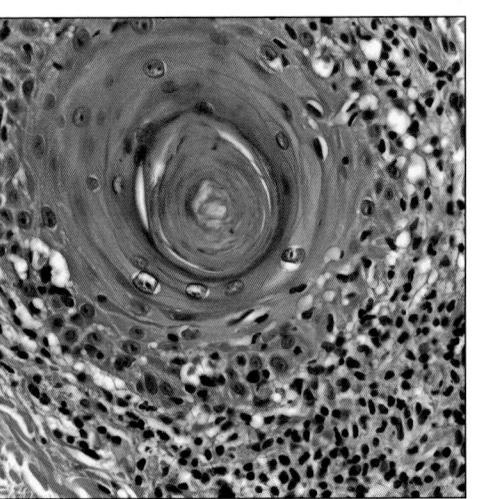

(Left) Folliculotropic mycosis fungoides shows atypical lymphocytes within and surrounding the follicular epithelium. (Right) A cornified hair follicle is infiltrated by atypical lymphocytes in folliculotropic mycosis fungoides on high-power examination.

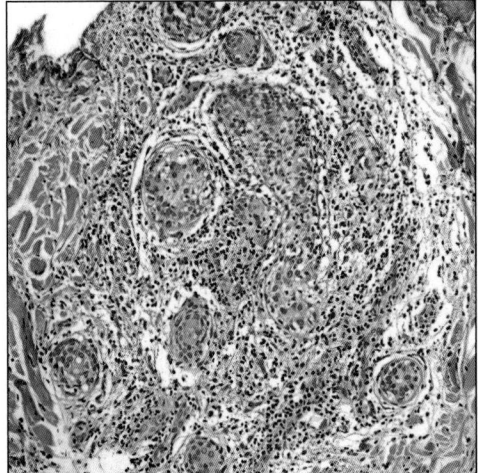

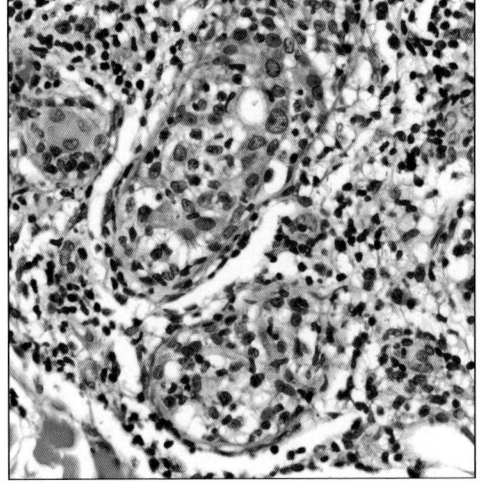

(Left) A case of the syringotropic variant of mycosis fungoides shows a lymphocytic infiltrate predominantly involving eccrine sweat glands. (Right) Higher magnification of the syringotropic type of mycosis fungoides shows atypical small cerebriform lymphocytes involving and surrounding eccrine glands.

Variant Microscopic Features

(Left) Granulomatous slack skin disease is a rare variant of mycosis fungoides. This is an advanced-stage lesion and shows a dense lymphohistiocytic infiltrate in the dermis. *(Right)* Granulomatous slack skin disease shows a dense lymphohistiocytic infiltrate extending to the deep dermis, with many giant cells ⇗ easily identified.

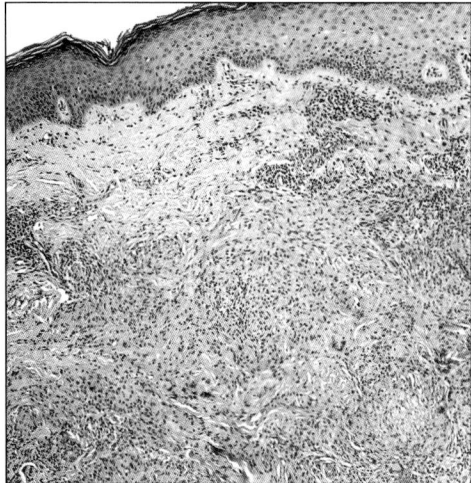
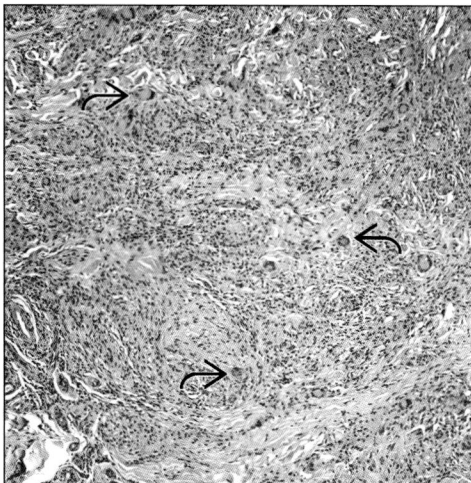

(Left) Granulomatous slack skin disease often shows giant cells containing 20-30 nuclei. Some of the giant cells have nuclei localized in the periphery of the cytoplasm. Focal elastophagocytosis is present ⇗. The lymphocytes between the giant cells are small without pronounced cytological atypia. *(Right)* Immunohistochemistry in granulomatous slack skin disease shows that the infiltrating lymphocytes are strongly CD3(+).

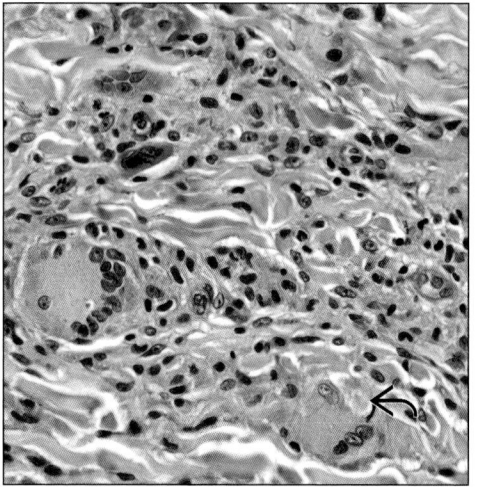
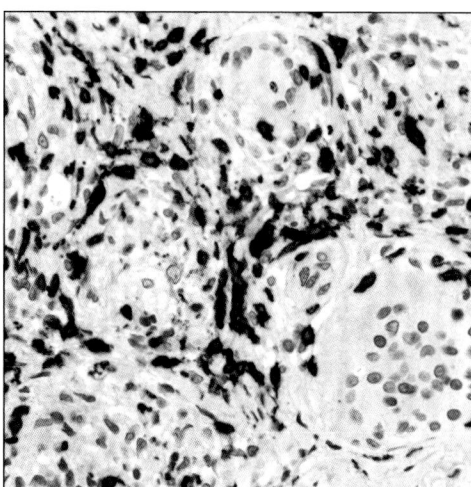

(Left) Pagetoid reticulosis is a slow-growing, psoriasiform, crusty patch or plaque typically found on the distal limb. Note the hyperkeratotic, crusty epithelium with a lymphocytic infiltrate that shows vacuolar interface changes. *(Right)* High magnification of pagetoid reticulosis shows that the infiltrating lymphocytes are atypical and small to medium in size with perinuclear halos.

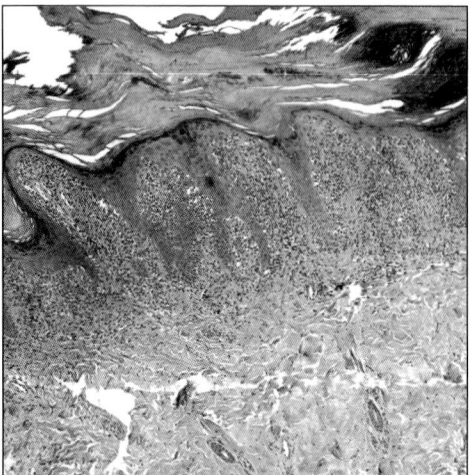
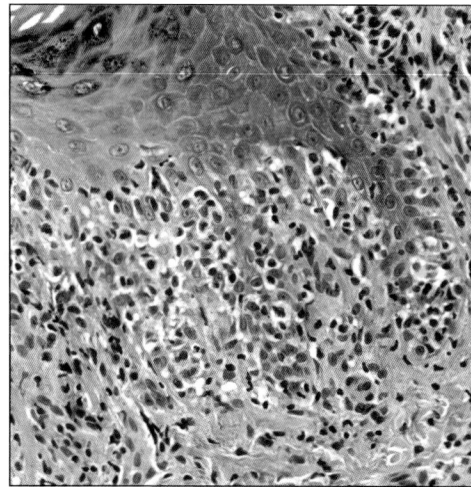

MYCOSIS FUNGOIDES (AND SUBTYPES)

Variants of Mycosis Fungoides and Lymph Node

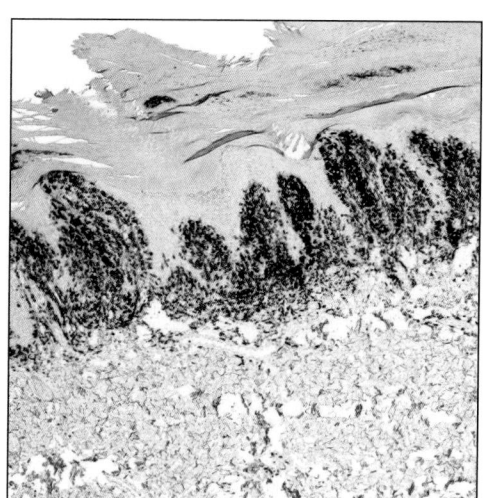
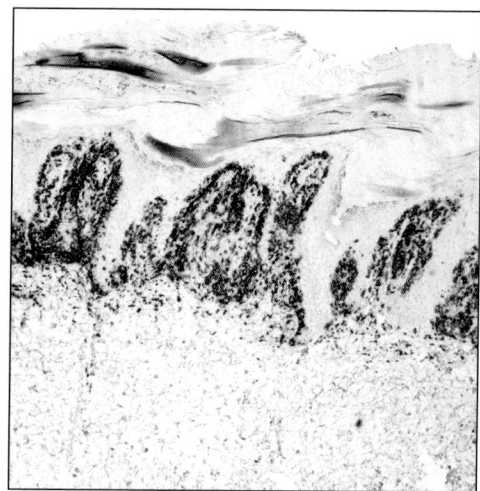

(Left) As is this CD3(+) staining, the lymphocytes in pagetoid reticulosis are typically CD3(+) and CD8(+) (not shown) in most cases, although CD8(-) pagetoid reticulosis is not uncommon. (Right) Pagetoid reticulosis lymphocytes are strongly and diffusely CD8(+).

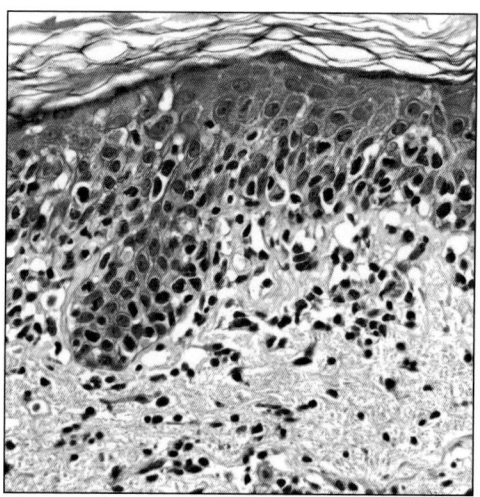
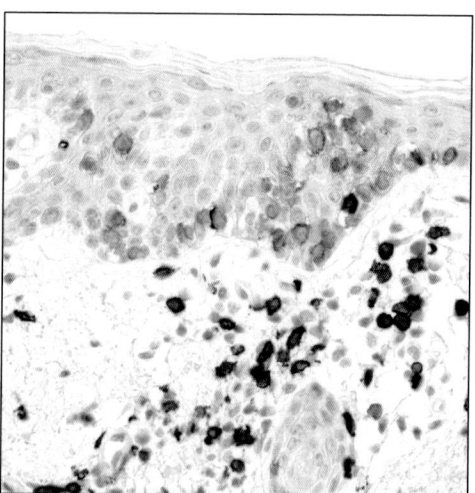

(Left) This case of otherwise typical mycosis fungoides was CD8(+). The histologic features are identical to conventional CD4(+) mycosis fungoides, and they differ from pagetoid reticulosis and primary cutaneous aggressive epidermotropic CD8(+) cytotoxic T-cell lymphoma. (Right) This case of otherwise typical mycosis fungoides is CD8(+). The CD8 immunostain highlights the neoplastic intraepidermal T cells that express CD8 more dimly than reactive CD8(+) T cells in this field.

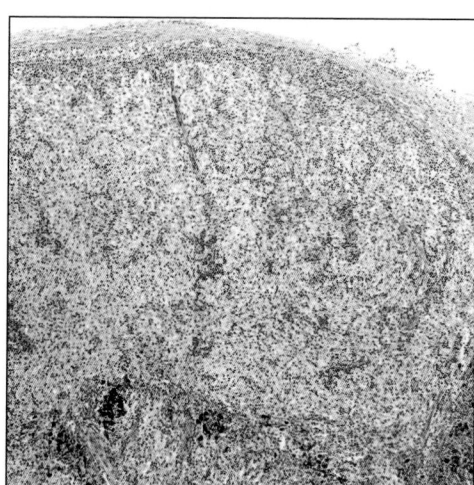
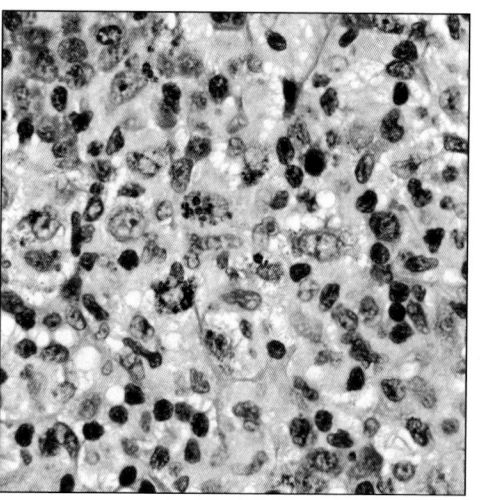

(Left) Lymph node biopsy specimen from a patient with mycosis fungoides shows marked dermatopathic changes and maintained nodal architecture. (Right) Lymph node biopsy specimen from a patient with mycosis fungoides shows many interdigitating dendritic cells, Langerhans cells, and melanin-containing macrophages. The lymphocytes are not atypical. This would be interpreted as no histologic evidence of mycosis fungoides (N1).

Nonmelanocytic Tumors of the Skin: Lymphomas and Hematopoietic Proliferations

Lymph Node, Blood, and Bone Marrow

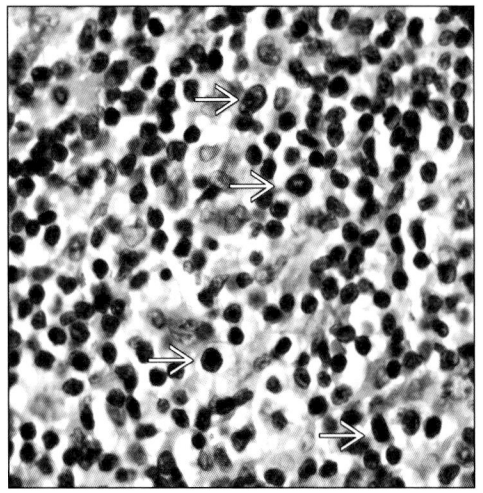 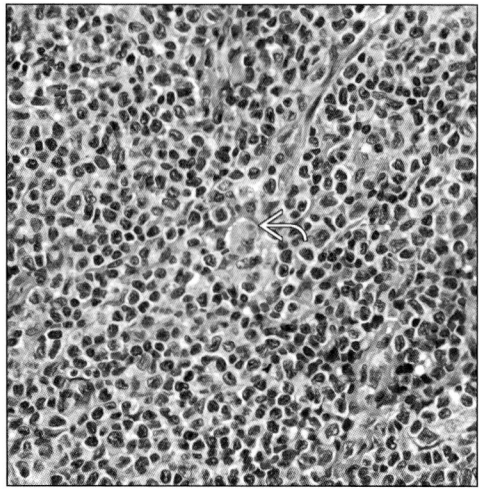

(Left) Lymph node biopsy specimen from a patient with mycosis fungoides shows a few scattered, larger, atypical cells ➡. The histological grading of this involvement is still N1. (Right) Lymph node biopsy specimen from a patient with mycosis fungoides shows sheets of tumor cells present (N3). Macrophages containing melanin pigment ➡ are also present focally.

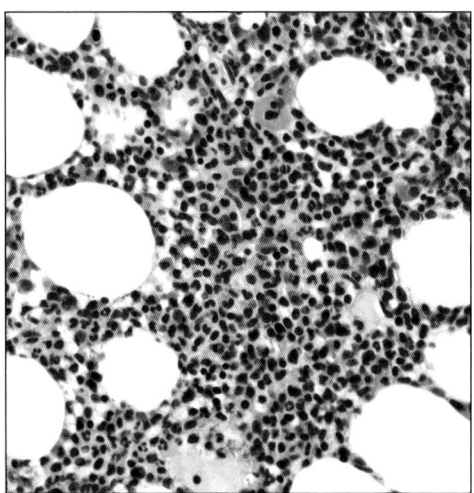 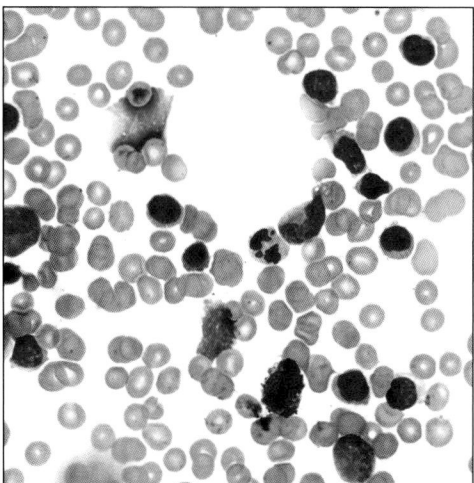

(Left) Bone marrow involvement by mycosis fungoides is uncommon. When the bone marrow is involved, there often is an interstitial pattern of infiltration. (Right) Bone marrow aspirate smear reveals many atypical small to medium-sized lymphocytes, consistent with bone marrow involvement by mycosis fungoides.

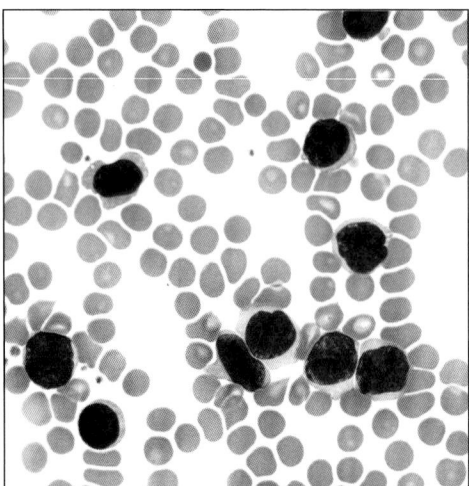 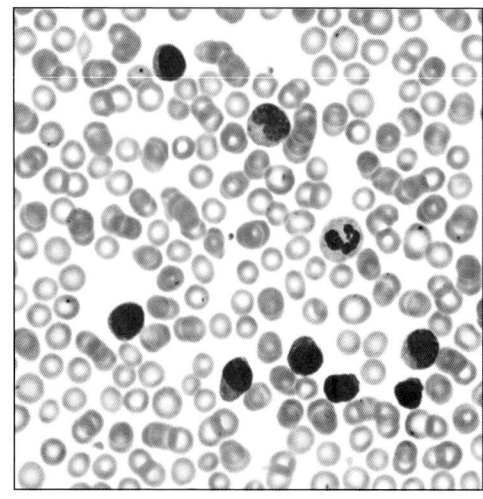

(Left) Peripheral blood smear shows many large cerebriform (Sézary) cells, consistent with mycosis fungoides in the leukemic phase (so-called secondary Sézary syndrome). (Right) Peripheral blood smear in a case of mycosis fungoides shows lymphocytosis. The lymphocytes are small with round nuclei and lack typical Sézary cell morphology. However, flow cytometry and molecular studies confirmed the lymphocytes to be neoplastic T cells.

MYCOSIS FUNGOIDES (AND SUBTYPES)

Differential Diagnosis

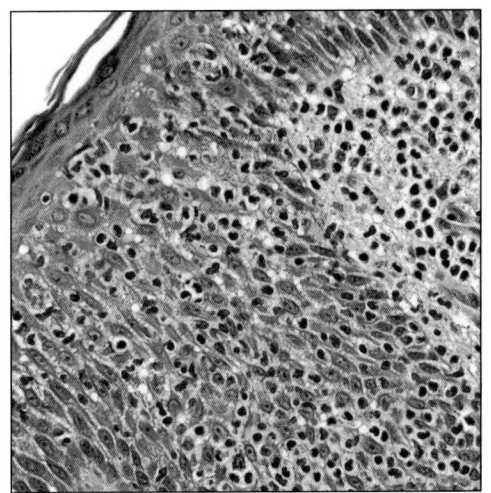
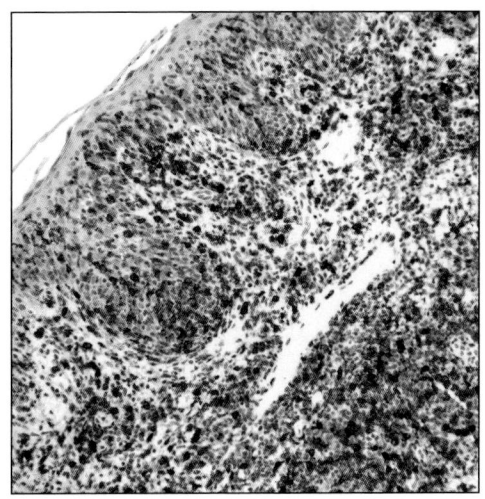

(Left) Primary cutaneous aggressive epidermotropic CD8(+) cytotoxic T-cell lymphoma shows that the lymphoma cells are small to medium-sized, with irregular nuclear contours, and diffusely infiltrate the epidermis. *(Right)* Immunohistochemistry in primary cutaneous aggressive epidermotropic CD8(+) cytotoxic T-cell lymphoma shows that the lymphoma cells are very strongly CD8(+).

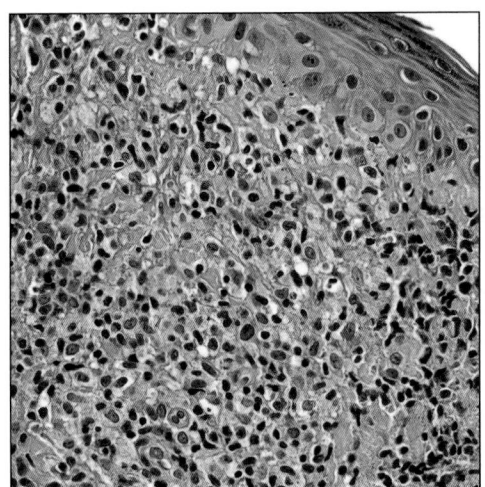
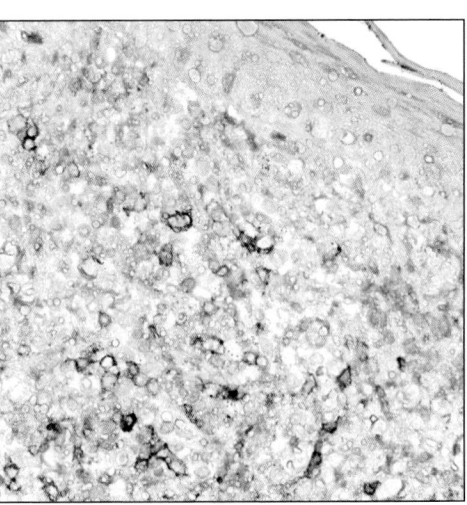

(Left) This is an example of a primary cutaneous CD30(+) T-cell lymphoproliferative disorder, consistent with lymphomatoid papulosis, type A. A dermal infiltrate consisting of a mixture of small lymphocytes, histiocytes, and scattered large cells is present. *(Right)* In primary cutaneous CD30(+) T-cell lymphoproliferative disorder consistent with lymphomatoid papulosis, type A, CD30 highlights scattered large cells.

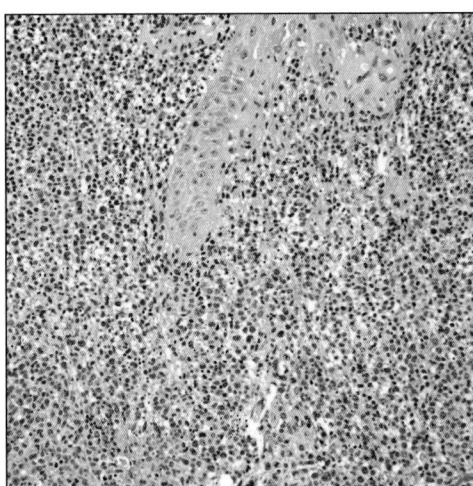
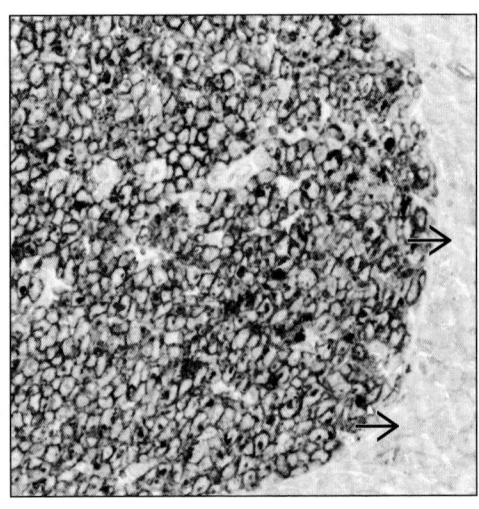

(Left) This is an example of a cutaneous anaplastic large cell lymphoma (C-ALCL). Some cases of mycosis fungoides (MF) with large cell transformation can be uniformly CD30(+) and mimic C-ALCL. A history of MF or evidence of MF elsewhere in the patient, or at the margins of the lesion in the biopsy specimen, is helpful in this differential diagnosis. *(Right)* The neoplastic cells in C-ALCL are strongly and uniformly CD30(+); note the epidermis present at the right ⮕.

ADULT T-CELL LEUKEMIA/LYMPHOMA

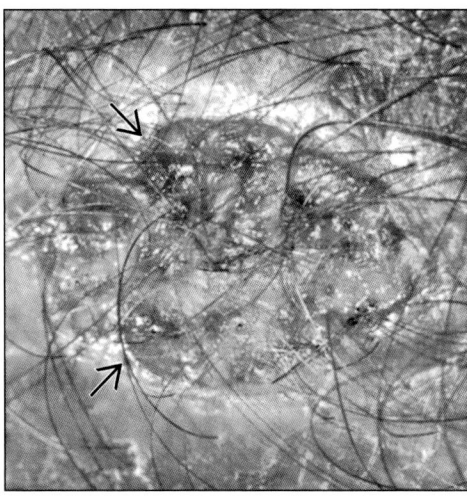

This clinical photograph shows an ulcerating lesion ➡, which is 2.5 cm in greatest dimension, from the foot of a person from the Caribbean region with ATLL, HTLV-1(+).

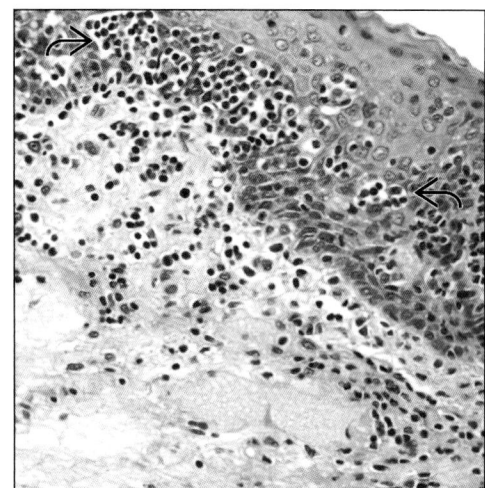

This ATLL involves the mucosa. Note the small lymphocytes with irregular hyperchromatic nuclei infiltrating squamous mucosa, forming Pautrier-like microabscesses ➡. (Courtesy C. Bueso-Ramos, MD.)

TERMINOLOGY

Abbreviations
- Adult T-cell leukemia/lymphoma (ATLL)

Synonyms
- Adult T-cell leukemia

Definitions
- T-cell lymphoma/leukemia of regulatory T cells (CD4[+], CD25[+], FOXP3[+]) caused by human T-cell leukemia virus type 1 (HTLV-1)

ETIOLOGY/PATHOGENESIS

Infectious Agents
- Human T-cell leukemia virus type 1
  - Progresses to leukemia/lymphoma in < 5% of infected individuals
  - Long latency period
    - Most exposed as infants/children
    - Tumor often after 20 years of viral exposure
  - Transmitted through blood or breast milk
  - Also causes tropical spastic paraparesis
  - Encodes Tax (a viral oncoprotein)
    - Plays a role in development of ATLL
    - Activates transcription factors for T-cell proliferation genes

CLINICAL ISSUES

Epidemiology
- Age
  - Adults, most commonly in 50s or 60s
- Gender
  - Male:female = 1.5:1.0
- Ethnicity
  - Endemic to southwest Japan, Caribbean islands, South America, and central Africa

Presentation
- Skin lesions
  - Develop in 50% of ATLL patients
  - Usually multiple nodules/tumors, papules, plaques, or macules
    - Papules may cover large segments of body
  - Rarely, erythroderma, purpura, prurigo, or erythema multiforme
- Other sites of disease include lymph nodes, peripheral blood, bone, spleen and sometimes lung, liver, and CNS
  - Most patients have generalized lymphadenopathy
  - Hypercalcemia from increased osteoclast bone resorption
- 4 clinical presentations: Acute, chronic, lymphoma, and smoldering
  - Acute subtype
    - Most common subtype
    - Severe peripheral blood lymphocytosis, ↑ WBC, ↑ LDH, skin lesions, lymphadenopathy
    - Hypercalcemia and lytic bone lesions
    - Immunodeficiency leads to other opportunistic infections
  - Chronic subtype
    - Lymphocytosis, but ↓ WBC than acute subtype
    - No hypercalcemia, exfoliative skin rash
  - Lymphomatous subtype
    - ↑ lymphadenopathy; usually no peripheral blood involvement
    - Less hypercalcemia than acute subtype; skin often involved
  - Smoldering subtype
    - > 5% tumor cells in peripheral blood, even though normal WBC count
    - Tumor cells small with less pleomorphism and lobation
    - No hypercalcemia or lymphadenopathy

Treatment
- Adjuvant therapy

ADULT T-CELL LEUKEMIA/LYMPHOMA

Key Facts

Etiology/Pathogenesis

- Long latency period between HTLV-1 infection and tumor development
- Small risk of ATLL in HTLV-1 infected people
- Tax viral oncoprotein linked to tumorigenesis

Clinical Issues

- 4 clinical presentations: Acute, chronic, lymphoma, and smoldering

Microscopic Pathology

- Skin with T-cell infiltrate in epidermis, dermis, &/or subcutis
  - Epidermotropism &/or Pautrier microabscesses
- Peripheral blood with multilobated "flower" cells
- Lymph nodes with effaced architecture and diffuse infiltrate

Ancillary Tests

- Confirmation of HTLV-1 infection by serology
- Immunophenotype: Regulatory T cells CD3(+), CD4(+), CD25(+), FOXP3(+), CCR4(+); often loses CD7; cytotoxic markers negative
- Clonal T-cell receptor gene rearrangement
- Complex chromosomal abnormalities; no one abnormality is characteristic of ATLL

Top Differential Diagnoses

- *Mycosis fungoides*
  - Similar clinical picture with epidermotropism and peripheral blood lymphocytosis
  - Also CD4(+), CD8(-) T cells, but CD25(-), FOXP3(-), and CD30(-)
- Anaplastic large cell lymphoma

- Multiagent chemotherapy
- Some indolent cases followed with only "watchful waiting"
- Allogenic hematopoietic stem cell transplant used in select patients

Prognosis

- Better in chronic and smoldering variants than acute and lymphomatous variants
  - < 10% 5-year survival for acute and lymphomatous variants
  - 1/4 of chronic and smoldering variants transform to acute and lymphomatous variants
- Better if skin infiltrate is superficial and not deep
- Worse if hypercalcemia or ↑ LDH
- Worse in tumors as compared to papules

IMAGE FINDINGS

Radiographic Findings

- Osteolytic bone lesions

MICROSCOPIC PATHOLOGY

Histologic Features

- Skin
  - Atypical lymphoid infiltrate in epidermis, dermis, &/or subcutis
    - Frequent epidermotropism &/or Pautrier microabscesses
  - Eosinophils present (usually absent in MF)

Cytologic Features

- Usually medium to large-sized pleomorphic T cells with marked atypia, coarse clumped chromatin, and small/absent nucleoli
  - "Flower" cells (a.k.a. cauliflower cells) are multilobated T cells
    - More easily seen in peripheral blood

Rare Morphologic Variants

- Small cell
- Anaplastic
- Reed-Sternberg-like variant
  - Reed-Sternberg-like cells are B cells, not T cells, and are CD30(+) and EBV(+)
    - EBV(+) B cells in ATLL patients probably due to immunosuppression
- Angioimmunoblastic-like variant
  - Proliferation of high endothelial venules
  - Inflammatory cells such as plasma cells and eosinophils
  - Malignant T cells negative for CD10, CXCL13
  - No increased CD21 positive follicular dendritic cells

Lymph Nodes

- Low power
  - Effaced architecture and diffuse infiltrate
- High power
  - Medium to large T cells, often with multilobated nuclei

Bone Marrow

- Diffuse, interstitial, or sinusoidal collections of tumor cells

ANCILLARY TESTS

Immunohistochemistry

- T-cell antigens positive (CD3, CD5)
  - CD7 is often lost
- Usually CD4(+), CD8(-)
  - Rarely CD4(-), CD8(+) or CD4(+),CD8(+)
- CD25(+) (almost always), FOXP3(+), CCR4(+), CD30 often scattered (+) in large cells, but ALK1(-)
- Cytotoxic markers (TIA1 and granzyme-B) negative
- Adult T-cell leukemia lymphoma-associated antigen positive
  - Specific antibody for human T-cell lymphotropic virus type 1

ADULT T-CELL LEUKEMIA/LYMPHOMA

ATLL Subtypes

	Acute	Chronic	Smoldering
Abnormal T cells in blood	Yes	Very little	> 5%
Bone marrow involved	Sometimes	No	No
Calcium	Sometimes increased	Normal	Normal
Hepatosplenomegaly	Sometimes	Mild	No
LDH	Increased	+/-	Usually normal
Lymphadenopathy	Often	Sometimes	No
Lymphocytosis	Increased	Sometimes increased	No
Skin lesions	Sometimes	Sometimes	Sometimes

Molecular Genetics

- Clonal T-cell receptor gene rearrangement
- Cytogenetics
  - Numerous complex chromosomal abnormalities
  - No single diagnostic chromosomal abnormality

Serologic Testing

- Diagnosis requires confirmation of HTLV-1 infection

DIFFERENTIAL DIAGNOSIS

Mycosis Fungoides/Sézary Syndrome

- Skin lesions with epidermotropism and Pautrier microabscesses like ATLL
- Circulating atypical lymphocytes, as in ATLL
  - Cerebriform nuclei of *Mycosis fungoides* fold inward, whereas "flower" cells of ATLL have outward nuclear projections
- Immunophenotypic CD4(+), CD8(-) T cells, like ATLL
  - But not CD25(+), FOXP3(+), or CD30(+)
  - Patients not infected with HTLV-1

Anaplastic Large Cell Lymphoma (ALCL)

- CD30(+) T-cell lymphoma with large cells like ATLL
- FOXP3(-), CCR4(-); ALK1 and EMA(+/-)

Hodgkin Lymphoma

- ATLL with Hodgkin-like cells contains Reed-Sternberg-like cells that are CD30(+), EBV(+)
- No aggregates of malignant T cells in Hodgkin lymphoma
- Usually no malignant cells in peripheral blood, no skin lesions, and no hypercalcemia in Hodgkin lymphoma

Angioimmunoblastic-like T-cell Lymphoma (AITL)

- ↑ high endothelial venules, plasma cells, and eosinophils
- Tumor cells CD10(+), Bcl-6(+), and CXCL13(+), unlike ATLL
- ↑ follicular dendritic cells expressing CD21

T-cell Large Granular Lymphocytic Leukemia

- Also peripheral blood involved with variable absolute lymphocyte count and large granular lymphocytes in blood
- Large granular lymphocytes

  - Different morphology from ATLL T cells, with increased pale cytoplasm and prominent azurophilic granules
  - Mild nuclear indenting, but no polylobated nuclei as in ATLL
- Immunohistochemistry
  - Differs from ATLL
    - T-LGL is CD8(+), CD16(+), CD57(+)

T-cell Prolymphocytic Leukemia

- Involves blood at presentation with ↑ WBC
- Some nuclear irregularity, but no "flower" cell morphology as in ATLL

Reactive Cutaneous Infiltrates

- Usually less atypia, no epidermotropism, and no T-cell gene receptor γ chain rearrangements

SELECTED REFERENCES

1. Amano M et al: Epstein-Barr virus-associated primary central nervous system lymphoma in a patient with adult T-cell leukemia/lymphoma. J Dermatol. 38(6):575-80, 2011
2. Kim NH et al: Prominent apoptosis in pautrier microabscesses: a distinctive finding in adult T-cell leukemia/lymphoma? Am J Dermatopathol. 33(5):530-1, 2011
3. Sawada Y et al: Type of skin eruption is an independent prognostic indicator for adult T-cell leukemia/lymphoma. Blood. 117(15):3961-7, 2011
4. Venkataraman G et al: Adult T-cell leukemia/lymphoma with Epstein-Barr virus-positive Hodgkin-like cells. Hum Pathol. 42(7):1042-6, 2011
5. Hishizawa M et al: Transplantation of allogeneic hematopoietic stem cells for adult T-cell leukemia: a nationwide retrospective study. Blood. 116(8):1369-76, 2010
6. Santos JB et al: The importance of flower cells for the early diagnosis of acute adult T-cell leukemia/lymphoma with skin involvement. Acta Oncol. 49(2):265-7, 2010
7. Bittencourt AL et al: Adult T-cell leukemia/lymphoma (ATL) presenting in the skin: clinical, histological and immunohistochemical features of 52 cases. Acta Oncol. 48(4):598-604, 2009
8. Karube K et al: Adult T-cell lymphoma/leukemia with angioimmunoblastic T-cell lymphomalike features: Report of 11 cases. Am J Surg Pathol. 31(2):216-23, 2007
9. Mesnard JM et al: Multiple control levels of cell proliferation by human T-cell leukemia virus type 1 Tax protein. Virology. 257(2):277-84, 1999

ADULT T-CELL LEUKEMIA/LYMPHOMA

Microscopic and Immunohistochemical Features

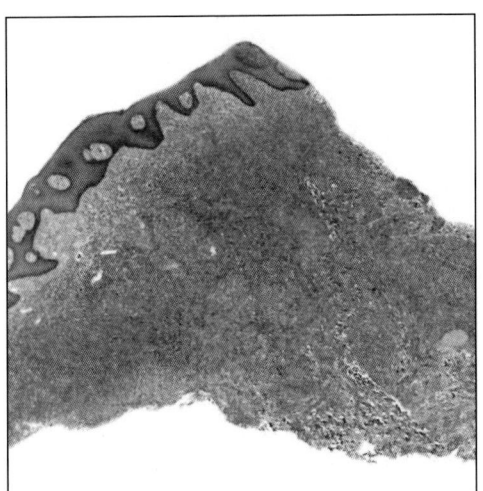

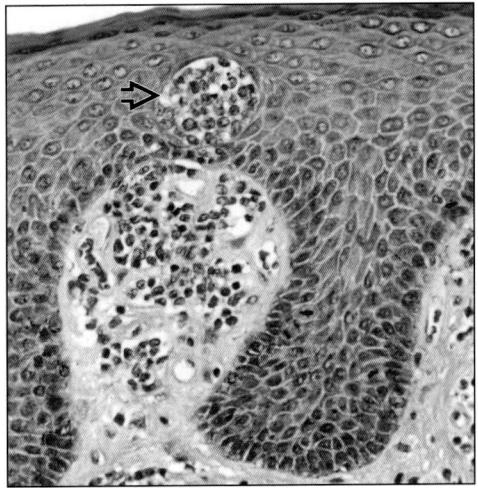

(Left) ATLL involving skin shows diffuse multinodular lymphoid aggregates throughout the dermis. (Courtesy C. Bueso-Ramos, MD.) (Right) High magnification of ATLL shows atypical cells in the epidermis forming a well-circumscribed, Pautrier-like microabscess ➡. Smaller and less-cellular aggregates are more characteristic of mycosis fungoides, although sometimes the distinction is not possible. (Courtesy C. Bueso-Ramos, MD.)

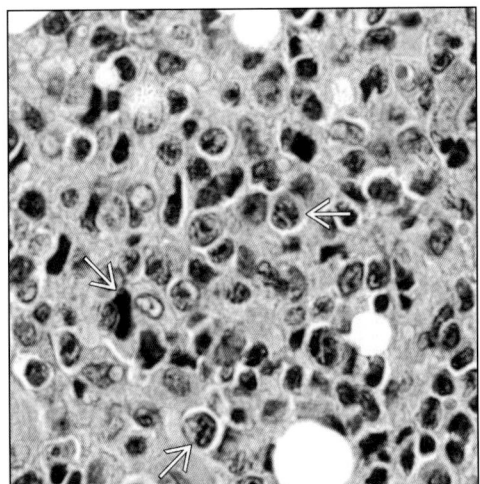

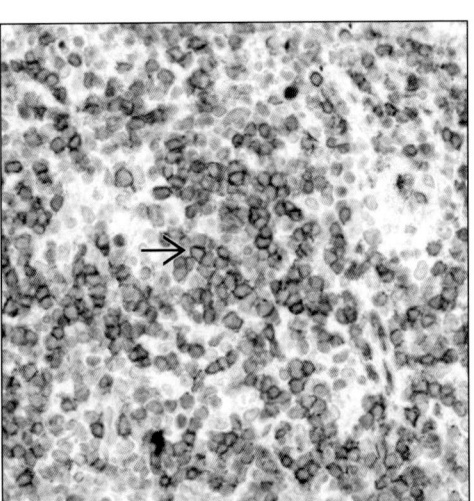

(Left) In this high magnification of ATLL, there is a diffuse infiltrate of medium-sized pleomorphic-appearing cells ➡ with hyperchromasia, atypical nuclear contours, focally prominent nucleoli, and vesicular chromatin. (Right) The malignant T cells are strongly positive for the CD25 antibody in a membranous/cytoplasmic distribution pattern ➡. FOXP3 and HTLV1 antibodies are also immunoreactive (not shown).

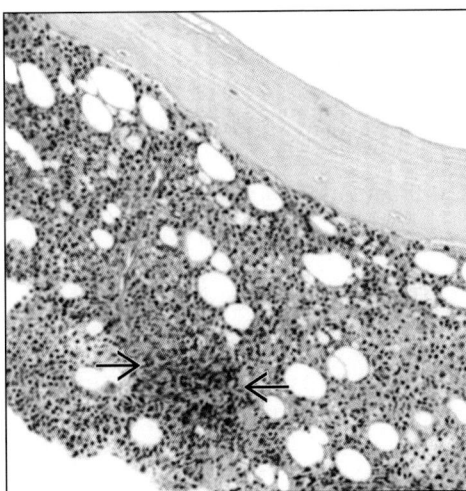

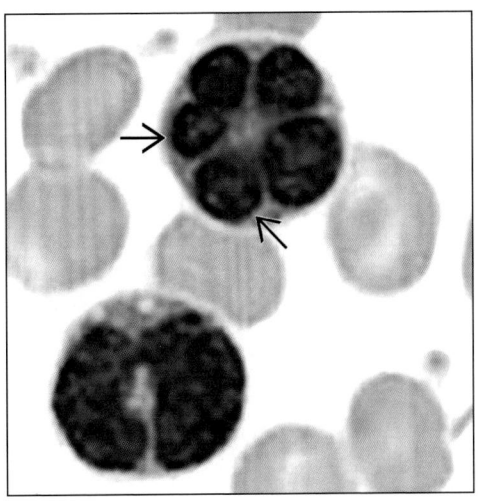

(Left) This image shows malignant T cells in the bone marrow of a patient with ATLL. There is a patchy distribution pattern with malignant T cells in clusters ➡. The T cells are CD25(+) and FOXP3(+) (not shown). The acute subtype shows the most severe bone marrow involvement. (Right) High-magnification image (oil) of peripheral blood shows medium to large lymphocytes with irregular nuclei. These cells are called "flower" cells because of the multiple nuclear lobules or convolutions ➡.

SUBCUTANEOUS PANNICULITIS-LIKE T-CELL LYMPHOMA

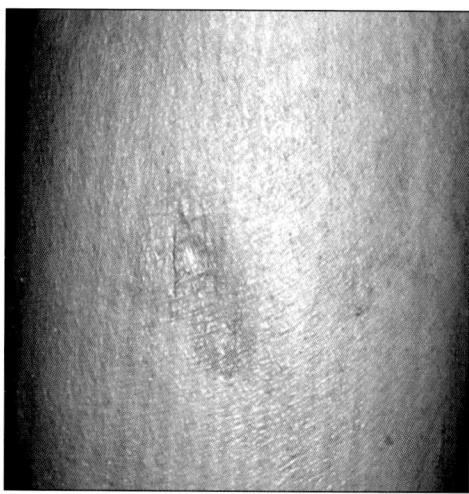

This clinical photograph shows a single nonulcerated subcutaneous nodule on the arm of a 35-year-old patient. Upon excision, the nodule was diagnosed as SPTCL. (Courtesy M. Tomaszewsky, MD.)

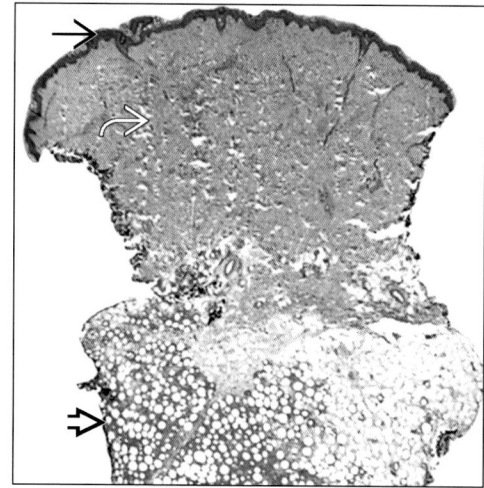

Low-power view of SPTCL shows malignant T cells confined to subcutaneous tissue ➔. The dermis ➔ and epidermis ➔ are both spared and are morphologically unremarkable. (Courtesy M. Tomaszewsky, MD.)

TERMINOLOGY

Abbreviations

- Subcutaneous panniculitis-like T-cell lymphoma (SPTCL)

Definitions

- T-cell lymphoma of αβ cells involving subcutaneous tissue with prominent karyorrhexis and cytotoxic phenotype
  - Cases composed of γδ cells are reclassified as cutaneous γδ T-cell lymphoma in the WHO Classification of Hematopoietic and Lymphoid Tumors
  - Subcutaneous T-cell lymphomas of γδ type are more aggressive than αβ cases

ETIOLOGY/PATHOGENESIS

Autoimmune Disease

- Autoimmune disease present in ~ 20% of patients
  - Systemic lupus erythematosus (SLE) most common
    - Microscopic findings of SPTCL overlap with lupus profundus panniculitis

Viral Infection

- Rarely, SPTCL is seen with Epstein-Barr virus infection
  - May be due to immunosuppression

CLINICAL ISSUES

Epidemiology

- Incidence
  - < 1% of all non-Hodgkin lymphoma
    - Presents sporadically without familial involvement
- Age
  - Median: ~ 35 years (range: 5 months to 84 years)
    - 20% < 20 years old

- Rarely, children < 2 years old
- Gender
  - Men = women
- Ethnicity
  - No ethnic predisposition

Site

- Extremities and trunk most common
- Uncommonly disseminates
  - Can involve lymph nodes, but not at initial diagnosis

Presentation

- Single or multiple erythematous subcutaneous nodules or plaques
  - Painless mass, rarely ulcerates
  - Symptoms due to mass effects
- B symptoms in up to 50%
  - Diagnosis often not discovered until months to years after onset of symptoms
- Hemophagocytic syndrome (HPS) in up to 20%
  - Related to release of cytotoxic molecules
  - May occur up to 5 years after presenting diagnosis

Laboratory Tests

- Cytopenias (anemia, leukopenia, thrombocytopenia)
- ↑ liver function tests
- ↑ erythrocyte sedimentation rate, ↑ C-reactive protein

Treatment

- Surgery
  - Sometimes excision of single lesion with no further recurrence
- Immunosuppressive agents
  - Often given, at least initially
  - High-dose systemic corticosteroids
- Chemotherapy
  - Recurrence or resistant cases treated with CHOP or CHOP-like therapy
- Radiation
  - Sometimes for localized disease

SUBCUTANEOUS PANNICULITIS-LIKE T-CELL LYMPHOMA

Key Facts

Terminology

- T-cell lymphoma of αβ cells usually involving subcutaneous tissue with prominent karyorrhexis and cytotoxic phenotype
- Cases composed of γδ cells are reclassified as cutaneous γδ T-cell lymphomas

Clinical Issues

- 20% hemophagocytic syndrome
- Excellent prognosis

Microscopic Pathology

- Atypical lobular panniculitic T-cell infiltrate confined to subcutis
- Malignant T cells rim around adipocytes
- Prominent necrosis/apoptosis and angioinvasion
- Vacuolated histiocytes

Ancillary Tests

- Immunohistochemistry, TCR-βF1(+), TCR-δ(-), CD8(+), CD4(-), CD56(-), EBER(-)
- (+) for cytotoxic markers
- T-cell receptor gene rearrangement

Top Differential Diagnoses

- Cutaneous γ/δ T-cell lymphoma
  - Panniculitis, but also in dermis &/or epidermis with ulceration, TCR-βF1(-), TCR-δ(+)
  - Worse prognosis than SPTCL
- Lupus profundus panniculitis
  - Similar inflammation in subcutis in panniculitic pattern
  - Lobular panniculitis, but shows plasma cells and germinal centers unlike SPTCL

- Stem cell transplant
  - Can be considered for refractory/recurrent disease

Prognosis

- Indolent disease
  - 5-year overall survival ~ 80%
  - Mostly stage I (confined to skin)
  - Rare systemic spread
    - Including lymph nodes
    - Often years after diagnosis
- HPS poor prognostic indicator
  - Medium survival ~ 2 years

IMAGE FINDINGS

CT Findings

- Enhancing nodules in subcutaneous tissue

MICROSCOPIC PATHOLOGY

Histologic Features

- Atypical T-cell infiltrate of subcutaneous fat lobules
  - Involves lobules, usually spares septa
    - Uncommon septal pattern represents spilling of T cells from lobules
    - Typically, no tumor in overlying dermis or epidermis
  - Malignant T cells rim individual adipocytes
    - Characteristic, but not specific for SPTCL
  - Neoplastic cells
    - Small to large in size
    - Mild to marked atypia with irregular nuclear contours
    - Hyperchromatic nuclei
    - Pale, clear cytoplasm
- Karyorrhexis (apoptosis) and fat necrosis characteristic
  - Necrosis from released cytotoxic molecules
- Initial biopsy commonly shows minimal T-cell atypia
  - Later biopsies show more atypia
- Angioinvasion in some cases
  - Poor prognostic indicator

- Reactive inflammatory cells
  - Histiocytes
    - Vacuolated foamy cytoplasm from imbibed material/lipid
    - Erythrophagocytosis or cytophagocytosis
    - Sometimes poorly formed granulomas with multinucleated giant cells
  - Usually lacks plasma cells, eosinophils, or neutrophils

ANCILLARY TESTS

Immunohistochemistry

- T-cell antigens (+) (CD2, CD3, CD5, CD7)
  - May lack 1 or more T-cell antigens
- CD8(+)/CD4(-) in > 95% of SPTCL
  - CD4(-)/CD8(-) and CD4(+)/CD8(-) rarely
- TCR-βF1(+), TCR-δ-1(-) (alpha-beta T cells)
- Cytotoxic markers (+) (perforin, TIA1, and granzyme)
  - But GZM-M negative, unlike other T-cell lymphomas
- CD56(-), CD30(-), Bcl-2(-)

Cytogenetics

- No specific cytogenetic abnormalities

In Situ Hybridization

- Epstein-Barr encoded receptor (EBER) usually negative
  - Rare EBER(+) associated with immunocompromised and Asian patients

Molecular Genetics

- Monoclonal T-cell receptor gene rearrangement

DIFFERENTIAL DIAGNOSIS

Cutaneous γ/δ T-cell Lymphoma

- Panniculitic pattern of tissue involvement, like SPTCL
  - Dermal and epidermal involvement, unlike SPTCL
  - Ulcerated epidermis, contrary to SPTCL
- γδ cells, not αβ cells of SPTCL
  - Immunophenotype

SUBCUTANEOUS PANNICULITIS-LIKE T-CELL LYMPHOMA

SPTCL Compared to Primary Cutaneous γ/δ T-cell Lymphoma

	SPTCL	PC γ/δ T-cell Lymphoma
Age	Younger; median age: 30s	Older; mean age: 50s
Ulceration	Usually not present	Usually present
Clinical	B symptoms (+) or (-)	Usually B symptoms and HPS
Histology	Subcutaneous infiltrate with pleomorphism	Similar, but also in dermis and massive necrosis
Immunohistochemistry	CD3(+), CD8(+), TIA1(+), CD56(-), TCR-βF1(+), TCR-δ-1(-)	CD3(+), CD8(-), TIA1(+), CD56(+), TCR-βF1(-), TCR-δ-1(+)
Prognosis	Excellent prognosis without HPS	Poor prognosis with HPS and sometimes metastasis
Treatment	High-dose corticosteroids, or CHOP if recurrences	Multiagent chemotherapy, allogeneic stem cell transplantation
5-year survival	82%	11%

- TCR-βF1(-), TCR-δ-1(+), CD56(+), unlike SPTCL
- Usually CD4(-), CD8(-) (double negative)
- Clinical presentation compared to SPTCL
  - Older median age of diagnosis (~ 60 years)
  - Generalized lesions
  - More B symptoms
  - More often HPS ~ 50% (of patients)
  - Worse prognosis than SPTCL ~ 10% 5-year survival
  - More often given multiagent chemotherapy, systemic corticosteroids often given in SPTCL

Other Hematopoietic Neoplasms

- Usually involve epidermis or dermis, contrary to SPTCL
  - **Anaplastic large cell lymphoma**
    - Superficial nodules, rarely panniculitic, CD30(+)
  - **Blastic plasmacytoid dendritic cell neoplasm**
    - Different phenotype than SPTCL, with CD4(+), CD56(+), CD123(+), cytotoxic markers negative
  - **Enteropathy associated T-cell lymphoma**
    - Can have subcutis dissemination
    - But will typically present with gastrointestinal mass, &/or other features of celiac disease
  - **Diffuse large B-cell lymphoma**
    - Can have subcutaneous involvement
    - But will have a B-cell phenotype and Ig heavy chain immunoglobulin gene rearrangement

Reactive Panniculitis

- **Lupus profundus panniculitis**
  - Difficult to differentiate from SPTCL in some cases
    - Patients can have both lupus profundus panniculitis and SPTCL
  - Similarities to SPTCL
    - Inflammation in subcutis in panniculitic pattern
    - No/minimal lymphocyte atypia, like early lesions of SPTCL
    - Self-heal and improve with steroids, like many SPTCL cases
  - Differences from SPTCL
    - Plasma cells and germinal centers
    - Mixed inflammatory infiltrate with histiocytes, eosinophils, and neutrophils
    - Less T-cell atypia, minimal rimming of fat cells
    - B-cell aggregates
    - Mix of CD4(+) and CD8(+) T cells
    - T cells negative for cytotoxic markers
    - Vacuolar epidermal change and interstitial mucin

- Usually polyclonal *TCR* rearrangement, but rarely oligoclonal T-cell populations are present
  - Other features of lupus
    - History of SLE
    - Laboratory tests: ANA(+), antidouble stranded DNA antibodies, rheumatoid factor(+), ↓ C4 levels
    - Superficial epidermal and dermal findings including interface inflammation and perivascular and periadnexal infiltrates
- **Atypical lymphocytic lobular panniculitis**
  - Clonal lymphoid infiltrate without histologic criteria for lymphoma
  - Chronic condition that spontaneously regresses
  - Lobular T-cell infiltrate of small to medium-sized cells without atypia
    - Less rimming of fat cells
    - No karyorrhexis
    - Can have CD4(+) cells
  - ↑ numbers of histiocytes
  - May develop into SPTCL
- **Histiocytic cytophagic panniculitis (HCP)**
  - Most cases are reclassified as SPTCL
    - Few HCP cases still remain
    - Rarely if ever progresses to SPTCL
  - ↑ histiocytes
  - No clonal T-cell receptor gene rearrangement

SELECTED REFERENCES

1. Parveen Z et al: Subcutaneous panniculitis-like T-cell lymphoma: redefinition of diagnostic criteria in the recent World Health Organization-European Organization for Research and Treatment of Cancer classification for cutaneous lymphomas. Arch Pathol Lab Med. 133(2):303-8, 2009
2. Pincus LB et al: Subcutaneous panniculitis-like T-cell lymphoma with overlapping clinicopathologic features of lupus erythematosus: coexistence of 2 entities? Am J Dermatopathol. 31(6):520-6, 2009
3. Kong YY et al: Subcutaneous panniculitis-like T-cell lymphoma: a clinicopathologic, immunophenotypic, and molecular study of 22 Asian cases according to WHO-EORTC classification. Am J Surg Pathol. 32(10):1495-502, 2008
4. Willemze R et al: Subcutaneous panniculitis-like T-cell lymphoma: definition, classification, and prognostic factors: an EORTC Cutaneous Lymphoma Group Study of 83 cases. Blood. 111(2):838-45, 2008

SUBCUTANEOUS PANNICULITIS-LIKE T-CELL LYMPHOMA

Microscopic Features

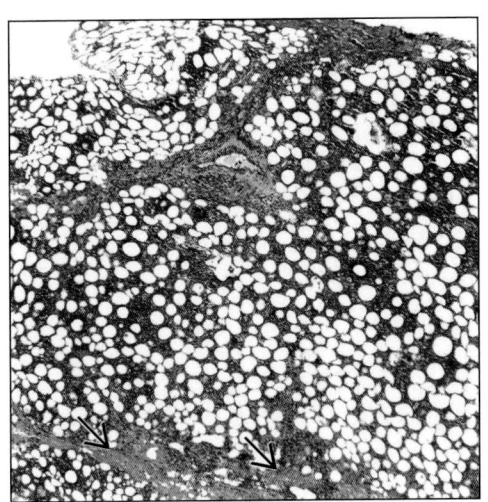

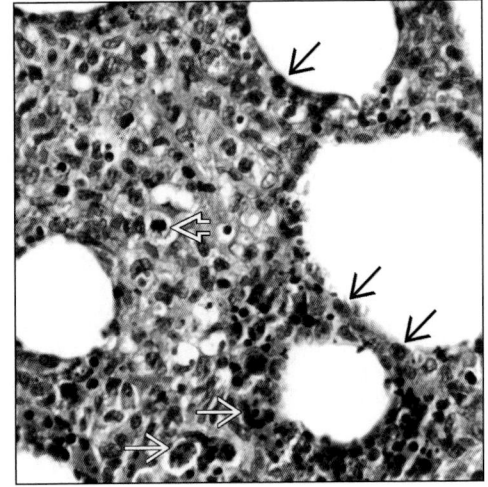

(Left) Even at low-power examination, this SPTCL shows infiltration of the fat lobules by atypical lymphoid cells. However, the septae ➡ are relatively uninvolved. *(Right)* Higher power shows a lobular pattern of atypical T cells rimming fat cells ➡. There are also numerous histiocytes containing apoptotic debris ("bean bag cells") ➡ and markedly atypical lymphocytes present between the fat cells, with a mitotic figure ➡.

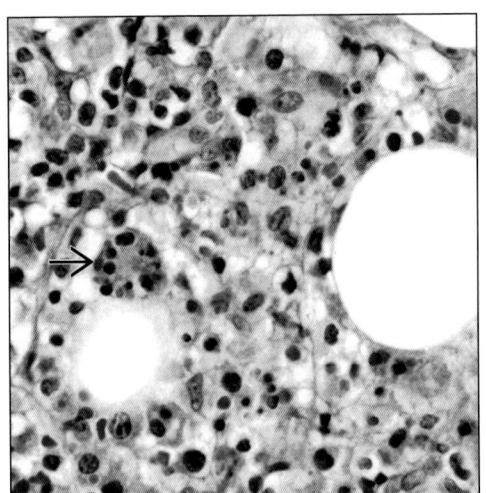

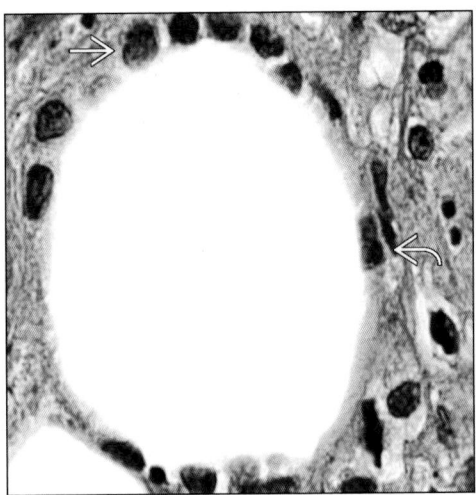

(Left) In this high-power view of SPTCL, there are abundant histiocytes ➡ containing apoptotic cellular debris, a finding typical of SPTCL. Sometimes these histiocytes have a vacuolated appearance. *(Right)* This fat cell is surrounded by T cells that are medium to large in size ➡ and that show some nuclear irregularity ➡. The atypia in these T cells is not typically seen in reactive lesions with panniculitis.

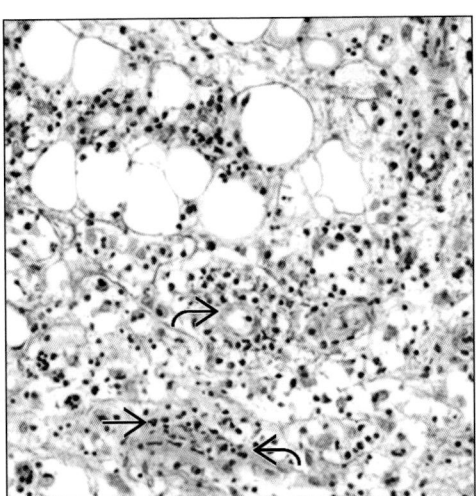

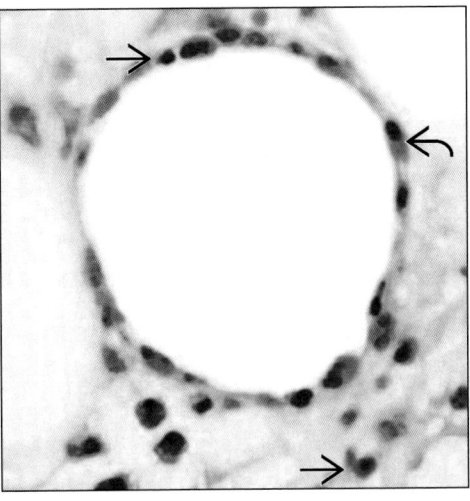

(Left) This SPTCL shows prominent karyorrhexis and angiocentricity. There is prominent karyorrhexis ➡ and focal necrosis in this tumor. The malignant cells also appear to surround and involve small blood vessels ➡. *(Right)* This is an unusual case of SPTCL with eosinophils. Malignant T cells ➡ rim the fat. It is unusual that eosinophils ➡ also surround this fat lobule, since eosinophils, plasma cells, and neutrophils are more common in reactive panniculitis than SPTCL.

SUBCUTANEOUS PANNICULITIS-LIKE T-CELL LYMPHOMA

Ancillary Techniques

(Left) In this CD3(+) SPTCL, the CD3 immunostain strongly highlights the numerous malignant T cells diffusely infiltrating and rimming the fat cells ⊡. *(Right)* This image is a composite picture with a CD8 stain on the left and a CD4 stain on the right. In this case of SPTCL, the malignant T cells strongly express CD8 ⊡ but are nonimmunoreactive for CD4 ⇗ (only scattered histiocytes and reactive T cells are marking CD4[+]).

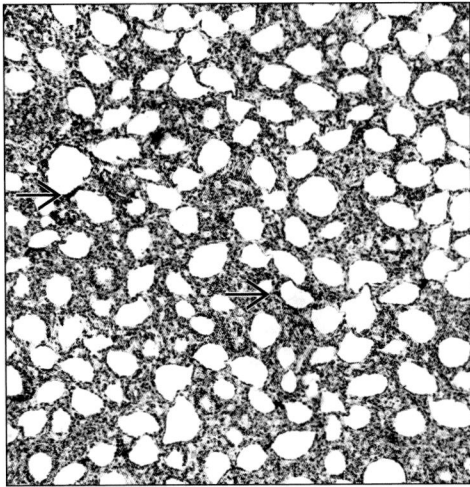
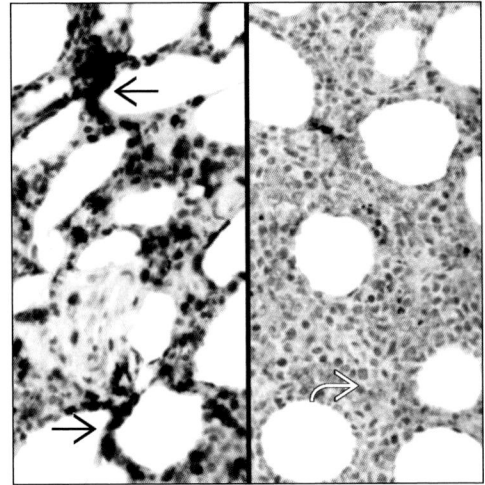

(Left) TCR-β-F1 immunohistochemical stain is expressed in the malignant T cells rimming the fat ⊡, similar to the CD3 and CD8 stains. This is evidence that the cells in SPTCL are αβ T cells and not γδ T cells. *(Courtesy T. Muzzafar, MD.)* *(Right)* Granzyme-B is a cytotoxic marker that is typically strongly and diffusely positive in SPTCL. Note the staining of areas of fat-rimming ⇗. These cells were also positive for other cytotoxic markers, including TIA-1 and perforin (not shown).

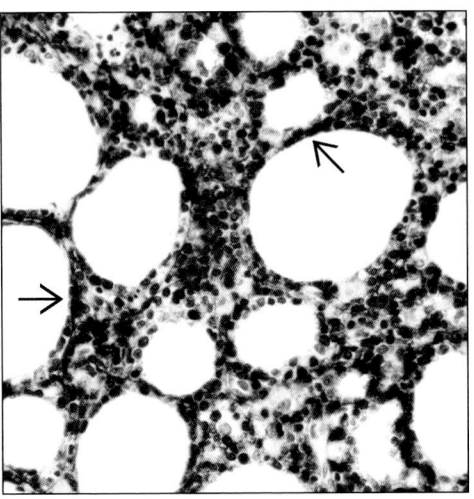
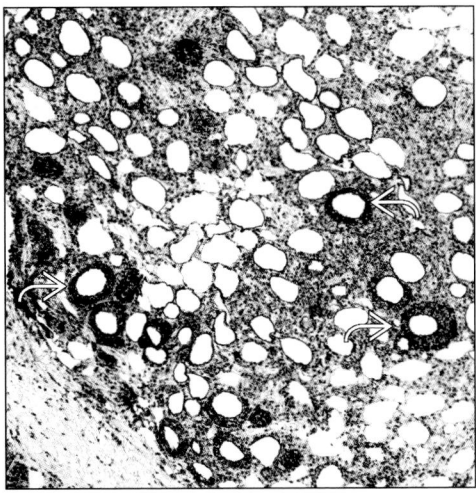

(Left) This CD56 immunohistochemical stain is negative in the malignant cells of the SPTCL. In cases of cutaneous γδ T-cell lymphoma, CD56 is typically positive. *(Right)* This test is a PCR T-cell receptor gene rearrangement performed on a case of SPTCL. The appearance of a blue peak between 180 and 280 base pairs in size is suggestive of a clonal T-cell rearrangement, as is commonly seen in this tumor.

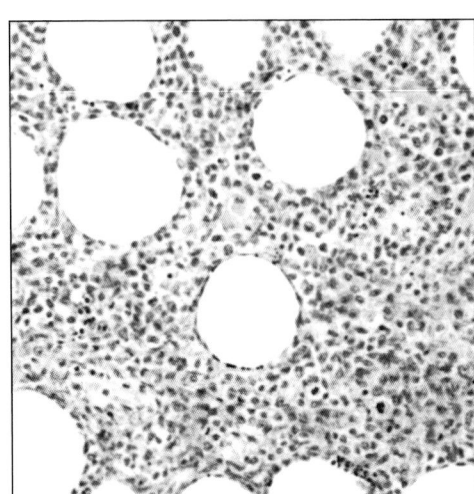
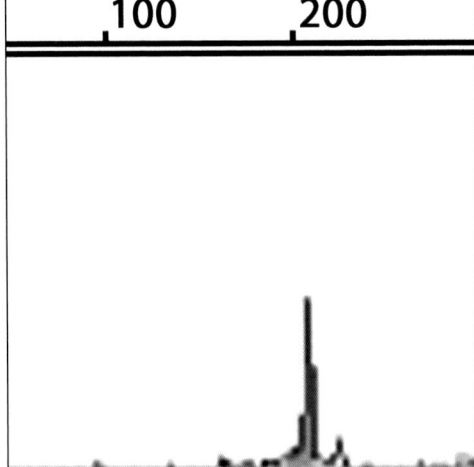

I

12

SUBCUTANEOUS PANNICULITIS-LIKE T-CELL LYMPHOMA

Differential Diagnosis

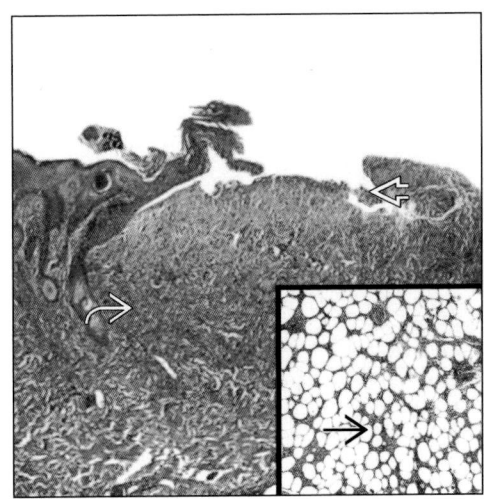

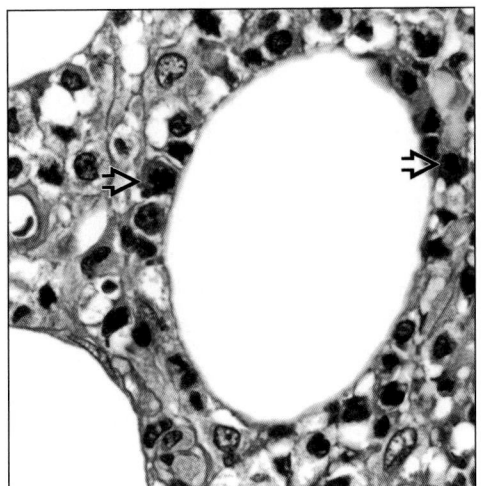

(Left) Primary cutaneous γδ T-cell lymphoma (PCGDTCL) is the main differential diagnosis of SPTCL. In this cutaneous γδ T-cell lymphoma, T cells rim fat (lower right inset ➡), similar to SPTCL. However, there is an overlying ulcer ➡ and dermal infiltrate ➡, unlike SPTCL. *(Right)* In this PCGDTCL, the neoplastic cells exhibit greater cytologic atypia than those of SPTCL and rim the adipocytes in this field. Mitotic figures are present ➡. *(Courtesy L. J. Medeiros, MD.)*

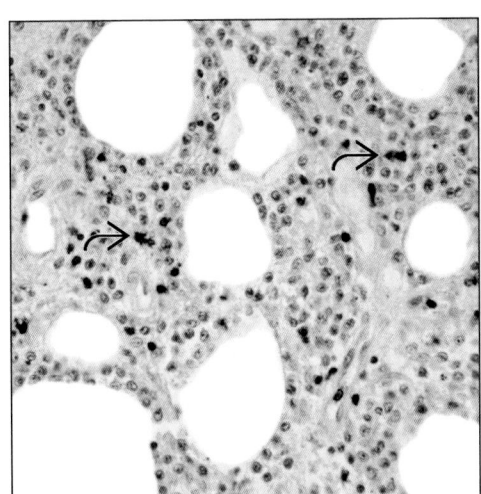

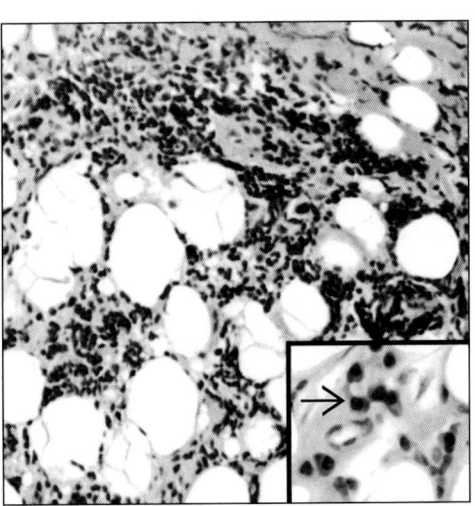

(Left) This is a βF1 stain done on a PCGDTCL. The neoplastic T cells are negative for TCR-βF1, although a few scattered reactive T cells are positive ➡. Absence of TCR-βF1 is presumptive evidence that the neoplastic cells express the TCR-γδ. *(Courtesy L. J. Medeiros, MD.)* *(Right)* This case of lupus profundus shows a lobular panniculitis. Scattered plasma cells are seen ➡. Plasma cells are a component of lupus profundus, but are not commonly seen in SPTCL.

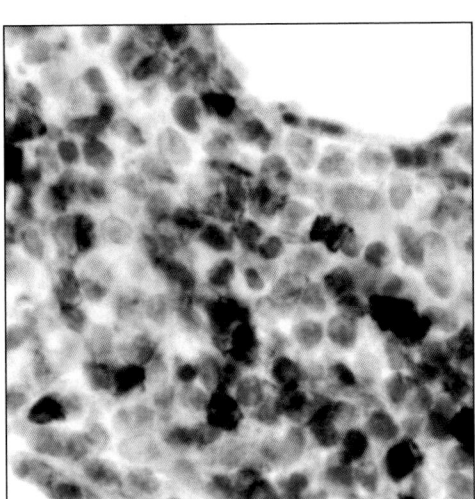

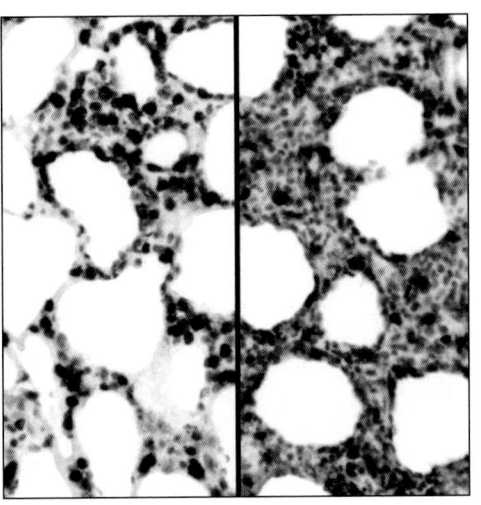

(Left) This is a case of lupus profundus with CD20(+) B cells. This CD20 immunohistochemical stain shows several clusters of B cells. This finding favors lupus profundus over SPTCL, which usually does not show B-cell aggregates. *(Right)* Unlike SPTCL, which consists of CD8(+) T cells, lupus profundus (as seen here) usually has a mixture of CD4(+) and CD8(+) cells. In this image, the CD4 stain (left) and the CD8 stain (right) both show clusters of positive cells in the subcutis.

EXTRANODAL NK/T-CELL LYMPHOMA, NASAL TYPE

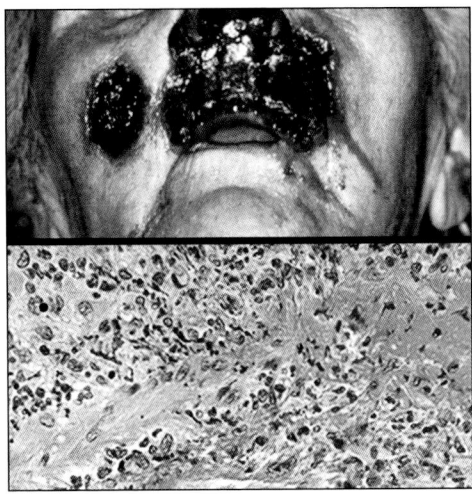

Clinical photograph of ENNKTCL, nasal type shows extensive destruction of the nasolabial region (above). High magnification of this lesion shows an atypical lymphoid infiltrate with vascular destruction.

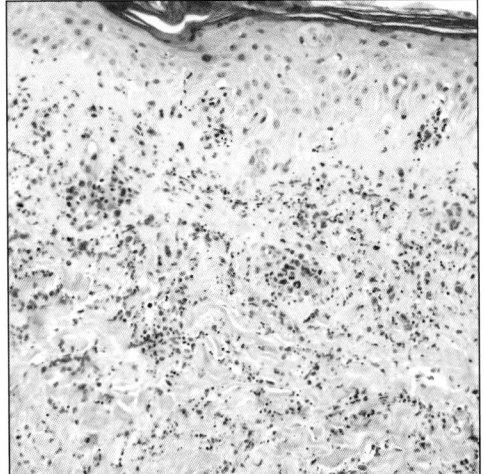

This is a nasal-type extranodal NK/T-cell lymphoma of NK cell lineage involving the skin. The neoplastic cells are enlarged and show nuclear hyperchromasia. (Courtesy L. J. Medeiros, MD.)

TERMINOLOGY

Abbreviations
- Extranodal NK/T-cell lymphoma, nasal type (ENNKTCL)

Synonyms
- Angiocentric T-cell lymphoma, malignant midline reticulosis, lethal midline granuloma, polymorphic reticulosis

Definitions
- Lymphoma composed of NK cells or T cells that is characterized by necrosis, Epstein-Barr virus infection, and often angioinvasion
  - Usually extranodal

ETIOLOGY/PATHOGENESIS

Infectious Agents
- Epstein-Barr virus
  - Epstein-Barr virus antigens are identified by immunohistochemistry and in situ hybridization
- Immunosuppression
  - Subset of patients are immunosuppressed
    - Including post transplant

CLINICAL ISSUES

Epidemiology
- Incidence
  - Rare in United States; more common in South America, Central America, and Asia
- Age
  - Usually adults

Site
- Nasal
  - Most common location of disease

- Anywhere in upper aerodigestive tract
    - Includes nasal cavity, nasopharynx, sinuses, and palate
- Extranasal
  - Skin
    - Most common extranasal site
    - Skin can be primary disease or secondary to disease elsewhere
    - Often extremities or torso
  - Other sites include gastrointestinal tract, lymph nodes, and testes

Presentation
- Skin
  - Nodules &/or plaques on skin
    - Often ulcerated
- Nasal
  - Obstruction or epistaxis
- Gastrointestinal tract
  - Perforation or mass
- B symptoms including fever &/or weight loss
- Hemophagocytic syndrome in some cases

Laboratory Tests
- EBV DNA can be assessed to check disease activity

Natural History
- Can spread to regional lymph nodes
  - Tumor only in lymph nodes and not other anatomic sites is uncommon
  - Primary lymph node involvement is very rare
- Can involve bone marrow

Treatment
- Chemotherapy and radiation therapy

Prognosis
- Median survival < 15 months
  - Better survival with intense radiotherapy and chemotherapy
- Poor prognostic indicators

EXTRANODAL NK/T-CELL LYMPHOMA, NASAL TYPE

Key Facts

Terminology
- Tumor of NK cells or T cells, with necrosis, Epstein-Barr virus infection, and angioinvasion

Etiology/Pathogenesis
- Epstein-Barr virus

Clinical Issues
- Common in adults in South America, Central America, and Asia
- Nasopharynx most common site, skin is 2nd

Microscopic Pathology
- Diffuse dermal/subcutaneous infiltrate of variably sized tumor cells, angiocentric with necrosis
- Dense chromatin, can be vesicular in large cells
- Coagulative necrosis in most cases

Ancillary Tests
- Epstein-Barr virus antigen (+)
- Mostly NK-cell markers phenotype
  - βF1(-), CD2(+), cytoplasmic CD3-ε(+), CD56(+/-), cytotoxic markers(+)
- Less often T-cell marker phenotype
  - βF1(+), CD2(+), cytoplasmic CD3-ε(+), CD56(-/+), cytotoxic markers(+)
- No specific cytogenetic abnormalities

Top Differential Diagnoses
- Wegener granulomatosis
- Infection
- B-cell lymphomas (DLBCL, lymphomatoid granulomatosis)
- PTCL-NOS, NK-cell leukemia

- High stage of disease
- Bone marrow with EBV(+) cells
- High International or Korean Prognostic Index
  - B symptoms, serum LDH, regional lymph nodes, stage
- ↑ EBV DNA
- ↑ C-reactive protein, thrombocytopenia
- ↑ Ki-67 > 50%
- Better prognostic indicators
  - More favorable for nasal disease than extra-nasal
  - High absolute lymphocyte count
  - CD56(+), CD30(+) coexpression has been reported

IMAGE FINDINGS

General Features
- Mass lesion that can destroy bone, especially in nasal tumors

MACROSCOPIC FEATURES

General Features
- 1 or more firm nodules

MICROSCOPIC PATHOLOGY

Histologic Features
- Skin/mucosa
  - Diffuse pattern of infiltration
    - Mostly dermal infiltrate, sometimes subcutis
    - Rare foci of epidermotropism in 30%
  - Tumor cells can be small, medium, or large
    - Irregular nuclear shapes
    - Dense chromatin, can be vesicular in large cells
    - Sometimes ↑ clear cytoplasm
  - Coagulative necrosis in most cases
  - Tumor cells are angiocentric and angiodestructive
  - Overlying epithelium/mucosa
    - ± ulceration
    - Often shows pseudoepitheliomatous hyperplasia

- ↑ mitoses
- Erythrophagocytosis is sometimes seen
- Lymph node
  - Tumor tends to involve paracortical areas
- Bone marrow
  - Usually interstitial infiltrate
    - Lacking large tumor aggregates
  - Involved in 15% of cases

Cytologic Features
- Rarely, diagnosis can be made by fine needle aspirate
  - Azurophilic granules in some tumor cells

ANCILLARY TESTS

In Situ Hybridization
- In situ hybridization for EBV small-encoded RNA (EBER)

Immunohistochemistry
- Epstein-Barr virus antigens positive
  - Immunohistochemistry for latent membrane protein (LMP)
    - LMP is less sensitive than EBER
  - EBV antigens can be found in patients before tumor develops
- NK-cell markers
  - 75% of cases
    - βF1(-), CD2(+), cytoplasmic CD3-ε(+), surface CD3(-), CD4(-), CD5(-), CD8(-), CD56(+/-), cytotoxic markers(+)
- T-cell markers
  - 25% of cases
    - βF1(+), CD2(+), cytoplasmic CD3-ε(+), CD5(+), CD8(+/-), CD43(+), CD56(-/+), cytotoxic markers(+)
- CD56(-) cases should be EBER(+) or cytotoxic markers(+)

Cytogenetics
- No specific abnormalities identified
  - Del(6)(q21q25), i(6)(p10) reported

EXTRANODAL NK/T-CELL LYMPHOMA, NASAL TYPE

PCR
- T-cell receptor gene rearrangements
  - Found in T-cell tumors
  - Not found in NK-cell tumors

Molecular Genetics
- No specific abnormalities
  - But many have been reported
    - Mutation of *FAS*, β-catenin, *KRAS*, *P53*, *KIT*, *KRAS* genes

Electron Microscopy
- Electron-dense membrane-bound granules

DIFFERENTIAL DIAGNOSIS

Wegener Granulomatosis
- Also found in upper airways
  - But patients also usually have disease in kidneys and lungs
- Morphology classically shows triad of necrosis, vasculitis, and granulomas
  - All 3 components only seen in < 25% of cases
- Usually more of a mixed inflammatory infiltrate than ENNKTCL
  - Neutrophils, eosinophils, lymphocytes, plasma cells, histiocytes

Infection
- Similarities to ENNKTCL
  - Common in upper airways
    - Necrosis can be seen
- Differences from ENNKTCL
  - No large atypical tumor cells
  - More mixed inflammatory infiltrate with neutrophils
  - No *TCR* gene rearrangements
  - No EBER or LMP
  - Organisms can be identified
- EBV infection
  - Also EBV(+), but usually no mass lesion, no clonality and no metastasis, good prognosis

Non-Hodgkin B-cell Lymphomas
- Similarities to ENNKTCL
  - Can be in upper airways
    - Diffuse large B-cell lymphoma is most common
  - Large atypical cells, similar to ENNKTCL
- Differences from ENNKTCL
  - Less angiocentric than ENNKTCL
  - Different phenotype than ENNKTCL
    - B-cell markers(+) (CD19, CD20, CD79, pax-5) and NK/T-cell markers(-)
  - Monoclonal *IgH* gene rearrangement
  - Epstein-Barr virus antigens negative (EBER and LMP)
- Lymphomatoid granulomatosis
  - Also an EBV(+) neoplasm that is angiocentric
  - B-cell markers (+) and *IgH* gene rearrangement, unlike ENNKTCL

T-cell or Other NK-cell Neoplasms
- Peripheral T-cell lymphoma, NOS (PTCL, NOS)

  - Overlapping histologic features with ENNKTCL
    - Both can have necrosis and angioinvasion
  - Different immunophenotype
    - Often CD3(+), CD56(-), and EBV(-)
- Hydroa vacciniforme-like lymphoma
  - Also, EBER(+), cytotoxic markers(+), T cells &/or NK cells
  - Also, necrosis and angioinvasion
  - Usually in children, unlike ENNKTCL
  - Patients present with papulovesicular eruption on sun-exposed areas
- NK-cell leukemia
  - Presents more as leukemia with primary involvement of bone marrow and peripheral blood, but
    - Also EBV(+) and can have skin lesions
- Post-transplant lymphoproliferative disorder (PTLD), extranodal NK/T-cell lymphoma, nasal type
  - Rarely, tumors can develop post transplant that morphologically and phenotypically mimic ENNKTCL
  - Necrosis and angioinvasion
  - EBER(+), CD56(+), CD3(+), cytotoxic markers(+)
- Anaplastic large cell lymphoma (ALCL)
  - Both ALCL and ENNKTCL can be CD30(+), CD56(+)
    - ALCL is usually not necrotic or angiocentric
    - ALCL has much better clinical course
- Primary cutaneous CD4(+) small/medium pleomorphic T-cell lymphoma (SMPTCL)
  - Both can present with dermal T-cell infiltrate
  - SMPTCL is EBER(-), CD4(+), CD8(-)
    - Less necrosis and angioinvasion than ENNKTCL
- Angioimmunoblastic T-cell lymphoma (AITL)
  - Also presents as a dermal T-cell infiltrate and is EBER(+)
  - Less necrosis and angioinvasion than ENNKTCL
  - Increased follicular dendritic cells, unlike ENNKTCL
  - PD1(+), CXCL13(+), unlike ENNKTCL

SELECTED REFERENCES

1. Berti E et al: Cutaneous extranodal NK/T-cell lymphoma: a clinicopathologic study of 5 patients with array-based comparative genomic hybridization. Blood. 116(2):165-70, 2010
2. Huang Y et al: Gene expression profiling identifies emerging oncogenic pathways operating in extranodal NK/T-cell lymphoma, nasal type. Blood. 115(6):1226-37, 2010
3. Au WY et al: Clinical differences between nasal and extranasal natural killer/T-cell lymphoma: a study of 136 cases from the International Peripheral T-Cell Lymphoma Project. Blood. 113(17):3931-7, 2009
4. Choi YL et al: Extranodal NK/T-cell lymphoma with cutaneous involvement: 'nasal' vs. 'nasal-type' subgroups-- a retrospective study of 18 patients. Br J Dermatol. 160(2):333-7, 2009
5. Natkunam Y et al: Co-expression of CD56 and CD30 in lymphomas with primary presentation in the skin: clinicopathologic, immunohistochemical and molecular analyses of seven cases. J Cutan Pathol. 27(8):392-9, 2000
6. Chan JK et al: Nonnasal lymphoma expressing the natural killer cell marker CD56: a clinicopathologic study of 49 cases of an uncommon aggressive neoplasm. Blood. 89(12):4501-13, 1997

EXTRANODAL NK/T-CELL LYMPHOMA, NASAL TYPE

Imaging and Microscopic Features

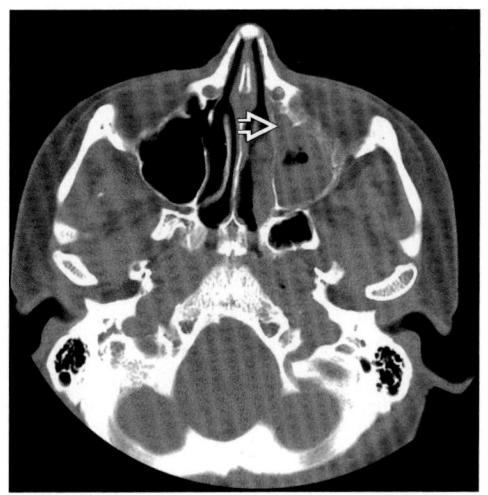

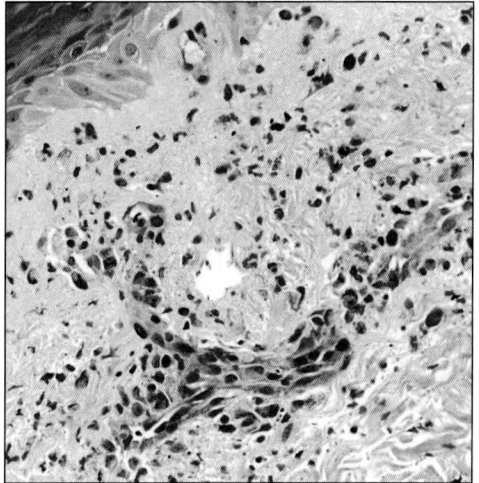

(Left) This is a CT scan of extranodal NK/T-cell lymphoma, nasal type that shows an almost completely opacified maxillary sinus and thickening of mucosa in the nasopharynx ➡. *(Courtesy L. J. Medeiros, MD.)* *(Right)* High-magnification view of ENNKTCL shows focal necrosis, hemorrhage, and atypical lymphoid cells surrounding a blood vessel. *(Courtesy L. J. Medeiros, MD.)*

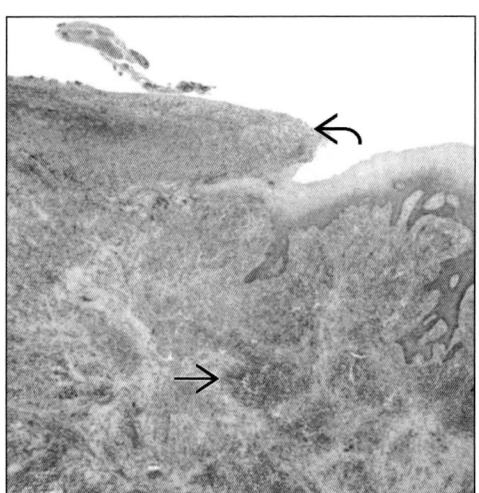

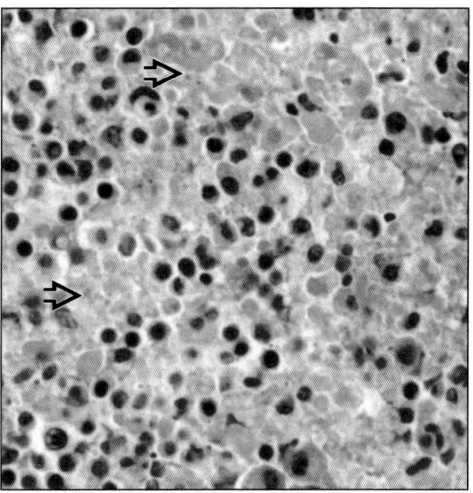

(Left) The surface of this example of ENNKTCL is extensively ulcerated ➡. Beneath the ulcerated surface, the tumor ➡ replaces the normal dermal architecture. *(Right)* There is extensive coagulative necrosis ➡ in this case of ENNKTCL. Necrosis is a classic morphologic feature in these tumors.

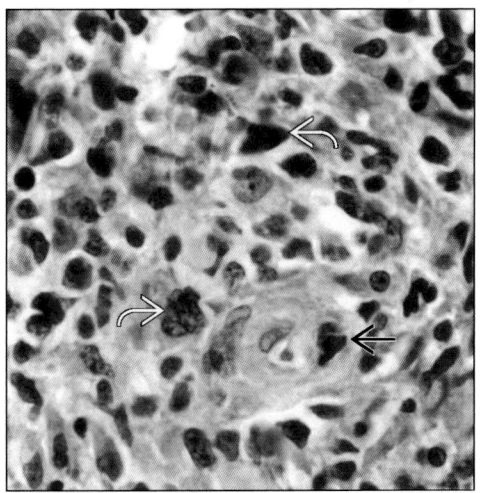

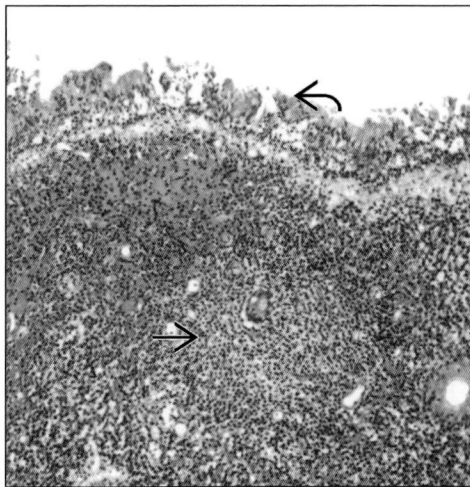

(Left) The tumor cells in ENNKTCL tend to be angiocentric and angioinvasive. The blood vessel is surrounded by frankly atypical tumor cells ➡ and shows malignant cells invading its wall ➡. *(Right)* The nasopharynx is the most common site of presentation for ENNKTCL. In this case, there is a diffuse/nodular infiltrate ➡ deep to the mucosal surface ➡.

Ancillary Techniques

(Left) This is a CD3(+) stain in a case of ENNKTCL. This antibody detects the epsilon chain of CD3 within the cell cytoplasm. Expression of CD3-ε chain is (+) in both T cells & NK cells. (Courtesy L. J. Medeiros, MD.) *(Right)* CD56 shows many positive neoplastic cells in ENNKTCL. CD56 is commonly (but not invariably) expressed, and CD56 is highly suggestive of, but not specific for, NK cell lineage. (Courtesy L. J. Medeiros, MD.)

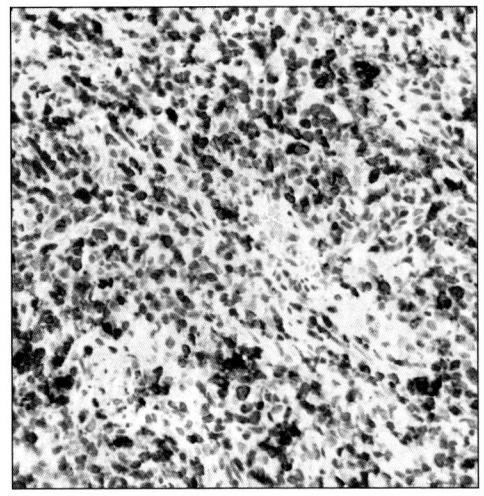
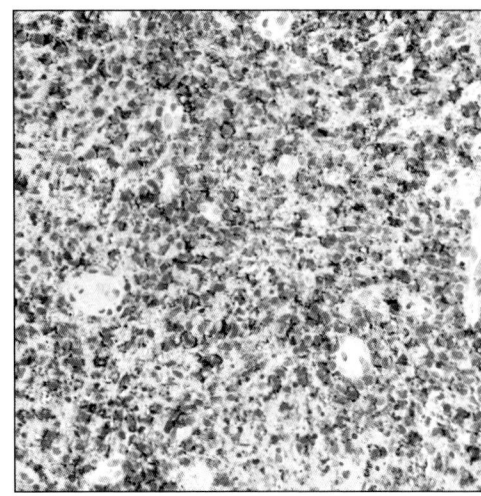

(Left) TIA-1 immunohistochemical stain shows that essentially all of the neoplastic cells in ENNKTCL are strongly (+). TIA, as well as granzyme-B and perforin, are cytotoxic markers that are usually expressed in ENNKTCL. (Courtesy L. J. Medeiros, MD.) *(Right)* Granzyme-B immunohistochemical stain highlights numerous neoplastic cells supporting cytotoxic lineage in ENNKTCL. (Courtesy L. J. Medeiros, MD.)

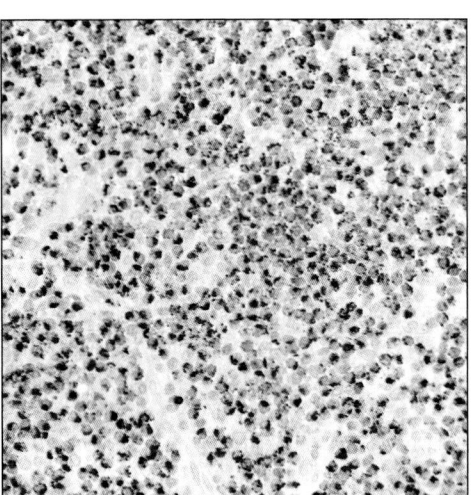
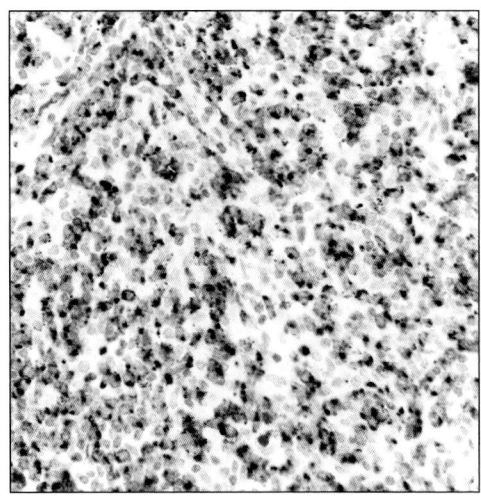

(Left) This CD8 immunohistochemical stain shows that the neoplastic cells are CD8(+), supporting T-cell lineage. (Courtesy L. J. Medeiros, MD.) *(Right)* This in situ hybridization test for Epstein-Barr virus small-encoded RNA (EBER) is strongly positive. EBV infection is an invariable feature of extranodal NK/T-cell lymphoma, nasal type as defined in the 2008 WHO Classification of Lymphoid Tumors. (Courtesy L. J. Medeiros, MD.)

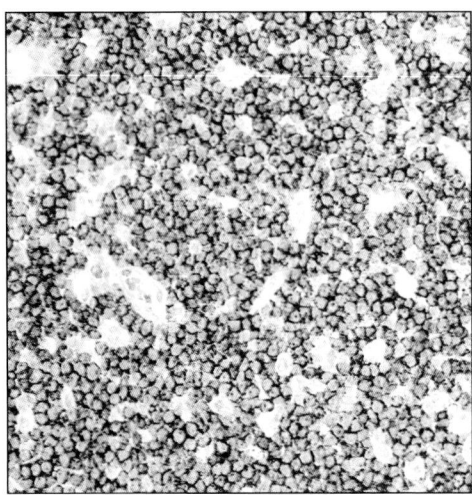
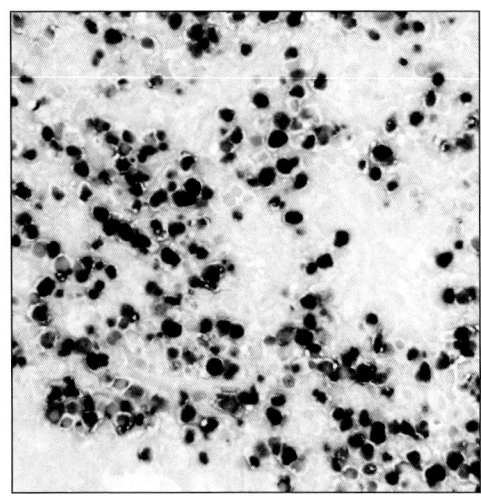

Differential Diagnosis

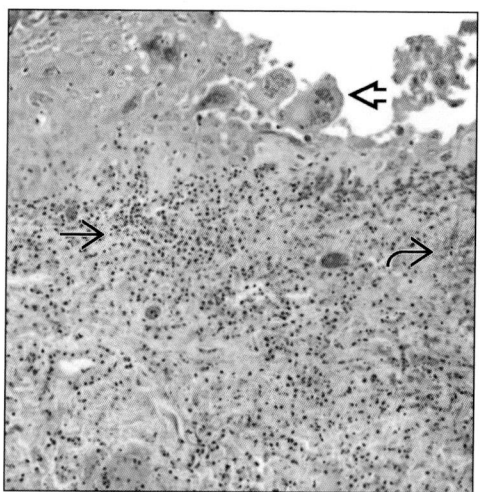

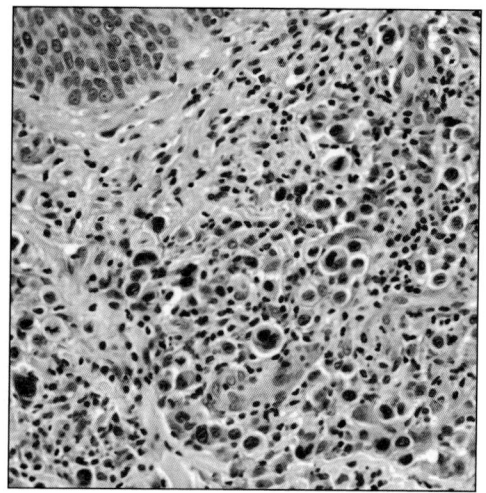

(Left) Herpes infection can mimic ENNKTCL. Many infections involve the nasal region. This herpes infection shows necrosis ⇥, like ENNKTCL, but has more acute inflammation ⇥, and virus-infected cells with multinucleation, chromatin margination, and moulding are identified ⇥. *(Right)* Histologic section from a patient with cutaneous ALCL shows large anaplastic cells with abundant cytoplasm and irregular multilobated nuclei, admixed with inflammatory cells.

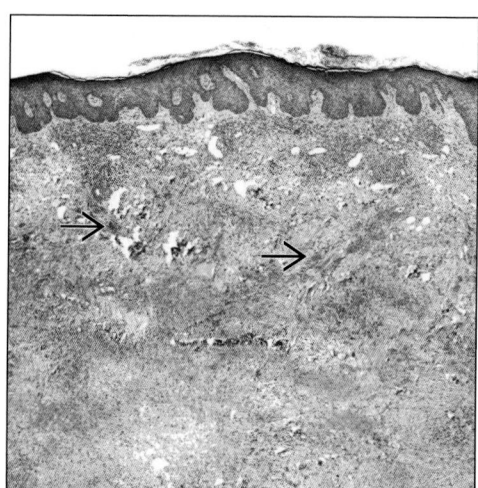

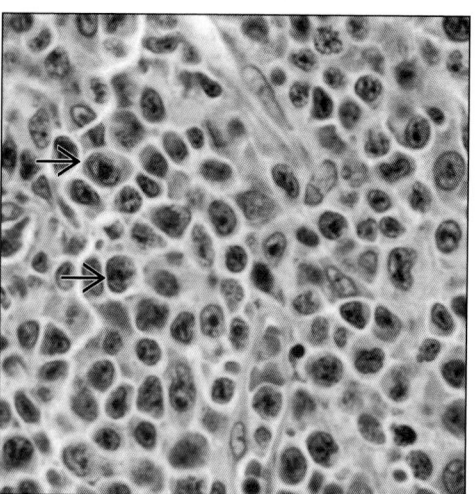

(Left) Lymphomatoid granulomatosis of skin is angiocentric ⇥, angiodestructive, and EBER(+), like ENNKTCL. However, this is a B-cell neoplasm and expresses multiple B-cell antigens. *(Right)* Diffuse large B-cell lymphoma (DLBCL) can also involve the upper airways like ENNKTCL. This DLBCL involves the maxillary sinuses. The tumor cells ⇥ are large and morphologically indistinguishable from ENNKTCL, but are CD20(+), CD19(+), and pax-5(+).

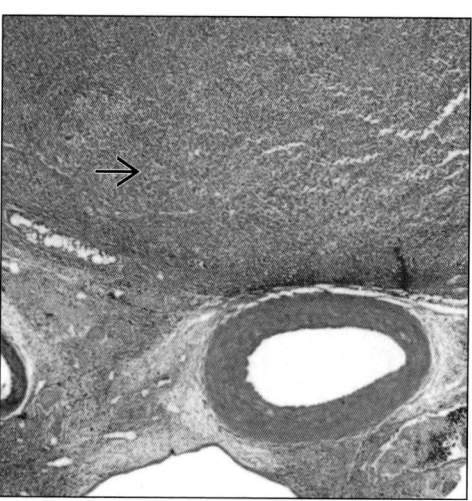

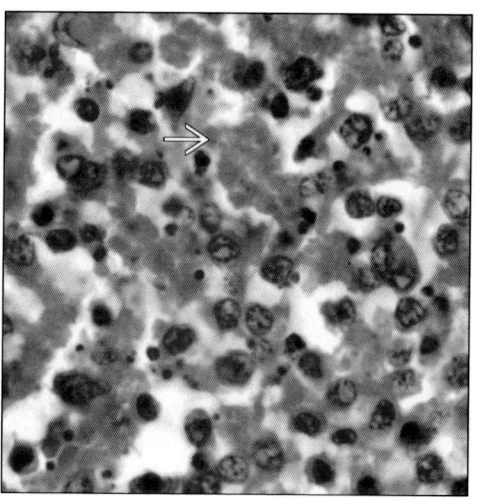

(Left) Here is a post-transplant lymphoproliferative disorder with an extranodal NK/T-cell lymphoma type. This patient developed a soft tissue/cutaneous lesion after transplant. The tumor shows a nodular aggregate of malignant cells in the soft tissue ⇥. *(Right)* This case of PTLD, extranodal NK/T-cell lymphoma type shows medium-sized tumor cells with extensive necrosis ⇥ that are CD3(+), CD56(+), TIA(+), granzyme-B(+), and EBER(+).

LYMPHOMATOID PAPULOSIS

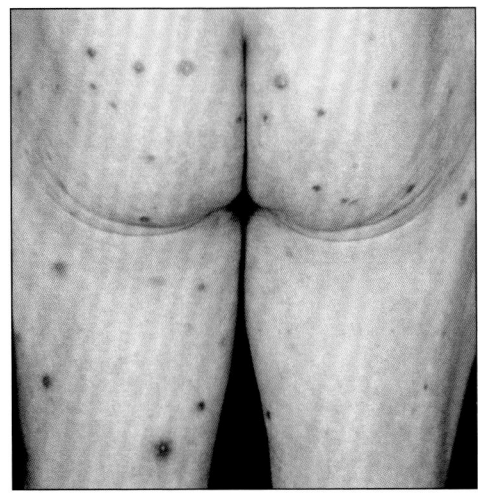

In this clinical photograph of LyP, there are papules around the buttocks and lower legs at different stages of evolution. (Courtesy R. Willemze, MD.)

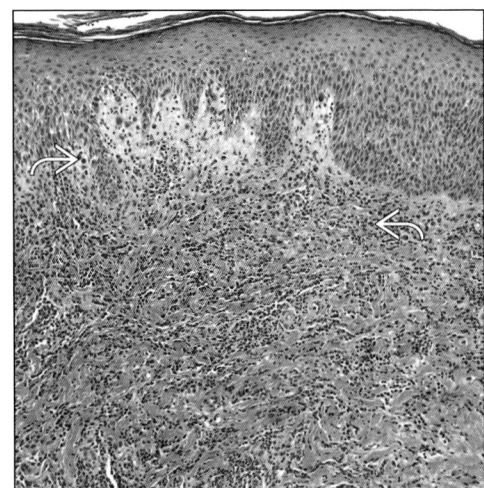

Low magnification of LyP type A shows epidermal acanthosis, spongiosis, and a mixed dermal infiltrate containing scattered large, hyperchromatic-staining atypical lymphocytes ➋.

TERMINOLOGY

Abbreviations
- Lymphomatoid papulosis (LyP)

Definitions
- Recurrent, self-healing cutaneous lesions composed of CD30(+) atypical T cells in polymorphous inflammatory background
  - One of the CD30(+) T-cell lymphoproliferative disorders (LyP, primary cutaneous anaplastic large cell lymphoma [C-ALCL], and borderline cases)

ETIOLOGY/PATHOGENESIS

Idiopathic
- Viral infection, chronic antigenic stimulation, and immunosuppression have all been implicated as factors in some cases

CLINICAL ISSUES

Epidemiology
- Incidence
  - 0.1-0.2 cases per 100,000
- Age
  - Mostly adults (30s to 50s), median age 45, less common in children
- Gender
  - Male:female = 3:1

Site
- Disease usually confined to skin
  - Common on trunk and extremities

Presentation
- Multiple erythematous papules or nodules
  - ± ulceration
  - Lesions at different stages of development

- New lesions simultaneously occur at multiple anatomic sites
- New lesions develop as old lesions regress
- May form vesicular, crusted, or hemorrhagic lesions

Natural History
- Lesions spontaneously heal with scarring
  - Individual skin lesions regress within 3-12 weeks
- Duration of disease
  - Waxing/waning clinical course; may persist for up to 40 years
- LyP-associated malignant lymphoma
  - Up to 20% of patients with LyP have another lymphoma
    - LyP may precede, proceed, or occur simultaneously with associated malignant lymphoma
    - Mycosis fungoides (MF), ALCL, Hodgkin lymphoma most common

Treatment
- Adjuvant therapy
  - No specific treatment for most patients other than follow-up to monitor changes in skin lesions
  - Sometimes low-dose methotrexate ± irradiation and psoralen ultraviolet A

Prognosis
- Excellent
  - ~ 100% 5-year survival
- 2% of associated lymphomas lead to death

MICROSCOPIC PATHOLOGY

Histologic Features
- Dermal infiltrate, often wedge-shaped or band-like, of medium- to large-sized T cells
  - Sometimes angiocentric
  - Folliculotropic if CD30(+) cells around hair follicles

LYMPHOMATOID PAPULOSIS

Key Facts

Terminology
- One of the CD30(+) T-cell lymphoproliferative disorders
- Recurrent lymphoproliferative cutaneous disorder
- Disorder with self-healing lesions that regress without treatment and have atypical CD30(+) T cells in polymorphous background

Clinical Issues
- Papules or nodules at different stages of development that regress
- 20% have LyP-associated malignant lymphoma
- Excellent prognosis

Microscopic Pathology
- Often wedge-shaped infiltrate; large atypical T cells
- Polymorphous background infiltrate

- 4 types: A, B, C, and D

Ancillary Tests
- CD3(+), CD30(+), CD4(+), CD8(-), cytotoxic markers(+)
- t(2;5)(p23;q35) negative
- Clonal T-cell receptor gene rearrangement in 40%

Top Differential Diagnoses
- Primary and systemic anaplastic large cell lymphoma
  ○ Differentiated from LyP based on morphology and clinical course
- Reactive conditions
  ○ Infection and drug reaction can mimic LyP by showing clusters of atypical CD30(+) cells
- Mycosis fungoides
  ○ Similar to type B LyP with epidermotropism

- Epidermis may show ulceration, hyperkeratosis, and parakeratosis
- Variable histology with 4 subtypes (A, B, C, D) representing spectrum of disease
  ○ **Type A (mixed infiltrate)**
    ▪ Few scattered large atypical Reed-Sternberg-like or multinucleated cells
    ▪ Abundant reactive polymorphous inflammatory cells
  ○ **Type B (mycosis fungoides-like)**
    ▪ Epidermotropism of small T cells showing cerebriform nuclei
    ▪ Only 10% of LyP cases
    ▪ Cannot be separated from MF by histology or immunohistochemistry
    ▪ Type B LyP spontaneously regresses, unlike MF
  ○ **Type C (ALCL-like)**
    ▪ Monotonous sheets of large atypical cells
    ▪ Scant polymorphous background infiltrate
    ▪ Cannot be separated from ALCL by histology or immunohistochemistry
  ○ **Type D (cytotoxic T-cell variant)**
    ▪ Marked epidermotropism and CD8(+)
- Polymorphous background infiltrate
  ○ Histiocytes, neutrophils, eosinophils, and lymphocytes
- Biopsy may show overlapping features of type A, B, or C

ANCILLARY TESTS

Immunohistochemistry
- T-cell antigens expressed: CD2(+), CD3(+), CD5(+), CD7(+)
  ○ ± loss of T-cell antigens (CD7 most common)
- CD30(+) necessary for diagnosis of type A and type C
  ○ CD30 often (-) in type B
  ○ ALK(-), EMA(-)
- Usually CD4(+), CD8(-), rarely CD8(+) cases (type D)
- Sometimes (+) for CD15, CD56 (10%), CD25, MUM1, TRAF, and Bcl-2

- Cytotoxic markers (+) (TIA-1, granzyme-B, perforin)

Cytogenetics
- No specific abnormalities

In Situ Hybridization
- t(2;5)(p23;q35) negative

PCR
- Clonal T-cell receptor gene rearrangement
  ○ In ~ 40% of LyP cases
  ○ Identical T-cell clone in LyP lesions and LyP-associated lymphoma in same patient by sequencing studies

DIFFERENTIAL DIAGNOSIS

Primary and Systemic ALCL
- Also CD30(+) T-cell lymphoproliferative disorders
- Similar morphology to LyP
  ○ Both show proliferation of large atypical T cells
  ○ Both have similar immunophenotype
    ▪ CD30 expression in LyP and ALCL
    ▪ CD4(+) and cytotoxic markers(+)
    ▪ ALK is negative in LyP and cutaneous (C-ALCL), (+) in systemic ALCL
- Differentiated from LyP based on morphology and clinical course
  ○ ALCL usually single nodular lesion
  ○ Polymorphous background infiltrate not as prominent
  ○ t(2;5)(p23;q35) can be positive in systemic ALCL, unlike LyP

Borderline Lesions
- Overlapping features of LyP and C-ALCL
- Unusual clinical features or discrepancy between clinical features and histology &/or immunophenotype
  ○ Multiple papules that do not regress
  ○ 1 or more nodular lesions that show mixed inflammatory infiltrate

LYMPHOMATOID PAPULOSIS

Comparison of Lymphomatoid Papulosis and Anaplastic Large Cell Lymphoma

Feature	Lymphomatoid Papulosis	Anaplastic Large Cell Lymphoma
Lesions	Multiple papules and nodules	Often 1 nodule, less often several nodules or occasionally papules
Natural history	Papules regress	May rarely regress, but generally recur
Lymph node involvement	No	Sometimes
Systemic involvement	No, only if LyP-associated malignant lymphoma develops	Rare
Morphology	Large atypical T cells	Large atypical T cells
Polymorphous background infiltrate	Often prominent	Not prominent
CD30	Positive, but lower % of CD30(+) cells (except type C)	Positive, with higher % of CD30(+) cells, often in sheets or nodules
ALK	Negative	Cutaneous type negative, systemic type positive
CD4	Positive	Positive
Cytotoxic markers	Positive	Positive
t(2;5)(p23;q35)	Negative	Rarely (+) in skin, commonly (+) in systemic cases
Treatment	Often no treatment, or low-dose methotrexate and psoralen ultraviolet A	Skin targeted therapy (local excision &/or radiation) for low-stage disease, chemotherapy for systemic disease

Mycosis Fungoides
- Similar to type B LyP
  - Both LyP and MF present with epidermotropism
- Different clinical course than LyP
  - Lacks self-regressing skin lesions
  - Clinical course: Patches → plaques → tumor stage

Reactive Conditions
- Viral infections can mimic LyP
  - HSV, VZV, EBV, HPV
  - Dense infiltrate in dermis with CD30(+) T cells
  - Resolves in a few weeks
  - ± viral inclusions
  - IHC for viral antigens
  - PCR for viral DNA may be needed for definite diagnosis
- Arthropod bite reactions and dermatophyte infections can also mimic LyP
- Drug reactions can mimic LyP
  - Histology shows clusters of large CD30(+) cells in dermal T-cell infiltrate
  - History of drug use
  - Resolves after discontinuation of drug
- Pityriasis lichenoides et varioliformis acuta (PLEVA)
  - Common in children/young adults
  - Scaly erythematous/hemorrhagic lesions
  - Interface dermatitis with necrotic keratinocytes and Civatte/colloid bodies
  - CD8(+), CD30(-) (usually)

Classic Hodgkin Lymphoma
- Similarities to LyP
  - Hodgkin-like cells can be seen in LyP type A
  - Both tumors have polymorphous background infiltrate
  - Both are CD30(+)
- Differences from LyP
  - Rarely involves skin
  - Often CD15(+), EBER(+)
  - B-cell lymphoma, whereas LyP is a T-cell proliferation

- Classic Hodgkin lymphoma is often pax-5(+)

Primary Cutaneous Aggressive Epidermotropic CD8(+) Cytotoxic T-cell Lymphoma (AEC-TCL)
- Can be morphologically indistinguishable from cytotoxic variant of LyP (type D)
  - Both are CD8(+), CD30(+), cytoxic markers(+)
  - Worse prognosis with AEC-TCL than LyP

SELECTED REFERENCES

1. Saggini A et al: A variant of lymphomatoid papulosis simulating primary cutaneous aggressive epidermotropic CD8+ cytotoxic T-cell lymphoma. Description of 9 cases. Am J Surg Pathol. 34(8):1168-75, 2010
2. de Souza A et al: Clinical, histopathologic, and immunophenotypic features of lymphomatoid papulosis with CD8 predominance in 14 pediatric patients. J Am Acad Dermatol. 61(6):993-1000, 2009
3. El Shabrawi-Caelen L et al: Lymphomatoid papulosis: reappraisal of clinicopathologic presentation and classification into subtypes A, B, and C. Arch Dermatol. 140(4):441-7, 2004
4. Kempf W et al: Fascin expression in CD30-positive cutaneous lymphoproliferative disorders. J Cutan Pathol. 29(5):295-300, 2002
5. Bekkenk MW et al: Primary and secondary cutaneous CD30(+) lymphoproliferative disorders: a report from the Dutch Cutaneous Lymphoma Group on the long-term follow-up data of 219 patients and guidelines for diagnosis and treatment. Blood. 95(12):3653-61, 2000
6. Kummer JA et al: Most primary cutaneous CD30-positive lymphoproliferative disorders have a CD4-positive cytotoxic T-cell phenotype. J Invest Dermatol. 109(5):636-40, 1997

LYMPHOMATOID PAPULOSIS

Microscopic and Immunohistochemical Features

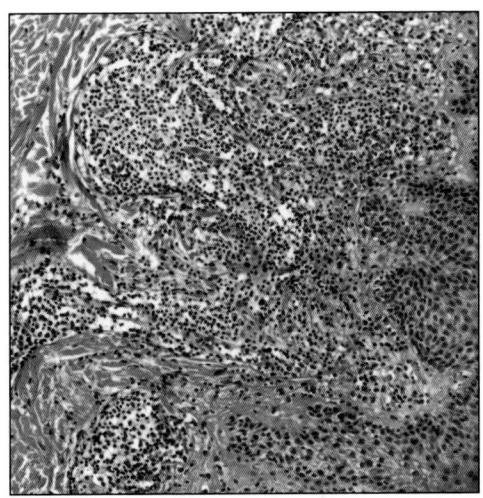

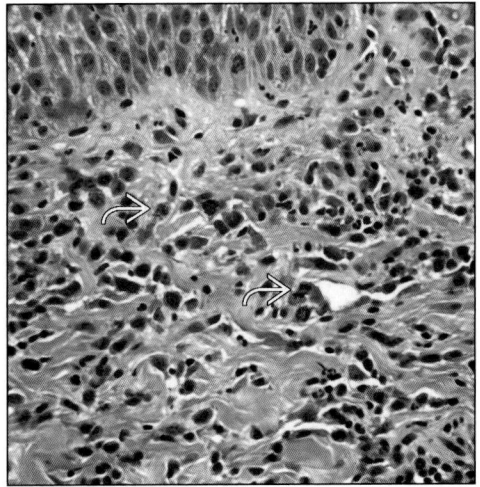

(Left) Histologic section shows lymphomatoid papulosis (LyP) type A. The lesion involves the dermis and is composed of a mixed population of small to medium-sized lymphocytes with scattered large cells. (Courtesy C. Yin, MD.) (Right) Higher magnification of LyP type A shows that the lesion involves the dermis and is composed of a mixed population of small to medium-sized lymphocytes with scattered large cells. Note the presence of mitotic figures ⟹.

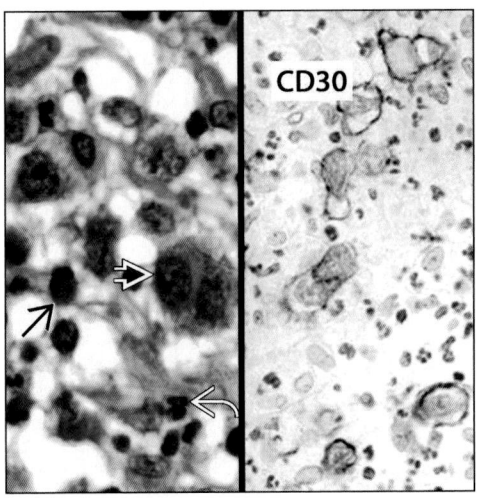

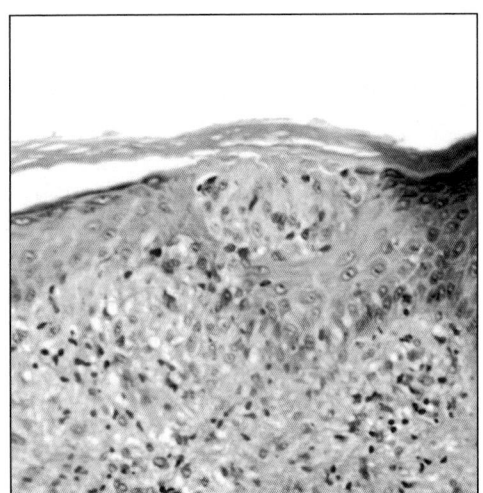

(Left) This lymphomatoid papulosis shows a type A pattern with scattered large atypical cells ⟹ and a mixed background infiltrate of eosinophils ⟶ and neutrophils ⟹. The CD30 stain highlights the large atypical cells. (Courtesy M. Tomaszewski, MD.) (Right) This case of LyP has a type B pattern of infiltration with epidermotropism. There are small T cells in the epidermis with cerebriform nuclei. CD30 is negative, as expected in type B.

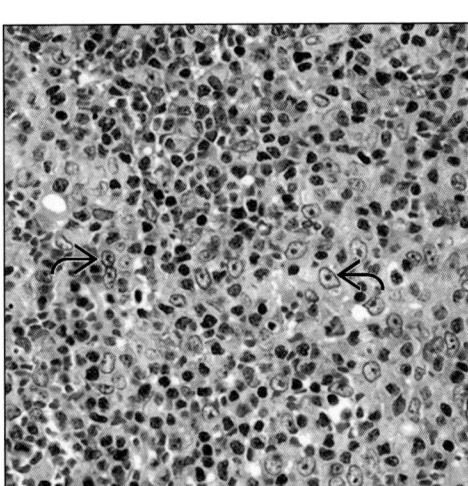

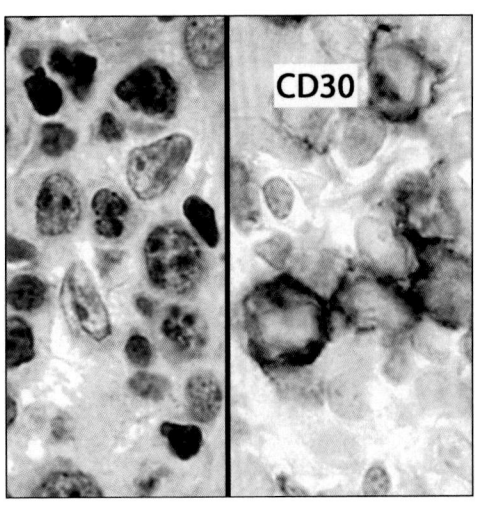

(Left) In this case of lymphomatoid papulosis type C, there are sheet-like aggregates of large atypical cells with vesicular chromatin, prominent nucleoli ⟹, and pale cytoplasm, with only a sparse lymphocytic background. (Right) This high-power image of type C LyP shows that the large atypical cells express CD30 by immunohistochemical staining. The aggregates of CD30(+) T cells are similar to anaplastic large cell lymphoma. (Courtesy M. Tomaszewski, MD.)

Ancillary Techniques

(Left) Immunohistochemical study for CD30 in a case of LyP type A shows large atypical cells that are CD30(+), usually singly scattered, and represent a minority cell population in type A cases. (Courtesy C. Yin, MD.) *(Right)* CD3 is also expressed in the T-cell infiltrate, as expected in LyP. T-cell antigens including CD2(+), CD3(+), CD5(+), and CD7(+) are immunoreactive in LyP. Sometimes there can be loss of one of the T-cell antigens, with CD7 being most common. (Courtesy C. Yin, MD.)

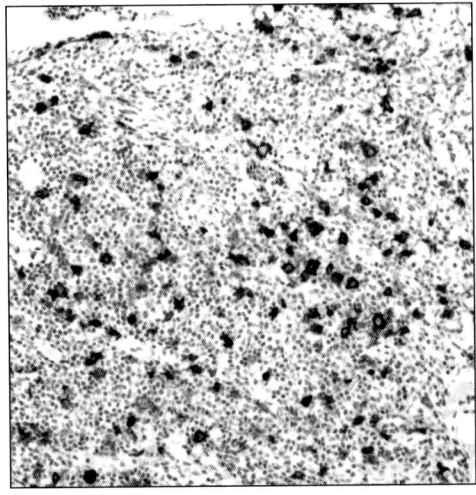
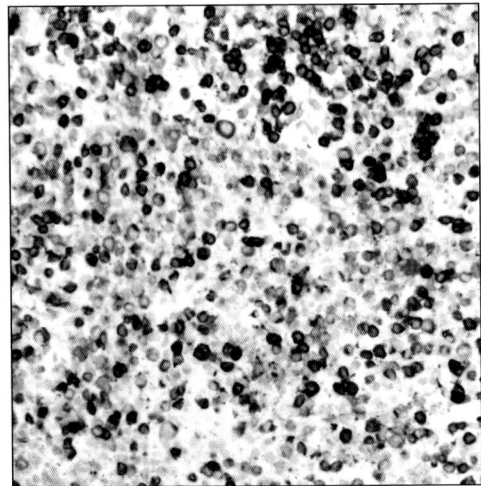

(Left) The CD30 immunohistochemical stain is strongly and diffusely positive in the infiltrate in this case of LyP type C. CD30(+) is also seen in anaplastic large cell lymphoma and in other reactive conditions including infections and some drug reactions. (Courtesy C. Yin, MD). *(Right)* Immunohistochemical study for Ki-67 in a case of LyP type C shows that lymphoid cells of LyP usually have a high proliferative rate. (Courtesy C. Yin, MD.)

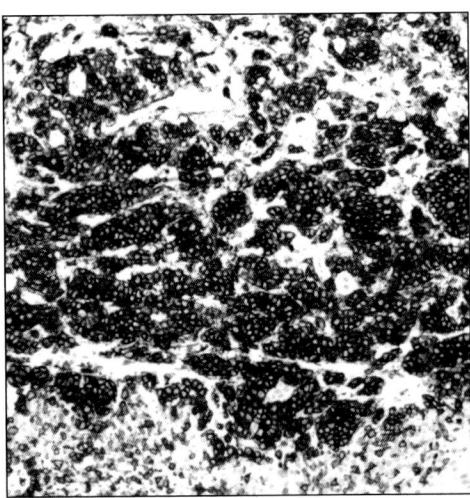
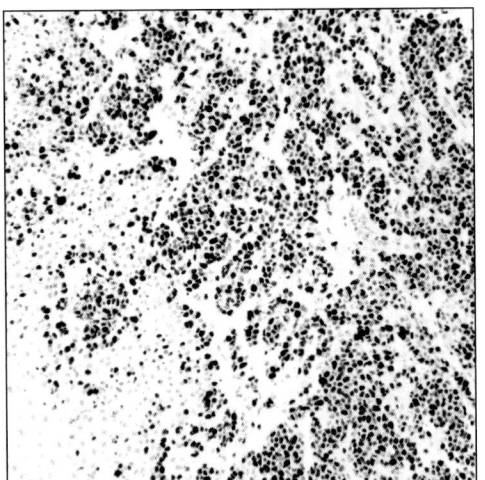

(Left) This break-apart probe FISH for 2p23(ALK) shows the lack of ALK rearrangement in a patient with LyP. A blue signal ➤ represents the ALK 5' region, and a pink signal ➜ represents the ALK 3' region. Two combined yellow signals indicate that ALK has not rearranged. (Courtesy N. Potter, MD and G. Nichols, MD.) *(Right)* In this case of LyP, the blue peak between 180 and 280 base pairs in size is suggestive of a clonal T-cell rearrangement, as is seen in 40% of cases of LyP.

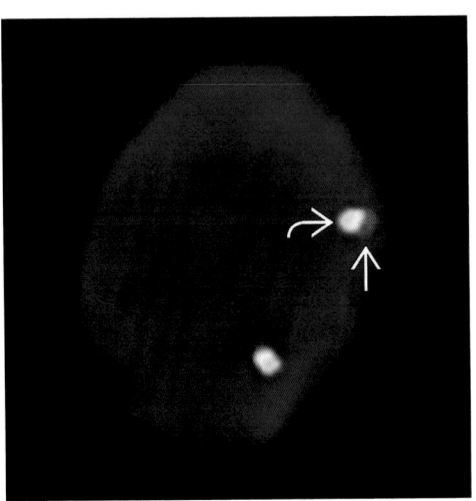
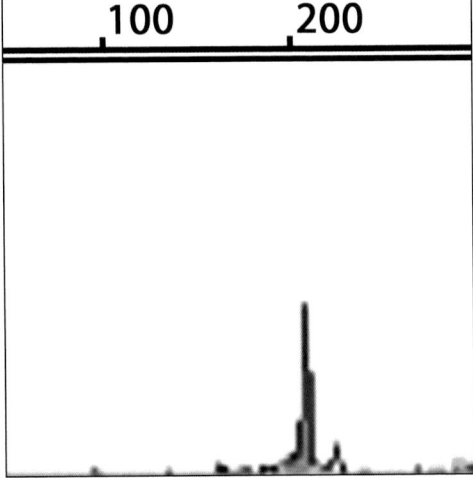

Differential Diagnosis

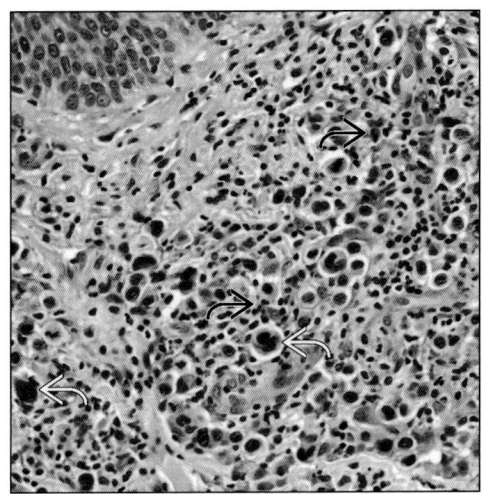
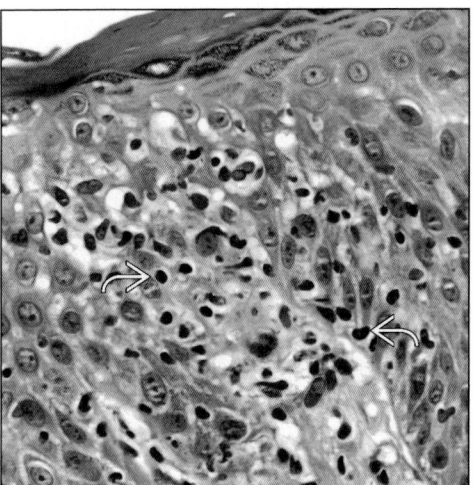

(Left) ALCL shows large anaplastic cells with abundant cytoplasm and irregular multilobated nuclei ⇗, admixed with inflammatory cells including a few eosinophils ⇗. The histologic findings are essentially identical to those in LyP, and clinical findings are essential to distinguish these entities. (Courtesy C. Yin, MD.) (Right) This case of mycosis fungoides shows epidermotropism of numerous small but hyperchromatic-staining T cells ⇗ in the epidermis, similar to type-B LyP.

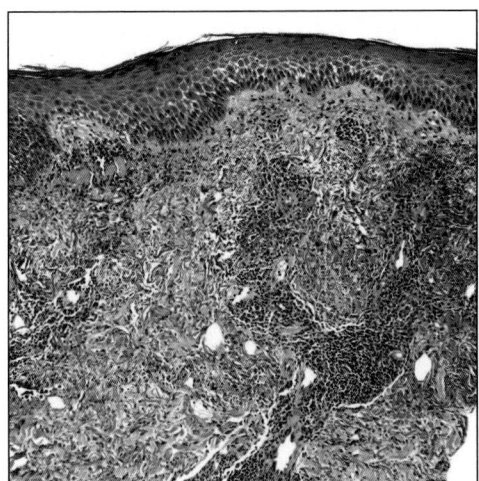
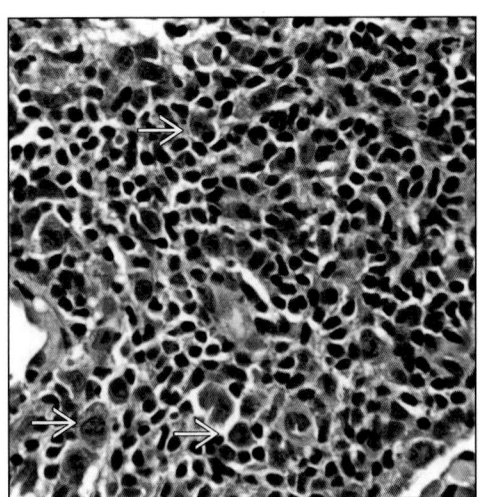

(Left) Dermatophyte infection mimicking LyP. At low power, there is a dense, atypical inflammatory infiltrate involving the entire dermis. These mononuclear cells with atypia appear similar to the atypical T cells in LyP. Many reactive conditions can mimic LyP, but the most common are infections and drug reactions. (Right) At higher power, large atypical cells ⇒ in the dermis form aggregates and appear identical to those seen in LyP.

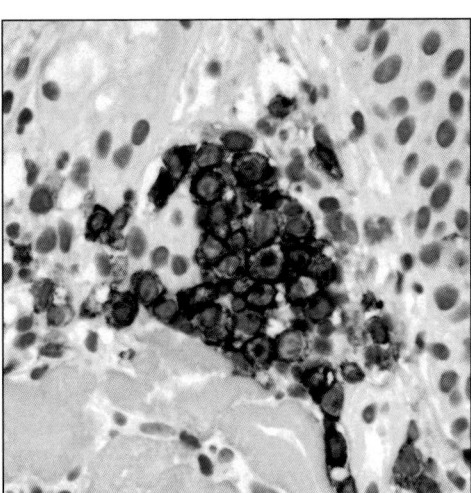
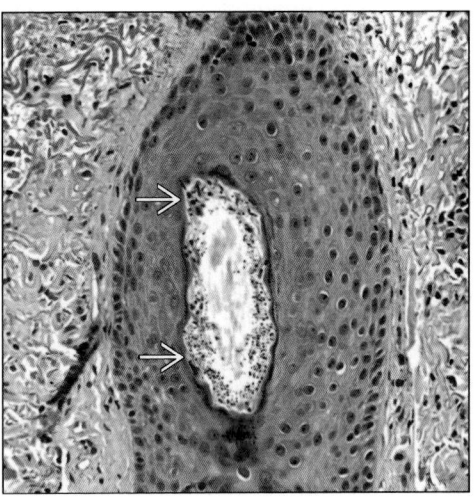

(Left) CD30(+) cells in dermatophyte infection. In the same case of dermatophyte infection, high magnification of a CD30 IHC stain shows that the large atypical cells are strongly immunoreactive for CD30, just like the T cells of LyP. (Right) Also in the same case, this hair follicle contains numerous hyphal organisms ⇒, which is diagnostic for a dermatophyte infection. Infections and arthropod bite reactions can mimic LyP, especially when they show increased CD30(+) cells.

PRIMARY CUTANEOUS ANAPLASTIC LARGE CELL LYMPHOMA

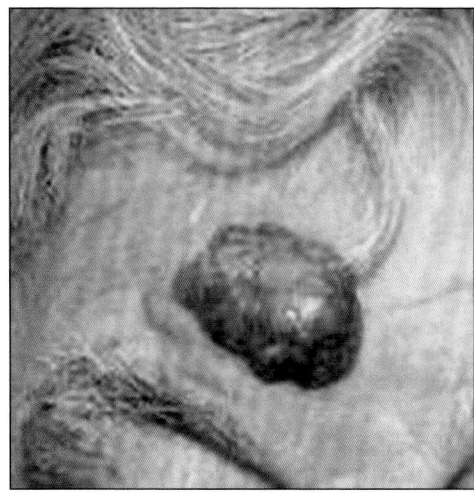

This is a solitary raised nonulcerated tumor nodule on the forehead of a man diagnosed with primary cutaneous anaplastic large cell lymphoma. (Courtesy R. Willemze, MD.)

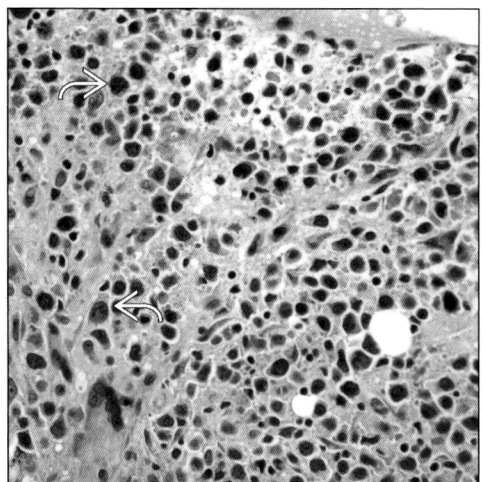

Histologic section of cutaneous ALCL shows large atypical cells with abundant cytoplasm and irregular multilobated nuclei ➡, admixed with a background of small inflammatory cells.

TERMINOLOGY

Abbreviations
- Primary cutaneous anaplastic large cell lymphoma (PCALCL)

Synonyms
- Regressing atypical histiocytosis
- Primary cutaneous large cell T-cell lymphoma, CD30(+)

Definitions
- CD30(+) T-cell lymphoma consisting of atypical, usually large cells, without evidence of mycosis fungoides
  - One of the primary cutaneous CD30(+) T-cell lymphoproliferative disorders, including lymphomatoid papulosis (LyP) and borderline lesions

ETIOLOGY/PATHOGENESIS

Idiopathic
- Viral infection, chronic antigen stimulation, and immunosuppression may play a role
- Mechanism may involve CD30/TRAF1 upregulation of NF-κB

CLINICAL ISSUES

Epidemiology
- Incidence
  - 2nd most common cutaneous T-cell lymphoma after mycosis fungoides
    - 0.1-0.2 per 100,000 people
    - 20% of systemic ALCL cases involve skin
- Age
  - Median age: 60s, but can occur in children
- Gender

- Male:female = 2-3:1

Site
- Often trunk, face, and extremities

Presentation
- Solitary or localized nodules, tumors, or papules
  - ± ulceration
  - Multifocal ~ 20%
- Usually no symptoms other than mass effect

Natural History
- Partial or complete spontaneous regression (40%), but frequently recur
- Extracutaneous dissemination ~ 10%
  - Usually to regional lymph nodes

Treatment
- Adjuvant therapy
  - Radiation for localized nodules
  - Methotrexate for multifocal lesions
  - Chemotherapy for systemic disease

Prognosis
- Better than most T-cell lymphomas
  - ~ 90% 10-year survival
  - Age < 60 years and spontaneous regression are good prognostic indicators
  - Systemic disease is poor prognostic indicator
    - Multifocal skin lesions and local lymph node involvement do not yield worse prognosis

MICROSCOPIC PATHOLOGY

Histologic Features
- Diffuse sheets of large T cells in the dermis ± subcutis
  - Infrequent epidermotropism ± ulceration
  - Can involve lymphatic spaces
- Tumor cells
  - Large anaplastic, pleomorphic, or immunoblastic appearance

PRIMARY CUTANEOUS ANAPLASTIC LARGE CELL LYMPHOMA

Key Facts

Terminology
- One of the primary cutaneous CD30(+) T-cell lymphoproliferative disorders
  - T-cell lymphoma of atypical, usually large CD30(+) cells, without evidence of mycosis fungoides

Clinical Issues
- Solitary or localized nodules that can regress but frequently occur
- Can involve regional lymph nodes
- Treated with skin-targeted therapy for low-stage disease, chemotherapy for systemic disease
- Good prognosis, ~ 90% 10-year survival

Microscopic Pathology
- Polymorphic background infiltrate not prominent
- Diffuse sheets of large T cells in the dermis ± subcutis

- Hallmark cells with multiple nuclei (horseshoe-shaped), helpful if present

Ancillary Tests
- Immunohistochemistry: CD30(+), CD15(-), CD3(+), cytotoxic markers(+), EMA(-), ALK(-), CLA(+)
- Molecular: No *ALK* gene translocations on chromosome 2

Top Differential Diagnoses
- Systemic ALCL with cutaneous involvement
  - EMA(+), ALK(+) and *ALK* gene translocations, unlike primary cutaneous ALCL
- Lymphomatoid papulosis (LyP)
  - Groups of papules that regress and recur
  - Wedge-shaped and prominent polymorphous background infiltrate

---

- Anaplastic cells with roundish shapes ± abundant cytoplasm
  - Small cell and histiocyte-rich variants are rare
- Mitotic figures
- Hallmark cells with multiple nuclei (horseshoe-shaped), often not seen, but helpful if present
- Polymorphic background infiltrate (eosinophils and plasma cells) uncommon, unlike LyP
  - Exceptions
    - Ulcerating ALCL has polymorphic infiltrate, fewer CD30(+) cells, and epidermal hyperplasia
    - Neutrophil-rich (pyogenic ALCL) shows clusters of neutrophils with only scattered CD30(+) cells

ANCILLARY TESTS

Immunohistochemistry
- CD30(+) (> 75% of tumor cells), CD15(-)
- T-cell antigens expressed (CD2[+], CD3[+], CD5[+], CD7[+])
  - But can show loss of T-cell antigens
    - CD7 most common
- CD4(+)/CD8(-)
  - CD8(+) and CD4(-)/CD8(-) rarely
- Cytotoxic markers positive
  - Granzyme-B, perforin, TIA
- EMA(-) and ALK(-) in PCALCL
  - Usually EMA(+) and ALK(+) in systemic ALCL
  - ALK(+) skin tumor likely indicates secondary cutaneous ALCL
- Cutaneous lymphocyte antigen (CLA[+]) and HOXC5(+) in PCALCL
  - But CLA(-) in systemic ALCL
- Negative for B-cell markers (CD20 and CD79)
  - Rarely positive for pax-5

Cytogenetics
- No specific findings

Molecular Genetics
- Clonal T-cell receptor gene rearrangement ~ 90%
- No translocations of *ALK* gene on chromosome 2p23

DIFFERENTIAL DIAGNOSIS

Systemic ALCL with Cutaneous Involvement
- Similar morphologic features and overlapping phenotype with PCALCL
- Separate disease from PCALCL, with different molecular findings and prognosis
  - Primary tumor in extracutaneous site that secondarily involves skin
- Differences from PCALCL
  - Systemic ALCL also found in extracutaneous sites
  - Typically EMA(+) and ALK(+), unlike PCALCL
  - Translocations involving *ALK* gene
  - Less favorable prognosis (especially ALK[-] systemic ALCL)

Lymphomatoid Papulosis (LyP)
- Also CD30(+) T-cell lymphoproliferative disorder, but with more polymorphic background infiltrate
- Both often present with large atypical T cells
- Both have similar immunophenotype
  - CD30(+) in LyP and ALCL
  - CD4(+) and cytotoxic markers(+)
  - ALK is negative in both, except for systemic ALCL
- Differentiated from ALCL based on morphology and clinical course
  - Usually more of a wedge-shaped infiltrate
  - Polymorphic background infiltrate is prominent
  - Groups of papules that regress without treatment and often recur
  - Better prognosis than ALCL
  - Sometimes only clinical findings can differentiate ALCL from LyP

Borderline Lesions
- Another type of primary cutaneous CD30(+) T-cell lymphoproliferative disorder
- Discrepancy between clinical features and histology/ immunophenotype
  - Examples of borderline lesions
    - Case with clinical features of LyP (multiple papules/nodules), which are present with a

PRIMARY CUTANEOUS ANAPLASTIC LARGE CELL LYMPHOMA

Translocations in Systemic Anaplastic Large Cell Lymphoma

Translocation	Percentage of Cases	Gene Partner	IHC Staining
t(2;5)(p23;q35)	84	NPM	Nuclear, cytoplasmic
t(1;2)(q25;p23)	13	TPM3	Cytoplasmic
inv(2)(p23;q35)	1	ATIC	Cytoplasmic
t(X;2)(q11-12;p23)	< 1	MSN	Membrane
t(2;3)(p23;q12)	< 1	TFG	Cytoplasmic
t(2;17)(p23;q25)	< 1	ND	Cytoplasmic
t(2;17)(p23;q23)	< 1	CLTC	Granular cytoplasmic
t(2;19)(p23;p13.1)	< 1	TPM4	Cytoplasmic
t(2;22)(p23;q11.2)	< 1	MYH9	Cytoplasmic

CD30(+) Skin Diseases

	PCALCL	LyP	Systemic ALCL
Morphology	Dermal anaplastic cells, few inflammatory cells	Variable numbers of anaplastic cells with mixed inflammatory background cells	Same as PCALCL
Dissemination	Can be in regional lymph nodes	Confined to skin	LN and extranodal sites can be involved
IHC	EMA(-), ALK(-)	EMA(-), ALK(-)	EMA(±), ALK(±)
Prognosis	10-year survival ~ 90%	10-year survival ~ 100%	10-year survival ~ 35%

morphology more typical of ALCL (sheets of large atypical cells)
  - Case with clinical features of ALCL (solitary nonregressing lesion) with histology more like LyP (fewer atypical cells and polymorphous background infiltrate)

Large Cell Transformation of Mycosis Fungoides (MF)
- Patient with history/clinical evidence of MF
  o Patches, plaques, or tumors
- Large atypical T cells with similar phenotype to ALCL
  o CD4(+), CD30(±)
- ≥ 25% large T cells in tumor
  o Can look identical to neoplastic cells in ALCL
- Often loses epidermotropism

Reactive Conditions Expressing CD30
- Viruses, arthropod bites, and drugs are the most common reactive conditions that mimic ALCL
  o They can show clusters of large CD30(+) cells
  o Diagnosis may need clinical correlation or PCR for viral DNA

Classic Hodgkin Lymphoma
- Similarities to ALCL
  o Both have CD30(+) cells
  o Both have large, atypical tumor cells
  o Pax-5(+) in 50% of classic Hodgkin lymphoma and rare cases of ALCL
- Differences from ALCL
  o Rare in skin
  o CD15(+)
  o EBER(+)
  o LCA(-)
  o Malignant cells not in aggregates

Diffuse Large B-cell Lymphoma
- Similar large, atypical cells as in ALCL, and can be CD30(+)
- However, strongly expresses B-cell antigens (CD20, CD19, pax-5)

SELECTED REFERENCES

1. Feldman AL et al: PAX5-positive T-cell anaplastic large cell lymphomas associated with extra copies of the PAX5 gene locus. Mod Pathol. 23(4):593-602, 2010
2. Burg G et al: Pyogenic lymphoma of the skin: a peculiar variant of primary cutaneous neutrophil-rich CD30+ anaplastic large-cell lymphoma. Clinicopathological study of four cases and review of the literature. Br J Dermatol. 148(3):580-6, 2003
3. Bekkenk MW et al: Primary and secondary cutaneous CD30(+) lymphoproliferative disorders: a report from the Dutch Cutaneous Lymphoma Group on the long-term follow-up data of 219 patients and guidelines for diagnosis and treatment. Blood. 95(12):3653-61, 2000
4. Boulland ML et al: Primary CD30-positive cutaneous T-cell lymphomas and lymphomatoid papulosis frequently express cytotoxic proteins. Histopathology. 36(2):136-44, 2000
5. Stein H et al: CD30(+) anaplastic large cell lymphoma: a review of its histopathologic, genetic, and clinical features. Blood. 96(12):3681-95, 2000
6. Gascoyne RD et al: Prognostic significance of anaplastic lymphoma kinase (ALK) protein expression in adults with anaplastic large cell lymphoma. Blood. 93(11):3913-21, 1999

PRIMARY CUTANEOUS ANAPLASTIC LARGE CELL LYMPHOMA

Microscopic Features

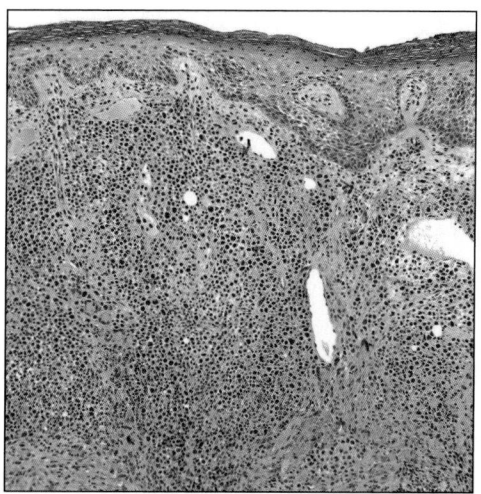

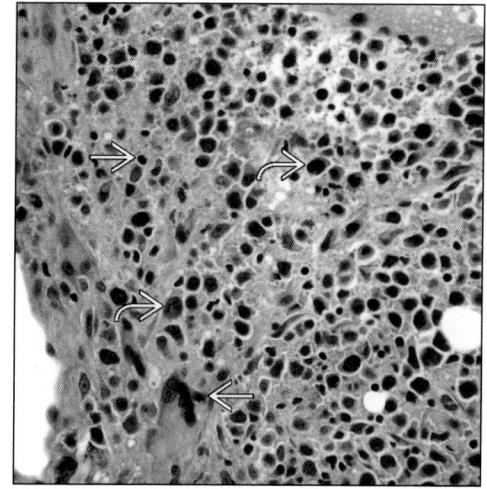

(Left) Low magnification histologic section from a patient with primary cutaneous ALCL shows a diffuse, sheet-like proliferation of numerous large atypical cells with abundant cytoplasm and hyperchromatic nuclei admixed with smaller inflammatory cells. (Right) Higher magnification of ALCL shows large atypical cells with abundant cytoplasm and irregular multilobated nuclei ➡, admixed with a background of small inflammatory cells including eosinophils ➡.

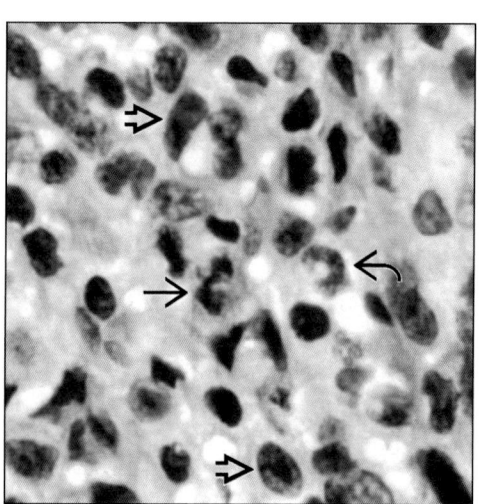

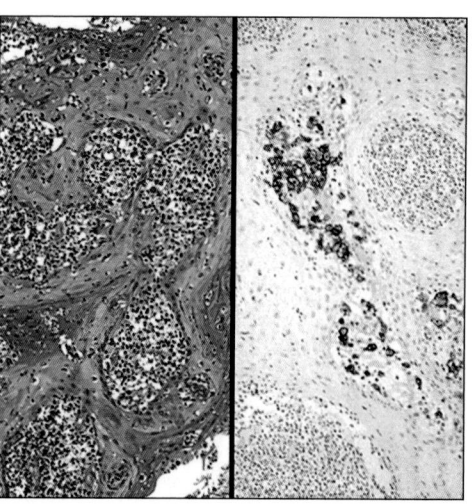

(Left) At high power, the malignant T cells ➡ are large with dense chromatin and irregular nuclear shapes. Scattered mitotic figures ➡ are easily seen. Rare cells have the horseshoe-shaped nuclei of so-called hallmark cells ➡. No neutrophils or eosinophils are seen. (Right) This case of ALCL is primarily involving the lymphatic spaces. The right side of the image is a CD30 immunohistochemical stain, which marks the tumor cells within the lymphatics. (Courtesy M. Tomaszewski, MD.)

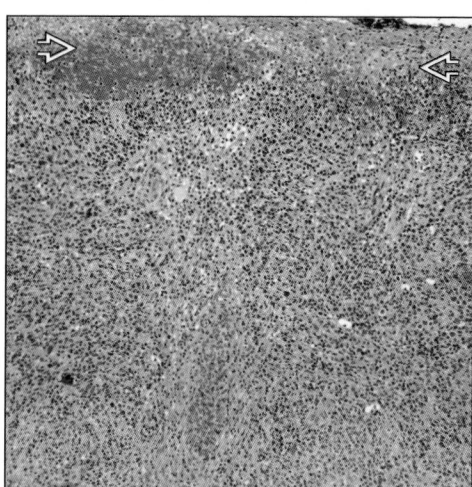

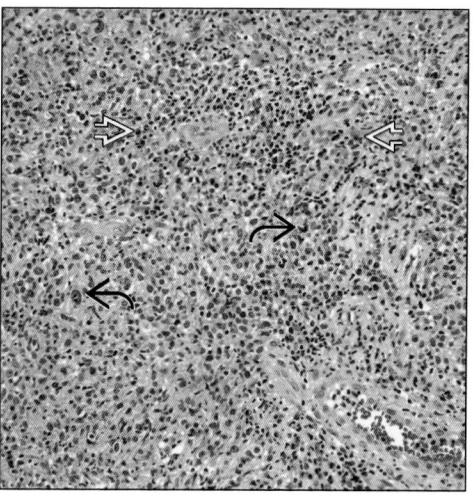

(Left) Ulcerated lesion of primary cutaneous ALCL shows dense serum crusting ➡ overlying a dense mixed inflammatory infiltrate with eosinophils, which can be numerous in a small number of cases. (Right) Higher magnification of an ulcerated lesion of primary cutaneous ALCL shows a dense mixed inflammatory infiltrate with scattered large, atypical cells ➡ and numerous eosinophils ➡, mimicking LyP.

Ancillary Techniques

(Left) In this case of ALCL, on the left-sided H&E, one can see the large anaplastic-appearing malignant cells. On the right is a CD3 immunohistochemical stain that shows the malignant cells immunoreactive for CD3, as expected in this T-cell lymphoma. **(Right)** This high-power image of a CD4 IHC stain shows that the tumor cells are CD4(+). CD8 (not shown) was negative. Most cases of ALCL are CD4(+)/CD8(-), and only 5% are CD4(-)/CD8(+).

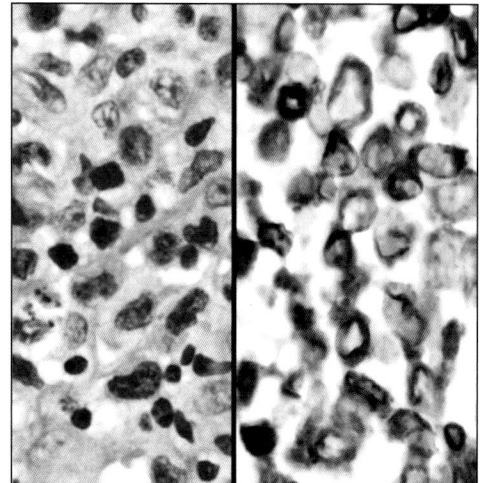
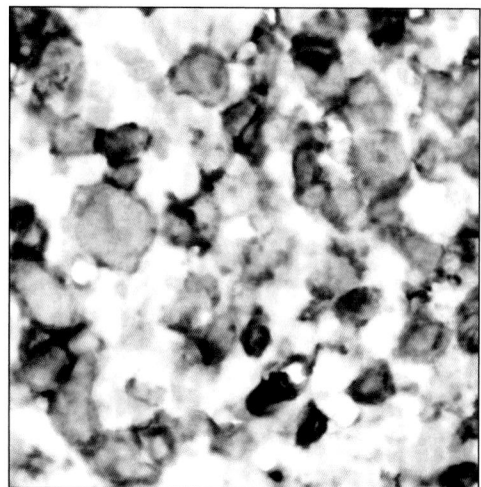

(Left) Negative ALK immunohistochemical stain in a primary cutaneous ALCL is shown, which is typically ALK negative. **(Right)** Positive ALK immunohistochemical stain. This is a systemic ALCL with secondary cutaneous involvement, which is often ALK positive. Currently, systemic ALCL is either classified as ALK(+) or ALK(-) and are considered different diseases.

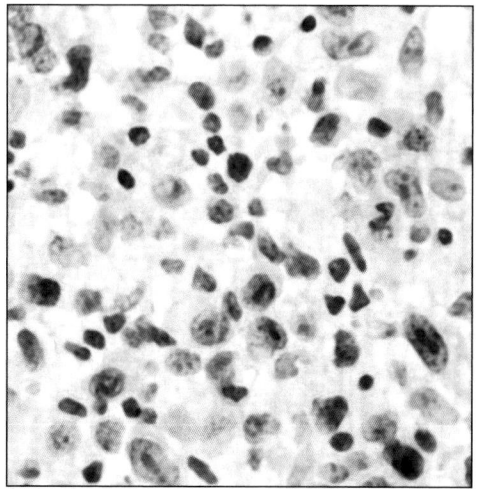
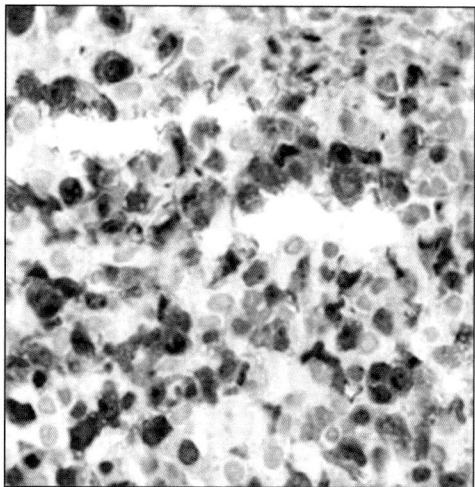

(Left) Positive EMA immunohistochemical stain. This is a case of systemic ALCL with secondary involvement of skin, which is often EMA positive. Cases of primary cutaneous ALCL are EMA negative. **(Right)** A break-apart probe FISH test for 2p23 (ALK). The ALK rearrangement most commonly seen in ALCL shows a blue signal ➡ representing the 5' region of ALK and a pink signal ➡ representing the 3' region of ALK.

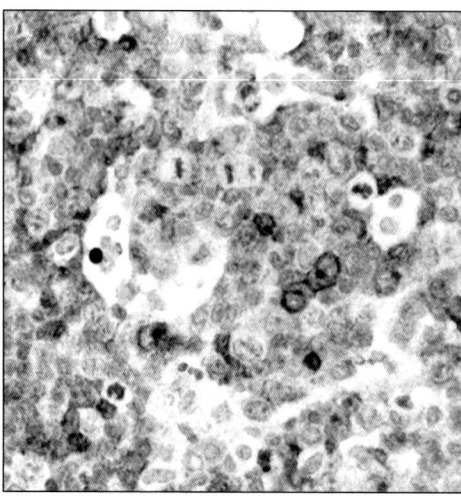
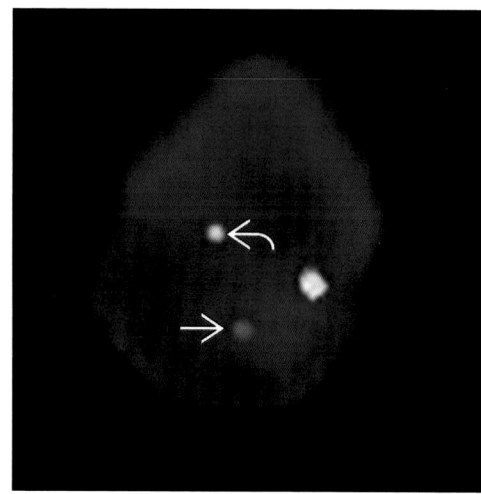

I

12

PRIMARY CUTANEOUS ANAPLASTIC LARGE CELL LYMPHOMA

Differential Diagnosis

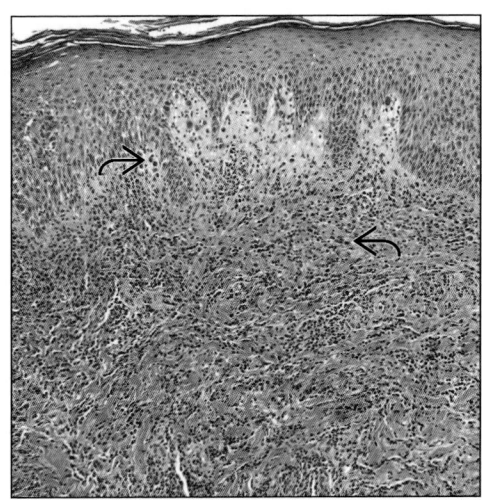

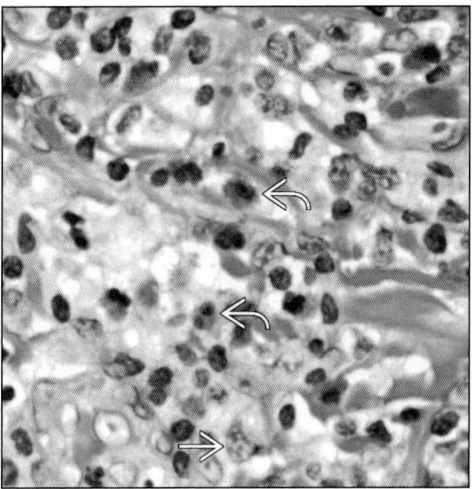

(Left) ALCL can be difficult to distinguish from LyP, especially type C. Low magnification of LyP shows epidermal acanthosis, spongiosis, and a mixed dermal infiltrate containing scattered large, hyperchromatic-staining atypical lymphocytes ➡. *(Right)* This case of lymphomatoid papulosis has scattered large atypical cells ➡ as seen in ALCL but has a prominent polymorphous background infiltrate with eosinophils ➡ and histiocytes, which are not a common feature of ALCL.

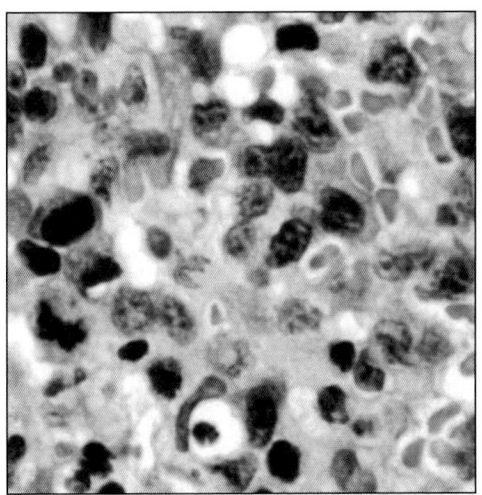

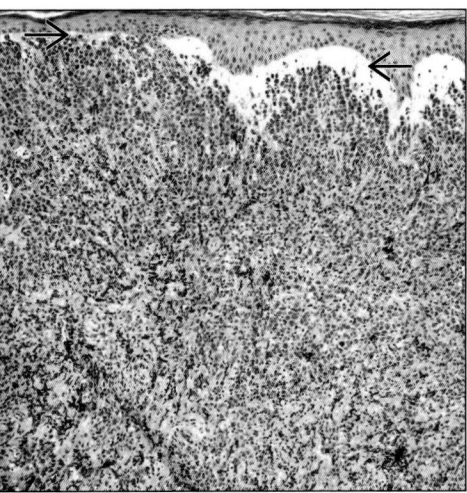

(Left) Systemic ALCL involving the skin. These are essentially indistinguishable from primary cutaneous ALCL without clinical history and immunohistochemistry for ALK and EMA. *(Right)* Primary cutaneous diffuse large B-cell lymphoma, leg type can be difficult to distinguish from ALCL without immunohistochemistry. Low magnification shows a diffuse, sheet-like infiltrate replacing the dermis with a thin grenz zone ➡ and sparing of the epidermis.

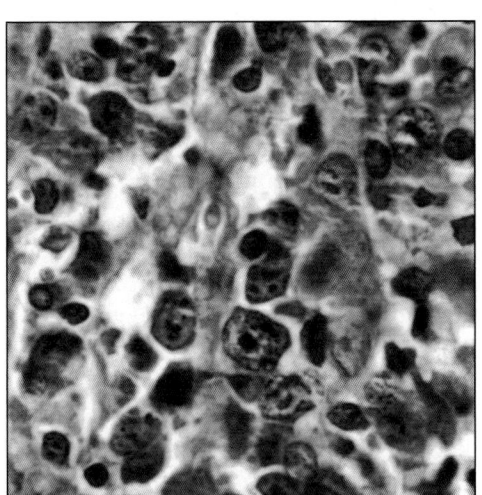

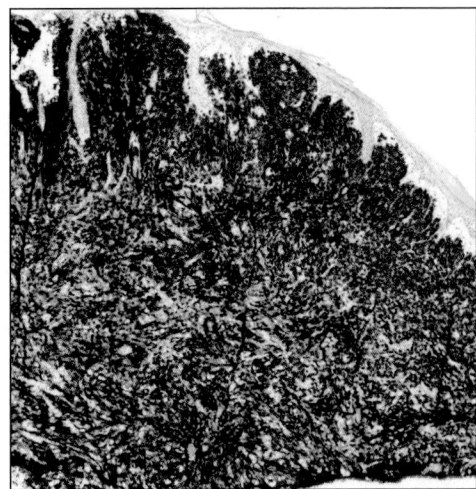

(Left) This diffuse large B-cell lymphoma has large atypical malignant cells with morphology akin to ALCL and is CD30(+). Unlike ALCL, this case is CD20(+), CD79(+), and is t(14;18)(+) by FISH. *(Right)* CD20 shows very strong and diffuse staining in this primary cutaneous diffuse large B-cell lymphoma, leg type. This finding excludes ALCL and is diagnostic of a B-cell lymphoma.

AGGRESSIVE EPIDERMOTROPIC CD8+ CYTOTOXIC T-CELL LYMPHOMA

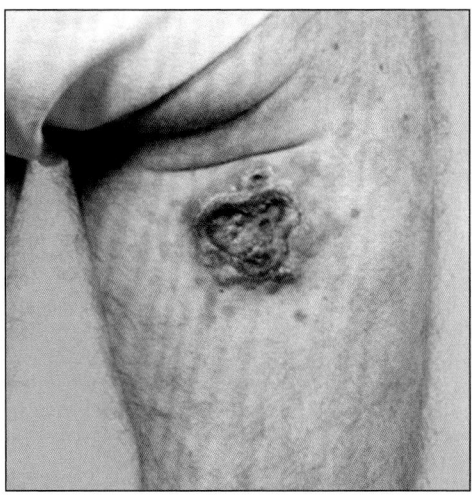

This is a clinical photograph of a large tumor on the posterior leg of a person with AECTCL. As is typical of this disease, the lesion is extensively ulcerated. (Courtesy R. Willemze, MD.)

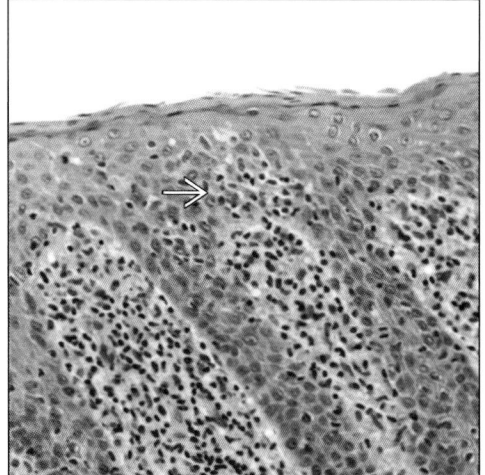

This is a medium magnification of a case of AECTCL with considerable epidermotropism ➡. The T cells in the epidermis are medium in size with moderate atypia and coarse chromatin.

TERMINOLOGY

Abbreviations
- Aggressive epidermotropic cytotoxic T-cell lymphoma (AECTCL)

Synonyms
- Primary cutaneous aggressive epidermotropic cytotoxic T-cell lymphoma

Definitions
- T-cell lymphoma consisting of CD8(+) cytotoxic αβ T cells prominently involving the epidermis and exhibiting aggressive clinical behavior
  - Provisional entity in the 2008 WHO Classification of Hematopoietic and Lymphoid Tissues
  - Previously included in cases of peripheral T-cell lymphoma, not otherwise specified (PTCL, NOS)
  - Often separated from other CD8(+) lymphomas based on clinical behavior

CLINICAL ISSUES

Epidemiology
- Incidence
  - Rare
    - < 1% of cutaneous T-cell lymphomas
- Age
  - Adults
    - Median age: 53
- Gender
  - Male:female = 1.4:1.0

Presentation
- Skin lesions
  - Often tumors, nodules, and papules
    - Less often patches or plaques
  - Usually ulceration &/or necrosis
  - Often widespread disseminated lesions
- Rapid extracutaneous spread

  - Fairly frequent
  - Lungs, testes, brain, and oral cavity involved
  - Lymph nodes are usually spared

Treatment
- Adjuvant therapy
  - Often multiagent chemotherapy

Prognosis
- Aggressive clinical course
  - 32-month median survival
  - No difference in prognosis if tumor cells are smaller or larger
  - 1 study suggests that CD2(-)/CD7(+) cases have worse prognosis

MICROSCOPIC PATHOLOGY

Histologic Features
- T-cell infiltrate in dermis
  - Can involve superficial dermis or deeper tissues
    - Sometimes angiocentric
    - Sometimes lichenoid
    - Destroys adnexa
- Epidermotropism
  - Can be pagetoid spread with linear colonization of basal epidermis
- Epidermis
  - Ulceration, necrosis, or blister common
  - Can be acanthotic or atrophic
    - Variable apoptotic keratinocytes and spongiosis
- Variable numbers of histiocytes
  - Rare eosinophils and plasma cells

Cytologic Features
- Small to medium-sized T cells with moderate to marked atypia, coarse or blastic chromatin

AGGRESSIVE EPIDERMOTROPIC CD8+ CYTOTOXIC T-CELL LYMPHOMA

Key Facts

Terminology

- Provisional diagnosis in the 2008 WHO, T-cell lymphoma consisting of CD8(+) cytotoxic αβ T cells in epidermis, exhibiting aggressive clinical behavior
- Previously included in cases of peripheral T-cell lymphoma, not otherwise specified
- Often separated from other CD8(+) lymphomas based on clinical behavior

Clinical Issues

- Rare
- Often disseminated tumors, nodules, and papules with ulceration/necrosis
- Rapid spread to lungs, testes, brain, and oral cavity
- Often spares lymph nodes
- Often treated with multiagent chemotherapy
- Aggressive clinical course

Microscopic Pathology

- T-cell infiltrate in dermis with epidermotropism
- Small to medium-sized T cells with moderate to marked atypia

Ancillary Tests

- CD3(+), CD2(+), βF1(+), CD4(-), CD8(+), LMP1(-), CD15(-/+), CD56(+/-)
- Clonal for T-cell receptor gene gamma rearrangement

Top Differential Diagnoses

- Mycosis fungoides
  - Is rarely CD8(+), but progression to tumor stage often takes years
- Lymphomatoid papulosis
  - More banal clinical course with papules that spontaneously regress

---

ANCILLARY TESTS

Immunohistochemistry

- T-cell antigens (+) (CD3, CD2, CD7)
  - Sometimes 1 or more T-cell antigens lost
    - CD5 is most commonly lost
- Positive for cytotoxic markers
  - Granzyme-B, perforin, and TIA1(+)
- αβ T cells
  - βF1(+), TCR-δ-1(-)
- Cytotoxic cells
  - CD4(-), CD8(+)
- Negative for Epstein-Barr virus markers (LMP1), CD15(-/+), CD56(+/-)
- High proliferative rate by MIB-1 (> 90% of tumor cells)

Cytogenetics

- No specific abnormalities identified

Molecular Genetics

- Clonal for T-cell receptor gene gamma rearrangement

DIFFERENTIAL DIAGNOSIS

Mycosis Fungoides

- Vast majority of cases: CD4(+)/CD8(-), unlike AECTCL
  - Slower natural history of disease
    - Progression from patch to plaque to tumor often takes years
  - Less necrosis by morphology

Pagetoid Reticulosis

- Localized
  - Woringer-Kolopp disease
    - CD8(+) cases are reported, which appear histologically and immunophenotypically similar to AECTCL
    - Has a different clinical picture, with much less aggressive disease, a protracted clinical course, and less necrosis than AECTCL
- Disseminated
  - Ketron-Goodman disease

- Currently considered a form of AECTCL and is not separately classified

Lymphomatoid Papulosis (LyP)

- Similarities to AECTCL
  - Can rarely present with epidermotropism and CD8(+) T cells (type D LyP)
  - Both CD8(+) LyP and AECTCL lack eosinophils and plasma cells
  - Both present with markedly atypical T cells with angiocentric growth pattern
- Differences from AECTCL
  - Presents with papules, usually non-ulcerating, that often regress
  - No extracutaneous systemic involvement
  - CD30(+), which is uncommon in AECTCL

Adult T-cell Lymphoma/Leukemia

- Also epidermotropic T-cell infiltrate
  - However, patients show serology for HTLV-1 and the cells usually are CD4(+)

Extranodal NK/T-cell Lymphoma, Nasal Type

- Both show angiocentric infiltrates, CD56(+), and necrosis
  - Different phenotype with CD16(+) and EBER(+)

SELECTED REFERENCES

1. Saggini A et al: A variant of lymphomatoid papulosis simulating primary cutaneous aggressive epidermotropic CD8+ cytotoxic T-cell lymphoma. Description of 9 cases. Am J Surg Pathol. 34(8):1168-75, 2010
2. Csomor J et al: Rare provisional entity: primary cutaneous aggressive epidermotropic CD8+ cytotoxic T-cell lymphoma in a young woman. J Clin Pathol. 61(6):770-2, 2008
3. Magro CM et al: CD8+ lymphomatoid papulosis and its differential diagnosis. Am J Clin Pathol. 125(4):490-501, 2006
4. Berti E et al: Primary cutaneous CD8-positive epidermotropic cytotoxic T cell lymphomas. A distinct clinicopathological entity with an aggressive clinical behavior. Am J Pathol. 155(2):483-92, 1999

AGGRESSIVE EPIDERMOTROPIC CD8+ CYTOTOXIC T-CELL LYMPHOMA

Microscopic and Immunohistochemical Features

(Left) At scanning magnification of an AECTCL, there is a dense dermal lymphoid infiltrate, which also involves the epidermis. The dermal infiltrate is angiocentric, which is a common infiltration pattern in AECTCL. *(Right)* At medium magnification, one is more able to see the dermal infiltrate ➡ extending into the epidermis ➡. The T cells in the epidermis are seen singly and in small clusters, disrupting much of the epidermis.

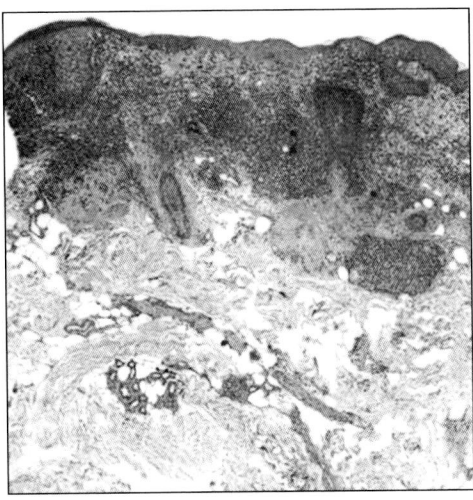
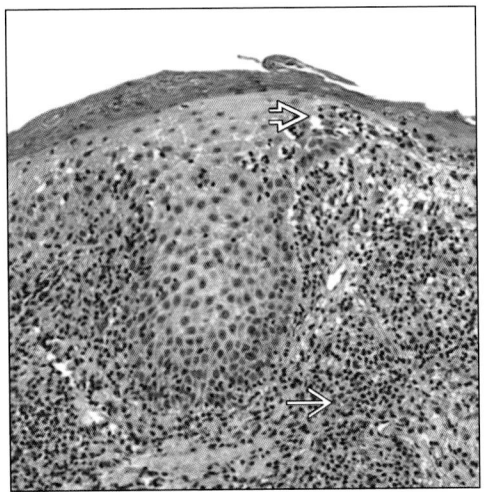

(Left) At high magnification, the epidermotropic lymphocytes have coarse chromatin and irregular nuclear contours. There is moderate atypia. *(Right)* Another case of AECTCL at high magnification demonstrates T cells that are larger in size with marked atypia ➡ and somewhat vesicular chromatin. There is a large amount of necrosis ➡ in the background, as is often found in AECTCL. Skin ulceration was also present in some sections.

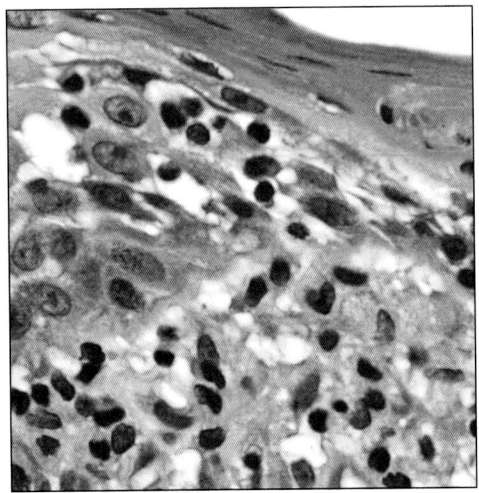
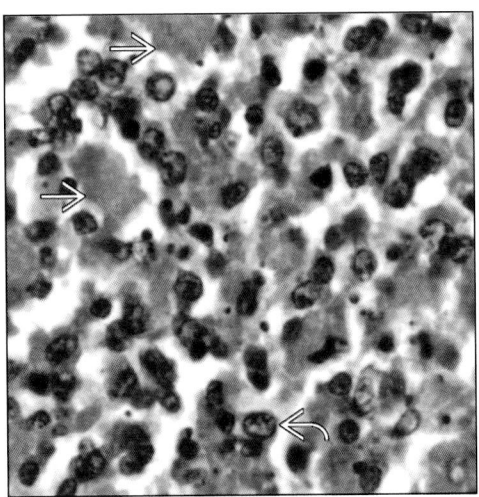

(Left) CD8 shows strong cytoplasmic immunoreactivity in the malignant T cells in this case of AECTCL. The atypical CD8(+) cells are located in the dermis ➡ and epidermis ➡. *(Right)* This βF1 immunohistochemical stain strongly marks the malignant T cells in the epidermis in a case of AECTCL, indicating that these are αβ T cells. This tumor is also CD3(+), CD4(-), LMP1(-), CD15(-), and CD56(-) (not shown).

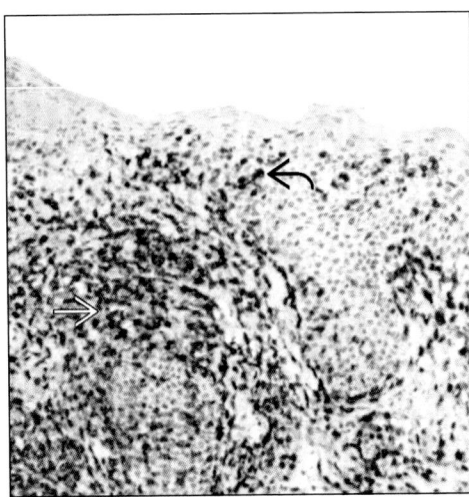
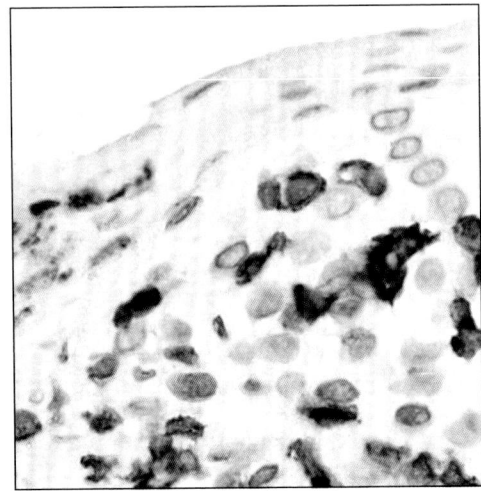

AGGRESSIVE EPIDERMOTROPIC CD8+ CYTOTOXIC T-CELL LYMPHOMA

Differential Diagnosis

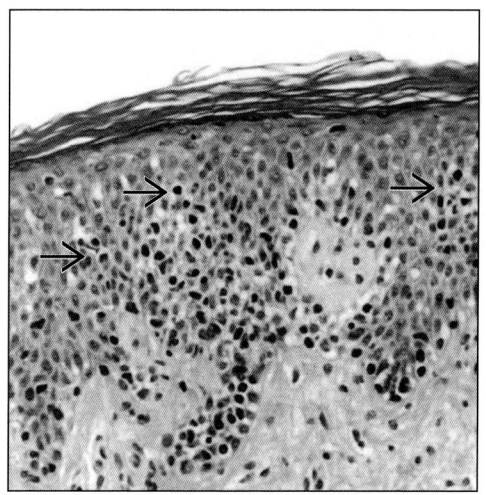

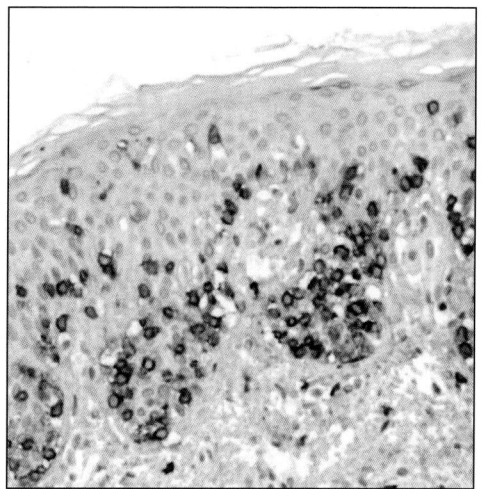

(Left) This is a case of CD8(+) mycosis fungoides. There are malignant T cells ⇨ singly and scattered in the epidermis, a morphologic pattern identical to AECTCL. *(Right)* In the same case of CD8(+) mycosis fungoides, a CD8 immunohistochemical stain marks the T cells in the epidermis. A minority of cases of mycosis fungoides are CD4(-)/CD8(+), unlike the vast majority of AECTCL. Mycosis fungoides shows less necrosis than AECTCL and has a slower natural history of disease.

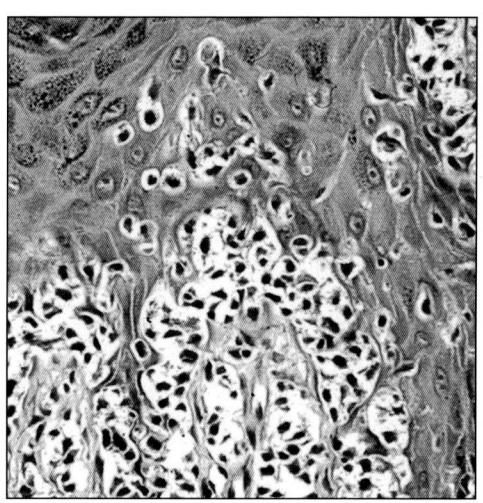

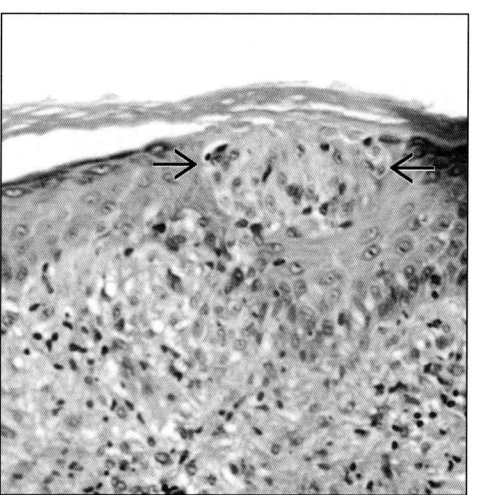

(Left) Pagetoid reticulosis (PR) shows prominent spongiosis and haloed T cells. This extensive epidermotropism can be confused with AECTCL, but PR would be a single lesion. *(Courtesy M. Tomaszewski, MD.)* *(Right)* This case of lymphomatoid papulosis, type B shows clusters of atypical T cells ⇨ in the epidermis, similar to AECTCL. Both diseases present with atypical T cells, but LyP presents with self-healing, non-ulcerating papules without extracutaneous involvement.

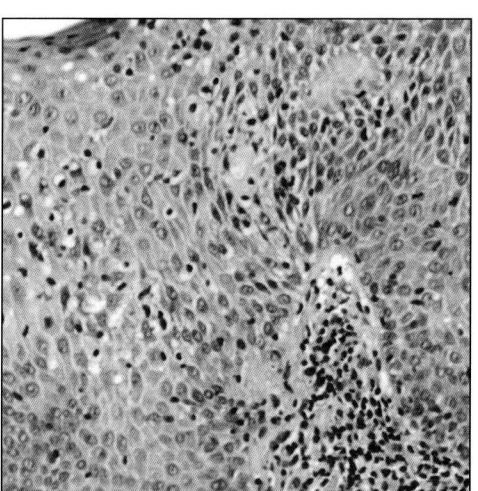

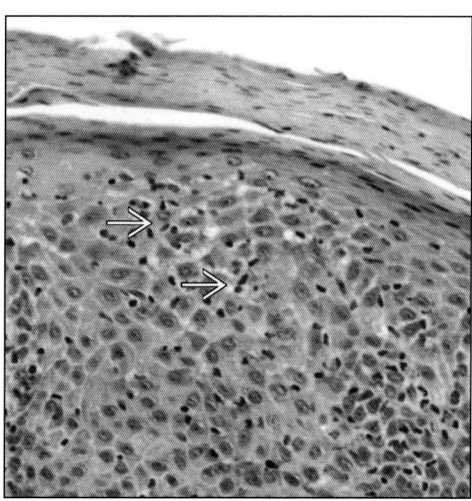

(Left) This case of cutaneous adult T-cell leukemia/lymphoma (ATLL) is similar to AECTCL with significant epidermotropism. While both tumors show malignant epidermotropic T cells, ATLL has CD4(+) T cells, and AECTCL has CD8(+) T cells (and presents in HTLV1(-) patients). *(Right)* In this case of a spongiotic dermatitis, there are scattered lymphocytes ⇨ in the spongiotic areas, mimicking epidermotropism. The lymphocytes are small and lack significant atypia.

PRIMARY CUTANEOUS CD4+ SMALL/MEDIUM PLEOMORPHIC T-CELL LYMPHOMA

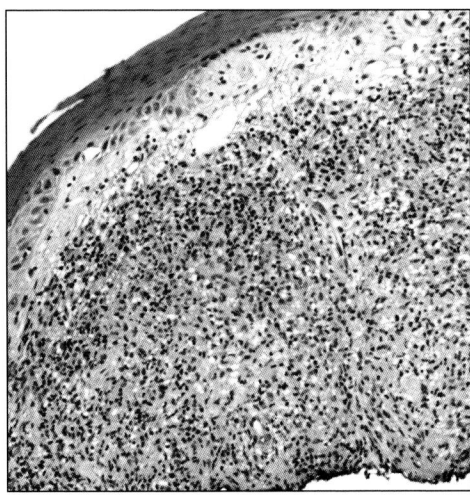

Low-power view of a primary cutaneous CD4(+) small/medium pleomorphic T-cell lymphoma shows a dense lymphoid infiltrate filling the dermis in a diffuse pattern of infiltration.

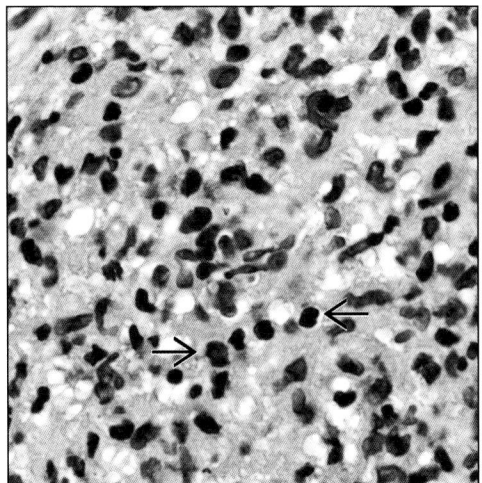

At higher power magnification, the lymphocytes are small to medium in size and show moderate atypia and pleomorphism ➡.

TERMINOLOGY

Abbreviations
- Primary cutaneous CD4(+) small/medium pleomorphic T-cell lymphoma (SMPTCL)

Synonyms
- Idiopathic T-cell lymphomatoid hyperplasia

Definitions
- T-cell lymphoma of skin with small to medium-sized CD4(+) T cells, and usually indolent clinical course
  - Without typical patches/plaques of mycosis fungoides
- Provisional entity in 2008 WHO Classification of Tumors of Hematopoietic and Lymphoid Tissue
  - Nonaggressive natural history, but worrisome histologic and molecular features

ETIOLOGY/PATHOGENESIS

Idiopathic
- Cause of this lymphoma unknown

Postulated Normal Cell Counterpart
- CD4(+) helper T cell

CLINICAL ISSUES

Epidemiology
- Incidence
  - Rare
    - 2% of cutaneous T-cell lymphomas in the Dutch and Austrian Cutaneous Lymphoma Group Registry
- Age
  - Median: 53 years; range: 3-90 years
- Gender
  - M:F = 0.5:1

Site
- Head and neck area most common
  - Upper torso often
  - Lower extremities rare

Presentation
- Single plaque or tumor
  - Less commonly > 1 tumor nodule
  - Less commonly ≥ 1 papules
  - No lesions (patches/plaques) typical of mycosis fungoides
- Usually asymptomatic other than skin lesions
  - No lymphadenopathy
  - No systemic disease

Laboratory Tests
- No known laboratory abnormalities

Natural History
- Does not usually disseminate
  - Rarely, local recurrence is seen

Treatment
- Excision
- Radiation therapy
- Usually nonaggressive therapy
  - Especially if single lesion

Prognosis
- Mostly favorable outcome, especially if solitary lesion or localized to skin
  - Better prognosis than secondary cutaneous T-cell lymphomas
  - Better prognosis than primary cutaneous peripheral T-cell lymphoma, not otherwise specified
- Nonaggressive disease
  - Overall 5-year survival: 60-80%
  - Disease-specific 5-year survival up to 75%
- Good prognostic indicators
  - Solitary lesion
  - Disease localized to skin

Key Facts

Terminology

- T-cell lymphoma of skin with small to medium-sized CD4(+) T cells and usually indolent clinical course
  - Provisional entity in 2008 WHO Classification of Tumors of Hematopoietic and Lymphoid Tissue
  - Lacks lesions typical of mycosis fungoides

Clinical Issues

- Usually single plaque or tumor
- Good prognosis, especially if single lesion

Microscopic Pathology

- Dense dermal and subcutaneous infiltrate of small/medium-sized pleomorphic T cells
- Sometimes focal epidermotropism
- Scattered large T cells (< 30% of total)
- Background reactive infiltrate

- Granulomatous inflammation may be present

Ancillary Tests

- CD3(+), CD4(+), CD8(-), CD30(-)
- Loss of T-cell antigens
- Positive follicular helper T-cell markers (PD1, CXCL13)
- Clonal T-cell receptor gene rearrangements
- Cytogenetics: No known abnormalities
- Epstein-Barr virus small-encoded RNA(-)

Top Differential Diagnoses

- Pseudolymphoma of the skin
- Mycosis fungoides
- Angioimmunoblastic T-cell lymphoma
- Peripheral T-cell lymphoma unspecified
- Cutaneous B-cell lymphoma

- Worse prognostic indicators
  - Multiple lesions
  - Large lesions

MACROSCOPIC FEATURES

General Features

- Usually single, less often multiple firm lesion(s)

MICROSCOPIC PATHOLOGY

Histologic Features

- Dense dermal infiltrate
  - Sometimes involves subcutaneous tissue
  - Usually nonepidermotropic
    - Rarely focal epidermotropism
- Growth pattern
  - Diffuse
  - Nodular
- Size of T cells
  - Small or medium in most cases
  - Large cells can also be seen
    - When present, < 30% of total cells
- Pleomorphic with some nuclear irregularity
- Other features
  - Background reactive infiltrate is fairly common
    - Small reactive lymphocytes, eosinophils, and histiocytes
  - ↑ reactive-appearing B cells also often present
  - Granulomatous inflammation can be seen

Cytologic Features

- Rarely diagnosed by cytology

ANCILLARY TESTS

Immunohistochemistry

- T-cell antigens positive
  - CD2(+), CD3(+), CD5(+), CD7(+)
  - Rarely loss of 1 or more T-cell antigens

  - CD7 > CD5, CD2
  - CD4(+), CD8(-)
- Expresses follicular helper T-cell markers
  - PD1(+), CXCL13(+), Bcl-6(+)
- Cytotoxic markers negative
  - TIA, GZM-B, and perforin
- CD30(-), LMP1(-)

Cytogenetics

- No known specific abnormalities

In Situ Hybridization

- Epstein-Barr virus small-encoded RNA (EBER) negative

PCR

- *TCR* gene rearrangement clonal
  - 60% in one series
- *IgH* immunoglobulin gene rearrangements polyclonal

DIFFERENTIAL DIAGNOSIS

Atypical Reactive Lymphoid Infiltrates ("Pseudolymphomas") of the Skin

- Similarities to SMPTCL
  - Overlapping morphology with atypical dermal infiltrates
  - Reactive B cells and plasma cells in SMPTCL are difficult to distinguish from reactive conditions
- Differences from SMPTCL
  - More CD8(+) T cells in pseudolymphoma
  - Lack of clonality in T-cell receptor gene rearrangement favors pseudolymphoma over SMPTCL
  - Pseudolymphoma may resolve without treatment
  - Loss of T-cell antigens favors SMPTCL

Mycosis Fungoides

- Similarities to SMPTCL
  - Morphology is akin to SMPTCL with an infiltrate of mostly small/medium-sized pleomorphic T cells
  - Similar phenotype to SMPTCL
    - T-cell markers(+), with loss of some T-cell antigens

- ▪ CD4(+), CD8(-), CD30(-)
- Differences from SMPTCL
  - o Mycosis fungoides presents with significant epidermotropism, contrary to SMPTCL
  - o Usually negative for follicular helper T-cell markers
    - ▪ PD1, CXCL13, Bcl-6

Angioimmunoblastic T-cell Lymphoma (AITL)

- Similarities to SMPTCL
  - o Also presents with a dermal-based T-cell infiltrate
  - o Also expresses follicular T-helper cell markers
    - ▪ PD1, CXCL13, Bcl-6
- Differences from SMPTCL
  - o Often presents with lymph node involvement or systemic disease
  - o Morphology shows increased vasculature
  - o CD21(+), CD23(+) in follicular dendritic cells
  - o Worse prognosis than SMPTCL

Anaplastic Large Cell Lymphoma (ALCL)

- Similar phenotype to SMPTCL
  - o T-cell infiltrate in the dermis
- Differences from SMPTCL
  - o Often has > 30% large atypical cells, unlike SMPTCL
    - ▪ Except small cell variant of ALCL
  - o CD30(+) in ALCL

Primary Cutaneous Peripheral T-cell Lymphoma, Not Otherwise Specified

- Similar phenotype to SMPTCL
  - o T-cell infiltrate in dermis
- Differences from SMPTCL
  - o Often has > 30% large atypical cells, unlike SMPTCL
  - o Worse prognosis than SMPTCL
  - o Polymorphous infiltrate favors SMPTCL

Cutaneous B-cell Lymphoma

- Including primary cutaneous marginal zone lymphoma, primary cutaneous follicle center lymphoma, and CLL
- Similar morphology to SMPTCL
  - o Also presents with dermal lymphoid nodules
  - o SMPTCL can have prominent B-cell component
- Differences from SMPTCL
  - o B-cell markers positive
    - ▪ CD19(+), CD20(+), CD79a(+), pax-5(+)
  - o Monoclonal *IgH* immunoglobulin gene rearrangements in B-cell lymphomas
    - ▪ Polyclonal *IgH* immunoglobulin gene rearrangement in SMPTCL

Granulomatous Dermatitis

- Granulomatous inflammation can also be seen in SMPTCL, but should be focal
- Atypical/pleomorphic T-cell infiltrate favors SMPTCL over granulomatous dermatitis

DIAGNOSTIC CHECKLIST

Clinically Relevant Pathologic Features

- Tissue distribution (less aggressive cases are usually solitary lesions and confined to skin)

Pathologic Interpretation Pearls

- Remember immunophenotype: CD3(+), CD4(+), CD8(-), CD30(-), EBV(-)

SELECTED REFERENCES

1. Cetinözman F et al: Expression of programmed Death-1 in primary cutaneous CD4-positive small/medium-sized pleomorphic T-cell lymphoma, cutaneous pseudo-T-cell lymphoma, and other types of cutaneous T-cell lymphoma. Am J Surg Pathol. Epub ahead of print, 2011
2. Weaver J et al: Non-mycosis fungoides cutaneous T-cell lymphoma: reclassification according to the WHO-EORTC classification. J Cutan Pathol. 37(5):516-24, 2010
3. Beltraminelli H et al: Primary cutaneous CD4+ small-/medium-sized pleomorphic T-cell lymphoma: a cutaneous nodular proliferation of pleomorphic T lymphocytes of undetermined significance? A study of 136 cases. Am J Dermatopathol. 31(4):317-22, 2009
4. Boussault P et al: Primary cutaneous CD4+ small/medium-sized pleomorphic T-cell lymphoma associated with an annular elastolytic giant cell granuloma. Br J Dermatol. 160(5):1126-8, 2009
5. Ferenczi K: Could follicular helper T-cells play a role in primary cutaneous CD4+ small/medium-sized pleomorphic T-cell lymphomas? J Cutan Pathol. 36(6):717-8, 2009
6. Rodríguez Pinilla SM et al: Primary cutaneous CD4+ small/medium-sized pleomorphic T-cell lymphoma expresses follicular T-cell markers. Am J Surg Pathol. 33(1):81-90, 2009
7. Grogg KL et al: Primary cutaneous CD4-positive small/medium-sized pleomorphic T-cell lymphoma: a clonal T-cell lymphoproliferative disorder with indolent behavior. Mod Pathol. 21(6):708-15, 2008
8. Khamaysi Z et al: The applicability of the new WHO-EORTC classification of primary cutaneous lymphomas to a single referral center. Am J Dermatopathol. 30(1):37-44, 2008
9. Burg G et al: WHO/EORTC classification of cutaneous lymphomas 2005: histological and molecular aspects. J Cutan Pathol. 32(10):647-74, 2005
10. Slater DN: The new World Health Organization-European Organization for Research and Treatment of Cancer classification for cutaneous lymphomas: a practical marriage of two giants. Br J Dermatol. 153(5):874-80, 2005
11. Bekkenk MW et al: Peripheral T-cell lymphomas unspecified presenting in the skin: analysis of prognostic factors in a group of 82 patients. Blood. 102(6):2213-9, 2003
12. Scarabello A et al: Cutaneous lymphomas with prominent granulomatous reaction: a potential pitfall in the histopathologic diagnosis of cutaneous T- and B-cell lymphomas. Am J Surg Pathol. 26(10):1259-68, 2002
13. von den Driesch P et al: Localized cutaneous small to medium-sized pleomorphic T-cell lymphoma: a report of 3 cases stable for years. J Am Acad Dermatol. 46(4):531-5, 2002
14. Grange F et al: Prognostic factors in primary cutaneous lymphomas other than mycosis fungoides and the Sézary syndrome. The French Study Group on Cutaneous Lymphomas. Blood. 93(11):3637-42, 1999
15. Beljaards RC et al: Primary cutaneous T-cell lymphoma: clinicopathological features and prognostic parameters of 35 cases other than mycosis fungoides and CD30-positive large cell lymphoma. J Pathol. 172(1):53-60, 1994

PRIMARY CUTANEOUS CD4+ SMALL/MEDIUM PLEOMORPHIC T-CELL LYMPHOMA

Microscopic Features

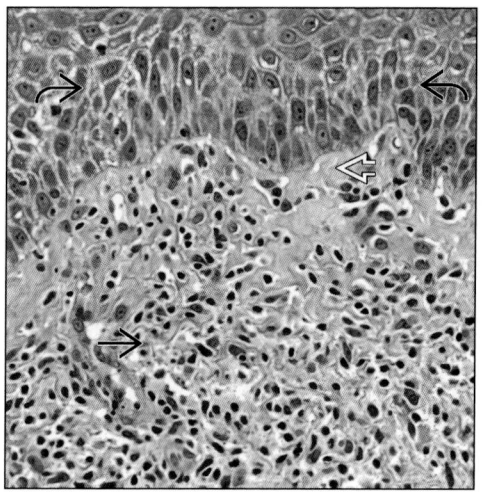

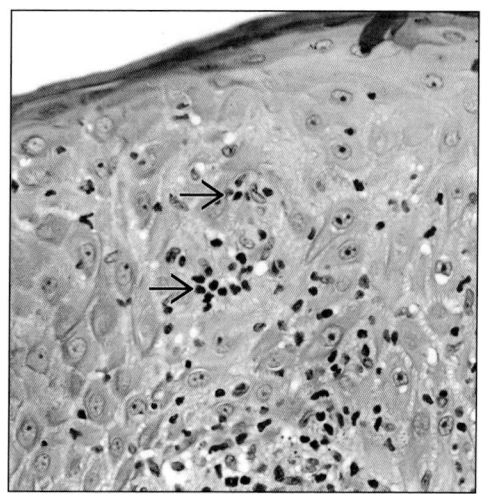

(Left) In this case of SMPTCL, the tumor is seen in the superficial dermis ➡ but is separated from the uninvolved epidermis ➡ by a thin grenz zone ⇨. In most cases, SMPTCL does not infiltrate the epidermis. *(Right)* Scattered pleomorphic T cells ➡ are found in the epidermis in this case of SMPTCL. Up to 30% of cases can show focal epidermotropism.

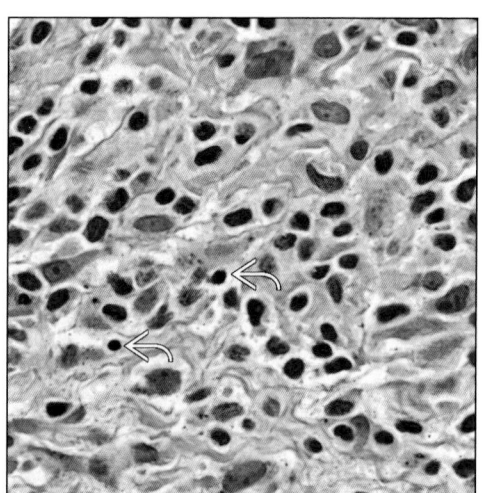

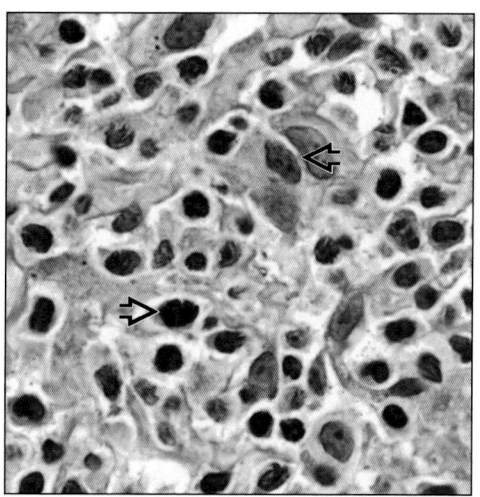

(Left) Higher power examination of a SMPTCL shows the T cells are mostly small to medium in size and show considerable pleomorphism. Small reactive lymphocytes ➡ can be used as a reference in determining the size of the tumor cells. *(Right)* High-power view shows there are scattered cells that are large in size ⇨ with marked atypia. When present, large cells will make up less than 30% of the total cells.

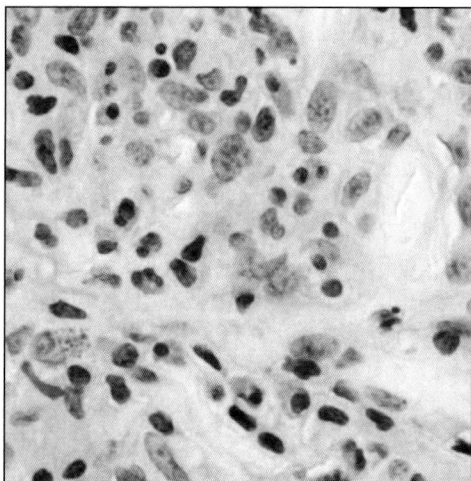

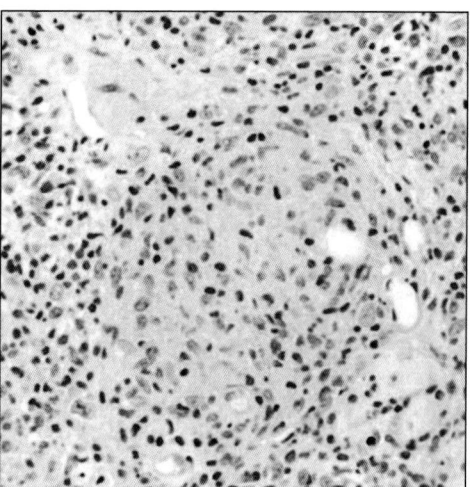

(Left) At high power there are scattered eosinophils in this case of SMPTCL. The background infiltrate can also contain neutrophils, plasma cells, and histiocytes. *(Right)* In this same case of SMPTCL, there are focal areas with granulomatous inflammation. Granulomatous inflammation is not uncommonly seen in these lesions, and can be confused with a reactive process including infection.

Immunohistochemical Features

(Left) CD3 immunohistochemical stain at high magnification shows that SMPTCL is a dermal T-cell infiltrate, which is strongly and diffusely positive for CD3. *(Right)* CD20 is only positive in a few scattered B cells in this case of SMPTCL. In some cases of SMPTCL, B cells are more numerous. SMPTCL has a T-cell lineage, but is often accompanied by reactive B cells.

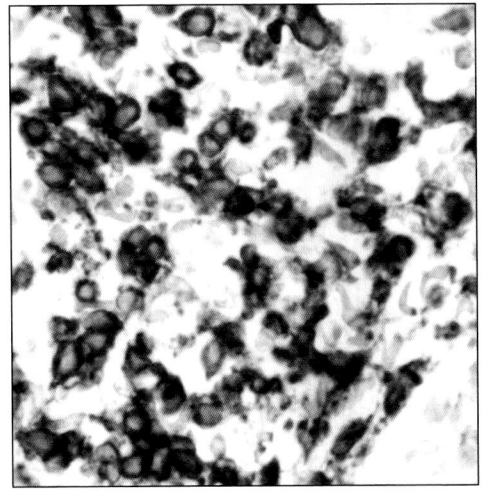
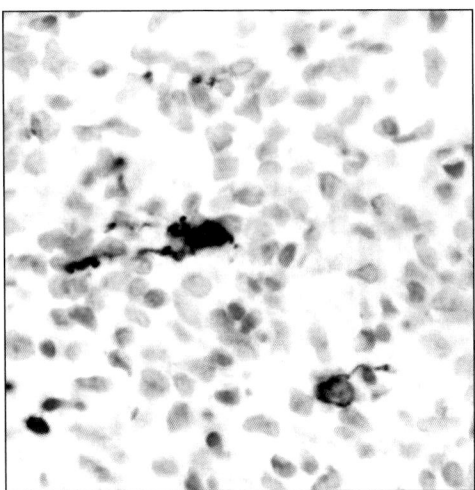

(Left) There is strong CD4 expression in nearly all of the T cells, as is typical of this T-cell lymphoma. *(Right)* As compared to the previous CD4 stain, CD8 is essentially negative, with only rare cells showing a slight blush of staining ⊳. This lymphoma typically has a CD4(+), CD8(-) phenotype.

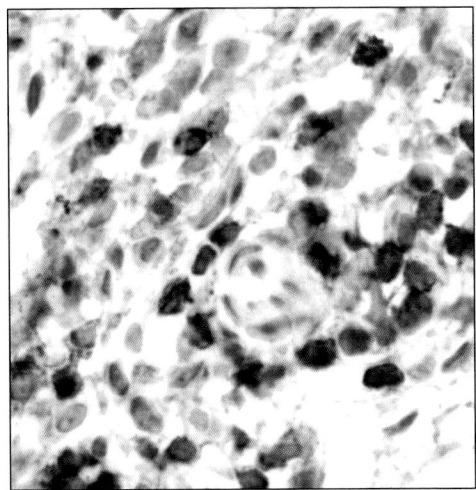
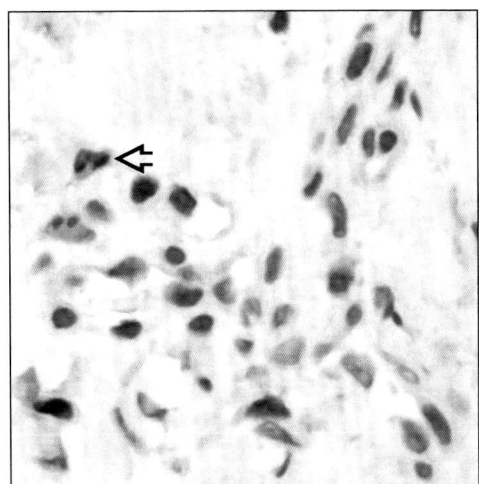

(Left) PD1, a marker of follicular T cells, is strongly positive in this case of SMPTCL. CXCL13 is another follicular T-cell antibody·that is often expressed in SMPTCL. *(Right)* Medium magnification depicts loss of CD7 in most of the T cells with only rare cells → weakly expressing CD7. CD7 is the T-cell antigen most frequently lost, and CD2 is the 2nd most commonly lost.

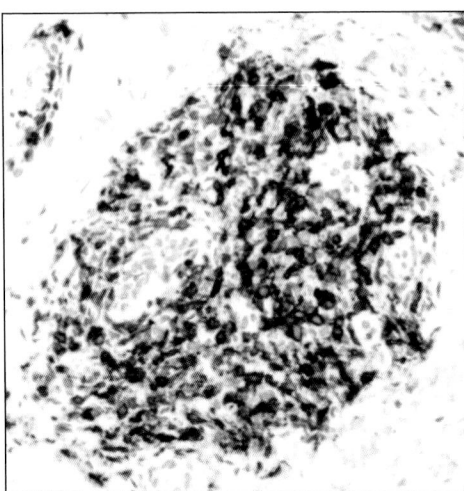
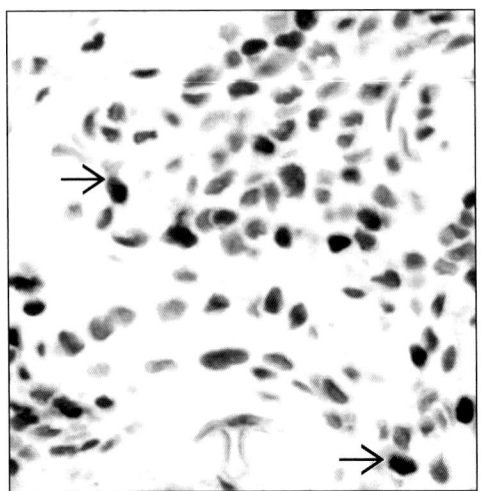

PRIMARY CUTANEOUS CD4+ SMALL/MEDIUM PLEOMORPHIC T-CELL LYMPHOMA

Differential Diagnosis

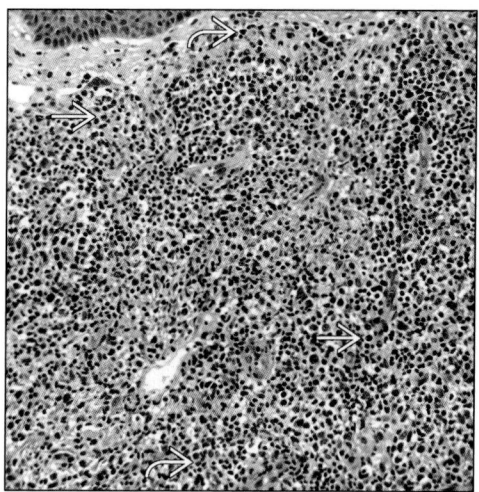
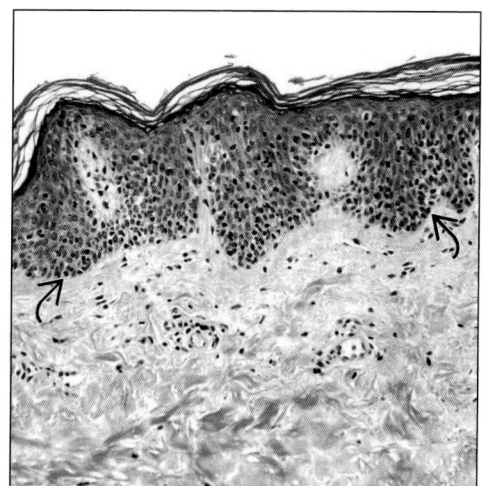

(Left) *This case of pseudolymphoma developed after taking captopril. As in SMPTCL, the dermis has a diffuse lymphoid infiltrate. However, the infiltrate contained scattered eosinophils ➡ & plasma cells ➡ & spontaneously resolved after discontinuing medication.* **(Right)** *Mycosis fungoides (MF) has similar phenotype as SMPTCL with CD4(+), CD8(-) T cells. However, MF presents with more epidermotropism. Note numerous T cells in the epidermis ➡.*

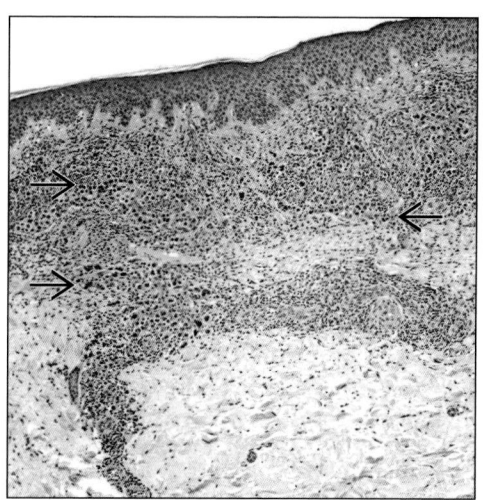
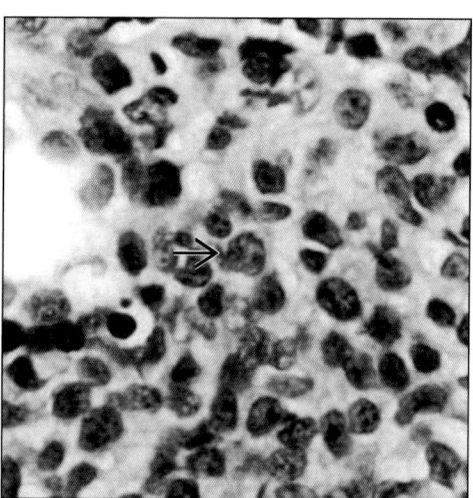

(Left) *Primary cutaneous anaplastic large cell lymphoma (ALCL) is shown with tumor cells diffusely involving the dermis ➡. The tumor cells are larger than expected for SMPTCL. (Courtesy C. Yin, MD.)* **(Right)** *The tumor cells in PTCL-NOS are also large in size and show marked atypia. PTCL-NOS often contains tumor cells that are larger in size ➡ than SMPTCL. Less than 30% of the tumor cells in SMPTCL are large.*

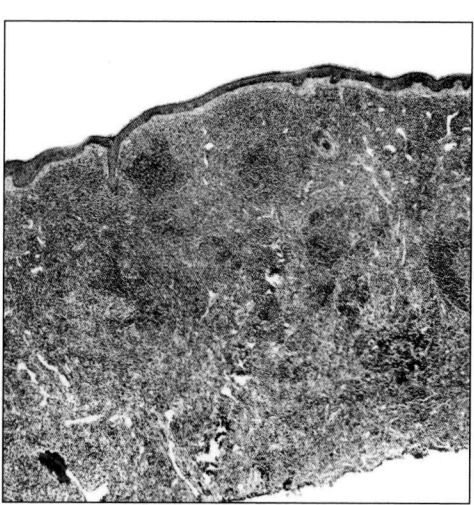
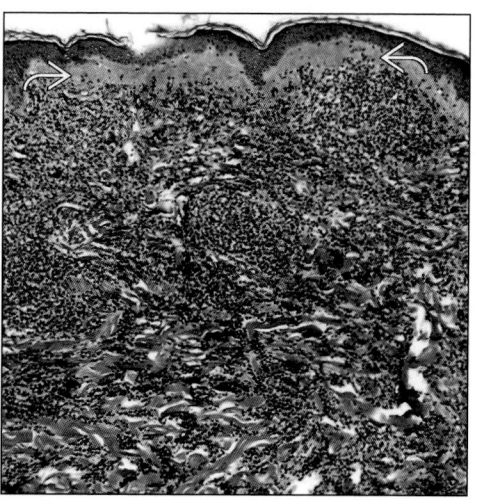

(Left) *Primary cutaneous follicle center lymphoma also presents with nodular/ diffuse dermal infiltrates. However these lymphocytes are B cells, are CD20(+), CD10(+), and show Ig heavy chain gene rearrangement. (Courtesy R. Miranda, MD.)* **(Right)** *Chronic lymphocytic leukemia is also a dermal-based infiltrate composed of B cells, which typically involves the superficial and deep dermis. The epidermis is uninvolved and separated from the malignant B cells by a thin grenz zone ➡.*

CUTANEOUS GAMMA-DELTA T-CELL LYMPHOMA

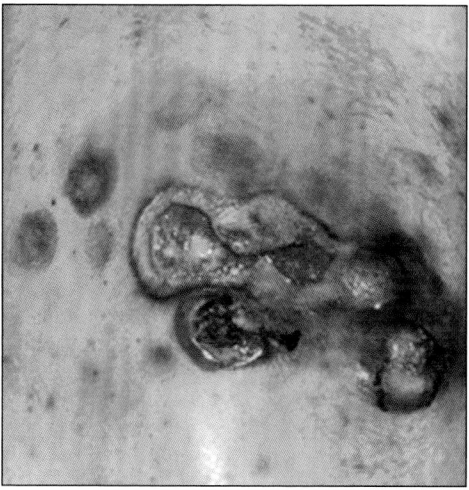

Cutaneous γδ T-cell lymphoma shows a large raised lesion with ulcer and satellite lesions. (Courtesy C. Sander, MD.)

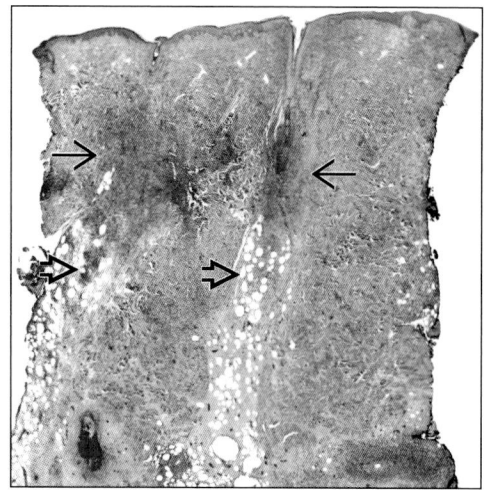

Primary cutaneous γδ T-cell lymphoma involves the epidermis, dermis ➡, and subcutaneous tissue ⇨ with the most extensive disease in the dermis and subcutis. (Courtesy L. J. Medeiros, MD.)

TERMINOLOGY

Abbreviations
- Cutaneous gamma-delta T-cell lymphoma (CGDTCL)

Synonyms
- Subcutaneous panniculitis-like T-cell lymphoma with γδ cells

Definitions
- T-cell lymphoma arising in the skin, which is composed of cytotoxic γδ T cells
  - Does not include subcutaneous panniculitis-like T-cell lymphoma composed of αβ cells
    - May encompass mucocutaneous γδ cell T-cell lymphoma, but further study is needed

ETIOLOGY/PATHOGENESIS

Immunosuppression or Dysregulation of T Cells
- Found in many of the patients

Chronic Antigenic Stimulation
- Speculative, but possibly involved in pathogenesis

Cell of Origin
- γδ T cells
  - Involved with mucosal and epithelial immune system function

CLINICAL ISSUES

Epidemiology
- Incidence
  - Rare tumor, < 100 cases reported in literature
    - < 1% of all cutaneous T-cell lymphomas
- Age
  - Commonly adults

- Gender
  - No gender preponderance

Site
- Mostly extremities
  - Sometimes mucosal sites, where normal γδ T cells are found
  - Metastasis common
    - Spread to lungs, liver, kidneys, oral mucosa, and brain
    - Usually not in bone marrow, lymph node, or spleen

Presentation
- 1 or multiple skin lesions
- Patches or plaques due to epidermal infiltrates
  - Tumors or nodules due to dermal infiltrates
    - ± ulcerated epidermis
- Hemophagocytic syndrome (HPS) may be present in 45% of cases
  - More often in subcutaneous lesions
    - Related to release of cytotoxic molecules

Laboratory Tests
- Cytopenias
- ↑ liver function tests

Treatment
- Adjuvant therapy
  - Multiagent chemotherapy ± radiotherapy
    - Poor response to allogenic stem cell transplant

Prognosis
- Poor prognosis
  - 5-year survival: ~ 11%
  - Subcutaneous disease is a poor prognostic indicator
    - Better prognosis if only disease in dermis or epidermis
  - HPS is a poor prognostic indicator

CUTANEOUS GAMMA-DELTA T-CELL LYMPHOMA

Key Facts

Terminology
- T-cell lymphoma of mature γδ cells
- Separately classified from SPTCL in WHO (2008)

Clinical Issues
- Hemophagocytic syndrome in 45%
- Poor prognosis
- Treated with multiagent chemotherapy

Macroscopic Features
- Skin nodules with ulceration

Microscopic Pathology
- 3 patterns of disease: Epidermotropic, dermal, and subcutaneous
  - Malignant T cells rim around adipocytes
  - Prominent karyorrhexis/apoptosis and angioinvasion

Ancillary Tests
- Immunohistochemistry: TCRδ1(+), βF1(-), CD56(+), CD4(-), CD8(-), EBER(-), cytotoxic markers (+)
- T-cell receptor gene rearrangement

Top Differential Diagnoses
- Subcutaneous panniculitis-like T-cell lymphoma
  - Panniculitis, but not in dermis or epidermis; lacks ulceration; TCRδ1(-), βF1(+)
  - Much better prognosis than CGDTCL
- Peripheral T-cell lymphoma, not otherwise specified
- Lupus profundus panniculitis
  - Similar inflammation in the subcutis in panniculitic pattern
  - Lobular panniculitis, but contains plasma cells and germinal centers, unlike CGDTCL

MICROSCOPIC PATHOLOGY

Histologic Features
- 3 patterns of disease
  - **Epidermotropic**
    - Ranges from mild to marked
    - Can mimic mycosis fungoides or pagetoid reticulosis
  - **Dermal**
    - More dermal and epidermal involvement typically present than in subcutaneous panniculitis-like T-cell lymphoma
  - **Subcutaneous**
    - Lobules mostly involved
    - Septae less frequently involved and represents secondary spilling of T cells from lobules
    - Subcutis involvement can appear identical to subcutaneous panniculitis-like T-cell lymphoma of αβ cells, including rimming of fat cells
- Often more than 1 pattern of disease in a patient
  - Different patterns of disease in a single biopsy or in different biopsies
- Malignant T cells with nuclear atypia, hyperchromasia
- Frequent necrosis/apoptosis and vascular invasion
  - Necrosis may be caused by released cytotoxic molecules
- ↑ reactive histiocytes
  - Vacuolated foamy cytoplasm from imbibed material/lipid
  - With erythrophagocytosis or cytophagocytosis

Cytologic Features
- Medium to large T cells with coarse, hyperchromatic-staining chromatin, sometimes vesicular nuclei, and variably prominent nucleoli

ANCILLARY TESTS

Immunohistochemistry
- T-cell antigens (CD2, CD3, CD5, CD7) positive
  - May lose 1 or more T-cell antigens
- Most cases: CD4(-)/CD8(-)
  - Few cases: CD4(-)/CD8(+)
- TCRδ1(+), βF1(-)
  - If TCRδ1 antibody is unavailable, βF1 can be used instead
    - Negative βF1 may serve to assume γδ cell origin
- CD56 usually positive, unlike subcutaneous panniculitis-like T-cell lymphoma
- Cytotoxic markers (perforin, TIA1, granzyme) positive

Cytogenetics
- No specific reproducible chromosomal abnormalities

In Situ Hybridization
- Epstein-Barr encoded receptor (EBER) negative
  - But may be positive in mucocutaneous γδ T-cell lymphoma

Molecular Genetics
- Clonal rearrangement of *TCRγ* gene and *TCRδ* and sometimes rearranged *TCRβ*

DIFFERENTIAL DIAGNOSIS

Subcutaneous Panniculitis-like T-cell Lymphoma (SPTCL)
- Previously included cases of CGDTCL until reclassification in the WHO Classification of Hematopoietic and Lymphoid Tumors (2008)
- Presents with panniculitic pattern of tissue involvement similar to CGDTCL
  - Differs in morphology as subcutaneous panniculitis-like T-cell lymphoma is typically confined to subcutis
    - Does not invade dermis or epidermis
    - Epidermis is not ulcerated, contrary to CGDTCL
- Shows the immunophenotype of αβ cells and not the γδ cells of CGDTCL
  - BF1(+), TCRδ1(-), CD56(-), unlike CGDTCL
  - Usually CD4(-), CD8(+)
- Much better prognosis than CGDTCL

CUTANEOUS GAMMA-DELTA T-CELL LYMPHOMA

Cutaneous γδ T-cell Lymphoma Compared to Subcutaneous Panniculitis-like T-cell Lymphoma

	CGDTCL	SPTCL
Age	Median age: 50s	Median age: 30s
Ulceration	Usually present	Usually not present
Clinical	Usually B symptoms and HPS	B symptoms positive or negative
Histology	Subcutaneous and dermal infiltrate with massive necrosis	Usually not in dermis and no necrosis
Immunohistochemistry	CD3(+), CD8(-), TIA1(+), CD56(+), βF1(-), TCRδ1(+)	CD3(+), CD8(+), TIA1(+), CD56(-), βF1(+), TCRδ1(-)
Prognosis	Poor prognosis with HPS and sometimes metastasis	Excellent prognosis without HPS
Treatment	Multiagent chemotherapy, sometimes allogenic stem cell transplant	Systemic corticosteroids, CHOP for recurrent/resistant cases
5-year survival	11%	82%

- 5-year survival: ~ 85%
- Hemophagocytic syndrome less prevalent than in CGDTCL
- Patients younger than in CGDTCL and less B symptoms
- Often treated with systemic corticosteroids
  - Whereas CGDTCL is often treated with multiagent chemotherapy

Other Primary Cutaneous Lymphomas
- Usually involve epidermis or dermis unlike SPTCL
  - **Peripheral T-cell lymphoma, not otherwise specified**
    - Similar morphology, often with dermal and subcutis involvement
    - Both diseases often have pleomorphic tumor cells
    - Often CD4(+) and CD8(+) cells, whereas CGDTCL is usually CD4(-)/CD8(-)
    - Usually βF1(+), unlike CGDTCL, which is βF1(-)
  - **Anaplastic large cell lymphoma** (ALCL)
    - Usually in dermis and only rarely in subcutis
    - CD30(+), unlike CGDTCL
  - **Enteropathy-associated T-cell lymphoma**
    - Can have subcutis dissemination
    - But will typically present with gastrointestinal mass and show features of celiac disease
  - **Mycosis fungoides**
    - Atypical T cells in the epidermis with lining up and clustering of cells
    - CD4(+)/CD8(-) T cells; cytotoxic markers (-)
  - **Pagetoid reticulosis**
    - CGDTCL with marked epidermotropism resembles pagetoid reticulosis
    - Unlike CGDTCL, pagetoid reticulosis often occurs on feet
    - Usually CD4(-)/CD8(+), whereas CGDTCL is usually CD4(-)/CD8(-)
  - **Diffuse large B-cell lymphoma**
    - Can have subcutaneous dissemination
    - But will have B-cell phenotype and Ig heavy chain immunoglobulin gene rearrangement
  - **Blastic plasmacytoid dendritic cell neoplasm**
    - Diffuse, atypical infiltrate of CD56(+) cells, like CGDTCL

- Different phenotype than CGDTCL with cytotoxic markers negative; usually CD3(-), CD123(+), TCL1(+), CD4(+), and CD8(-)

Reactive Panniculitis
- **Lupus profundus panniculitis**
  - Also inflammation in the subcutis in lobular panniculitis pattern
  - Can be difficult to differentiate reactive panniculitis from CGDTCL or subcutaneous panniculitis-like T-cell lymphoma
  - Features favoring lupus panniculitis over SPTCL
    - Plasma cells and germinal centers
    - Mixed inflammatory infiltrate with histiocytes, eosinophils, and neutrophils
    - Lymphocytes do not show atypia and do not rim fat cells
    - B-cell aggregates
    - Mixture of CD4(+) and CD8(+) cells
    - Vacuolar epidermal change and interstitial mucin
    - T-cell receptor rearrangements are usually not clonal, but rarely oligoclonal T-cell populations are present
    - Other clinical or lab evidence of autoimmune disease

DIAGNOSTIC CHECKLIST

Pathologic Interpretation Pearls
- Atypical lobular panniculitic gamma-delta T-cell infiltrate with karyorrhexis and fat necrosis rimming individual fat cells
- Dermal and epidermal involvement with ulceration, unlike subcutaneous panniculitis-like T-cell lymphoma

SELECTED REFERENCES

1. Garcia-Herrera A et al: Nonhepatosplenic γδ T-cell lymphomas represent a spectrum of aggressive cytotoxic T-cell lymphomas with a mainly extranodal presentation. Am J Surg Pathol. 35(8):1214-25, 2011
2. Nakashima H et al: Cutaneous gamma/delta T-cell lymphoma treated with retinoid and narrowband ultraviolet B. Clin Exp Dermatol. 34(7):e345-6, 2009
3. Tripodo C et al: Gamma-delta T-cell lymphomas. Nat Rev Clin Oncol. 6(12):707-17, 2009

CUTANEOUS GAMMA-DELTA T-CELL LYMPHOMA

Microscopic and Immunohistochemical Features

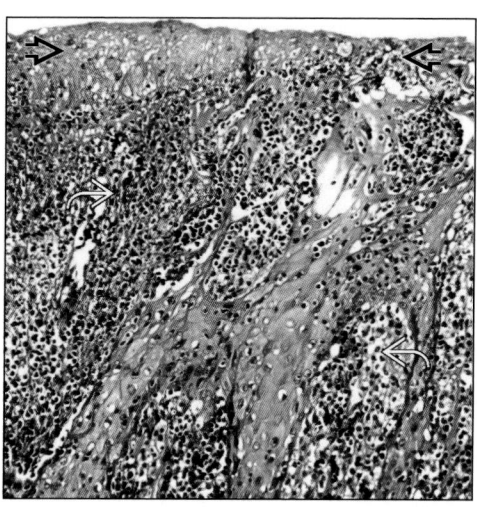

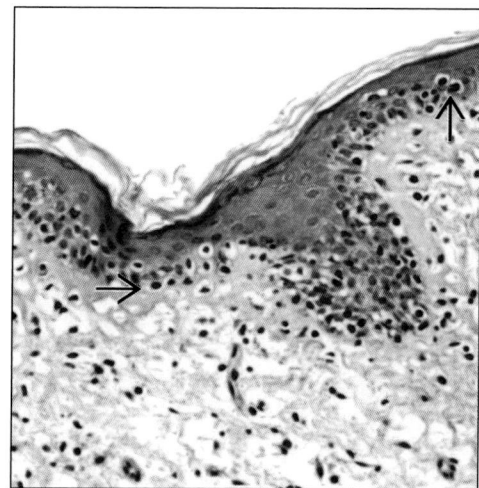

(Left) There is ulceration of the epidermis ➡ due to prominent infiltration by the neoplastic cells, which is commonly seen in CGDTCL. The atypical lymphoid infiltrate also diffusely involves the superficial dermis ➡. *(Right)* This is an example of CGDTCL with much milder epidermal involvement. The infiltrate of malignant cells involves the epidermis ➡ in small clusters and single cells, mimicking mycosis fungoides.

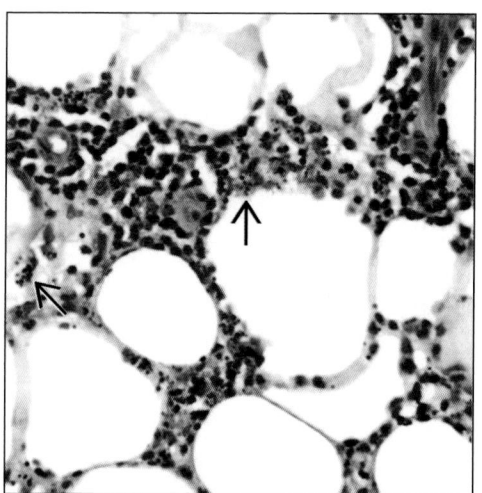

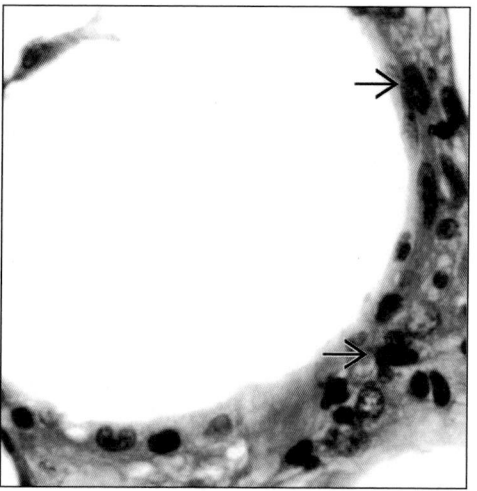

(Left) In the same case with ulcerated epidermis, there is a deep infiltrate showing lobular panniculitis composed of atypical T cells rimming fat lobules with prominent apoptosis/karyorrhexis ➡. *(Right)* A higher power image of the subcutaneous tissue shows that there are atypical T cells ➡ that line individual fat cells. These cells are more atypical than would be expected in a reactive panniculitis.

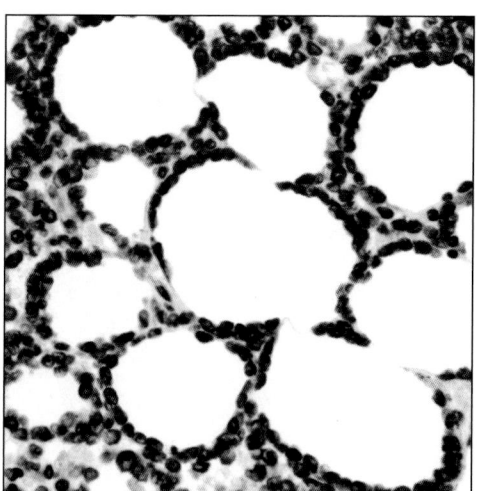

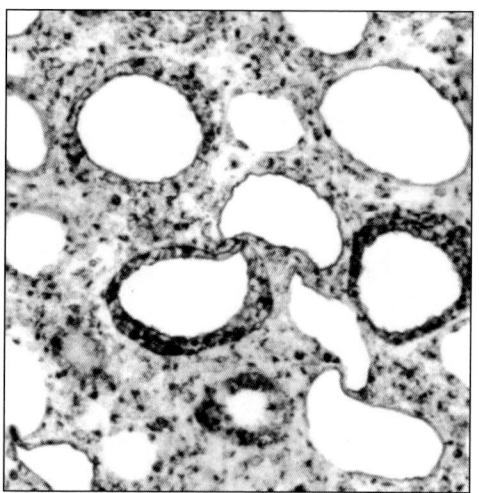

(Left) At high power, this CD3 immunohistochemical stain highlights atypical T cells that are lining fat cells. This feature is common to CGDTCL and to subcutaneous panniculitis-like T-cell lymphoma. *(Courtesy L. J. Medeiros, MD.)* *(Right)* This is a medium-power TIA-1 immunohistochemical stain in CGDTCL. Atypical neoplastic cells rimming the fat strongly express TIA-1. These cells were also positive for other cytotoxic markers including granzyme-B and perforin.

Immunohistochemical Features

(Left) In this example of CGDTCL, most of the malignant T cells are not immunoreactive for CD4. The few positive cells are likely histiocytes. Often cases of CGDTCL are CD4(-)/CD8(-), whereas most of the cases of subcutaneous panniculitis-like T-cell lymphoma are CD4(-)/CD8(+). **(Right)** This a medium-power magnification of a CD8 immunostain in a case of CGDTCL. The malignant T cells show no expression of CD8.

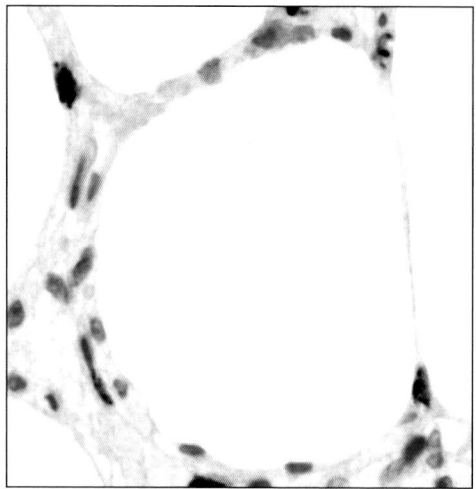
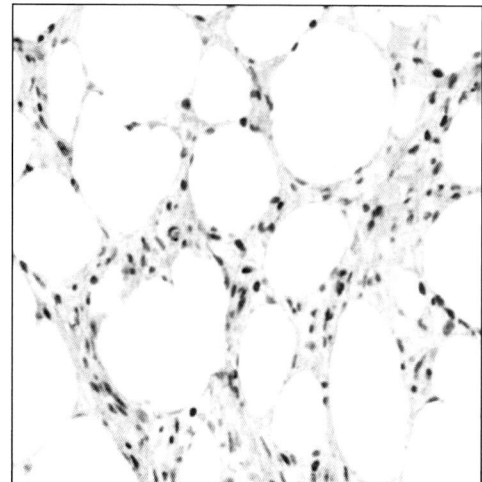

(Left) PCGDTCL involving the dermis. A subset of the neoplastic cells in this case are strongly CD8(+). Most cases of PCGDTCL are CD8(-), but a subset of neoplasms can show partial or diffuse CD8 expression. (Courtesy L. J. Medeiros, MD.) **(Right)** CD56 immunohistochemical stain marks the malignant T cells ➡ in this case of CGDTCL. CD56 is differentially expressed in CGDTCL and subcutaneous panniculitis-like T-cell lymphoma, as it is usually positive in CGDTCL and negative in SPTCL.

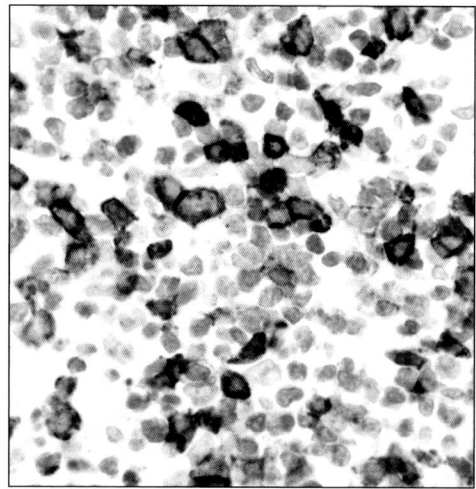
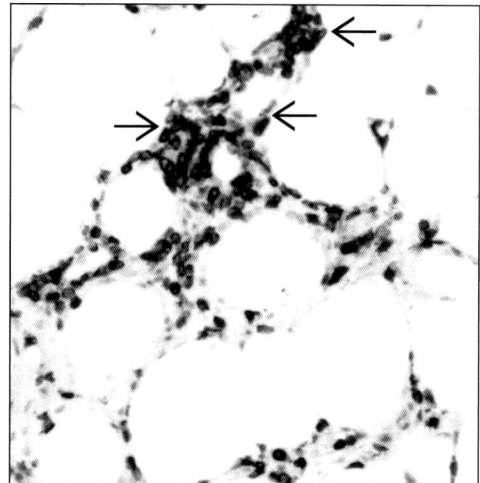

(Left) The malignant T cells encircling fat are positive for TCRδ-1 ➡, as expected, since the tumor is composed of γδ T cells. **(Right)** This βF-1 stain is negative in the T cells rimming the fat. Lack of βF1 is presumptive evidence that the T cells express the γδTCR. CGDTCL is βF1(-), whereas subcutaneous panniculitis-like T-cell lymphoma is βF1(+).

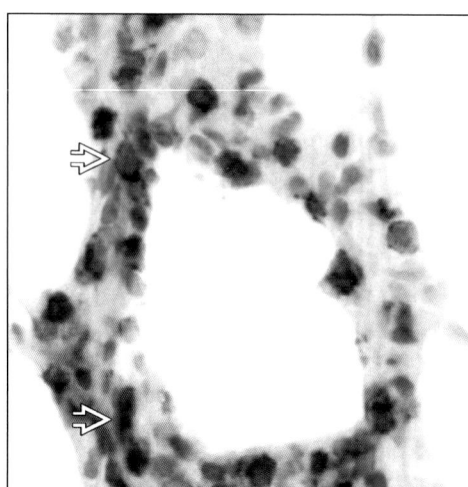
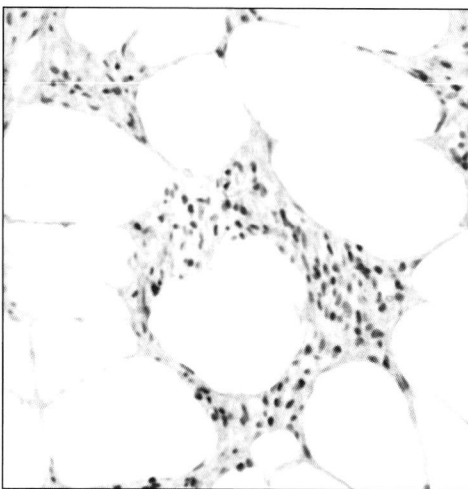

Differential Diagnosis

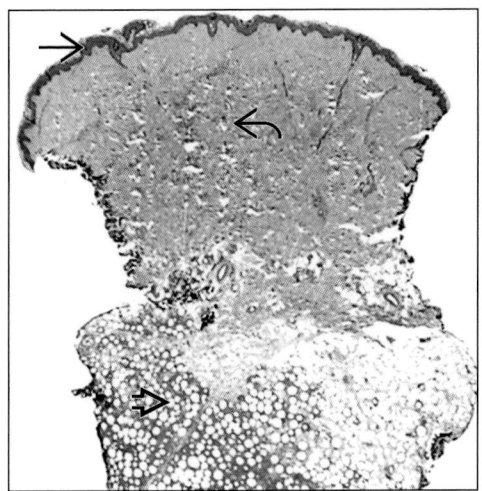

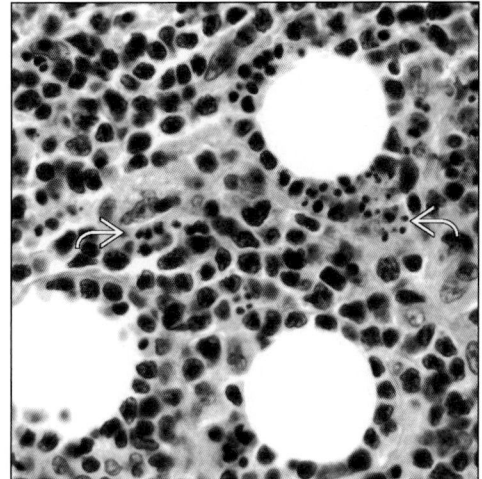

(Left) SPTCL, which is the main differential diagnosis of subcutaneous γδ T-cell lymphoma, shows malignant T cells that are confined to the subcutis ⊡, but the dermis ⊡ and epidermis ⊡ are not involved. (Courtesy M. Tomaszewsky, MD.) **(Right)** High magnification of SPTCL shows a population of atypical, hyperchromatic-staining neoplastic cells infiltrating between and around adipocytes. Apoptosis and karyorrhexis are present ⊡. (Courtesy L. J. Medeiros, MD.)

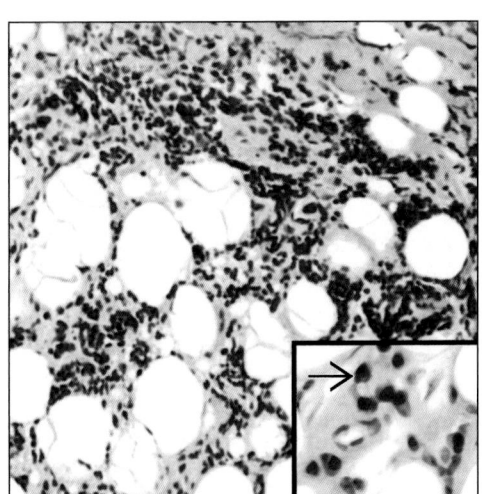

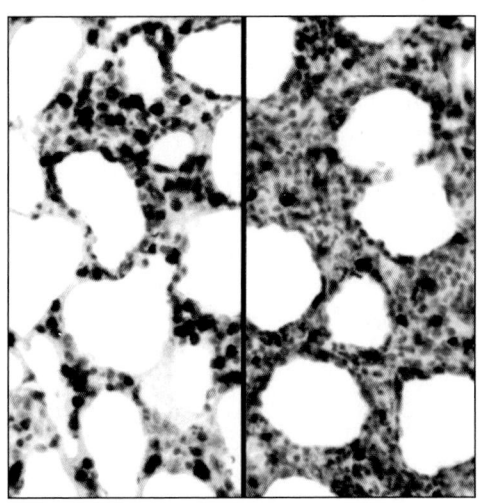

(Left) This case of lupus profundus shows a lobular panniculitis. Scattered plasma cells are seen ⊡ (lower right insert). Plasma cells are a component of lupus profundus, but not expected in CGDTCL. **(Right)** Lupus profundus usually has a mixture of CD4(+) and CD8(+) cells, whereas CGDTCL is usually CD4(-)/CD8(-) or CD4(-)/CD8(+). In this image of lupus profundus, the CD4 stain (left) and the CD8 stain (right) both show clusters of positive cells.

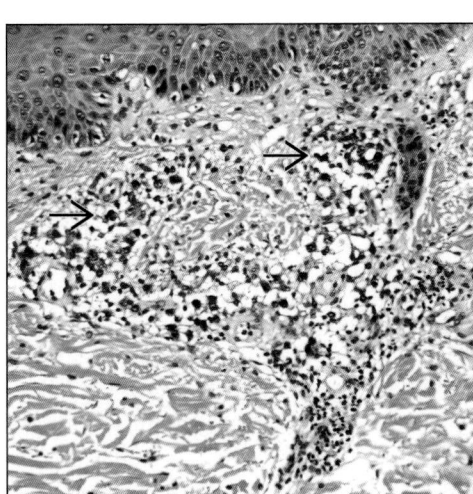

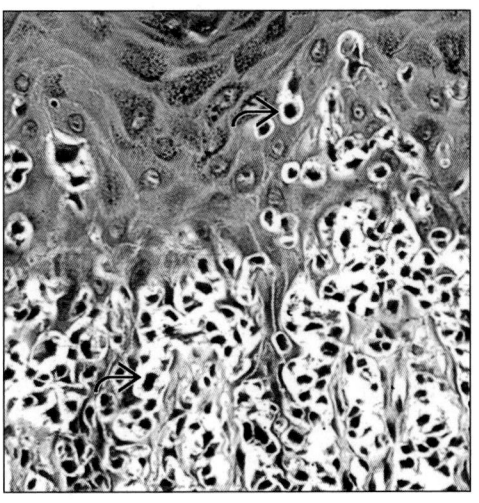

(Left) This case of peripheral T-cell lymphoma, not otherwise specified, shows some similarities to CGDTCL with an epidermal and dermal ⊡ infiltrate of atypical T cells. However, the T cells in this case are CD4(+)/βF1(+), unlike CGDTCL, which is usually CD4(-)/βF1(-). **(Right)** Pagetoid reticulosis (PR) can also appear similar to CGDTCL with pleomorphic cells ⊡ in the epidermis. However, PR differs by having an acral distribution in most cases and a CD4(-)/CD8(+) immunophenotype.

ANGIOIMMUNOBLASTIC T-CELL LYMPHOMA

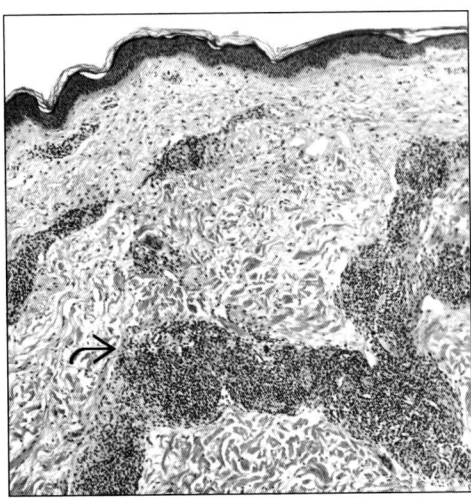

Cutaneous involvement by angioimmunoblastic T-cell lymphoma often shows a nonspecific dense dermal perivascular ➔ infiltrate at low magnification. (Courtesy S. Wang, MD.)

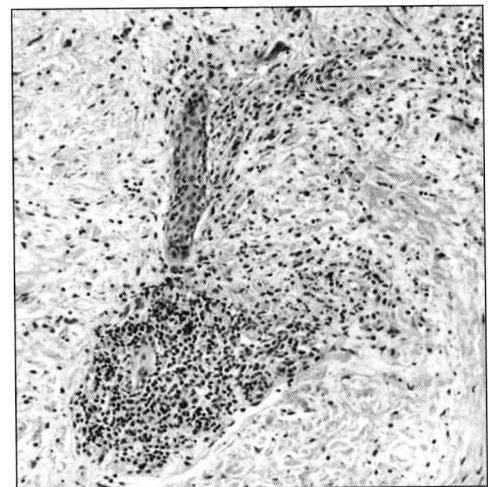

At higher magnification, the T cells in the infiltrate only show mild atypia. In cutaneous lesions of AITL patients, the lymphocytes may or may not show significant atypia.

TERMINOLOGY

Abbreviations
- Angioimmunoblastic T-cell lymphoma (AITL)

Synonyms
- Angioimmunoblastic lymphadenopathy with dysproteinemia
- Immunoblastic lymphadenopathy
- Immunodysplastic disease
- Lymphogranulomatous X

Definitions
- T-cell lymphoma of follicular helper T cells associated with
  - Systemic disease, polymorphous infiltrate, and proliferating high endothelial venules

ETIOLOGY/PATHOGENESIS

Viral Infection
- Epstein-Barr virus
  - EBV(+) B cells are frequently seen in AITL
  - Neoplastic T cells are EBV(-)
- Other viruses
  - Cytomegalovirus, herpes, and HIV also may be associated with AITL
    - PCR for human herpes virus 6B found in many AITL cases
  - Infections may be secondary to tumor

Dysfunction of the Immune System
- Patients with AITL have hypergammaglobulinemia and other immune dysfunctions
  - Possible mechanism
    - Follicular helper T cells upregulate CXCL13 and CXCR5
    - CXCL13 involved with B-cell recruitment
- Cytokine dysregulation

- Patients with AITL show abnormal cytokine dysregulation
- Debated whether skin represents tumor or secondary reaction to cytokines

Drugs
- Implicated as a causative agent in some cases (never proven)

Postulated Normal Cell Counterpart
- CD4(+) follicular helper T cell

CLINICAL ISSUES

Epidemiology
- Incidence
  - Comprises 1-2% of all non-Hodgkin lymphoma
  - 18% of all peripheral T-cell lymphomas
    - 1,000 new cases per year in USA
- Age
  - Mostly adults, middle-aged to elderly
    - Rarely seen in children
  - Median age: 63
- Gender
  - Equal male/female distribution
- Ethnicity
  - Most common in Caucasians
  - More common in Europe than in North America

Site
- Skin
  - Frequent extranodal site
    - ~ 50% of cases have skin lesions
    - Usually secondary to systemic disease
    - Rarely, skin lesion can be 1st manifestation of disease
- Lymph node
  - Nearly all cases involve lymph nodes
- Other sites of disease
  - Often in spleen, liver, and bone marrow

ANGIOIMMUNOBLASTIC T-CELL LYMPHOMA

Key Facts

Terminology
- T-cell lymphoma of follicular helper T cells

Clinical Issues
- Uncommon
- Mostly adults, no gender preference
- Skin rash (50%)
- Generalized lymphadenopathy
- Autoimmune hemolytic anemia
- Polyclonal hypergammaglobulinemia
- Treatment: Chemotherapy
- Median survival: 1-2 years

Microscopic Pathology
- Skin
  - Nonspecific superficial dermal lymphocytic infiltrate with eosinophils
  - ± atypia and hyperplastic capillaries
  - May be tumor cells in skin, or a secondary reactive-appearing rash from cytokine production
- Lymph node
  - Tumor cells with clear cytoplasm, arborizing high endothelial vessels, and disrupted follicular dendritic meshworks
  - Polymorphic background inflammatory cells

Ancillary Tests
- Immunophenotype
  - CD4(+) T cells, CD10(±), Bcl-6(+), CXCL13(+), PD1(+)
  - CD21, in disrupted follicular dendritic meshworks
- Molecular
  - EBER(+) in lymph nodes, and usually (-) in skin
  - Clonal *TCR* gene rearrangement

- No follicular dendritic cells in bone marrow AITL, so bone marrow AITL is CD21(-)
- No CXCL13 in bone marrow AITL

Presentation
- Skin
  - Rash, usually pruritic
    - Maculopapular eruption most common
    - Purpura, erythroderma, papulovesicular, nodules, and urticarial lesions are less common
  - Often generalized lesions
    - Frequently on trunk or extremities
  - Rash can be before, after, or same time as initial diagnosis of AITL
- Extracutaneous presentation
  - Generalized lymphadenopathy
  - Hepatomegaly
  - Splenomegaly
  - B symptoms
  - Arthritis/arthralgia
  - Ascites

Laboratory Tests
- Complete blood cell count
  - Anemia
    - Autoimmune hemolytic anemia
    - Cryoglobulins/cold agglutinins
    - Sometimes positive Coombs test
  - Lymphocytes
    - Lymphopenia more often
    - Lymphocytosis less often
  - Thrombocytopenia
  - Eosinophilia
- Hypergammaglobulinemia or hypogammaglobulinemia
  - Polyclonal
  - Hypoalbuminemia
- ↑ erythrocyte sedimentation rate
- ↑ serum lactate dehydrogenase
- ↑ β-2-microglobulin
- Autoantibodies are sometimes positive
  - Rheumatoid factor
  - Anti-smooth muscle antibody

Natural History
- AITL-related secondary lymphomas
  - Increased risk of developing 2nd lymphoma in patients with AITL
    - Diffuse large B-cell lymphoma is most common 2nd lymphoma
    - Diffuse large B-cell lymphoma usually has positive EBER cells

Treatment
- Adjuvant therapy
  - Combined chemotherapy
    - Treatment in most cases
  - Steroids
    - In patients who do not receive chemotherapy
- Autologous stem cell transplant
  - Sometimes follows treatment with chemotherapy

Prognosis
- Aggressive disease
  - Median survival 1-2 years
- Poor prognostic indicators
  - Males
  - Anemia
  - Mediastinal lymphadenopathy

IMAGE FINDINGS

General Features
- Generalized lymphadenopathy
- Internal organ involvement

MICROSCOPIC PATHOLOGY

Histologic Features
- Skin
  - Usually nonspecific, variable histologic patterns
    - Often superficial dermal infiltrates with lymphocytes and eosinophils
    - Sometimes perivascular lymphocytic infiltrate

ANGIOIMMUNOBLASTIC T-CELL LYMPHOMA

- Sometimes sheet-like lymphocytic infiltrate
- Lymphocytes ± atypia
- Hyperplastic capillaries
- Usually no epidermotropism present
  - Leukocytoclastic vasculitis is rarely seen
  - Necrotizing granulomas are occasionally present
  - May be tumor cells in skin, or secondary reactive infiltrate from cytokine production
- Lymph node
  - Effaced architecture
    - Partial or complete
  - Tumor usually involves paracortical areas
    - Early disease, tumor may be only in paracortex
    - Peripheral cortical sinuses of lymph node are often patent
  - Tumor cells
    - Small to medium in size
    - Increased clear cytoplasm
  - High endothelial venules
    - ↑ vessels in tumor
    - Usually branching blood vessels
    - Follicular dendritic cells located near blood vessels
    - Periodic acid-Schiff stain highlights blood vessels
  - Follicular dendritic cell meshworks
    - Expanded and disrupted in tumor
    - Associated with high endothelial venules
  - Polymorphic background inflammatory cells
    - Often prominent
    - Eosinophils, reactive small lymphocytes, plasma cells
    - Epithelioid histiocytes give granulomatous appearance
    - B immunoblasts in paracortex
    - EBV(+) B cells
  - Lymph node follicles have variable appearance
    - Hyperplastic follicles
    - Atretic follicles (can be mistaken for Castleman lymphadenopathy)
    - No follicles

ANCILLARY TESTS

Immunohistochemistry
- Malignant T cells
  - T-cell antigens positive (CD2, CD3, CD5, CD7)
    - Can aberrantly lose 1 or more T-cell antigens
    - Most commonly lost T-cell antigen is CD7
  - Helper T cells (usually CD4[+], CD8[-], βF1[+])
  - Follicular helper T-cell phenotype
    - CD10(±), Bcl-6(+), CXCL13(+), PD1(+)
    - CXCL13 usually (+) in cutaneous AITL
    - CD10 often (-) in cutaneous AITL
- Follicular dendritic cell meshworks
  - CD21, CD23, CD35 and clusterin positive
- ↑ reactive B cells
  - Express B-cell markers (CD19, CD20, pax-5, CD79a)

Flow Cytometry
- Loss of 1 or more T-cell antigens
  - Most commonly lost T-cell antigen is CD7
- CD10 coexpressed on subset of T cells

Cytogenetics
- No specific chromosomal abnormalities
  - Trisomy of chromosomes 3, 5, 21 reported
  - Loss of 6q and gain of X reported, 1p alterations

In Situ Hybridization
- EBV small-encoded RNA (EBER)
  - 80-90% of lymph nodes positive
    - Usually negative in skin lesions

PCR
- Clonal *TCR* gene rearrangement in 87% of lymph nodes with AITL
  - Some skin infiltrates show clonal *TCR* gene rearrangement
    - Identical clones can be seen in skin and lymph node
- Clonal *IgH* gene rearrangement in 25% of lymph nodes with AITL

DIFFERENTIAL DIAGNOSIS

Cutaneous Infiltrates with Reactive T Cells
- Variety of entities can show nonspecific perivascular T-cell infiltrates in skin
  - Differential diagnosis includes
    - Infections
    - Drug reactions
    - Lymphocytic vasculitis
    - Granulomatous disease if granulomatous inflammation is seen
  - T cells have minimal atypia
  - Usually no clonal *TCR* gene rearrangements
  - No increase in CD21(+) follicular dendritic cells
  - T cells will not coexpress CD10 and will be EBER(-)
  - Clinical history is helpful in making diagnosis

Anaplastic Large Cell Lymphoma (ALCL)
- Common in skin (primary cutaneous ALCL)
- CD30(+); ALK/EMA(-)
- EBER(-)

Peripheral T-cell Lymphoma, Not Otherwise Specified (PTCL-NOS)
- Similarities to AITL
  - Both are malignant T-cell lymphomas, expressing T-cell antigens
  - Some PTCL-NOS have follicular T-cell profile, similar to AITL in gene expression arrays
  - Sometimes increased high endothelial venules
- Differences from AITL
  - No increased follicular dendritic cells by immunohistochemistry
  - EBER(-)

Classic Hodgkin Lymphoma
- Similarities to AITL
  - AITL can sometimes have Reed-Sternberg-like cells that look similar to classic Hodgkin lymphoma
  - Both can be EBER(+)
- Differences from AITL
  - No malignant T cells

ANGIOIMMUNOBLASTIC T-CELL LYMPHOMA

Clinical and Laboratory Findings in AITL

Clinical Finding	% of Cases	Laboratory Finding	% of Cases
B symptoms	68-85	Anemia	40-47
Generalized lymphadenopathy	94-97	Other cytopenias	20
Splenomegaly	70-73	Eosinophilia	39
Hepatomegaly	52-72	Hypergammaglobulinemia	50-83
Rash	48-58	Hypogammaglobulinemia	9-27
Arthritis	18	Autoantibodies	66-77
Ascites/effusions	23-37	↑ LDH	70

AITL vs. Peripheral T-cell Lymphoma, Not Otherwise Specified (PTCL-NOS)

Feature	AITL	PTCL-NOS
High endothelial venules	Increased and arborizing	Normal
Follicular dendritic cells	Increased and disrupted	Normal or decreased
Phenotype	Positive for CD10 and CXCL13	Negative for CD10 and CXCL13
EBV cells	Positive	Variable

- o No increased high endothelial venules
- o No increased follicular dendritic cell meshworks
- o No clonal *TCR* gene rearrangements
- o Rare in skin
- o CD45(-), CD15(+), CD30(+)

T-cell/Histiocyte-rich Large B-cell Lymphoma

- Similarities to AITL
  - o Both tumors have more T cells than B cells
- Differences from AITL
  - o Large atypical B cells and small reactive-appearing T cells in TCRLBCL
    - Often large atypical T cells and small B cells in AITL
  - o Clonal *IgH* gene rearrangement
  - o No increased follicular dendritic cells
  - o EBER(-)

EBV(+) Diffuse Large B-cell Lymphoma of the Elderly

- Both are EBV(+) malignant tumors
- Differences from AITL
  - o Usually polyclonal *TCR* gene rearrangement and clonal *IgH* gene rearrangement
  - o No increased follicular dendritic cells
  - o EBV(+) in sheets of large B cells, and far fewer in number in AITL
  - o No aberrant T-cell antigens

DIAGNOSTIC CHECKLIST

Clinically Relevant Pathologic Features

- Hypergammaglobulinemia and autoimmune hemolytic anemia

Pathologic Interpretation Pearls

- T-cell lymphoma with arborizing high endothelial venules and increased background inflammatory cells
- CD3(+), CD10(+), CXCL13(+)

SELECTED REFERENCES

1. Dorfman DM et al: CD200 (OX-2 membrane glycoprotein) is expressed by follicular T helper cells and in angioimmunoblastic T-cell lymphoma. Am J Surg Pathol. 35(1):76-83, 2011
2. Hatanaka K et al: Methotrexate-associated lymphoproliferative disorders mimicking angioimmunoblastic T-cell lymphoma. Pathol Res Pract. 206(1):9-13, 2010
3. Smithberger ES et al: Primary cutaneous angioimmunoblastic T-cell lymphoma histologically mimicking an inflammatory dermatosis. J Drugs Dermatol. 9(7):851-5, 2010
4. Rodriguez-Justo M et al: Angioimmunoblastic T-cell lymphoma with hyperplastic germinal centres: a neoplasia with origin in the outer zone of the germinal centre? Clinicopathological and immunohistochemical study of 10 cases with follicular T-cell markers. Mod Pathol. 22(6):753-61, 2009
5. Yoon GS et al: Angioimmunoblastic T cell lymphomas: frequent cutaneous skin lesions and absence of human herpes viruses. Ann Dermatol. 21(1):1-5, 2009
6. Ortonne N et al: Characterization of CXCL13+ neoplastic t cells in cutaneous lesions of angioimmunoblastic T-cell lymphoma (AITL). Am J Surg Pathol. 31(7):1068-76, 2007
7. Jayaraman AG et al: Cutaneous involvement by angioimmunoblastic T-cell lymphoma: a unique histologic presentation, mimicking an infectious etiology. J Cutan Pathol. 33 Suppl 2:6-11, 2006
8. Brown HA et al: Cutaneous involvement by angioimmunoblastic T-cell lymphoma with remarkable heterogeneous Epstein-Barr virus expression. J Cutan Pathol. 28(8):432-8, 2001
9. Martel P et al: Cutaneous involvement in patients with angioimmunoblastic lymphadenopathy with dysproteinemia: a clinical, immunohistological, and molecular analysis. Arch Dermatol. 136(7):881-6, 2000
10. Frizzera G et al: Angio-immunoblastic lymphadenopathy. Diagnosis and clinical course. Am J Med. 59(6):803-18, 1975

Cutaneous AITL

(Left) Low-power magnification of a skin biopsy from a patient with AITL who had a maculopapular rash shows a nonspecific, mostly perivascular ➡ lymphocytic infiltrate. **(Right)** In contrast, this AITL skin lesion shows diffuse, large sheets of malignant lymphocytes ➡. This sheet-like distribution pattern is less common.

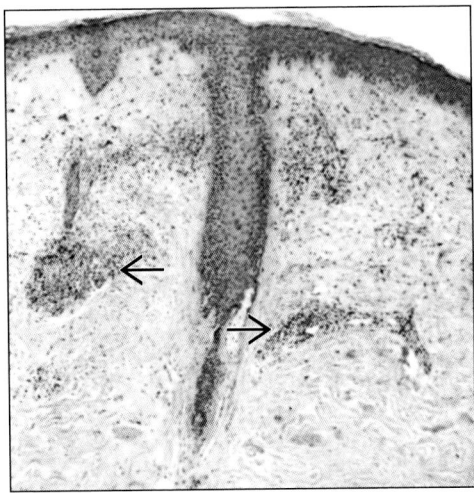
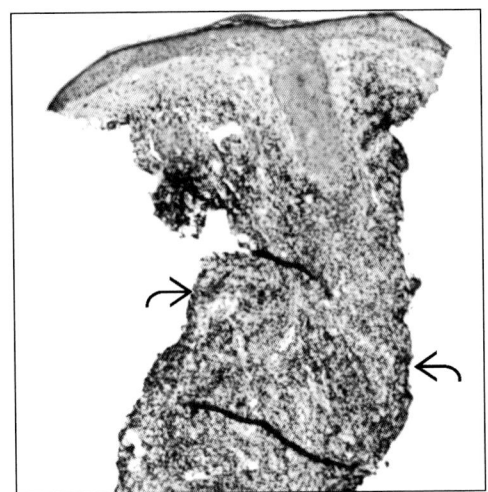

(Left) In another case of cutaneous AITL, the infiltrate is confined to the dermis ➡ and the epidermis ➡ is uninvolved. Most skin lesions in patients with AITL do not show epidermotropism. **(Right)** This CD3 immunohistochemical stain shows strongly positive staining of the dermal T cells. CD20 only marks rare scattered B cells (not shown).

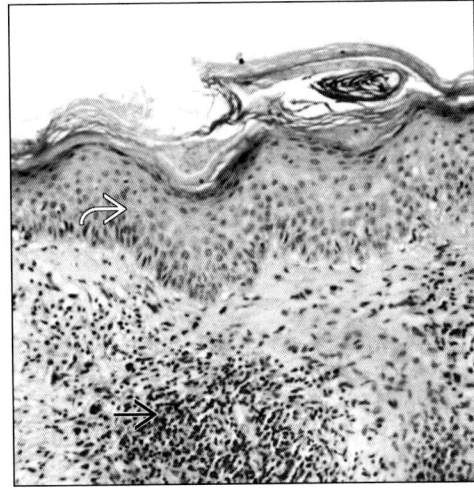
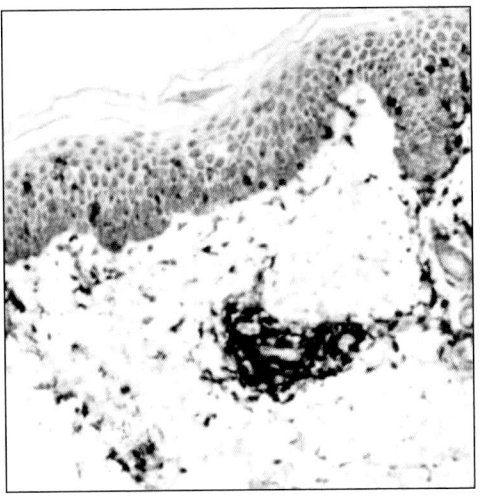

(Left) CD4 immunohistochemical stain shows strong cytoplasmic expression in cutaneous AITL. The T cells are positive for CD4, but negative for CD8 (not shown). **(Right)** CXCL13 is typically positive in cutaneous AITL. This CXCL13 immunostain shows that the T cells are strongly immunoreactive. Cutaneous lesions in patients with AITL are often CXCL13(+), but may be negative for CD10 (not shown).

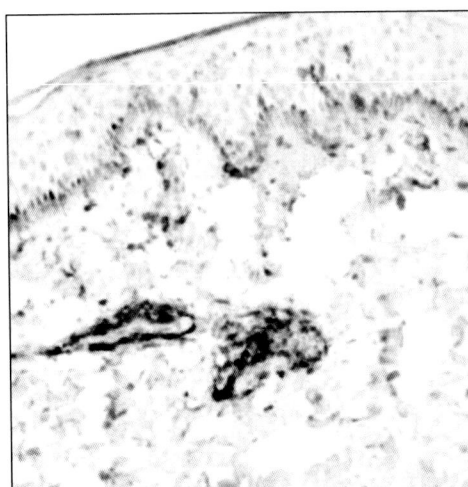
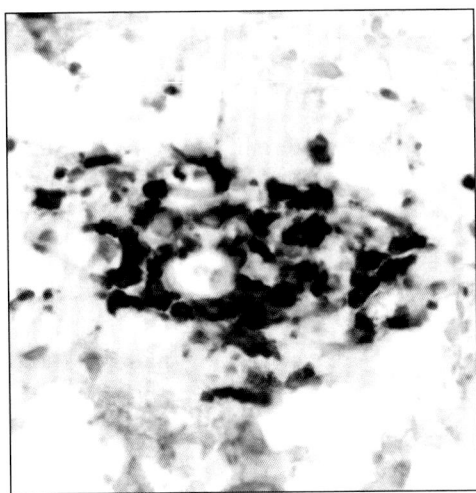

Systemic Disease in AITL

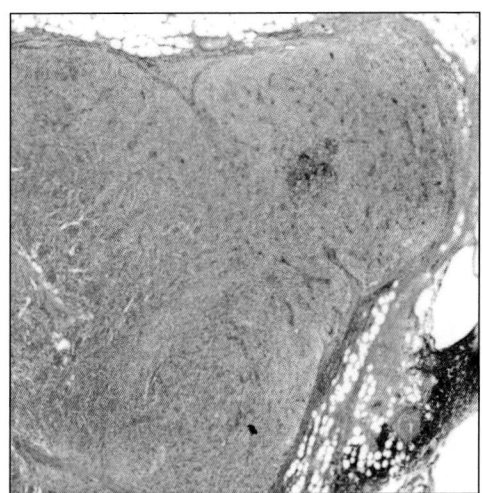
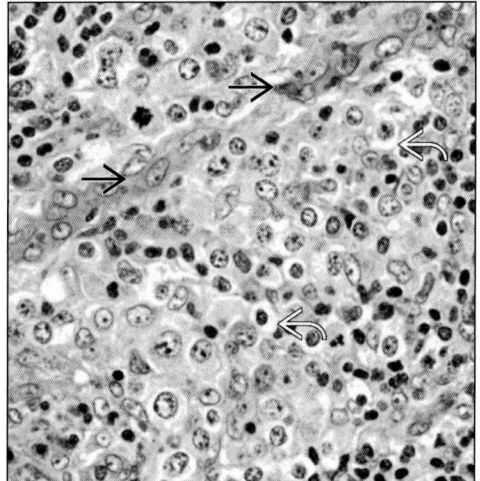

(Left) This lymph node is involved with AITL. At low power, the architecture is effaced by the tumor. Sometimes residual follicles, open subcapsular sinuses, and a paracortical tumor distribution are seen. *(Right)* At high-power magnification, there are increased high endothelial venules ⮕ surrounded by neoplastic cells with clear-staining cytoplasm ⮕.

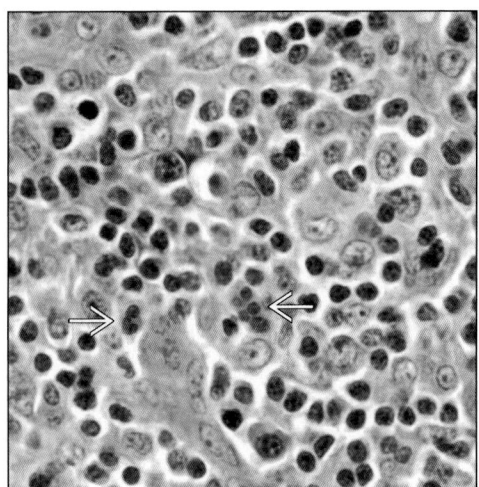
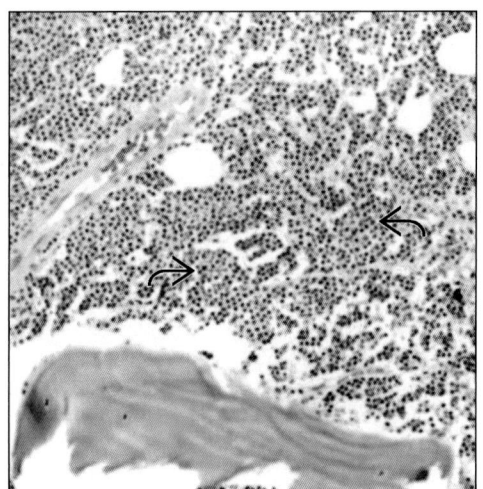

(Left) In AITL, the tumor cells are often accompanied by a mixed inflammatory infiltrate. In this image, there are scattered eosinophils ⮕. *(Right)* Bone marrow involvement in AITL often presents as a nodular infiltrate, either paratrabecular or nonparatrabecular. In the bone marrow, collections of tumor cells ⮕, as well as small lymphocytes, eosinophils, and histiocytes, are present.

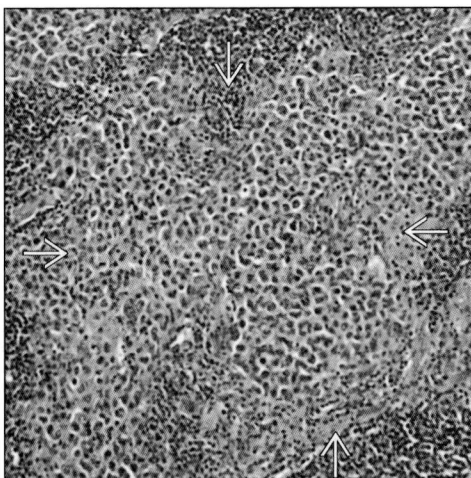
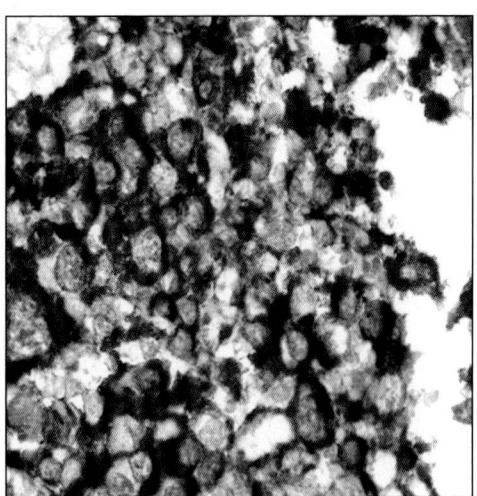

(Left) Histologic examination shows diffuse large B-cell lymphoma (DLBCL) in a patient with AITL. Patients with AITL can also develop B-cell lymphomas, which are thought to arise from B-cell immunoblasts in the AITL. In this image, the lymph node shows a nodular collection of large, atypical B cells ⮕. *(Right)* In this case of DLBCL in a patient with AITL, CD20 strongly highlights the large, atypical B cells of the DLBCL.

Ancillary Techniques for Lymph Nodes with AITL

(Left) High magnification of a lymph node involved by AITL shows that there are arborizing high endothelial venules ➡ amidst medium-sized neoplastic clear cells ➡. *(Right)* PD1 is strongly positive in this case of AITL. PD1 is one of the antigens found in follicular helper T cells that is expressed in AITL. (Courtesy S. Wang, MD.)

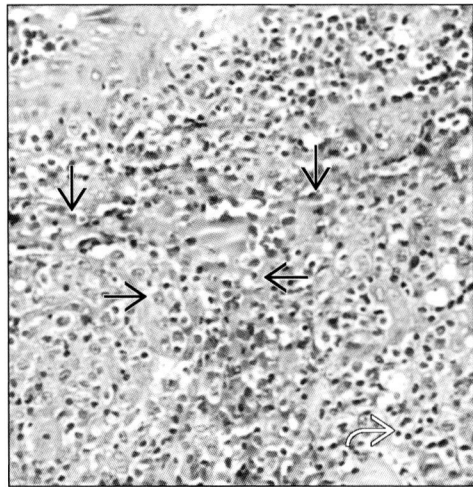
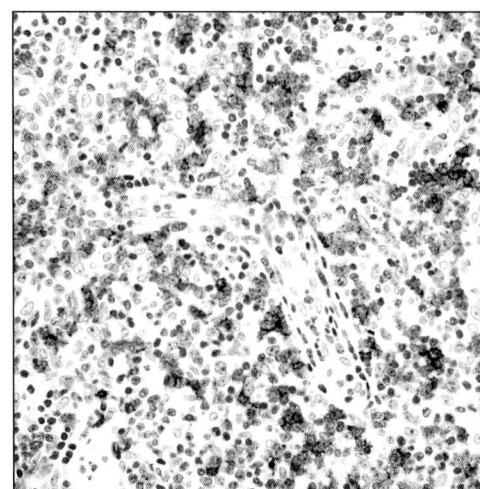

(Left) At high magnification, this CD3 immunostain is positive in the tumor cells of AITL. AITL often expresses multiple T-cell antigens, but may aberrantly lose more T-cell markers. *(Right)* This CD10 immunostain is coexpressed on the same T cells as in the previous CD3 image. CD10(+) and CD3(+) cells are commonly seen in AITL.

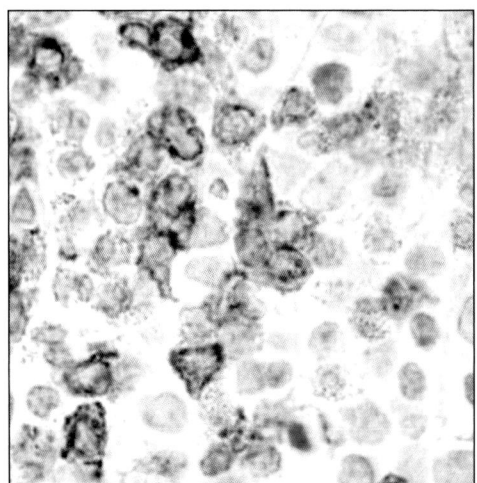
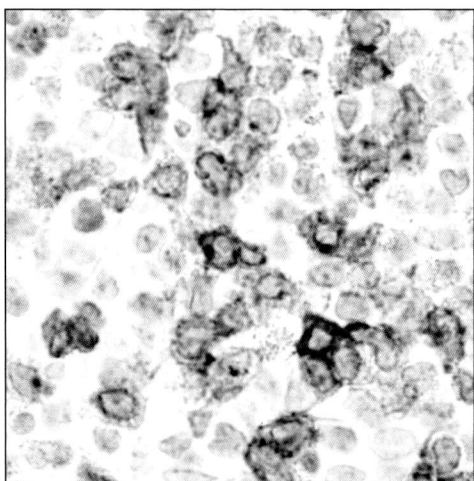

(Left) This EBER stain by in situ hybridization is positive ➡ in scattered cells in this case of AITL. ~ 80-90% of lymph nodes with AITL show EBER(+) cells, but skin lesions are often negative. *(Right)* This CD21 stain marks the follicular dendritic cells ➡, which surround blood vessels in AITL ➡. Lymph nodes with AITL typically show expanded and disrupted FDCs.

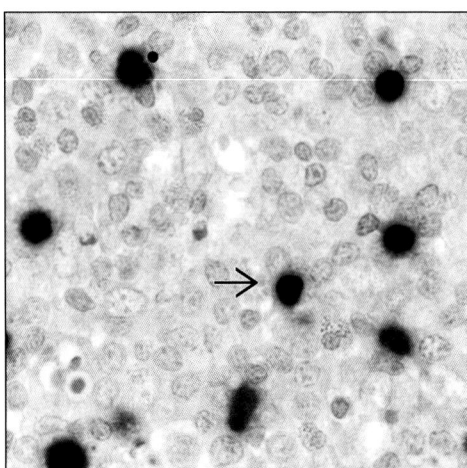
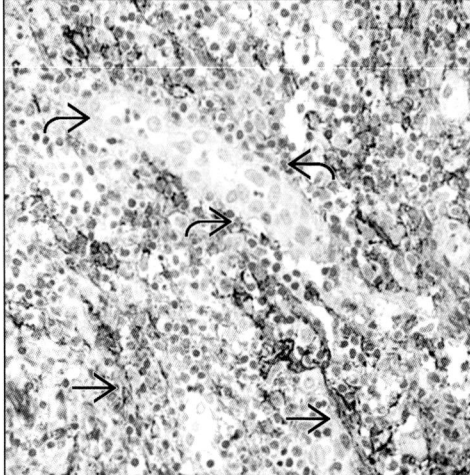

ANGIOIMMUNOBLASTIC T-CELL LYMPHOMA

Differential Diagnosis

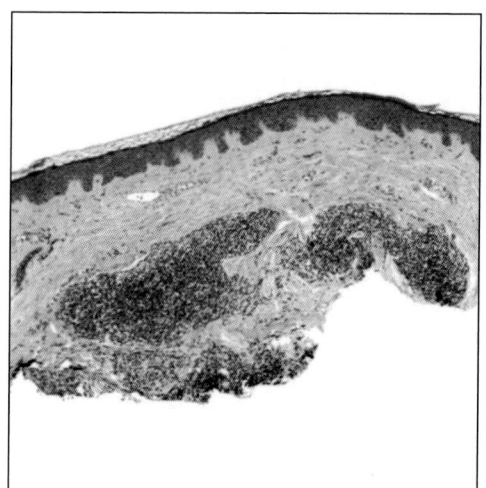

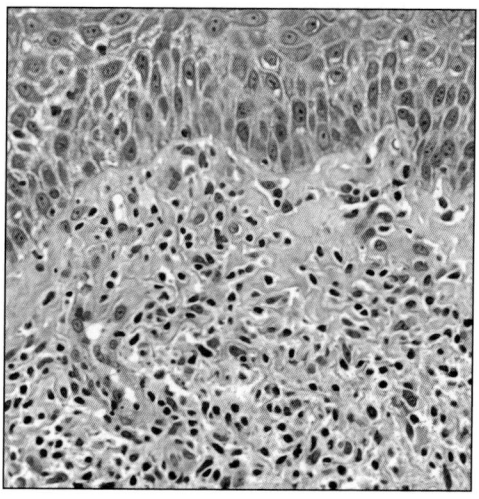

(Left) In this drug reaction from a patient on chlorambucil, there is a prominent angiocentric T-cell infiltrate. Angiocentric dermal infiltrates are also commonly seen in AITL. To differentiate between these diagnoses requires an appropriate clinical history. (Right) This primary cutaneous small medium pleomorphic CD4(+) T-cell lymphoma (SMPTCL) has a superficial perivascular T-cell infiltrate like AITL. However, in SMPTCL, the T cells are negative for CD10 and EBER.

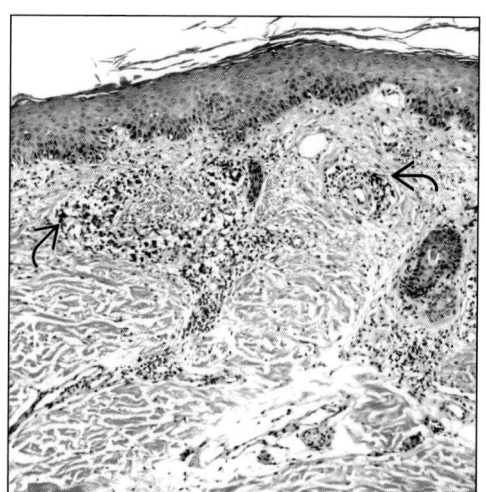

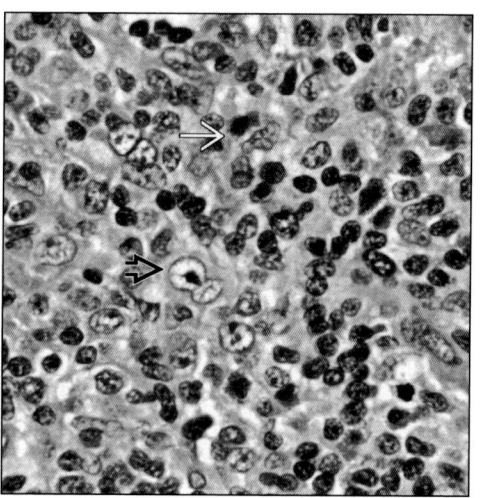

(Left) Peripheral T-cell lymphoma, not otherwise specified (PTCL-NOS) shows an atypical T-cell infiltrate ➔ surrounding the superficial blood vessels and adnexal structures. PTCL-NOS is often in the differential diagnosis of AITL. (Right) Hodgkin lymphoma (HL) can look like AITL with large atypical cells ➔ and mixed inflammation ➔, but the large atypical cells in HL are CD45(-), CD30(+), CD15(+). (Courtesy S. Wang, MD.)

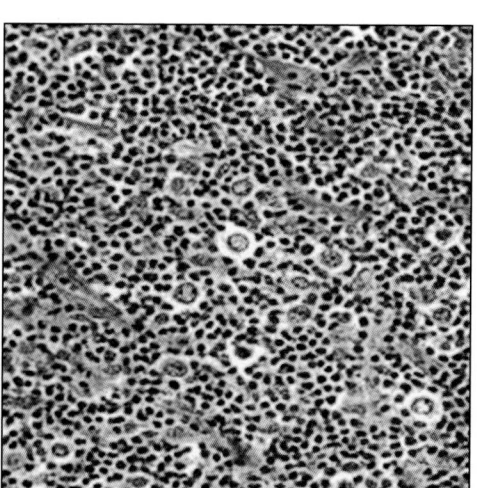

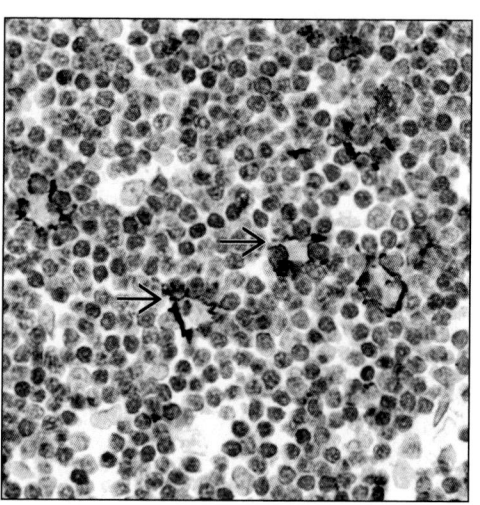

(Left) T-cell/histiocyte-rich large B-cell lymphoma (TCRLBCL) can look similar to AITL. In this case of TCRLBCL, there are scattered large neoplastic cells in a background of small lymphocytes and histiocytes. (Right) CD20 highlights the large neoplastic B cells ➔ in TCRLBCL. In AITL, the atypical cells would be CD20(-) and CD3(+). The large B cells are usually EBV(-), unlike many cases of AITL.

SYSTEMIC T-CELL AND NK-CELL LYMPHOMAS INVOLVING THE SKIN

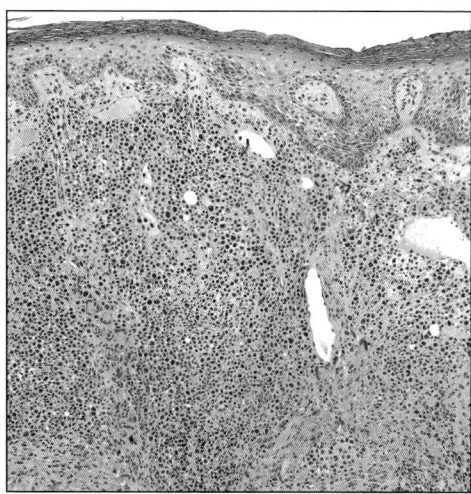

This is an example of a systemic anaplastic large cell lymphoma (ALCL) secondarily involving the skin. The lymphoid infiltrate diffusely fills the superficial and deep dermis.

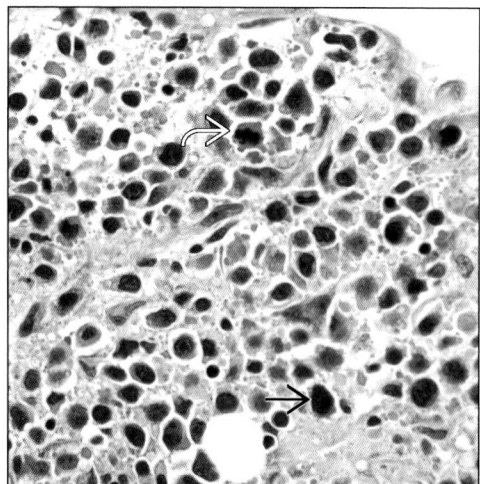

At higher power, tumor cells in systemic ALCL are large and pleomorphic appearing ➡. Mitotic figures are seen ➡.

TERMINOLOGY

Abbreviations
- Systemic T-cell lymphoma (STCL) involving skin

Synonyms
- Secondary cutaneous T-cell lymphoma

Definitions
- T-cell or NK-cell lymphoma that has spread to the skin as a secondary site of disease
  - Lymphoma originates systemically, but involves skin
  - Morphology of primary and secondary skin lymphomas are similar
    - Clinical behavior and treatment of each is divergent, however

ETIOLOGY/PATHOGENESIS

Depends on Type of NK/T-cell Lymphoma
- Can be therapy related
- Epstein-Barr virus infection in some lymphomas
  - Including angioimmunoblastic T-cell lymphoma and extranodal NK/T-cell lymphoma, nasal type

CLINICAL ISSUES

Epidemiology
- Incidence
  - Secondary cutaneous lymphomas make up 50% of all cutaneous lymphomas, excluding mycosis fungoides
  - Secondary T-cell lymphoma in skin is less common than systemic B-cell lymphoma in skin
  - 20-30% of peripheral T-cell lymphoma, unspecified, has cutaneous involvement
    - Represents ~ 14% of all secondary skin lymphomas

  - ~ 50% of angioimmunoblastic T-cell lymphoma (AILT) have cutaneous lesions
  - ~ 8-20% of extranodal NK/T-cell lymphoma, nasal type involve skin
- Age
  - Any age, but mostly adults
    - Systemic anaplastic large cell lymphoma (ALCL) displays a bimodal distribution that includes children, whereas primary cutaneous ALCL is primarily found in adults
- Gender
  - Occurs in both males and females

Presentation
- Often multiple lesions, less often single lesions
  - Usually tumors or nodules
  - Any cutaneous site, no site of predilection
  - Skin involvement may present at time of initial diagnosis or develop later

Treatment
- Usually adjuvant therapy
  - Frequently aggressive chemotherapy, contrary to many primary cutaneous T-cell lymphomas, which are treated with more conservative therapy

Prognosis
- Depends on type of T cell, but usually poor prognosis
  - Higher stage than primary cutaneous lymphoma
  - Usually much worse prognosis than primary cutaneous lymphoma
- ALK(-) ALCL has a worse prognosis than primary cutaneous ALCL or systemic ALK(+) ALCL

MICROSCOPIC PATHOLOGY

Histologic Features
- Morphology and immunophenotype sometimes identical to systemic disease

SYSTEMIC T-CELL AND NK-CELL LYMPHOMAS INVOLVING THE SKIN

Key Facts

Terminology

- Systemic T-cell or NK-cell lymphoma that has spread to the skin
- Morphology of primary and secondary skin lymphomas are similar

Etiology/Pathogenesis

- Epstein-Barr virus infection in some lymphomas

Clinical Issues

- Often multiple lesions, less often single lesion
- Most commonly in adults
- Usually much worse prognosis than primary cutaneous lymphoma
- Frequently aggressive chemotherapy, contrary to many primary cutaneous T-cell lymphomas, which are treated with more conservative therapy

Microscopic Pathology

- Peripheral T-cell lymphoma, unspecified, includes any T-cell lymphomas that do not fit into a better defined subtype of T-cell lymphoma
- Systemic ALK(+) anaplastic large cell lymphoma (ALCL): Often large atypical tumor cells in dermis, sometimes hallmark cells with multiple (horseshoe-shaped nuclei)
- Angioimmunoblastic T-cell lymphoma presents as superficial perivascular T-cell infiltrates with increased reactive inflammatory cells and high endothelial venules
- Extranodal NK/T-cell lymphoma, nasal type, presents as medium to large cells with necrosis and angiocentricity that express T-cell and NK markers and are EBER(+)

- **Peripheral T-cell lymphoma, not otherwise specified (PTCL, NOS)**
  - All T-cell lymphomas that do not fit into a better defined subtype of T-cell lymphoma
    - Other types of T-cell lymphoma must 1st be excluded
  - Wide variety of morphologic appearances
  - Usually an atypical nodular or diffuse dermal T-cell infiltrate sparing epidermis, which may extend to subcutis
    - Medium to large T cells, often with markedly pleomorphic nuclei
    - Sometimes immunoblastic T cells or Reed-Sternberg-like T cells
  - Background reactive infiltrate including small lymphocytes, plasma cells, and eosinophils
  - Can be confused with infection, granuloma annulare, lupus or dermatomyositis, panniculitis and vasculitis
- **Systemic ALK(+) anaplastic large cell lymphoma (ALCL)**
  - 30% involve skin
  - Often large atypical tumor cells in dermis, sometimes hallmark cells with multiple (horseshoe-shaped) nuclei
  - Usually no epidermotropism
  - Can involve lymphatic spaces
- **Systemic ALK(-) anaplastic large cell lymphoma**
  - Same histology as systemic ALK(+) ALCL but considered a different disease than primary cutaneous ALCL
- **Angioimmunoblastic T-cell lymphoma (AITL)**
  - Superficial perivascular infiltrates with lymphocytes, eosinophils, often plasma cells and histiocytes
  - Less often, may show more sheet-like, destructive dermal T-cell infiltrates
  - Increased numbers of high endothelial venules
- **Extranodal NK/T-cell lymphoma, nasal type**
  - Dense dermal infiltrate
    - ~ 30% of cases show rare foci of epidermotropism
  - Perivascular/periadnexal

- Medium/large irregular cells, sometimes with blastic chromatin
- Coagulative necrosis in most cases
- Tumor cells are angiocentric and angiodestructive

Cytologic Features

- Depend on subtype of systemic T-cell or NK-cell lymphoma

ANCILLARY TESTS

Immunohistochemistry

- **Peripheral T-cell lymphoma, unspecified**
  - Expresses some T-cell antigens, but may lack 1 or more T-cell antigens
  - Usually CD4(+)/CD8(-)
    - Rarely CD8(+)/CD4(-) or CD4(+)/CD8(+) or CD4(-)/CD8(-)
  - CD30 (+/-), CXCL13(-), PD-1(-), CD10(-), Bcl-6(-)
  - Cytotoxic antigens are usually negative
  - EBER is only rarely positive
- **Systemic ALK(+) ALCL**
  - CD30(+), usually CD4(+)
  - ALK and EMA are positive by IHC, whereas primary cutaneous ALCL is almost always negative for ALK and EMA
    - ALK(+) in skin lymphoma should warrant clinical evaluation for extracutaneous ALCL
    - Lack of ALK in skin lymphoma is not definite evidence for primary cutaneous ALCL, however
  - Clusterin expression may be seen in noncutaneous ALCL (not confirmed in later studies)
  - Cutaneous lymphocyte antigen (CLA) and HOXC5 are (-) in systemic ALCL, but (+) in primary cutaneous ALCL
- **Angioimmunoblastic T-cell lymphoma**
  - T-cell antigen positive (CD2, CD3, CD5, CD7)
    - Can lose 1 or more T-cell antigens
    - CD7 most commonly lost
  - Helper T cells
    - Usually CD4(+)/CD8(-)/TCR-βF1(+)

Molecular Abnormalities in T-cell Lymphomas and Leukemias

Lymphoma or Leukemia	Molecular Abnormality
Anaplastic large cell lymphoma	*ALK* translocations, t(2;5)(p23;q35), t(1;2)(q25;p23)
Angioimmunoblastic T-cell lymphoma	Trisomies, loss of 6q, gain of x
Enteropathy-associated T-cell lymphoma	9q34 amplifications
Hepatosplenic T-cell lymphoma	Isochromosome 7q
Peripheral T-cell lymphoma	*ITK/SYK* translocations
T-cell prolymphocytic leukemia	*TCL1A* translocations, t(14;14)(q11;q32), inv(14)(q11;q32), t(X;14)(q28;q11), i(8)(q10), t(8;8)(p12;q11)

- Follicular helper T-cell phenotype
  - CD10(-/+), Bcl-6(+), CXCL13(+), PD-1(+)
  - CD10 is often negative in cutaneous AITL
  - CXCL13 is usually positive in cutaneous AITL
- Follicular dendritic T-cell meshworks
  - Usually CD21, CD23, CD35, and clusterin positive
- ↑ reactive B cells
  - Express B-cell markers (CD20, CD79, pax-5)
- Often EBER positive
- **Extranodal NK/T-cell lymphoma, nasal type**
  - T-cell antigens positive (CD2, CD3, CD7)
  - CD56(+)
  - Cytotoxic markers positive
  - EBER(+) and LMP(+)

Molecular Tests
- *TCR* gene rearrangements are seen in all T-cell lymphomas
- Systemic ALCL
  - Translocations involving *ALK* are common t(2;5), unlike primary cutaneous ALCL
- *IRF4* translocations are found in primary cutaneous ALCL, but not in systemic ALCL or lymphomatoid papulosis

DIFFERENTIAL DIAGNOSIS

Primary Cutaneous T-cell Lymphomas
- May show overlapping features
- Often have to prove there is no extracutaneous lymphoma by clinical and imaging studies

B-cell Lymphomas
- Express B-cell antigens

DIAGNOSTIC CHECKLIST

Pathologic Interpretation Pearls
- SCTLs have a higher stage and worse prognosis than most primary cutaneous T-cell lymphomas
- SCTLs are treated more aggressively with chemotherapy than most primary cutaneous T-cell lymphomas

SELECTED REFERENCES

1. Kinney MC et al: Anaplastic large cell lymphoma: twenty-five years of discovery. Arch Pathol Lab Med. 135(1):19-43, 2011
2. Pan ST et al: Cutaneous peripheral T-cell lymphoma of cytotoxic phenotype mimicking extranodal NK/T-cell lymphoma. Am J Dermatopathol. 33(2):e17-20, 2011
3. Sánchez-Schmidt JM et al: Primary cutaneous CD30+ anaplastic large-cell lymphomas show a heterogeneous genomic profile: an oligonucleotide arrayCGH approach. J Invest Dermatol. 131(1):269-71, 2011
4. Wada DA et al: Specificity of IRF4 translocations for primary cutaneous anaplastic large cell lymphoma: a multicenter study of 204 skin biopsies. Mod Pathol. 24(4):596-605, 2011
5. Berti E et al: Cutaneous extranodal NK/T-cell lymphoma: a clinicopathologic study of 5 patients with array-based comparative genomic hybridization. Blood. 116(2):165-70, 2010
6. Liao JB et al: Clinicopathologic analysis of cutaneous lymphoma in taiwan: a high frequency of extranodal natural killer/t-cell lymphoma, nasal type, with an extremely poor prognosis. Arch Pathol Lab Med. 134(7):996-1002, 2010
7. Park S et al: Primary cutaneous Epstein-Barr virus-associated T-cell lymphoproliferative disorder-2 cases with unusual, prolonged clinical course. Am J Dermatopathol. 32(8):832-6, 2010
8. Querfeld C et al: Primary cutaneous and systemic anaplastic large cell lymphoma: clinicopathologic aspects and therapeutic options. Oncology (Williston Park). 24(7):574-87, 2010
9. Choi YL et al: Extranodal NK/T-cell lymphoma with cutaneous involvement: 'nasal' vs. 'nasal-type' subgroups--a retrospective study of 18 patients. Br J Dermatol. 160(2):333-7, 2009
10. Feldman AL et al: Recurrent translocations involving the IRF4 oncogene locus in peripheral T-cell lymphomas. Leukemia. 23(3):574-80, 2009
11. Schwartz EJ et al: Immunohistochemical characterization of nasal-type extranodal NK/T-cell lymphoma using a tissue microarray: an analysis of 84 cases. Am J Clin Pathol. 130(3):343-51, 2008
12. Lachenal F et al: Angioimmunoblastic T-cell lymphoma: clinical and laboratory features at diagnosis in 77 patients. Medicine (Baltimore). 86(5):282-92, 2007
13. Jayaraman AG et al: Cutaneous involvement by angioimmunoblastic T-cell lymphoma: a unique histologic presentation, mimicking an infectious etiology. J Cutan Pathol. 33 Suppl 2:6-11, 2006

SYSTEMIC T-CELL AND NK-CELL LYMPHOMAS INVOLVING THE SKIN

Systemic Peripheral T-cell Lymphoma, NOS

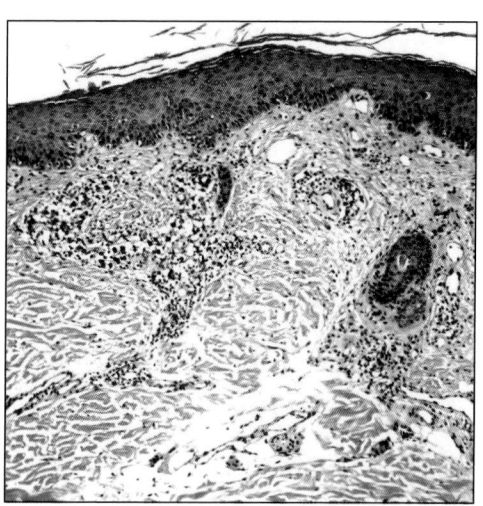

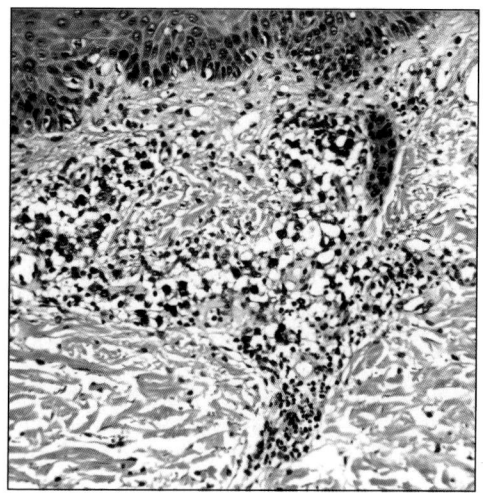

(Left) *This is an example of systemic peripheral T-cell lymphoma, not otherwise specified (PTCL, NOS) involving the skin. Several years ago, the patient was diagnosed with peripheral T-cell lymphoma of the cervical and inguinal lymph nodes, and now presents with multiple tumor nodules on his thigh.* *(Right)* *At higher magnification, this PTCL, NOS presents as a superficial and deep, mostly perivascular lymphoid infiltrate.*

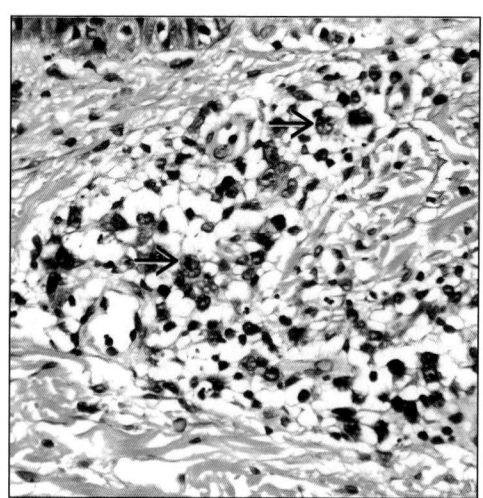

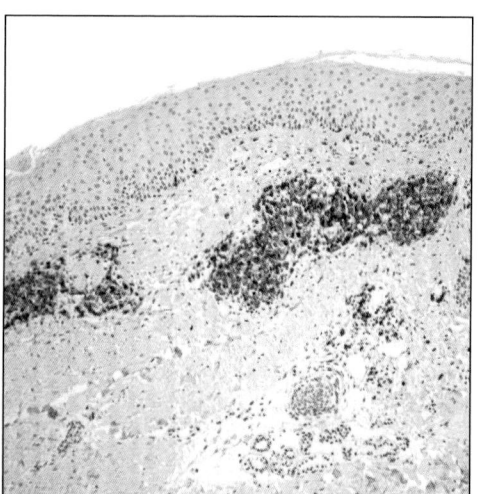

(Left) *On high magnification, the malignant T cells in PTCL, NOS range from medium to large in size. Some of the larger cells have coarse chromatin and enlarged nucleoli* ➡️. *(Right)* *CD3 immunohistochemical stain is strongly positive in this PTCL, NOS. PCR also showed TCR gamma gene rearrangement.*

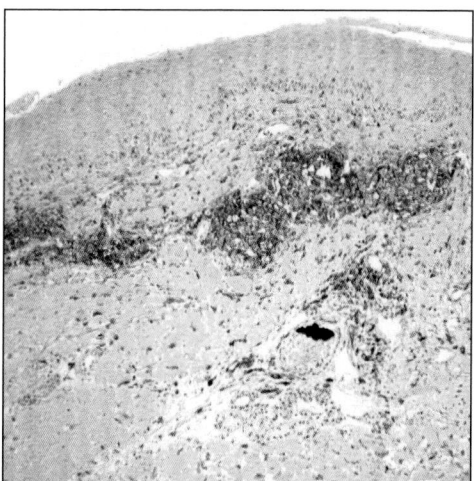

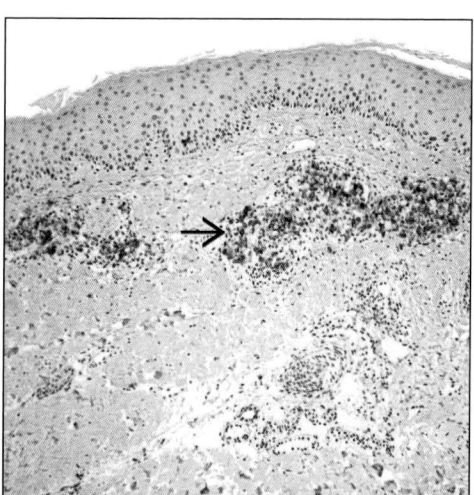

(Left) *CD4 immunohistochemical stain shows that the same CD3(+) T cells also strongly express CD4. CD8 (not shown) was negative.* *(Right)* *CD30 marker was positive* ➡️ *in this PTCL, NOS, even though it was negative in the original lymph node biopsies. Gain of CD30 expression can be seen in many cases, and does not indicate that this is ALCL. No ALK translocations were identified in the lymph nodes or skin biopsies.*

Systemic Anaplastic Large Cell Lymphoma

(Left) This is a case of systemic anaplastic large cell lymphoma involving the skin. Two years ago, the patient had been diagnosed with anaplastic large cell lymphoma in the lymph nodes. There is a diffuse dermal lymphoid infiltrate of large, markedly atypical cells. *(Right)* This case of ALCL is primarily involving lymphatic spaces. The image on the right is a CD30 immunohistochemical stain, which marks the tumor cells. *(Courtesy M. Tomaszewski, MD.)*

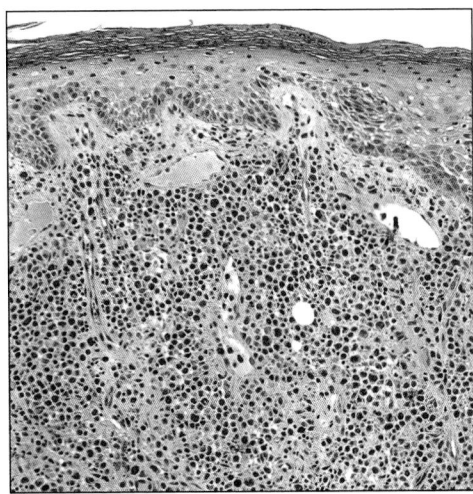
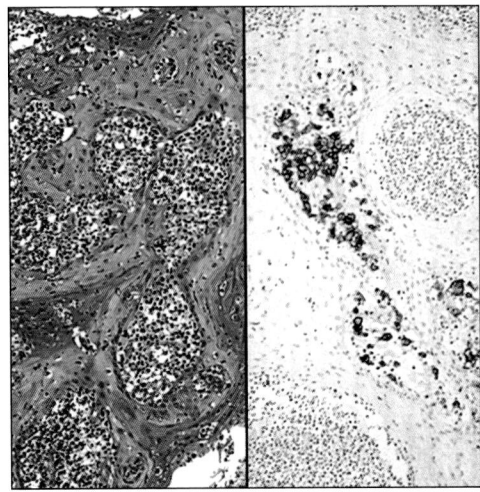

(Left) This high-power image of a CD4 IHC stain shows that the tumor cells are strongly CD4(+). CD8 (not shown) was negative. Most cases of ALCL are CD4(+)/CD8(-), and only 5% are CD4(-)/ CD8(+). *(Right)* This is a positive EMA stain in a case of systemic ALCL with secondary involvement of skin. Systemic cases are often positive for EMA, whereas primary cutaneous ALCL is usually EMA negative.

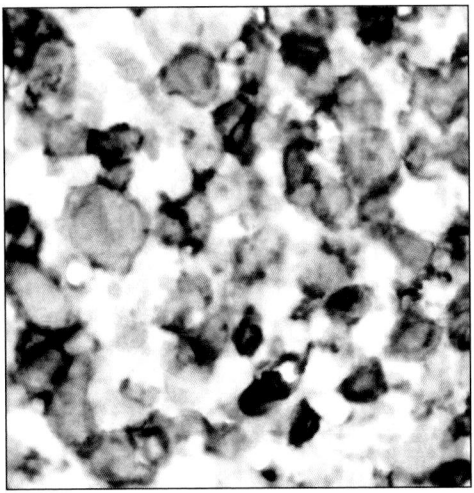
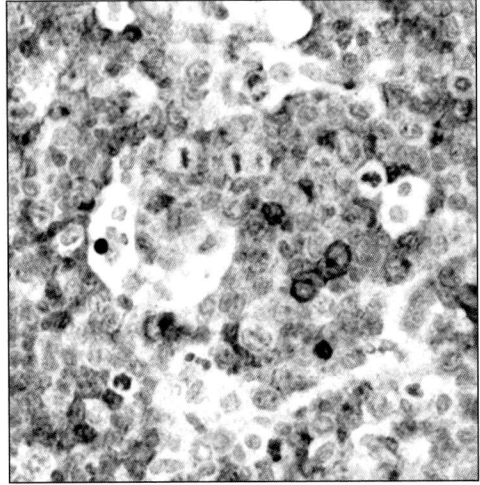

(Left) This systemic ALCL with secondary cutaneous involvement strongly expresses ALK by immunostaining ➡. Currently, systemic ALCL is either classified as ALK(+) or ALK(-), and these are considered different diseases. *(Right)* This is a break-apart probe FISH test for 2p23 (ALK). The blue signal ➡ represents the 5' region of ALK and a pink signal ➡ represents the 3' region of ALK. ALK rearrangements are usually seen in systemic ALCL, but not primary cutaneous ALCL.

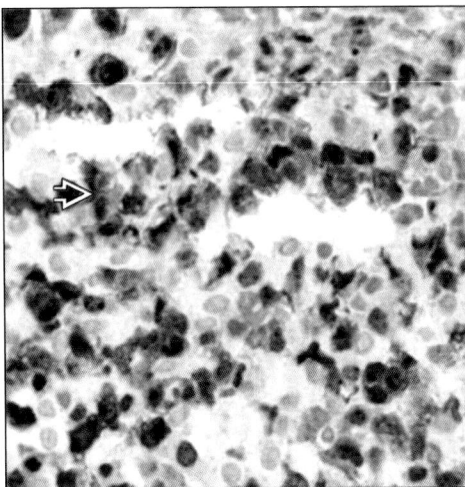
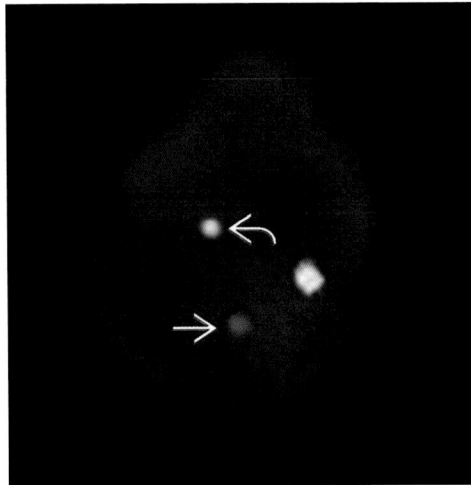

Angioimmunoblastic T-cell Lymphoma

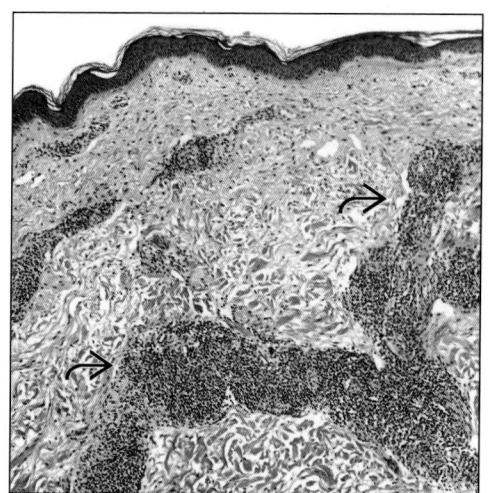

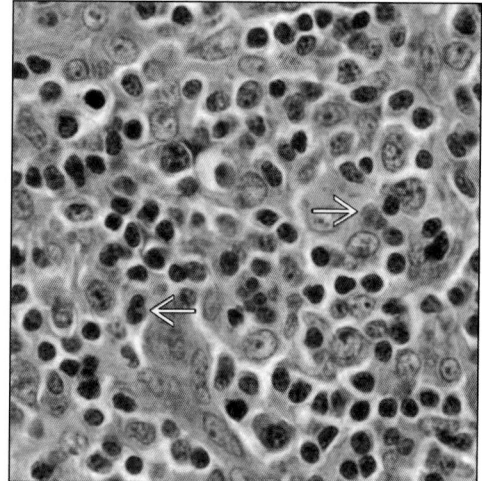

(Left) Cutaneous involvement by angioimmunoblastic T-cell lymphoma (AITL) often shows a nonspecific dense dermal perivascular ➡ infiltrate at low magnification. *(Courtesy S. Wang, MD.)* *(Right)* In AITL, the tumor cells are often accompanied by a mixed inflammatory infiltrate. In this image, there are scattered eosinophils present ➡.

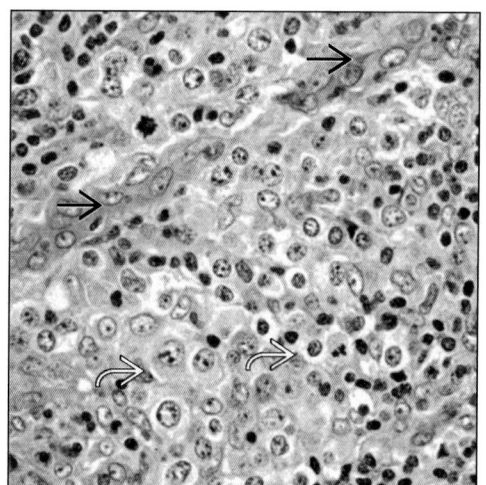

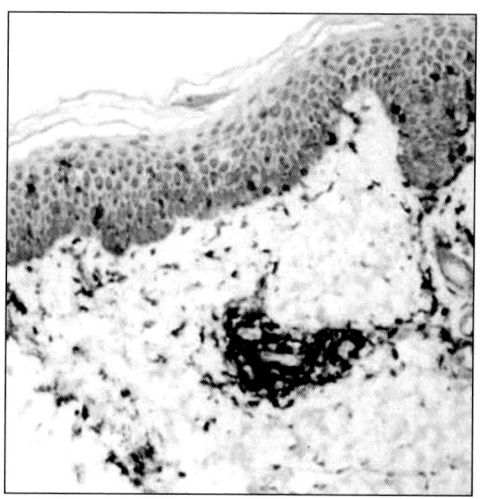

(Left) At higher power, there are increased high endothelial venules ➡ surrounded by neoplastic cells with clear cytoplasm ➡. *(Right)* In this CD3 immunohistochemical stain, CD3 is strongly positive in the dermal T cells. CD20 only marked rare scattered B cells (not shown).

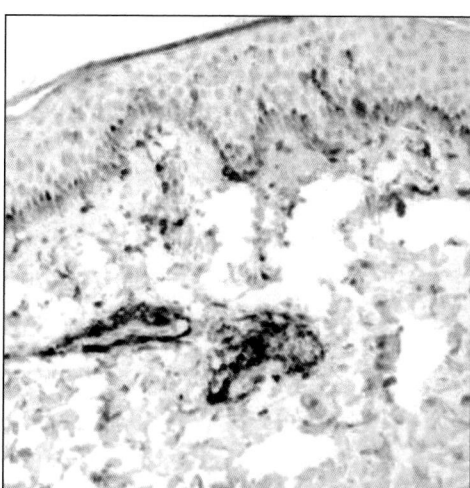

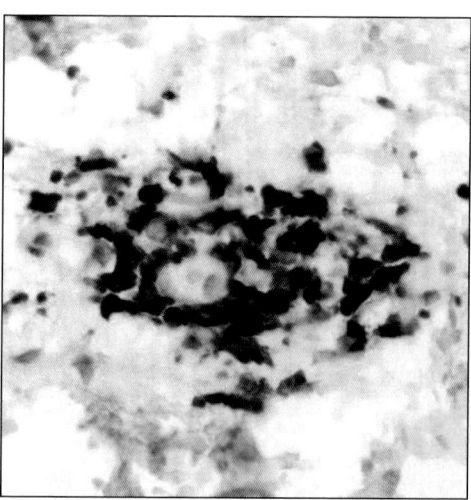

(Left) This is a CD4(+) immunohistochemical stain showing strong cytoplasmic expression in cutaneous AITL. The T cells are positive for CD4, but negative for CD8 (not shown). *(Right)* CXCL13 is positive in cutaneous AITL. The T cells are strongly immunoreactive for CXCL13. Cutaneous lesions in patients with AITL are often CXCL13(+), but are often negative for CD10 (not shown).

LEUKEMIA CUTIS

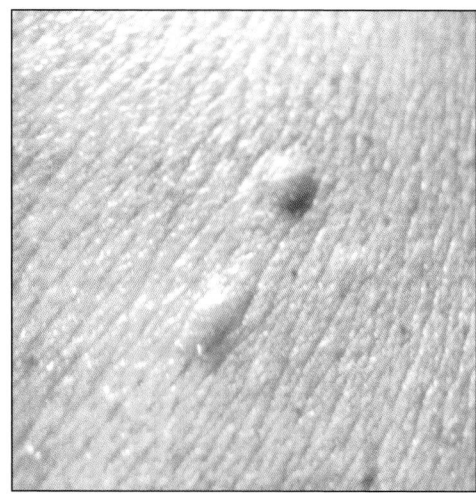

Clinical image shows 2 small papules in a patient with acute myeloid leukemia. Histologic examination confirmed leukemic infiltrates consistent with myeloid sarcoma. (Courtesy V. Tonkovic-Capin, MD.)

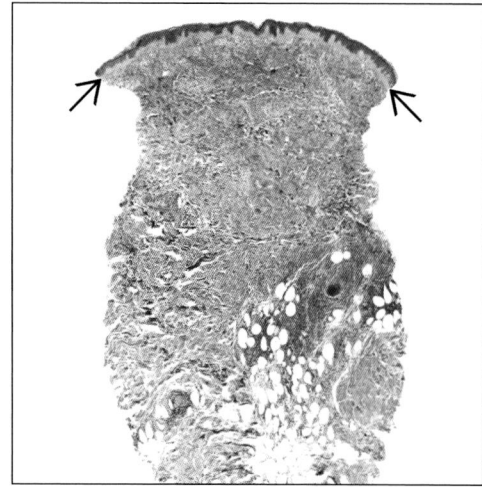

A punch biopsy shows leukemic infiltrates in the superficial and deep dermis, extending into the subcutaneous adipose tissue. Sparing of the epidermis with a thin Grenz zone ⇨ is noted.

TERMINOLOGY

Abbreviations
- Leukemia cutis (LC)

Synonyms
- Myeloid sarcoma (MS), granulocytic sarcoma, extramedullary myeloid cell tumor, chloroma
  - When composed of myeloid cells
- Monoblastic sarcoma
  - When composed of monocytic precursors
- Primary extramedullary leukemia

Definitions
- Clinically identifiable cutaneous lesions secondary to cutaneous infiltration by neoplastic leukocytes (myeloid or lymphoid)
- Leukemia cutis commonly used to describe lymphocytic leukemias involving skin
  - Designated by precursor B- or T-cell lineage and chronic lymphocytic leukemia
  - "Myeloid sarcoma" is preferred term when leukemic cells are of myeloid or monocytic lineage

ETIOLOGY/PATHOGENESIS

Mechanisms of Skin Homing
- Underlying process has not been defined
  - May involve coexpression of cutaneous lymphocyte antigen (CLA) and its interaction with specific chemokines
  - Other factors may include CCR4, TARC, and CCL22
- Predilection for sites with cutaneous inflammation (e.g., Sweet syndrome, psoriasis)

CLINICAL ISSUES

Epidemiology
- Incidence

- Acute monocytic, myelomonocytic, and T-cell leukemias show highest incidence of leukemia cutis
- LC can be observed in all forms of acute myeloid leukemia (AML)
- Occurs in 10-15% of patients with AML
  - Varies widely with AML subtype
  - Up to 50% of patients with acute myelomonocytic and monocytic types
- Less frequent in patients with myeloproliferative and myelodysplastic neoplasms
  - Rare reports of CML with LC presentation
  - Usually related to disease progression &/or transformation
- Is seen in up to 25% of chronic lymphocytic leukemia/small lymphocytic lymphoma (CLL/SLL) cases
- Occurs in 20-70% of mature T-cell leukemias
  - 40-70% of adult T-cell leukemia/lymphoma (ATLL)
  - 25-30% of T-cell prolymphocytic leukemia (T-PLL)
- Unusual in patients with precursor B- or T-cell lymphoblastic leukemia/lymphomas (LBL) and plasma cell leukemia
- Occurs in 25-30% of infants with congenital leukemia
- Age
  - Frequency higher among children than adults

Site
- Most commonly involves extremities (legs > arms)
- Back, chest, scalp, and face may also be involved
- Preferential involvement at sites of previous or concomitant inflammation
  - Sweet syndrome
  - Herpes zoster
  - Insect bites
  - Psoriasis

Presentation
- Presentation may precede (aleukemic LC), coincide with, or manifest as recurrence of acute leukemia

LEUKEMIA CUTIS

Key Facts

Terminology

- Clinically identifiable cutaneous lesions secondary to cutaneous infiltration by neoplastic leukocytes (myeloid or lymphoid)

Clinical Issues

- Presentation may precede (aleukemic LC), coincide, or manifest as recurrence of leukemia
- Acute monocytic, myelomonocytic, and T-cell leukemias show the highest incidence of leukemia cutis
  - Occurs in 10-15% of patients with AML
  - Occurs in 20-70% of mature T-cell leukemias
  - Occurs in up to 25% of chronic lymphocytic leukemia/small lymphocytic lymphoma (CLL/SLL) cases

Microscopic Pathology

- Perivascular, periadnexal, diffuse, and nodular infiltrates can be seen

Top Differential Diagnoses

- Inflammatory dermatoses
- Mature B-cell lymphomas
- Mature T-cell lymphomas
- Poorly differentiated carcinoma
- Blastic plasmacytoid dendritic cell neoplasm

Diagnostic Checklist

- Diagnosis requires
  - Careful histologic and immunohistochemical examination
  - Correlation with clinical data, bone marrow, and peripheral blood findings

---

- Most cases present after diagnosis of systemic leukemia
- < 10% present prior to blood or bone marrow involvement (aleukemic LC or primary extramedullary leukemia)
- Single or multiple skin lesions
  - Violaceous, red-brown, or hemorrhagic papules, nodules, and plaques of varying sizes
  - Erythematous papules and nodules most commonly reported
  - Eczematous lesions
  - Ulcers
  - "Blueberry muffin" appearance
    - Firm blue, red, or purple nodules in generalized distribution
    - Term historically used to describe cutaneous involvement in children with congenital leukemia
- Oral petechiae
- Thickening of the gums
  - Oral lesions more common in adults
    - Rare in congenital leukemias
- Other sites of extramedullary involvement are frequent (e.g., meninges)

Laboratory Tests

- Lactate dehydrogenase and β2-microglobulin
  - Higher levels reported in patients with leukemia cutis
- Serology for HTLV-1 in cases of ATLL

Treatment

- Options, risks, complications
  - Managed by treating underlying leukemia
    - Systemic chemotherapy
    - Bone marrow transplantation
  - Local therapy (e.g., radiation)
  - Aleukemic LC should not be managed differently from patients with known leukemia

Prognosis

- Poor prognosis
  - Generally a manifestation of disease progression

- Leukemia cutis in context of congenital myelogenous leukemia is an exception
  - Not associated with worse prognosis
  - Spontaneous regression of LC without treatment has been observed
- Prognosis in CLL patients is good
  - Exception of blastic transformation (Richter syndrome) is associated with poor prognosis

MICROSCOPIC PATHOLOGY

General Histologic Features

- Low-power patterns of involvement
  - Perivascular &/or periadnexal
  - Dense and diffuse
  - Nodular
  - Subtle superficial interstitial infiltrate (rare)
- Stromal fibrosis
- Lineage assignment unreliable with histology alone

Myeloid and Monoblastic Sarcoma

- Perivascular, periadnexal, diffuse, and nodular infiltrates can be seen
- Epidermotropism is very rare
- Myeloid blasts and granulocytic precursors predominate
  - Large cells with oval to convoluted nuclei, immature finely dispersed chromatin, occasional nucleoli
  - Nuclei may appear more cleaved/convoluted and cytoplasm more abundant with monocytic differentiation
    - Atypical monocytoid cells
  - Mitotic figures and apoptotic cells

Precursor B- or T-cell LBL

- Deep-seated infiltrates
  - Perivascular &/or diffuse
- Cells typically appear monomorphous
  - Intermediate-sized round nuclei, immature dispersed chromatin, inconspicuous nucleoli, scant cytoplasm
- Cytomorphologic features of B- and T-LBL are nearly identical

- Lack epidermotropism
- Frequent mitotic figures and apoptotic bodies
  - "Starry sky" pattern may be present
- Stromal fibrosis

Mature B-cell Lymphoproliferative Neoplasms

- Most commonly, chronic lymphocytic leukemia/small lymphocytic lymphoma (CLL/SLL)
  - Patterns of involvement
    - Perivascular and periadnexal
    - Nodular and diffuse
    - Band-like
    - Pseudoproliferation centers may be visible in large lesions
  - Monotonous population of small lymphoid cells
    - Round nuclei
    - Mature heterogeneous chromatin
  - Lesions may occur at sites previously involved by inflammatory &/or infectious agents or epithelial malignancies

Mature T-cell Lymphoproliferative Neoplasms

- **Adult T-cell leukemia/lymphoma (ATLL)**
  - Superficial band-like infiltrate with epidermotropism and Pautrier-like microabscesses
  - Often resembles mycosis fungoides (MF)
  - Perivascular infiltrate ± angioinvasion
  - Heterogeneous infiltrates
    - Small, intermediate, large, and pleomorphic T cells
- **T-cell prolymphocytic leukemia (T-PLL)**
  - Perivascular &/or periadnexal infiltrate
  - Focal epidermotropism
  - Stromal edema
  - Heterogeneous cytomorphology
    - Typically larger than normal lymphocytes
    - Round to irregular nuclei
    - ± prominent nucleoli
- **Sézary syndrome (SS)**
  - Perivascular &/or interstitial dermal infiltrates
  - Upper and mid-dermal infiltrates are most common
  - Epidermotropism often present, but may be focal
    - May be absent in significant proportion of cases
    - Lack of epidermotropism does not exclude diagnosis
  - Patterns can be indistinguishable from MF
  - Cytomorphology
    - Small to medium-sized cells
    - Often have irregular, twisted nuclear contours
    - Larger perivascular lymphocytes more common in SS

ANCILLARY TESTS

Flow Cytometry

- Evaluation of suspected lesions can be helpful
- Aberrant antigen expression patterns helpful in defining but not always specific to neoplasia

PCR

- T- and B-cell clonality studies
  - May be helpful
  - False positive results can occur in reactive infiltrates
  - Tests should be interpreted with caution
    - Always interpret in context of clinicopathologic findings
  - Monoclonal rearrangements for *JH* gene
    - Present in majority of B-LBL, CLL
  - Monoclonally rearranged T-cell receptor genes
    - Present in majority of T-LBL

Molecular Genetics

- Molecular abnormalities reflect those of the respective leukemia type
- **Myeloid sarcoma**
  - FISH probes to evaluate for WHO 2008 defined recurrent cytogenetic abnormalities are available in some specialized labs
    - Can be performed on paraffin-embedded tissue
    - May aid in the classification of aleukemic MS
  - Chromosome 8 abnormalities
    - Common in AML patients with leukemia cutis (30-40%)
- Molecular genetic studies in other subtypes of leukemia cutis are limited

DIFFERENTIAL DIAGNOSIS

Inflammatory Dermatoses

- Requires careful histologic and immunohistochemical examination
  - Immature B- or T-cell phenotype (TdT, CD1a, CD34) excludes inflammatory disorder
- Flow cytometry can be helpful
  - Neoplastic processes more likely to show antigen loss &/or aberrant antigen expression patterns
  - Additional tissue held for possible flow cytometry studies can be valuable
- Distinction with B- and T-cell clonality studies can be problematic
- Clinicopathologic correlation is essential

Mature B-cell Lymphomas

- Extranodal B-cell lymphomas may involve skin as primary site
- Nodal B-cell lymphomas may involve skin as secondary site of extension
- Express multiple B-cell antigens
  - CD19, CD20, CD79a, pax-5, MUM1
  - May express CD10, Bcl-2, and Bcl-6 (follicular lymphomas)
- Lack TdT, CD34, MPO, lysozyme

Mature T-cell Lymphomas

- Nodal and extranodal T-cell lymphomas may involve skin as secondary site of extension
- May show bone marrow involvement but lack peripheral blood involvement
- Express mature T-cell antigens without TdT or CD1a

LEUKEMIA CUTIS

Immunohistochemical Patterns of Leukemia Cutis

Diagnostic Type	Positive	Variable	Negative	Comments
Myeloid (granulocytic) sarcoma	CD34, CD43, CD117, MPO, lysozyme	CD4, CD45	CD68(PG-M1), CD10	MPO and lysozyme are often most helpful in demonstrating myeloid lineage
Myeloid (monoblastic) sarcoma	CD4, CD43, CD68(PG-M1), lysozyme	CD10, CD45, MPO, CD117	CD34	MPO and lysozyme are often most helpful in demonstrating myeloid lineage
Precursor B-ALL	CD10, CD19, CD34, CD43, CD79a, TdT	CD20, CD45		
Precursor T-ALL	CD1a, CD2, CD3, CD5, CD10, CD99, TdT	CD4, CD8		Surface CD3 may be absent; CD99 is nonspecific; combination of CD3 with TdT &/or CD1a considered most specific
Chronic lymphocytic leukemia/small lymphocytic lymphoma	CD5, CD19, CD20(dim), CD23, CD43, CD45, CD79a, pax-5			
Adult T-cell leukemia/lymphoma	CD2, CD3, CD4, CD5, CD25(+)	CD7	CD1a, TdT, TIA1, granzyme-B	Diminished or loss of CD7 is common
T-cell prolymphocytic leukemia	CD3, CD4, CD45RO, TCL1		CD1a, CD34, TdT	CD4 and CD8 coexpressed in 25% of cases
Sézary syndrome	CD3, CD4, CD25, CD45RO			Loss of diminished CD7 and CD26 are common; rare cases may express CD8; larger cells may express CD30

Blastic Plasmacytoid Dendritic Cell Neoplasm (BPDCN)

• Usually presents with solitary or multiple skin lesions
• 10-20% associated with or develop into AML
• Resembles myeloid sarcoma
• Expresses CD4, CD43, CD45RA, CD56, and plasmacytoid dendritic cell antigens (CD123, CD303, TCL1)
  ○ CD7 and CD33 expression is relatively common
  ○ CD68(+) in 50% of cases
  ○ Lysozyme(-) and MPO(-)
• CD4 and CD56 alone cannot be used to differentiate from MS
  ○ MS commonly expresses CD4, and rarely expresses CD56

Langerhans Cell Histiocytosis (LCH)

• Langerhans cells have abundant eosinophilic cytoplasm and coffee bean-shaped nuclei with nuclear grooves
• Frequently accompanied by numerous eosinophils
• Complete phenotypic analysis should be performed
  ○ Express CD1a and S100

Histiocytic Sarcoma

• Substantial overlap between monocytic and histiocytic sarcoma
• Composed of frankly atypical and pleomorphic-appearing histiocytes by morphology and IHC
• By definition, no evidence of blood or bone marrow involvement

Poorly Differentiated Carcinoma

• May present with large aggregates of tumor cells in dermis
• Glandular differentiation (±)
• History of carcinoma may be known
• Should show expression of at least some cytokeratins

Merkel Cell Carcinoma

• Histomorphologic features may overlap
• Express cytokeratins, CK20 (perinuclear dot-like pattern), and neuroendocrine markers, including chromogranin and synaptophysin
• Lack expression of lymphoid and myeloid markers

DIAGNOSTIC CHECKLIST

Pathologic Interpretation Pearls

• Diagnosis requires
  ○ Careful histologic and immunohistochemical examination
  ○ Correlation with clinical data, bone marrow, and peripheral blood findings
• Aleukemic leukemia cutis is frequently misdiagnosed as atypical lymphoid infiltrate or lymphoma
  ○ Immunophenotyping is essential to make distinction
  ○ Although rare, LC can precede a true leukemic presentation by weeks to months

SELECTED REFERENCES

1. Cho-Vega JH et al: Leukemia cutis. Am J Clin Pathol. 129(1):130-42, 2008
2. Robak E et al: Skin lesions in chronic lymphocytic leukemia. Leuk Lymphoma. 48(5):855-65, 2007
3. Barzilai A et al: Aleukemic monocytic leukemia cutis. Cutis. 69(4):301-4, 2002
4. Ratnam KV et al: Leukemia cutis. Dermatol Clin. 12(2):419-31, 1994
5. Su WP: Clinical, histopathologic, and immunohistochemical correlations in leukemia cutis. Semin Dermatol. 13(3):223-30, 1994
6. Resnik KS et al: Leukemia cutis in congenital leukemia. Analysis and review of the world literature with report of an additional case. Arch Dermatol. 129(10):1301-6, 1993

12

Clinical, Microscopic, and Immunohistochemical Features

(Left) Clinical photograph shows an adult male with a known history of AML who later presented with multiple violaceous plaques on the left side of the face. Histologic examination revealed findings of MS consistent with recurrent AML. (Courtesy M. Jackson, MD.) *(Right)* Diffuse dermal cellular infiltrates composed of large pleomorphic cells with sparing of the epidermis are shown in this example of cutaneous MS. This finding represents the initial manifestation of recurrent AML.

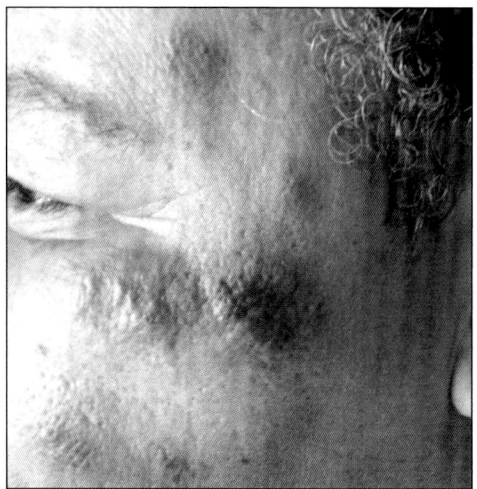
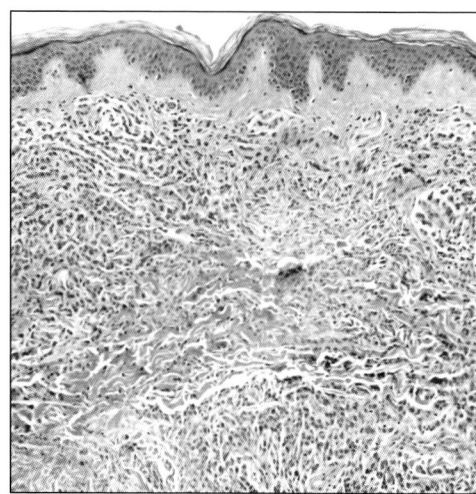

(Left) High-power view highlights the cytomorphologic detail of the leukemic blasts in this case of cutaneous MS. Note the variably pleomorphic large nuclei with dispersed chromatin and inconspicuous nucleoli. Occasional mitotic figures are noted ➡. *(Right)* IHC staining by lysozyme in this section of skin highlights numerous leukemic blasts in a patient with previously diagnosed and treated AML. The findings are consistent with recurrent AML.

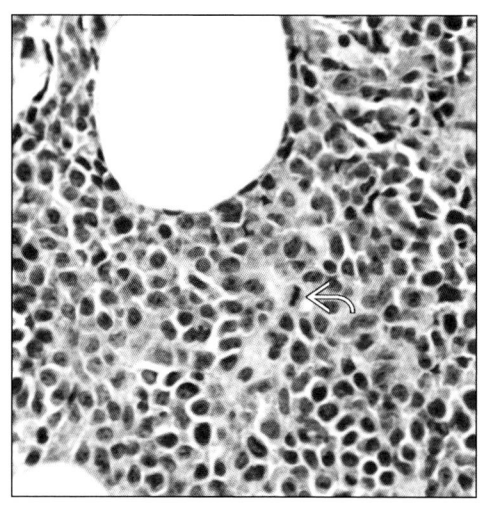
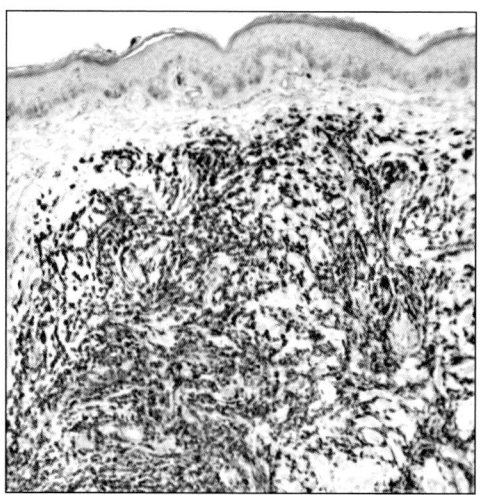

(Left) IHC staining with CD68 in this section at high-power magnification highlights numerous leukemic blasts with monocytic differentiation in a patient with previously diagnosed and treated AML. *(Right)* IHC staining by CD34 highlights the vascular structures ➡, but is negative in the leukemic blasts. Leukemic blasts with monocytic differentiation are frequently negative for CD34; however, this finding alone should not be used to exclude a diagnosis of MS.

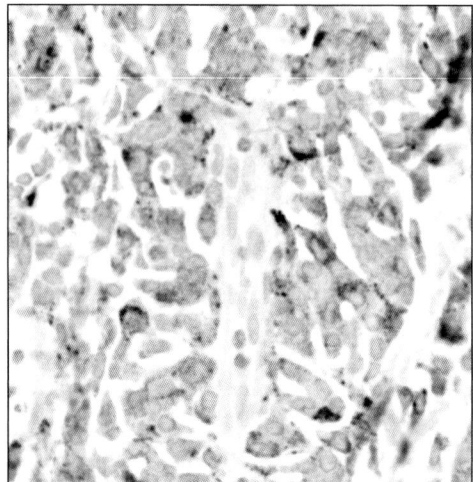
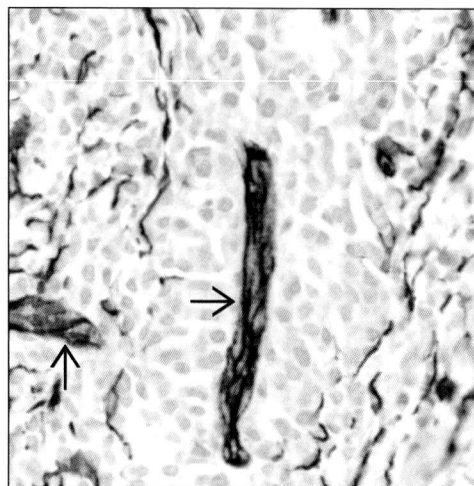

LEUKEMIA CUTIS

Microscopic Features and Differential Diagnosis

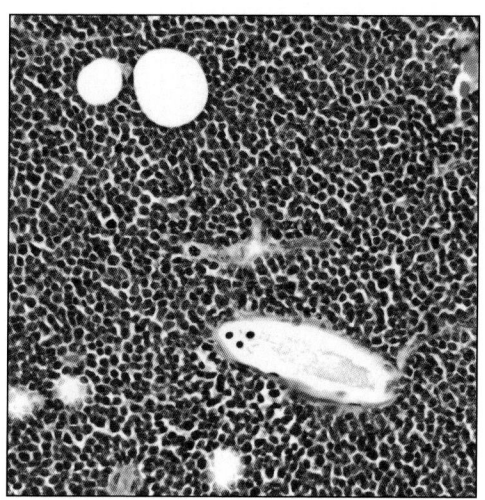

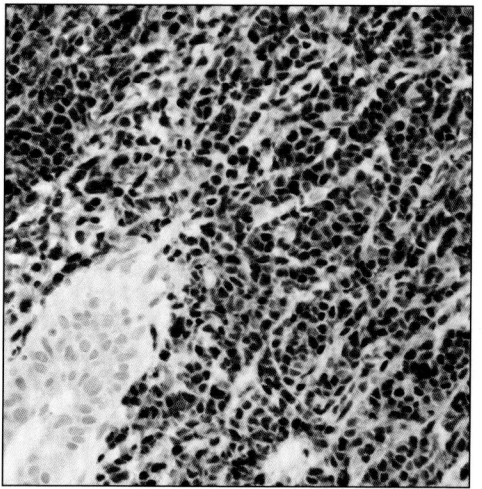

(Left) B-LBL involving skin. In this field, the lymphoblasts fill the dermis and surround blood vessels. Note the monomorphic cytomorphology is more typical of B- and T-LBL. (Courtesy C. Bueso-Ramos, MD, PhD.) (Right) IHC for TdT shows positive nuclear staining consistent with B-LBL. This pattern of staining is also observed in T-LBL. Additional B- and T-cell lineage markers are necessary to determine the lineage of the tumor. (Courtesy C. Bueso-Ramos, MD, PhD.)

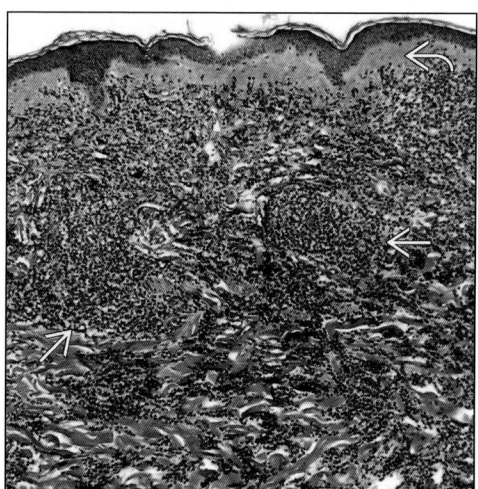

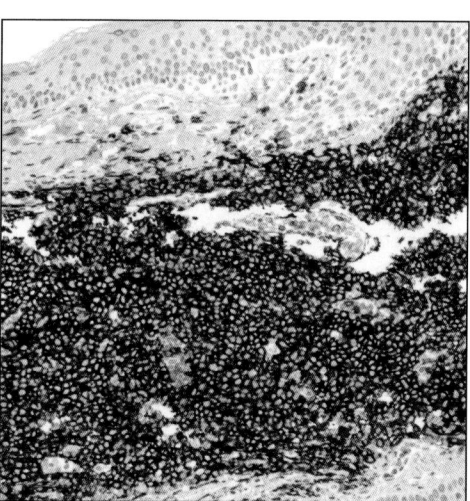

(Left) Skin with involvement by CLL/SLL. The B cells ➡ are in the superficial and deep dermis and show a dense, sheet-like growth pattern. The epidermis is uninvolved and separated from the malignant B cells by a thin grenz zone ➡. No germinal centers are present. (Right) CD20 is very strongly positive, showing that the cutaneous infiltrate in this patient with CLL/SLL consists of aggregates of B cells.

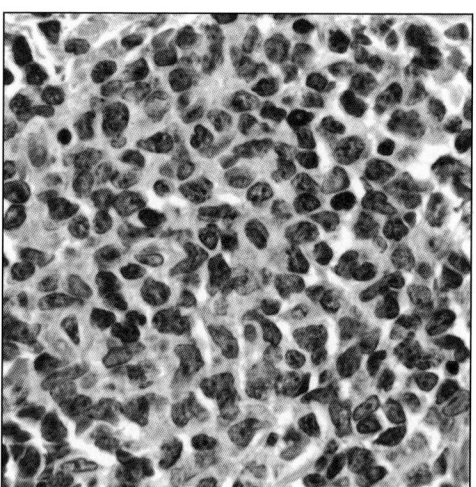

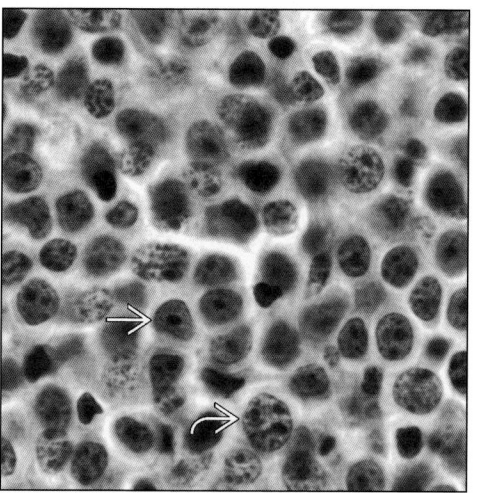

(Left) A case of BPDCN shows neoplastic cells with prominent pleomorphism and blastic-appearing chromatin. The cytologic features suggest a differential of MS with monocytic differentiation. The lack of lysozyme, CD33, and CD68 in BPDCN help make this distinction. (Right) A mixture of both centroblasts ➡ & immunoblasts ➡ are seen in this diffuse large B-cell lymphoma. A mature B-cell phenotype with negative MPO and lysozyme makes the distinction from LC.

BLASTIC PLASMACYTOID DENDRITIC CELL NEOPLASM

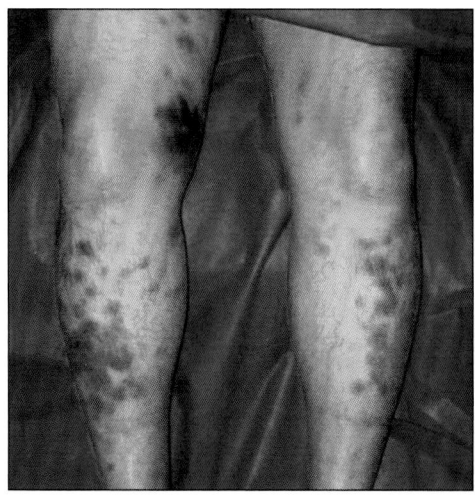

This patient rapidly developed generalized, indurated, purplish-red, well-defined papules and coalescent plaques over his legs. (Courtesy J. Alonso, MD.)

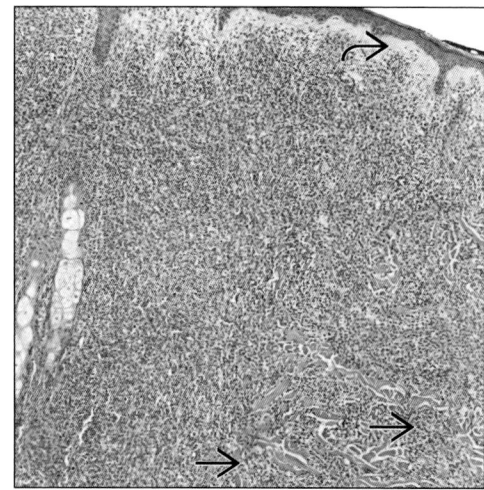

BPDCN shows the dermis replaced by a diffuse infiltrate of tumor cells with an infiltrative pattern, dissecting between collagen bundles ➡. The epidermis is spared, with a grenz zone ➡. (Courtesy L. J. Medeiros, MD.)

TERMINOLOGY

Abbreviations
- Blastic plasmacytoid dendritic cell neoplasm (BPDCN)
  - Terminology in 4th edition of World Health Organization classification

Synonyms
- CD4(+)/CD56(+) hematodermic neoplasm
- CD4(+)/CD56(+) blastic tumor of skin
- Blastic NK-cell lymphoma
- Agranular CD4(+) natural killer cell leukemia

Definitions
- Aggressive tumor of precursor plasmacytoid dendritic cells, which usually involves the skin; frequently culminates in leukemia
  - Included in the T-cell/NK-cell neoplasm section of the WHO classification, even though it is a tumor of plasmacytoid dendritic cells

ETIOLOGY/PATHOGENESIS

Plasmacytoid Dendritic Cells (PDCs)
- PDCs are found in T-cell areas of hematopoietic tissue
  - Found in lymph node, bone marrow, blood, and spleen (subcapsular)
    - Enter lymph node and mucosa in response to immune activation
- Functions of plasmacytoid dendritic cells
  - Interferon-γ production
  - IL-3α expression
  - Dendritic cell differentiation following exposure to IL3 and CD40
- Immunophenotype of plasmacytoid dendritic cells
  - Positive for
    - CD4, CD123, BDCA-2, CLA, TCL1, HLA-DR, CD43, CD68
  - Negative for
    - CD56, TdT, TIA-1, perforin
- Diseases with ↑ plasmacytoid dendritic cells
  - Castleman lymphadenopathy
  - Kikuchi-Fujimoto disease
  - Classic Hodgkin lymphoma
  - Chronic granulomatous inflammation
  - Psoriasis
  - Lupus erythematosus

CLINICAL ISSUES

Epidemiology
- Incidence
  - Rare
    - < 1% of all acute leukemias
    - < 1% of cutaneous lymphomas
- Age
  - Usually middle age to elderly
    - Can occur in children
  - Median: 65 years
    - Range: 8-96 years
- Gender
  - M:F = 3.3:1.0
- Ethnicity
  - No association

Site
- Often presents in > 1 anatomic site
  - Skin
    - Most common 1st manifestation of disease
    - Eventually skin involvement in nearly all patients
    - 50% confined to skin at initial staging
  - Bone marrow and peripheral blood
    - 60-90% of cases
    - There are rare leukemia variants without skin involvement that are recognized with intensive immunophenotyping
    - Can be subtle infiltrates in bone marrow
  - Lymph node

BLASTIC PLASMACYTOID DENDRITIC CELL NEOPLASM

Key Facts

Terminology
- Tumor of plasmacytoid dendritic cells, often involves the skin and bone marrow, and disseminates to blood

Clinical Issues
- Incidence
  - Rare
- Natural history
  - Clinically aggressive
- Gender/sex
  - Middle age to elderly, male predominance
- Multiple skin lesions
  - Usually eventually disseminated disease
- Prognosis and therapy
  - Poor response to lymphoma chemotherapy
  - Therapy for acute lymphoblastic leukemia is most effective

Microscopic Pathology
- Diffuse dermal infiltrate, spares epidermis, of medium-sized cells with blastic chromatin

Ancillary Tests
- Immunohistochemistry: CD123(+), CD4(+), CD56(+), TCL1(+), TdT(+) (sometimes)
- Molecular tests
  - All *IgH* gene rearrangement studies are nonclonal
  - Most T-cell receptor gene rearrangement studies are nonclonal
  - EBV-encoded small nuclear RNA (EBER) negative

Top Differential Diagnoses
- Leukemia cutis
- Extranodal NK/T-cell lymphoma, nasal type
- Peripheral T-cell lymphoma, NOS

- 45% of cases
- Other organs that have been reported to be involved by BPDCN
  - Liver, spleen, tonsils, nasopharynx, conjunctiva, kidneys, central nervous system

Presentation
- Generalized, localized, or solitary cutaneous lesions
  - Macules, plaques, &/or tumors
    - Sometimes erythema &/or purpura
- Lymphadenopathy
- Rarely B symptoms present

Laboratory Tests
- Cytopenias
  - Thrombocytopenia most common
- Monocytosis is sometimes present

Natural History
- Relapse and metastasis in most cases
  - Soft tissue and CNS frequently at relapse, but rare at diagnosis
- Leukemia
  - Often relapses as leukemia
    - 10-20% of cases develop into acute myeloid leukemia
    - Often myelomonocytic leukemia
  - Presents more like leukemia than lymphoma

Treatment
- Adjuvant therapy
  - Multiagent chemotherapy
    - Poor response to non-Hodgkin lymphoma chemotherapy (R-CHOP)
    - 90% of cases relapse after chemotherapy
  - Acute lymphoblastic leukemia protocols
    - Intrathecal chemotherapy followed by allogeneic bone marrow transplantation
    - Most effective therapy, especially in children

Prognosis
- Poor
  - Median survival ~ 13 months

- Less aggressive in children with median survival of 3 years
- Often favorable initial response to chemotherapy, but eventual relapse

MACROSCOPIC FEATURES

General Features
- Nodules, tumors, or plaques of skin, which may have ulceration

MICROSCOPIC PATHOLOGY

Histologic Features
- Skin
  - Dermal infiltrate
    - Typically extends into subcutaneous tissue
    - Spares the epidermis with grenz zone
  - Growth pattern
    - Diffuse, if extensive involvement
    - Perivascular
    - Periadnexal
  - Increased mitotic figures
  - Extravasated erythrocytes
  - Scattered reactive T cells amidst tumor cells
- Lymph node
  - Effacement of lymph node architecture
    - Often interfollicular and medullary involvement by tumor
    - Sometimes tumor in sinuses
- Bone marrow
  - Aggregates of tumor cells or scattered tumor cells
    - Often interstitial distribution
  - Residual bone marrow often shows dysplasia
- Peripheral blood
  - Tumor cells can have vacuoles in the cytoplasm
    - Pseudopods
    - Resemble monoblasts

Cytologic Features
- Medium-/large-sized atypical cells

BLASTIC PLASMACYTOID DENDRITIC CELL NEOPLASM

- o Usually fine blastic chromatin, resembling lymphoblast or myeloblast
  - 1 or more small nucleoli
- o Sometimes tumor cells have more atypia and coarse chromatin
- o Sparse cytoplasm

ANCILLARY TESTS

Histochemistry
- MPO
  - o Reactivity: Negative
  - o Staining pattern
    - Cytoplasmic
- NSE
  - o Reactivity: Negative
  - o Staining pattern
    - Cytoplasmic

Immunohistochemistry
- Plasmacytoid dendritic cell antibodies
  - o CD123(+), BDCA-2/CD303(+)
    - These are the 2 most specific markers
  - o CD4(+)
    - May be weakly positive
  - o CD56(+)
    - May be weakly positive
    - Rarely CD56 is negative, and does not exclude the diagnosis
  - o TCL1(+)
    - Also positive in some lymphomas, but negative in AML
    - Can differentiate BPDCN from AML
  - o CD68(+)
    - 50% of cases with cytoplasmic dot positivity
  - o MxA(+)
    - Marker for interferon-γ
  - o CD45RA(+/-), CD43(+)
- Other positive antibodies
  - o CLA(+), Bcl-6(+/-)
- Negative immunohistochemical markers
  - o Negative for blast markers
    - CD34(-), CD117(-)
    - TdT(+) in 1/2 of cases, but usually in only a fraction of the tumor cells
  - o Most myeloid markers are negative
    - CD13(-), CD15(-), lysozyme(-), CD163(-), myeloperoxidase(-)
    - But CD33 and CD43 can be positive
  - o Most B-cell markers are negative
    - CD19(-), CD20(-), CD79a(-)
    - Pax-5 and MUM1 can be positive
  - o Most T-cell markers negative
    - CD3(-), CD5(-)
    - CD2, CD45RA, and CD7 can rarely be positive

Flow Cytometry
- Similar findings to immunohistochemistry
  - o Except cytotoxic markers (granzyme B, TIA-1, perforin)
    - Positive by flow cytometry
    - Negative by immunohistochemistry

Cytogenetics
- Complex chromosomal abnormalities (2/3 of cases)
- But no single abnormality is specific
  - o Hypodiploidy
  - o 5q, 6q, 9, 12p, 13q, and 15q

In Situ Hybridization
- EBV-encoded small nuclear RNA (EBER) negative

PCR
- All *IgH* gene rearrangement studies are nonclonal
- Most T-cell receptor gene rearrangement studies are nonclonal

DIFFERENTIAL DIAGNOSIS

Acute Myeloid Leukemia/Myeloid Sarcoma
- AML with monocytic differentiation has similar presentation to BPDCN
  - o Both skin and bone marrow disease
- Similarities to BPDCN
  - o Blastic tumor cells
  - o Both tumors may express CD56, CD4, CD33, CD123, TdT
    - CD123(+), but weak in AML
- Multiple myeloid markers favor acute myeloid leukemia
  - o i.e., MPO, CD13, and CD33
  - o MPO(+) and lysozyme(+) in AML, but negative in BPDCN
- Multiple plasmacytoid dendritic cell markers favors BPDCN over acute myeloid leukemia
  - o i.e., CD123, BDCA-2
  - o CD123 is only weakly positive in AML
  - o TCL1 can be positive in BPDCN but is negative in AML

Myeloid Neoplasms with Increased Plasmacytoid Dendritic Cells
- Form nodules
- CD123(+), CD4(+), **TdT(-)**, **CD56(-)**
  - o These are not the same as PDCs in BPDCN
  - o BPDCN: CD123(+), CD4(+), **TdT(+)**, **CD56(+)**

Precursor T Lymphoblastic Leukemia/Lymphoma (T-ALL)
- Similarities to BPDCN
  - o Tumor cells with blastic chromatin like BPDCN
  - o May express CD56 ± CD4
  - o Both are often TdT(+)
- Differences from BPDCN
  - o Multiple B-cell antigens or T-cell antigens favor B-ALL or T-ALL, respectively
  - o TdT is usually strongly positive in all tumor cells in ALL
  - o Younger age of patients in ALL
  - o Often mediastinal mass in T-ALL
  - o Clonal T-cell receptor gamma gene rearrangements
  - o CD10(+) in ALL
    - CD1a can be positive
    - CD123 usually negative
    - BDCA-2 usually negative

BLASTIC PLASMACYTOID DENDRITIC CELL NEOPLASM

Immunophenotype of Blastic Plasmacytoid Dendritic Cell Neoplasm

CD4	CD56	CD123	TCL	TdT	MPO	CD3
Positive	Positive	Positive	Positive	Sometimes positive	Negative	Negative

Extranodal NK-/T-cell Lymphoma, Nasal Type

- May express CD56 ± CD4
  - Prominent necrosis, angioinvasion, CD2(+), EBER(+), and cytotoxic markers(+)
  - CD123(-) and TCL1(-)
  - **T-cell receptor gamma** rearrangements clonal
  - Tumor cells usually do not have blast-like chromatin

Peripheral T-cell Lymphoma, NOS

- May express CD56 ± CD4
- Differences from BPDCN
  - T-cell lymphomas express more T-cell antigens than just CD43 and CD4
  - Clonal T-cell receptor gene rearrangement common in T-cell lymphoma

Mature B-cell Lymphomas

- Diffuse large B-cell lymphoma and Burkitt lymphoma both present with aggregates of malignant cells like BPDCN
- Differences from BPDCN
  - B-cell lymphomas express multiple B-cell antigens
    - CD20, CD19, pax-5, CD79a, MUM1
    - B-cell lymphomas are often CD10 and Bcl-6 positive
  - Molecular findings
    - B-cell lymphomas have clonal *IgH* gene rearrangements
    - t(14;18) in diffuse large B-cell lymphoma
    - t(8;14) and other *MYC* translocations in Burkitt lymphoma

Metastatic Malignant Melanoma

- Similarities to BPDCN
  - Often presents with large aggregates of tumor cells in the dermis
  - Tumor cells are large, atypical, and may show diffuse, sheet-like pattern
- Differences from BPDCN
  - Melanin pigment may be seen microscopically
  - Expresses melanoma markers by immunohistochemistry
    - S100, MART-1/Melan-A, HMB-45, tyrosinase, BKA-62

Poorly Differentiated Carcinoma

- Similarities to BPDCN
  - Can present with large aggregates of tumor cells in the dermis
  - Tumor cells are large, atypical, and may not form glands
- Differences from BPDCN
  - Any glandular differentiation favors carcinoma
  - History of carcinoma
  - Typically express at least some cytokeratins, dependent on type of tumor

DIAGNOSTIC CHECKLIST

Clinically Relevant Pathologic Features

- Skin lesions
  - Usually macules, nodules, or plaques
  - May be disseminated
- Can be associated with dysplasia or leukemia

Pathologic Interpretation Pearls

- Typically tumor cells with blast-like chromatin
- Needs extensive immunophenotyping
  - CD123(+), CD4(+), CD56(+), TCL1(+), TdT(+), MPO(-)

SELECTED REFERENCES

1. Choi KW et al: CD4-/CD56+/CD123+ Hematodermic neoplasm showing early liver metastasis. Ann Dermatol. 22(2):186-90, 2010
2. Cota C et al: Cutaneous manifestations of blastic plasmacytoid dendritic cell neoplasm-morphologic and phenotypic variability in a series of 33 patients. Am J Surg Pathol. 34(1):75-87, 2010
3. Eros N et al: Central nervous system involvement in CD4+/CD56+ hematodermic neoplasm: a report of two cases. J Neurooncol. 97(2):301-4, 2010
4. Jegalian AG et al: Blastic plasmacytoid dendritic cell neoplasm in children: diagnostic features and clinical implications. Haematologica. 95(11):1873-9, 2010
5. Magro CM et al: Cutaneous CD4+ CD56+ hematologic malignancies. J Am Acad Dermatol. 63(2):292-308, 2010
6. Su O et al: A case of CD4+/CD56+ hematodermic neoplasm (plasmacytoid dendritic cell neoplasm). Dermatol Online J. 16(4):8, 2010
7. Alencar AJ et al: Hematodermic tumor presenting with generalized skin involvement. J Clin Oncol. 27(18):3059-61, 2009
8. Jegalian AG et al: Plasmacytoid dendritic cells: physiologic roles and pathologic states. Adv Anat Pathol. 16(6):392-404, 2009
9. Kaune KM et al: Solitary cutaneous nodule of blastic plasmacytoid dendritic cell neoplasm progressing to overt leukemia cutis after chemotherapy: immunohistology and FISH analysis confirmed the diagnosis. Am J Dermatopathol. 31(7):695-701, 2009
10. Kohrt H et al: Extranodal natural killer/T-cell lymphoma: current concepts in biology and treatment. Leuk Lymphoma. 50(11):1773-84, 2009
11. Dijkman R et al: Gene-expression profiling and array-based CGH classify CD4+CD56+ hematodermic neoplasm and cutaneous myelomonocytic leukemia as distinct disease entities. Blood. 109(4):1720-7, 2007
12. Pilichowska ME et al: CD4+/CD56+ hematodermic neoplasm ("blastic natural killer cell lymphoma"): neoplastic cells express the immature dendritic cell marker BDCA-2 and produce interferon. Am J Clin Pathol. 128(3):445-53, 2007

12

Microscopic Features

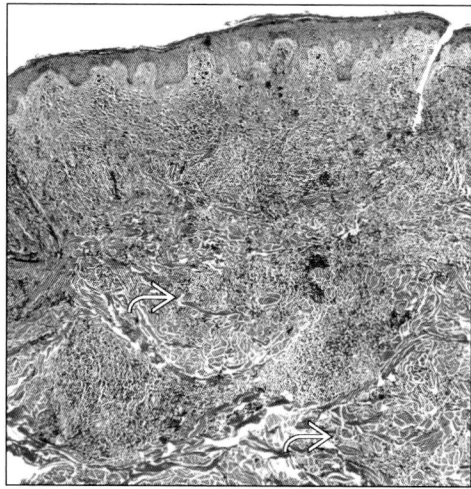
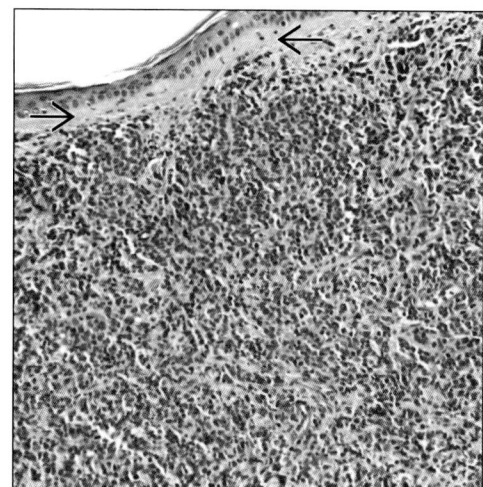

(Left) This case of BPDCN shows the dermis nearly entirely replaced by a diffuse infiltrate of tumor cells. There is an infiltrative pattern with tumor cells dissecting between collagen bundles ➡. *(Courtesy L. J. Medeiros, MD.)* *(Right)* Higher magnification of BPDCN shows the superficial dermis replaced by the neoplasm. The epidermis is uninvolved, and a distinct grenz zone ➡ can be appreciated. *(Courtesy L. J. Medeiros, MD.)*

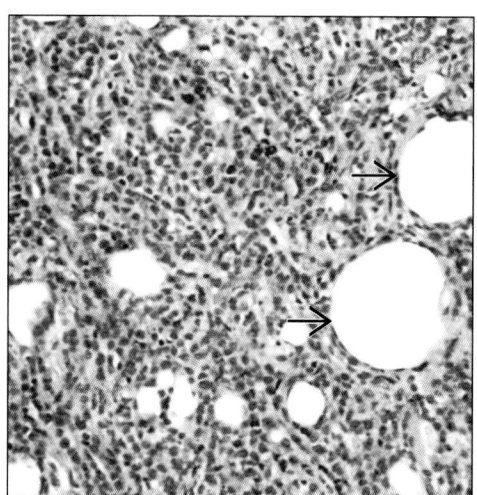
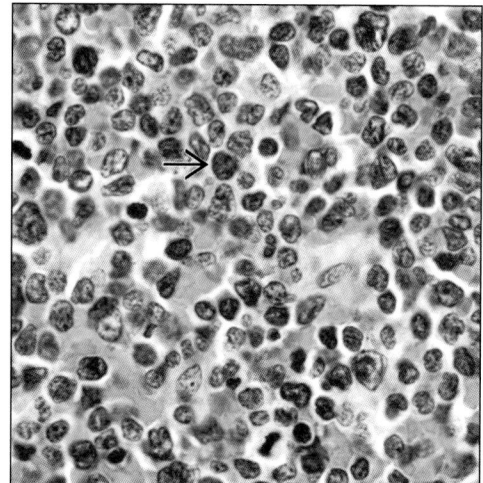

(Left) Deep involvement in BPDCN shows the tumor cells extending into the deep subcutaneous fat. Tumor is seen infiltrating around individual fat cells ➡. *(Right)* At high magnification, the tumor cells have a fine homogeneous blast-like chromatin pattern ➡. One or more small nucleoli can be seen in some of the cells. This is the classic morphology of the tumor cells in BPDCN.

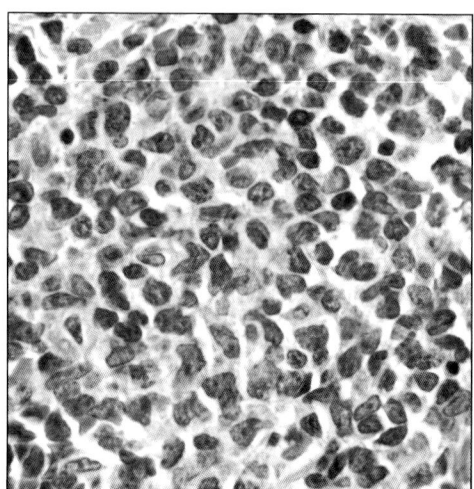
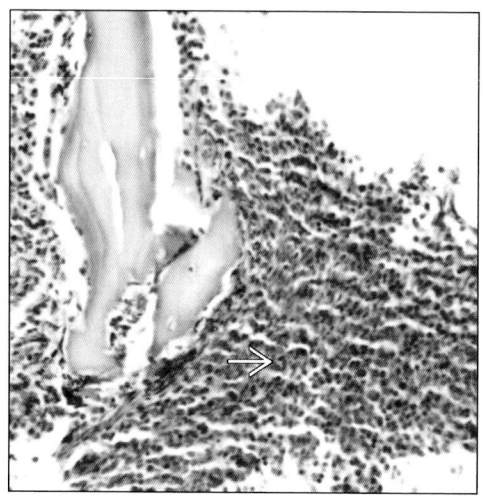

(Left) High magnification of another case of BPDCN shows that the neoplastic cells are small to intermediate in size. These cytologic features suggest a differential diagnosis with lymphoblastic lymphoma and small cell T-cell lymphomas. *(Right)* BPDCN can often disseminate to other anatomic sites. In this case, sheets of malignant cells ➡ are found in the bone marrow. Sometimes the bone marrow infiltrate is subtle, requiring phenotyping.

BLASTIC PLASMACYTOID DENDRITIC CELL NEOPLASM

Ancillary Techniques

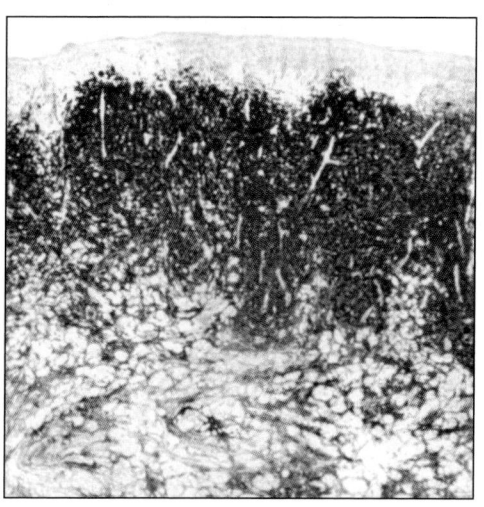
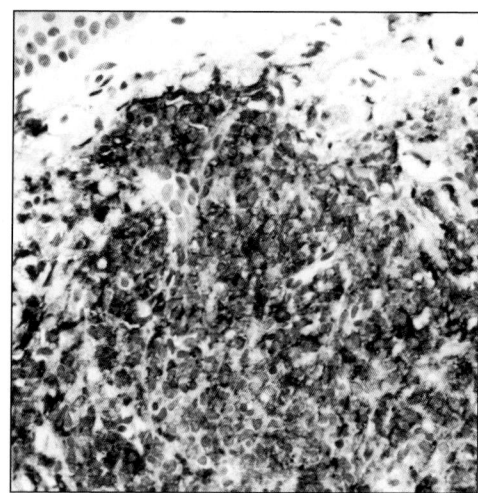

(Left) In this TCL1 immunostain, the tumor cells are strongly and diffusely positive. TCL1 is also expressed in T-cell prolymphocytic leukemia. (Right) High magnification of BPDCN involving the dermis shows the neoplastic cells strongly CD56(+). (Courtesy L. J. Medeiros, MD.)

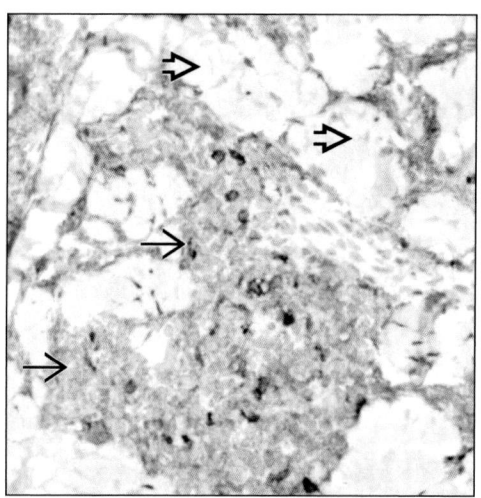
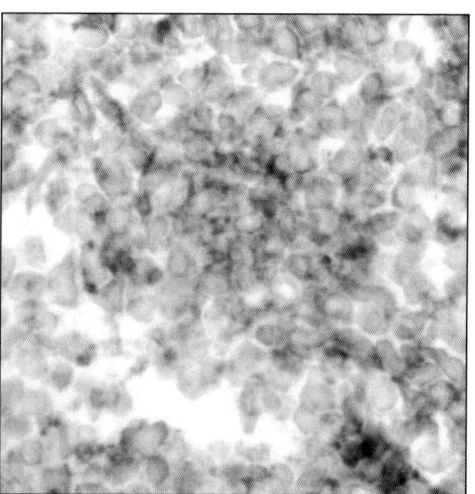

(Left) This CD4 stain weakly highlights tumor cells ⇨ that are infiltrating between muscle ⊳. The combination of CD4(+)/CD56(+) is characteristic of BPDCN, but can also be seen in acute leukemias, especially those with monocytic differentiation. (Right) BPDCN can be labeled with CD123, since CD123 is a marker of plasmacytic dendritic cells. BDCA-2 and MXA are other plasmacytic dendritic cell markers that are often positive in BPDCN.

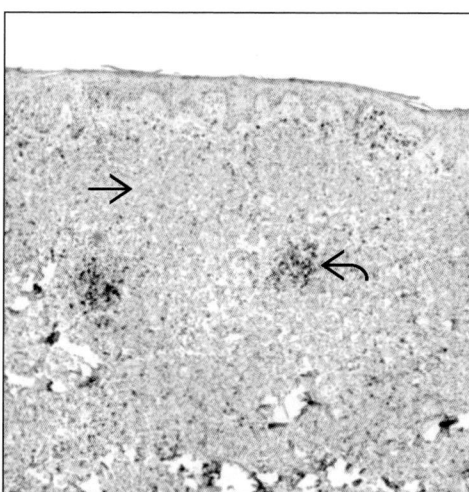
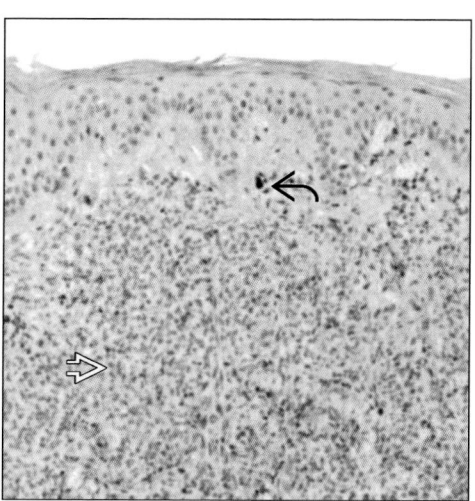

(Left) CD3 is negative in the tumor cells ⇨ in this case of BPDCN. Reactive T cells ⤷ singly and in clusters express CD3. (Right) In this case of BPDCN, CD20 is negative in the tumor cells ⇨. Scattered reactive B cells ⤷ are present expressing CD20. BPDCN is a diagnosis of exclusion, and thus B-cell and T-cell markers should be performed to rule out other types of B-cell or T-cell lymphomas.

BLASTIC PLASMACYTOID DENDRITIC CELL NEOPLASM

Lymph Node Findings

(Left) In this case of blastic plasmacytoid dendritic cell neoplasm (BPDCN) involving lymph node, the neoplasm completely replaces the lymph node and has a diffuse pattern. (Courtesy L. J. Medeiros, MD.) (Right) At higher magnification, the tumor cells are small and have immature chromatin resembling, in part, lymphoblasts. (Courtesy L. J. Medeiros, MD.)

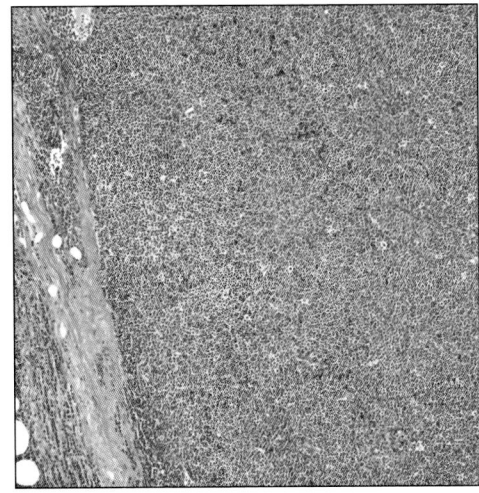
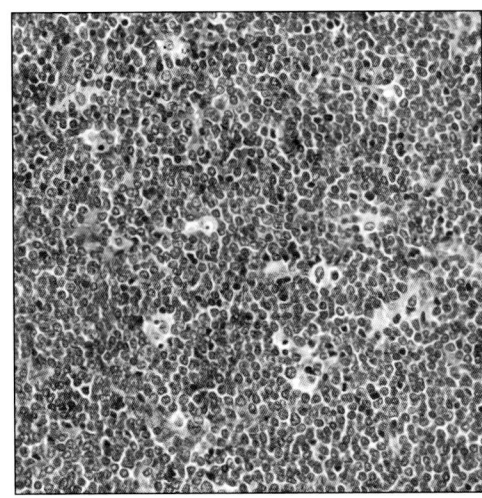

(Left) The neoplastic cells in this case of BPDCN express CD4 with dim intensity and a cytoplasmic staining pattern. (Courtesy L. J. Medeiros, MD.) (Right) The neoplastic cells are CD56(+). A residual follicle ➡ is CD56(-). (Courtesy L. J. Medeiros, MD.)

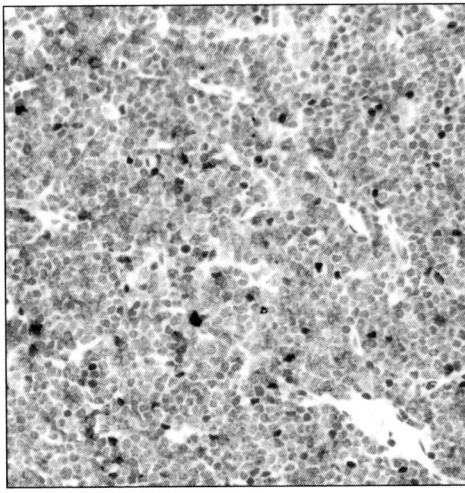
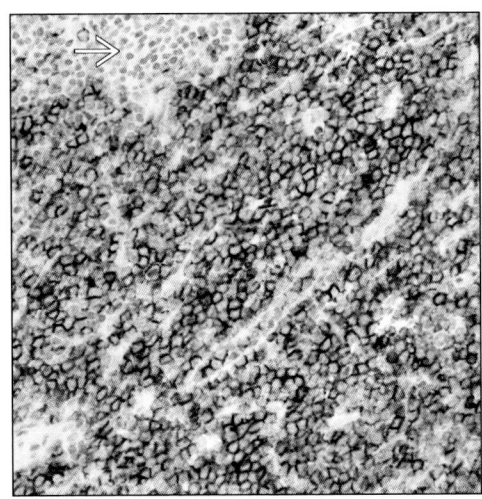

(Left) The neoplastic cells are strongly TCL1(+) with a nuclear pattern of expression. TCL1 expression is present in these neoplasms and helpful in the differential diagnosis. (Courtesy L. J. Medeiros, MD.) (Right) The neoplastic cells are strongly CD123(+). Expression of CD123 is characteristic of this neoplasm and very helpful in the differential diagnosis. (Courtesy L. J. Medeiros, MD.)

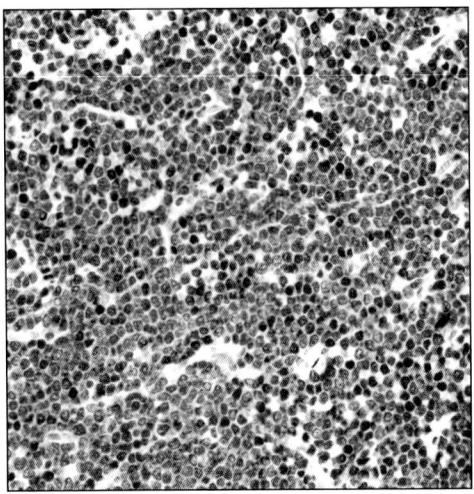
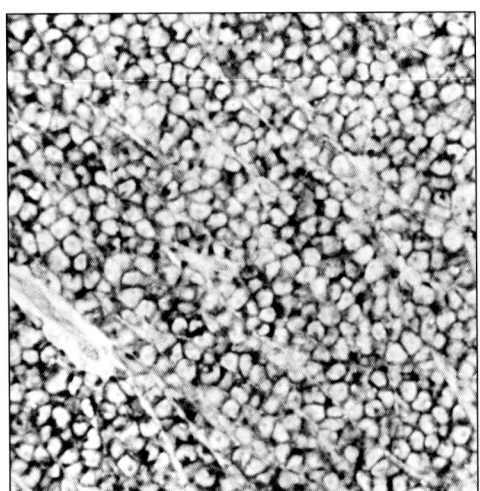

BLASTIC PLASMACYTOID DENDRITIC CELL NEOPLASM

Differential Diagnosis

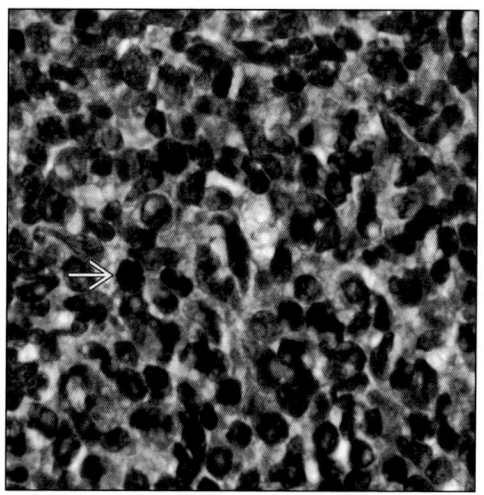

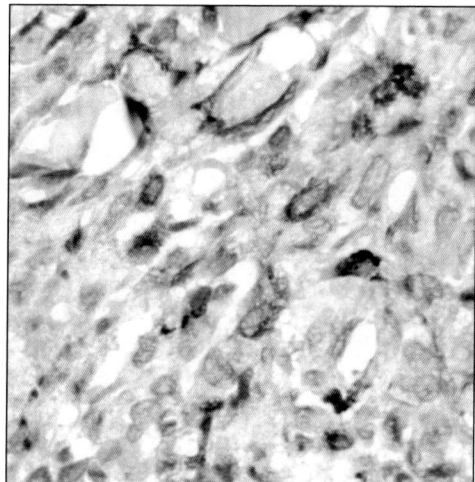

(Left) Leukemia cutis must be excluded in all cases of BPDCN. In this case of leukemia cutis, the infiltrate filled the dermis. At high power, the tumor cells are large ➡ with fine blastic chromatin. (Right) In this MPO stain of leukemia cutis, the tumor cells are myeloperoxidase positive. The tumor cells were also CD15(+), CD68(+), and CD4(+), showing monocytic differentiation.

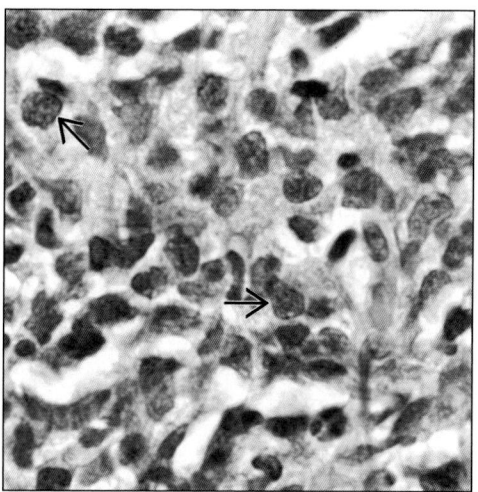

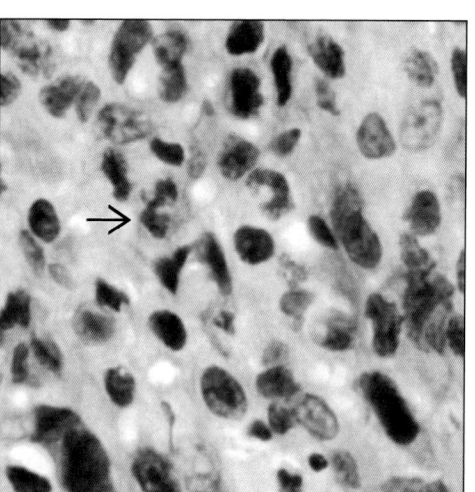

(Left) Diffuse large B-cell lymphoma is in the differential diagnosis of BPDCN. This case shows a diffuse dermal infiltrate with large malignant cells with coarse chromatin ➡. This case had a different immunophenotype from BPDCN expressing pax-5, CD20, and was positive for t(14;18). (Right) This case of anaplastic large cell lymphoma has a similar morphology to BPDCN with a diffuse dermal infiltrate of large malignant cells ➡, but a different phenotype (CD30[+], ALK[+/-]).

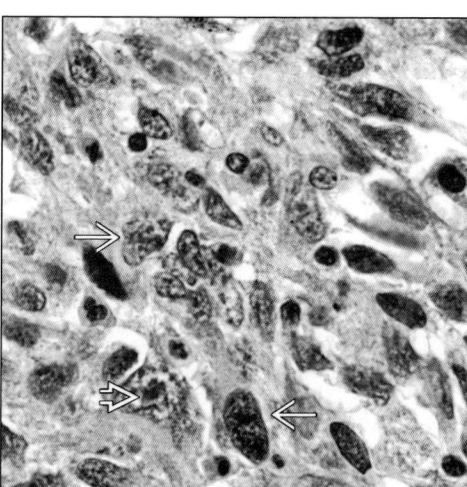

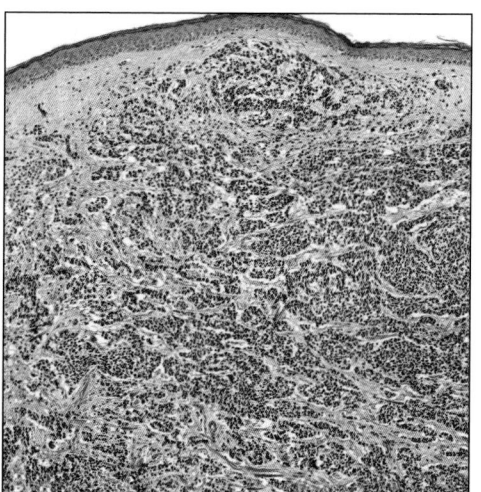

(Left) Melanoma can also be mistaken for BPDCN. In this case of melanoma, the tumor cells show more atypia ➡ and prominent nucleoli ➡ and are typically S100(+), HMB-45(+), MART-1/Melan-A(+), and tyrosinase(+). (Right) Metastatic small cell carcinoma of the lung shows a diffuse, infiltrative pattern in the dermis, with sparing of the epidermis and separation from it by a grenz zone. However, the tumor cells are typically strongly CK7(+) and TTF-1(+).

EXTRAMEDULLARY HEMATOPOIESIS

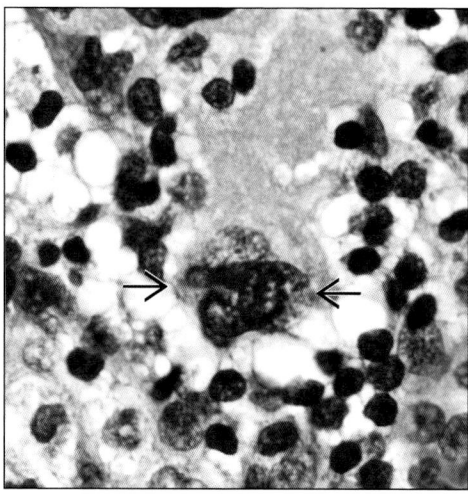

This is a skin biopsy specimen with extramedullary hematopoiesis, as evidenced by the large megakaryocyte ⇨.

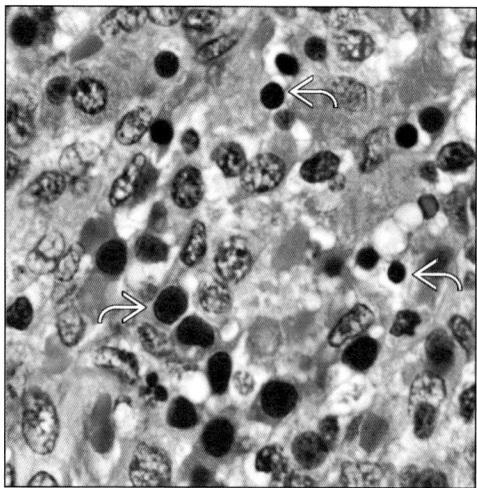

The skin contains small clusters of nucleated red blood cells ⇨, which were positive for a hemoglobin A immunostain (not shown).

TERMINOLOGY

Abbreviations
- Extramedullary hematopoiesis (EMH)

Definitions
- Formation of blood cells (including nucleated red blood cells, lymphocytes, and megakaryocytes) outside of bone marrow
  - Occurs most commonly in liver and spleen
    - Also found in other organs including lymph nodes, kidney, adrenal, gastrointestinal tract, lung, breast, central nervous system
  - Hematopoiesis occurs in skin early in embryonic life

ETIOLOGY/PATHOGENESIS

Viral Infection
- Has been reported in skin in neonates with intrauterine viral infections including
  - Cytomegalovirus (CMV)
  - Coxsackievirus
  - Rubella

Hematopoietic Disorders
- In neonates, EMH occurs in congenital hematologic disorders including
  - Hemolytic disease of newborn
  - Twin transfusion syndrome
- In adults, EMH is seen with hematopoietic disorders
  - All myeloproliferative neoplasms are associated with EMH
    - Primary myelofibrosis is most common, especially in patients who have had splenectomy
    - Essential thrombocythemia, polycythemia vera, and chronic myelogenous leukemia have also been reported

Neoplasms
- Can also develop in a variety of tumors
  - Pilomatrixomas can rarely show EMH

CLINICAL ISSUES

Presentation
- Variable and depends on associated disease
  - Erythema, single lesions, plaques, ulcers, or bullae
  - EMH can develop in surgical wounds
  - "Blueberry muffin" appearance is multiple violaceous papulonodular lesions in neonates with EMH
- Patients with EMH in spleen develop splenomegaly

Treatment
- Usually, underlying disorder is treated rather than EMH

Prognosis
- Depends on aggressiveness of patient's underlying disorder

MICROSCOPIC PATHOLOGY

Histologic Features
- Occurs in superficial and deep dermis
- Polymorphic infiltrate with myeloid cells, erythroid cells, and megakaryocytes
  - Cells are at all stages of maturation; thus, can present with myelocytes, promyelocytes, bands, and neutrophils
  - Megakaryocytes are often the most easily seen elements
- Often a perivascular distribution
- Can cause fibrosis in skin, liver, and spleen
- Peripheral blood can often show leukoerythroblastosis, especially if patient has primary myelofibrosis
- In liver, EMH occurs in sinusoids

EXTRAMEDULLARY HEMATOPOIESIS

Key Facts

Terminology

- Formation of blood cells (erythroid cells, myeloid cells, megakaryocytes) outside bone marrow
- Most common in liver and spleen
- Hematopoiesis occurs in skin in early embryonic life

Etiology/Pathogenesis

- Associated with viral infections, hematopoietic disorders, and neoplasms

Microscopic Pathology

- Dermis with myeloid cells, erythroid cells, and megakaryocytes at all stages of maturation

Ancillary Tests

- Myeloid cells positive for CD33, CD13, CD43, and CD15
- Erythroid cells positive for hemoglobin A
- Megakaryocytes express factor VIII and CD61

ANCILLARY TESTS

Immunohistochemistry

- Myeloid cells can be highlighted by myeloperoxidase (MPO), CD33, CD13, CD43, MAC387, and CD15
- Erythroid cells are immunoreactive with hemoglobin A and glycophorin
- Megakaryocytes express factor VIII, CD61, CD34, and LMP
- CD45RB is positive in all myeloid cells, erythroid cells, and megakaryocytes

Special Stains

- Leder stain is positive in myeloid cells

DIFFERENTIAL DIAGNOSIS

Leukemia

- Early myeloid cells of EMH can rarely be mistaken for acute myeloid leukemia
- Early erythroid cells could be confused with acute erythroid leukemia

Chronic Myeloproliferative Neoplasms

- Similarly can present with proliferations of myeloid cells, erythroid cells, &/or megakaryocytes

SELECTED REFERENCES

1. Rajiah P et al: Extramedullary hematopoiesis in unusual locations in hematologically compromised and noncompromised patients. Skeletal Radiol. 40(7):947-53, 2011
2. Smith J et al: Extramedullary haematopoiesis secondary to hereditary spherocytosis. Br J Haematol. 154(5):543, 2011
3. Miyata T et al: Cutaneous extramedullary hematopoiesis in a patient with idiopathic myelofibrosis. J Dermatol. 35(7):456-61, 2008
4. Haniffa MA et al: Cutaneous extramedullary hemopoiesis in chronic myeloproliferative and myelodysplastic disorders. J Am Acad Dermatol. 55(2 Suppl):S28-31, 2006
5. Fernández Aceñero MJ et al: Extramedullary hematopoiesis in an adult. J Am Acad Dermatol. 48(5 Suppl):S62-3, 2003
6. Revenga F et al: Cutaneous extramedullary hematopoiesis. Int J Dermatol. 39(12):957-8, 2000
7. Patel BM et al: Cutaneous extramedullary hematopoiesis. J Am Acad Dermatol. 32(5 Pt 1):805-7, 1995
8. Mizoguchi M et al: Cutaneous extramedullary hematopoiesis in myelofibrosis. J Am Acad Dermatol. 22(2 Pt 2):351-5, 1990
9. Schofield JK et al: Cutaneous extramedullary hematopoiesis with a preponderance of atypical megakaryocytes in myelofibrosis. J Am Acad Dermatol. 22(2 Pt 2):334-7, 1990
10. Hocking WG et al: Cutaneous extramedullary hematopoiesis following splenectomy for idiopathic myelofibrosis. Am J Med. 76(5):956-8, 1984
11. Kuo T: Cutaneous extramedullary hematopoiesis presenting as leg ulcers. J Am Acad Dermatol. 4(5):592-6, 1981
12. Sarma DP: Extramedullary hemopoiesis of the skin. Arch Dermatol. 117(1):58-9, 1981

IMAGE GALLERY

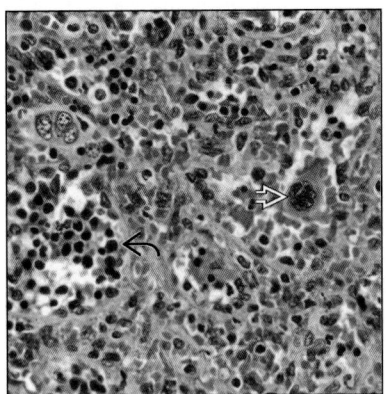
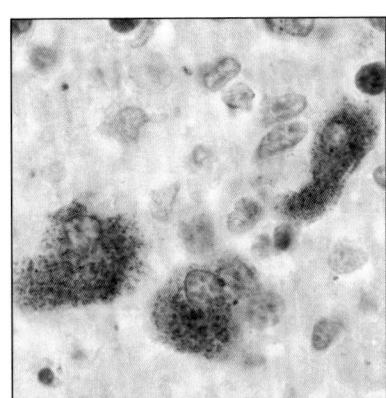
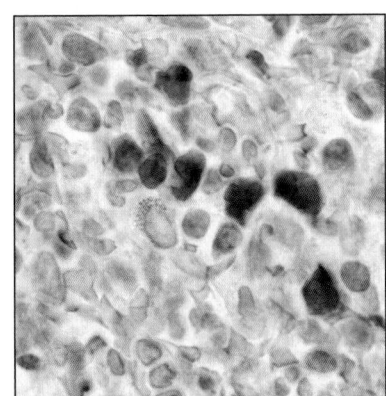

(Left) This is a spleen with extensive EMH. There are clusters of nucleated red blood cells ➡ on the left and 1 megakaryocyte ➡ on the right. *(Center)* This is a factor VIII immunostain in a patient with EMH of the skin. The megakaryocytes are positive for factor VIII. Other megakaryocyte markers include CD61, CD34, and LMP. *(Right)* This is a hemoglobin A immunostain in a skin biopsy specimen with EMH; the stain is highlighting erythroid cells.

CUTANEOUS AND SYSTEMIC MASTOCYTOSIS

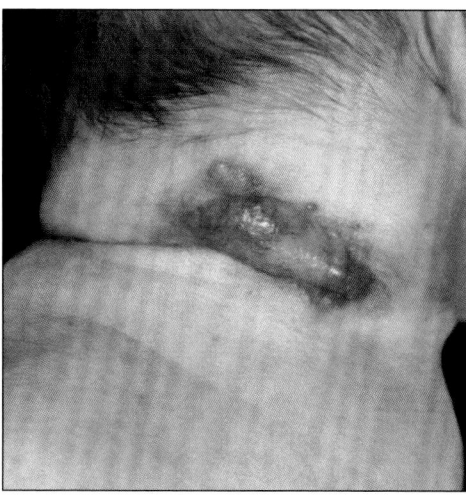

This mastocytoma of the skin was present at birth on the right neck of this newborn. Mastocytomas of the skin occur almost exclusively in infants. (Courtesy S. Vanderhooft, MD.)

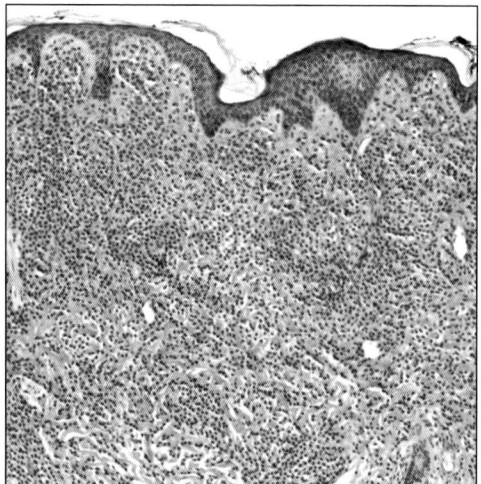

Mastocytoma of the skin in an infant shows a dense infiltrate of mast cells with epidermal sparing that showed round nuclei with abundant basophilic-staining cytoplasm at high power.

TERMINOLOGY

Abbreviations
- Cutaneous mastocytosis (CM)
- Systemic mastocytosis (SM)

Synonyms
- Mast cell disease

Definitions
- Heterogeneous group of clonal, neoplastic mast cell proliferations that accumulate in 1 or more organ systems
- Subtypes based mainly on distribution of disease and clinical manifestations
  - **Cutaneous mastocytosis** (CM): Mast cell infiltrates confined to skin
    - Urticaria pigmentosa (UP)/maculopapular cutaneous mastocytosis (MPCM)
    - Diffuse cutaneous mastocytosis
    - Mastocytoma of skin
  - **Systemic mastocytosis** (SM): Involvement of at least 1 extracutaneous organ ± skin lesions
    - Indolent systemic mastocytosis (ISM)
    - Systemic mastocytosis with associated clonal hematological non-mast cell lineage disease (SM-AHNMD)
    - Aggressive systemic mastocytosis (ASM)
    - Mast cell leukemia (MCL)
    - Mast cell sarcoma (MCS)
    - Extracutaneous mastocytoma

ETIOLOGY/PATHOGENESIS

Molecular Background
- Frequently associated with somatic activating point mutations within *c-KIT* protooncogene
  - Encodes tyrosine kinase receptor for stem cell factor (SCF)

- Various mutations result in ligand-independent activation of c-KIT tyrosine kinase
  - Constitutively activated c-KIT leads to clonal proliferation of mast cells
- Most common mutation: D816V in exon 17 encoding tyrosine kinase domain
  - Identified in ≥ 95% of adults with SM when sensitive methods are used
  - Present in 35% of pediatric CM cases
  - Provides relative resistance to prototypical tyrosine kinase inhibitor imatinib
- Other activating point mutations: D816Y, D816H, D816F, and D816I in exon 17 (rarely seen)
  - Frequency significantly higher in CM than in SM
- Activating point mutations in exons 8, 9, and 11 (mutually exclusive with codon 816 mutations)
  - 44% of pediatric CM cases
- Pediatric CM historically regarded as reactive condition with transient dysregulation of local growth factors
  - Increasing evidence supports neoplastic nature associated with activating *c-KIT* mutations (as in adults)
    - Despite high rate of spontaneous regression (mechanism unknown)
- Rare familial cases with germline mutations of c-*KIT* have been reported
- In patients with SM-AHNMD, additional genetic defects are detected depending on type of AHNMD
- About 30% of SM cases associated with *TET2* mutations
  - *TET2* acts as putative tumor suppressor gene
  - 50% of those cases also carry *c-KIT* D816V mutation

CLINICAL ISSUES

Epidemiology
- Incidence
  - Very rare

CUTANEOUS AND SYSTEMIC MASTOCYTOSIS

Key Facts

Terminology

- Heterogeneous group of clonal neoplastic proliferations of mast cells in ≥ 1 organ system
  ○ Cutaneous mastocytosis: Confined to skin
  ○ Systemic mastocytosis: Involvement of at least 1 organ ± skin lesions

Etiology/Pathogenesis

- Frequently associated with somatic activating point mutations within *c-KIT* protooncogene
- About 30% of SM cases associated with *TET2* mutations

Clinical Issues

- 2/3 of cases occur in children
- Prognosis depends on disease category
  ○ Pediatric onset CM has favorable outcome

- Approximately 80% of patients with mastocytosis have evidence of skin involvement

Microscopic Pathology

- Multifocal compact or diffuse compact mast cell infiltrates
- Diffuse interstitial infiltration pattern
- Cytology varies, but abnormal features are almost always detected, including spindling and hypogranularity
- Frequent bi- or multilobated nuclei usually indicate aggressive disease

Top Differential Diagnoses

- Reactive mast cell hyperplasia
- Cutaneous lymphoma
- Myeloid and lymphoid neoplasms with eosinophilia

- Lack exact numbers with regard to frequency
- Calculated incidence of 5-10 new cases per 1,000,000 population per year in various studies
  ○ CM
    - UP: Most common CM variant
    - Mastocytoma of skin (10-15% of pediatric CM cases)
    - Diffuse CM (rare)
  ○ SM
    - ISM: Most common SM variant (46% of SM cases)
    - SM-AHNMD (40% of SM cases)
    - ASM (12% of SM cases)
    - MCL, MCS, and extracutaneous mastocytoma are extremely rare
- Age
  ○ Occurs at any age
    - 2/3 occur in children in 1st 2 years of life
  ○ CM most common in children, less frequent in adults
    - 50% of affected children develop typical skin lesions before 6 months of age
    - May present at birth
  ○ SM generally diagnosed after 2nd decade of life, rare in pediatric population
- Gender
  ○ Slight male predominance in CM
  ○ M:F = 1:1-1:3 in SM

Site

- Approximately 80% of patients with mastocytosis have evidence of skin involvement
- CM: Mast cell infiltrates confined to skin
- SM: Involvement of at least 1 extracutaneous organ ± skin lesions
  ○ Bone marrow (BM) almost always involved
  ○ Skin lesions occur in ≥ 50% of cases, more often in those with indolent disease
  ○ Spleen, lymph nodes, liver, and gastrointestinal tract mucosa
  ○ Rarely peripheral blood (PB) shows leukemia
  ○ Any tissue may be affected

Presentation

- CM
  ○ Includes 3 distinct clinicohistopathologic entities
  ○ Characterized by 2 main groups of symptoms
  ○ Skin lesions due to mast cell infiltrate and release of mediators (flushing, blistering, pruritus)
    - Lesions can urticate when stroked ("Darier" sign) in 1/2 of cases
  ○ Systemic symptoms due to release of mast cell mediators (histamine most significant)
    - Headache
    - GI manifestations including acid reflux disease, peptic ulcer disease, and diarrhea
    - Respiratory symptoms including shortness of breath and asthma exacerbations
    - Cardiovascular symptoms including tachycardia, hypotension, syncope, or rarely, even shock
- UP/MPCM
  ○ Widespread distribution of tan macules and occasionally nodules or plaques
    - In children, lesions tend to be larger and papular
  ○ Most lesions show intraepidermal accumulation of melanin pigment
  ○ Sparing of palms, soles, face, and scalp
  ○ In children, typically involving head and lateral face
  ○ Number of lesions varies, but does not predict presence of systemic disease
  ○ Rare special forms
    - Plaque form: Nonpigmented, plaque-forming lesions in young children
    - Nodular form: Brown nodules
    - Telangiectasia macularis eruptiva perstans (TMEP): Brown macules and erythema with telangiectasias on trunk and extremities
    - Blistering variant ("bullous mastocytosis"): Exaggeration of urticaria due to chymase cleaving dermal-epidermal junction
- Diffuse CM
  ○ Diffusely thickened skin with "orange peel" appearance and yellow-red discoloration
  ○ No discernible individual lesions

CUTANEOUS AND SYSTEMIC MASTOCYTOSIS

- o In more severe variant, blistering may precede mast cell infiltration
  - ▪ Differential diagnosis with congenital bullous diseases
- o More likely associated with severe systemic symptoms (higher concentrations of mast cells)
  - ▪ GI manifestations (including severe diarrhea), hypotension, or even shock
- **Mastocytoma of skin**
  - o Single indurated red-brown macule, papule, plaque, or tumor measuring ≤ 4 cm in diameter
    - ▪ Multiple mastocytomas in different locations have been reported
  - o Almost exclusively in infants
  - o Slight predilection for trunk, but also occurs on extremities, head and neck
- **Systemic mastocytosis**
  - o Includes 6 distinct clinicohistopathologic entities
  - o Symptoms grouped into few categories
  - o Constitutional symptoms
    - ▪ Fatigue, weight loss, fever, diaphoresis
  - o Skin manifestations
    - ▪ Pruritus, urticaria, dermographism
  - o Mediator-related systemic events (due to release of histamine, eicosanoids, proteases, and heparin)
    - ▪ Same as CM systemic symptoms
  - o Musculoskeletal complaints
    - ▪ Bone pain, osteopenia/osteoporosis, fractures, arthralgias, myalgias
  - o Symptoms related to organ impairment due to mast cell infiltrates (absent in indolent but present in aggressive variants)
    - ▪ Splenomegaly (often minimal)
    - ▪ Lymphadenopathy and hepatomegaly (less frequent)
  - o Hematological abnormalities
    - ▪ Anemia, leukocytosis, eosinophilia (frequent), neutropenia, and thrombocytopenia
    - ▪ BM failure only in aggressive or leukemic variants
    - ▪ Significant numbers of circulating mast cells are suggestive of MCL
    - ▪ 30-40% of SM has associated clonal hematological non-mast cell lineage disease (AHNMD) diagnosed before, simultaneously with, or after SM diagnosis
    - ▪ Any defined myeloid or lymphoid malignancy possible, myeloid predominates (chronic myelomonocytic leukemia [CMML] most common)

Laboratory Tests

- Serum total tryptase
  - o Persistently elevated (> 20 ng/mL suggestive of SM, used as minor criterion for diagnosis)
    - ▪ Criterion not valid in SM-AHNMD
  - o Normal to slightly elevated in patients with CM
    - ▪ Usually reserved for adult work-up of CM
- Histamine
  - o May be very elevated in diffuse CM, but are rarely part of routine work-up for CM

Treatment

- CM

- o Alleviate symptoms with antihistamines and topical steroids
- o Prevent episodes by avoiding mast cell degranulators
  - ▪ Physical stimuli (temperature changes, rubbing/friction, intense physical exertion)
  - ▪ Foods (spicy foods, citrus fruits, cheese, alcohol)
  - ▪ Medications (antibiotics, aspirin, lidocaine, etc.)
- o Educate and reassure families
- SM
  - o Currently no cure
  - o PKC412 tyrosine kinase inhibitor may be effective in treating SM with mutated *KIT*
- ASM, MCL, and MCS
  - o Candidates for cytoreductive therapies

Prognosis

- Depends on disease category
- Pediatric-onset CM has favorable outcome
  - o Majority of cases have improvement of symptoms over time
    - ▪ Complete regression by adolescence in > 50%
    - ▪ Very low likelihood of progressive disease
  - o Transformation to SM rare, but more likely in diffuse CM than UP
- In adults, cutaneous lesions generally do not regress and are often associated with SM (usually ISM)
- SM
  - o Usually normal life expectancy
  - o Patients with aggressive variants may survive only a few months
  - o SM-AHNMD depends on the associated hematological disorder
  - o Predictors of poorer prognosis for SM
    - ▪ Late onset of symptoms, absence of CM, thrombocytopenia, elevated LDH, anemia, BM hypercellularity, abnormal myeloid maturation patterns, PB smear abnormalities, elevated alkaline phosphatase, and hepatosplenomegaly
    - ▪ Percentage and morphology of mast cells in BM smears is independent predictor of survival

MICROSCOPIC PATHOLOGY

General Microscopic Features

- Normal mast cells in tissue sections (H&E)
  - o Loosely scattered
  - o Round to oval nuclei with clumped chromatin and inconspicuous nucleoli
  - o Low nuclear to cytoplasmic ratio with numerous basophilic cytoplasmic granules
- Normal mast cells on smear preparations (Romanowsky stains)
  - o Medium-sized round to oval cells with round to oval nuclei and plentiful cytoplasm, containing densely packed metachromatic granules
    - ▪ Basophils: Smaller cells with segmented nuclei and larger and fewer granules
- Neoplastic mast cells
  - o Cytology varies, but abnormal features (including spindling and hypogranularity) are almost always detected

CUTANEOUS AND SYSTEMIC MASTOCYTOSIS

- More pronounced in high-grade lesions; occurrence of metachromatic blast cells is usual feature of mast cell leukemia
  - Frequent bi- or multilobated nuclei ("promastocytes") usually indicates aggressive mast cell proliferation
  - Mitotic figures in mast cells do occur but are infrequent even in aggressive or leukemic variants
  - Pattern of infiltrate may vary depending on tissue
  - Multifocal compact or diffuse compact mast cell infiltrates
    - Highly compatible with diagnosis
    - Additional immunohistochemical and molecular studies are still recommended
  - Diffuse interstitial infiltration pattern
    - Loosely scattered mast cells in absence of compact aggregates
    - Also observed in reactive mast cell hyperplasia and myelomastocytic leukemia
    - Additional immunohistochemical and molecular studies are necessary to establish diagnosis

Microscopic Features of CM

- **UP**
  - Aggregates of round to spindle-shaped mast cells in papillary and reticular dermis
  - Often in perivascular and periadnexal location
  - Mast cells are fewer in adults than in children
- **Diffuse CM**
  - Band-like infiltrate of mast cells in papillary and upper reticular dermis
- **Mastocytoma of skin**
  - Dense sheets of mature-appearing highly metachromatic mast cells in papillary and reticular dermis
  - May extend into subcutaneous tissues
  - Abundant cytoplasm
  - No cytologic atypia (distinguishes it from extremely rare mast cell sarcoma of skin)
  - Highest concentration of mast cells compared with other types of CM

Microscopic Features of SM

- Bone marrow: 4 types of infiltrates
  - Multifocal, sharply demarcated compact infiltrates of mast cells
    - Paratrabecular, perivascular, &/or parafollicular in location
    - "Mixed infiltrates" composed of mast cells, intermingled with lymphocytes, eosinophils, histiocytes, and fibroblasts
  - Monomorphic infiltrate with spindle-shaped mast cells that abut or stream along bony trabeculae
    - Significant reticulin fibrosis and thickening of adjacent bone are frequent
  - Diffuse replacement of BM by compact mast cell infiltrates
    - Usually mixture of spindle-shaped and round mast cells
    - Resembles sheets of fibroblasts
  - Compact infiltrates composed exclusively of round hypergranular mast cells (rare)

- Tryptase positive round cell infiltration of BM (TROCI-BM)
  - Careful examination of BM not involved by mastocytosis is crucial
    - Unremarkable: ISM with skin and BM involvement or isolated BM mastocytosis
    - Extremely hypercellular due to proliferation of cells of non-mast cell lineages (reactive or coexisting hematopoietic neoplasm)
  - Reactive, nonclonal mast cell hyperplasia may accompany variety of hematological disorders (lymphoplasmacytic lymphoma and hairy cell leukemia)
- Lymph node
  - Focal or diffuse infiltrates, often paracortical
  - Total effacement of lymph node architecture is rare
  - Hyperplasia of germinal centers, angioneogenesis, tissue eosinophilia, plasmacytosis, and reticulin/collagen fibrosis may be present
- Spleen
  - Red &/or white pulp may be involved
  - Eosinophilia and fibrosis are frequent
- Liver
  - Small granulomatoid foci of mast cells within periportal tracts and loosely scattered mast cells within sinusoids
  - Widening and fibrosis of periportal areas
- Gastrointestinal (GI) tract mucosa
  - Involvement frequently suspected clinically
  - Various patterns may be seen

Diagnostic Criteria

- CM
  - Skin lesions show typical clinical features of UP/MPCM, diffuse cutaneous mastocytosis, or solitary mastocytoma
  - Mast cells in multifocal or diffuse pattern
  - Lack features/criteria of SM
- SM
  - Major criterion and 1 minor criterion or at least 3 minor criteria are present

ANCILLARY TESTS

Immunohistochemistry

- Normal mast cells express CD9, CD33, CD45, CD68, and CD117
  - Lack several myelomonocytic antigens including CD14, CD15, and CD16
  - Lack most T- and B-cell-related antigens
  - Tryptase expressed in virtually all mast cells irrespective of stage of maturation or neoplastic state
  - Chymase expressed in subpopulation of mast cells
    - Highly specific but less sensitive for atypical and immature mast cells than CD117
- Neoplastic mast cells have similar antigen profile to normal mast cells
  - In contrast, coexpress CD2 &/or CD25
    - Distinguish from CD2 positive T cells
    - CD25 expression may be inconsistent or even undetectable in well-differentiated SM or subgroup of MCL

CUTANEOUS AND SYSTEMIC MASTOCYTOSIS

Diagnostic Criteria for Systemic Mastocytosis*

Major Criterion**

Multifocal, compact, dense mast cell infiltrates (≥ 15 mast cells in aggregates) in bone marrow or tissue sections

Minor Criteria**

> 25% of mast cells show atypical, spindled, or immature morphologies in smears or tissue sections

D816V KIT mutation present

Mast cells show aberrant expression of CD2 &/or CD25

Total serum tryptase level > 20 ng/mL***

*Adapted from WHO 2008 classification. **Diagnosis of SM made when major and 1 minor criterion or ≥ 3 minor criteria are present. ***Parameter not valid If associated clonal hematological non-mast cell lineage disease (AHNMD) is present.*

Classification of Mastocytosis*

Categories	Comments
Cutaneous mastocytosis	Lacks features/criteria of SM
Systemic mastocytosis	1 major and 1 minor or ≥ 3 minor criterion are present
Mast cell leukemia	≥ 20% mast cells in bone marrow; usually ≥ 10% mast cells in peripheral blood
Mast cell sarcoma	High-grade cytology; unifocal lesion; destructive; no evidence for SM
Extracutaneous mastocytoma	Low-grade cytology; unifocal lesion; nondestructive; no evidence for SM
Indolent systemic mastocytosis	Low mast cell burden; skin lesions typical
Aggressive systemic mastocytosis	≥ 1 of the following: Bone marrow dysfunction, hepatomegaly with liver function impairment, ascites, portal hypertension, skeletal involvement, splenomegaly, malabsorption, and weight loss
Systemic mastocytosis with associated clonal hematological non-mast cell lineage disease	Meets SM criteria and meets WHO criteria for a clonal hematopoietic non-mast cell lineage disorder (i.e., MDS, MPN, AML, lymphoma)

Adapted from WHO 2008 classification.

DIFFERENTIAL DIAGNOSIS

Reactive Mast Cell Hyperplasia
- Lacks compact mast cell infiltrates, no atypical cytology, and no aberrant antigen expression
- May be seen in BM following toxic or inflammatory exposures

Congenital Bullous Diseases
- Blistering variants of UP and diffuse CM can clinically resemble bullous diseases
- No significant mast cell infiltrate on skin biopsy

Cutaneous Lymphoma
- Mast cells only mildly increased, if any
- Evaluate with appropriate IHC panel

Myelomastocytic Leukemia
- Advanced myeloid neoplasm with elevated numbers of immature atypical mast cells
- Criteria for SM not met

Myeloid and Lymphoid Neoplasms with Eosinophilia
- Exclude *FIP1L1-PDGFRA* rearrangement in cases with PB and BM eosinophilia
- Serum tryptase and BM mast cells may be increased but typically less than SM
- Mast cells do not form large compact aggregates as in SM

Child Abuse
- CM can clinically resemble multiple bruises

SELECTED REFERENCES

1. Bodemer C et al: Pediatric mastocytosis is a clonal disease associated with D816V and other activating c-KIT mutations. J Invest Dermatol. 130(3):804-15, 2010
2. Klco JM et al: Molecular pathology of myeloproliferative neoplasms. Am J Clin Pathol. 133(4):602-15, 2010
3. Parker RI: Pediatric mast cell disease: what's the big (hematologic) deal? Pediatr Blood Cancer. 53(4):527-8, 2009
4. Uzzaman A et al: Pediatric-onset mastocytosis: a long term clinical follow-up and correlation with bone marrow histopathology. Pediatr Blood Cancer. 53(4):629-34, 2009
5. Briley LD et al: Cutaneous mastocytosis: a review focusing on the pediatric population. Clin Pediatr (Phila). 47(8):757-61, 2008
6. Metcalfe DD: Mast cells and mastocytosis. Blood. 112(4):946-56, 2008

CUTANEOUS AND SYSTEMIC MASTOCYTOSIS

Clinical and Microscopic Features

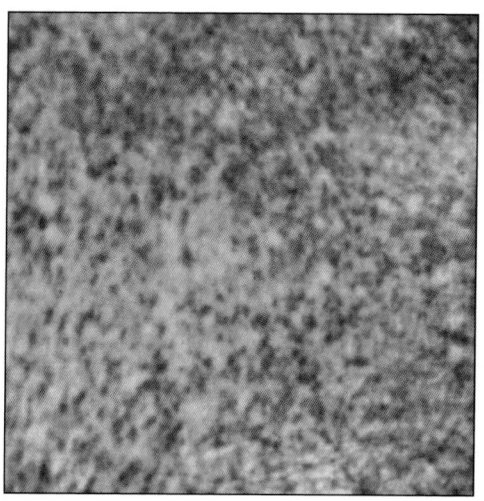
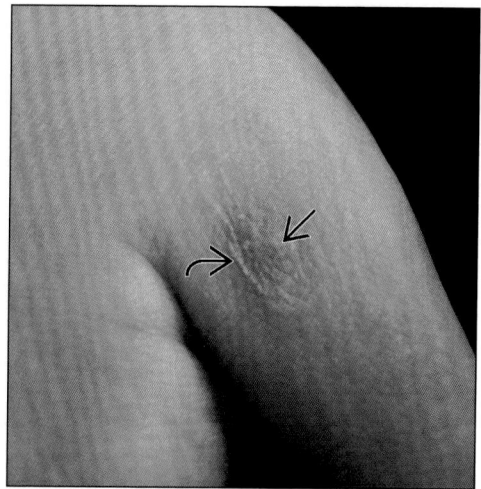

(Left) Clinical image of maculopapular cutaneous mastocytosis is shown. Note the macular and maculopapular brown skin lesions. The pigmentation is usually caused by an intraepidermal accumulation of melanin. (Courtesy C. Bueso-Ramos, MD, PhD.) *(Right)* Brownish-red plaque ➡ on the thumb of a 5-year-old boy shows a positive Darier sign where a linear wheal ➡ has formed at the site of a scratch by the wooden end of a cotton swab. (Courtesy J. Hall, MD.)

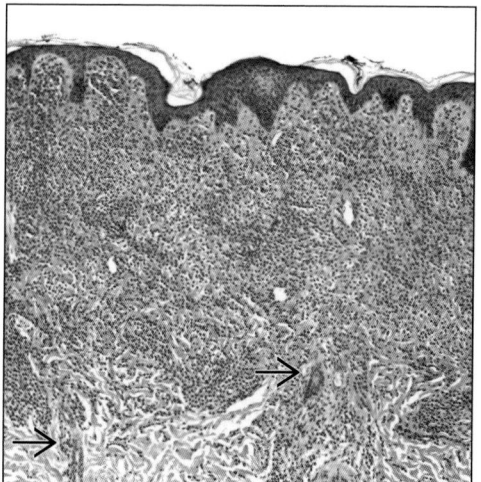
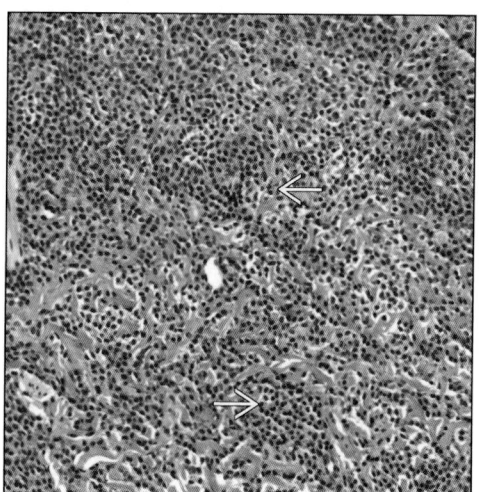

(Left) Cutaneous mastocytosis is shown at low power to highlight the patchy mast cell infiltrates within the dermis. Some of the infiltrate is seen surrounding adnexal structures ➡. *(Right)* Cutaneous mastocytosis is shown at medium power to highlight the dermal mast cell infiltrate ➡. The mast cells show variable cytologic features with some showing spindled nuclei and other areas showing more round nuclei. All contain abundant basophilic cytoplasm.

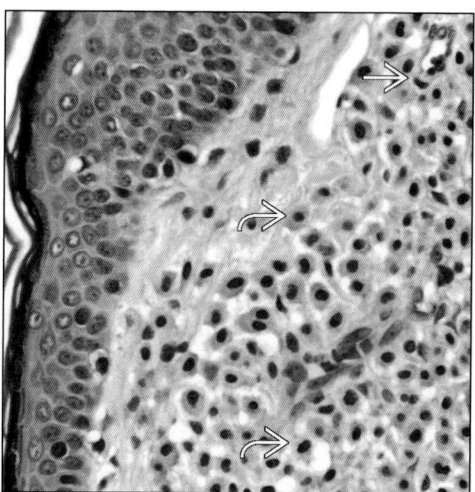
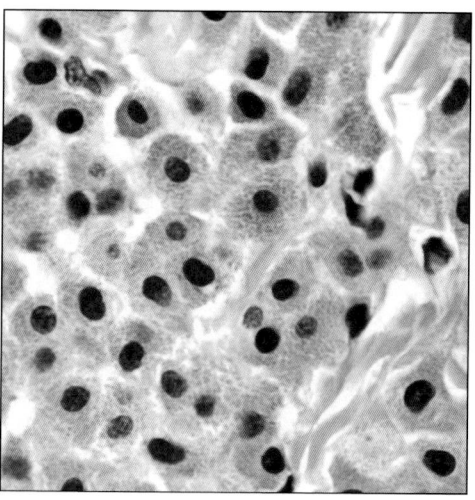

(Left) High magnification of cutaneous mastocytosis displays a dense dermal mast cell infiltrate. This infiltrate in an adult should prompt staging to exclude systemic mastocytosis. Note the variable cytologic features, which include both spindled ➡ and round to oval nuclei ➡. *(Right)* High-power view of mastocytoma highlights the cytologic features, which include enlarged round to oval nuclei with abundant basophilic granular cytoplasm.

CUTANEOUS AND SYSTEMIC MASTOCYTOSIS

Microscopic Features and Ancillary Techniques

(Left) A bone marrow aspirate in a patient with SM shows scattered mast cells ⮕. Mast cells were readily identified away from the spicules, whereas in many patients with a clinical suspicion of SM, careful inspection of the spicules for mast cells is required. *(Right)* A core biopsy from a patient with SM shows a cohesive aggregate of atypical mast cells ⮕. This finding meets both major (>15 mast cells in aggregate) and minor (> 25% are of spindle-shaped) criteria for SM.

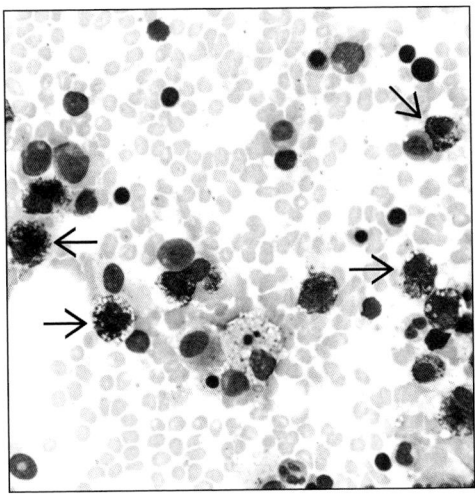

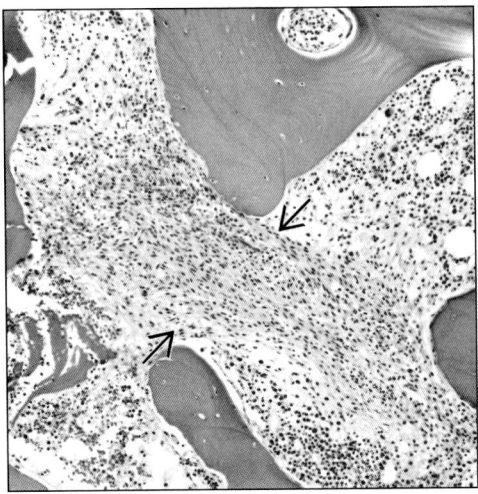

(Left) Atypical mast cells forming a cohesive aggregate in a bone marrow core biopsy are shown at high power. Note the spindle-shaped nuclei ⮕ and the prominent cell borders ⮕ that are typical of mast cell infiltrates. *(Right)* Mast cell tryptase shows positive cytoplasmic reactivity in the mast cells that are forming an atypical cohesive aggregate in this core biopsy specimen. The findings are consistent with a diagnosis of SM.

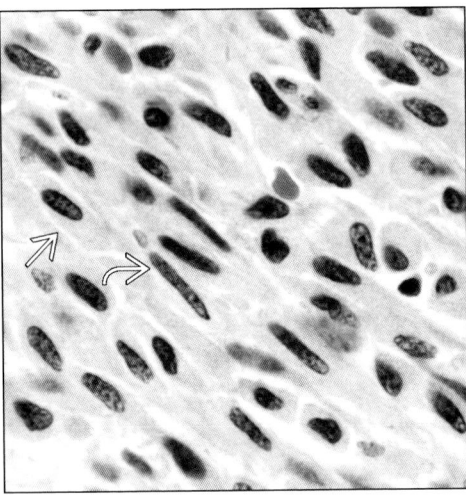

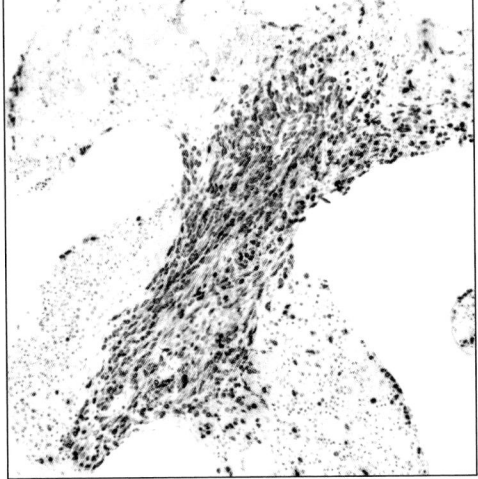

(Left) Extracutaneous mastocytoma involving soft tissue of the shoulder is shown. Immunohistochemistry for CD2 highlights the mast cells. CD2 expression by mast cells is aberrant and supports mast cell neoplasia. (Courtesy C. Bueso-Ramos, MD, PhD.) *(Right)* IHC for CD25 shows a compact cluster of mast cells in this bone marrow biopsy specimen. Reactivity of mast cells with CD25 fulfills a minor diagnostic criterion for the diagnosis of SM. (Courtesy C. Bueso-Ramos, MD, PhD.)

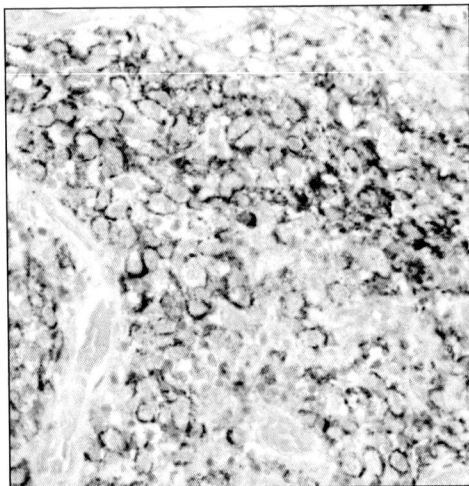

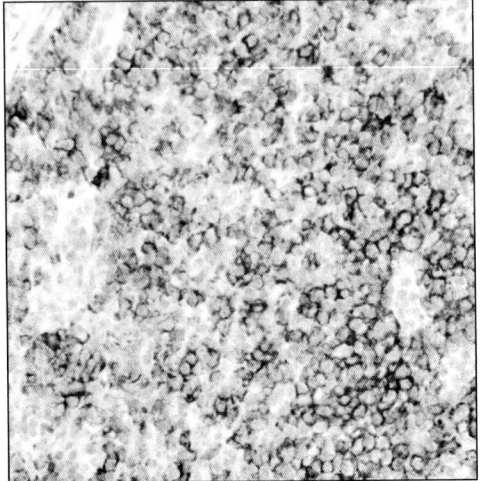

Microscopic Features and Differential Diagnosis

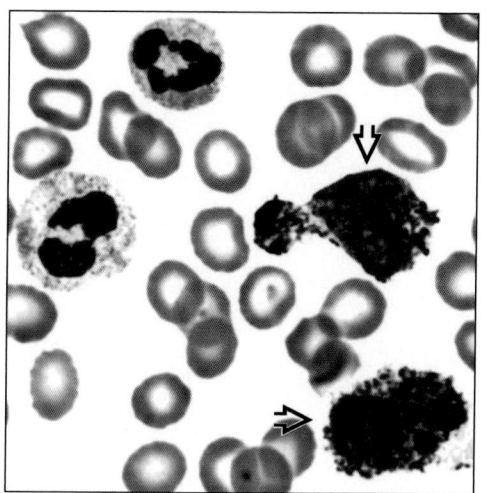

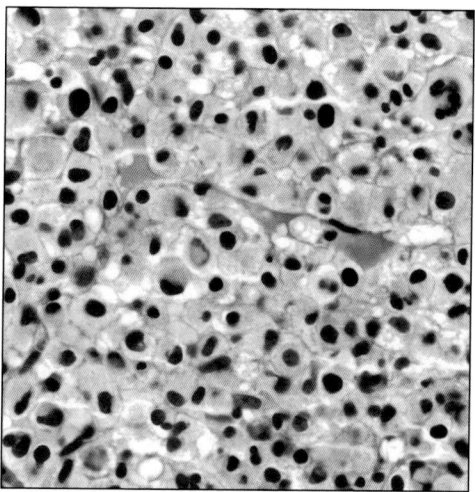

(Left) Two circulating, well-granulated mast cells ⮕ are seen in this PB smear from a patient with mast cell leukemia (MCL). "Leukemic" MCL typically shows > 10% circulating mast cells. *(Courtesy K. Reichard, MD.)* *(Right)* MCL is an aggressive form of mastocytosis and often a differential diagnostic consideration. In contrast to SM, the mast cells are more often round rather than spindled and account for ≥ 20% of BM aspirate nucleated cells. *(Courtesy K. Reichard, MD.)*

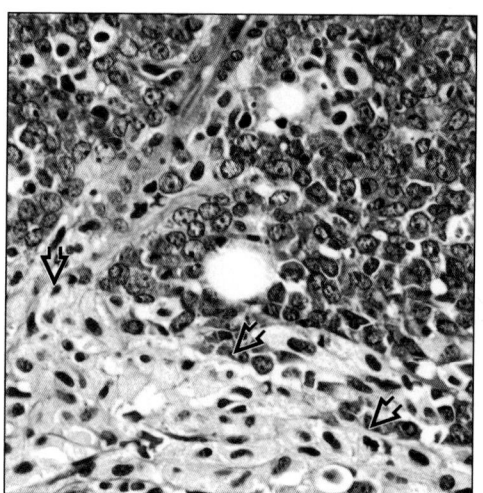

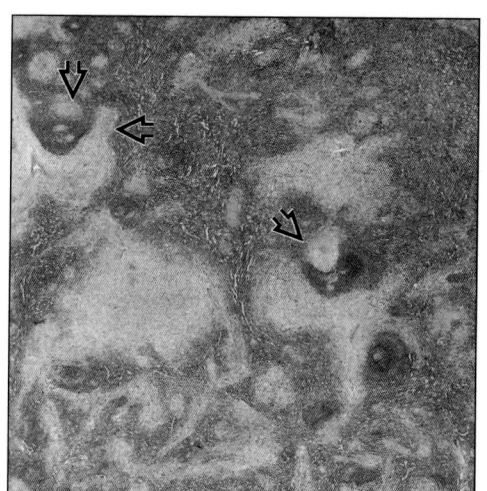

(Left) The bone marrow shows a mast cell cluster ⮕ adjacent to acute myeloid leukemia (AML) with t(8;21)(q22;q22), consistent with AHNMD. *(Courtesy K. Reichard, MD.)* *(Right)* Spleen in a patient with systemic mastocytosis (SM) is shown. Note perifollicular pale mast cell aggregates ⮕. Characteristically patchy fibrosis is associated with and can obscure mast cells. *(Courtesy C. Bueso-Ramos, MD, PhD.)*

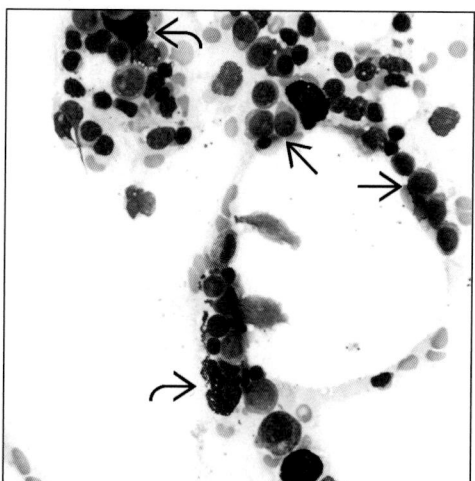

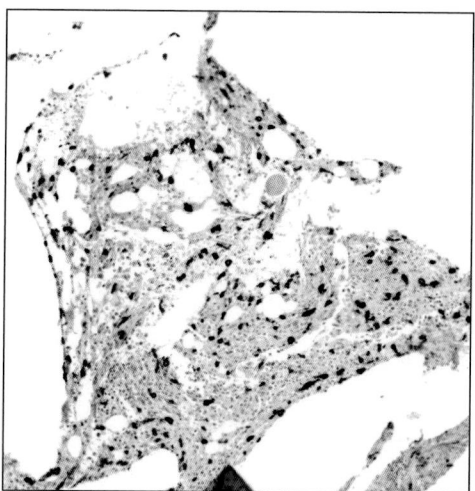

(Left) Myelomastocytic leukemia is an exceedingly rare diagnosis. Myeloid blasts ⮕ are a key component of the diagnosis along with neoplastic mast cells ⮕. *(Courtesy K. Reichard, MD.)* *(Right)* Mast cells are highlighted by CD117. Mast cell hyperplasia may occur after potent myeloablative chemotherapy or other massive toxic insult. In contrast to SM, the mast cells do not form compact aggregates. *(Courtesy K. Reichard, MD.)*

Benign Melanocytic Tumors (Nevi)

CONGENITAL MELANOCYTIC NEVI

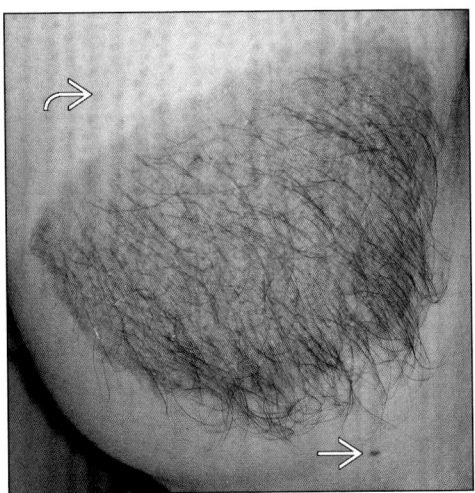

This light tan, medium-sized congenital melanocytic nevus, 10 x 8 cm, has coarse terminal hairs within it. The patient also has keratosis pilaris ⇒ and an acquired melanocytic nevus ⇒.

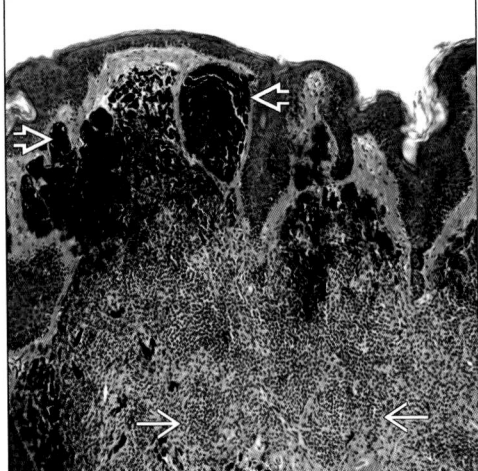

This congenital nevus has nests of larger, heavily pigmented superficial cells ⇒ progressing to small nonpigmented cells deeper in the dermis ⇒, consistent with maturation with dermal descent.

TERMINOLOGY

Synonyms
- Giant/bathing suit/garment-type melanocytic nevus

CLINICAL ISSUES

Epidemiology
- Incidence
  - 1% of newborns
- Age
  - Present at birth, by definition
  - However, some congenital melanocytic nevi may be "tardive"
    - Not readily noticeable at birth; becomes more obvious with age (generally by age 2)

Presentation
- Categorized by size
  - Small
    - < 1.5 cm diameter
    - Round to oval, symmetric
    - Color is variation of brown; may be speckled
    - Surface may be pebbled &/or hairy
  - Medium
    - > 1.5 cm, < 20 cm diameter
    - Round to oval, symmetric; color brown to black, may be speckled
    - Surface may be pebbled &/or hairy
  - Large
    - > 20 cm diameter
    - Often involves the back; dark color, brown to black
    - Surface thickened with increased hair; may make it difficult to follow these lesions for changes over time
    - Satellite nevi often present
    - Underlying soft tissue hypertrophy may be present

- Proliferative nodules, usually < 5 mm in diameter, may develop with time

Treatment
- Sometimes completely excised (if possible) for cosmetic purposes or to reduce risk of melanoma
- Nodules developing within congenital melanocytic nevi
  - At the least: Should be biopsied and followed clinically
  - May be judicious to conservatively excise and follow clinically

Prognosis
- Risk of developing cutaneous malignant melanoma in congenital melanocytic nevi
  - Risk highest for large subtype, estimated at ~ 5%; median age ~ 5 years (average age ~ 13 years)
  - Risk quite low (to possibly none) in small to medium subtypes
- Patients with large congenital melanocytic nevi on head/neck/trunk
  - At risk for neurocutaneous melanosis with risk of primary central nervous system melanoma

MICROSCOPIC PATHOLOGY

Histologic Features
- May be heterogeneous within 1 lesion
- Epidermis may be normal or hyperplastic
  - Lentiginous array of melanocytes may be seen
  - Focal pagetoid scatter may be present
- Small congenital melanocytic nevi may be junctional only
- Most nevi extend into lower reticular dermis and sometimes subcutaneous tissue
- Dermal involvement
  - Occasionally periadnexal or perivascular predominant in small nevi
  - Generally diffuse and interstitial

CONGENITAL MELANOCYTIC NEVI

Key Facts

Clinical Issues

- Present at birth, by definition
- However, some congenital melanocytic nevi may be "tardive" and not readily noticeable at birth
- Categorized by size: < 1.5 cm = small; > 1.5 cm to < 20 cm = medium; > 20 cm = large
- Risks, particularly for large congenital melanocytic nevus: ~ 5% risk of developing cutaneous melanoma; at risk for neurocutaneous melanosis

Microscopic Pathology

- Melanocytes usually extend into lower reticular dermis and sometimes subcutaneous tissue with infiltration of arrector pili muscle, adnexal structures, nerves, and clustering around vessels
- Cells become smaller with depth and less dense
- Nodular proliferations (more common in large nevi): Based superficially in dermis, no epidermal involvement or necrosis

---

- ○ Rows of single melanocytes between collagen bundles
- ○ Infiltration of arrector pili muscle, adnexal structures, and nerves, with clustering around vessels
- ○ Cells become smaller with depth and less dense (maturation)
- Nodular proliferations (more common in large nevi)
  - ○ Variable morphology of melanocytes (spindled, epithelioid, round)
  - ○ Based superficially in dermis
  - ○ Nodule not well demarcated from (blends into) surrounding nevus
  - ○ Lack of epidermal involvement and necrosis
  - ○ Mitoses may be prominent
  - ○ Cytologic atypia usually not prominent
- Large lesions may contain bone, cartilage, fat, vascular proliferation

Cytologic Features

- Melanocytes, particularly junctional, may show slightly enlarged nuclei with small nucleoli

DIFFERENTIAL DIAGNOSIS

Acquired Melanocytic Nevi

- History (not present at birth) may be key
- Generally do not extend as deeply as congenital nevi (i.e., limited to upper 1/2 of reticular dermis)

- Dermal involvement with only periadnexal/perivascular clusters of melanocytes seen more commonly in congenital nevi

Atypical (Dysplastic/Clark) Melanocytic Nevi

- History (not present at birth) may be key
- Junctional component shows cytologic atypia, bridging, and lateral extension beyond intradermal cells
- Generally limited to upper 1/2 of reticular dermis

Malignant Melanoma Arising in Congenital Nevus

- In differential diagnosis of dermal nodular proliferation
- Very rare if age is < 1 year
- Well-demarcated, highly cellular nodules of atypical epithelioid to spindled cells with cytologic atypia
- Nuclear pleomorphism and necrosis often present

SELECTED REFERENCES

1. Shah KN: The risk of melanoma and neurocutaneous melanosis associated with congenital melanocytic nevi. Semin Cutan Med Surg. 29(3):159-64, 2010
2. Tokuda Y et al: Histogenesis of congenital and acquired melanocytic nevi based on histological study of lesion size and thickness. J Dermatol. 37(12):1011-8, 2010
3. van Houten AH et al: Proliferative nodules in a giant congenital melanocytic nevus-case report and review of the literature. J Cutan Pathol. 37(7):764-76, 2010

IMAGE GALLERY

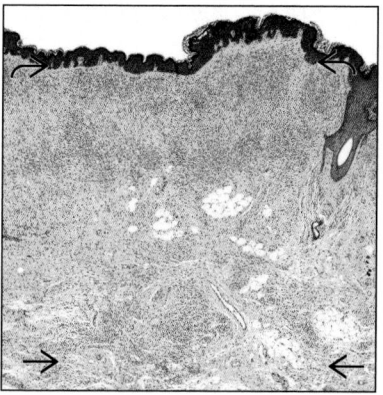
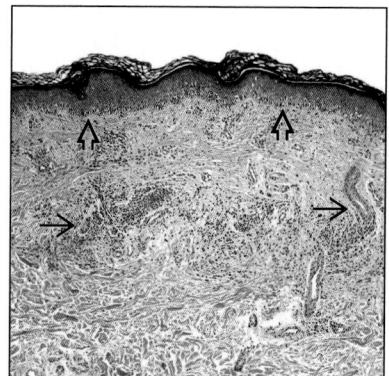
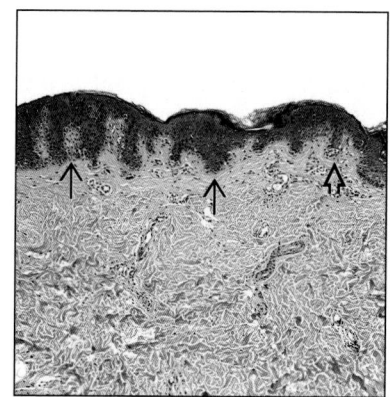

(Left) This congenital melanocytic nevus has a subtle lentiginous melanocytic proliferation at the junction ➡. Melanocytes are superficially nested and become smaller and dispersed deeply ➡. *(Center)* Congenital nevi may show melanocytes singly in the basal layer ➡ and clustered around vessels and adnexal structures ➡. *(Right)* Some congenital nevi, especially if small, may be purely junctional with scattered nests ➡ and single melanocytes ➡ at the tips and sides of rete, mimicking an acquired junctional melanocytic nevus.

COMMON ACQUIRED MELANOCYTIC NEVI

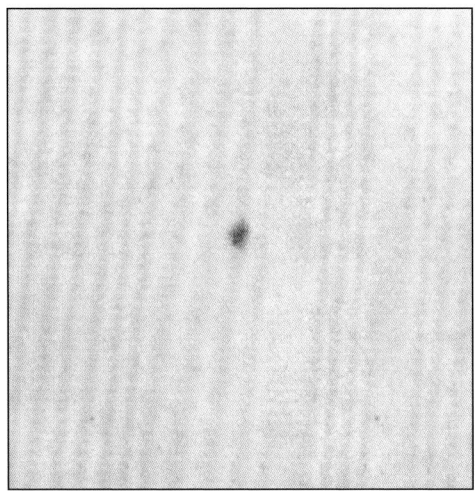

This junctional melanocytic nevus is an oval macule of even, light brown pigment. There is overall symmetry with a smooth border; the size was measured to be 2 x 1 mm.

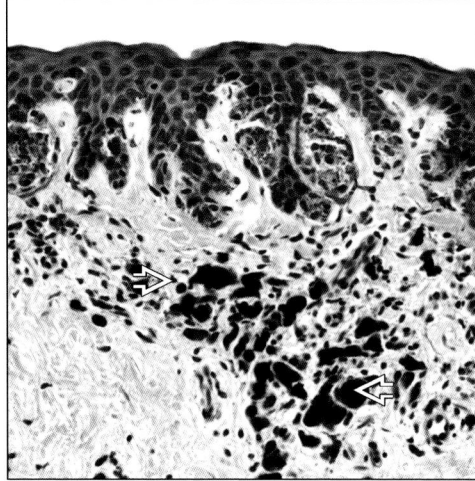

This junctional melanocytic nevus shows nests at the tips and sides of rete ridges. The presence of pigmented parakeratosis and pigment incontinence ➡ likely corresponds to a dark color clinically.

TERMINOLOGY

Synonyms
- Benign melanocytic nevus, junctional melanocytic nevus, compound melanocytic nevus, intradermal melanocytic nevus, common mole, common melanocytic nevus, nevocellular nevus

ETIOLOGY/PATHOGENESIS

Exact Etiology Unknown
- Believed by some to arise from intraepidermal melanocytes
- Others suggest that melanocytic nevi arise from nerves or pluripotential cells

Tumor vs. Hamartoma?
- Still debated
- Evidence for tumor
  - Studies showing that some nevi are clonal
  - Growth advantage of nevus cells over epidermal, dendritic melanocytes in cell culture
  - Similar expression of different markers by nevi and malignant melanoma
  - Presence of mutations in *BRAF* oncogene in majority of nevi
- Evidence for hamartoma
  - Other proliferative elements: Epidermal, follicular, connective tissue
  - Studies showing that some nevi are polyclonal

CLINICAL ISSUES

Epidemiology
- Incidence
  - Number of acquired nevi
    - Increases with age up to 3rd decade
    - May be related to familial predisposition
    - Sun exposure in childhood also linked to development of nevi
    - More common in lighter skinned individuals
- Age
  - Not present at birth
  - Majority develop in adolescence
  - Density of nevi generally decreases after 4th decade

Presentation
- Junctional lesions
  - Flat to minimally raised macule/very thin papule
  - Generally < 6 mm, but may be larger
  - Color often a variation of brown
- Compound lesions
  - Slightly raised papule
  - Variable color (brown, flesh-colored, pink)
  - May contain hair
- Intradermal lesions
  - Papule, may be pedunculated
  - Variable color (brown, flesh-colored, pink)
  - May contain hair

Natural History
- Abtropfung hypothesis of Unna
  - Melanocytes are initially junctional
  - With chronologic time (aging), melanocytes "drop off" into dermis, creating compound melanocytic lesions
  - With more time, the junctional melanocytes have all "dropped off," creating intradermal melanocytic lesions
  - Intradermal melanocytic lesions may eventually "shed" or become acrochordons
    - Degenerative changes include balloon cell change and fatty change
- Alternative hypothesis
  - Nevi begin in the dermis
- Not all melanocytic nevi display progressive changes; some arrest at a given stage indefinitely

COMMON ACQUIRED MELANOCYTIC NEVI

Key Facts

Clinical Issues
- Majority develop in adolescence

Microscopic Pathology
- Flat surface to slightly raised to polypoid
- Epidermis varies (e.g., thin or seborrheic keratosis-like)
- Well-circumscribed
- Melanocytes arranged in regular clusters/nests, particularly at junction of epidermis and dermis and superficial dermis
- Nest defined as 3-5 clustered melanocytes
- Generally symmetrical from side to side
- Orderly arrangement of nests at junction and in superficial dermis
- Mitoses generally absent

- Melanin pigment often limited to junctional or superficial dermal nests
- Dermal maturation: Type A nevus cells superficially, type B and C nevus cells with descent into dermis
  - Type A nevus cells: Epithelioid
  - Type B nevus cells: Lymphocytoid
  - Type C nevus cells: Spindled, neuroid
  - May see pseudonuclear inclusion: Lighter staining round area within nucleus

Top Differential Diagnoses
- Atypical/"dysplastic"/Clark nevus
- Congenital melanocytic nevus
- DDx of junctional lentiginous melanocytic nevus
  - Lentigo (simple)
- DDx of intradermal nevus (especially neurotized)
  - Neurofibroma

Treatment
- Not necessary
- Conservative removal (e.g., shave removal) generally sufficient
  - Residual dark pigment may remain
  - Pigment may recur irregularly within scar (recurrent nevus)

Prognosis
- Benign

MICROSCOPIC PATHOLOGY

Histologic Features
- Flat surface to slightly raised to polypoid
- Well-circumscribed
- Melanocytes arranged in nests, particularly at junction of epidermis and dermis and superficial dermis
- Nest defined as cluster of at least 3 (some authors) or 5 (other authors) melanocytes
- Generally symmetrical from side to side
- Orderly arrangement of nests at junction and in superficial dermis
- Nest size regular
- Cell and nest size sometimes enlarged in younger patients
- Junctional component, when present
  - Often ends peripherally with nests
  - Nests centered at tips and sometimes sides of rete
  - Variable numbers of single, rounded melanocytes present in basal layer (may predominate in junctional lentiginous melanocytic nevus)
  - Pagetoid spread unusual (may be seen in nevi of special sites and irritated/traumatized nevi)
- Intradermal component, when present, matures with depth
  - Melanocytes near base are smaller in diameter (type B) than those in superficial dermis (maturation)
    - Superficial dermis: Type A cells: Epithelioid with pink to finely pigmented cytoplasm and oval to round nuclei, sometimes with small nucleoli;

multinucleate cells (with clustered nuclei or wreath-like arrangement of nuclei) may also be seen
    - Toward base of lesion: Type B cells: Lymphocyte-like with round, blue nuclei and little cytoplasm
    - Base of lesion may be composed of Type C cells: Spindled and neural in appearance (these cells predominate in neurotized nevus)
- Mitoses generally absent
- Melanin pigment often limited to junctional or superficial dermal nests
- Specific patterns that may be present
  - Pseudovascular pattern
    - Melanocytes line empty spaces, giving appearance of vessels
  - "Degenerative" pattern
    - Also known as fatty change
    - Lipocytes are interspersed among melanocytes
    - Degeneration may also manifest with "balloon" cells or sebocyte-like cells; such cells have prominent, vacuolated cytoplasm
- Additional findings that may be seen include
  - Dermal ossification
    - Termed "nevus of Nanta"
  - Epidermal spongiosis
    - Termed "Meyerson nevus"
  - Epidermal hyperplasia that resembles seborrheic keratosis
    - Term "keratotic melanocytic nevus" proposed by some
  - Stromal desmoplasia
    - Termed "desmoplastic (sclerotic) melanocytic nevus"
  - Bizarre cells with enlarged nuclei in dermis with generally absent mitoses
    - Termed "ancient melanocytic nevus"

Cytologic Features
- Type A nevus cells
  - Epithelioid
    - Pink to light blue cytoplasm
    - Oval, pale nucleus

COMMON ACQUIRED MELANOCYTIC NEVI

- ■ May see pseudonuclear inclusion: Lighter staining around area within nucleus
- Type B nevus cells
  - ○ "Lymphocytoid"
    - ■ Little cytoplasm
    - ■ Round, blue nucleus
    - ■ May see pseudonuclear inclusion: Lighter staining round area within nucleus
- Type C nevus cells
  - ○ Spindle-shaped with pink cytoplasm (can appear neural)
- Multinucleate cells
  - ○ Arrangement of nuclei
    - ■ Wreath-like (Touton giant cell-like)
    - ■ Clumped, termed "mulberry-type"

DIFFERENTIAL DIAGNOSIS

Atypical ("Dysplastic" or Clark) Nevus
- In compound lesions, junctional component extends beyond dermal component (shoulder phenomenon)
- Bridging of nests across rete ridges
- Nest size variable and irregular
- Single melanocytes often seen between nests
- May be asymmetric side to side
- Papillary dermal fibrosis (lamellar and concentric)
- Perivascular lymphocytes
- Dermal component, if present, shows maturation
- Deep mitoses absent
- Cytologically, melanocytes may show enlarged nuclei with nucleoli and increased cytoplasm; cytoplasm may be finely pigmented (smoky)

Congenital Melanocytic Nevus
- History (present at birth) may be key
- Often deeper than acquired melanocytic nevi
- Melanocytes
  - ○ May involve arrector pili muscle
  - ○ May cluster around vessels/adnexal structures
  - ○ Often splay singly through collagen toward base

Combined Nevus
- Banal or "ordinary" junctional, compound, or intradermal melanocytic nevus
- Additionally, 2nd type of nevus (most commonly blue nevus, but may also be deep-penetrating or Spitz nevus type) present

Lentigo (Simplex or Solar)
- In differential diagnosis of junctional lentiginous melanocytic nevus
- Increased number of single melanocytes in basal layer of epidermis may be seen in some cases
- Nests of melanocytes absent

Neurofibroma
- In differential of intradermal nevus with extensive neurotization
- Fragmented collagen like "shredded carrots," darker than stroma
- Short, spindled cells with tapered nuclei in light pink stroma

- Lacks nests/clusters of melanocytic cells

Malignant Melanoma
- In differential of ancient melanocytic nevus
- Presence of significant atypia, pleomorphism, and mitotic activity; lack of maturation
- Mitoses and inflammation uncommonly present in ancient melanocytic nevus

Desmoplastic Melanoma
- In differential of desmoplastic (sclerotic) melanocytic nevus
- Overlying changes of melanoma in situ often present
- Atypical spindled cells with hyperchromatic nuclei infiltrate dermis
- Perivascular and interstitial lymphocytes often present

DIAGNOSTIC CHECKLIST

Pathologic Interpretation Pearls
- Junctional nevus
  - ○ Well-circumscribed, symmetric from side to side
  - ○ Generally ends in nests peripherally
  - ○ Orderly arrangement of nests
  - ○ Melanocytes with round nuclei and pink to finely pigmented cytoplasm
  - ○ Nuclear atypia and mitoses not present
- Compound melanocytic nevus
  - ○ Junctional component
    - ■ Similar to that of junctional melanocytic nevus: Well-circumscribed, symmetric, ends in nests peripherally, nest size regular and orderly, melanocytes have round nuclei and pink to finely pigmented cytoplasm
    - ■ Does not usually extend laterally past intradermal component
  - ○ Dermal component matures
    - ■ Type A (epithelioid) cells and multinucleate cells superficially
    - ■ Type B (lymphocytoid) cells &/or type C (spindled) cells deeper
- Intradermal melanocytic nevus
  - ○ Well-circumscribed, symmetric
  - ○ Often polypoid in shape; otherwise, dermal component similar to that of compound nevi
  - ○ Note: Some intradermal melanocytic nevi, particularly from centrofacial location, have overlying single melanocytes arrayed in basal layer

SELECTED REFERENCES

1. Barnhill RL et al: State of the art, nomenclature, and points of consensus and controversy concerning benign melanocytic lesions: outcome of an international workshop. Adv Anat Pathol. 17(2):73-90, 2010
2. Tokuda Y et al: Histogenesis of congenital and acquired melanocytic nevi based on histological study of lesion size and thickness. J Dermatol. 37(12):1011-8, 2010
3. Takata M et al: Genetic alterations in melanocytic tumors. J Dermatol Sci. 43(1):1-10, 2006

Microscopic Features

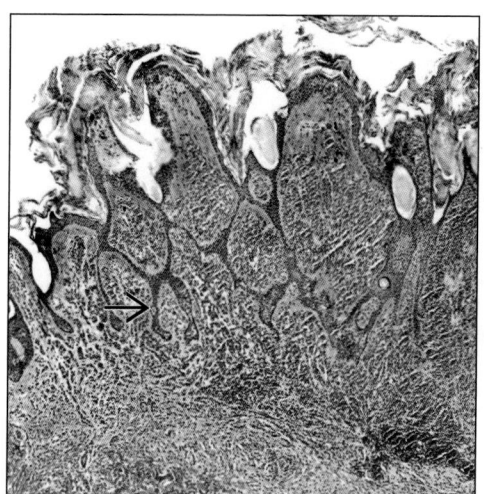

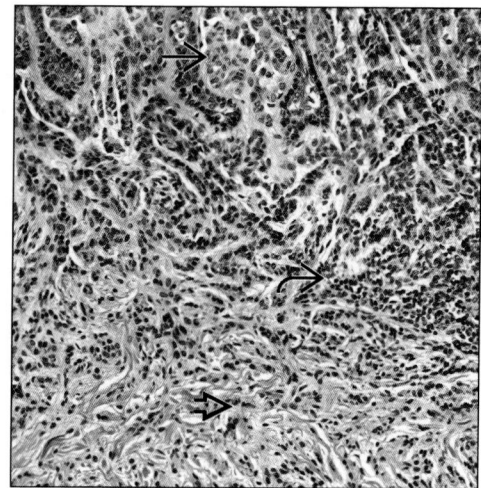

(Left) This compound melanocytic nevus shows epidermal hyperplasia. There are occasional nests in the epidermis ➡. Melanocytes are nested in the superficial dermis and mature with depth, becoming smaller and more dispersed. (Right) Higher magnification view of a compound melanocytic nevus shows a dermal component that matures from superficial type A (epithelioid) nested cells ➡ to type B (lymphocytoid) cells ➡ to type C (spindled/neuroid) cells ➡ at the base.

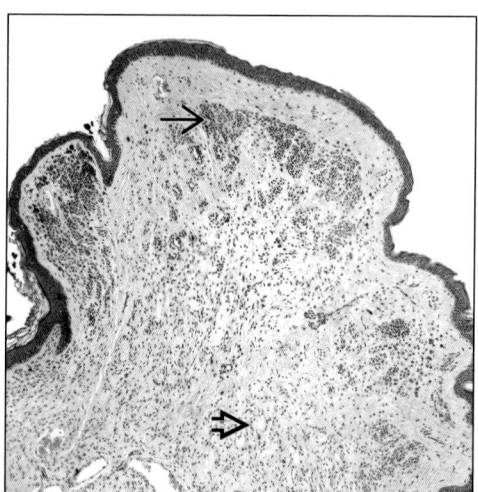

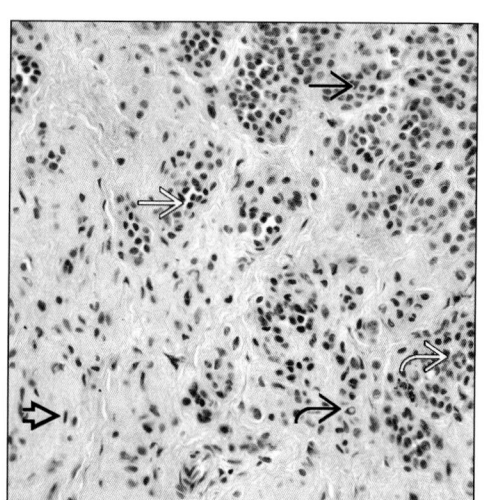

(Left) This polypoid intradermal melanocytic nevus shows dermal melanocytes with a "congenital pattern" and maturation. There are nested, larger melanocytes ➡ at the surface and more spindled melanocytes ➡ toward the base. (Right) Type A (epithelioid) ➡, type B (lymphocytoid) ➡, and type C (spindled) ➡ cells are shown. Varying proportions of these cells compose any given melanocytic nevus. Note pseudonuclear inclusions ➡ and multinucleate cells ➡.

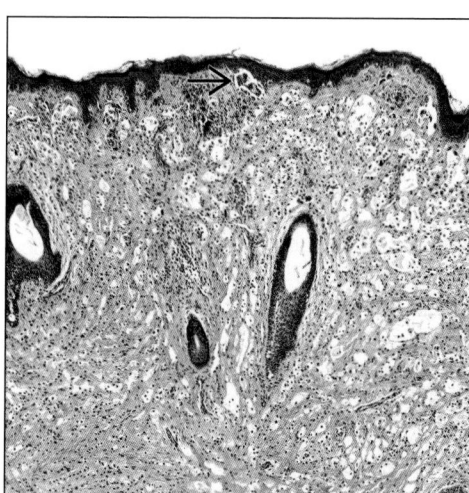

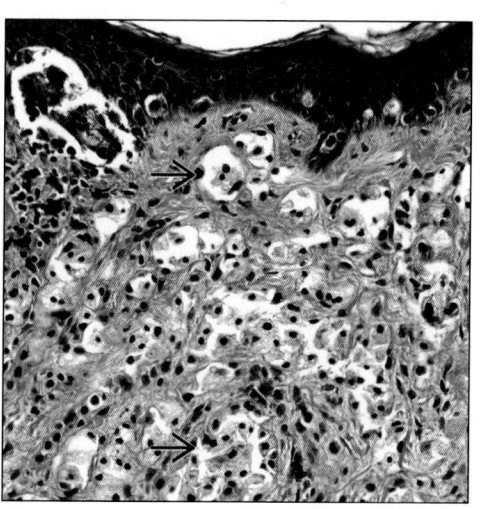

(Left) This is a balloon cell nevus: A compound melanocytic nevus with prominent balloon cells. Balloon cells (or sebocyte-like cells) are a degenerative phenomenon. There are a few remaining junctional nests ➡ of pigmented melanocytes. (Right) Higher magnification shows the balloon cells (sebocyte-like cells) have foamy/vacuolated cytoplasm. The balloon cells may be clustered/nested ➡.

CONVENTIONAL BLUE NEVI

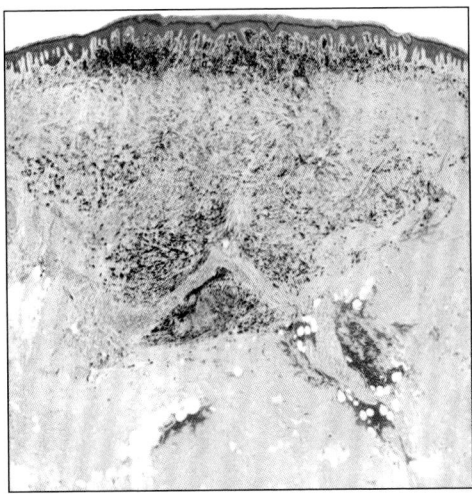

Scanning magnification of a BN shows a symmetrical, wedge-shaped, and evenly pigmented melanocytic tumor present throughout the dermis.

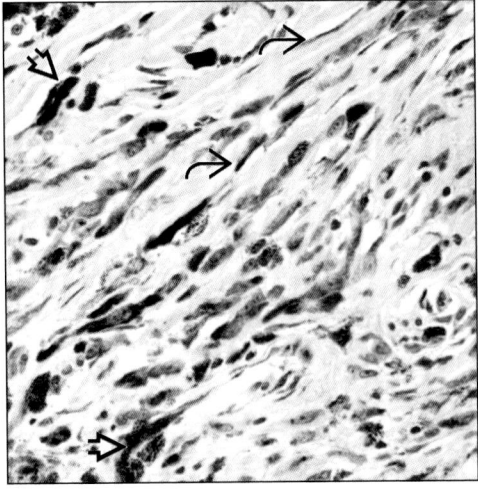

High-power magnification of a conventional BN shows 2 cell types: Spindled to dendritic melanocytes ⤏ and melanophages ⧁.

TERMINOLOGY

Abbreviations
- Blue nevus (BN)

Synonyms
- Dendritic blue nevus, common blue nevus, Jadassohn-Tièche-type nevus

Definitions
- Heterogeneous group of acquired and congenital melanocytic tumors
- Composed predominantly of spindled to dendritic-shaped melanocytes
- Varying degrees of cellularity, intra- and extracellular melanin content, and dermal sclerosis

ETIOLOGY/PATHOGENESIS

Developmental Anomaly
- May represent aberrant melanocytic precursor migration in development

CLINICAL ISSUES

Epidemiology
- Incidence
  - Very common
- Age
  - Principally in children
  - However, can occur later in life at any age

Site
- Most occur in skin, commonly on extremities and face
- Other documented extracutaneous anatomic sites include
  - Subungual region, orbit, conjunctiva, oral cavity
  - Sinusoidal mucosa, bronchus, esophagus
  - Lymph nodes, vagina, uterine cervix, endometrium, penis, and prostate

Presentation
- Well-demarcated, slightly raised papules (< 1 cm in diameter)
- Range in color from blue to gray to blue-black to black

Treatment
- Surgical approaches
  - Simple excision

Prognosis
- Excellent; no significant malignant potential

MICROSCOPIC PATHOLOGY

Histologic Features
- Can grow in short fascicles with intervening grenz zone
- Dermal sclerosis with variable amount of collagen in tumor stroma
- Ill-defined dermal or submucosal proliferation of 2 cell types
  - Elongated melanocytes with fine dendritic processes
  - Melanophages with coarse, cytoplasmic melanin pigment
- Variants
  - Amelanotic BN (lack of significant pigmentation)
  - Sclerotic BN (prominent stromal sclerosis)
  - Agminated BN (multiple adjacent similar satellite lesions)

Cytologic Features
- Melanocyte
  - Bipolar, spindled-shaped
  - Elongated dendritic processes
  - Variable amount of granular melanin in cytoplasm and within dendritic processes
  - Minimal nuclear atypia

CONVENTIONAL BLUE NEVI

Key Facts

Terminology
- Benign melanocytic tumor composed of spindle-shaped and dendritic melanocytes and melanophages

Clinical Issues
- Occurs in any age, in wide range of locations
- Well-demarcated, slightly raised papule (< 1 cm in diameter)
- Color ranges from blue to gray to blue-black to black

- Excellent prognosis; no significant malignant potential

Microscopic Pathology
- Well-demarcated, wedge-shaped dermal melanocytic tumor with variable amount of collagenosis
- 2 cell types: Slender melanocytes and round melanophages
- Heavy to sometimes light mixture of melanophages

  ○ Mitotic figures are almost always absent
- Melanophages
  ○ Round, ample cytoplasm
  ○ Abundant, coarse cytoplasmic melanin pigment
  ○ Nuclei difficult to see due to heavy melanin pigment

DIFFERENTIAL DIAGNOSIS

DDx of Sclerosing (Desmoplastic) BN
- Desmoplastic Spitz nevus
- Desmoplastic acquired melanocytic nevus
- Desmoplastic melanoma
  ○ Immunostains for HMB-45 and MART-1/Melan-A are usually negative in desmoplastic melanoma, but positive in BN
- Dermatofibroma
  ○ Mixture of spindled and histiocytic-appearing cells with vacuolated cytoplasm
  ○ Overlying epidermal hyperplasia with basilar hyperpigmentation
  ○ Pigmented cells can be present, but contain hemosiderin (Fe[+]), not melanin

DDx of Amelanotic BN
- Dermatofibroma
  ○ Mixture of spindled and histiocytic-appearing cells with vacuolated cytoplasm
  ○ Overlying epidermal hyperplasia with basilar hyperpigmentation

DIAGNOSTIC CHECKLIST

Clinically Relevant Pathologic Features
- Slate gray to blue round papule/macule

Pathologic Interpretation Pearls
- Typically heavily pigmented, search for ill-defined dermal spindle cell proliferation associated with sclerotic collagen
- Under high-power magnification, search for dendritic processes originating from elongated cells

SELECTED REFERENCES

1. Zembowicz A et al: Blue nevi and variants: an update. Arch Pathol Lab Med. 135(3):327-36, 2011
2. Murali R et al: Blue nevi and related lesions: a review highlighting atypical and newly described variants, distinguishing features and diagnostic pitfalls. Adv Anat Pathol. 16(6):365-82, 2009
3. Massi G et al: Histological Diagnosis of Nevi and Melanoma. Darmstadt, Germany: Steinkopff Verlag, 2004
4. Zembowicz A et al: Dermal dendritic melanocytic proliferations: an update. Histopathology. 45(5):433-51, 2004
5. Crowson AN et al: The Melanocytic Proliferations: A Comprehensive Textbook of Pigmented Lesions. New York: Wiley-Liss, 2001
6. del Río E et al: Blue nevus with satellitosis mimicking malignant melanoma. Cutis. 65(5):301-2, 2000
7. Levene A: On the natural history and comparative pathology of the blue naevus. Ann R Coll Surg Engl. 62(5):327-34, 1980

IMAGE GALLERY

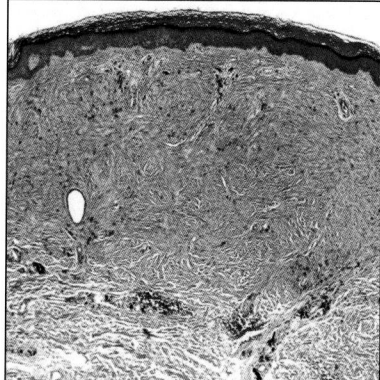 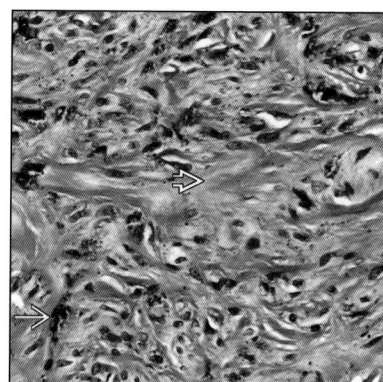 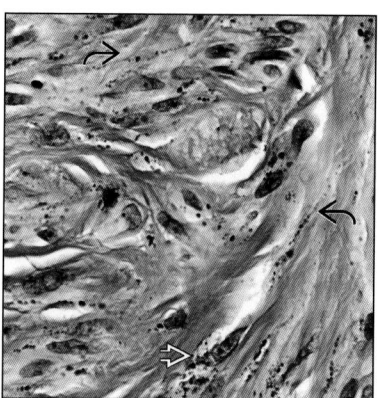

(Left) Another example of a BN shows more pronounced hyalinizing collagenosis in the stroma. *(Center)* Medium-power magnification of a BN demonstrates more abundant collagen in the tumor stroma ⮊ and scattered melanophages ⮊. *(Right)* High-power magnification shows numerous melanocytes with very fine dendritic processes ⮕ and fine granular melanin pigment in their cytoplasm ⮊.

CELLULAR BLUE NEVI

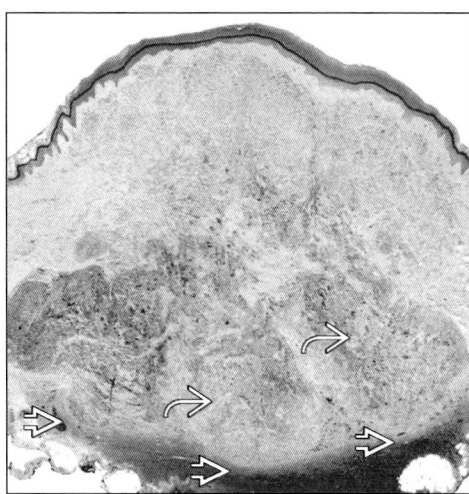

Scanning magnification of a CBN shows symmetrical hypercellular lobules resembling "dumbbells" ➡. These nodules push evenly and deeply beyond the reticular dermis into the subcutis ➡.

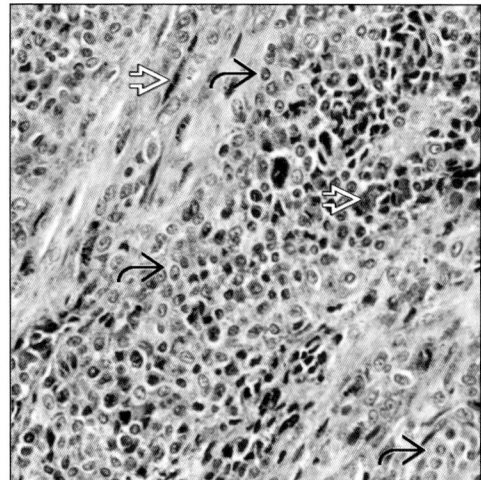

High-power examination of a hypercellular fascicle shows oval-to-spindled cells; when cut en face, these cells appear more cuboidal ➡. There are few scattered melanophages ➡.

TERMINOLOGY

Abbreviations
- Cellular blue nevus (CBN)

Definitions
- Cellular variant of blue nevus
- Presents as large blue to blue-black, well-circumscribed, multilobulated tumor composed of oval to spindle-shaped melanocytes

CLINICAL ISSUES

Epidemiology
- Incidence
  - All races
- Age
  - Occurs in childhood and young adult life
    - Mean: 33 years
- Gender
  - Female predominance (female:male ~ 2:1)

Site
- Mostly occurs on sacrococcygeal regions and buttock, but may also be located on the scalp, neck, face, hands, and extremities (especially dorsal foot)

Presentation
- Heavily pigmented black or blue nodule or a plaque ranging from 1-2 cm in diameter (even up to 6 cm)
- Ulceration may be seen in lesions appearing in area with growth restriction, such as dorsal foot

Treatment
- Surgical approaches
  - Simple excision

Prognosis
- Benign lesion but may rarely recur

- Regional lymph node involvement and appearance of "benign" metastases to regional lymph nodes by CBN are rare, but well documented
  - Resulting lymphadenopathy is prone to misdiagnosis as metastatic malignant tumor or melanoma
- CBN has potential for malignant transformation, and affected patients have poor clinical outcome

MICROSCOPIC PATHOLOGY

Histologic Features
- Architecture consists of central mass with adjacent ramifications
  - These have a dumbbell or peninsula-like shape occupying place of effaced hair follicles (follicular epithelium is usually absent)
- In addition, there is zonal sequence; in higher portion, near epidermis, desmoplasia is conspicuous
- Lesion is much more cellular in center with ovoid and spindled pale cells in large solid sheets or roundish nests
- Collagen bundles between cells are thickened
- CBN exhibits classic features of common blue nevus in areas, i.e., dendritic, heavily pigmented melanocytes with numerous densely pigmented melanophages
  - These features of "common" blue nevus are usually found around outer edges of the lesion
- Margins are usually pushing

Cytologic Features
- Ovoid, clear cells are abundant
- Cells have small, monomorphous nucleus with evenly speckled and margined chromatin
- Cells have finely eosinophilic or clear cytoplasm, with vesicular nuclei and small nucleoli
- Heavily pigmented spindled and dendritic cells alternate with clear cells
  - They may rarely be amelanotic

CELLULAR BLUE NEVI

Key Facts

Terminology
- Cellular variant of blue nevus

Clinical Issues
- Occurs in children and young adults
- Heavily pigmented black/blue nodule or plaque ranging from 1-2 cm; tends to occur on buttocks and sacrococcygeal region
- Has low incidence of transformation into melanoma

Microscopic Pathology
- Dumbbell-shaped architecture
- Oval and spindle-shaped cells with bland cytology
- Lack of mitoses or necrosis

Top Differential Diagnoses
- Atypical cellular blue nevus
- Melanoma developing in cellular blue nevus and malignant blue nevus
- Desmoplastic melanoma

- There is no/minimal atypia, no nuclear pleomorphism

DIFFERENTIAL DIAGNOSIS

Atypical Cellular Blue Nevus (ACBN)
- CBN that exhibits atypia insufficient for diagnosis of malignancy
- Cytologic atypia can be focal or diffuse
- No necrosis, and mitotic rate of < 2 per mm²

Melanoma Developing in Cellular Blue Nevus and Malignant Blue Nevus
- Malignant cytology in areas, often with benign blue nevus component
  - Atypia with hyperchromatic nuclei and obvious nucleoli in majority of cells
- Sarcoma-like solid sheets of atypical spindle cells
- Large sheets or nodules of atypical cells with epithelioid shape
- Prominent mitoses (increased numbers, often atypical)
- Presence of areas of cellular necrosis

Desmoplastic Melanoma
- Lymphocytic infiltrate often prominent
- Desmoplastic melanoma often is achromic, in contrast to CBN, which has many melanophages
- Desmoplastic melanoma typically only positive for S100; CBN show diffuse HMB-45 and MART-1/Melan-A staining as well

DIAGNOSTIC CHECKLIST

Clinically Relevant Pathologic Features
- Heavily pigmented black or blue nodule or a plaque ranging from 1-2 cm in diameter (even up to 6 cm)

Pathologic Interpretation Pearls
- Look for multiple mitoses and necrosis, both of which favor malignancy

SELECTED REFERENCES

1. Zembowicz A et al: Blue nevi and variants: an update. Arch Pathol Lab Med. 135(3):327-36, 2011
2. Murali R et al: Blue nevi and related lesions: a review highlighting atypical and newly described variants, distinguishing features and diagnostic pitfalls. Adv Anat Pathol. 16(6):365-82, 2009
3. Zembowicz A et al: Dermal dendritic melanocytic proliferations: an update. Histopathology. 45(5):433-51, 2004
4. Crowson AN et al: The Melanocytic Proliferations: A Comprehensive Textbook of Pigmented Lesions. New York: Wiley-Liss, 2001
5. Rodriguez HA et al: Cellular blue nevus. Clinicopathologic study of forty-five cases. Cancer. 21(3):393-405, 1968

IMAGE GALLERY

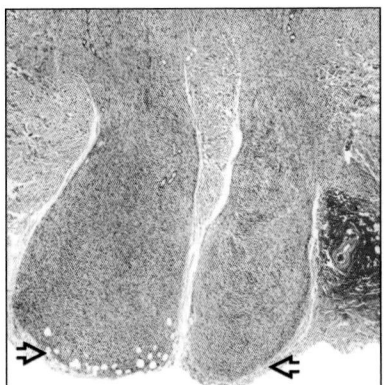 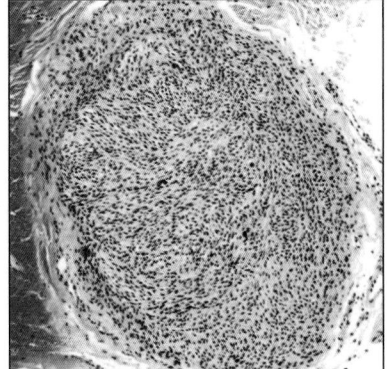 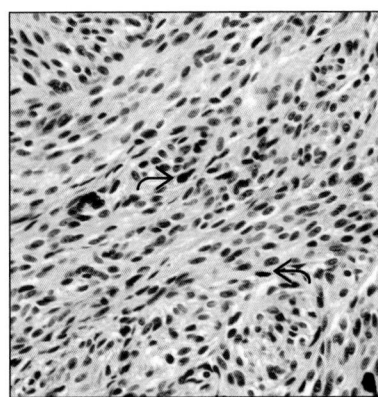

(Left) Scanning magnification of another CBN exhibits dumbbell-appearing hypercellular lobules extending into the subcutis ⊳. *(Center)* Medium-power magnification shows a hypercellular lobule composed of ovoid to spindle-shaped cells with mild nuclear hyperchromasia. *(Right)* Higher examination of a cellular lobule reveals oval to spindle cells with relatively uniform, hyperchromatic nuclei ⊅. There is only mild nuclear pleomorphism, and no mitoses are identified.

COMBINED NEVI

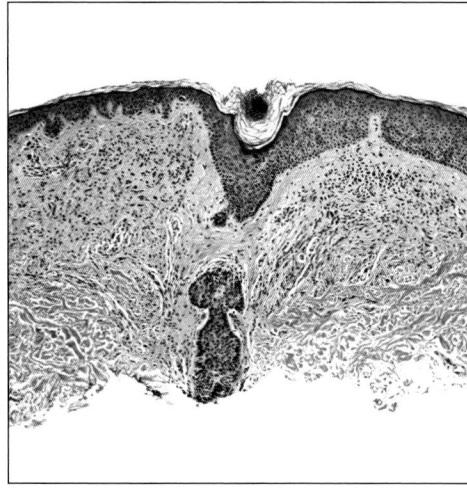

This is an example of a combined nevus of the most common type, i.e., composed of an "ordinary" intradermal melanocytic nevus and a blue nevus. The lesion is symmetric and orderly appearing.

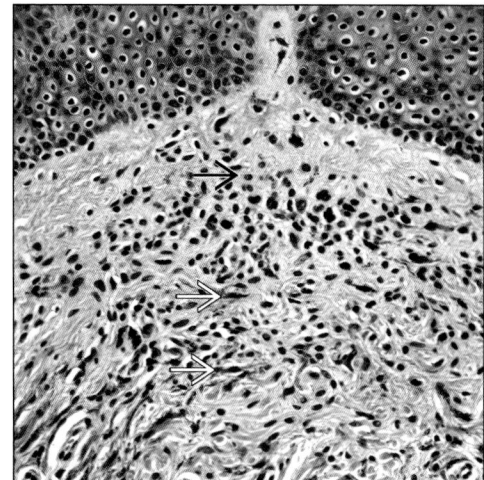

This higher magnification view shows the admixed melanocytic cell types. There are bland epithelioid (type A) nevus cells ⇨ interspersed with pigmented spindled to dendritic melanocytes ⇢.

TERMINOLOGY

Synonyms
- Melanocytic nevus with phenotypic heterogeneity, clonal nevus, nevus with focal epithelioid component, combined Spitz nevus, inverted type A nevus

Definitions
- Presence of 2 or more distinct populations of melanocytes (i.e., type A melanocytic nevus cells, and spindled dendritic cells) **or**
- Presence of 2 or more types of melanocytic nevi (i.e., intradermal melanocytic, blue)

CLINICAL ISSUES

Presentation
- Generally in young adults
- Any site, but may be more common on head and neck
- Pigment of lesion often very dark brown to black or blue-black
- Lesion may have small focus of blue to blue-black color in background of lighter pigment
- Size usually < 6 mm

Prognosis
- No significant malignant potential

MICROSCOPIC PATHOLOGY

Histologic Features
- All combined nevi
  - Lesion overall symmetric
  - Well-circumscribed
  - Orderly arrangement of melanocytes
- Most common type of combined nevus
  - Intradermal or compound melanocytic nevus plus blue nevus

- Blue nevus component: Variable composition of dendritic melanocytes, melanophages, and fibrosis; may extend deeply &/or have plexiform configuration
- Another type of combined nevus: Compound or intradermal melanocytic plus pigmented spindle cells or spitzoid/epithelioid cells
  - Pigmented spindle cells in nests/fascicles **or**
  - Spitzoid/epithelioid cells in nests/fascicles
    - Large cells with round to oval nuclei, often with melanin pigment

Cytologic Features
- Most common type of combined nevus
  - Intradermal melanocytes
    - Type A: Round cells with pink cytoplasm, round nuclei, small nucleoli may be visible (epithelioid)
    - Type B: Resemble lymphocytes with round, blue nuclei and little cytoplasm
    - Mulberry-type giant cells: Molded, tightly packed nuclei with little cytoplasm
    - Giant cells with wreath-like arrangement of nuclei at periphery of cells
  - Blue nevus-type melanocytes
    - Melanocytes with dendritic processes and cytoplasmic melanin

DIFFERENTIAL DIAGNOSIS

DDx of Combined Nevus (Compound or Intradermal Melanocytic Plus Blue Nevus)
- Blue nevus (common)
  - Lacks junctional component and type A/B melanocytic cells
- Compound blue nevus
  - Rare lesion
  - Junctional component composed of nonnested dendritic melanocytes
- Congenital melanocytic nevus

COMBINED NEVI

Key Facts

Terminology
- Presence of 2 or more distinct populations of melanocytes **or**
- Presence of 2 or more types of melanocytic nevi

Clinical Issues
- Generally in young adults, size < 6 mm
- Pigment of lesion often very dark brown to black or blue-black
- Site: May be more common on head and neck

Microscopic Pathology
- Lesion overall orderly, symmetric, and well-circumscribed
- Most commonly: Compound/intradermal melanocytic nevus plus blue nevus

Top Differential Diagnoses
- Blue nevus (common and cellular types)
- Deep penetrating nevus
- Congenital melanocytic nevus

- o Lacks dendritic and spindle-shaped melanocytes
- Cellular blue nevus
  - o Lacks junctional component
  - o Melanophages, pigmented dendritic melanocytes, and cellular nests or lobules of spindled melanocytes (often with little melanin pigment)
  - o Architecture often bulbous/pushing into subcutaneous fat
- Deep penetrating nevus
  - o Wedge-shaped architecture
  - o Often deep extension into dermis/subcutaneous
  - o Junctional nests may be present
  - o Dermal component composed of pigmented spindled melanocytes in nests bordered by melanophages
  - o Nests/fascicles of cells may be centered around adnexal/neurovascular structures in dermis
  - o Occasionally, bulbous/pushing margin is present

DDx of Combined Compound or Intradermal Melanocytic Plus Spitzoid/Epithelioid Nevus
- Melanoma arising in dermis of melanocytic nevus
  - o Large expansile nests/sheets of atypical cells (pleomorphic, enlarged, hyperchromatic)
  - o Mitoses often common
    - Atypical &/or deep

DIAGNOSTIC CHECKLIST

Pathologic Interpretation Pearls
- Combined nevi
  - o Either the combination of 2 or more types of melanocytic nevi **or** combination of 2 or more melanocytic cell types in 1 lesion
  - o Types of melanocytic nevi
    - "Ordinary" (junctional/compound/intradermal melanocytic) nevus
    - Congenital melanocytic nevus
    - Dysplastic/atypical melanocytic nevus
    - Blue nevus (any type: Common, cellular, epithelioid, deep penetrating, etc.)
    - Spitz nevus
    - Pigmented spindle cell nevus
  - o Types of melanocytes
    - Type A ("epithelioid") or B ("lymphocytoid") "ordinary" melanocytic nevus cells
    - Dendritic
    - Epithelioid with enlarged nuclei and prominent nucleoli
    - Spindled (pigmented or amelanotic)

SELECTED REFERENCES
1. Barnhill RL et al: State of the art, nomenclature, and points of consensus and controversy concerning benign melanocytic lesions: outcome of an international workshop. Adv Anat Pathol. 17(2):73-90, 2010

IMAGE GALLERY

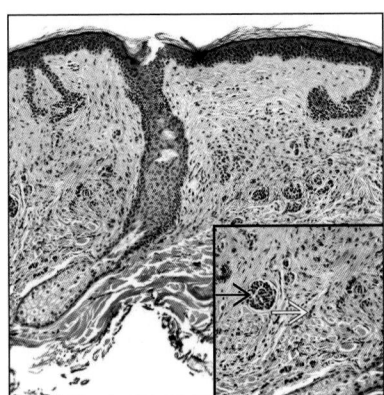 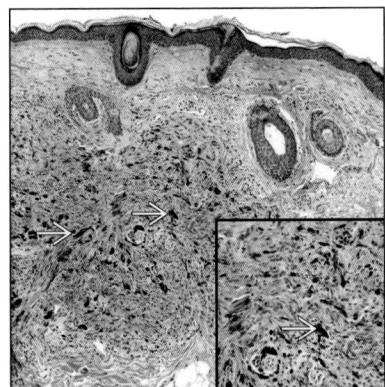 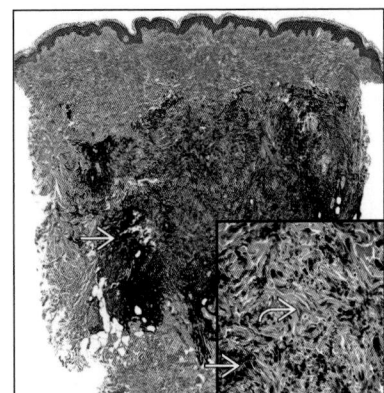

(Left) This combined nevus has an "ordinary" compound melanocytic nevus and a blue nevus. Inset shows banal, nested melanocytes ➔ and dendritic melanocytes ➔ at higher magnification. *(Center)* This deep penetrating nevus has nodular collection of finely pigmented spindled to epithelioid cells in fascicles with interspersed melanophages ➔. *(Right)* This blue nevus has numerous melanophages ➔ and scattered dendritic melanocytes ➔.

HALO NEVI

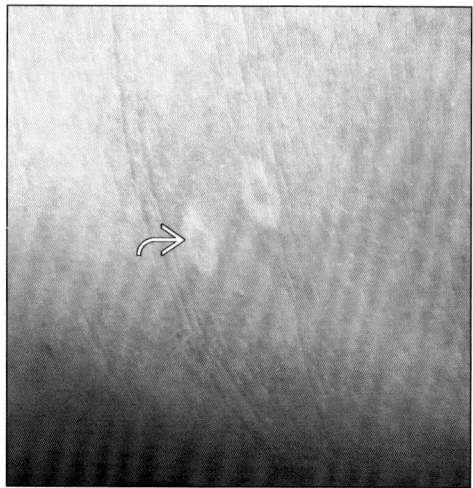

Two halo nevi seen on the back of a young adult are oval, well demarcated, and depigmented (skin colored or paler). With time, the white area may replace the nevus entirely ➦.

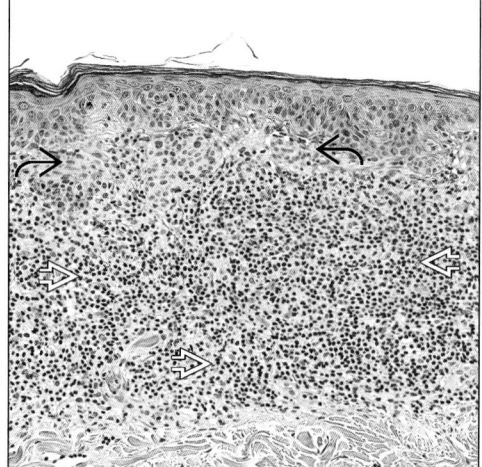

Halo nevus is characterized by a dense, band-like lymphohistiocytic infiltrate in the dermis ⬌. Junctional and superficial nests of melanocytes can be appreciated upon close inspection ➶.

TERMINOLOGY

Synonyms
- Sutton nevus
- Nevus depigmentosa centrifugum

Definitions
- Nevus with clinically depigmented halo surrounding pigmented area
- Dense inflammatory infiltrate typically present
  - Histologically heavily inflamed nevi that lack a clinical halo may be said to show "halo reaction/phenomenon," but they are not true halo nevi

ETIOLOGY/PATHOGENESIS

Inflammatory Process
- Thought to be a reaction to melanocytic antigens
- Infiltrate includes numerous T cells, including cytotoxic CD8(+) cells that may induce melanocyte apoptosis

CLINICAL ISSUES

Epidemiology
- Age
  - Usually young patients (children and young adults)
  - Patients over 40 years old uncommon
    - Should raise concern for the possibility of melanoma at another site

Site
- Most common on the back, but may occur at any site

Presentation
- Pigmented lesion
  - Depigmented halo surrounds lesion
  - Central lesion eventually loses pigmentation
- Often multiple

Natural History
- Progressively loses pigmentation over several months
  - Central nevus
    - Initially pigmented; may show erythema before regressing
    - May remain depigmented after regression or show repigmentation

Treatment
- Surgical approaches
  - Complete conservative excision is curative

Prognosis
- Excellent
- May be associated with melanoma, typically at another site, in older patients

MICROSCOPIC PATHOLOGY

Histologic Features
- Compound nevus associated with dense inflammatory infiltrate
- Infiltrate typically shows a lichenoid (band-like) pattern in dermis
  - Composed mostly of lymphocytes with scattered histiocytes and melanophages
  - Rarely, clinically typical-appearing halo nevi can lack significant inflammation
- Nevus may be of any type, but usually a conventional compound nevus
  - Junctional and dermal nests are surrounded by dense inflammatory infiltrate
  - Nests predominate in early lesions, single cells in later lesions
    - May be completely absent in late-stage lesions
  - Dermal component should show evidence of maturation with descent
  - Reactive atypia may be present, but should be low grade (mild/moderate)

HALO NEVI

Key Facts

Terminology
- Nevus with clinically depigmented halo surrounding pigmented area

Clinical Issues
- Usually young patients (children and young adults)
- In older patients, should raise concern for melanoma

Microscopic Pathology
- Nevus associated with dense inflammatory infiltrate

- Infiltrate typically shows a lichenoid pattern in dermis
- Nests predominate in early lesions, single cells later
- Melanocytic markers may be useful to confirm presence of melanocytes
- Reactive atypia may be present

Top Differential Diagnoses
- Melanoma
- Myerson nevus (eczematous nevus)

- ■ Severe atypia should raise suspicion for melanoma
- ○ Mitoses should be rare to absent
  - ■ May be difficult to determine if a mitosis is in an inflammatory or stromal cell vs. a melanocyte
- ○ Spitzoid features may be present in some cases ("halo Spitz nevi")
- Epidermis shows loss of pigmentation and normal melanocytes at periphery of lesion
  - ○ Can be confirmed by melanin stain

ANCILLARY TESTS

Immunohistochemistry
- Melanocytic markers may be useful to confirm presence of melanocytes if not obvious on histologic sections
  - ○ S100, MART-1/Melan-A, HMB-45, and tyrosinase
    - ■ S100 also stains Langerhans cells and dermal dendritic cells, limiting its usefulness
    - ■ HMB-45 often positive in junctional cells, but negative in dermal component (may be useful in favoring a nevus over melanoma)
  - ○ Combined MART-1/Melan-A and Ki-67 stain may be useful to determine if there is melanocytic proliferative activity

DIFFERENTIAL DIAGNOSIS

Melanoma
- May be heavily inflamed in some cases

- ○ But usually shows more of a patchy infiltrate than halo nevi
- Shows greater degree of cytologic and architectural atypia
- Pagetoid scatter also usually present
- Lack of maturation (if invasive)
- Lack of symmetry and circumscription
- Dermal mitotic figures and elevated Ki-67 proliferative rate often seen

Myerson Nevus (Eczematous Nevus)
- Eczematous (spongiotic) reaction involving a nevus
- May show eczematous halo clinically
- Milder inflammation with eosinophils usually present

SELECTED REFERENCES

1. Ohtsuka T: Multiple Sutton nevi: Hypomelanocytic halo development around 28 melanocytic nevi. J Dermatol. 36(6):355-7, 2009
2. Moretti S et al: Fibrosis in regressing melanoma versus nonfibrosis in halo nevus upon melanocyte disappearance: could it be related to a different cytokine microenvironment? J Cutan Pathol. 34(4):301-8, 2007
3. Sotiriadis D et al: Does halo nevus without halo exist? J Eur Acad Dermatol Venereol. 20(10):1394-6, 2006
4. Cui Z et al: Halo naevus: a visible case of immunosurveillance in humans? Lancet Oncol. 5(7):397-8, 2004
5. Epstein WL et al: Halo nevi and melanoma. JAMA. 225(4):373-7, 1973
6. Frank SB et al: The halo nevus. Arch Dermatol. 89:367-73, 1964

IMAGE GALLERY

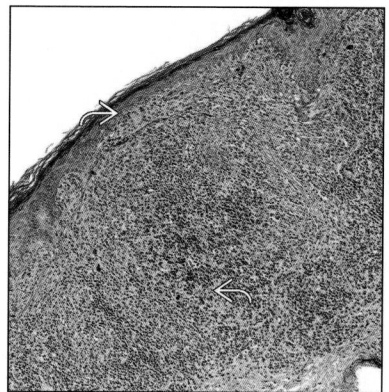 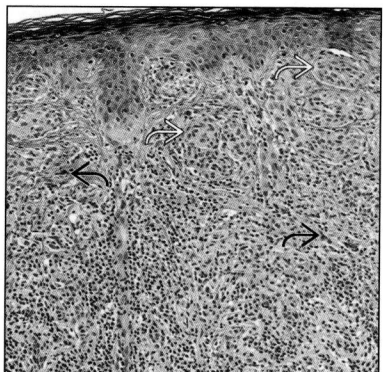 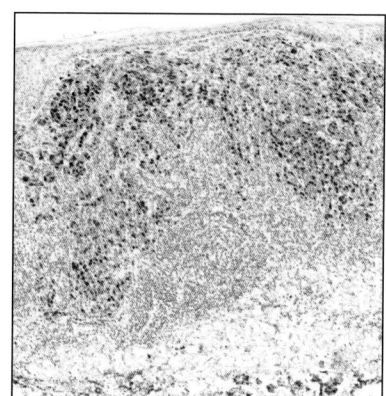

(Left) Low magnification of a halo nevus shows a dense infiltrate surrounding scattered junctional and dermal nests of melanocytes ➡. *(Center)* Higher magnification shows a dense lymphohistiocytic infiltrate with scattered melanophages ➡. The melanocytes are mildly enlarged and atypical-appearing ➡ but show no mitotic activity. *(Right)* Melan-A shows strong and diffuse staining of the residual melanocytes; it is often more useful than S100, given its greater specificity.

DERMAL MELANOCYTOSES (NEVUS OF OTA AND ITO, MONGOLIAN SPOT)

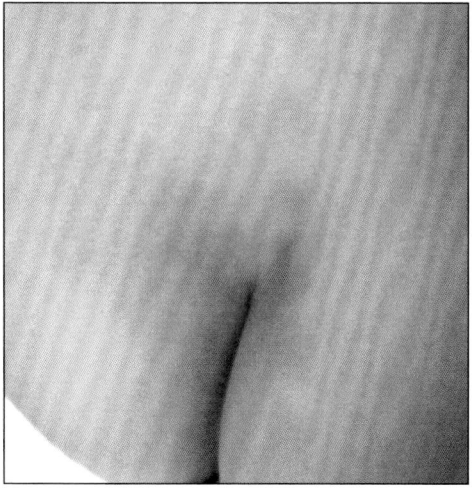

This is the typical location for a Mongolian spot, over the sacral area. There may also be patches in other areas of the back.

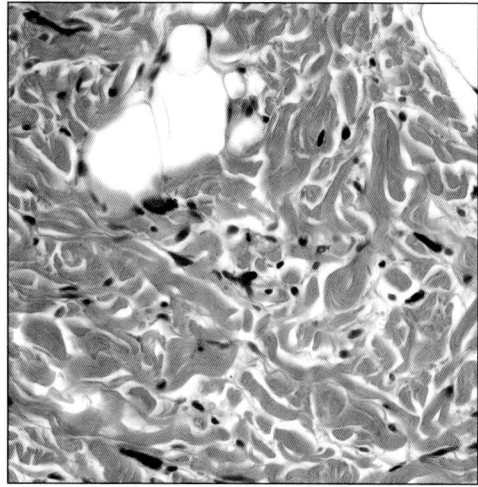

This high-magnification view of a Mongolian spot shows dendritic melanocytes with cytoplasmic melanin pigment in the deep dermis.

CLINICAL ISSUES

Epidemiology
- Age
  - Often evident at birth, but occasionally manifest later
- Ethnicity
  - More common in Asians

Site
- Nevus of Ota
  - Located near/involving the eye (conjunctiva)
    - In distribution of trigeminal nerve (ophthalmic/maxillary)
- Nevus of Ito
  - Located on shoulder/deltoid area
- Mongolian spot
  - Located most commonly on the back, especially lumbosacral
  - Rarely, in so-called "aberrant" form, may involve extremities
    - When located in areas other than the back, overlaps with blue nevi

Presentation
- Nevus of Ota/Ito
  - Often unilateral
  - Color often blue to gray
  - Variably sized mottled patch
- Mongolian spot
  - Generally 1 or more patches of blue to gray
  - Evident at birth
  - May be associated with nevus flammeus (capillary malformation), nevus spilus, &/or nevus anemicus (so-called phacomatosis pigmentovascularis)

Natural History
- Nevus of Ota and Ito generally stable over time
- Mongolian spots generally fade by age 5
  - "Aberrant" Mongolian spots may not fade

Treatment
- Benign, no treatment necessary
- Laser may be used if treatment is desired for cosmetic purposes

Prognosis
- Very rarely, malignancy has been reported to develop within nevus of Ota and Ito
- Rarely, nevus of Ota associated with deafness
- Rarely, extensive Mongolian spots associated with inheritable storage disease

MICROSCOPIC PATHOLOGY

Histologic Features
- Nevus of Ota and Ito and Mongolian spot show similar histologic features
  - Dendritic melanocytes in dermis, may cluster around adnexal structures/vessels/nerves
    - Nevus of Ota/Ito: Melanocytes may be sparse to more numerous, usually in upper dermis
    - Mongolian spot: Melanocytes may be sparse, usually in deeper dermis, often arranged parallel to epidermis
  - Dermis generally otherwise normal (without sclerosis)
  - Melanophages generally absent

Cytologic Features
- Melanocytes
  - Not atypical, dendritic, melanin pigment in cytoplasm

DIFFERENTIAL DIAGNOSIS

DDx of Nevus of Ota
- Blue nevus
  - Clinically, confluent macule or patch of blue pigmentation, generally not present at birth

DERMAL MELANOCYTOSES (NEVUS OF OTA AND ITO, MONGOLIAN SPOT)

Key Facts

Clinical Issues
- Nevus of Ota and Ito and Mongolian spot
  - Often evident at birth
  - Occasionally manifest later in life
  - Generally stable over time (nevus of Ota and Ito); resolution with time (Mongolian spot)
  - Blue to gray macule/patch
- Nevus of Ota: Near/involving eye
- Nevus of Ito: Shoulder area

- Mongolian spot: Generally on back

Microscopic Pathology
- Dendritic melanocytes in dermis
- Dermis generally otherwise normal (without sclerosis)

Top Differential Diagnoses
- Blue nevus
- Hori nevus
- Becker nevus
- Child abuse

  - Histologically spindled melanocytes in dermis with variable numbers of melanophages
- Hori nevus
  - Clinically
    - Generally bilateral
    - Acquired in adulthood
    - Female predominance
    - More common in Asian populations
    - Similar to nevus of Ota, involves malar cheeks
    - Often composed of numerous hyperpigmented macules
    - Usually becomes more gray over time
  - Histologically similar to nevus of Ota or Ito
- Sun nevus
  - Clinically acquired in adulthood, unilateral hyperpigmented macules in malar area
  - Histologically similar to nevus of Ota or Ito

DDx of Nevus of Ito
- Becker nevus
  - Clinically tan to brown patch on shoulder/upper back area; may show hypertrichosis within lesion
  - Histologically
    - Basal layer may show increased melanin pigment
    - Increased smooth muscle bundles in dermis
    - Hair follicles may be increased in number
- Macular amyloid
  - Clinically on shoulder/upper back area with rippled pattern of hyperpigmentation
  - Histologically
    - Deposits of amyloid in papillary dermis

    - ± pigment incontinence
    - No melanocytes

DDx of Mongolian Spot
- Child abuse
  - In contrast to bruising from child abuse, Mongolian spots present at birth, shows uniform blue-gray color
- Patch-like blue nevus
  - "Aberrant" Mongolian spot may be indistinguishable clinically from patch-like blue nevus
  - Histologically similar, although patch-like blue nevus is more cellular

DIAGNOSTIC CHECKLIST

Pathologic Interpretation Pearls
- Dendritic melanocytes in dermis
- Usually no dermal sclerosis
- Absent melanophages

SELECTED REFERENCES

1. Wise SR et al: Malignant melanoma transformation within a nevus of Ito. J Am Acad Dermatol. 62(5):869-74, 2010
2. Park JM et al: Acquired bilateral nevus of Ota-like macules (Hori nevus): etiologic and therapeutic considerations. J Am Acad Dermatol. 61(1):88-93, 2009
3. Ashrafi MR et al: Extensive Mongolian spots: a clinical sign merits special attention. Pediatr Neurol. 34(2):143-5, 2006

IMAGE GALLERY

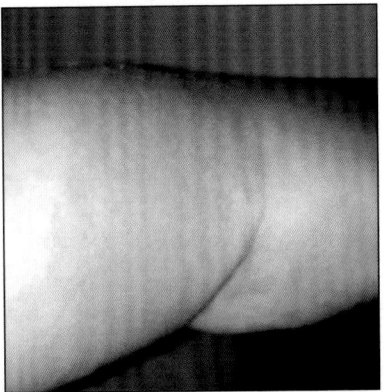 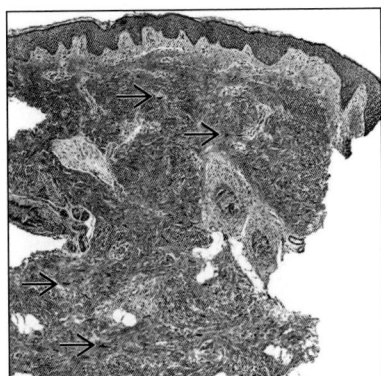 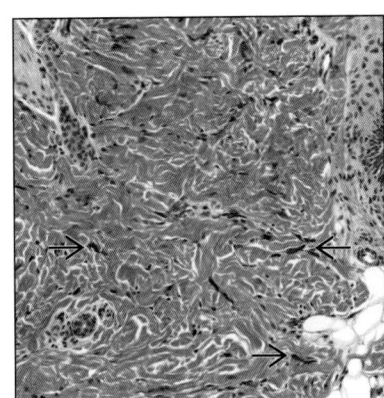

(Left) This Mongolian spot on the wrist is termed "aberrant," overlaps with patch-like blue nevus, and has less tendency to spontaneously resolve. *(Center)* This low-magnification view of a Mongolian spot shows a normal epidermis and pigmented cells ➡ scattered through the dermis. *(Right)* This intermediate-magnification view of a Mongolian spot shows dermal dendritic melanocytes ➡, some oriented parallel to the epidermal surface.

PARAGANGLIOMA-LIKE DERMAL MELANOCYTIC TUMOR

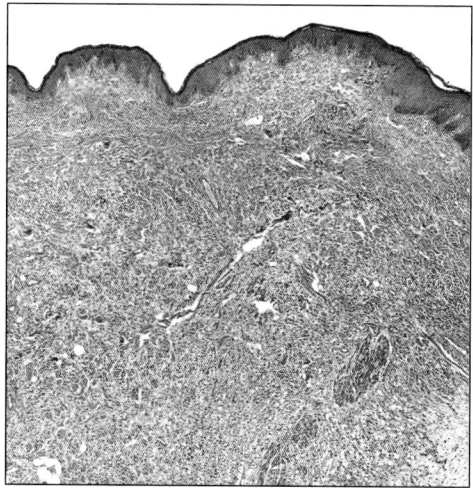

Histologic sections show a diffuse proliferation of clear cells located in the dermis. PLDMT is often a well-circumscribed, but unencapsulated, dermal-based tumor that can extend into the subcutis.

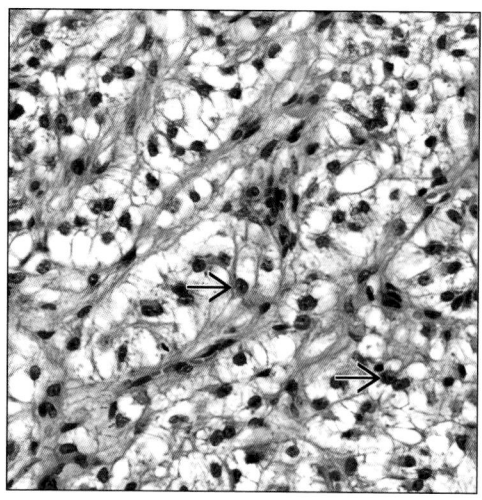

High magnification shows that the tumor is composed of closely packed nests of cells with clear or granular cytoplasm and round to oval nuclei with small nucleoli ➡.

TERMINOLOGY

Abbreviations
- Paraganglioma-like dermal melanocytic tumor (PLDMT)

Definitions
- Dermal-based low-grade melanocytic tumor with histologic similarities to paraganglioma

CLINICAL ISSUES

Epidemiology
- Incidence
  ○ Very rare tumors; only 10 cases reported to date
- Age
  ○ Typically occur in young adults
    ▪ Range: 18-53 years
    ▪ Mean: 35 years
- Gender
  ○ More common in females

Site
- Usually occur on extremities
  ○ Mostly lower limb
    ▪ Thigh, knee, lower leg

Presentation
- Dermal-based mass lesion
  ○ Clinically amelanotic in most cases

Treatment
- Surgical approaches
  ○ Complete excision should be recommended, given uncertain biologic potential of these tumors

Prognosis
- Local recurrences rare
- No metastases reported to date

MACROSCOPIC FEATURES

General Features
- Circumscribed dermal-based nodule

MICROSCOPIC PATHOLOGY

Histologic Features
- Nodular dermal-based melanocytic tumor
  ○ Relatively well-circumscribed, nonencapsulated, and symmetric-appearing tumor
    ▪ Focal infiltrative features at edges of tumor may be seen in some cases
- Typically composed of well-formed packets of bland pale to clear-staining oval-shaped cells, mimicking paraganglioma
  ○ Cells are surrounded by thin fibrous septa
  ○ Cells show moderate amounts of clear cytoplasm
  ○ Only focal, fine cytoplasmic melanin pigment may be found in some cases
- Mitotic activity may be present, but is usually low (1-4/10 HPF)

Cytologic Features
- Uniform oval to spindle-shaped nuclei
- Small nucleoli
- Abundant clear cytoplasm
- No high-grade cytologic atypia described

ANCILLARY TESTS

Immunohistochemistry
- Positive for S100, variably so for MART-1/Melan-A and HMB-45

Molecular Genetics
- *EWS/ATF1* gene rearrangement absent

PARAGANGLIOMA-LIKE DERMAL MELANOCYTIC TUMOR

Key Facts

Terminology

- Paraganglioma-like dermal melanocytic tumor (PLDMT)
- Rare dermal-based, low-grade melanocytic tumor with histologic similarities to paraganglioma

Microscopic Pathology

- Typically composed of packets of oval to spindle-shaped cells surrounded by thin fibrous septa
- Uniform nuclei, small nucleoli, clear cytoplasm

Ancillary Tests

- Positive for S100; MART-1/Melan-A, and HMB-45 (variable)

Top Differential Diagnoses

- Clear cell/balloon cell melanoma
- Clear cell sarcoma
- Perivascular epithelioid cell tumor (PEComa)
- Primary dermal melanoma

DIFFERENTIAL DIAGNOSIS

Clear Cell/Balloon Cell Melanoma

- Atypical proliferation of melanocytes, often with overlying intraepidermal component
- Pagetoid spread and lentiginous hyperplasia in junctional component
- Dermal component shows greater cytologic atypia and mitotic activity than PLDMT

Clear Cell Sarcoma of Soft Parts

- Typically based in deep subcutis, but may invade dermis
- Young adults, often on lower extremity
- Immunohistochemistry similar to that of PLDMT
  - Multiple melanocytic markers typically expressed
- t(12;22), *EWS/ATF1* fusion

Perivascular Epithelioid Cell Tumor (PEComa)

- Rare tumors composed of nests and sheets of bland-appearing clear cells
- HMB-45 and MART-1/Melan-A(+), usually only weakly/focally (+) for S100
- SMA(+) and variably so for desmin and CK (unlike in PLDMT)

Primary Dermal Melanoma

- Very rare variant of melanoma located in dermis &/or subcutaneous tissues

- Well-circumscribed, large, cellular nodule, which mimics metastatic melanoma in most cases
- Cytologic atypia, mitotic activity, sometimes necrosis
- S100 protein, MART-1/Melan-A, and HMB-45 positive
- Lacks t(12;22), *EWS/ATF1* fusion

DIAGNOSTIC CHECKLIST

Clinically Relevant Pathologic Features

- Mitotic rate may be important if higher than usual

Pathologic Interpretation Pearls

- Dermal melanocytes in small nests in fibrous septa

SELECTED REFERENCES

1. Cimpean AM et al: Paraganglioma-like dermal melanocytic tumor: a case report with particular features. Int J Clin Exp Pathol. 3(2):222-5, 2009
2. Walsh SN et al: PEComas: a review with emphasis on cutaneous lesions. Semin Diagn Pathol. 26(3):123-30, 2009
3. Cassarino DS et al: Primary dermal melanoma: distinct immunohistochemical findings and clinical outcome compared with nodular and metastatic melanoma. Arch Dermatol. 144(1):49-56, 2008
4. Sarma DP et al: Paraganglioma-like dermal melanocytic tumor: a case report. Cases J. 1(1):48, 2008
5. Deyrup AT et al: Paraganglioma-like dermal melanocytic tumor: a unique entity distinct from cellular blue nevus, clear cell sarcoma, and cutaneous melanoma. Am J Surg Pathol. 28(12):1579-86, 2004

IMAGE GALLERY

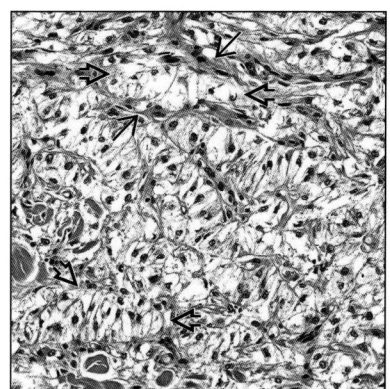 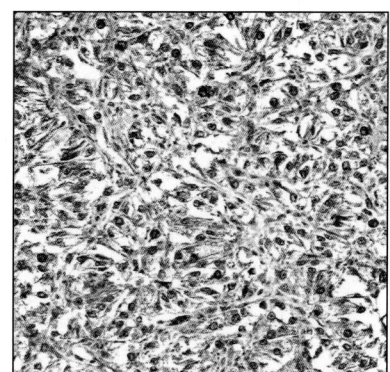 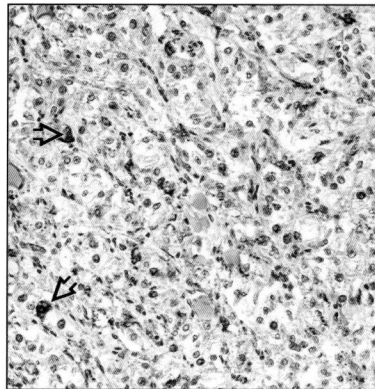

(Left) The paraganglioma-like tumor nests ⧩ are separated by delicate fibrous septa ⧩. *(Center)* Immunostaining for S100 shows diffuse nuclear and cytoplasmic positivity. This helps in the distinction from perivascular epithelioid cell tumor (PEComa), which is usually negative or only very focally positive for S100 (but positive for other melanocytic markers including HMB-45 and MART-1/Melan-A). *(Right)* The lesional cells show focal cytoplasmic positivity for HMB-45 ⧩.

ATYPICAL (DYSPLASTIC) MELANOCYTIC NEVI

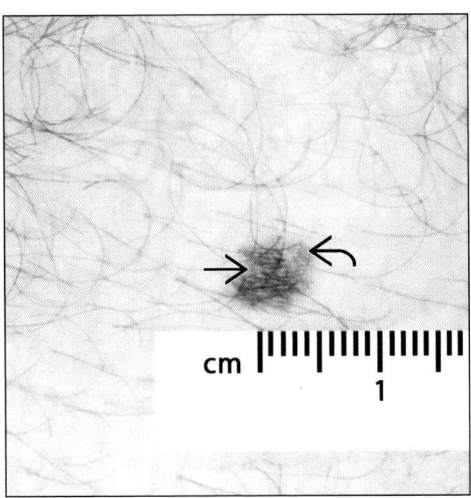

Clinical photograph of an atypical compound nevus shows a pigmented lesion with somewhat irregular borders. Note the central papular area ➡ surrounded by a macular periphery ➡. (Courtesy P. Duray, MD.)

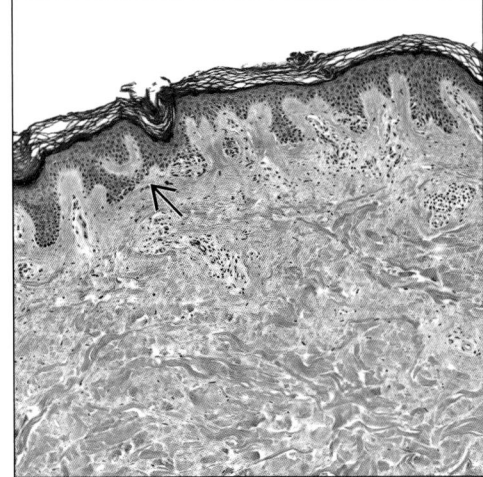

Mildly atypical compound nevus shows a proliferation of scattered small nests and a few single cells along the dermal-epidermal junction with focal bridging across rete ridges ➡.

TERMINOLOGY

Abbreviations
- Atypical melanocytic nevus (AMN)

Synonyms
- Dysplastic nevus, B-K mole, Clark nevus

Definitions
- Pigmented lesion with clinical, architectural, and cytologic atypia, which may be separated into familial and sporadic atypical/dysplastic nevi
- Controversial entity, as some believe that it may represent only another type of nevus, given the overlapping clinicopathological features that exist between it and common acquired melanocytic nevi

CLINICAL ISSUES

Epidemiology
- Age
  - Adolescents to young and old adults

Site
- Any location may be involved (especially those with familial type)
  - Including scalp, doubly covered areas (breasts in women and bathing trunk area in men and women), and lower legs

Presentation
- Papule, typically 8-10 mm
- Irregular borders
- Variegate pigmentation
- Central papule with peripheral macular flare or fuzzy border

Treatment
- Surgical approaches

- Simple excision for moderately atypical melanocytic nevi
- Excision with 5 mm clinical margins for severely atypical nevi

Prognosis
- Once adequately excised, should have very low risk of local recurrence; little, if any, risk of melanoma

MICROSCOPIC PATHOLOGY

Histologic Features
- Junctional or compound nevus with architectural disorder and asymmetry
  - Presence (extension) of peripheral nests beyond dermal component (shoulder phenomenon) in compound nevi, typically 3 rete ridges beyond center of lesion
  - Lentiginous proliferation of melanocytes that fuse (bridge across) adjacent rete ridges via proliferation of single cells and nests
  - Pagetoid scatter may be focally present, but usually limited to center of lesion
- Subepidermal lamellar (stacked) fibroplasia parallel to epidermis
- Circumferential fibroplasia surrounding nests
- Vascular proliferation in reticular dermis
- Chronic inflammation with melanophages in dermis

Cytologic Features
- Ample brown-gray cytoplasm
- Nuclear pleomorphism (greater in more moderate- and severe-grade lesions)
- Nuclear diameter larger than mid-layer epidermal keratinocyte, especially in moderately to severely atypical lesions
- Densely hyperchromatic chromatin pattern
- Nucleolar prominence (greater in higher grade lesions)

ATYPICAL (DYSPLASTIC) MELANOCYTIC NEVI

Key Facts

Terminology

- Pigmented lesion with clinical, architectural, and cytologic atypia, characterized into familial and sporadic dysplastic nevi
- Dysplastic nevus, B-K mole, Clark nevus

Clinical Issues

- Typically > 6 mm in diameter (range: 8-10 mm)
- Variegate pigmentation with irregular borders
- Central papule with peripheral macular flare or fuzzy appearance

Microscopic Pathology

- Presence of shouldering phenomenon
- Lamellar and concentric fibroplasia
- Range of cytologic atypia
  - Enlarged cells with dusky, abundant cytoplasm
  - Nuclear pleomorphism (mild to severe)
  - Small to prominent nucleoli

Top Differential Diagnoses

- Common acquired nevus
  - May show some shouldering, but no melanocytes proliferating to peripherally expand rete
- Congenital melanocytic nevus
  - Often have a greater intradermal than junctional component
  - Band-like distribution of intradermal cells surrounded by adnexal structures
- Malignant melanoma
  - Lack of symmetry and circumscription
  - Lack of maturation with increasing dermal depth
  - Often show mitoses and marked nuclear atypia, with irregular chromatin and large nucleoli

Grading Criteria for Cytologic Atypia in AMN

Features	Mildly Dysplastic	Moderately Dysplastic	Severely Dysplastic
Nuclear size	Same as a keratinocyte	1.5-2x keratinocyte	> 2x keratinocyte
Chromatin	Hyperchromatic	Hyperchromatic to vesicular	Vesicular
Nucleolus	Absent	Usually absent	Prominent
Dusky cytoplasm	Little	Little to abundant	Usually abundant

Atypia is determined subjectively by comparing the nuclear features of AMN to those of mid-layer epidermal keratinocytes. Modified from Weinstock MA et al: Reliability of the histopathologic diagnosis of melanocytic dysplasia. The Dysplastic Nevus Panel. Arch Dermatol. 133(8):953-8, 1997 and McKee PH et al: Diagnostic Atlas of Melanocytic Pathology. Philadelphia: Elsevier, 2009.

DIFFERENTIAL DIAGNOSIS

Common Acquired Nevus

- May exhibit some shouldering of junctional component
- No melanocytes proliferating to peripherally expand rete
- Lacks significant cytological atypia and mitotic activity

Congenital Melanocytic Nevus

- Often have greater intradermal than junctional component
- Band-like distribution of intradermal cells surrounded by adnexal structures and splaying of collagen bundles
- May show neurotization and pseudovascular spaces, especially in larger lesions
- Lacks cytologic atypia and mitotic activity

Malignant Melanoma

- Lack of symmetry and circumscription
- Shows significant cytologic atypia
  - Often marked nuclear atypia, with irregular chromatin and large nucleoli
- Lack of maturation with increasing dermal depth
- Mitoses often present; may be deep in dermal component

DIAGNOSTIC CHECKLIST

Clinically Relevant Pathologic Features

- Large pigmented macule with shades of tan and brown with irregular and fuzzy borders
- Presence of AMN is important risk factor for developing cutaneous melanoma

Pathologic Interpretation Pearls

- Search for shoulder phenomenon and cytological atypia

SELECTED REFERENCES

1. Brenn T: Atypical genital nevus. Arch Pathol Lab Med. 135(3):317-20, 2011
2. Sommer LL et al: Persistent melanocytic nevi: a review and analysis of 205 cases. J Cutan Pathol. 38(6):503-7, 2011
3. Zembowicz A et al: Nevus/Melanocytoma/Melanoma: an emerging paradigm for classification of melanocytic neoplasms? Arch Pathol Lab Med. 135(3):300-6, 2011
4. McKee PH et al: Diagnostic Atlas of Melanocytic Pathology. Philadelphia: Elsevier, 2009
5. Crowson AN et al: The Melanocytic Proliferations: A Comprehensive Textbook of Pigmented Lesions. New York: Wiley-Liss, 2001
6. Weinstock MA et al: Reliability of the histopathologic diagnosis of melanocytic dysplasia. The Dysplastic Nevus Panel. Arch Dermatol. 133(8):953-8, 1997

ATYPICAL (DYSPLASTIC) MELANOCYTIC NEVI

Microscopic Features

(Left) Low-power magnification of a mildly atypical junctional nevus shows fusion of rete ridges ➡ and concentric fibroplasia ➡ that surrounds the nests of junctional melanocytes. *(Right)* High-power magnification shows the junctional melanocytic proliferation fusing 2 adjacent rete ridges ➡. The concentric fibroplasia ➡ prominently hugs the junctional AMN.

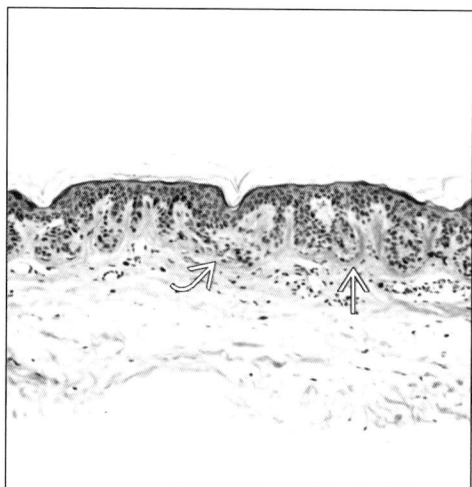 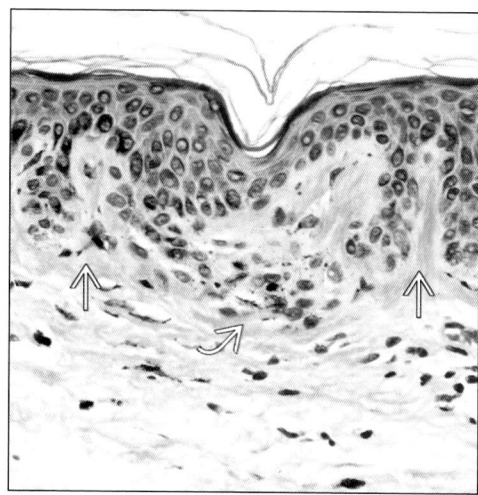

(Left) Moderately atypical compound nevus shows a junctional proliferation that extends laterally beyond the intradermal component ➡. The intraepidermal component is composed of scattered nests ➡ and single lentiginous cells ➡ along the dermal-epidermal junction. *(Right)* Higher magnification of the junctional component of a moderately atypical compound nevus shows lentiginous hyperplasia of single atypical junctional melanocytes and bridging across multiple rete ridges ➡.

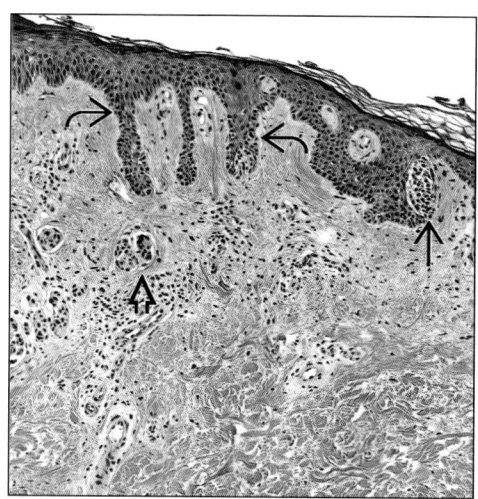 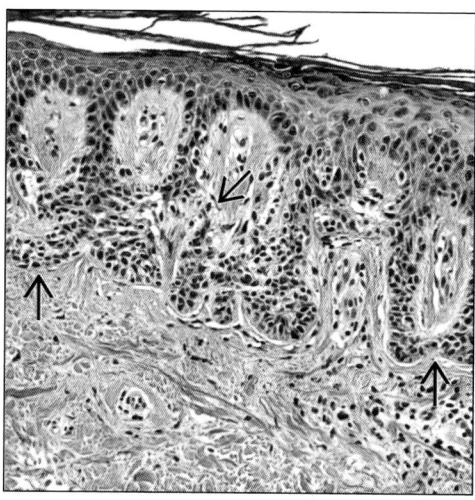

(Left) In another example of a moderately atypical junctional nevus, the nuclei of junctional melanocytes ➡ are the same size as those in the mid-level keratinocytes ➡. *(Right)* In this severely atypical compound nevus, the nuclei of junctional melanocytes ➡ are 2x larger than those in mid-level keratinocytes ➡.

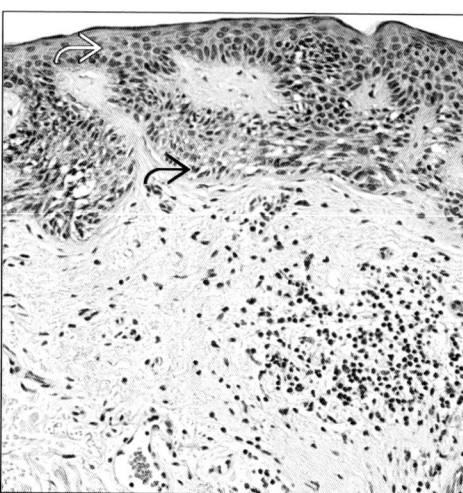 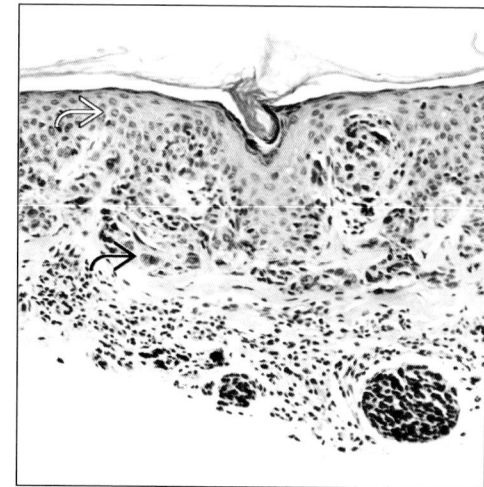

ATYPICAL (DYSPLASTIC) MELANOCYTIC NEVI

Differential Diagnosis

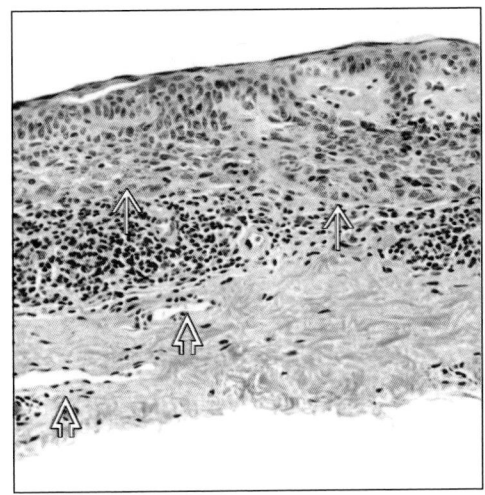
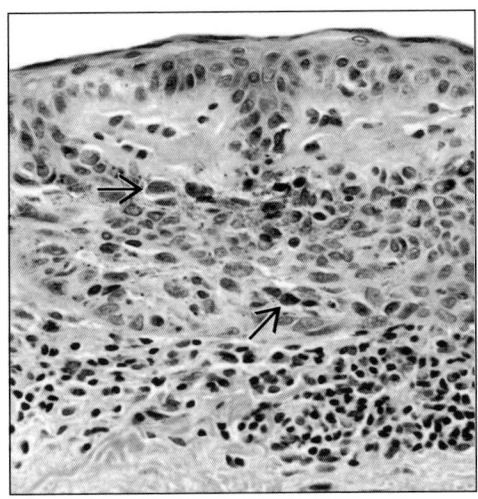

(Left) Severely atypical compound nevus exhibits a junctional proliferation of atypical melanocytes ➡, which fuse the rete ridges together. A chronic inflammatory infiltrate and a few slightly dilated blood vessels ➡ are noted in the dermis. Pagetoid upward spread is lacking. *(Right)* High-power magnification shows atypical melanocytes with gray-brown ample cytoplasm and pleomorphic, hyperchromatic-staining nuclei ➡.

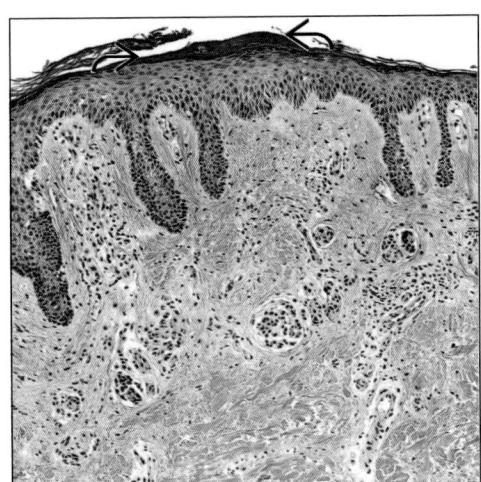
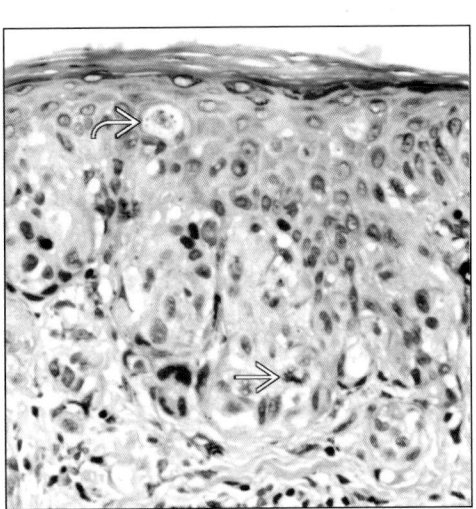

(Left) Traumatized moderately atypical compound nevus with recurrent nevus features shows dermal fibrosis and focal overlying parakeratosis and serum crusting ➡. *(Right)* Melanoma in situ, superficial spreading type shows a prominent atypical intraepidermal proliferation of large, epithelioid-shaped melanocytes with pagetoid spread ➡ and junctional mitotic figures ➡.

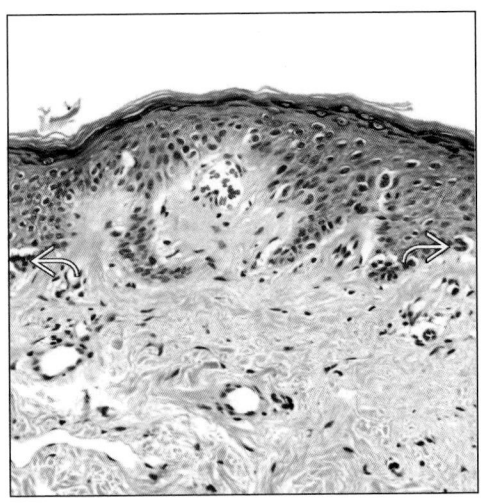
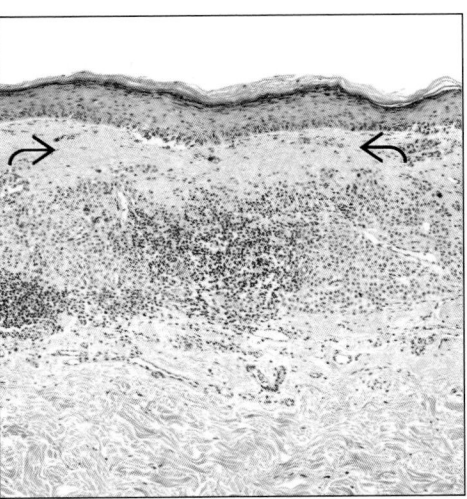

(Left) Melanoma in situ, lentigo maligna type shows a proliferation of atypical single lentiginous cells along the dermal-epidermal junction. Note the presence of multinucleated melanocytic cells ➡, which are often seen in lentigo maligna. *(Right)* Nevoid melanoma with regression shows a dense band of dermal fibrosis ➡ between the dermal melanocytic population and the overlying epidermis.

SPITZ (SPINDLE AND EPITHELIOID CELL) NEVI

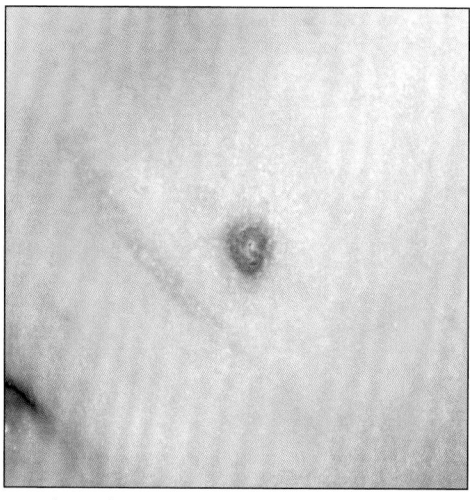

A pink papule, typical of a Spitz nevus, is shown on the face of a child. (Courtesy R. J. Antaya, MD.)

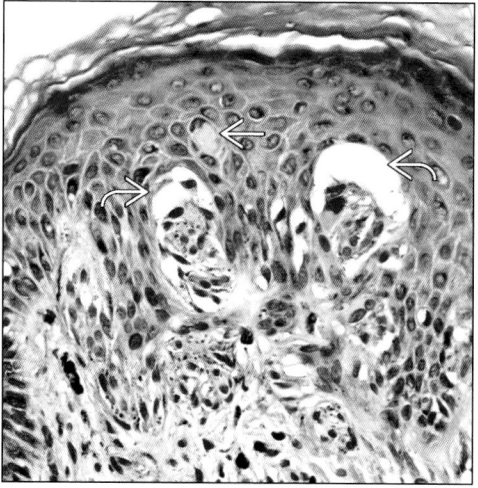

High-power examination of a Spitz nevus shows small nests of epithelioid to spindled melanocytes with overlying artifactual clefting ⇨ and an eosinophilic Kamino body ⇨.

TERMINOLOGY

Synonyms
- Spindle and epithelioid cell nevus
- Spindle cell nevus
- Epithelioid cell nevus
- Nevus of large spindle &/or epithelioid cells
- Benign juvenile melanoma (outdated term)

CLINICAL ISSUES

Site
- Extremities, especially thigh
- Trunk
- Head and neck

Presentation
- Most common in children and young adults
  - 0.5-1% of all nevi in children and adolescents
  - May occur at all ages
- Solitary
  - Can be clustered or disseminated

Treatment
- Complete conservative excision

Prognosis
- Benign
- Low recurrence rate, even after incomplete excision

MACROSCOPIC FEATURES

General Features
- Dome-shaped dermal nodule
- Pink or flesh-colored
- Often misdiagnosed clinically as hemangioma or pyogenic granuloma

Size
- Usually < 1 cm

MICROSCOPIC PATHOLOGY

Histologic Features
- Junctional, compound, and dermal forms
  - Most common type is compound with prominent dermal component
- Symmetric, well-circumscribed proliferation
  - Usually no lateral extension of junctional nests beyond dermal component
- Varying proportions of spindled and epithelioid melanocytes
  - Spindle cells more common in most cases
    - Completely spindle cells in ~ 45% of Spitz nevi
    - Mixed spindle and epithelioid cells in ~ 35%
    - Only epithelioid cells in ~ 20%
  - Epithelioid cells usually dispersed individually throughout lesion
- Spindle cells are arranged in fascicles perpendicular to epidermis
- Small clusters of melanocytes can be seen in epidermis
  - Can see pagetoid spread of a few single melanocytes
- Artifactual clefting of junctional nests from overlying epidermis
- Kamino bodies
  - Eosinophilic globules at dermal-epidermal junction
  - Important diagnostic clue, but may need step sections to find
  - PAS and trichrome positive
- Melanocytes "mature" by becoming smaller from superficial to deep
  - Melanocytes taper to narrow point in deep dermis, forming upside-down triangle
  - Deep melanocytes may resemble ordinary nevus cells
  - Important clue for differentiating from melanoma
- Other unique features

SPITZ (SPINDLE AND EPITHELIOID CELL) NEVI

Key Facts

Clinical Issues
- Benign melanocytic tumor
- Most common in children and young adults
- Common sites: Extremities, especially thigh
- Pink or flesh-colored, dome-shaped dermal papule or nodule

Microscopic Pathology
- Junctional, compound, and dermal forms
- Symmetric, well circumscribed
- Varying proportions of spindled and epithelioid melanocytes
  - Spindle cells much more common
  - Epithelioid cells usually dispersed individually throughout lesion
- Melanocytes "mature" by becoming smaller from superficial to deep

- Kamino bodies: Eosinophilic globules at dermal-epidermal junction
- Artifactual clefting of papillary dermal nests from overlying epidermis often present
- Can show atypical features (atypical Spitz nevus/tumor)

Top Differential Diagnoses
- Spitzoid melanoma; findings suspicious for melanoma include
  - Patient > 10 years old
  - Lesion > 1 cm
  - Ulceration and increased mitoses present
  - Asymmetry and poor circumscription
  - Subcutaneous involvement
- Pigmented spindle cell nevus of Reed
- Conventional melanocytic nevi

- Vascular and sometimes edematous stroma
- Pseudoepitheliomatous hyperplasia
- Giant nevus cells may be present and may be multinucleated
- **Halo Spitz nevus**
  - Nevus with depigmented rim
  - Heavy lymphocytic infiltrate with sparing of adjacent basal melanocytes
  - Often seen in combined Spitz and melanocytic nevus
- **Desmoplastic Spitz nevus**
  - Tend to occur in young adults on extremities
  - Usually dermal-based lesions
  - Predominantly spindle-shaped cells
  - Dense, hyalinized collagenous stroma
- **Atypical Spitz nevus/tumor**
  - Some cases show features in continuum between typical Spitz nevus and spitzoid melanoma
  - Atypical features include
    - Large, irregular nuclei with prominent eosinophilic nucleoli
    - Increased numbers of (typical) mitoses
    - Extreme cellular pleomorphism
  - Uncertain malignant potential

Predominant Pattern/Injury Type
- Nested

Predominant Cell/Compartment Type
- Spindle and epithelioid

DIFFERENTIAL DIAGNOSIS

Spitzoid Melanoma
- Asymmetry and poor circumscription at low magnification
- No "maturation" of melanocytes with dermal descent
- Cells typically show more coarse chromatin, anaplastic nuclear features
- Deep &/or atypical mitoses
- Findings that should raise suspicious for melanoma include

- Patient > 10 years of age
- Lesion > 1 cm
- Ulceration present
- Subcutaneous involvement

Pigmented Spindle Cell Nevus of Reed
- Typically considered a variant of Spitz nevus
- Usually occur in young adult females on extremities (especially thigh)
- Predominantly junctional proliferation, with only small superficial dermal component in most cases
- Cells show prominent pigmentation, unlike most Spitz nevi

Conventional Melanocytic Nevi
- Conventional nevi are composed of small, round to epithelioid-appearing cells
- Lack streaming together (or "raining down") of cells
- Kamino bodies and characteristic clefting around junctional nests are not present

SELECTED REFERENCES

1. Requena C et al: Spitz nevus: a clinicopathological study of 349 cases. Am J Dermatopathol. 31(2):107-16, 2009
2. Situm M et al: Nevus Spitz--everlasting diagnostic difficulties--the review. Coll Antropol. 32 Suppl 2:171-6, 2008
3. Massi G: Melanocytic nevi simulant of melanoma with medicolegal relevance. Virchows Arch. 451(3):623-47, 2007
4. Schaffer JV: Pigmented lesions in children: when to worry. Curr Opin Pediatr. 19(4):430-40, 2007
5. Sulit DJ et al: Classic and atypical Spitz nevi: review of the literature. Cutis. 79(2):141-6, 2007
6. Mooi WJ: Spitz nevus and its histologic simulators. Adv Anat Pathol. 9(4):209-21, 2002
7. Paniago-Pereira C et al: Nevus of large spindle and/ or epithelioid cells (Spitz's nevus). Arch Dermatol. 114(12):1811-23, 1978
8. Weedon D et al: Spindle and epithelioid cell nevi in children and adults. A review of 211 cases of the Spitz nevus. Cancer. 40(1):217-25, 1977
9. Allen AC et al: Histogenesis and clinicopathologic correlation of nevi and malignant melanomas; current status. AMA Arch Derm Syphilol. 69(2):150-71, 1954

SPITZ (SPINDLE AND EPITHELIOID CELL) NEVI

Microscopic Features

(Left) Low magnification of a compound Spitz nevus shows epidermal hyperplasia ⇗ associated with a compound melanocytic proliferation composed of a mixed population of spindled and epithelioid cells. *(Right)* Higher magnification shows a junctional nest of melanocytes with an overlying artifactual cleft ➡. While clefting is typical of a Spitz nevi, it is not always seen or may only be present in focal areas.

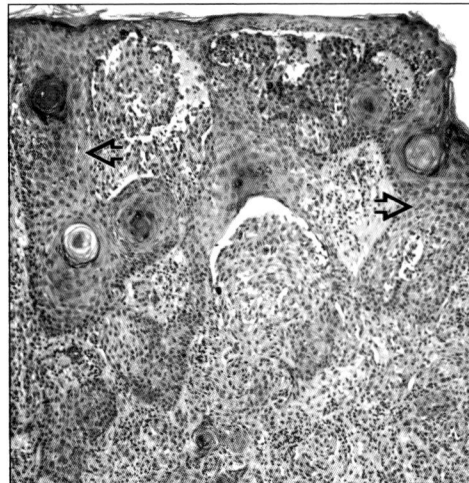
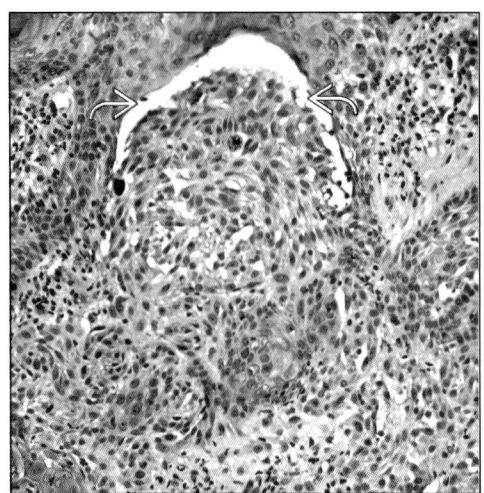

(Left) Spitz nevus shows nests of spindled melanocytes at the dermal-epidermal junction, which become smaller with depth in the dermis ➡. This is the "maturation" of melanocytes that is an important feature to distinguish Spitz nevus from melanoma. Scattered heavily pigmented melanophages are also present ⇗. *(Right)* High power shows a nest of melanocytes with a small artifactual cleft. While clefting is typical of a Spitz nevus, it is not always seen or may only be present in focal areas.

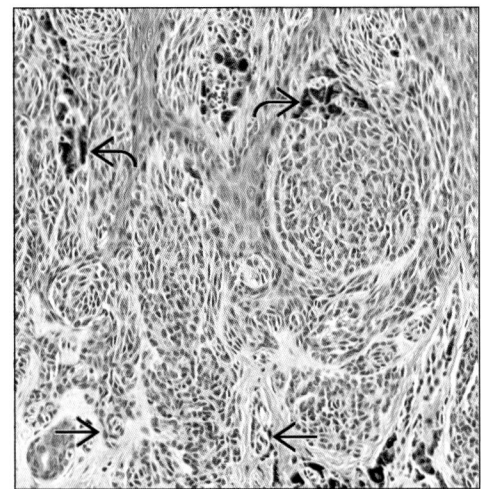
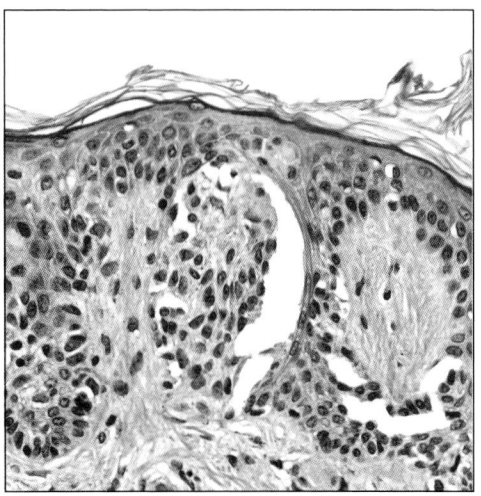

(Left) Histologic section at high power shows a small, densely eosinophilic-staining Kamino body ➡, which is an eosinophilic globule found at the dermal-epidermal junction. These are typical of Spitz nevi, but may be difficult to find. *(Right)* High-power view shows mildly atypical epithelioid melanocytes at the dermal-epidermal junction. Note the presence of a junctional mitosis ➡, which can be seen in benign Spitz nevi.

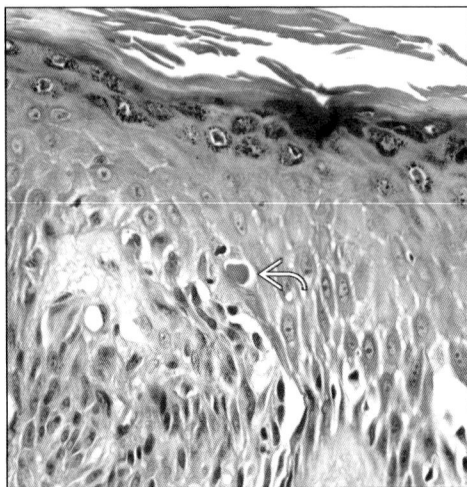
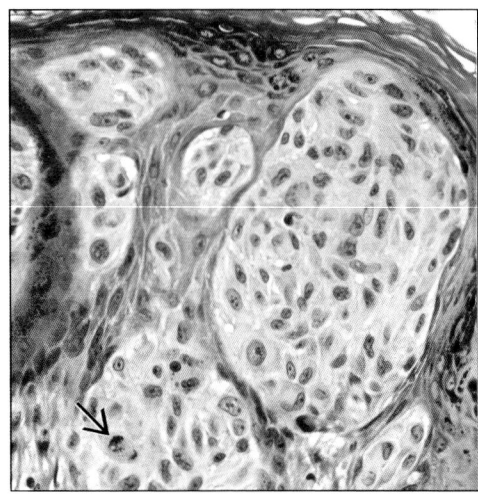

SPITZ (SPINDLE AND EPITHELIOID CELL) NEVI

Variant Microscopic Features and Differential Diagnosis

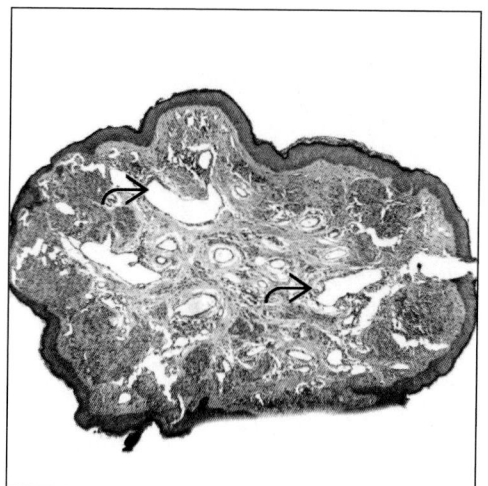

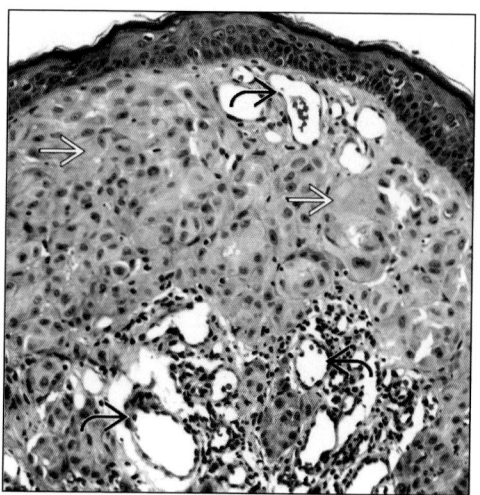

(Left) Polypoid Spitz nevus associated with prominent telangiectasia ➡. This case was thought to be a pyogenic granuloma clinically. *(Right)* High magnification of the superficial portion of a polypoid Spitz nevus shows a population of enlarged, epithelioid-appearing melanocytes in the dermis. The cells exhibit abundant amphophilic-staining cytoplasm ➡. Note the numerous blood vessels ➡ and inflammatory infiltrate present.

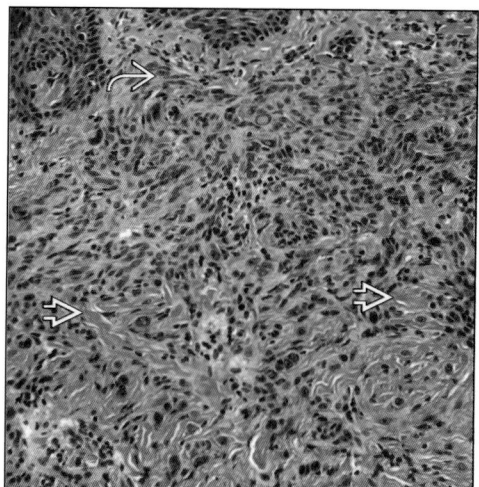

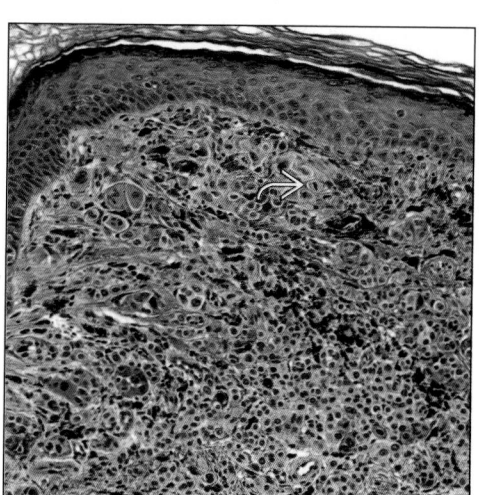

(Left) Desmoplastic Spitz nevus is a rare variant that is typically dermal-based. The tumor cells are arrayed in irregular nests, short fascicles ➡, and cords in a dense, hyalinized-appearing stroma ➡. *(Right)* An example of an atypical Spitz tumor shows a predominantly dermal proliferation of atypical epithelioid cells, many of which show abundant dusky gray pigmented cytoplasm, which is uncommon in most Spitz nevi. Scattered mitotic figures are present ➡, but are superficial.

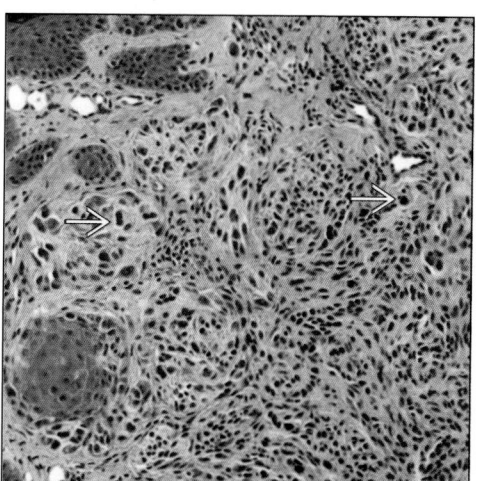

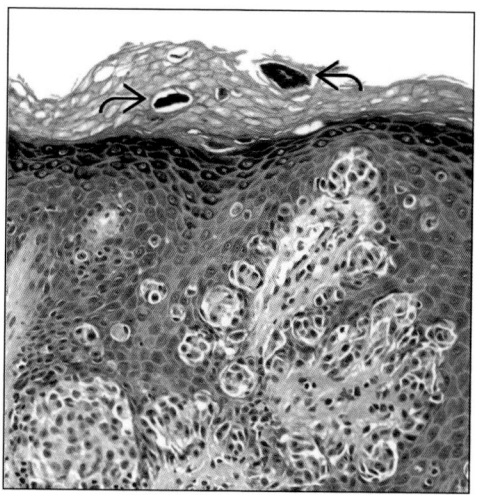

(Left) Atypical Spitz tumor shows a proliferation of enlarged and markedly atypical-appearing melanocytes. Many of the cells show atypical nuclei with prominent nuclear hyperchromasia ➡. *(Right)* This is an example of a spitzoid melanoma occurring in a young adult. Note the very prominent, irregular pagetoid upward spread, extending completely through the stratum corneum ➡.

PIGMENTED SPINDLE CELL NEVUS (REED NEVUS)

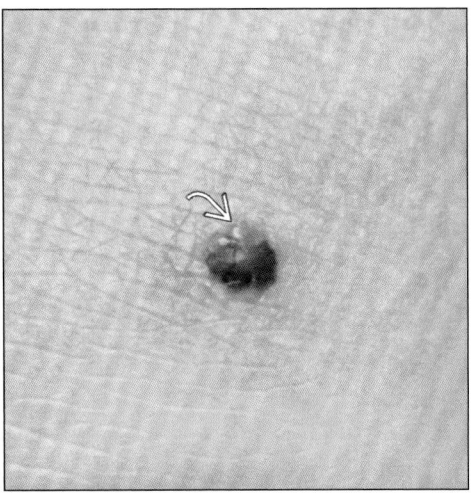

Clinical photograph shows a pigmented spindle cell nevus on the knee of a young adult patient. This case shows dark pigmentation, except 1 area at the top of the lesion with depigmentation ➡. (Courtesy P. Hsu, MD.)

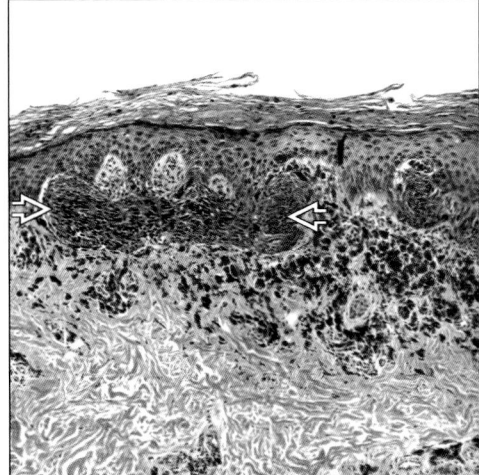

Histologic examination of a Reed nevus shows fusion of rete ridges by a proliferation of junctional pigmented spindle cells, which show a characteristic "streaming together" ➡ pattern.

TERMINOLOGY

Abbreviations
- Pigmented spindle cell nevus (PSCN)

Synonyms
- Pigmented spindle cell nevus of Reed

Definitions
- Melanocytic proliferation that is typically predominantly junctional and composed of a population of spindle-shaped cells with heavy cytoplasmic melanin pigmentation
- Controversial, but often considered a variant of Spitz nevus, which occurs more frequently in adults

ETIOLOGY/PATHOGENESIS

Unknown
- May be related to solar exposure in some cases

CLINICAL ISSUES

Epidemiology
- Incidence
  - Relatively uncommon tumors
- Age
  - Typically young adults (usually < 35 years old)
- Gender
  - More common in females
- Ethnicity
  - Caucasian patients in most cases

Site
- Most often presents on extremities, especially leg
  - Classic presentation is on thigh of a young woman

Presentation
- Pigmented lesion
  - Usually papular, but can be nodular

Treatment
- Surgical approaches
  - Complete excision is curative
    - Typically recommended in partially sampled lesions
    - To allow for complete evaluation to exclude more atypical areas
    - To prevent recurrence

Prognosis
- Excellent; may recur if incompletely excised, but very low risk of developing melanoma

MACROSCOPIC FEATURES

Size
- Usually small (< 1 cm)

MICROSCOPIC PATHOLOGY

Histologic Features
- Compound, predominantly junctional (in most cases) melanocytic proliferation
  - Symmetric, well-circumscribed lesion
  - Junctional nests often large and show bridging across several rete ridges
  - Composed of spindle-shaped melanocytes with "streaming together" appearance
    - Overlapping features with junctional Spitz nevi, but conventional Spitz nevi not as heavily pigmented
  - Pagetoid upward scatter may be seen, similar to Spitz nevi
  - Dermal component is usually small and superficial and composed of a few single cells &/or small nests in papillary dermis

PIGMENTED SPINDLE CELL NEVUS (REED NEVUS)

Key Facts

Terminology
- Pigmented spindle cell nevus (PSCN)
- Pigmented spindle cell nevus of Reed
- Melanocytic proliferation that is typically predominantly junctional and composed of a population of spindle-shaped cells with heavy cytoplasmic pigmentation

Clinical Issues
- Typically young adults (usually < 35 years old)
- More common in females
- Most often presents on extremities, especially leg

Microscopic Pathology
- Compound, predominantly junctional (in most cases) melanocytic proliferation

- Composed of spindle-shaped melanocytes with "streaming together" appearance
- Pagetoid upward scatter may be seen
- Dermis shows numerous melanophages in most cases
- Cells are moderately enlarged, spindle-shaped melanocytes
  - Typically show hyperchromatic-staining nuclei with small nucleoli
  - Cytoplasm with prominent melanin pigmentation
- **Atypical Reed nevus**
  - Often larger, more cellular lesions
  - Increased mitotic activity, especially in junctional component

Top Differential Diagnoses
- Spitz nevus
- Melanoma

- Overlying hyperkeratosis and pigmented parakeratosis are usually present
- Often associated with dermal inflammation
  - Dermis shows numerous melanophages in most cases
- **Atypical Reed nevus**
  - Pigmented spindle cell nevus with atypical features
    - Still shows features such as symmetry, circumscription, and lack of dermal mitoses
  - Often larger, more cellular lesions
  - Cytologic atypia and pleomorphism present
  - Increased mitotic activity, especially in junctional component
    - Dermal mitoses &/or atypical mitoses should raise suspicion for melanoma

Cytologic Features
- Cells are moderately enlarged, spindle-shaped melanocytes
  - Typically show hyperchromatic-staining nuclei with small nucleoli
  - Moderate to abundant amounts of cytoplasm with prominent melanin pigmentation
  - Scattered junctional mitotic figures often present

DIFFERENTIAL DIAGNOSIS

Spitz Nevus
- Conventional Spitz nevus typically occurs in children, not adults (as in Reed nevus)
- More common on head and neck and trunk region, as opposed to extremities (as is typical of Reed nevus)
- Composed of a mixed population of spindled and epithelioid cells (almost all spindled in Reed nevus)
- Lacks prominent pigmentation in most cases
- Larger dermal component usually present

Melanoma
- Typically occurs in older patients in areas of sun-damaged skin

- Predominance of epithelioid cells in most cases, especially superficial spreading type of melanoma (as opposed to spindled cells in Reed nevus)
  - Lentigo maligna and acral lentiginous types of melanoma are composed mostly of spindled-shaped cells, but
    - Show predominantly single lentiginous cells, not nests, along junction
    - Lack streaming together of cells, which is seen in Reed nevi
    - Lack symmetry and show poorly circumscribed borders with peripheral trailing off of single atypical cells
- Immunohistochemistry: Increased proliferative rate by Ki-67 and loss of p16 expression often seen

DIAGNOSTIC CHECKLIST

Pathologic Interpretation Pearls
- Compound, predominantly junctional, heavily pigmented, spindle cell melanocytic proliferation

SELECTED REFERENCES

1. Webber SA et al: Pigmented spindle cell naevus of Reed: a controversial diagnostic entity in Australia. Australas J Dermatol. 52(2):104-8, 2011
2. Requena C et al: Hypopigmented Reed nevus. J Cutan Pathol. 35 Suppl 1:87-9, 2008
3. Sau P et al: Pigmented spindle cell nevus: a clinicopathologic analysis of ninety-five cases. J Am Acad Dermatol. 28(4):565-71, 1993
4. Barnhill RL et al: The histologic spectrum of pigmented spindle cell nevus: a review of 120 cases with emphasis on atypical variants. Hum Pathol. 22(1):52-8, 1991
5. Barnhill RL et al: Pigmented spindle cell naevus and its variants: distinction from melanoma. Br J Dermatol. 121(6):717-25, 1989
6. Smith NP: The pigmented spindle cell tumor of Reed: an underdiagnosed lesion. Semin Diagn Pathol. 4(1):75-87, 1987

PIGMENTED SPINDLE CELL NEVUS (REED NEVUS)

Microscopic and Immunohistochemical Features

(Left) Low-magnification examination of a pigmented spindle cell nevus shows a compound, predominantly junctional proliferation of heavily pigmented melanocytes. There are numerous superficial dermal melanophages ➡. *(Right)* Reed nevus typically shows a proliferation of spindle-shaped cells in nests along the junction and in the superficial dermis. The spindle cells show a "streaming together" pattern ➡, similar to conventional Spitz nevi.

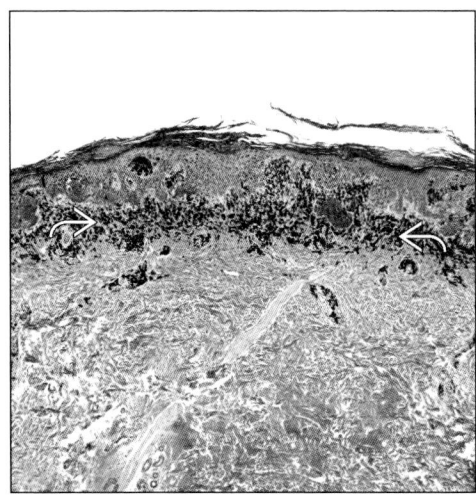
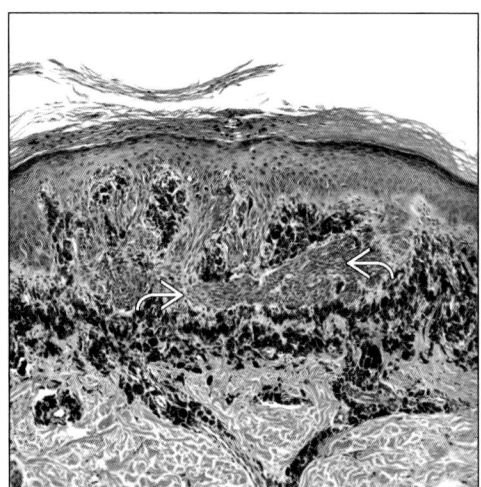

(Left) Intermediate magnification of a large nest ➡ of melanocytes shows pigmented spindle-shaped cells with hyperchromatic nuclei and heavily pigmented cytoplasm. Note the numerous darkly pigmented melanophages in the superficial dermis ➡. *(Right)* Higher magnification of the junctional nests of melanocytes shows relatively uniformly pigmented cells with hyperchromatic, oval to spindle-shaped nuclei, and pigmented cytoplasm.

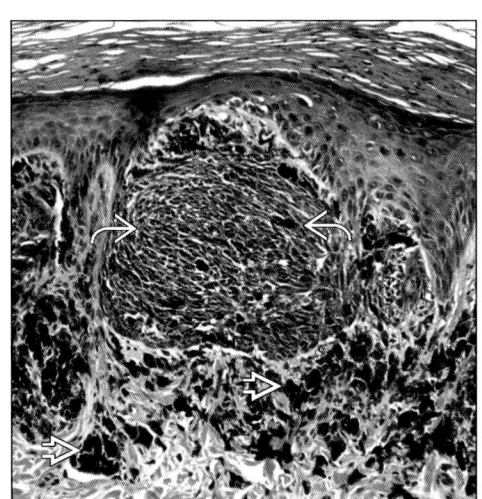
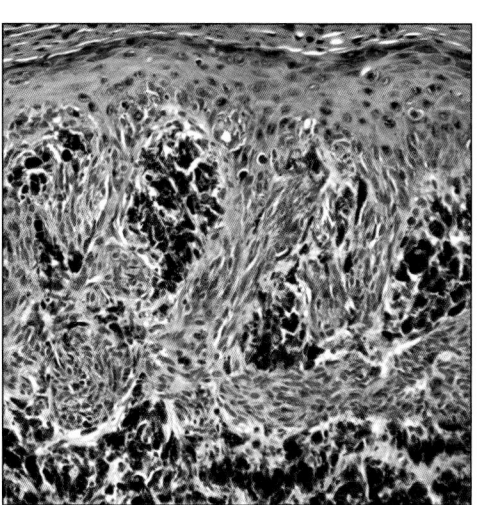

(Left) High magnification of the intraepidermal component shows elongated spindle-shaped cells with pigmented cytoplasmic processes ➡. Overlying pigmented parakeratosis is commonly seen ➡. *(Right)* Immunohistochemistry for HMB-45 shows strong staining of the intraepidermal melanocytes, including pagetoid cells ➡, in this atypical Reed nevus. However, the dermal cells show weaker ➡ to negative expression with dermal descent, consistent with maturation.

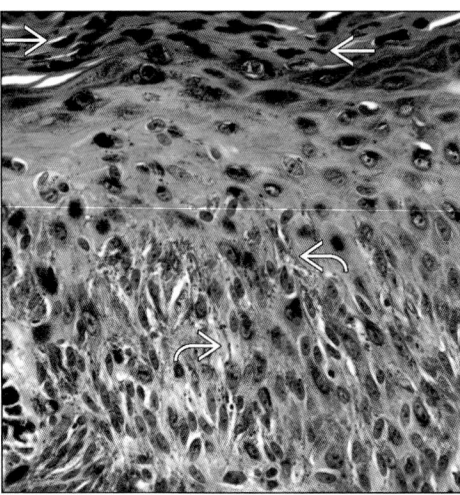
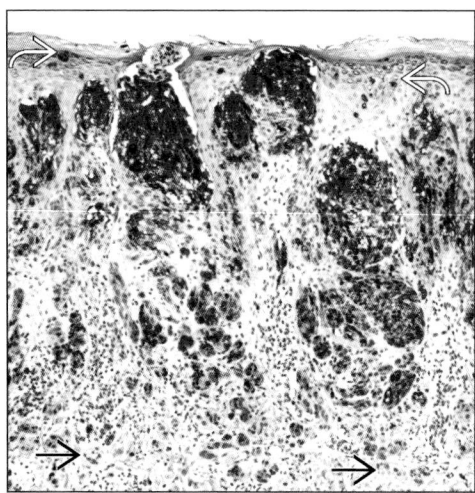

PIGMENTED SPINDLE CELL NEVUS (REED NEVUS)

Differential Diagnosis

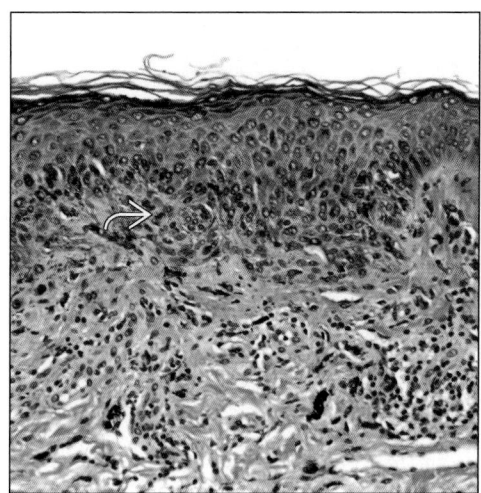

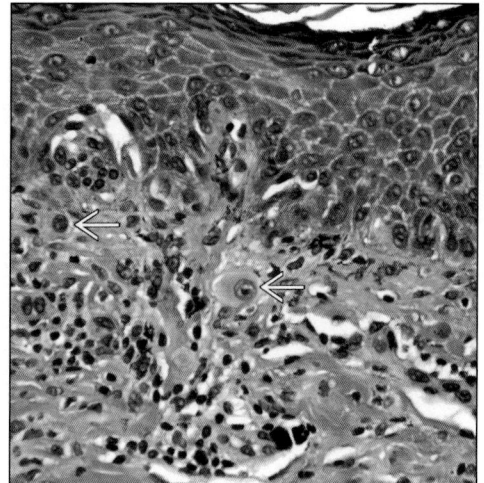

(Left) Severely atypical melanocytic proliferation with Reed nevus features shows small nests of enlarged, atypical-appearing cells along the junction. Note the presence of a junctional mitotic figure ➤. *(Right)* Another area of an atypical Reed-like proliferation shows a small population of atypical-appearing cells along the junction and in the superficial dermis. Note that some of the cells have an epithelioid appearance ➤, which is considered an atypical finding in Reed nevi.

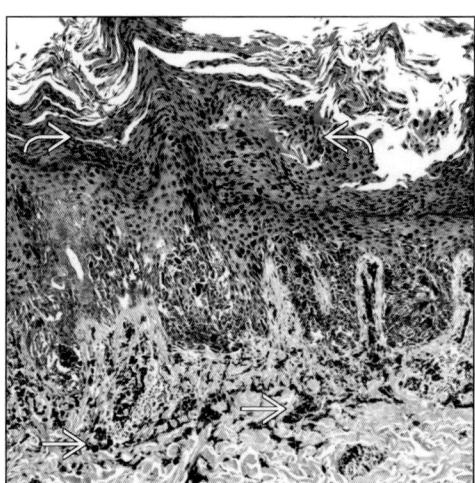

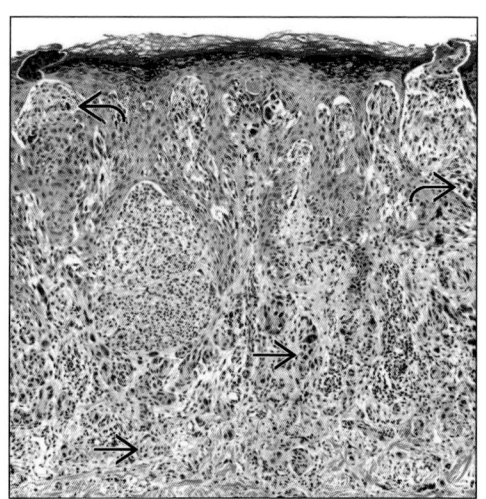

(Left) Melanoma in situ with Reed-like features shows an irregular proliferation of heavily pigmented junctional melanocytes with severe cytologic atypia, pagetoid spread, and marked pigmented parakeratosis ➤. The dermis shows numerous melanophages ➤. *(Right)* This conventional Spitz nevus shows some mild pigmentation of scattered cells ➤ but lacks the heavy and diffuse pigmentation typical of Reed nevi. Many of the cells are also more epithelioid-shaped ➤ in the dermis.

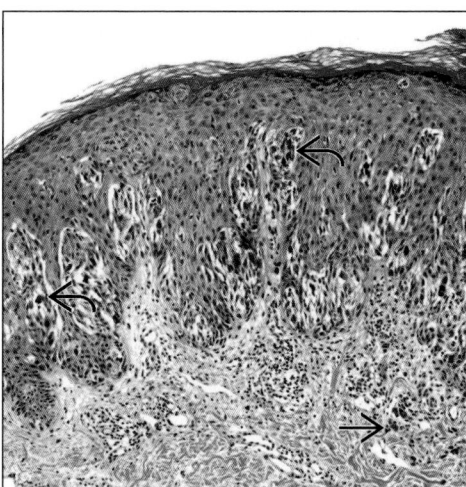

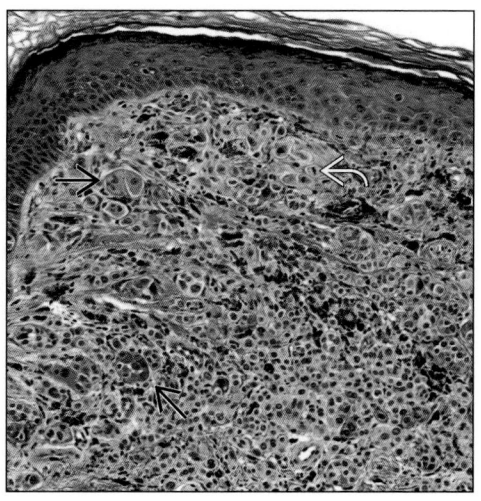

(Left) This atypical junctional Spitz nevus in a child shows some cytoplasmic pigment ➤ but lacks the heavy pigmentation of a Reed nevus. A few melanophages are seen in the dermis ➤, but they are also less numerous than those seen in Reed nevi. *(Right)* This severely atypical Spitz tumor shows prominent cytoplasmic pigmentation of some of the cells ➤, but is based in the dermis, as opposed to the junctional predominance of Reed nevi. Note the superficial mitotic figures ➤.

ATYPICAL/BORDERLINE AND MALIGNANT SPITZ TUMORS

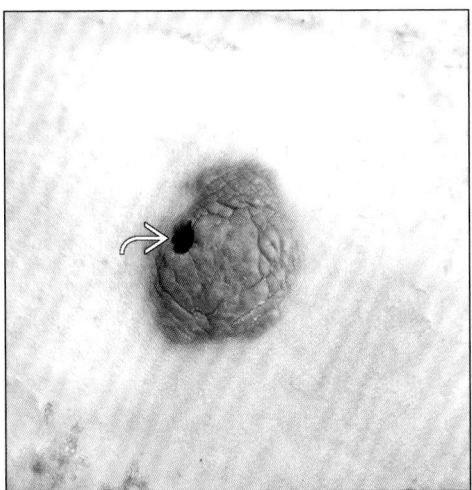

Clinical photograph shows an atypical compound Spitz tumor in a child. The tumor is large and somewhat nodular appearing. The focal epidermal defect ➥ represents a biopsy site. (Courtesy J. Wu, MD.)

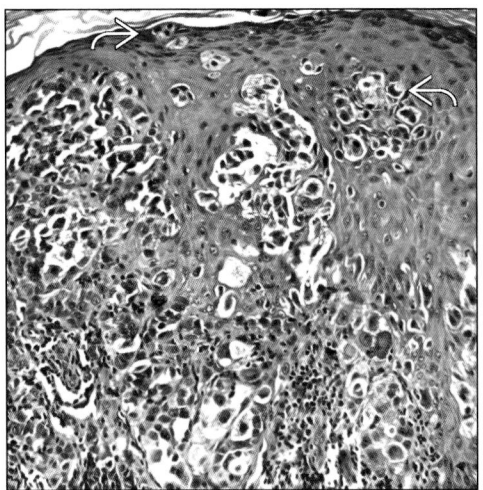

Spitzoid melanoma in a young adult patient shows very marked atypia and pleomorphism, as well as prominent pagetoid scatter ➥ extending throughout the full thickness of the epidermis.

TERMINOLOGY

Abbreviations
- Atypical Spitz tumor (AST)

Synonyms
- Atypical spitzoid melanocytic proliferation
- Spitz tumor of borderline/uncertain malignant potential
- Spitzoid melanoma

Definitions
- Atypical/borderline Spitz tumor: Severely atypical melanocytic proliferation with features intermediate between benign Spitz nevus and spitzoid melanoma
- Spitzoid melanoma: Malignant melanocytic proliferation with spitzoid features

ETIOLOGY/PATHOGENESIS

Unknown
- Typically occur in young patients without any known risk factors for melanoma
- Sun exposure may be a risk factor in some cases

Possible Genetic Role
- Suggested by chromosome 11p amplification in a minority of cases

CLINICAL ISSUES

Epidemiology
- Incidence
  - Very rare tumors
- Age
  - Mostly young patients, range: 2-30 years
  - Malignant tumors more common in post-puberty age group

Presentation
- Dermal papule or nodule

Treatment
- Surgical approaches
  - Complete and wide excision is standard therapy
    - Typically ≥ 5 mm clinical margins for atypical/borderline tumors
    - Spitzoid melanomas should be treated with same margins as invasive melanomas of similar Breslow depth
  - Sentinel lymph node biopsy is highly controversial
    - Should be considered a prognostic rather than therapeutic procedure at this time
    - Likely should not be routinely used (especially for atypical/borderline tumors) until validated by extensive clinical studies

Prognosis
- Difficult to predict
  - Most patients have relatively good prognosis, with only a minority of cases progressing to death
  - Even patients with lymph node involvement have a relatively good prognosis, as most tumors do not disseminate further

MICROSCOPIC PATHOLOGY

Histologic Features
- **Severely atypical/borderline Spitz tumor**
  - Typically, large and deep cellular compound melanocytic tumor
  - May appear symmetric and well-circumscribed at low power
  - Composed of nests, fascicles, and often sheet-like collections of melanocytes
  - Junctional component is variable
    - May show irregular nesting, confluence, and areas of pagetoid upward scatter

ATYPICAL/BORDERLINE AND MALIGNANT SPITZ TUMORS

Key Facts

Terminology
- Atypical Spitz tumor (AST)
- Spitz tumor of borderline/uncertain malignant potential
- Spitzoid melanoma

Clinical Issues
- Mostly young patients, age range: 2-30 years
- Prognosis difficult to predict
  - Most patients have a good prognosis, with only a minority of cases progressing to systemic disease or death

Microscopic Pathology
- **Severely atypical/borderline Spitz tumor**
  - Typically, large and deep cellular compound melanocytic tumors

- May appear symmetric and well-circumscribed at low power
- Cells show severe cytologic atypia with nuclear hyperchromasia, enlarged nucleoli, irregular chromatin, and abundant amphophilic or dense eosinophilic cytoplasm
- Mitotic figures often present, increased compared to conventional Spitz nevi
- **Spitzoid melanoma**
  - Also large and deep tumors
  - Frank atypia and pleomorphism present
  - Junctional component often shows irregular nesting, confluence, and prominent pagetoid upward scatter
  - Multiple mitotic figures usually present
  - Often atypical &/or deep

- Dermal melanocytes often do not show maturation with dermal descent (unlike most typical Spitz nevi)
- Composed of a variable mixture of spindled &/or epithelioid melanocytes
- Cells show severe cytologic atypia with nuclear hyperchromasia, enlarged nucleoli, irregular chromatin, and abundant amphophilic or dense eosinophilic cytoplasm
- Mitotic figures often present, increased compared to conventional Spitz nevi
  - Deep &/or atypical mitoses may be seen, but not numerous
- **Spitzoid melanoma**
  - Also large and deep tumors
  - Frank atypia and pleomorphism present
  - Junctional component often shows irregular nesting, confluence, and prominent pagetoid upward scatter
  - Multiple mitotic figures usually present
    - More numerous than in AST
    - Often deep &/or atypical
  - Lymphovascular invasion may be present

DIFFERENTIAL DIAGNOSIS

Spitz Nevus
- Typically smaller, more well-circumscribed and symmetric-appearing melanocytic proliferation
- Conventional Spitz nevi do not show marked cytologic atypia and pleomorphism
- Mitotic figures may be present, but are typically superficial and non-atypical appearing
  - Rare deep mitoses may be seen in some cases, especially in larger and more cellular lesions, and do not necessarily indicate malignancy by themselves

Conventional Melanoma
- Less likely to be considered in the differential diagnosis than spitzoid melanoma
- Usually shows mostly epithelioid cells, rather than mixture of spindled and epithelioid cells in AST and spitzoid melanoma

- Spindle cell-predominant lesions can be seen in invasive lentigo maligna melanoma, acral lentiginous melanoma
- Lack clefting artifact, epidermal hyperplasia, and Kamino bodies

DIAGNOSTIC CHECKLIST

Pathologic Interpretation Pearls
- Large lesion composed of nests, fascicles, and often sheet-like collections of atypical spindled and epithelioid melanocytes
- Dermal melanocytes do not show maturation with dermal descent (unlike most typical Spitz nevi)
- Mitotic figures often present, increased in numbers, and may be atypical (especially in spitzoid melanomas)

SELECTED REFERENCES

1. Berk DR et al: Melanoma and melanocytic tumors of uncertain malignant potential in children, adolescents and young adults--the Stanford experience 1995-2008. Pediatr Dermatol. 27(3):244-54, 2010
2. Cerroni L et al: Melanocytic tumors of uncertain malignant potential: results of a tutorial held at the XXIX Symposium of the International Society of Dermatopathology in Graz, October 2008. Am J Surg Pathol. 34(3):314-26, 2010
3. Ferrara G et al: Pediatric atypical spitzoid neoplasms: a review with emphasis on 'red' ('spitz') tumors and 'blue' ('blitz') tumors. Dermatology. 220(4):306-10, 2010
4. Ludgate MW et al: The atypical Spitz tumor of uncertain biologic potential: a series of 67 patients from a single institution. Cancer. 115(3):631-41, 2009
5. Murali R et al: Sentinel lymph node biopsy in histologically ambiguous melanocytic tumors with spitzoid features (so-called atypical spitzoid tumors). Ann Surg Oncol. 15(1):302-9, 2008
6. Sulit DJ et al: Classic and atypical Spitz nevi: review of the literature. Cutis. 79(2):141-6, 2007
7. Barnhill RL: The Spitzoid lesion: rethinking Spitz tumors, atypical variants, 'Spitzoid melanoma' and risk assessment. Mod Pathol. 19 Suppl 2:S21-33, 2006

ATYPICAL/BORDERLINE AND MALIGNANT SPITZ TUMORS

Microscopic Features

(Left) Severely atypical compound Spitz tumor shows a predominantly intradermal population of atypical spindled cells with nuclear hyperchromasia ➔. (Right) This is an example of a severely atypical Spitz tumor with an intradermal component composed mostly of atypical epithelioid cells with cytoplasmic pigmentation. Note the presence of mitotic figures ➔.

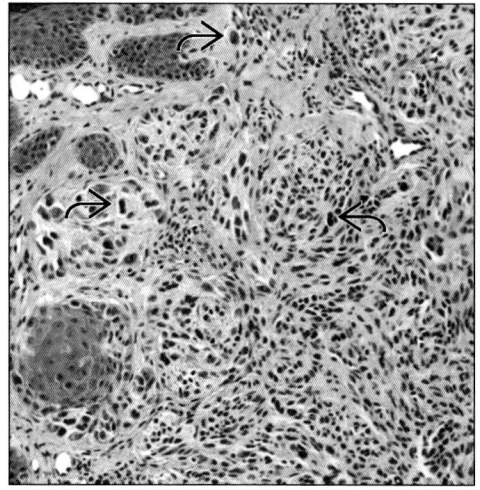
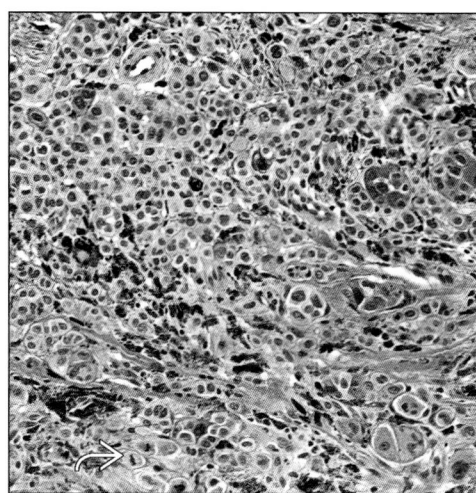

(Left) This is an example of an atypical desmoplastic Spitz tumor, which shows a predominantly dermal distribution and associated dense stromal sclerosis. Even at this low magnification, scattered enlarged, pleomorphic, and hyperchromatic-staining nuclei are evident ➔. (Right) High magnification of atypical desmoplastic Spitz tumor shows several enlarged, bizarre-appearing nuclei with multiple nucleoli ➔.

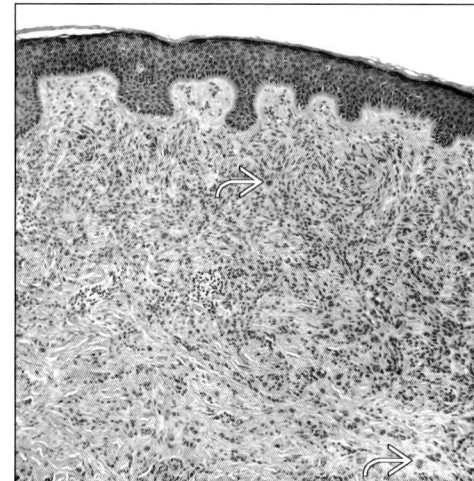
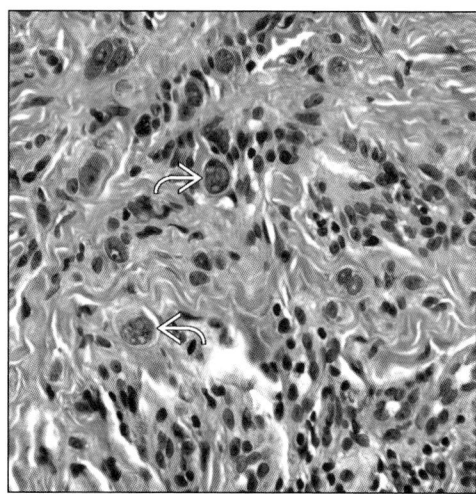

(Left) This severely atypical, compound, predominantly intradermal Spitz tumor is composed of pleomorphic epithelioid and spindle-shaped cells with hyperchromatic-staining nuclei. Only a few mitotic figures are present, and the cells show some evidence of maturation with dermal descent ➔. (Right) High magnification of a severely atypical compound Spitz tumor shows pleomorphic epithelioid and spindle-shaped cells with hyperchromatic-staining nuclei and focal mitotic figures ➔.

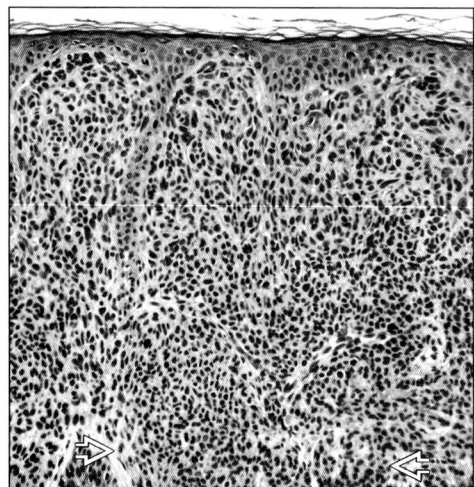
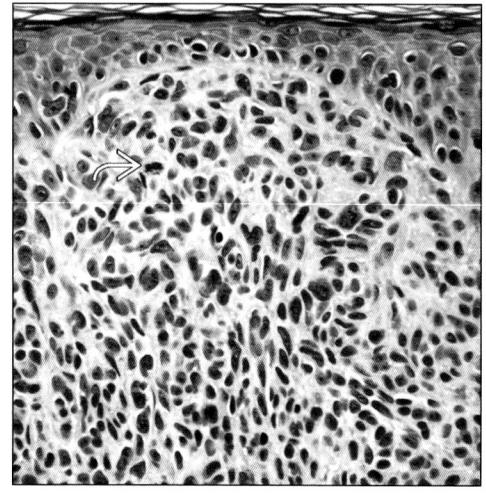

ATYPICAL/BORDERLINE AND MALIGNANT SPITZ TUMORS

Microscopic and Immunohistochemical Features

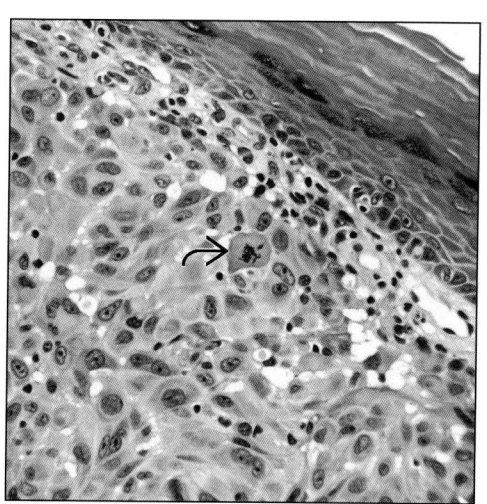
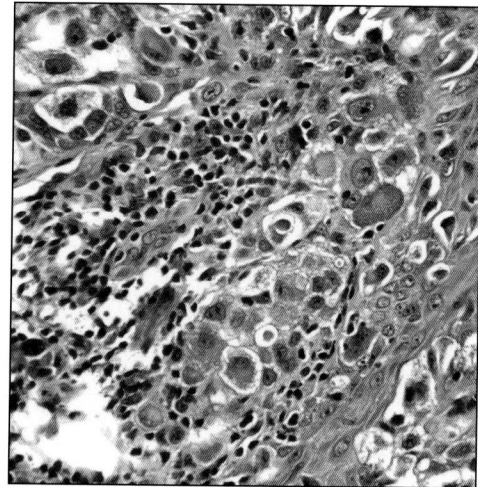

(Left) This is a high-magnification view of a spitzoid melanoma involving the dermis that shows severe cytologic atypia, marked pleomorphism, and an atypical mitotic figure ➔. *(Right)* High magnification in a case of spitzoid melanoma shows the presence of frank atypia and pleomorphism, with an associated lymphohistiocytic infiltrate.

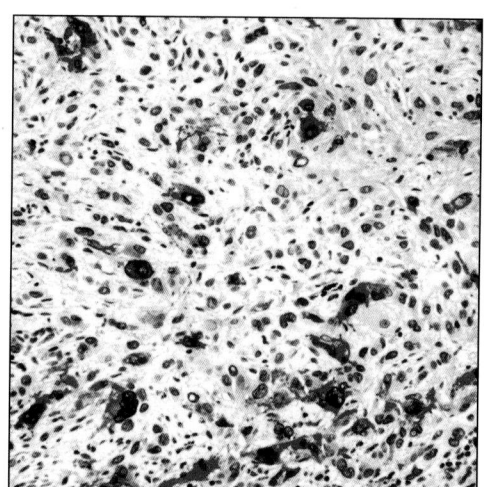
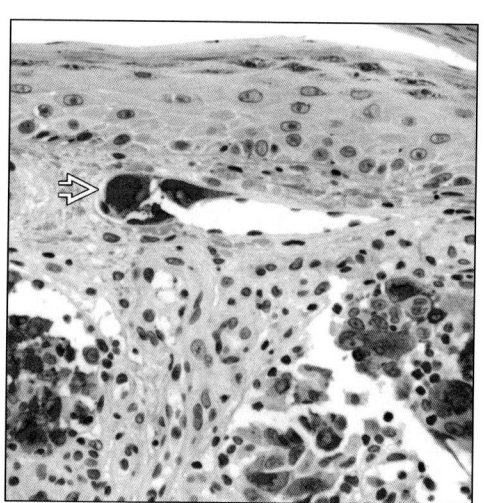

(Left) HMB-45 in a spitzoid melanoma shows strong cytoplasmic staining of many of the enlarged, markedly atypical-appearing cells in the dermis. *(Right)* A Melan-A stain highlights a focus of superficial lymphatic invasion ⊟ in a spitzoid melanoma.

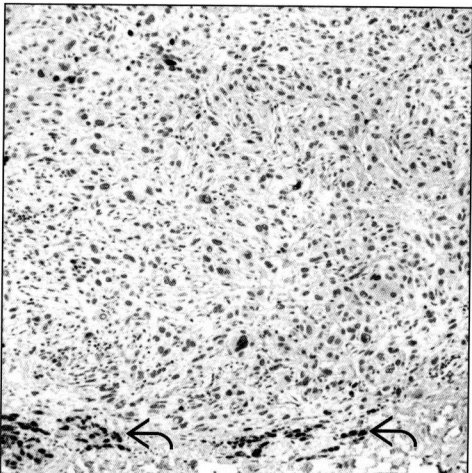
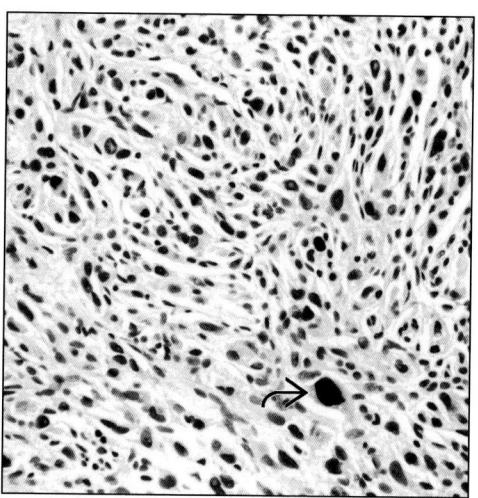

(Left) p16 immunohistochemistry shows loss of expression in most of the cells in this case of spitzoid melanoma arising in a large congenital nevus. The surrounding benign nevus cells show strong nuclear and cytoplasmic staining ➔. *(Right)* Ki-67 immunohistochemistry shows a low proliferative rate, but strong staining of a few large, bizarre-appearing nuclei ➔.

Malignant Tumors (Melanomas and Related Lesions)

Melanoma In Situ

Invasive Melanoma

MELANOMA IN SITU, LENTIGO MALIGNA TYPE

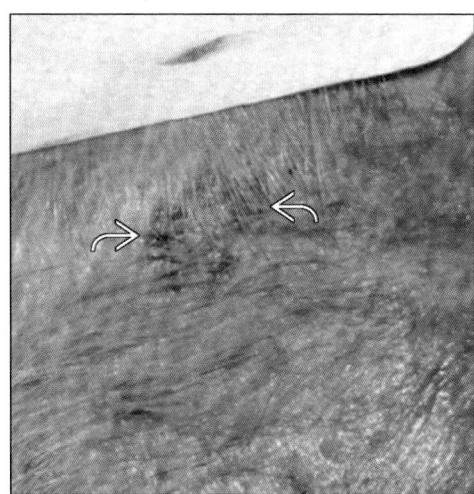

Clinical photograph of a lentigo maligna type of melanoma in situ shows an irregularly shaped and unevenly pigmented ➡ lesion on the scalp of an elderly patient.

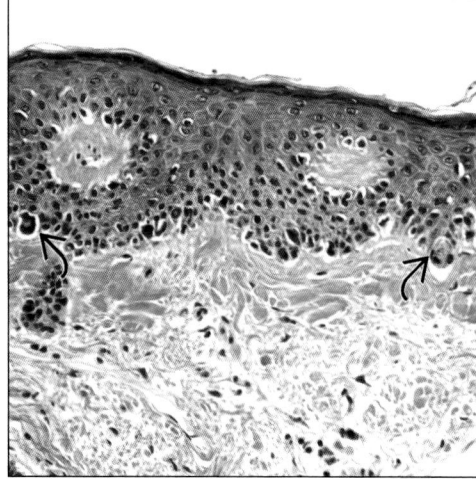

Histologic examination of MIS-LMT shows a junctional melanocytic proliferation, which is composed of atypical, hyperchromatic-staining single cells, including several multinucleated tumor cells ➡.

TERMINOLOGY

Abbreviations
- Melanoma in situ, lentigo maligna type (MIS-LMT)

Synonyms
- Hutchinson melanotic freckle
- Precancerous melanosis of Dubreuilh

Definitions
- Slowly evolving, indolent melanoma subtype that usually presents on head and neck (sun-exposed regions) in older patients

ETIOLOGY/PATHOGENESIS

Environmental Exposure
- Long-term exposure to ultraviolet irradiation

CLINICAL ISSUES

Epidemiology
- Incidence
  - Very common subtype of melanoma in situ
  - Approximately 5% overall lifetime risk
- Age
  - Older adults, usually > 72 years
- Gender
  - Slight female predominance

Site
- Most common on face (in women) and on scalp, neck, and ears (in men)
- Extrafacial sites include forearms, lower legs (in women), and trunk (in men)

Presentation
- Nonpalpable, broad lesion (size > 1 cm), can sometimes cover large portion of affected area
- Strikingly variegated colors of tan, brown, dark brown, black admixed with gray or blue-black
- Irregular borders

Treatment
- Surgical approaches
  - Excision with clear margins (usually 5 mm clinical margins recommended)
  - Mohs surgery controversial but reportedly effective in some cases

Prognosis
- Surgical margins of at least 5 mm give cure rates of 90-95%
- Low incidence of associated invasive melanoma

MICROSCOPIC PATHOLOGY

Histologic Features
- Lentiginous proliferation of atypical melanocytes along dermal-epidermal junction replacing basal keratinocytes
  - Mostly single cells, but irregular nests may also be present
- Typically limited pagetoid upward scatter of melanocytes
- Ill-defined peripheral borders (trailing off of single cells)
- Extension of atypical melanocytes along adnexal structures
- Epidermal atrophy and effacement of rete ridges
- Predominantly lymphocytic dermal infiltrate can obscure dermal-epidermal junction
  - Melanophages can also be numerous
- Marked solar elastosis

Cytologic Features
- Nuclei are small, often angulated (may resemble lymphocytes)
- Nuclear hyperchromasia

MELANOMA IN SITU, LENTIGO MALIGNA TYPE

Key Facts

Terminology
- Melanoma in situ, lentigo maligna type (MIS-LMT)
- Hutchinson melanotic freckle

Clinical Issues
- Most common on face (in women) and on scalp, neck, and ears (in men)
- Nonpalpable broad, slowly evolving pigmented patch
- Strikingly variegated colors with irregular borders

Microscopic Pathology
- Ill-defined lentiginous proliferation of atypical melanocytes along dermal-epidermal junction replacing basal keratinocytes
- Epidermal atrophy accompanied by cytological atypia

Top Differential Diagnoses
- Invasive lentigo maligna melanoma
- Actinic (solar) melanocytic hyperplasia
- Atypical (dysplastic) nevus

- Scant cytoplasm, typically without melanin granules

DIFFERENTIAL DIAGNOSIS

Invasive Lentigo Maligna Melanoma
- Typically microinvasive, and dermal component can be difficult to identify
- Multiple deeper level sections (and, in more difficult cases, immunohistochemistry) should be used to exclude invasion

Actinic (Solar) Melanocytic Hyperplasia
- Seen in heavily sun-damaged skin
- Consists of scattered single atypical cells along dermal-epidermal junction
- Not nested or confluent; does not involve adnexal epithelium

Atypical (Dysplastic) Nevus
- Severely atypical junctional nevi can be difficult to distinguish from MIS-LMT
  - Especially on small, partial biopsy
- Features such as symmetry, circumscription, and lack of confluence favor nevus
  - Complete excision may be necessary to evaluate these features ·

Reed (Pigmented Spindle Cell) Nevus
- Hyperplastic (not atrophic) epidermis, lateral margins are sharply defined (no trailing off of single cells)

- Cells may be atypical, but are typically monomorphous (not pleomorphic as in MIS-LMT)

DIAGNOSTIC CHECKLIST

Clinically Relevant Pathologic Features
- Large pigmented patch, slowly evolving indolent melanoma subtype on chronically sun-exposed regions

Pathologic Interpretation Pearls
- Epidermal atrophy and effaced rete ridges, in background of solar elastosis
- Trace dermal-epidermal junction using medium to high magnification to look for cytological atypia

SELECTED REFERENCES

1. Crowson AN et al: The precursors of malignant melanoma. Recent Results Cancer Res. 160:75-84, 2002
2. . Tannous ZS et al: Progression to invasive melanoma from malignant melanoma in situ, lentigo maligna type. Hum Pathol. 31(6):705-8, 2000
3. Flotte TJ et al: Lentigo maligna and malignant melanoma in situ, lentigo maligna type. Hum Pathol. 30(5):533-6, 1999
4. Barnhill RL et al: The histopathology of cutaneous malignant melanoma. Semin Diagn Pathol. 10(1):47-75, 1993
5. Clark WH Jr et al: Lentigo maligna and lentigo-maligna melanoma. Am J Pathol. 55(1):39-67, 1969

IMAGE GALLERY

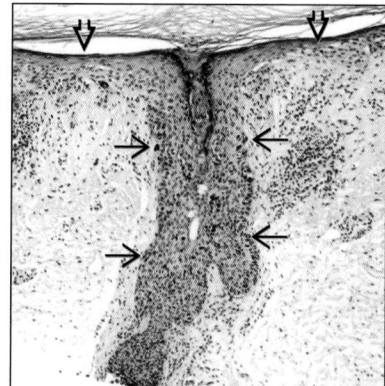 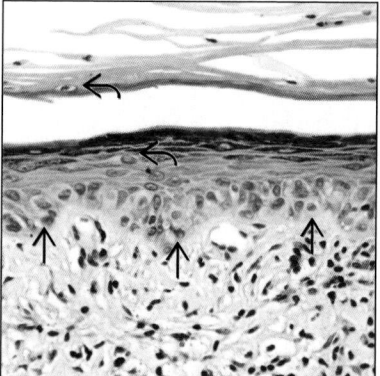 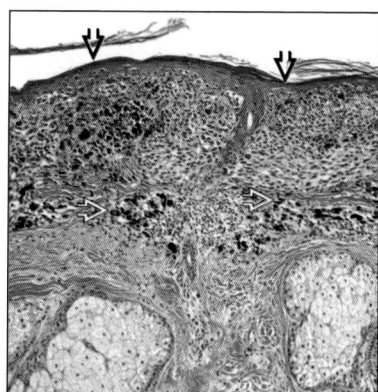

(Left) MIS-LMT shows atypical melanocytes replacing the basilar layer, thinning the epidermis ➡, and extending down the follicular epithelium ➡. *(Center)* High magnification shows almost complete replacement of the basal layer ➡. Focal pagetoid upward scatter is noted ➡. *(Right)* A hypercellular example of MIS-LMT shows an atypical junctional melanocytic proliferation replacing the basal keratinocytes. There is solar elastosis, dermal inflammation with melanophages ➡, and epidermal atrophy ➡.

MELANOMA IN SITU, SUPERFICIAL SPREADING TYPE

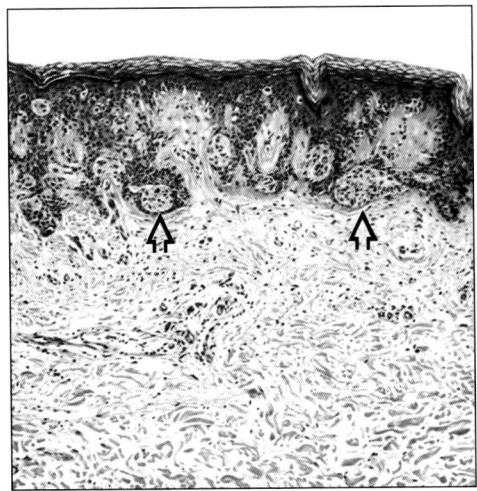

Low magnification of a MIS-SST shows an atypical intraepidermal melanocytic proliferation in all layers of the epidermis and irregular nests of atypical cells along the dermal-epidermal junction ⊵.

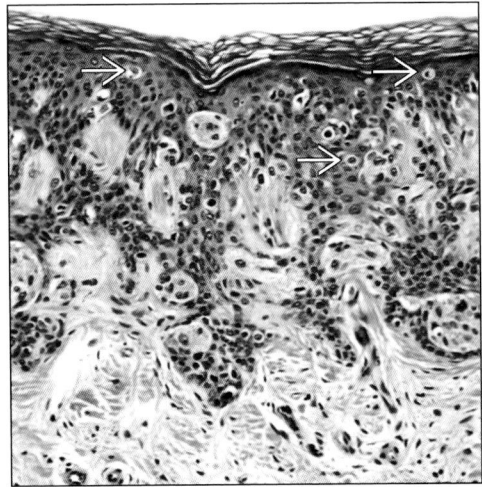

Higher power magnification reveals multifocal pagetoid scatter of atypical, epithelioid-shaped melanocytes throughout all layers of the epidermis ➔.

TERMINOLOGY

Abbreviations
- Melanoma in situ, superficial spreading (MIS-SST) type

Synonyms
- Superficial spreading melanoma in situ

Definitions
- Earliest stage of melanoma limited to epidermis, showing spread along dermoepidermal junction (radial growth phase)

CLINICAL ISSUES

Epidemiology
- Incidence
  - Most common variant of melanoma
- Age
  - Generally adults
- Gender
  - Males and females, different site predilections
- Ethnicity
  - Typically light-colored persons (especially red hair and skin type I/II)

Site
- Varies according to gender, on back (in men) and on legs (in women)
  - Intermittently sun-exposed areas (as opposed to chronically sun-exposed areas in lentigo maligna type of melanoma in situ)

Presentation
- Large dark brown macule (2.5 cm is average size)
- Variegated color with shades of tan, brown, black, blue-black, red (due to inflammation or vascular ectasia), gray and white (zones of regression)
- Irregular borders

Treatment
- Surgical approaches
  - Complete excision with 5 mm clear margins is standard treatment

Prognosis
- Excellent prognosis
- Almost all patients are cured with adequate excision
- 100% survival at 5 and 10 years has been reported

MICROSCOPIC PATHOLOGY

Histologic Features
- Asymmetric, poorly circumscribed lesion with lateral expansion of large nests of atypical melanocytes
  - Irregular distribution of nests, which can be confluent with indented borders
- Increased numbers of single atypical melanocytes involving both rete ridges and suprapapillary plates
- Typically abundant pagetoid spread of atypical melanocytes located in spinous layer
  - Pagetoid spread at periphery of lesion (as opposed to only central focal spread in atypical & irritated nevi)
- Large artifactual clefts between nests and epidermis above
- Dense but irregularly distributed inflammatory dermal infiltrate

Cytologic Features
- Large cells with ample cytoplasm
- Nuclear hyperchromasia and pleomorphism
  - Large eosinophilic or purple nucleoli
- Mitotic figures often present

ANCILLARY TESTS

Immunohistochemistry
- p16 often lost (expressed in nevi)

MELANOMA IN SITU, SUPERFICIAL SPREADING TYPE

Key Facts

Terminology

- Melanoma in situ composed mostly of irregular nests spreading along dermal-epidermal junction

Clinical Issues

- Most common variant of melanoma
- Broad pigmented macule, variegated colors, irregular borders
- Sites vary: Often back (in men), legs (in women)
- Excellent prognosis

Microscopic Pathology

- Spread of atypical single cells and nests along junction (radial growth phase)
- Abundant pagetoid scatter of atypical melanocytes into spinous layer

Top Differential Diagnoses

- Severely atypical (dysplastic) junctional nevus
- Traumatized nevus or of special site
- Reed (pigmented spindle cell) nevus

- Ki-67 often shows elevated nuclear proliferative rate (> 10-15%)

DIFFERENTIAL DIAGNOSIS

Atypical (Dysplastic) Junctional Melanocytic Nevus

- Should show symmetry and circumscription at low magnification
  - Can be difficult to assess on partial biopsy
- Typically shows less pagetoid upward scatter of melanocytes
  - If present, should be in center of lesion
- Mitoses should be rare or absent

Melanocytic Nevi Subjected to External Forces (Irritated/Traumatized or UV Light) or Nevi Located on Special Sites

- In cases of suspected trauma, search for parakeratosis &/or serum above focus of pagetoid spread
- Recognize clinical setting and anatomic site
- p16 typically positive; Ki-67 low

Reed (Pigmented Spindle Cell) Nevus

- Hyperplastic (not atrophic) epidermis, lateral margins are sharply defined (no trailing off of single cells)
- Composed mostly of spindle-shaped cells, which may be atypical but are often monomorphous (not pleomorphic as in MIS-SST)

Mammary and Extramammary Paget Disease

- Cells are not at junction but above basal keratinocytes
- May show glandular structures
- Immunohistochemistry positive for CK7, EMA, CEA; negative for S100 and MART-1/Melan-A

DIAGNOSTIC CHECKLIST

Clinically Relevant Pathologic Features

- Large macule with variegated colors and irregular borders

Pathologic Interpretation Pearls

- Large junctional lesion with lateral expansion of atypical melanocytes, often with abundant pagetoid spread

SELECTED REFERENCES

1. Duncan LM: The classification of cutaneous melanoma. Hematol Oncol Clin North Am. 23(3):501-13, ix, 2009
2. Massi G et al: Histological Diagnosis of Nevi and Melanoma. Darmstadt, Germany: Steinkopff Verlag, 2004
3. Crowson et al: The Melanocytic Proliferations: A Comprehensive Textbook of Pigmented Lesions. New York: Wiley-Liss, 2001
4. Lopansri S et al: Clinical and pathological correlation of malignant melanoma. J Cutan Pathol. 6(3):180-94, 1979

IMAGE GALLERY

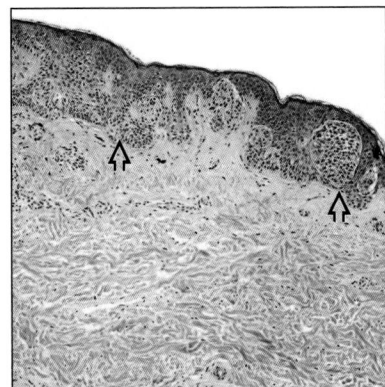 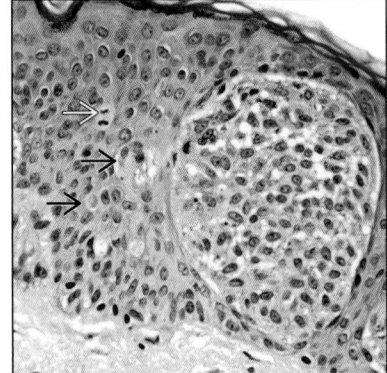 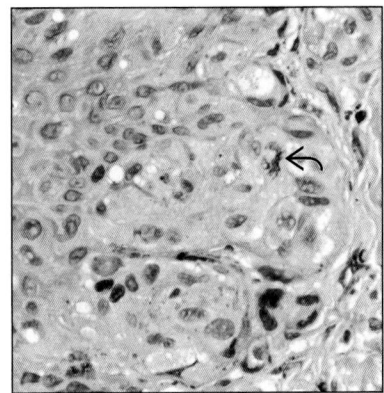

(Left) Low magnification of an example of MIS-SST shows spread of irregularly shaped nests along the junction ➥, the defining feature of superficial spreading type melanoma. *(Center)* High-power examination shows a large intraepidermal nest and pagetoid upward scatter of several single melanocytes ➥. A melanocyte is identified in mitosis ➥. *(Right)* High magnification of another case of MIS-SST shows nests of enlarged, atypical cells. Note the atypical (crab-like) mitosis ➥.

MELANOMA IN SITU, NOS

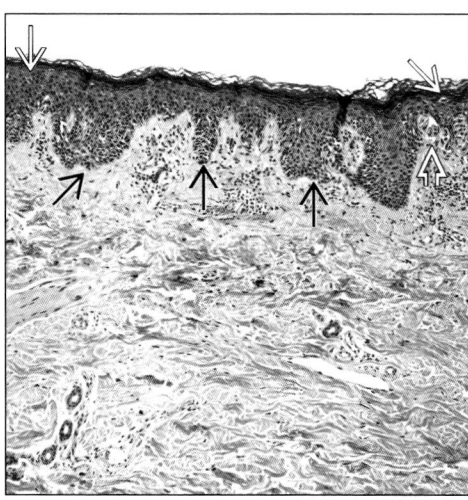

MIS-NOS shows numerous atypical lentiginous cells ➡ along the junction (similar to lentigo maligna), but there is also focal pagetoid scatter ➡ and irregular nesting ➡ (similar to MIS-SST).

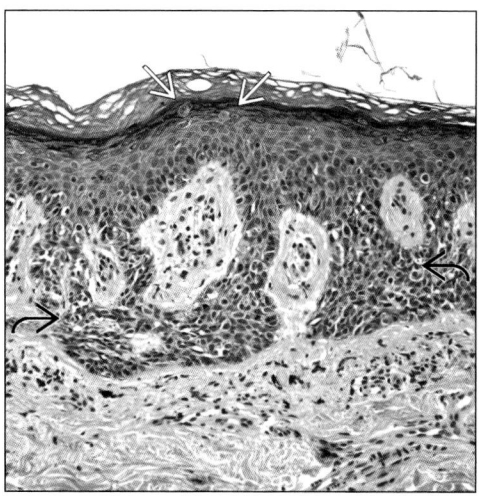

Higher power magnification shows a predominantly lentiginous proliferation of atypical cells along the junction, with bridging across rete ridges ➡ and limited pagetoid upward scatter of a few cells ➡.

TERMINOLOGY

Abbreviations
- Melanoma in situ, not otherwise specified (MIS-NOS)

Synonyms
- Melanoma in situ, unspecified type

Definitions
- Cases that cannot be clearly categorized as either lentigo maligna, acral lentiginous, or superficial spreading type of melanoma in situ

CLINICAL ISSUES

Epidemiology
- Incidence
  - Uncommon tumors
- Age
  - Typically occur in elderly patients

Site
- Usually located on sun-exposed areas, especially cheeks, upper trunk, and arms

Presentation
- Borders of lesions are irregular, asymmetric, and often notched
- Lesions are dark, broad macules about 0.8 cm in diameter
- Mottled pigmentation

Treatment
- Surgical approaches
  - Complete excision with 5.0 mm clear margins
  - Mohs surgery may also be effective, but is controversial

Prognosis
- Excellent: Little recurrence potential with adequate surgical margins

MICROSCOPIC PATHOLOGY

Histologic Features
- Melanocytic proliferation typically characterized by both lentiginous junctional spread (similar to lentigo maligna) and irregular nesting and pagetoid spread (similar to superficial spreading type of MIS)
- Asymmetric, poorly circumscribed junctional melanocytic lesion
  - Peripheral trailing off of single atypical cells
  - Melanocytes extend laterally beyond last nests
- Spitzoid features may be present in some cases
  - Cells are markedly enlarged and atypical to bizarre-appearing
  - Composed of mixture of spindled and epithelioid-shaped cells
  - Markedly atypical junctional spitzoid lesions in adults are much more likely to represent MIS than atypical Spitz nevus
- Dermis may show dense but irregularly distributed inflammatory dermal infiltrate
  - Can be difficult to exclude invasion in some cases without immunohistochemistry
    - Immunostains including MART-1/Melan-A, tyrosinase, and HMB-45 can be useful to exclude invasion

Cytologic Features
- Nuclear atypia and pleomorphism
  - Large eosinophilic or purple nucleoli
- Mitotic figures often present

DIFFERENTIAL DIAGNOSIS

Melanoma In Situ, Superficial Spreading Type (MIS-SST)
- Proliferation of predominantly nested and pagetoid melanocytes

Key Facts

Terminology

- In situ melanoma that cannot be neatly categorized as well-recognized type of MIS such as lentigo maligna or superficial spreading type

Microscopic Pathology

- Asymmetric, poorly circumscribed atypical junctional melanocytic proliferation
- Single atypical melanocytes with lentiginous spread and pagetoid upward scatter

- Peripheral trailing off of single atypical cells
- Spitzoid features may be present in some cases
  - Cells are markedly enlarged and atypical to bizarre-appearing

Top Differential Diagnoses

- Melanoma in situ, superficial spreading type
- Melanoma in situ, lentigo maligna type
- Atypical (dysplastic) junctional melanocytic nevus
- Irritated/traumatized nevi and nevi of special sites

- Broad, asymmetric junctional spread of irregularly shaped and irregularly sized nests

Melanoma In Situ, Lentigo Maligna Type (MIS, LMT)

- Proliferation of predominantly single lentiginous cells along dermal-epidermal junction
- Less nesting and pagetoid scatter than MIS, NOS and MIS-SST

Atypical (Dysplastic) Junctional Melanocytic Nevus

- Should show symmetry and circumscription at low magnification
  - Can be difficult, if not impossible, to assess on partial biopsy
- Typically shows less atypia and pagetoid upward scatter of melanocytes
  - If present, should be focal in center of lesion
- Immunohistochemistry typically shows p16 positive; Ki-67 low to negative

Irritated/Traumatized Junctional Nevi and Nevi of Special Sites

- Search for parakeratosis &/or serum above foci of pagetoid spread
- Important to recognize clinical setting and anatomic site
- Immunohistochemistry shows p16 positive; Ki-67 low/negative

Reed (Pigmented Spindle Cell) Nevus

- Usually occurs on extremities in young adults, more common in females
- Hyperplastic epidermis, lateral margins are sharply defined
- Composed mostly of spindle-shaped cells, which may be atypical, but are often monomorphous
  - Cells typically heavily pigmented, and numerous melanophages present in dermis

DIAGNOSTIC CHECKLIST

Pathologic Interpretation Pearls

- Single atypical melanocytes as well as irregular nesting and areas of limited pagetoid scatter

SELECTED REFERENCES

1. King R: Lentiginous melanoma. Arch Pathol Lab Med. 135(3):337-41, 2011
2. Erickson C et al: Treatment options in melanoma in situ: topical and radiation therapy, excision and Mohs surgery. Int J Dermatol. 49(5):482-91, 2010
3. Gerami P et al: Superficial melanocytic neoplasms with pagetoid melanocytosis: a study of interobserver concordance and correlation with FISH. Am J Surg Pathol. 34(6):816-21, 2010
4. Massi G et al: Histological Diagnosis of Nevi and Melanoma. Darmstadt, Germany: Steinkopff Verlag, 2004

IMAGE GALLERY

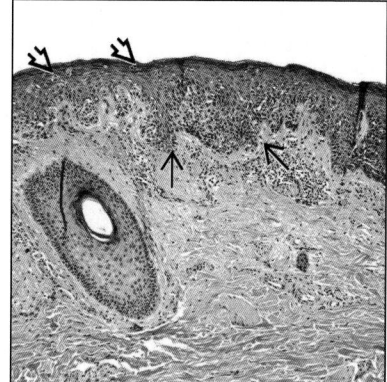 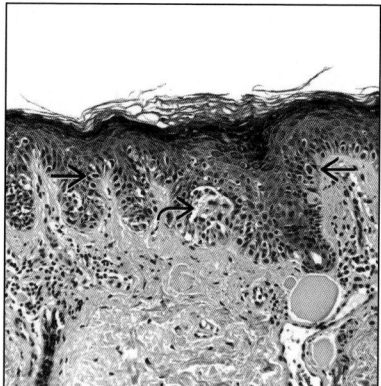 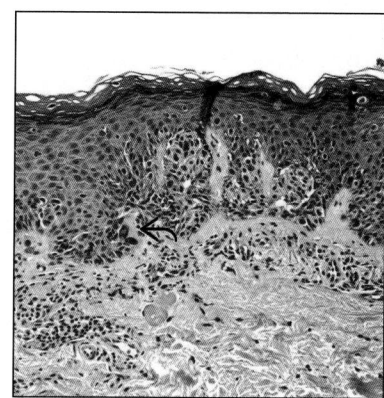

(Left) MIS is shown with overlapping features of lentigo maligna and superficial spreading types. There is relatively prominent pagetoid scatter ⊉ and irregular nesting, as well as a proliferation of atypical lentiginous cells ⊒ along the junction. *(Center)* Higher magnification shows numerous atypical single lentiginous cells ⊒ and a few irregular nests ⊅ along the junction. *(Right)* Focal, large, bizarre-appearing spitzoid cells ⊅ are present along the junction.

CHILDHOOD MELANOMA

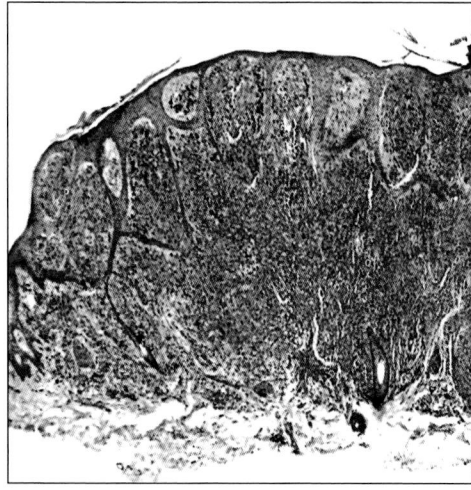

A nevoid melanoma arising in a 4-year-old child is shown. Although the cells appear to show some maturation at low magnification, there were deep atypical cells and mitoses present on high power.

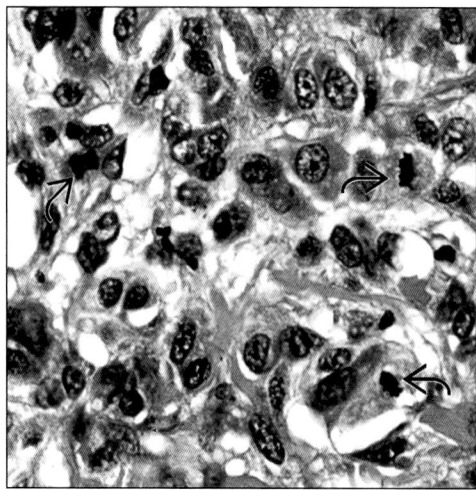

High magnification of a melanoma arising in a 4-year-old child shows an area with prominent cytologic atypia and multiple mitotic figures ⊿.

TERMINOLOGY

Abbreviations
- Malignant melanoma (MM)

Synonyms
- Melanoma of childhood

Definitions
- Malignant cutaneous melanocytic neoplasm arising in children

ETIOLOGY/PATHOGENESIS

Classification of Pediatric Melanoma
- Classified according to mode of occurrence and histology
  - Transformation from giant congenital melanocytic nevus (CMN)
  - In association with congenital predisposing conditions
  - Development from preexisting nevus
  - Transplacental melanoma

CLINICAL ISSUES

Epidemiology
- Incidence
  - Accounts for 1-3% of all childhood malignancies
  - Accounts for < 0.5% of all melanomas
  - 7x more frequent in 2nd decade than 1st decade of life
  - On the rise in children and teenagers
- Age
  - Prepubescent melanoma
    - Congenital and infantile melanomas are rare
    - Develops transplacentally, de novo, or within a CMN, especially giant congenital nevi
  - Postpubescent melanoma

- > 14 years of age
- Clinical features and prognosis tend to resemble adult counterparts
- Gender
  - Slight female predominance

Site
- Can occur anywhere on the skin
  - Rarely mucous membranes and meninges

Presentation
- 50% arise in association with preexisting lesion
  - 30% arise within a giant CMN (> 20 cm)
    - 50-70% before puberty
    - Tend to arise within dermis
    - Worse prognosis
  - 20% in association with other cutaneous nevi
    - Small to medium-sized CMNs
    - Acquired melanocytic nevi
    - More likely to occur after puberty
- 50% arise de novo
- May arise within neurocutaneous melanosis
  - Rare but carries a high risk of malignant transformation in children
  - Median age is 3 years old
  - Up to 2/3 of patients may develop primary intracranial melanomas
- Signs and symptoms may include
  - Rapid increase in size of lesion, hemorrhage, ulceration, change in color, loss of previously regular borders, pruritus, lymphadenopathy
- Important clinical signs ("ABCD" criteria)
  - Asymmetry
  - Border irregularity
  - Color/pigmentation irregularities
  - Diameter of 6 mm or greater
- **Risk factors**
  - Fair skin
  - Giant CMN (bathing trunk nevus)

CHILDHOOD MELANOMA

Key Facts

Clinical Issues

- Knowledge of clinical dimensions is of maximum importance
  - Ensure viewing of entire lesion before making a benign diagnosis
  - Can be difficult, especially in cases of giant congenital melanocytic nevus (CMN)

Microscopic Pathology

- Asymmetry of lesion
  - One of most powerful criteria for diagnosing melanoma
- Lack of circumscription
- Pagetoid spread of single melanocytes above basal layer, especially at periphery of lesion
- Lack of maturation
- Lack of dispersion
- Deep dermal mitoses
- Pigment deep in lesion
- Solitary epidermal melanocytes predominating over nests

Reporting Considerations

- Breslow thickness, not histologic subtype, is most important prognostic parameter
- Presence or absence of ulceration changes stage

Malpractice Considerations

- Expert consultation recommended before diagnosing melanoma in any pediatric patient
- Due to wide range of histologic features and subtypes of melanomas
  - Diagnosis of melanoma should be considered when encountering any unusual cutaneous malignancy

---

- Risk correlates with size, depth, and number of nevomelanocytes
- Occurs in 1 in 20,000 newborns
- ≥ 20 cm in largest diameter
- Up to 5-7% risk of malignant transformation
- Dysplastic nevus syndrome
- Numerous acquired melanocytic nevi
  - Independent risk factor
- Sporadic atypical nevi
  - Independent risk factor
- Xeroderma pigmentosum
- Albinism
- Immunosuppression
- Family history of melanoma (familial melanoma)
  - Occur at younger age
  - Often multifocal
  - Germline mutations of *CDKN2A* tumor suppressor gene

Treatment

- Options, risks, complications
  - Surgical resection with standard margins
    - Treatment of choice for primary disease
    - Potentially curative
    - May also include sentinel lymph node biopsy or regional lymphadenectomy
    - Both the NCCN and AAD publish online guidelines for surgical margins
  - Chemotherapy of minimal benefit
  - Experimental immunotherapy of unproven benefit
  - Treatment protocols based on adult population

Prognosis

- Most important prognostic factors
  - Depth of invasion
    - Clark level and Breslow thickness
    - Most accurately measured by Breslow thickness
    - Clark level is of questionable significance
  - Stage at diagnosis
    - Stage IV 5-year survival rate (34%)
    - Stage I-II 5-year survival rate (90%)
- Other poor prognostic indicators

- Previous nonmelanocytic malignancies, nodular type, fusiform cytology, vertical growth phase
- High dermal mitotic activity, ulceration, vascular invasion, age > 10 years, and presence of metastases at diagnosis
- Presence of ulceration upstages tumor (e.g., T2a to T2b)
- Overall 5-year survival ~ 79%
- Survival characteristics similar to adult population

MACROSCOPIC FEATURES

Size

- Usually > 7 mm

MICROSCOPIC PATHOLOGY

Histologic Features

- May or may not have ulceration
- Asymmetry
  - One of the most powerful histologic criteria
  - Nests showing
    - Variability in size and shape
    - Haphazard interval and array
  - Haphazard arrangement of solitary epidermal melanocytes
- Poor circumscription
  - Lesion does not start or end in nests
  - Difficult to discern where lesion begins and ends
  - Single melanocytes predominate at edge of lesion
- Solitary epidermal melanocytes predominate over nests
- Pagetoid spread of melanocytes
  - Ascent of single melanocytes above dermoepidermal (DE) junction
  - Can also be present in Spitz nevi (sometimes full nests) and acral nevi
  - Should not be at the periphery of Spitz or acral nevi
- Lack of maturation
  - Deeper melanocytes as large as superficial ones
- Deep dermal mitoses

CHILDHOOD MELANOMA

- Pigment present deep in lesion
- Atypical melanocytes
  - Atypical features not always present
  - May have marked nuclear pleomorphism
  - Melanocytes may be small and spindled or epithelioid
- Confluence of melanocytes
- Absence of Kamino bodies
- Melanomas arising in giant CMN
  - When arising in type 1 CMN, usually arises at DE junction
  - When arising in type 2 CMN, usually arises in dermal component
- Inflammatory infiltrate can be helpful, especially if asymmetrical
  - Often seen surrounding invasive component

Cytologic Features

- High nuclear to cytoplasmic ratio
- Prominent nucleoli, often appear "cherry red"
- Marked nuclear pleomorphism
- Hyperchromasia
- Dusty melanin

Histologic Subtypes

- **Superficial spreading melanoma**
  - Most common subtype
  - Found on non-sun-exposed skin
  - Characteristic radial (lateral) growth phase
  - Asymmetrical proliferation of atypical epithelioid-appearing melanocytes
    - Cells often have abundant cytoplasm, fine melanin pigmentation, pleomorphic vesicular nuclei, prominent "cherry red" nucleoli, and scattered mitotic figures
  - Pagetoid spread of single melanocytes common
  - Epidermal acanthosis with effacement of rete ridges
  - FISH and CGH studies less sensitive
- **Acral lentiginous melanoma**
  - Found on palms and soles
  - More common in Asian and black populations
  - Acanthosis and elongation of epidermal ridges infiltrated by atypical melanocytes
    - Often pleomorphism, hyperchromasia, conspicuous nucleoli, and mitoses
    - Fixation retraction artifact
  - Scattered foci of junctional nests
  - Lichenoid chronic inflammatory infiltrate
  - Includes subungual melanomas
    - Most often affect large toe
  - FISH and CGH studies more sensitive
- **Nodular melanoma**
  - Large nodules of oval to round epithelioid melanocytes
  - May be symmetrical in all directions
  - Lacks intraepidermal melanocytic proliferation
  - FISH and CGH studies more sensitive
- **Desmoplastic and neurotropic melanoma**
  - Spindle cells associated with dense desmoplastic stroma
  - S100 only reliable immunostain
    - HMB-45 and Mart-1/Melan-A usually negative

- p16 staining can be helpful in differentiating from desmoplastic Spitz nevus
  - p16 staining often lost in desmoplastic melanomas
- **Spindle cell melanoma**
  - Spindled cytology
  - S100 only reliable immunostain
    - Often HMB-45 and Mart-1/Melan-A negative
- **Lentigo maligna and lentigo maligna melanoma**
  - Do not occur in children
- Other rare melanoma variants
  - Spitzoid, amelanotic, balloon cell, pedunculated, nevoid, small cell, and myxoid

ANCILLARY TESTS

Immunohistochemistry

- S100 positive, considered the most sensitive marker
- HMB-45 and MART-1/Melan-A positive, more specific but less sensitive than S100
- MITF, SOX10, KBA62, and tyrosinase also usually positive

In Situ Hybridization

- FISH assays targeting most common chromosomal aberrations can be helpful
  - Probes vary from institution to institution, but 6p25, 6q23, Cep6, and 11q13 are often used

Array CGH

- Can be a very helpful adjunctive test, especially for most difficult cases
- Most benign nevi show no chromosomal aberrations
- Spitz nevi tend to demonstrate isolated gains of 11p
- > 96% of malignant melanomas demonstrate chromosomal aberrations
  - Most common are gains of chromosome 1q, 6p, 7p, 7q, 8q, 17q, and 20q or losses of 6q, 9p, 9q, 10q, 10p, and 11q
- Benign proliferations in CMNs can show chromosomal aberrations
  - These differ from aberrations found in melanomas arising in CMNs, which are similar to melanomas arising de novo

DIFFERENTIAL DIAGNOSIS

Spitz Nevus

- Preferentially involves head and neck of children
- Usually < 1 cm in diameter
- Characterized by large spindled or epithelioid cells
- Features that support diagnosis of Spitz nevus
  - Symmetry, maturation with depth, wedge-shaped silhouette
  - Melanocytic nests clutched by rete ridges or showing pagetoid spread
  - Clefts around nests
  - Kamino bodies
    - Dull pink globules often situated above tips of dermal papillae
    - No published case reports of well-formed Kamino bodies in a melanoma proven by metastatic spread

CHILDHOOD MELANOMA

Melanocytic Nevus
- Symmetrical and well-circumscribed nests of melanocytes
- Typically lacks cytologic atypia and pagetoid spread
  - Pagetoid spread can be seen in middle of Spitz and acral nevi
- Melanocytes mature with depth
- Lacks deep mitoses
- Usually lacks lymphocytes
  - Exceptions include irritated nevi, Spitz nevus, halo nevus, and dysplastic nevus

Atypical (Dysplastic) Nevus
- Pigmented papules, macules, and plaques
- Clinical features may resemble melanoma
- Features that support diagnosis of dysplastic nevus
  - Elongated clubbed rete ridges and bridging melanocytic nests
  - Concentric or lamellar fibroplasia in papillary dermis
  - Melanocytic maturation, well-nested melanocytes at dermoepidermal junction, no deep mitoses, and no pigment deep in lesion

Benign Proliferative Nodule in Giant CMNs
- Area of higher cell density and nuclear enlargement with higher mitotic activity in a CMN
- Can also be hamartoma arising in giant CMN
  - Nonmelanocytic cells such as smooth muscle, nerve, or sebaceous cells normally also present
- Typically become softer in time, stop growing, and subsequently become smaller or regress completely

Spindle Cell Malignancies
- Dermatofibrosarcoma protuberans (DFSP)
  - Densely cellular proliferation of spindle cells that deeply infiltrate fat in storiform pattern
  - CD34 extensively positive in almost all tumors
  - Negative for S100 and other melanoma markers
  - Pigmented DFSP is also referred to as Bednar tumor
- Malignant peripheral nerve sheath tumor (MPNST)
  - Can be focally S100 positive; usually not diffuse and strongly positive as in melanoma
  - Can be a very difficult differential diagnosis
  - By definition must arise from a nerve
- Cutaneous leiomyosarcoma
  - Extremely rare in children
  - Positive for smooth muscle markers (SMA, MSA, desmin, or H-caldesmon)
  - Typically S100 negative, rarely positive cases
- Spindle cell squamous cell carcinoma (SCC)
  - Very rare, but SCC may be seen in children with xeroderma pigmentosa and dystrophic epidermolysis bullosa
  - Usually cytokeratin (high molecular weight) and p63 positive

MALPRACTICE CONSIDERATIONS

Misdiagnosis
- Commonly occurs

- Up to 40% of pediatric melanomas initially misdiagnosed as benign
- Up to 60% of patients < 20 years experience a delay in treatment

Points of Diagnostic Confusion
- Similar histologic presentations as Spitz nevi
- Atypia in proliferative nodules of giant CMN

Uncertainty
- Is not uncommon in these difficult lesions and challenging patient population
- Consultation encouraged of any markedly atypical/ highly suspicious lesion
  - Expert review of cases often needed and improves patient care
- Often only true measure of malignancy in pediatric population is death or distant metastasis

STAGING

AJCC
- Staging does not differ from that for adults
- **Breslow thickness**
  - Measurement in mm from top of the granular layer to the deepest point of invasion
  - Extension along adnexal structures is not measured
  - Considered most important prognostic indicator and more accurate than Clark levels
- **Clark levels**
  - Officially removed from AJCC staging in 2009 (replaced by mitotic index for thin melanomas)
  - Can be used for subclassifying thin melanomas without ulceration when mitotic index cannot be determined
  - Level I: In situ within epidermis (not necessary to report)
  - Level II: Invades papillary dermis
  - Level III: Fills papillary dermis and extends to border with reticular dermis
  - Level IV: Invades reticular dermis
  - Level V: Invades subcutaneous fat
- Ulceration and mitotic index may increase stage and result in lymph node dissection
  - Presence will change stage from T1a to T1b
    - Sentinel lymph node examination

SELECTED REFERENCES

1. Ducharme EE et al: Pediatric malignant melanoma: an update on epidemiology, detection, and prevention. Cutis. 84(4):192-8, 2009
2. Jen M et al: Childhood melanoma. Clin Dermatol. 27(6):529-36, 2009
3. Downard CD et al: Melanoma in children and adolescents. Surg Oncol. 16(3):215-20, 2007
4. Krengel S et al: Melanoma risk in congenital melanocytic naevi: a systematic review. Br J Dermatol. 155(1):1-8, 2006
5. Ferrari A et al: Does melanoma behave differently in younger children than in adults? A retrospective study of 33 cases of childhood melanoma from a single institution. Pediatrics. 115(3):649-54, 2005

Clinical and Microscopic Features

(Left) Clinical photograph shows a large melanoma with variegated color, jagged border, and irregular surface, all of which are concerning clinical signs. *(Right)* H&E shows melanoma from the back of a 16-year-old girl. The lesion is composed of atypical epithelioid cells with several mitotic figures ➡, and there are atypical cells advancing up through the epidermis (pagetoid spread) ➡. *(Courtesy C. Cockerell, MD.)*

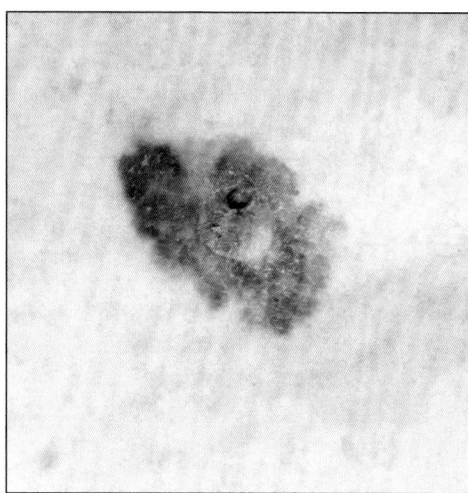
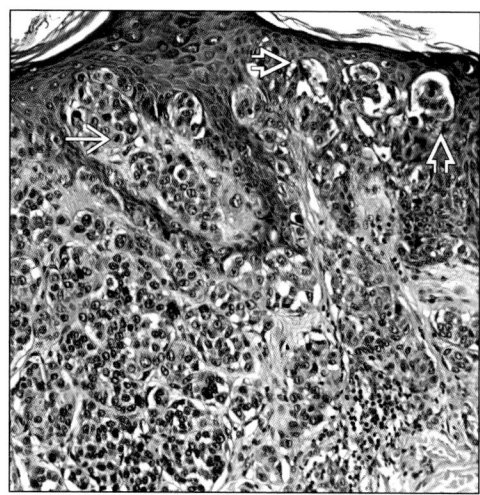

(Left) This preauricular superficial spreading melanoma is larger than 6 mm in diameter with an irregular border, asymmetry, and pseudopod of different color on the superior edge ➡. *(Right)* Superficial spreading melanoma shows prominent pagetoid spread ➡ and obvious atypia with nuclear hyperchromasia, pleomorphism, and cytologic atypia. An atypical mitosis is also present ➡.

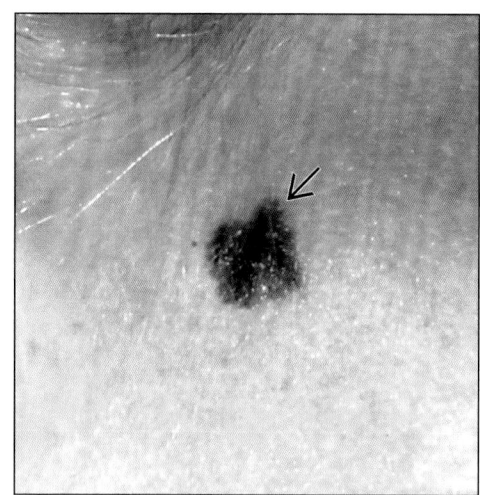
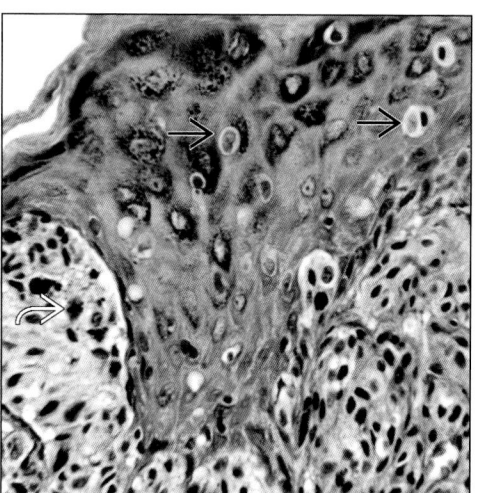

(Left) Nodular-type melanoma presents as a dark brown asymmetric nodule with irregular borders. *(Courtesy J. Wu, MD.)* *(Right)* Nodular melanoma demonstrates a characteristic pedunculated shape. These are usually sharply circumscribed and contain nests of oval to round atypical epithelioid melanocytes growing throughout the dermis. Lack of maturation (uniform cells throughout) and large irregular nests are other helpful features. *(Courtesy G. Fraga, MD.)*

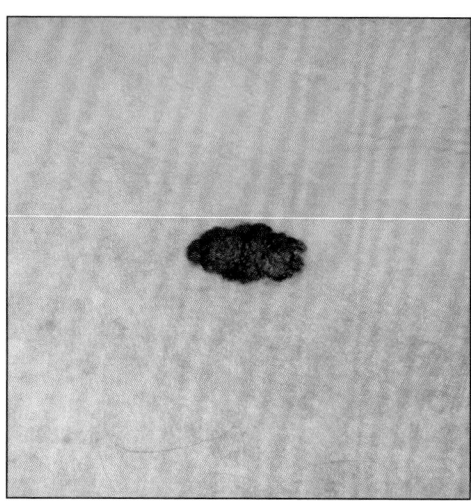
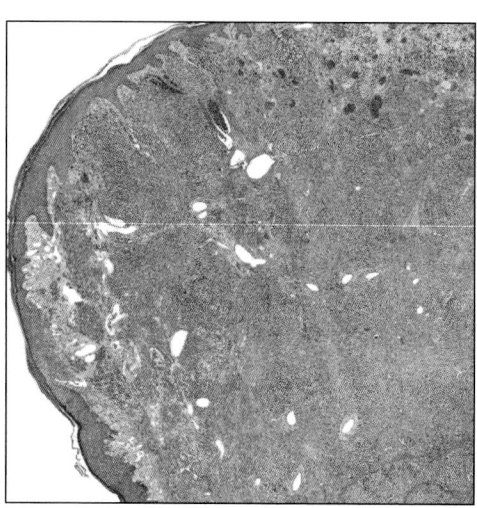

CHILDHOOD MELANOMA

Differential Diagnosis

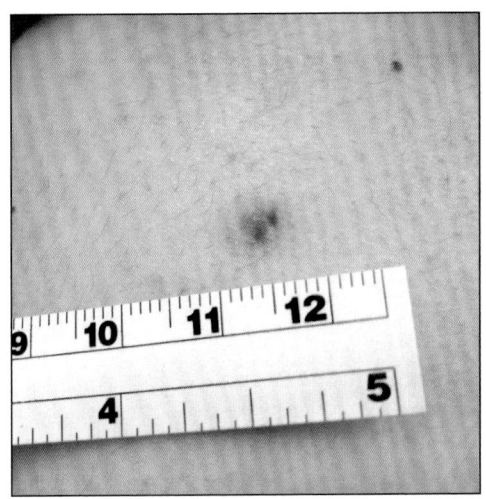

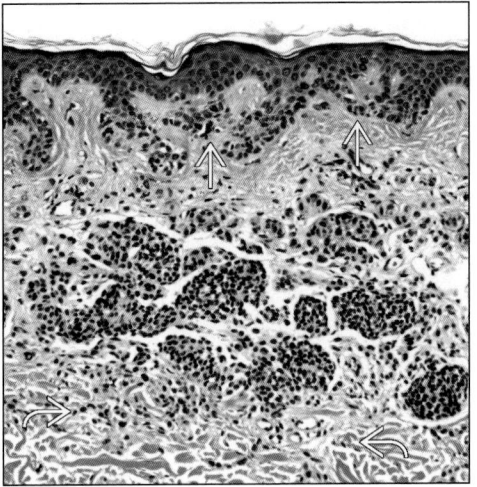

(Left) Clinical image of an atypical (dysplastic) nevus shows a multicolored, irregularly bordered, asymmetric nevus that mimics a melanoma, as it frequently does. *(Right)* Mildly atypical compound nevus shows a proliferation of small nests and a few single cells along the dermal-epidermal junction with focal bridging across rete ridges ➡. The dermal component is composed of small, relatively uniform-appearing cells that show dispersion (maturation) with dermal descent ➡.

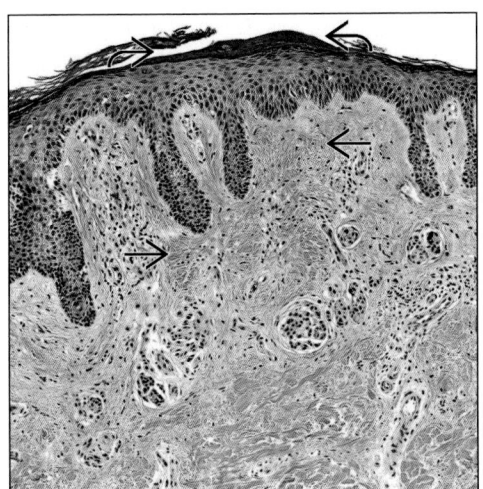

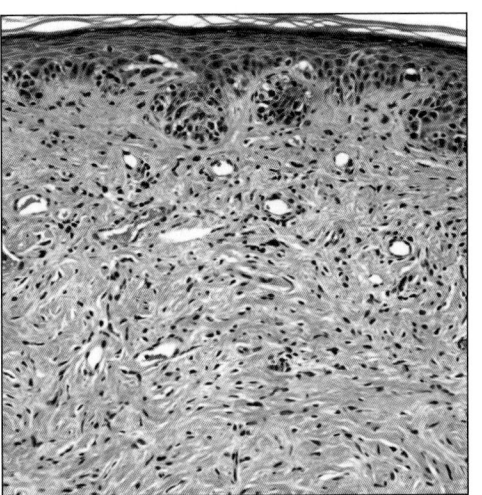

(Left) Traumatized atypical compound nevus with junctional lentiginous hyperplasia (consistent with recurrent nevus features) shows dermal fibrosis ➡ and focal overlying parakeratosis ➡ and serum crusting. *(Right)* An atypical combined nevus with a desmoplastic nevus (DN) component in dermis is seen. The junctional component is moderately atypical, but the dermal cells are small and bland appearing. Note lack of severe solar elastosis & lymphoid aggregates typical of DN.

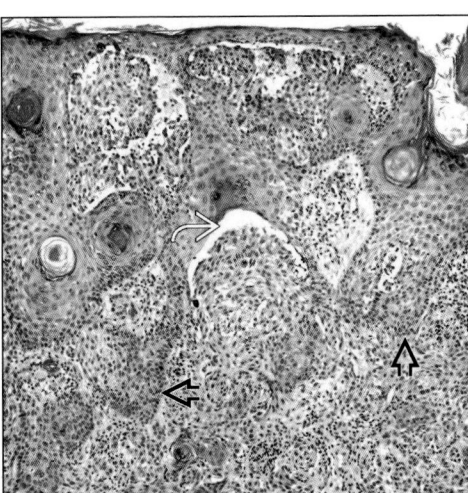

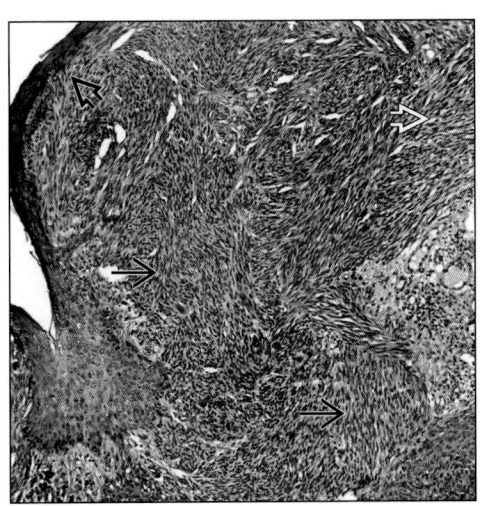

(Left) A compound Spitz nevus shows epidermal hyperplasia ➡ associated with a compound melanocytic proliferation composed of a mixed population of spindled and epithelioid cells. Note the clefting over some of the junctional nests ➡. *(Right)* This is a spitzoid melanoma from the ear of a 7-year-old girl. Note the spindled morphology of the melanocytes ➡. The cells do not appear to mature from the epidermis ➡ to the deeper dermis ➡. *(Courtesy C. Cockerell, MD.)*

MELANOMA, LENTIGO MALIGNA TYPE

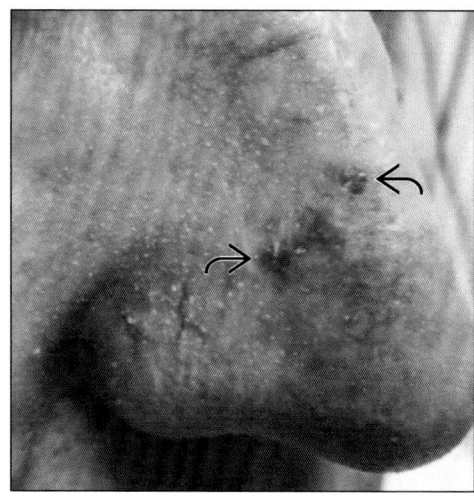

Clinical photograph of lentigo maligna melanoma on the nose of an elderly patient shows irregular pigmentation ➚. Both in situ and invasive melanoma were present on biopsy. (Courtesy P. Hsu, MD.)

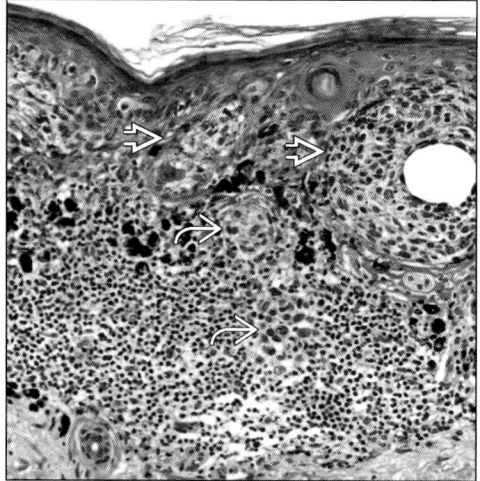

LMM shows epidermal atrophy, consumed rete ridges, and an atypical junctional melanocytic lesion ➚. The papillary dermis is obscured by a dense lymphocytic infiltrate, but focal invasion is present ➚.

TERMINOLOGY

Abbreviations
- Lentigo maligna melanoma (LMM)

Synonyms
- Invasive melanoma, lentigo maligna type
- Hutchinson freckle (clinical term, which typically refers to melanoma in situ, lentigo maligna type)

Definitions
- Indolent melanoma subtype that evolves slowly and usually presents on head and neck (sun-exposed regions) in older patients

CLINICAL ISSUES

Epidemiology
- Age
  - Older patients, typically > 60 years old

Site
- Usually on head and neck (sun-exposed regions)

Presentation
- Broad patch with a nodule, may grow 5-10 cm or larger
- Variegated colors
- Irregular borders

Natural History
- Slowly evolving, indolent but invasive type melanoma

Treatment
- Surgical approaches
  - Complete excision, margins depend on the depth of invasion
  - Mohs surgery if poorly defined margins; recurrence rates of < 1%
- Drugs

  - Imiquimod cream is controversial, but has shown promise for a subset of patients
    - Long-term follow-up and several post-treatment biopsies are encouraged, even with lack of clinical recurrence

Prognosis
- Surgical margins of at least 5 mm give cure rates of 90-95%

MICROSCOPIC PATHOLOGY

Histologic Features
- Severely atypical compound melanocytic proliferation with junctional lentiginous component (typical of lentigo maligna)
  - Confluence of melanocytes replacing basilar keratinocytes, often forming a cleft
  - Numerous solitary units and small nests of atypical cells along basilar layer
  - Extension of atypical melanocytes along adnexal structures
  - Epidermal atrophy and effacement of rete ridges
- Predominantly lymphocytic dermal infiltrate may obscure junctional component
- Invasion of dermis by atypical cells, usually in nests &/or fascicles
  - Dermal component often shows spindle cell &/or desmoplastic melanoma features
    - Desmoplastic melanoma can be difficult to recognize, especially if it is hypocellular
    - Can be composed primarily of single hyperchromatic-staining cells
    - Lymphoid aggregates and perineural invasion often present
  - Often deeply invasive with no evidence of maturation
- Solar elastosis present, typically severe

MELANOMA, LENTIGO MALIGNA TYPE

Key Facts

Terminology

- Indolent melanoma subtype that typically evolves slowly
- Invasive melanoma, lentigo maligna type

Clinical Issues

- Usually occurs on head and neck (sun-exposed regions) of elderly patients
- Broad patch with irregular, mottled pigmentation and irregular borders

Microscopic Pathology

- Confluence of atypical melanocytes replacing basilar keratinocytes forming a cleft
- Epidermal atrophy and loss of rete ridges
- Tumor cells extend along adnexal structures
- Invasion of dermis by atypical cells, usually in nests &/or fascicles
- Dermal component often shows spindle cell &/or desmoplastic melanoma features

Cytologic Features

- Cells are angulated and may be spindled
- Scant cytoplasm with only few if any melanin granules
- Nuclei are hyperchromatic and pleomorphic

DIFFERENTIAL DIAGNOSIS

Reed (Pigmented Spindle Cell) Nevus

- Hyperplastic epidermis, symmetry and well-defined peripheral margins
- Tumor cells are spindle-shaped and may show atypia but are usually monomorphous

Dysplastic Compound Melanocytic Nevus

- Less cytological atypia
- No basal confluence of nevus cells
- No adnexal extension
- Dermal component matures with increasing depth

Invasive Melanoma, Superficial Spreading Type

- Junctional component shows greater nesting and pagetoid spread compared to lentigo maligna
- Dermal component often nested and composed mostly of epithelioid-shaped cells
  - Not composed of oval to spindled cells of lentigo maligna melanoma
- Not associated with spindle cell/desmoplastic melanoma

DIAGNOSTIC CHECKLIST

Pathologic Interpretation Pearls

- Look for epidermal atrophy
- Confluent nesting along junction
- Adnexal extension
- Dermal invasion, often composed of spindled cells
  - May be difficult to identify, especially if desmoplastic type or heavily inflamed

SELECTED REFERENCES

1. Van Meurs T et al: Treatment of lentigo maligna with imiquimod cream: a long-term follow-up study of 10 patients. Dermatol Surg. 36(6):853-8, 2010
2. Raziano RM et al: Staged margin control techniques for surgical excision of lentigo maligna. G Ital Dermatol Venereol. 144(3):259-70, 2009
3. van Meurs T et al: Recurrence of lentigo maligna after initial complete response to treatment with 5% imiquimod cream. Dermatol Surg. 33(5):623-6; discussion 626-7, 2007
4. Massi G et al: Histological Diagnosis of Nevi and Melanoma. Darmstadt, Germany: Steinkopff Verlag, 2004
5. Crowson AN et al: The Melanocytic Proliferations: A Comprehensive Textbook of Pigmented Lesions. New York: Wiley-Liss, 2001
6. Tannous ZS et al: Progression to invasive melanoma from malignant melanoma in situ, lentigo maligna type. Hum Pathol. 31(6):705-8, 2000
7. Flotte TJ et al: Lentigo maligna and malignant melanoma in situ, lentigo maligna type. Hum Pathol. 30(5):533-6, 1999

IMAGE GALLERY

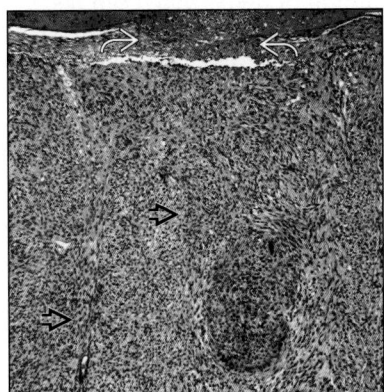 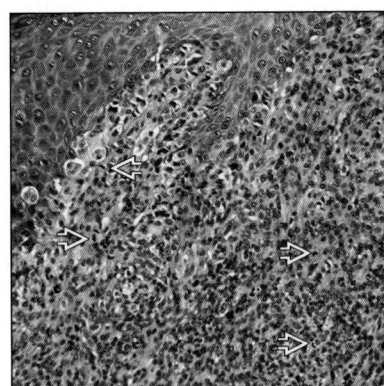 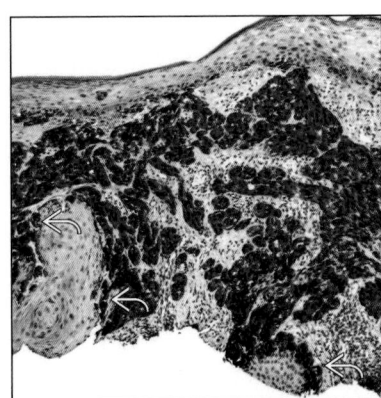

(Left) Low-power magnification of a LMM shows epidermal atrophy, focal ulceration ➤, and deep dermal invasion by fascicles and sheets of atypical spindle cells ➤. *(Center)* High-power examination reveals the invasive melanoma with numerous mitoses ➤ in the superficial dermis. *(Right)* HMB-45 immunohistochemistry shows strong and diffuse staining of the in situ and dermal cells, consistent with invasive melanoma. Note the florid surrounding of adnexal structures ➤.

MELANOMA, SUPERFICIAL SPREADING TYPE

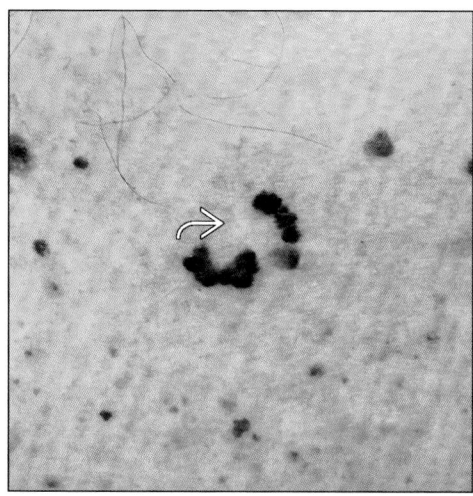

Clinical photograph of a melanoma, superficial spreading type shows darkly pigmented areas surrounding a central area of regression ➔. (Courtesy J. Wu, MD.)

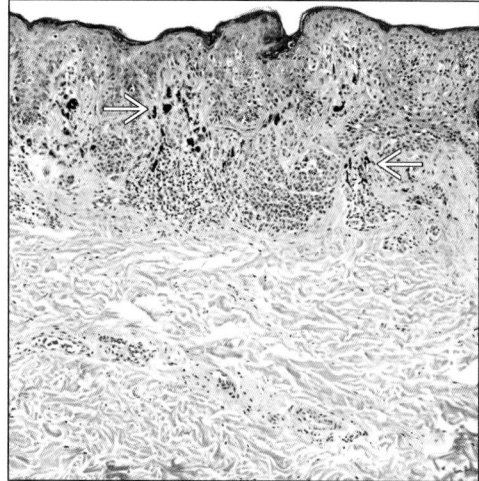

Low-power magnification of a MM-SST shows a highly atypical compound melanocytic proliferation with mild dermal inflammation with scattered melanophages ➔.

TERMINOLOGY

Abbreviations
- Malignant melanoma, superficial spreading type (MM-SST)

Definitions
- Most common variant of invasive melanoma
- Characterized histologically by lateral expansion of large dermal nests of atypical melanocytes, which appear similar to overlying melanoma in situ cells

CLINICAL ISSUES

Epidemiology
- Incidence
  - 6th most common cancer in USA with increasing incidence
- Gender
  - Both men and women, but more common overall in men
- Ethnicity
  - Typically persons with red hair and skin type I/II, but can occur in other ethnicities

Site
- Varies according to gender, on the back (in men) and on the legs (in women)

Presentation
- Large dark brown macule (2.5 cm is average size)
- Variegated color with shades of tan, brown, black, blue-black, red (inflammation or vascular ectasia), gray and white (zones of regression)
- Irregular borders
- Presence of distinctive nodule can signify vertical growth phase

Treatment
- Surgical approaches

  - Complete excision with clear margins
    - Peripheral margins are determined by depth of invasion (Breslow depth)

Prognosis
- Varies according to Breslow depth, ulceration, and mitotic index
  - 2010 AJCC criteria for determining prognosis

MACROSCOPIC FEATURES

Size
- Typically > 1 cm in diameter

MICROSCOPIC PATHOLOGY

Histologic Features
- Lateral expansion of large nests of atypical melanocytes in both epidermis and dermis, i.e., radial growth phase
  - Proliferation of single atypical melanocytes involving both rete ridges and suprapapillary plates
  - Abundant pagetoid spread of atypical melanocytes located in spinous layer
  - Irregular distribution of nests, which can be confluent with indented borders
  - Large artifactual clefts between nests and epidermis above
  - Highly atypical melanocytes form confluent nests or nodule in dermis
  - Nuclear to cytoplasmic ratio does not change with increasing dermal depth, i.e., dermal melanocytes fail to mature with increasing depth in dermis
- Dense but irregularly distributed inflammatory dermal infiltrate (mostly lymphocytes)
- Asymmetrical distribution of melanin pigment in dermis

MELANOMA, SUPERFICIAL SPREADING TYPE

Key Facts

Terminology
- Most common variant of invasive melanoma

Clinical Issues
- Most frequently occurs on back for males, legs for females
- Broad macule with variegated colors
- Irregular borders
- Presence of papule/nodule may represent invasive component

Microscopic Pathology
- Proliferation of single atypical melanocytes involving both rete ridges and suprapapillary plates
- Abundant pagetoid spread of atypical melanocytes located in spinous layer

- Broad invasive front in which invasive dermal cells appear similar to overlying melanoma in situ (radial growth phase)
- Highly atypical melanocytes form confluent nests or nodule in dermis
- Lack of maturation of dermal component
- Mitotic activity in deep dermal component
- Dense but irregularly distributed inflammatory dermal infiltrate (mostly lymphocytes)
- Asymmetrical distribution of melanin pigment

Top Differential Diagnoses
- Severely dysplastic compound melanocytic nevus
- Atypical Reed nevus
- Epidermotropic metastatic melanoma
- Paget disease

Cytologic Features
- Enlarged, atypical epithelioid cells
- Nuclear pleomorphism
- Thick, irregular nuclear membrane
- Large eosinophilic or purple nucleoli
- Presence of mitoses in dermal component

DIFFERENTIAL DIAGNOSIS

Severely Atypical (Dysplastic) Compound Melanocytic Nevus
- Typically appears symmetric and well-circumscribed at low magnification
  - May need excisional specimen in order to adequately evaluate these features
- Less cytological atypia and mitotic activity than melanoma
  - Dermal mitoses highly suspicious for melanoma
- Less pagetoid spread
- Dermal component should mature with increasing dermal depth

Atypical Reed Nevus
- Hyperplastic epidermis, lateral margins are sharply defined (no trailing off of single cells)
- Composed mostly of spindle-shaped cells, which may be atypical, but are often monomorphous (not pleomorphic as in MM-SST)
- Kamino bodies may be present

Metastatic Melanoma (with Epidermotropism)
- Dermal component that is much larger than intraepidermal component
- Uniform cytologic atypia in dermal component
- Lymphatic invasion typically present (may need levels &/or immunohistochemistry, i.e., D2-40/podoplanin or CD31 to identify)

Paget Disease
- Cells are not at junction, but above basal keratinocytes

- May find glandular structures

DIAGNOSTIC CHECKLIST

Clinically Relevant Pathologic Features
- Broad macule with variegated colors and papule; white area may signify regression

Pathologic Interpretation Pearls
- Pagetoid spread of atypical melanocytes throughout epidermis
- Lack of maturation (tumor cells stay same size) with increasing dermal depth
- Cytological atypia
- Lymphocytic infiltrate hugs dermal tumor cells
- Asymmetrical distribution of melanin pigment

SELECTED REFERENCES

1. Piris A et al: AJCC melanoma staging update: impact on dermatopathology practice and patient management. J Cutan Pathol. 38(5):394-400, 2011
2. Thompson JF et al: Prognostic significance of mitotic rate in localized primary cutaneous melanoma: an analysis of patients in the multi-institutional American Joint Committee on Cancer melanoma staging database. J Clin Oncol. 2011 Jun 1;29(16):2199-205. Epub 2011 Apr 25. Erratum in: J Clin Oncol. 29(21):2949, 2011
3. Balch CM et al: Multivariate analysis of prognostic factors among 2,313 patients with stage III melanoma: comparison of nodal micrometastases versus macrometastases. J Clin Oncol. 28(14):2452-9, 2010
4. Massi G et al: Histological Diagnosis of Nevi and Melanoma. Darmstadt, Germany: Steinkopff Verlag, 2004
5. Crowson AN et al: The Melanocytic Proliferations: A Comprehensive Textbook of Pigmented Lesions. New York: Wiley-Liss, 2001

MELANOMA, SUPERFICIAL SPREADING TYPE

Microscopic Features

(Left) Low-power examination shows melanoma in situ with pagetoid spread ⮕, superficial spreading type, overlying the invasive melanoma. This case was complicated by a preexisting intradermal melanocytic nevus ⮕. *(Right)* Medium-power examination readily exhibits abundant pagetoid upward scatter ⮕.

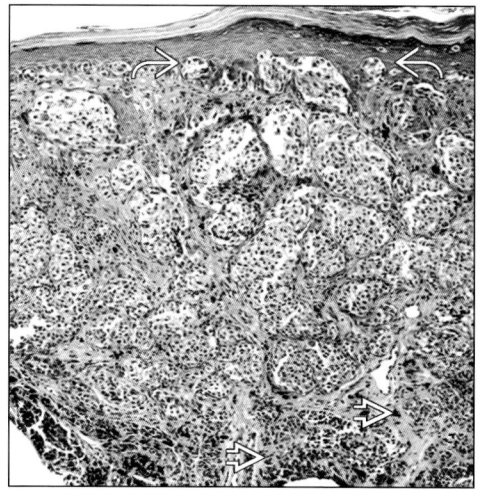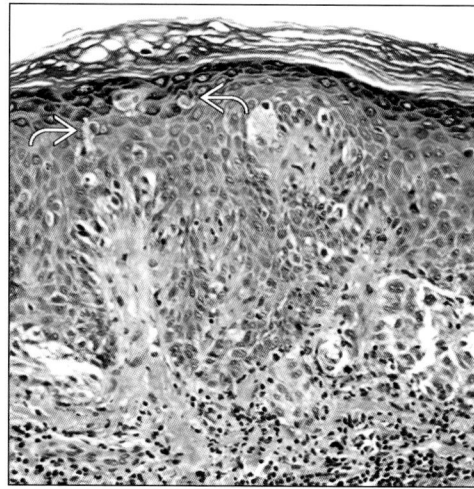

(Left) The dermal component fails to mature from the superficial to deeper dermis. Multiple mitoses ⮕ are easily found. *(Right)* High-power magnification shows the dermal component, which demonstrates prominent cytologic atypia and 2 adjacent mitoses ⮕.

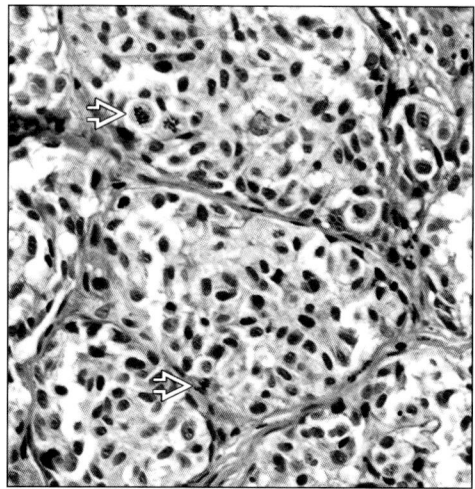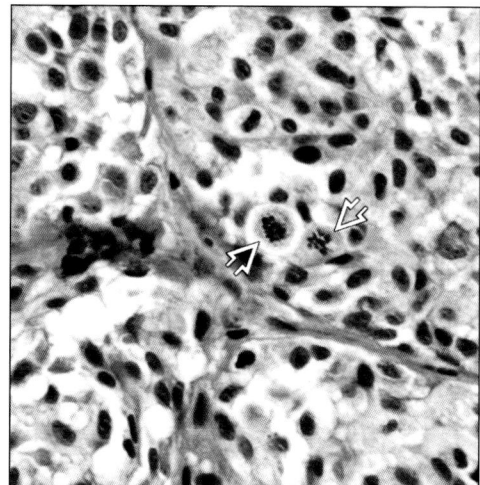

(Left) Low-power magnification of another example of MM-SST shows a dome-shaped, predominantly dermal-based tumor, raising the possibility of an epidermotropic melanoma metastasis. *(Right)* Higher magnification shows that the dermal component fails to mature with increasing dermal depth. The dermis also shows uneven melanin pigment even deep within the reticular dermis ⮕.

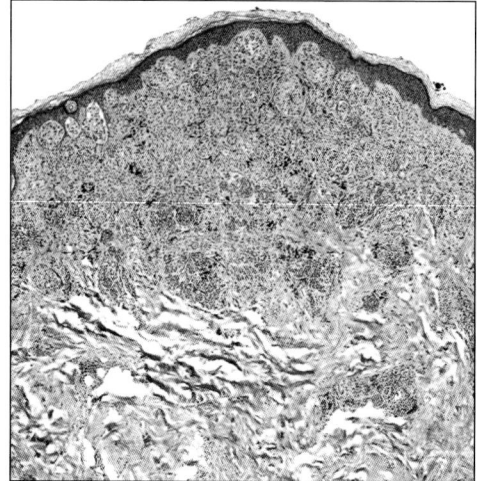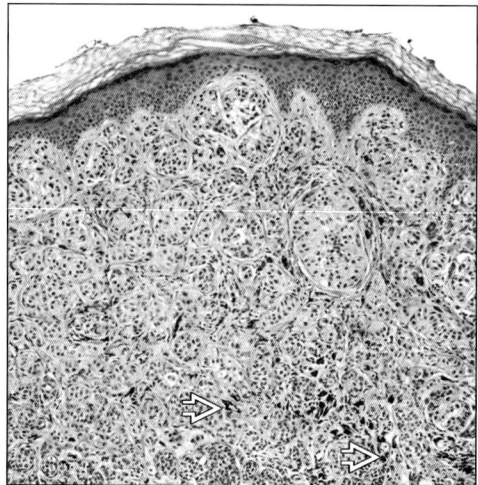

MELANOMA, SUPERFICIAL SPREADING TYPE

Microscopic Features and Differential Diagnosis

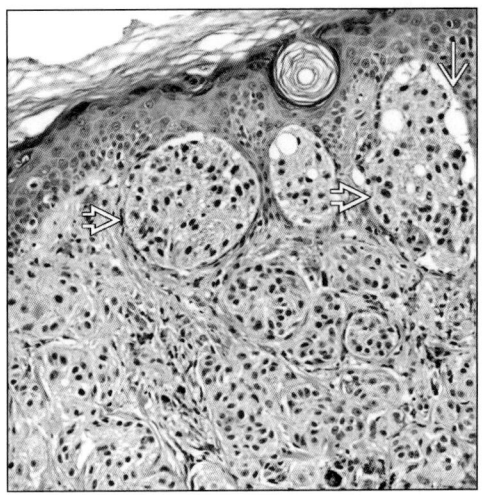

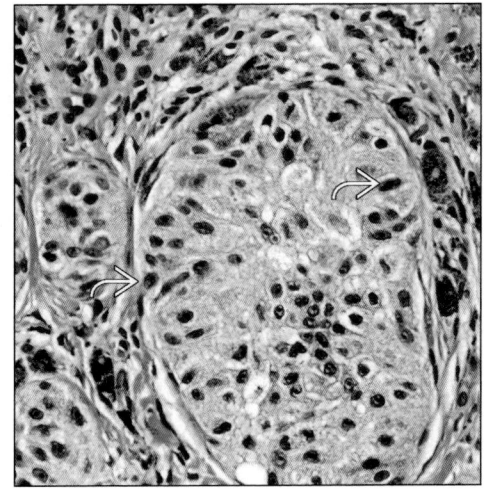

(Left) The presence of irregularly scattered intraepidermal nests ➡ with scalloped borders ➡ define the radial growth phase. (Right) High-power magnification shows atypical cells with ample gray-melanized cytoplasm with nuclear hyperchromasia and pleomorphism ➡.

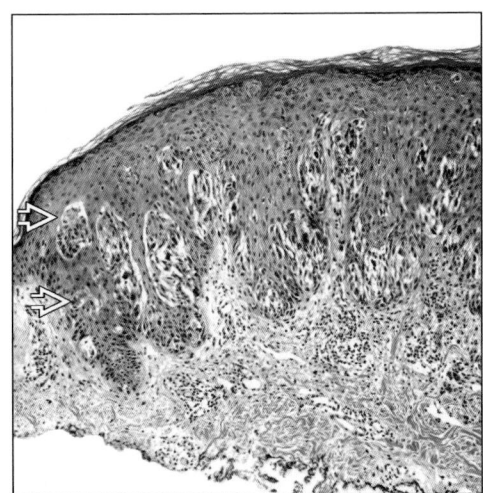

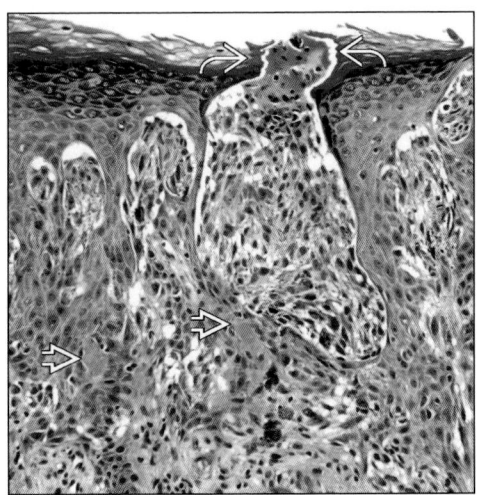

(Left) Atypical pigmented spindle cell nevus (of Reed) shows a predominantly junctional proliferation of atypical spindle-shaped cells in irregular nests. Note the sharp lateral circumscription ➡, as opposed to the trailing off of cells seen in MM-SST. (Right) High magnification of the center of an atypical Reed nevus shows pagetoid spread eroding through the granular layer ➡, but the cells are more uniform and spindled compared to MM-SST. Note the presence of Kamino bodies ➡.

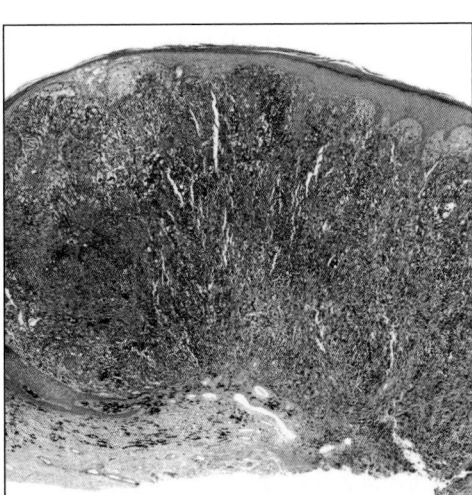

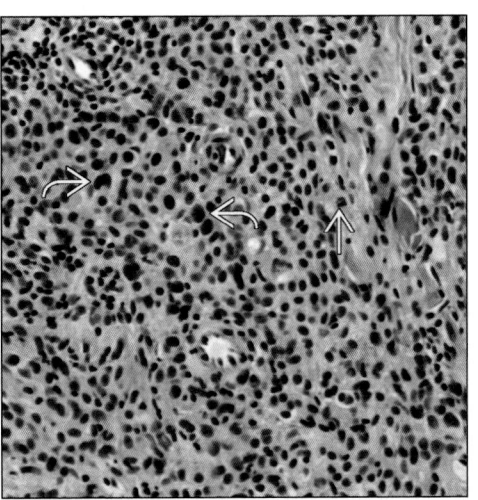

(Left) Nodular type invasive melanoma shows a predominantly dermal-based tumor with a nodular to sheet-like growth pattern in the dermis. (Right) Nevoid-type melanoma can also be considered in the differential diagnosis, although it is more often mistaken for a nevus. Despite the relatively small size and uniformity of the nuclei, they show significant hyperchromasia and focal pleomorphism ➡. Mitotic figures ➡ and lack of maturation are also important clues to the diagnosis.

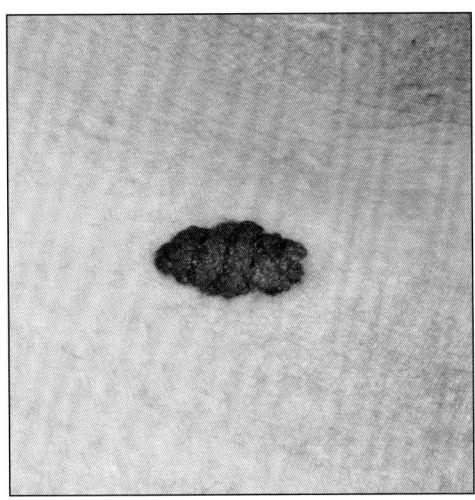

Clinical photograph of a nodular-type melanoma shows a darkly pigmented elevated lesion with irregular borders on the chest. (Courtesy J. Wu, MD.)

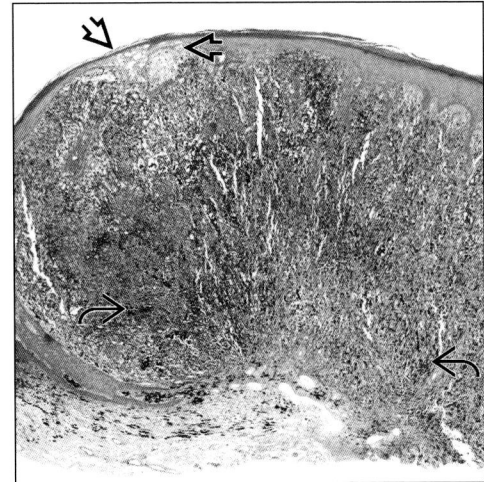

Low-power examination of a MM-NT shows a large, expansile dermal nodule with irregular pigmentation ➢ and areas of epidermal thinning and necrosis ➢ (but no complete ulceration in this section).

TERMINOLOGY

Abbreviations
- Melanoma, nodular type (MM-NT)

Definitions
- Invasive melanoma that histologically lacks a prominent junctional component (radial growth phase does not extend beyond 3 rete ridges of invasive vertical growth phase)

CLINICAL ISSUES

Epidemiology
- Incidence
  - 2nd most common subtype of invasive melanoma (after superficial spreading type)
- Age
  - Median age of onset is 49 years

Site
- Typically on backs of males and legs of females
- Usually found in sun-exposed areas; much less common in areas without sun exposure

Presentation
- Raised, firm, dome-shaped mass of varied color
  - May be black, reddish, partially pigmented, or even achromatic
  - May have unequal color distribution or be homogeneous in color
  - Dominant color is black, with brown being 2nd most common color
- Usually symmetrically shaped
- Ulceration and bleeding commonly occur

Natural History
- May grow very quickly and commonly are relatively new-onset lesions that lack a radial growth phase

- More commonly are deeply invasive than other types of melanoma

Prognosis
- Depends on depth of invasion (Breslow depth), ulceration, and mitotic index
- Lymphatic invasion and lymph node metastasis are significant poor prognostic indicators
  - Median survival with metastasis: 4.4 months
- Considerable Breslow depth, local invasion, and early metastases to vital organs lead to poor prognosis in most cases

MICROSCOPIC PATHOLOGY

Histologic Features
- Preferential growth in dermis, rather than epidermis
- Junctional component is tiny or absent, except at borders of lesion, and nodule may be separated from epidermis by thin rim of collagen
- At border of lesion, confluent nests of abnormal melanocytes may be seen
- Within lesion, nests have varying amounts of pigmentation; some lesions may even appear to completely lack pigment
  - However, small granules of melanin will be often found histologically (or with melanin stain) with complete search
- Smaller nodules, sheets of melanocytes, or closely apposed nests are usually found
- May find focal to sheet-like areas of necrosis

Cytologic Features
- Epithelioid cell morphology with vesicular nuclei
- Pleomorphic nuclei with hyperchromasia
- Prominent, cherry-red macronucleoli
- Mitoses present deep in dermal component

MELANOMA, NODULAR TYPE

Key Facts

Terminology
- Nodular, predominantly dermal invasive melanoma

Clinical Issues
- Elevated, firm, rapidly growing nodule

Microscopic Pathology
- Junctional component is small, and nodule may be separated from epidermis
- Areas of nodular/sheet-like growth pattern

- Epithelioid cell morphology with vesicular nuclei, prominent nucleoli
- Pleomorphic nuclei with hyperchromasia
- Mitoses often numerous, present deep in dermal component

Top Differential Diagnoses
- Superficial spreading type of invasive melanoma
- Spitz nevus
- Metastatic melanoma (with epidermotropism)

DIFFERENTIAL DIAGNOSIS

Superficial Spreading Type of Invasive Melanoma
- Shows broader atypical junctional component
  - Often extends laterally well beyond dermal component
- Dermal component often broader than that in MM-NT and composed mostly of irregular nests (less nodular/sheet-like areas)

Spitz Nevus
- Younger patients (children to young adults)
- Symmetrical, well-circumscribed architecture at low magnification
- Composed of mixture of spindled and epithelioid cells in most cases
- Hyperkeratotic epidermis (not irregular thinning), often with clefting around nests
- Kamino bodies
- Mitoses usually superficial and nonatypical

Metastatic Melanoma (with Epidermotropism)
- Dermal component that is much larger than the intraepidermal one
- Uniform atypical cytology in dermal component
- Lymphatic invasion almost always present (may need levels or immunohistochemistry, i.e., D2-40/podoplanin, to identify)

DIAGNOSTIC CHECKLIST

Clinically Relevant Pathologic Features
- Depth of invasion
- Ulceration
- Mitotic rate

Pathologic Interpretation Pearls
- Nodular, predominantly dermal-based lesion
- Prominent vertical growth phase with sheeting growth pattern

SELECTED REFERENCES

1. Erkurt MA et al: Nodular melanoma presenting with rapid progression and widespread metastases: a case report. J Med Case Reports. 3:50, 2009
2. Segura S et al: In vivo microscopic features of nodular melanomas: dermoscopy, confocal microscopy, and histopathologic correlates. Arch Dermatol. 144(10):1311-20, 2008
3. Warycha MA et al: Changes in the presentation of nodular and superficial spreading melanomas over 35 years. Cancer. 113(12):3341-8, 2008
4. Demierre MF et al: Early detection of thick melanomas in the United States: beware of the nodular subtype. Arch Dermatol. 141(6):745-50, 2005
5. Crowson AN et al: The Melanocytic Proliferations: A Comprehensive Textbook of Pigmented Lesions. New York: Wiley-Liss, 2001

IMAGE GALLERY

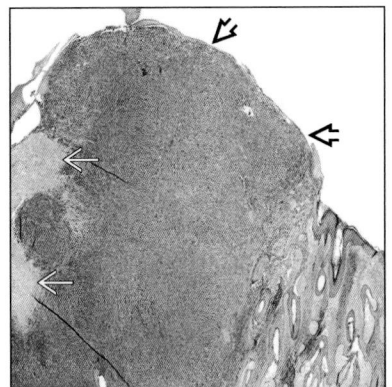 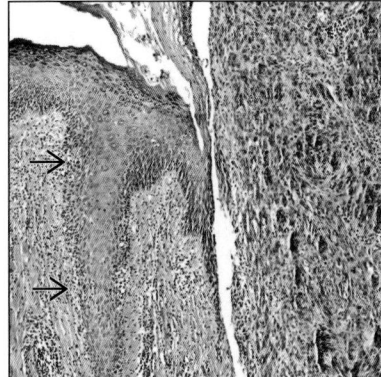 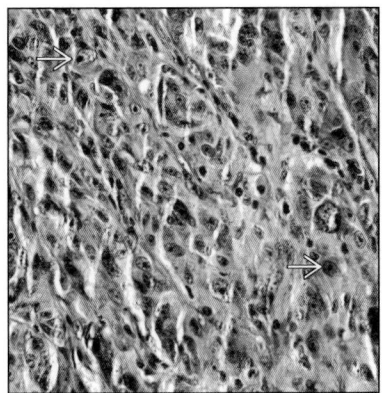

(Left) Scanning magnification of a nodular melanoma shows a large nodule with broad areas of overlying ulceration ⬘ and large areas of necrosis ➡. *(Center)* Medium-power magnification shows a lack of radial growth phase, but an adjacent minimal junctional component ➡ is found. *(Right)* High-power magnification shows sheets of melanoma cells with bizarre cytology (pleomorphic nuclei, thick and irregular nuclear membranes, and prominent nucleoli ➡).

DESMOPLASTIC MELANOMA

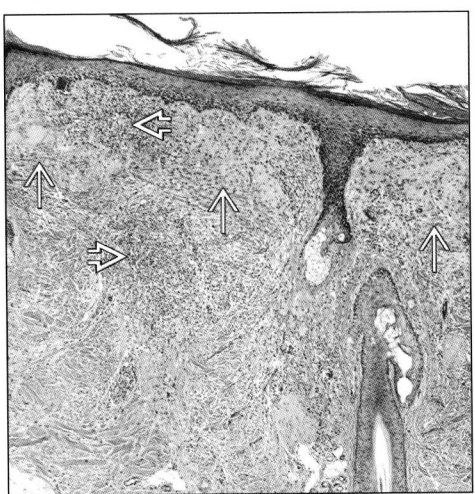

DM may resemble an inflamed scar on low-power examination. However, aggregates of lymphoid cells ➡ and prominent solar elastosis ➡ are usually identified and are helpful findings.

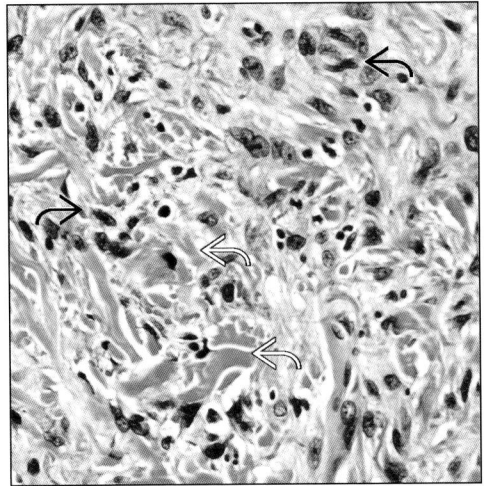

High-magnification examination shows hyperchromatic-staining atypical spindle cells ➡ surrounded by abundant collagen ➡ bundles.

TERMINOLOGY

Abbreviations
- Desmoplastic melanoma (DM)

Synonyms
- Desmoplastic/neurotropic melanoma

Definitions
- Form of invasive melanoma composed of spindle cells associated with dense stromal collagen, resembling a scar

CLINICAL ISSUES

Epidemiology
- Age
  - Presents in sun-damaged skin of elderly adults

Presentation
- Firm skin-colored, tan or pink plaque or nodule
- Sometimes depressed
- Often amelanotic

Treatment
- Surgical approaches
  - It is important to resect DM with clear surgical margins as early as possible for successful clinical management
  - There is increasing evidence that sentinel lymph node biopsy may not be indicated for "pure" variants of DM because of the low incidence of regional lymph node metastases

Prognosis
- Tumor thickness
- Clark level (IV vs. V)
- Histological subtype: "Pure" (longer disease-free survival) vs. "combined"
  - "Pure" subtype is defined as > 90% scar-like areas

- "Combined" subtype is defined as densely cellular spindle cell collections without significant scar-like areas (> 10%)
- Tumor mitotic rate

MICROSCOPIC PATHOLOGY

Histologic Features
- Ill-defined spindle cell neoplasm with highly infiltrative pattern of growth
- Overlying epidermis may show melanoma in situ (usually lentigo maligna type)
- Stromal collagen on scanning magnification resembles a scar
- Spindle cells are arranged in fascicles and merge with scar-like areas
- Cellular density and cytologic atypia can vary based on histologic subtype
- Discrete dermal lymphoid aggregates
- Solar elastosis

Cytologic Features
- "Pure" subtype shows
  - Spindle cells with often deceptively mild cytological atypia
  - Nuclear hyperchromasia
  - Irregular nuclear contours
  - Minimal nuclear pleomorphism
  - Inconspicuous mitotic activity
- "Combined" subtype shows
  - Greater cellularity and plump, elongated cells
  - Vesicular nuclei
  - Prominent nucleoli

ANCILLARY TESTS

Immunohistochemistry
- Typically strongly S100(+); negative for other melanocytic markers in most cases

DESMOPLASTIC MELANOMA

Key Facts

Terminology

- Invasive melanoma that often resembles an inflamed scar

Clinical Issues

- Firm skin-colored, tan or pink plaque or nodule
- Presents in sun-damaged skin of elderly adults

Microscopic Pathology

- Discrete dermal lymphoid aggregates admixed with abundant collagen
- Severe solar elastosis
- "Pure" and "combined" (more cellular) subtypes
- Ill-defined spindle cell neoplasm with highly infiltrative pattern of growth
- Overlying epidermis may show melanoma in situ (usually lentigo maligna type)

Ancillary Tests

- Immunostains for S100 and SOX10 usually positive

Top Differential Diagnoses

- Dermal scar
- Desmoplastic nevus
- Spindle cell squamous cell carcinoma (SCC)
  ○ Positive for HMWCKs, p63; S100(-)
- Atypical fibroxanthoma (AFX)
  ○ S100(-); CD10/CD68/CD99(+)
- Dermatofibroma: FXIIIa/CD10(+); S100(-)
- Dermatofibrosarcoma protuberans: CD34(+); S100(-)
- Neural tumors
  ○ S100/SOX10(+); CD34(+) (not in DM)
- Leiomyosarcoma
  ○ Actin/desmin (+), S100(-)

- SOX10 and KBA62 are often positive but also stain neural tumors

DIFFERENTIAL DIAGNOSIS

Fresh or Old Scar

- Dense collagen bundles, usually oriented parallel to the epidermis
- Verticalized blood vessels
- Clinical history of previous biopsy/procedure or trauma is helpful

Desmoplastic Nevi

- Desmoplastic Spitz nevus
  ○ Occurs in young adults, not elderly
  ○ Often shows scattered epithelioid cells
- Desmoplastic intradermal nevus

Spindle Cell Squamous Cell Carcinoma

- Spindle cell and desmoplastic SCC can histologically mimic DM
- Positive for HMWCKs, p63; S100(-)

Atypical Fibroxanthoma (AFX)

- Also occurs in heavily sun-damaged skin of elderly
- Usually more cellular proliferation of frankly atypical, enlarged pleomorphic cells
- Lacks stromal desmoplasia in most cases
- S100(-); CD10/CD68/CD99(+)

Fibrohistiocytic Tumors

- Dermatofibroma
  ○ Collagen entrapment and overlying epidermal hyperplasia
  ○ Lacks significant cytologic atypia
  ○ CD10/CD68/FXIIIa usually positive; S100(-)
- Dermatofibrosarcoma protuberans
  ○ Bland cellular spindle cell proliferation with storiforming
  ○ CD34(+); S100(-)

Neural Tumors

- Neurofibroma
  ○ Lacks significant cytologic atypia or lymphoid aggregates
  ○ S100/SOX10(+); CD34(+) (not in DM)
- Superficial malignant peripheral nerve sheath tumor
  ○ Rare, but shows similar immunohistochemical profile as DM (S100[+], SOX10[+/-]; negative for other melanocytic markers)

Leiomyosarcoma

- Fascicles of eosinophilic-staining cells
  ○ Actin/desmin (+), S100(-)

DIAGNOSTIC CHECKLIST

Pathologic Interpretation Pearls

- Extensive scar-like areas with prominent fibroblastic component and lymphoid aggregates should raise suspicion for DM
- If concerned about DM, examine the dermal-epidermal junction for the presence of an in situ component

SELECTED REFERENCES

1. Bernaba BN et al: Potentially useful markers for desmoplastic melanoma: an analysis of KBA.62, p-AKT, and ezrin. Am J Dermatopathol. 33(4):333-7; quiz 338-40, 2011
2. Busam KJ: Desmoplastic melanoma. Clin Lab Med. 31(2):321-30, 2011
3. Feng Z et al: Incidence and survival of desmoplastic melanoma in the United States, 1992-2007. J Cutan Pathol. 38(8):616-24, 2011
4. Murali R et al: Clinical and pathological features of metastases of primary cutaneous desmoplastic melanoma. Histopathology. 58(6):886-95, 2011
5. Ramos-Herberth FI et al: SOX10 immunostaining distinguishes desmoplastic melanoma from excision scar. J Cutan Pathol. 37(9):944-52, 2010
6. Busam KJ et al: Cutaneous desmoplastic melanoma: reappraisal of morphologic heterogeneity and prognostic factors. Am J Surg Pathol. 28(11):1518-25, 2004
7. Bruijn JA et al: Desmoplastic melanoma: clinicopathologic aspects of six cases. Dermatology. 185(1):3-8, 1992

DESMOPLASTIC MELANOMA

Microscopic Features

(Left) Aggregates of lymphoid infiltrate ⊃ and solar elastosis ➔ are readily found in most cases and are clues to suggest the diagnosis. *(Right)* Poorly nested, lentiginous growth of atypical melanocytes ⊃ in the epidermis and follicular epithelium is consistent with an in situ component. This finding is helpful in confirming the diagnosis.

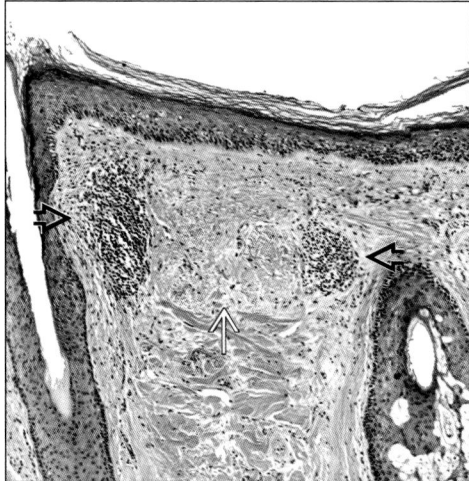
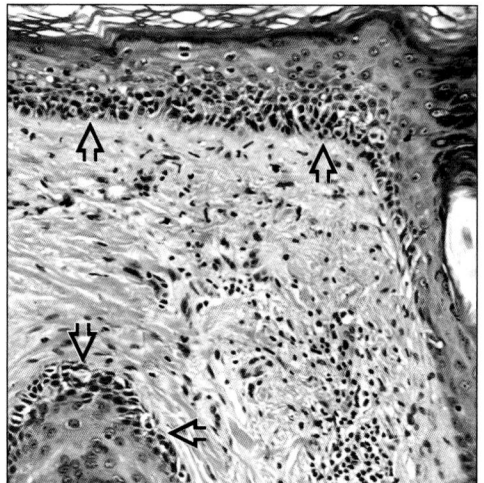

(Left) An example of DM arising in very severely solar-damaged skin, with a relatively dense chronic inflammatory infiltrate in the dermis ⬀, is shown. Note the small focus of overlying melanoma in situ ⊃. *(Right)* This desmoplastic melanoma shows a very dense lymphoid infiltrate at the deep aspect of the tumor. There is adjacent stromal desmoplasia with scattered atypical, hyperchromatic-staining spindle cells ➔ (which were strongly S100[+], not shown).

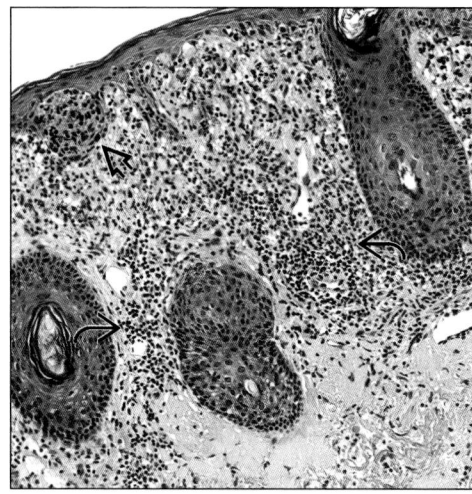
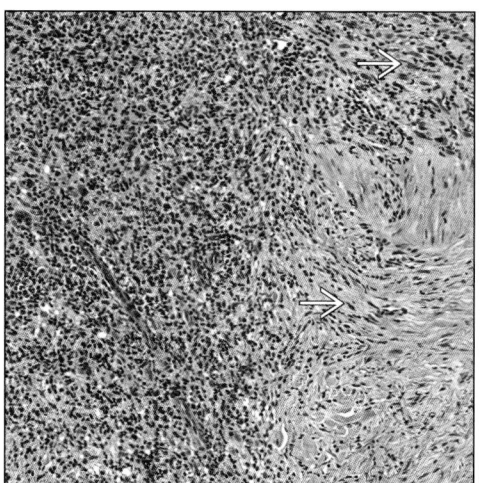

(Left) An area of desmoplastic melanoma shows stromal sclerosis with hyalinized balls of collagen resembling those seen in dermatofibromas. However, note the presence of atypical, hyperchromatic nuclei ➔ and adjacent lymphoid aggregates ⬀. *(Right)* Mitotic figures ➔ may be seen in DM, but they are usually sparse. Additional sections may be needed to search for mitotic activity.

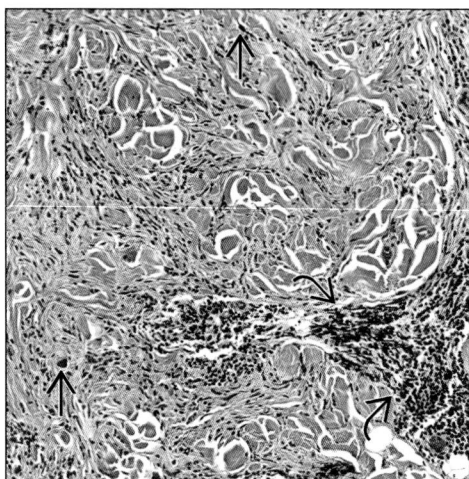
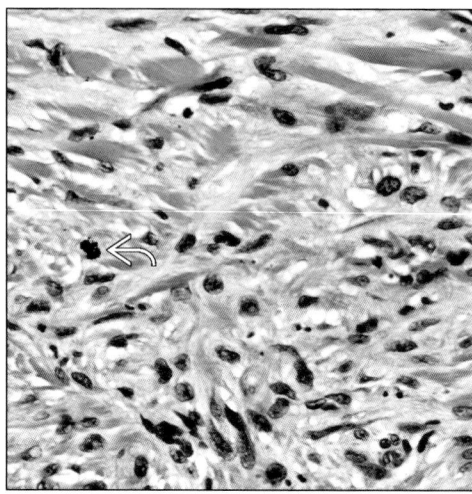

Immunohistochemical Features and Differential Diagnosis

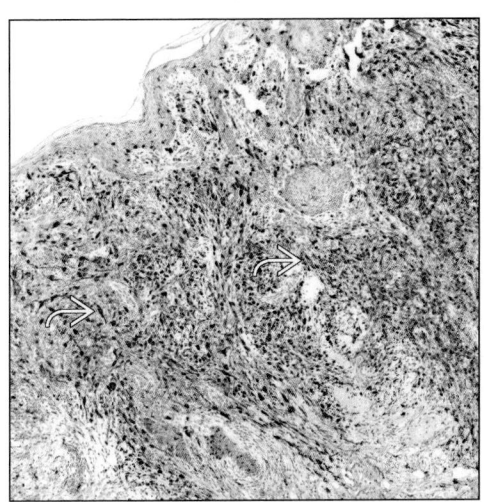

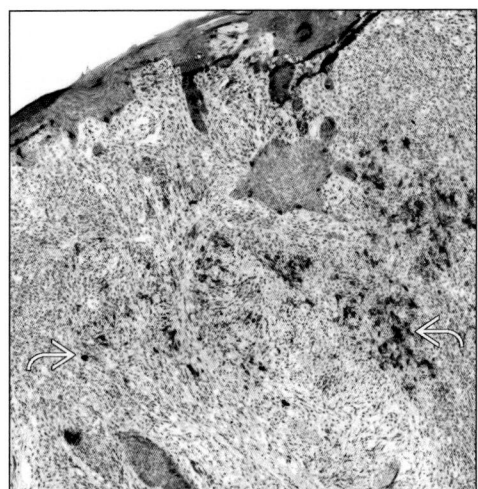

(Left) S100 immunohistochemistry shows strong and diffuse nuclear and cytoplasmic staining ⇗ of the dermal spindle cell population in DM. *(Right)* Melan-A stain shows patchy staining of a portion of tumor cells ⇗. Although most often negative in DM, markers such as MART-1/Melan-A, HMB-45, and tyrosinase can occasionally be positive (reportedly in up to 20-25% of cases).

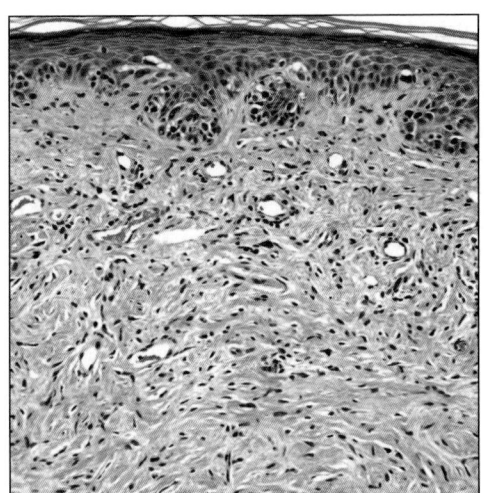

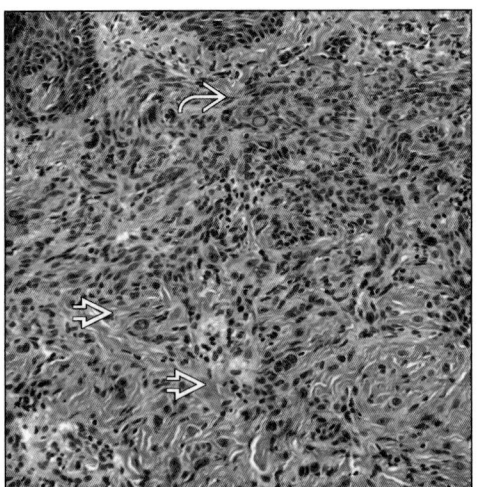

(Left) Atypical combined nevus with a desmoplastic nevus component in the dermis is shown. The junctional component is moderately atypical, but the dermal cells are small and bland-appearing. Note the lack of severe solar elastosis and lymphoid aggregates typical of DM. *(Right)* Desmoplastic Spitz nevus shows spindled and epithelioid cells arrayed in irregular nests, short fascicles ⇗, and cords in a dense, hyalinized-appearing stroma ⇗. These tumors typically occur in young adults.

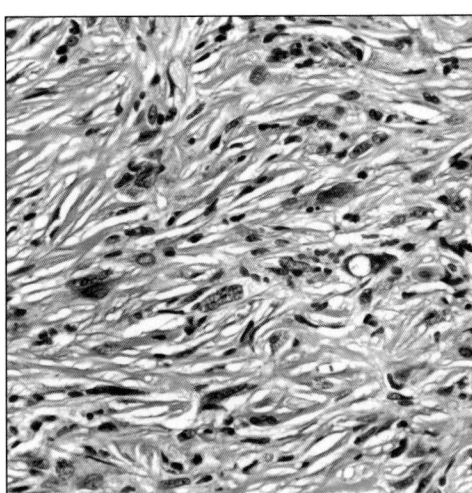

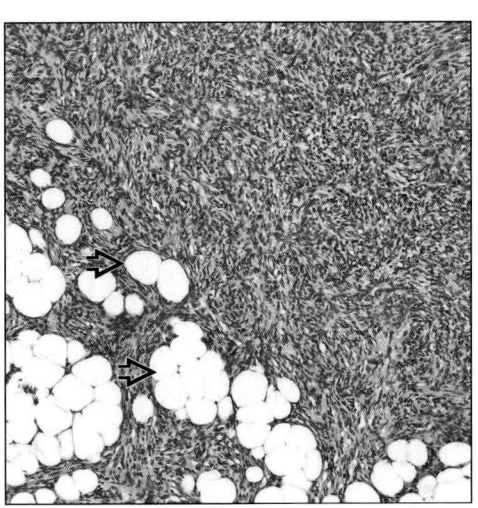

(Left) Atypical DF/fibrous histiocytoma shows a proliferation of enlarged and pleomorphic spindle-shaped and histiocytoid cells, which are larger than those typically seen in DM. In addition, the cells are S100(-) and CD10/CD68/FXIIIa(+). *(Right)* DFSP shows deep dermal and subcutaneous involvement by a cellular spindle cell tumor with honeycombing fat entrapment ⇗. These tumors are more cellular than DM typically is, lack the stromal desmoplasia, and are S100(-)/CD34(+).

NEVOID MELANOMA

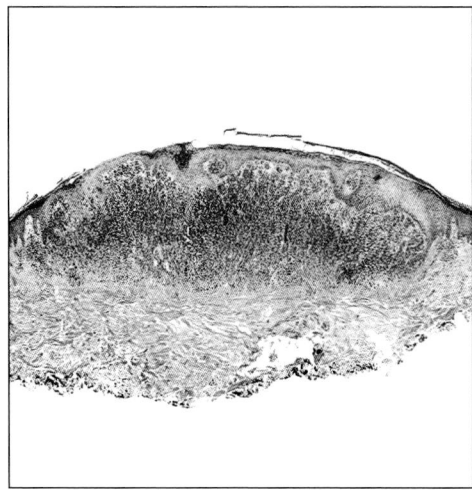

Nevoid melanoma is deceptively symmetrical appearing on low-power examination, mimicking a compound or intradermal nevus.

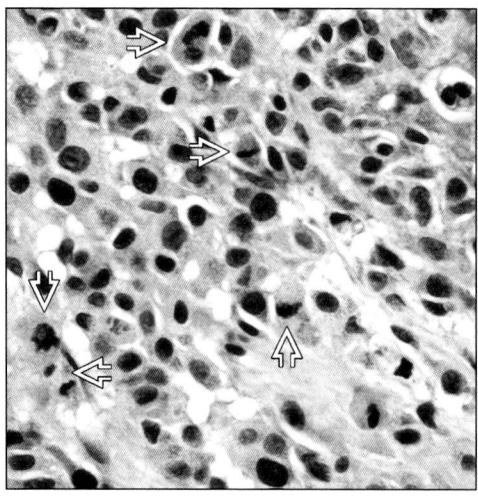

On high-power examination, numerous mitotic figures ▶ are easily found in this nevoid melanoma.

TERMINOLOGY

Synonyms
- Some cases have been described as "minimal deviation melanoma," but this term is very controversial and should be avoided

Definitions
- Uncommon variant of melanoma that shows histological features mimicking a nevus

ETIOLOGY/PATHOGENESIS

Environmental Exposure
- Likely solar/UV radiation related, similar to most types of melanoma

CLINICAL ISSUES

Presentation
- Occurs in wide age range
- Can be ubiquitous, but occurs more frequently on the back and extremities
- Dome-shaped papule or nodule, or a verrucous lesion
- Often not recognized clinically as melanoma
  - Can resemble a nevus or basal cell carcinoma

Treatment
- Surgical approaches
  - Complete excision with clear margins
  - Sentinel lymph node biopsy often performed for staging, especially if lesion is thicker than 1.0 mm or
    - Level IV
    - Ulcerated
    - Exhibits dermal mitotic figures

Prognosis
- Similar to conventional melanoma

- Determined by AJCC staging, especially the depth of invasion (Breslow depth), ulceration, and mitotic activity

MICROSCOPIC PATHOLOGY

Histologic Features
- At scanning magnification, there are 2 variants
  - Verrucous or papillated
    - Mimics polypoid intradermal melanocytic nevus
  - Flat or dome shaped
    - Mimics ordinary intradermal or compound melanocytic nevus
- Imparts "nevoid" appearance on initial examination
  - Cells mimic type A nevus cells
  - Can also mimic lymphocytes
- Tightly packed, it forms "sheets" of relatively banal-appearing nevoid cells
  - Hypercellular
  - Sheets, not nests, are often present
- Slightly asymmetric
- Predominantly intradermal
- May exhibit "pseudomaturation" with increasing dermal depth
  - At low-power examination, it may appear that intradermal cells mature
  - However, atypia and mitotic figures should be identified at high magnification

Cytologic Features
- Abundant eosinophilic cytoplasm
- Round to oval vesicular nuclei
- Prominent nucleoli seen at high magnification
- Nuclear pleomorphism, best appreciated at high magnification
- Mitotic activity present, often deep within lesion
- Atypical mitotic figures

NEVOID MELANOMA

Key Facts

Terminology
- Uncommon variant of conventional melanoma that looks deceptively benign

Clinical Issues
- Melanoma is not suspected clinically

Microscopic Pathology
- Dome shaped or verrucous
- Exhibits pseudomaturation

- Increased mitotic activity or proliferation index

Ancillary Tests
- Immunostaining for Ki-67 (or MIB-1) to determine proliferation index (> 5-10% supports the diagnosis)

Top Differential Diagnoses
- Intradermal melanocytic nevus
- Congenital melanocytic nevus
- Combined melanocytic nevus

DIFFERENTIAL DIAGNOSIS

Intradermal Melanocytic Nevus
- No sheeting
- Lack of prominent nucleoli and mitotic activity

Congenital Melanocytic Nevus
- Band-like proliferation of cells surrounding adnexal structures
- Matures properly with increasing dermal depth

Combined Melanocytic Nevus
- May show mixture of type A nevus cells with other cell types
  - Type B or C nevus cells
- Matures properly with increasing dermal depth

DIAGNOSTIC CHECKLIST

Clinically Relevant Pathologic Features
- Finding 1 dermal mitotic figure alone usually does not justify diagnosis of melanoma, especially if superficial; however it indicates need to look for other clues to support diagnosis of melanoma
- Nevoid melanoma is classic diagnostic trap
  - Diagnosis is not infrequently made retrospectively after appearance of metastases

Pathologic Interpretation Pearls
- Look for sheet-like growth pattern in dermis
- Beware of hypercellular areas in dermis

- Search for lack of cellular dispersion at bottom of lesion
- Examine for mitoses, especially multiple, deep, or atypical forms

SELECTED REFERENCES

1. Diwan AH et al: Nevoid melanoma. Clin Lab Med. 31(2):243-53, 2011
2. Massi G et al: Histological Diagnosis of Nevi and Melanoma. New York: Springer-Verlag, 2004
3. Zembowicz A et al: Morphological analysis of nevoid melanoma: a study of 20 cases with a review of the literature. Am J Dermatopathol. 23(3):167-75, 2001
4. McNutt NS: "Triggered trap": nevoid malignant melanoma. Semin Diagn Pathol. 15(3):203-9, 1998
5. McNutt NS et al: Nevoid malignant melanoma: morphologic patterns and immunohistochemical reactivity. J Cutan Pathol. 22(6):502-17, 1995
6. Wong TY et al: Nevoid melanoma: a clinicopathological study of seven cases of malignant melanoma mimicking spindle and epithelioid cell nevus and verrucous dermal nevus. Hum Pathol. 26(2):171-9, 1995
7. Blessing K et al: Verrucous naevoid and keratotic malignant melanoma: a clinico-pathological study of 20 cases. Histopathology. 23(5):453-8, 1993
8. Wong TY et al: Melanoma mimicking dermal and Spitz's nevus ("nevoid" melanoma). Semin Surg Oncol. 9(3):188-93, 1993
9. Muhlbauer JE et al: Minimal deviation melanoma: a histologic variant of cutaneous malignant melanoma in its vertical growth phase. J Invest Dermatol. 80 Suppl:63s-65s, 1983

IMAGE GALLERY

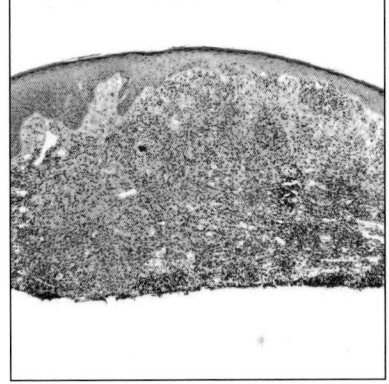 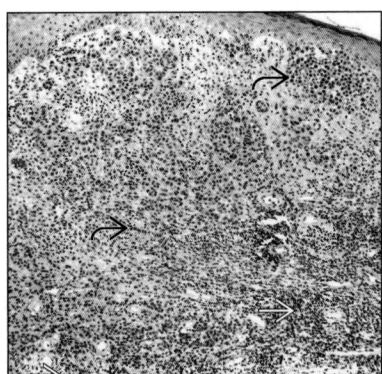 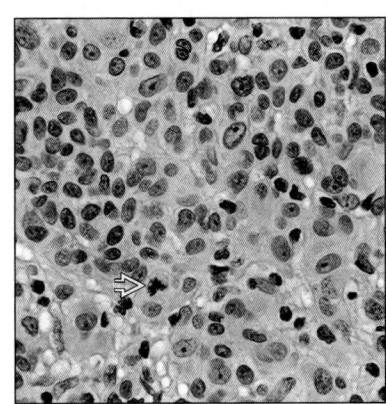

(Left) Low-power examination shows a deceptively bland-appearing compound, predominantly intradermal proliferation, mimicking a nevus. (Center) Higher magnification shows that the cells are hyperchromatic-staining ⬈ and do not show definite evidence of maturation with dermal descent. Note also the relatively dense surrounding lymphoid infiltrate ⬊. (Right) High magnification shows large cells with eosinophilic cytoplasm and a mitotic figure ⬊ is seen deep in the lesion.

ACRAL LENTIGINOUS MELANOMA

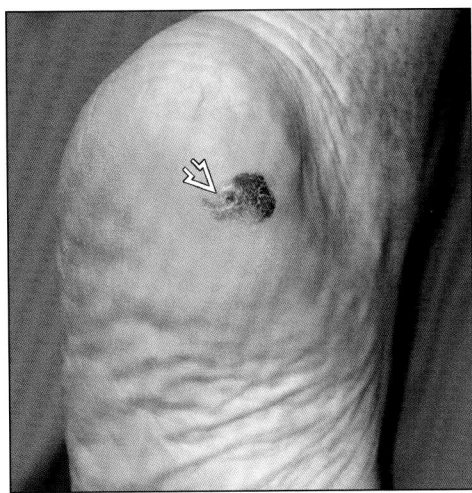

The heel of this patient shows a dark brown plaque with early depigmentation ➡. (Courtesy J. Finch, MD.)

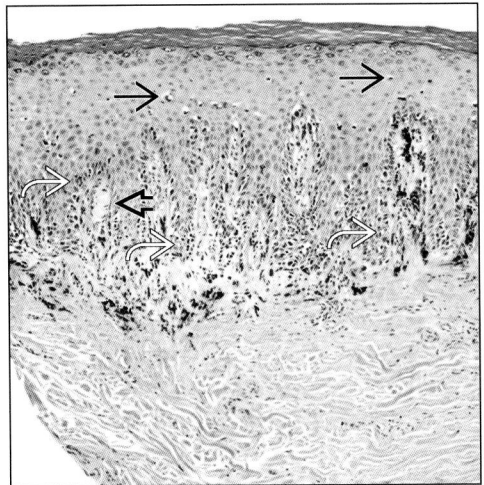

Lentiginous growth of atypical melanocytes ➡ is seen in this early in situ lesion. Only rare upward scatter ➡ of atypical melanocytes is identified. A Meissner corpuscle ➡ is seen in the dermis.

TERMINOLOGY

Abbreviations
- Acral lentiginous melanoma (ALM)

Definitions
- Form of cutaneous melanoma that microscopically grows in a lentiginous array and occurs on acral sites
  - Palms
  - Soles
  - Digits
  - Subungual regions

CLINICAL ISSUES

Presentation
- < 5% of all malignant melanomas
- More common on sole of foot or in subungual region of big toe or thumb
- Most frequently reported symptoms are change in size, bleeding, change in color, and becoming raised or nodular
  - May remain flat or present as large, pigmented macule
  - Lesion becomes darker and more irregular as it progresses
  - Invasive areas may be associated with hyperkeratotic plaques, papules, nodules, and even ulceration
  - Spreads rapidly
- Average age at diagnosis is between 60-70 years old
- Relatively uncommon in Caucasians, but most common subtype of melanomas in Asians and Africans

Treatment
- Surgical approaches
  - Wide surgical excision and amputation give comparable survival rates
  - In many cases of subungual melanomas, amputation is preferred due to relative lack of soft tissue between tumor and bone beneath nail

Prognosis
- Compared to other cutaneous melanomas, disease-specific survival rates are lower
  - 5-year melanoma-specific survival rates: 80.3%
  - 10-year melanoma-specific survival rates: 67.5%
- Compared to other melanomas matched for Breslow thickness, the prognosis is the same

MACROSCOPIC FEATURES

Dermoscopic Exam
- Shows parallel ridge pattern, where globules may be seen symmetrically along both sides of furrows

Areas of Regression
- Appear as gray-white coloration
- Become extensive in larger, invasive lesions

Epiluminescent Examination
- Differentiates benign from malignant
  - Benign lesions display pigmentation following the depressions between dermatoglyphic ridges
  - Melanomas display pigmentation overlying the dermatoglyphic ridges

MICROSCOPIC PATHOLOGY

Histologic Features
- Growth pattern of atypical melanocytes
  - Early lesions
    - Lentiginous array
    - Scattered among basal layer keratinocytes
  - Late lesions
    - Lentiginous array is no longer present
    - Confluent at dermal-epidermal junction

ACRAL LENTIGINOUS MELANOMA

Key Facts

Terminology
- Acral melanoma that grows in a lentiginous pattern

Clinical Issues
- < 5% of all malignant melanomas
- Most often on sole of foot or subungual region

Microscopic Pathology
- Lentiginous proliferation of atypical melanocytes with rare pagetoid scatter

- ALM in situ may present with very few atypical melanocytes
- Nesting at dermal-epidermal junction
  - Rare to absent in early lesions, prominent and confluent in late lesions
  - Nests are irregular in size and shape, randomly alternate with single melanocytes
- Cells show elongated, ovoid hyperchromatic nuclei with little cytoplasm

---

- Invasion of atypical cells into the dermis
- Nesting at dermal-epidermal junction
  - Early lesions
    - Absent to poorly formed
  - Late lesions
    - Prominent and confluent
    - Nests are irregular in size and shape, and they randomly alternate with single melanocytes
- ALM in situ may present with very few atypical melanocytes before progressing to invasive ALM
- Inflammatory response in superficial dermis
  - Lichenoid pattern with areas of subepidermal clefts
  - Leukocytes typically found in dermis except early lesions

Cytologic Features
- Elongated, ovoid shape with little cytoplasm
- Nuclei are
  - Hyperchromatic
  - Vertically oriented
  - Angulated
- Little nucleolar detail
- Pagetoid cells may appear epithelioid
- Invasive cells appear spindled

DIFFERENTIAL DIAGNOSIS

Acral Melanocytic Nevus
- Need to examine entire lesion, especially periphery, to differentiate acral melanocytic nevus from early lesion of ALM

Spindle Cell Melanoma
- Dermal component of ALM is frequently spindle-shaped
- Lacks overlying melanoma in situ with characteristic features of ALM in situ

Clinical Differential
- Tinea nigra (darkly pigmented macule with irregular borders)
- Subungual hematoma caused by trauma (talon noir)

DIAGNOSTIC CHECKLIST

Pathologic Interpretation Pearls
- Early lesions are difficult to diagnose
  - Very few neoplastic melanocytes may be present
- Exercise caution when evaluating partially sampled lesions

SELECTED REFERENCES

1. Pollack LA et al: Melanoma survival in the United States, 1992 to 2005. J Am Acad Dermatol. 65(5 Suppl 1):S78-86, 2011
2. Wu XC et al: Racial and ethnic variations in incidence and survival of cutaneous melanoma in the United States, 1999-2006. J Am Acad Dermatol. 65(5 Suppl 1):S26-37, 2011
3. Bradford PT et al: Acral lentiginous melanoma: incidence and survival patterns in the United States, 1986-2005. Arch Dermatol. 145(4):427-34, 2009

IMAGE GALLERY

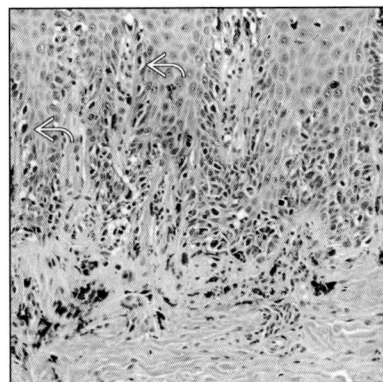 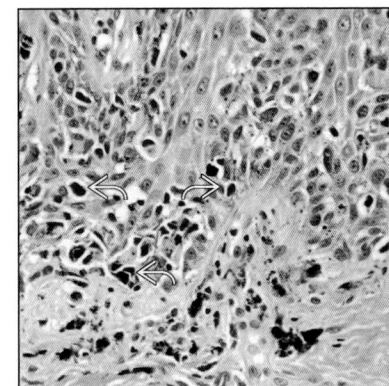 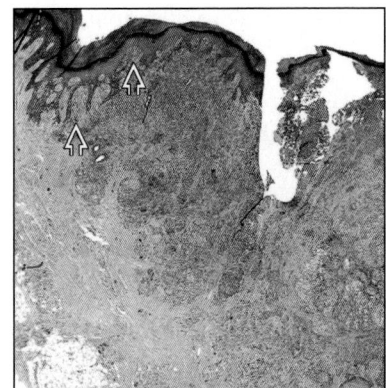

(Left) Lentiginous growth ➤ and lack of nesting at the dermal-epidermal junction are evident in this in situ lesion. (Center) Higher magnification of the same lesion shows angulated, hyperchromatic nuclei with scant amounts of cytoplasm ➤. (Right) A late invasive lesion is well nested ➤ at the dermal-epidermal junction. The lentiginous in situ growth phase may be identified in the periphery of the lesion.

ORAL MELANOMA

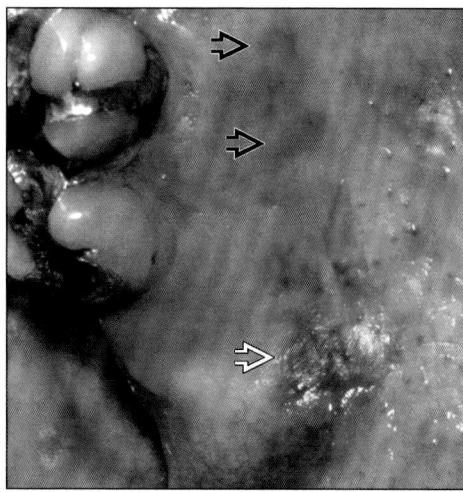

Primary melanoma of the hard palate presents as a diffuse, patchy area of heavy pigmentation with irregular borders ➡. Satellite lesions are noted away from the main area of pigmentation ➡.

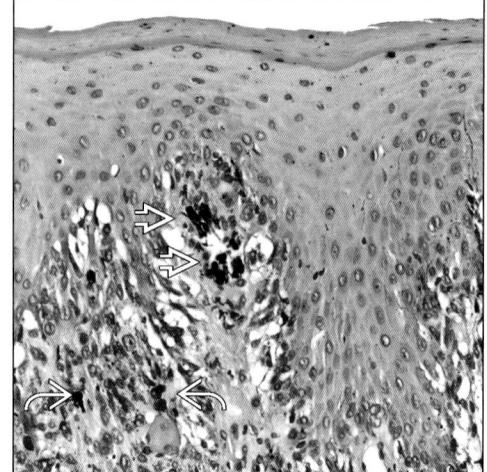

High magnification shows mucosal lentiginous melanoma of the hard palate with numerous atypical melanocytes present in the basal epithelium ➡ and invasion into the superficial submucosa ➡.

TERMINOLOGY

Definitions
- Malignant neural crest-derived neoplasm with melanocytic differentiation
  - Atypical melanocytes at epithelial-connective tissue interface with upward migration or connective tissue invasion

ETIOLOGY/PATHOGENESIS

Etiology
- Unknown (no ultraviolet exposure)

CLINICAL ISSUES

Epidemiology
- Incidence
  - Extremely rare, accounting for < 1% of all melanomas
    - 0.02/100,000 population/year in USA
  - Represent about 50% of all head and neck mucosal melanomas
  - Represent < 0.5% of all oral malignancies
  - Unlike cutaneous melanoma, oral melanoma incidence has been stable
- Age
  - Mean in 6th-7th decades
  - Rare in pediatric age group
- Gender
  - Male > female (2.5-3:1)
- Ethnicity
  - More common in Japan and western Africa

Site
- Hard palate and maxillary alveolus are most common sites of involvement (~ 80%)
- Remaining 20% include

  - Mandibular gingivae
  - Buccal mucosa
  - Floor of mouth and tongue

Presentation
- Most arise de novo although 1/3 are preceded by pigmented lesion for a few months or years
  - "Melanosis" reported before development of melanoma
- Asymmetric, painless, pigmented lesion
  - Irregular borders or outlines
  - Black, purple, red, gray
    - 15% of oral melanomas are amelanotic
  - Macular, with nodular areas
- Many patients present at advanced stage with pain, ulceration, loose teeth
- Cervical lymph nodes mets reported in up to 75% of cases at presentation
- Distant metastases present in about 50% at presentation

Treatment
- Surgical approaches
  - Radical surgical excision
    - Clear margins not always possible due to vital structures
  - Recommendation for regional lymph node dissection, even in clinically negative neck
- Adjuvant therapy
  - No clear cut evidence that chemotherapy or immunotherapy for oral melanoma provides any survival benefits
    - Generally used for palliative purposes
  - Not recommended as a single modality treatment
- Radiation
  - May provide prolonged palliation, but does not appear to provide any survival benefits

Prognosis
- Overall, poor prognosis
  - Median survival: 2 years

Key Facts

Terminology

- Malignant neural crest-derived neoplasm with melanocytic differentiation

Clinical Issues

- Extremely rare, accounting for < 1% of all melanomas
  - Represent < 0.5% of all oral malignancies
- Mean in 6th-7th decades
- Male > female (2.5-3:1)
- Hard palate and maxillary alveolus are most common sites of involvement (~ 80%)
- Cervical lymph nodes mets reported in > 50% of cases at presentation
- Asymmetric, painless, pigmented lesion with irregular borders
- Radical surgical excision
- Overall, poor prognosis (median: 2 years)

Image Findings

- Oral cavity mass with high T1WI on MR

Microscopic Pathology

- Pagetoid spread or in situ component with single or multiple melanoma cells in superficial epithelium
- Epithelioid or spindle-shaped morphology to melanocytes containing fine melanin granules
- 1/3 of cases have bone/cartilage invasion

Ancillary Tests

- Generally diffuse and strong staining for S100 protein, HMB-45, and vimentin

Top Differential Diagnoses

- Metastatic melanoma, spindle cell squamous cell carcinoma, pleomorphic sarcoma

---

- 5-year survival: 5-10%
- High rates of metastases to liver, brain, and lung
- Worse prognosis suggested by
  - Thickness of > 5 mm
  - Vascular invasion
  - Necrosis
  - Significant pleomorphism
  - Older age
  - High stage correlates with poor outcome

IMAGE FINDINGS

MR Findings

- Best imaging study is multiplanar MR imaging
- Oral cavity mass with high T1WI on MR
  - Melanotic melanomas show increased signal due to melanin, free radicals, metal ions, and hemorrhage, giving high or intermediate T1 signal

MACROSCOPIC FEATURES

General Features

- Brown to black pigmented lesion with irregular borders
- Flat macule extends laterally (radial growth phase); nodular lesion (vertical growth phase)
  - Some oral melanomas lack radial growth phase
- Satellite lesions of melanoma are common

Sections to Be Submitted

- Bone &/or cartilage for staging

Size

- Up to 4 cm generally

MICROSCOPIC PATHOLOGY

Histologic Features

- Radial growth phase similar to acral lentiginous melanoma

- Pagetoid spread (in situ): Single or multiple melanoma cells within epithelium above basal zone
- Atypical melanocytes in basal layer spreading laterally
- Superficial invasion of melanoma cells into lamina propria
- Prominent dendritic processes may be seen
- Nodular growth phase
  - Epithelioid or spindle-shaped morphology of melanocytes containing fine melanin granules
    - 15% of oral melanomas have little to no melanin
  - 1/3 of cases have bone/cartilage invasion
  - Vascular and perineural invasion not readily noted
  - Mitoses tend to be infrequent, but are increased in invasive tumors
  - Pleomorphic cells with atypical mitoses
  - Squamous surface ulceration or atrophy is common

ANCILLARY TESTS

Histochemistry

- Melanin can be highlighted with Masson-Fontana or Schmorl stains

Immunohistochemistry

- Generally diffuse and strong staining for S100, HMB-45, and vimentin
  - Tyrosinase, MART-1/Melan-A, and MITF are also positive
- Negative: Cytokeratin, myogenic markers, epithelial membrane antigen

Molecular Genetics

- NRAS and KIT mutations have been identified in mucosal melanomas
  - May be useful for targeted therapies

ORAL MELANOMA

Immunohistochemistry

Antibody	Reactivity	Staining Pattern	Comment
S100	Positive	Nuclear & cytoplasmic	Diffuse and strong
HMB-45	Positive	Cytoplasmic	Positive in most cases
Tyrosinase	Positive	Cytoplasmic	Variably reactive in most cases
melan-A103	Positive	Cytoplasmic	Positive in most cases
MITF	Positive	Nuclear	Positive in most cases
Vimentin	Positive	Cytoplasmic	All tumor cells positive
CD117	Positive	Cytoplasmic	Isolated tumor cells positive
CK-PAN	Negative		
Desmin	Negative		
CD45RB	Negative		

AJCC TNM Staging Criteria for Oral Melanoma (2010)

TNM	Stage Categories	Definition
Primary tumor (T)	pT3	Mucosal disease only
	pT4a	Moderately advanced disease
		Tumor involving deep soft tissue, cartilage, bone, or overlying skin
	pT4b	Very advanced disease
		Tumor involving brain, dura, skull base, lower cranial nerves (IX, X, XI, XII), masticator space, carotid artery, prevertebral space, or mediastinal structures
Regional lymph nodes (N)	NX	Regional lymph nodes cannot be assessed
	N0	No regional lymph node metastases
	N1	Regional lymph node metastasis present
Distant metastasis (M)		No distant metastasis (no pathologic M0; use clinical M to complete stage group)
	M1	Distant metastasis

Adapted from 7th edition AJCC Staging Forms.

AJCC Pathologic Prognostic Groups for Oral Melanoma (2010)

Group	T	N	M
III	T3	N0	M0
IVA	T4a	N0	M0
	T3-T4a	N1	M0
IVB	T4b	Any N	M0
IVC	Any T	Any N	M1

Adapted from 7th edition AJCC Staging Forms.

DIFFERENTIAL DIAGNOSIS

Metastatic Melanoma
- Extremely rare with very few reported cases of metastases to oral cavity
- Most common: Tongue, buccal mucosa, lip
- Clinical history necessary for distinction

Spindle Cell Squamous Cell Carcinoma
- Should be considered when there is no pigmentation
- Epithelial origin frequently present
- High-grade tumors with significant pleomorphism, increased mitoses
- Immunohistochemistry will separate these entities
  o Epithelial markers positive in up to 70% of cases
  o Lack melanoma markers

Pleomorphic Sarcoma
- High-grade spindled cell tumor
- Lacks surface origin or involvement
- By definition, lacks melanocytic and epithelial markers

SELECTED REFERENCES

1. Moreno MA et al: Management of mucosal melanomas of the head and neck: did we make any progress? Curr Opin Otolaryngol Head Neck Surg. 18(2):101-6, 2010
2. Bachar G et al: Mucosal melanomas of the head and neck: experience of the Princess Margaret Hospital. Head Neck. 30(10):1325-31, 2008
3. Femiano F et al: Oral malignant melanoma: a review of the literature. J Oral Pathol Med. 37(7):383-8, 2008

ORAL MELANOMA

Microscopic and Immunohistochemical Features

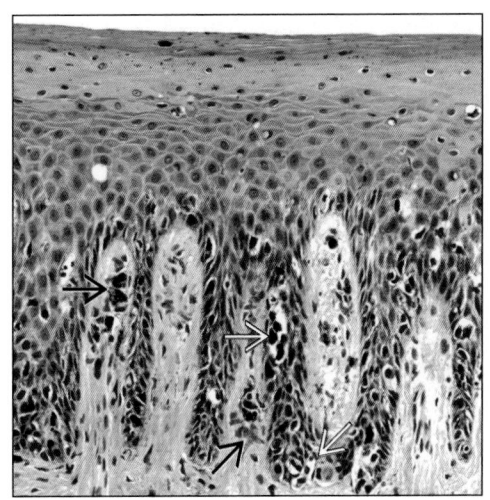
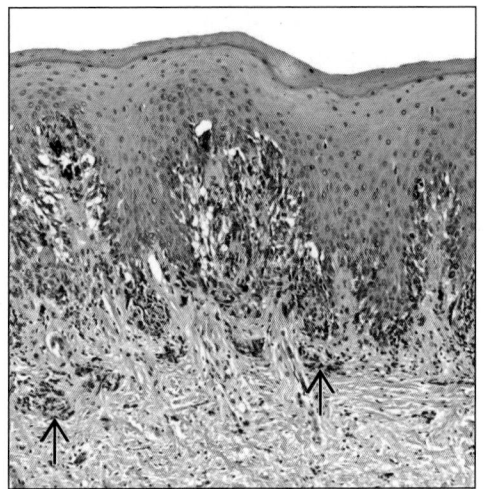

(Left) *In situ growth phase shows atypical and enlarged melanocytes at the epithelial-stromal junction. A number of pigmented melanophages ⊃ are present in the stroma. Small nests of atypical melanocytes ⇒ are present along the junction.* **(Right)** *The majority of the proliferation in this melanoma is noted at the epithelial-stromal junction. However, isolated nests of atypical melanocytes ⊃ are noted within the superficial region of the stroma. Inflammatory cells are inconspicuous.*

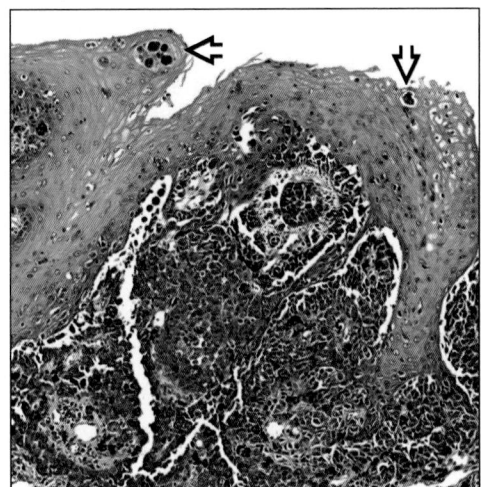
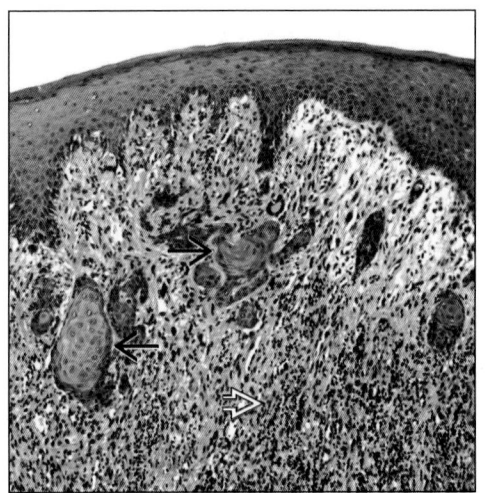

(Left) *Nodular melanoma of the hard palate is shown with epithelioid malignant melanocytes, some with melanin pigment present in the lamina propria. Individual melanocytes are invading into the upper level of the epithelium ⊃. **(Right)** Concurrent pseudoepitheliomatous hyperplasia ⇒ is present in association with atypical melanocytic proliferation. An inflammatory infiltrate is also present in the stroma ⊃. The melanoma may be missed or obscured by this process.*

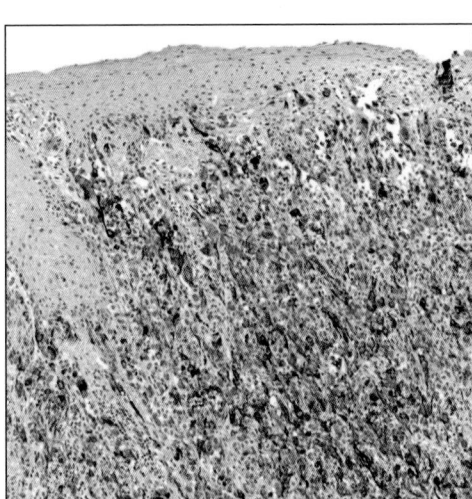
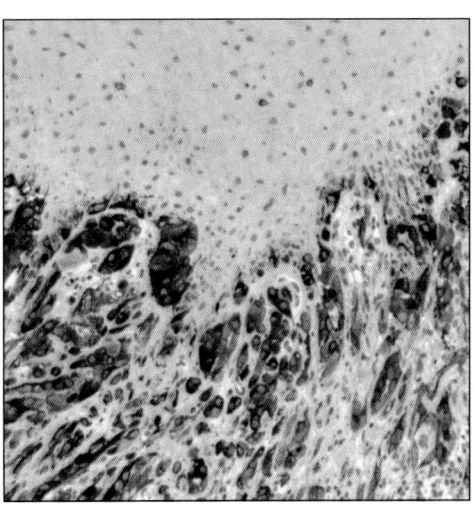

(Left) *S100 shows a very strong and diffuse nuclear and cytoplasmic reactivity in the neoplastic cells as they invade from the surface epithelium into the stroma. Depth of invasion is difficult to assess for oral melanoma. **(Right)** HMB-45 immunohistochemistry highlights the melanocytes present both in the basal layer as well as in the submucosa. This is one of the more specific markers for melanoma. It is important to know that staining can be patchy or focal.*

MUCOSAL MELANOMA (GENITAL)

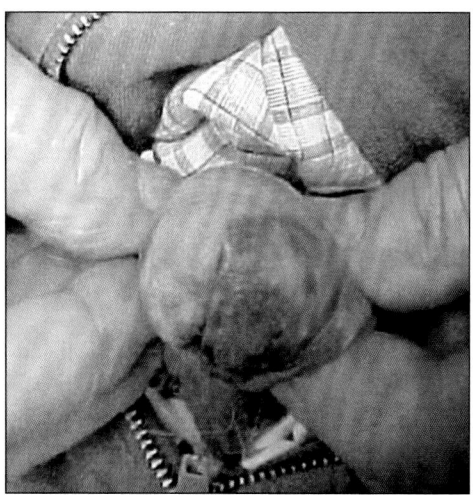

Clinical photograph shows a mucosal melanoma on the glans penis of an elderly patient. Histologic examination showed an invasive nodular type melanoma.

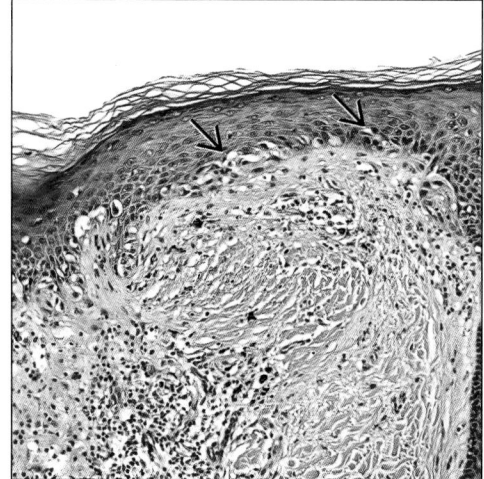

Mucosal melanoma in situ of the vulva shows a lentiginous and confluent pattern of growth without significant pagetoid spread (similar to lentigo maligna) ➡

TERMINOLOGY

Abbreviations
- Mucosal malignant melanoma (MMM)

Synonyms
- Vulvar melanoma, vaginal melanoma, penile melanoma, scrotal melanoma

Definitions
- Malignant tumor of melanocytes

ETIOLOGY/PATHOGENESIS

Unknown in Most Cases
- Alterations in *KIT* (~ 30% of cases)
- *NRAS* mutations have been reported
- 6% are associated with nevi
- Family history and genetic susceptibility

CLINICAL ISSUES

Epidemiology
- Incidence
  - Rare
    - ~ 2% of all melanomas in females
    - Even less frequent in males
- Age
  - 6th to 7th decade

Site
- Females
  - Vulva, vagina, and cervix
    - Labia majora and clitoris (most frequent sites)
- Males
  - Penis and scrotum
    - Glans (most frequent site)

Presentation
- Flat to nodular to polypoid lesions
- Irregular to well-defined borders
- Amelanotic, brown or black
  - 27% of vulvar MMM may be amelanotic
  - Such lesions mimic SCC or Paget disease
- Areas of regression may appear red, gray, or white

Treatment
- Surgical approaches
  - Surgical excision
  - Sentinel node biopsy for staging purposes
- Adjuvant therapy
  - Chemotherapy or immunotherapy (no definitive evidence of improved survival)
  - Molecularly targeted therapy (under investigation)

Prognosis
- Tumor thickness is most important parameter
- Similar to skin melanoma of comparable thickness

MACROSCOPIC FEATURES

General Features
- A few millimeters to several centimeters

MICROSCOPIC PATHOLOGY

Histologic Features
- Different histological variants may affect genital areas
  - Lentiginous (similar to lentigo maligna and acral lentiginous melanoma)
  - Superficial spreading
  - Nodular
  - Desmoplastic/neurotropic
- Neoplastic cells vary in morphology
  - Epithelioid, spindled, or nevoid
- Melanoma in situ
  - Confined to epidermis

MUCOSAL MELANOMA (GENITAL)

Key Facts

Clinical Issues
- Vulva (most frequent site in females)
- Glans penis (most common site in males)
- Flat to nodular to polypoid lesions
- Amelanotic, brown to black
  - Foci of regression appear red, gray, or white

Microscopic Pathology
- Different histological variants may affect genital area
  - Lentiginous
- Superficial spreading
- Nodular
- Desmoplastic/neurotropic

Top Differential Diagnoses
- Atypical genital nevi
- Nevi associated with lichen sclerosus
- SCC (in situ and invasive)
- Paget disease

- Lack of symmetry and circumscription
- Pagetoid spread from scant to prominent
- Invasive
  - Superficial or deep invasion
  - Lack of maturation with dermal descent
  - No mitoses may be seen in invasive component if superficial
- Variable amount of melanin pigment
- Ulceration &/or regression may be present

DIFFERENTIAL DIAGNOSIS

Atypical Genital Nevi
- Younger patients
- Architectural and cytologic atypia
- Focal pagetoid spread
- Maturation with descent (deep mitoses are absent)

Genital Nevi Arising in Lichen Sclerosus et Atrophicus
- Features reminiscent of "recurrent nevus phenomenon"
- Maturation (deep mitoses are absent)

SCC (In Situ and Invasive)
- Desmosomes may be evident
- Immunostains positive for keratins
- Negative for S100 and Mart-1

Paget Disease
- Atypical epithelioid cells with abundant cytoplasm

- Positive for PAS-D, CAM5.2, CK7, and CEA
- Negative for S100 and Mart-1

DIAGNOSTIC CHECKLIST

Pathologic Interpretation Pearls
- Deep mitosis is a feature of MM and not genital nevi

SELECTED REFERENCES

1. Omholt K et al: KIT pathway alterations in mucosal melanomas of the vulva and other sites. Clin Cancer Res. 17(12):3933-42, 2011
2. Gleason BC et al: Atypical genital nevi. A clinicopathologic analysis of 56 cases. Am J Surg Pathol. 32(1):51-7, 2008
3. Sugiyama VE et al: Vulvar melanoma: a multivariable analysis of 644 patients. Obstet Gynecol. 110(2 Pt 1):296-301, 2007
4. Sánchez-Ortiz R et al: Melanoma of the penis, scrotum and male urethra: a 40-year single institution experience. J Urol. 173(6):1958-65, 2005
5. Wechter ME et al: Vulvar melanoma: a report of 20 cases and review of the literature. J Am Acad Dermatol. 50(4):554-62, 2004
6. Carlson JA et al: Melanocytic proliferations associated with lichen sclerosus. Arch Dermatol. 138(1):77-87, 2002
7. Verschraegen CF et al: Vulvar melanoma at the M. D. Anderson Cancer Center: 25 years later. Int J Gynecol Cancer. 11(5):359-64, 2001
8. Ragnarsson-Olding BK et al: Malignant melanoma of the vulva in a nationwide, 25-year study of 219 Swedish females: predictors of survival. Cancer. 86(7):1285-93, 1999

IMAGE GALLERY

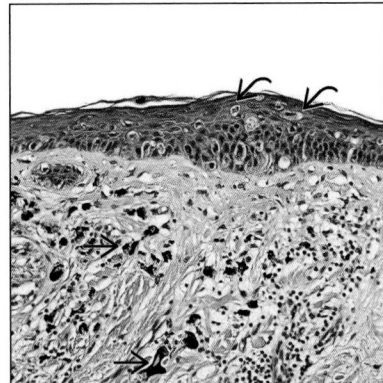
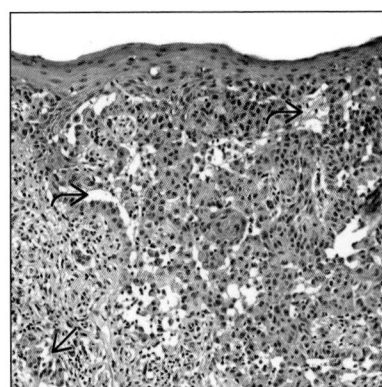
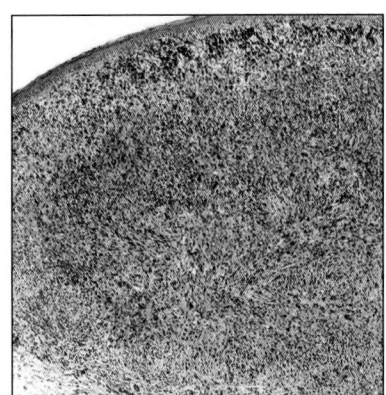

(Left) Melanoma in situ of the labia majora shows pagetoid spread ➡. Note the dermal fibrosis and pigment incontinence ➡ consistent with regression. *(Center)* Invasive mucosal melanoma shows dyscohesive growth of epithelioid melanocytes mimicking glandular structures ➡ similar to Paget disease. Note the invasive component ➡. *(Right)* This image shows genital nodular melanoma. Such deep tumors tend to have a poor prognosis due to their significant depth.

SINONASAL MELANOMA

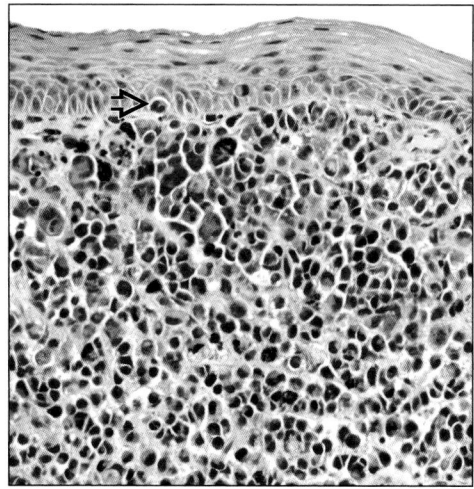

Isolated junctional neoplastic cells are noted ⊳ in this MMM. The neoplastic cells in the stroma show pleomorphism and a plasmacytoid appearance. Pigment is easily identified.

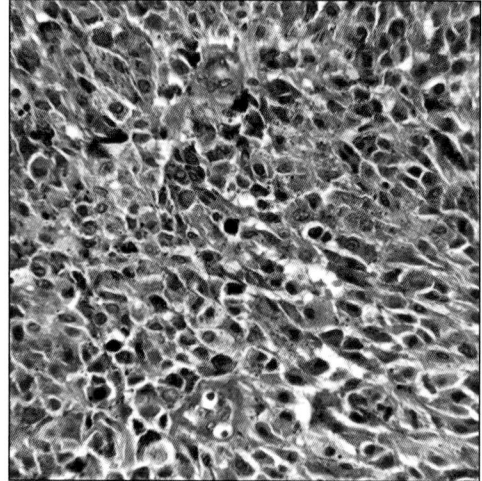

High magnification shows a spindled to polygonal population of highly atypical, pigmented neoplastic cells. These changes are characteristic of melanoma.

TERMINOLOGY

Synonyms
- Mucosal malignant melanoma (MMM)
- Sinonasal tract mucosal malignant melanoma (STMMM)

Definitions
- Neural crest-derived neoplasms originating from melanocytes and demonstrating melanocytic differentiation

ETIOLOGY/PATHOGENESIS

Environmental Exposure
- Formalin
- Possibly radiation
- UV exposure

CLINICAL ISSUES

Epidemiology
- Incidence
  - Rare
    - Represents < 1% of all melanomas
    - < 5% of all sinonasal tract neoplasms
    - 15-33% of all skin melanomas occur in head and neck
    - STMMM represent < 4% of all head and neck melanomas
- Age
  - Wide age range, usually in 5th-8th decades
- Gender
  - Equal gender distribution
- Ethnicity
  - Increased incidence in Japanese patients

Site
- About 15-20% of melanomas arise in head and neck

- 80% are cutaneous in origin
- Ocular origin account for majority of remaining MMM
- Sinonasal tract and oral cavity are next most common sites
- Anterior nasal septum > maxillary sinus

Presentation
- Nasal obstruction
- Epistaxis or nasal discharge
  - Melanorrhea: Black-flecked (melanin) discharge
- Polyp
- Pain is uncommon

Treatment
- Options, risks, complications
  - Metastatic melanoma to sinonasal tract can develop but is vanishingly rare
  - Breslow thickness and Clark level are not used in sinonasal tract
- Surgical approaches
  - Wide local excision is treatment of choice
- Radiation
  - Radiation can be used after surgery
    - In most cases, it is palliative

Prognosis
- Overall prognosis is poor
- 5-year survival: 17-47%
- Recurrences are common
- Poor prognosis associated with
  - Obstruction as presenting symptom
  - Nasopharynx or "mixed site" of involvement
  - Tumor ≥ 3 cm
  - Undifferentiated histology
  - High mitotic count
  - Recurrence
  - Stage of tumor
- Matrix metalloproteinases (MMPs: Proteolytic enzymes required for extracellular matrix degradation) expression may be associated with patient outcome

SINONASAL MELANOMA

Key Facts

Terminology

- Neural crest-derived neoplasms originating from melanocytes and demonstrating melanocytic differentiation

Clinical Issues

- Anterior nasal septum > maxillary sinus
- Overall prognosis is poor

Macroscopic Features

- Most are polyploid

Microscopic Pathology

- Protean histology, mimic of many other primary tumor types
- Junctional activity and epidermal migration (pagetoid spread) help to confirm primary tumor
- Many patterns of growth

- Variety of cell types can be seen
- Prominent, irregular, brightly eosinophilic, enlarged nucleoli
- Intranuclear cytoplasmic inclusions usually present
- Melanin-containing tumor cells can be seen

Ancillary Tests

- Positive: S100, HMB-45, MART-1/Melan-A, microphthalmia transcription factor, tyrosinase, vimentin

Top Differential Diagnoses

- Olfactory neuroblastoma
- Sinonasal undifferentiated carcinoma
- Melanotic neuroectodermal tumor of infancy
- Rhabdomyosarcoma
- Metastatic melanoma

- Decreased MMP2 expression associated with greater overall survival
- Positive MMP14 expression associated with poor survival

IMAGE FINDINGS

Radiographic Findings

- Usually identifies extent of tumor and bone invasion
- Positron emission tomography (PET) tends to show posterior nasal cavity and sinus tumors better than anterior nasal tumors
- Locoregional and metastatic disease can be detected

MACROSCOPIC FEATURES

General Features

- Most are polyploid
- White to gray, brown, or black
- Surface ulceration/erosion is common

Size

- Range up to 6 cm
- Mean: 2-3 cm

MICROSCOPIC PATHOLOGY

Histologic Features

- Protean histology, mimic of many other primary tumor types
- Junctional activity and intraepidermal migration (Pagetoid spread) help to confirm primary tumor
- Surface ulceration is common, obscuring "in situ" component
- Bone or soft tissue invasion is common
- Many patterns of growth
  - Nests
  - Solid
  - Organoid
  - Sheets

- Fascicles and interlacing bundles
- Storiform
- Meningothelial
- Papillary
- Hemangiopericytoma-like
- Peritheliomatous: Distinctive and unique for STMMM
- Variety of cell types can be seen
  - Undifferentiated
  - Epithelioid, polygonal
  - Small cell
  - Plasmacytoid
  - Rhabdoid
  - Giant cell
- Vesicular nuclei, although sometimes hyperchromatic
- Prominent, irregular, brightly eosinophilic, enlarged nucleoli
- Intranuclear cytoplasmic inclusions usually present
- Melanin-containing tumor cells can be seen
- Tumor cell necrosis is common
- Mitotic figures, including atypical forms, usually easily found
- Inflammation may be present, but not of consequence
- Desmoplastic type fibrosis can be seen, but is not common
- Perineural invasion, when present, is poor prognostic indicator
- Tumor depth of invasion (Clark) impossible to accurately assess
- Tumor thickness (Breslow) not meaningful in sinonasal tract

Lymphatic/Vascular Invasion

- Usually present but difficult to assess

Margins

- Difficult to assess, as samples are frequently fragmented and removed piecemeal

ANCILLARY TESTS

Histochemistry
- Fontana-Masson: Melanin bleach will confirm melanin in cytoplasm

Immunohistochemistry
- Positive: S100, HMB-45, MART-1/Melan-A, microphthalmia transcription factor, tyrosinase, vimentin
- p16 expression is lost in most MMM (74%)

Cytogenetics
- Comparative genomic hybridization (CGH) shows chromosome arm 1q is gained in nearly all tumors studied
- Gains of 6p (93%) and 8q (57%) are also identified

Electron Microscopy
- Premelanosomes and melanosomes confirms melanocytic origin

DIFFERENTIAL DIAGNOSIS

Olfactory Neuroblastoma
- Lobular architecture
- Fibrillary matrix material associated with rosettes and pseudorosettes
- CD56, chromogranin, synaptophysin, and sustentacular S100(+) reaction

Sinonasal Undifferentiated Carcinoma (SNUC)
- Small cells with high nuclear to cytoplasmic ratio
- Necrosis, destructive growth, and vascular invasion
- Strong, diffuse keratin immunoreactivity

Melanotic Neuroectodermal Tumor of Infancy
- Tumor of neonatal period, affecting gnathic bones
- Biphasic tumor with small and large cells, with pigment easily identified

Rhabdomyosarcoma
- Tends to develop in younger patients (although not alveolar type)
- Nests, alveolar patterns are similar
- Strap and rhabdoid patterns are helpful
- Cross striations can confirm diagnosis
- Immunoreactive with desmin, MYOD1, myogenin, SMA, MSA, CD56

Leiomyosarcoma
- Fascicular architecture, frequently associated with necrosis and high mitotic index
- Perinuclear vacuoles and cigar-shaped nuclei are rare in melanoma
- Muscle markers positive, while nonreactive with melanoma markers

Plasmacytoma
- Hematologic neoplasm giving sheet-like pattern of plasmacytoid cells
- Hoff-zone, paranuclear clearing, and rounded nuclei with clock face-like chromatin distribution
- CD138, CD79a, κ or λ, and other hematologic markers will be positive

Metastatic Melanoma
- While theoretic consideration, junctional/pagetoid spread helps to exclude this possibility
- Clinical and radiographic examination are really the only ways to make definitive separation

Mesenchymal Chondrosarcoma
- Small, undifferentiated cell appearance, but if enough sections are taken, cartilaginous features can be seen
- S100 protein will be positive (chondrocytic tumors are positive), but HMB-45, tyrosinase, Melan-A will not react

SELECTED REFERENCES

1. Wenig BM: Undifferentiated malignant neoplasms of the sinonasal tract. Arch Pathol Lab Med. 133(5):699-712, 2009
2. Bachar G et al: Mucosal melanomas of the head and neck: experience of the Princess Margaret Hospital. Head Neck. 30(10):1325-31, 2008
3. Dauer EH et al: Sinonasal melanoma: a clinicopathologic review of 61 cases. Otolaryngol Head Neck Surg. 138(3):347-52, 2008
4. Kim DK et al: Ki67 antigen as a predictive factor for prognosis of sinonasal mucosal melanoma. Clin Exp Otorhinolaryngol. 1(4):206-10, 2008
5. Kondratiev S et al: Expression and prognostic role of MMP2, MMP9, MMP13, and MMP14 matrix metalloproteinases in sinonasal and oral malignant melanomas. Hum Pathol. 39(3):337-43, 2008
6. McLean N et al: Primary mucosal melanoma of the head and neck. Comparison of clinical presentation and histopathologic features of oral and sinonasal melanoma. Oral Oncol. 44(11):1039-46, 2008
7. Cheng YF et al: Toward a better understanding of sinonasal mucosal melanoma: clinical review of 23 cases. J Chin Med Assoc. 70(1):24-9, 2007
8. Martin JM et al: Outcomes in sinonasal mucosal melanoma. ANZ J Surg. 74(10):838-42, 2004
9. Prasad ML et al: Clinicopathologic differences in malignant melanoma arising in oral squamous and sinonasal respiratory mucosa of the upper aerodigestive tract. Arch Pathol Lab Med. 127(8):997-1002, 2003
10. Thompson LD et al: Sinonasal tract and nasopharyngeal melanomas: a clinicopathologic study of 115 cases with a proposed staging system. Am J Surg Pathol. 27(5):594-611, 2003
11. van Dijk M et al: Distinct chromosomal aberrations in sinonasal mucosal melanoma as detected by comparative genomic hybridization. Genes Chromosomes Cancer. 36(2):151-8, 2003
12. Patel SG et al: Primary mucosal malignant melanoma of the head and neck. Head Neck. 24(3):247-57, 2002
13. Kardon DE et al: Sinonasal mucosal malignant melanoma: report of an unusual case mimicking schwannoma. Ann Diagn Pathol. 4(5):303-7, 2000
14. Regauer S et al: Primary mucosal melanomas of the nasal cavity and paranasal sinuses. A clinicopathological analysis of 14 cases. APMIS. 106(3):403-10, 1998

Immunohistochemistry

Antibody	Reactivity	Staining Pattern	Comment
S100	Positive	Nuclear & cytoplasmic	Diffuse and strong stain usually; identified in ~ 90% of cases
HMB-45	Positive	Cytoplasmic	Variably reactive in most cases (~ 75% of cases)
Tyrosinase	Positive	Cytoplasmic	Variably reactive in most cases (~ 75%)
melan-A103	Positive	Cytoplasmic	Variably reactive in majority of cases (~ 66%)
MITF	Positive	Nuclear	Positive in majority of cases (~ 55%)
NSE	Positive	Cytoplasmic	Positive in < 50% of tumor cells, often focal
CD117	Positive	Cytoplasmic	Positive in ~ 33% of cases
CD99	Positive	Cytoplasmic	Positive in ~ 25% of cases
Vimentin	Positive	Cytoplasmic	All tumor cells
CD56	Positive	Cell membrane & cytoplasm	~ 7% of cases
Synaptophysin	Positive	Cytoplasmic	Nonspecific, in ~ 10% of cases
EMA	Positive	Cytoplasmic	< 5% of tumor cells
Chromogranin-A	Negative		
CD45RB	Negative		
CK-PAN	Negative		
GFAP	Negative		
CD45RB	Negative		
Actin-HHF-35	Negative		
Actin-sm	Negative		
Desmin	Negative		
MYOD1	Negative		

Proposed Staging for Sinonasal Tract Melanomas

Classification	Description
Primary Tumor	
T1	Single anatomic site
T2	2 or more anatomic sites
Regional Lymph Nodes	
N0	No lymph node involvement
N1	Any lymph node metastases
Distant Metastasis	
M0	No distant metastases
M1	Distant metastasis
Stage Grouping	
I	T1 N0 M0
II	T2 N0 M0
III	Any T, N1, M0
IV	Any T, any N, M1

SINONASAL MELANOMA

Imaging and Microscopic Features

(Left) This MR image (T2-weighted axial) demonstrates high signal within the maxillary sinus, focally associated with fluid in the posterior portion ➡. This lesion was a maxillary sinus malignant melanoma, without associated involvement of the nasal cavity. *(Right)* The nasal septum cartilage ⊳ is being destroyed by the infiltrative neoplasm. The tumor forms a thick, sheet-like distribution. No pattern of growth can be seen at this magnification, although ulceration is present.

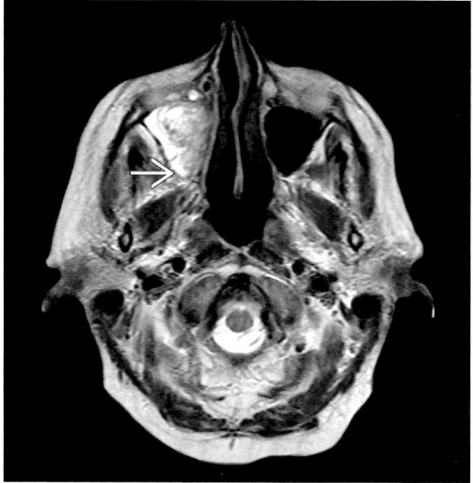
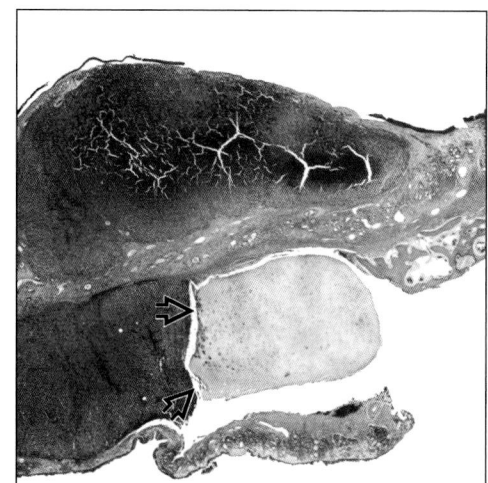

(Left) Atypical junctional melanocytes are noted within the respiratory epithelium, arranged in a pagetoid spread ➡. The tumor cells are also present within the stroma. *(Right)* This "peritheliomatous" or perivascular ➡ distribution of the neoplastic cells is quite characteristic of sinonasal melanoma. It is thought to represent viable tumor cells remaining around vessels. This pattern can be seen in other tumors, but not to the same frequency as it is in melanoma.

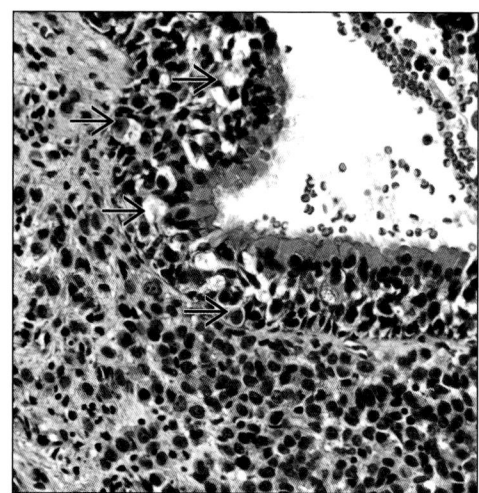
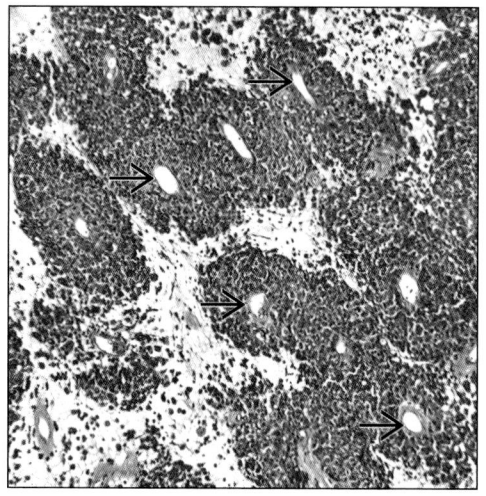

(Left) MMM can be arranged in a number of different architectural features, with a fascicular architecture seen here. The spindle cells are arranged in short, intersecting fascicles. The cells are somewhat syncytial in appearance. *(Right)* It is not uncommon to have an "undifferentiated" or "small round blue cell" appearance to MMM. There is a slightly plasmacytoid appearance to the cells. Note the very prominent nucleoli. Mitotic figures are noted ➡, but pigment is absent.

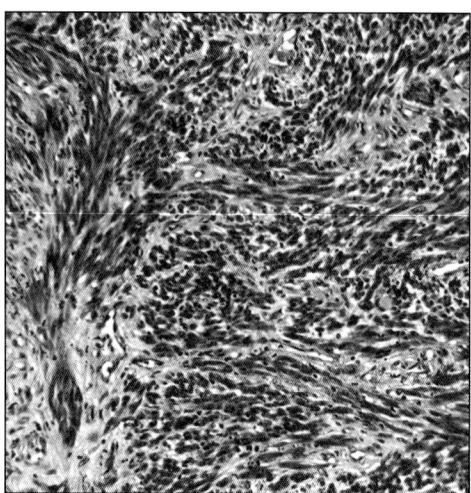
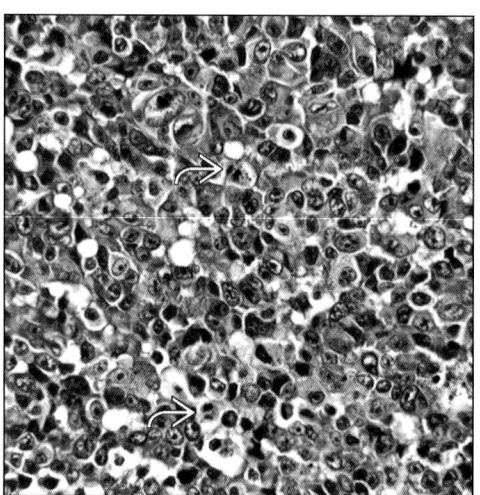

SINONASAL MELANOMA

Microscopic and Immunohistochemical Features

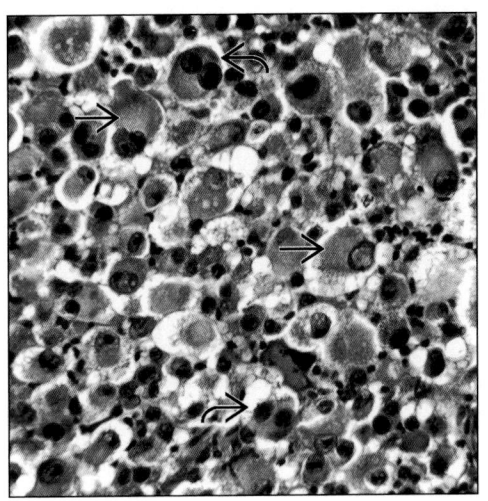

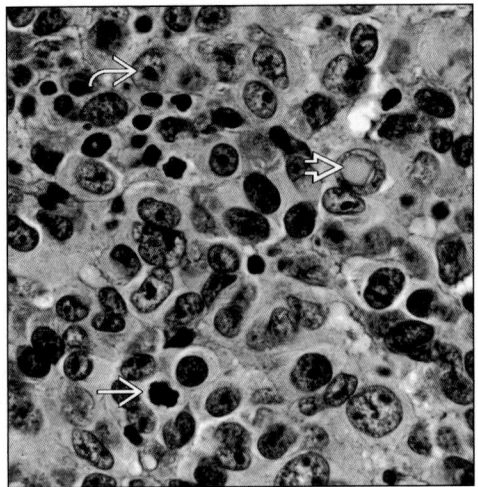

(Left) *This mucosal melanoma shows a very pronounced plasmacytoid appearance, including a "Hof-zone" adjacent to the nucleus ⇨. There are intranuclear cytoplasmic inclusions as well as binucleation ⇨. (Right) Pleomorphic epithelioid and polygonal cells comprise this melanoma. There is remarkable variability between cells. Prominent, eosinophilic nucleoli are present ➡, along with intranuclear cytoplasmic inclusions ⇨. Mitotic figures are also noted ➡.*

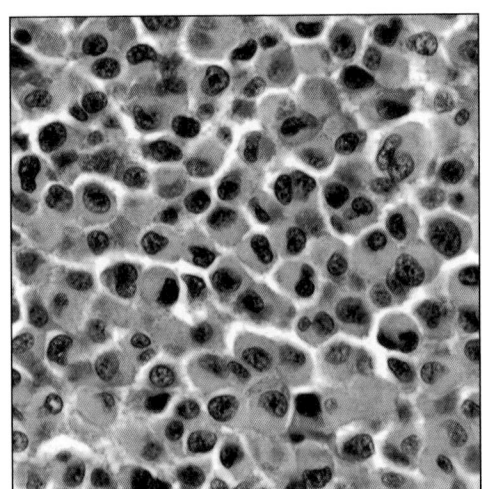

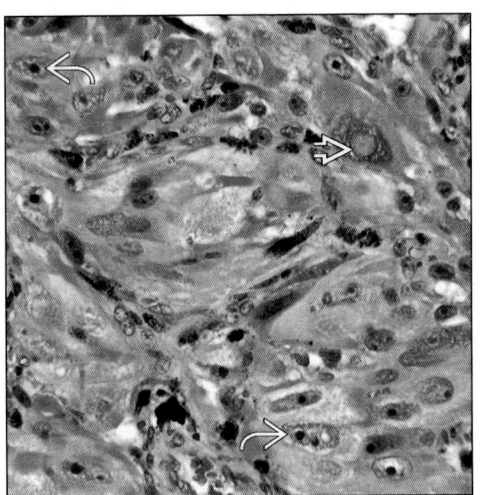

(Left) *A rhabdoid appearance with densely opacified, eosinophilic cytoplasm is the dominant pattern in this MMM. Nucleoli are not markedly enlarged. Mitotic figures, necrosis, and pigment are not appreciated. (Right) It is not uncommon to have a variable architecture and cellular morphology in a single tumor. Here a polygonal and spindled cell population shows melanin pigment, prominent nucleoli ➡, and intranuclear cytoplasmic inclusions ⇨.*

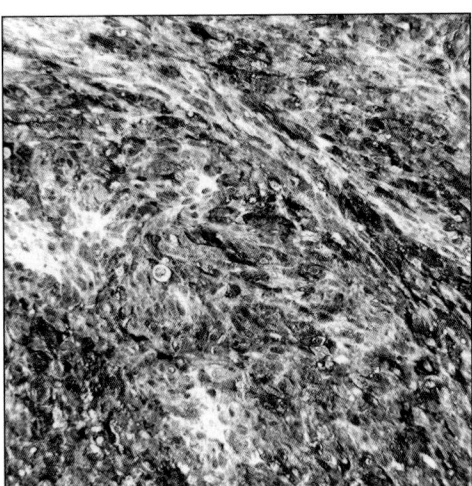

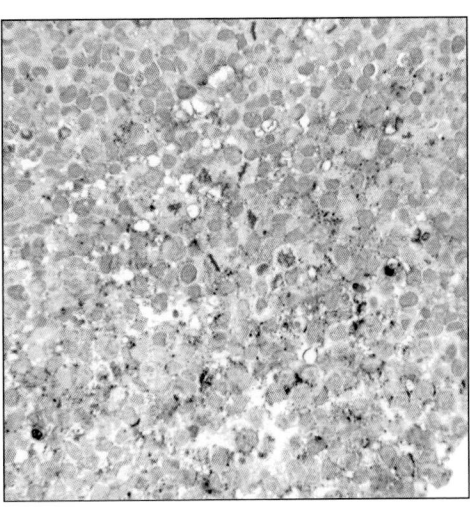

(Left) *S100 protein shows strong immunoreactivity in this spindled cell melanoma. There is both cytoplasmic and nuclear staining with this marker, which highlights nearly all of the cells. (Right) Positive HMB-45 in this "small round blue cell" type of melanoma demonstrates some of the variability that can be seen both within a tumor as well as between tumors. The intensity of the staining, as well as the number of positive cells, can be quite variable.*

MALIGNANT CELLULAR BLUE NEVUS (MELANOMA ARISING IN CELLULAR BLUE NEVUS)

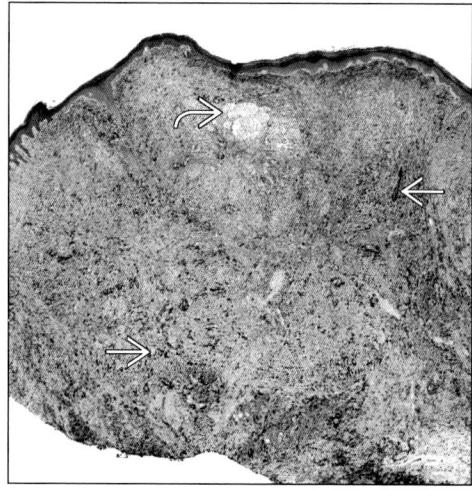

Malignant blue nevus at low magnification appears similar to a cellular blue nevus, with lobules of pale-staining cells ➡ surrounded by darker-staining pigmented spindle cells and melanophages ➡.

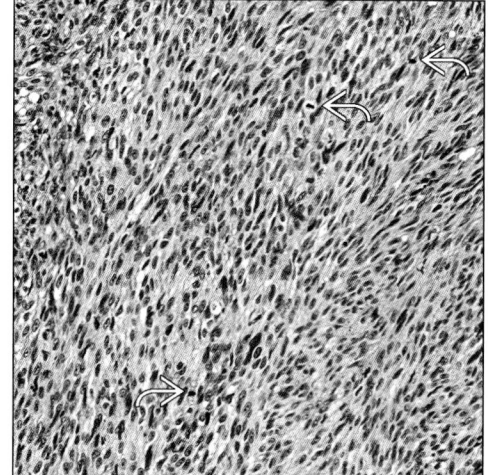

High magnification of a malignant cellular blue nevus shows a densely cellular area composed of fascicles of hyperchromatic-staining cells with multiple mitotic figures ➡.

TERMINOLOGY

Abbreviations
- Malignant cellular blue nevus (MCBN)

Synonyms
- Melanoma arising in cellular blue nevus
- Melanoma mimicking cellular blue nevus

Definitions
- Malignant dermal-based melanocytic neoplasm with associated cellular blue nevus or features simulating a cellular blue nevus

ETIOLOGY/PATHOGENESIS

Environmental Exposure
- May be related to solar damage

Genetics
- Multiple chromosomal abnormalities reported in some cases
- Mutations in *GNAQ* and *GNA11* have been reported
- 1 case reported to show a mutation in the hOGG-1 DNA repair enzyme

CLINICAL ISSUES

Epidemiology
- Incidence
  - Very rare tumor
- Age
  - Usually occurs in adults
- Gender
  - More common in males

Presentation
- Dermal mass/nodular lesion
  - May appear blue, bluish-gray, or bluish-black

Treatment
- Surgical approaches
  - Complete and wider surgical excision is necessary for local removal
  - Sentinel lymph node biopsy may be used for staging purposes, but is of doubtful therapeutic utility

Prognosis
- Controversial
  - Originally thought to be very aggressive, but recent reports may indicate a lower malignant potential

MICROSCOPIC PATHOLOGY

Histologic Features
- Cellular, dermal-based, nodular melanocytic tumor
  - Proliferation of atypical spindle-shaped cells in fascicles and lobules
  - Often asymmetric, appears poorly circumscribed at low magnification
  - May extend into the subcutis
  - Cytologic atypia is usually very marked
  - Mitotic figures present
    - Often atypical, and may be > 2/HPF
  - May show areas of necrosis
- Typically lacks epidermal involvement
- Areas of benign cellular blue nevus may be present
  - Some authorities require the presence of an associated nevus, but this is controversial

Cytologic Features
- Spindle-shaped cells with hyperchromatic-staining nuclei

ANCILLARY TESTS

Immunohistochemistry
- Elevated proliferative activity can be shown by Ki-67 and PCNA

MALIGNANT CELLULAR BLUE NEVUS (MELANOMA ARISING IN CELLULAR BLUE NEVUS)

Key Facts

Terminology
- Malignant dermal-based melanocytic neoplasm with associated cellular blue nevus or features simulating cellular blue nevus

Clinical Issues
- Very rare tumor
- Usually occurs in adults
- Complete and wider surgical excision is necessary for local removal

- Originally thought to be very aggressive, but recent reports may indicate a lower malignant potential

Microscopic Pathology
- Cellular, dermal-based, nodular melanocytic tumor
- Often asymmetric, appears poorly circumscribed
- Cytologic atypia is usually very marked
- Mitotic figures present, often atypical
- May show areas of necrosis
- Areas of benign cellular blue nevus may be present

- p16 often shows loss of expression (positive in cellular blue nevi)

DIFFERENTIAL DIAGNOSIS

Cellular Blue Nevus
- Dermal-based cellular melanocytic proliferation
  - Often symmetric and well-circumscribed at low magnification
- Lobules and fascicles of oval to spindle-shaped cells
- Often shows a "dumbbell-like" appearance at low-power examination
- Peripheral areas often show conventional blue nevus-like pattern with hypocellular areas of melanocytes associated with dermal fibrosis and melanophages
- Cells lack prominent cytologic atypia, mitotic activity, and necrosis
  - A few mitotic figures can be present, especially in cellular areas

Atypical Cellular Blue Nevus
- Shows overlapping features with cellular blue nevus but with increased atypia
- Lobules and fascicles of atypical spindled cells
- May show some asymmetry and infiltrative features
- Scattered mitotic figures may be present, but they are not as numerous or atypical-appearing as in malignant cellular blue nevus
- Necrosis should be lacking

Metastatic Melanoma
- Lacks a junctional component, similar to malignant blue nevus, but also shows
  - More epithelioid-appearing melanocytes, fewer spindled cells (most cases), and no dendritic cells
  - Fewer melanophages (unless regressing) and less surrounding dermal fibrosis
  - No associated benign blue nevus component
- Clinical history and complete examination may be necessary for distinction in some cases

SELECTED REFERENCES

1. Martin RC et al: So-called "malignant blue nevus": a clinicopathologic study of 23 patients. Cancer. 115(13):2949-55, 2009
2. Murali R et al: Blue nevi and related lesions: a review highlighting atypical and newly described variants, distinguishing features and diagnostic pitfalls. Adv Anat Pathol. 16(6):365-82, 2009
3. Barnhill RL et al: Atypical cellular blue nevi (cellular blue nevi with atypical features): lack of consensus for diagnosis and distinction from cellular blue nevi and malignant melanoma ("malignant blue nevus"). Am J Surg Pathol. 32(1):36-44, 2008
4. Hocevar M et al: Malignant blue nevus with lymph node metastases in five-year-old girl. Croat Med J. 46(3):463-6, 2005
5. Merkow LP et al: A cellular and malignant blue nevus: a light and electron microscopic study. Cancer. 24(5):888-96, 1969

IMAGE GALLERY

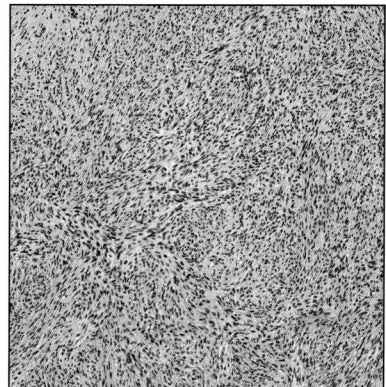 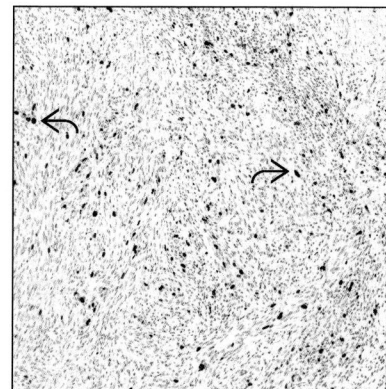 

(Left) This malignant blue nevus shows densely cellular areas of spindled melanocytes forming fascicular (sarcoma-like) arrangements. *(Center)* Ki-67 immunostaining shows increased nuclear positivity in this malignant cellular blue nevus, with scattered enlarged, atypical nuclei staining ➘. *(Right)* p16 immunohistochemistry shows almost complete loss of staining in this malignant cellular blue nevus. This marker is often lost in melanomas, but strongly expressed in nevi.

PIGMENTED EPITHELIOID MELANOCYTOMA ("ANIMAL-TYPE MELANOMA")

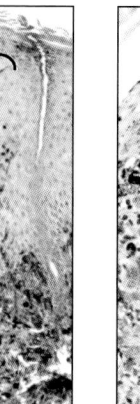

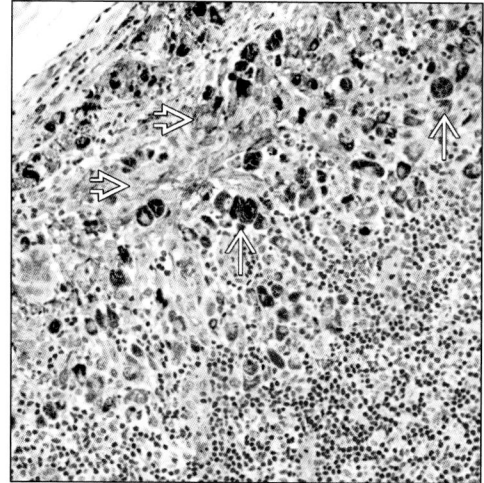

A punch biopsy specimen from an 11-year-old girl shows a heavily pigmented compound melanocytic tumor with epidermal hyperplasia, intraepidermal melanophages ➚, and large epithelioid cells ⏩.

A sentinel lymph node biopsy specimen from an 11-year-old girl with PEM shows melanophages ➡ and large epithelioid tumor cells ⏩. These cells colonized multiple foci throughout the lymph node.

TERMINOLOGY

Abbreviations
- Pigmented epithelioid melanocytoma (PEM)

Synonyms
- Animal-type melanoma
- Equine-type melanoma

Definitions
- Heavily pigmented, deeply invasive melanocytic proliferation with low-grade malignant potential
- Very controversial entity, not universally accepted (especially the inclusion of some epithelioid blue nevi in this category)

ETIOLOGY/PATHOGENESIS

Genetic Syndrome
- May occur sporadically or in association with Carney complex (CNC)

CLINICAL ISSUES

Site
- Extremities, trunk, and head and neck are most commonly affected sites

Presentation
- Heavily pigmented, dome-shaped, or verrucous nodule ≥ 1.0 cm in diameter
- Often of long duration

Treatment
- Surgical approaches
  - Complete excision necessary
  - Most experts recommend sentinel lymph node biopsy

- Systemic therapy may not be indicated, given lower malignant potential of PEM

Prognosis
- Has capacity to metastasize to lymph nodes, but with less frequent systemic spread
- Short-term follow-up suggested better prognosis for PEM than for conventional metastatic melanoma

MICROSCOPIC PATHOLOGY

Histologic Features
- Extends into deep reticular tissue and subcutaneous fat along adnexal structures or neurovascular bundles
- More cellular in center and shows infiltrative growth pattern at periphery
- Abuts epidermis and often associated with epidermal hyperplasia
  - However, some are separated from epidermis by grenz zone of uninvolved papillary dermis
- Composed of 3 principal cell types (listed from most to least abundant)
  - Medium-sized epithelioid cells with exorbitant intracellular coarse melanin
    - Unclear if these cells are all melanocytic in nature, as some have features of tumor-infiltrating macrophages
  - Spindled blue nevus-like cells
    - Found singly or in small groups penetrating among surrounding stromal collagen bundles
  - Large epithelioid cells
    - May be multinucleated
- Does not exhibit brisk dermal mitotic activity
- Rarely exhibits necrosis

Cytologic Features
- Depends on cell type
  - Medium-sized epithelioid cells have heavily pigmented cytoplasm obscuring nuclei

PIGMENTED EPITHELIOID MELANOCYTOMA ("ANIMAL-TYPE MELANOMA")

Key Facts

Clinical Issues
- Heavily pigmented, dome-shaped nodule
- Occur sporadically or in association with Carney complex
- Low-grade malignant potential
- Complete excision necessary

Microscopic Pathology
- Deep dermal tumor with frequent involvement of subcutis

- More cellular in center and shows infiltrative growth pattern at periphery
- Composed of 3 principal cell types
  - Medium-sized epithelioid cells, large epithelioid cells, and spindled cells

Top Differential Diagnoses
- Malignant blue nevus
- Atypical cellular blue nevus
- Cellular blue nevus

- Oval and regular nuclei contain multiple small eosinophilic nucleoli
- Spindled blue nevus-like cells have vesicular nuclei with amphophilic cytoplasm
- Large epithelioid cells have large vesicular nuclei with prominent macronucleoli and abundant cytoplasm
  - Melanin granules at periphery of cytoplasm, giving cells a "fried-egg" appearance

ANCILLARY TESTS

Immunohistochemistry
- Loss of expression for protein kinase A regulatory subunit 1-α

DIFFERENTIAL DIAGNOSIS

Malignant Blue Nevus
- Melanoma arising in or mimicking blue nevus
  - Has blue nevus (blue nevus-like) component
  - Dermal mitoses and tumor necrosis are common

Atypical Cellular Blue Nevus
- Usually shows areas of cellular blue nevus
- Tumor necrosis and ulceration are rare
- Atypical mitoses not observed

Cellular Blue Nevus
- Shows dumbbell-shaped cellular dermal lobules of bland-appearing melanocytes
- Often shows surrounding areas of more conventional blue nevus

Common Blue Nevus
- Does not show pigmented epithelioid cells of PEM
- Dermal sclerosis, common in blue nevus, is rarely seen in PEM

DIAGNOSTIC CHECKLIST

Clinically Relevant Pathologic Features
- Melanin-bleached sections are helpful in evaluation of cytological details

Pathologic Interpretation Pearls
- Finding "fried-egg" cells can be helpful

SELECTED REFERENCES

1. Mandal RV et al: Pigmented epithelioid melanocytoma: favorable outcome after 5-year follow-up. Am J Surg Pathol. 33(12):1778-82, 2009
2. Scolyer RA et al: Pigmented epithelioid melanocytoma. Am J Surg Pathol. 28(8):1114-5; author reply 1115-6, 2004

IMAGE GALLERY

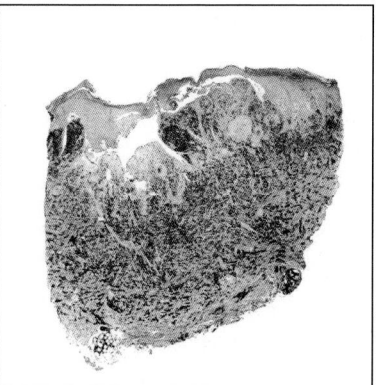 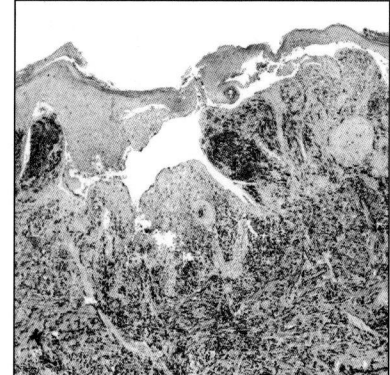 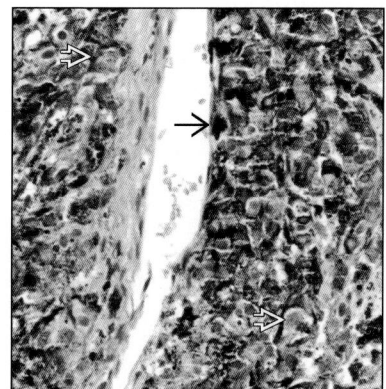

(Left) A punch biopsy specimen from the arm of a 5-month-old boy shows a heavily pigmented compound melanocytic tumor with epidermal hyperplasia extending deep into the dermis. *(Center)* The tumor is composed of an admixture of uniform epithelioid tumor cells, pigmented dendritic cells, and melanophages. *(Right)* High magnification shows large epithelioid cells ⇨ and melanophages ⇨ around blood vessels and lymphatics. No definitive lymphovascular invasion is identified.

PRIMARY DERMAL MELANOMA

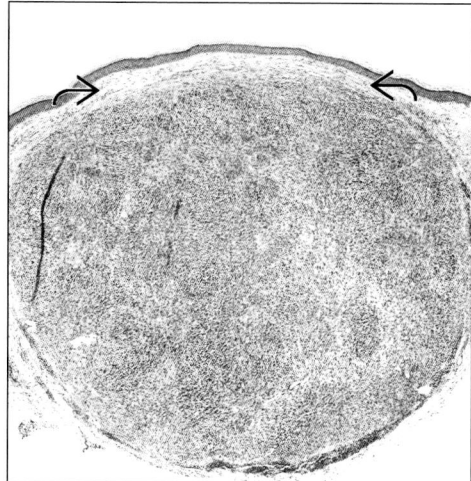

Low magnification of a PDM shows a well-circumscribed, dermal-based nodule, mimicking metastatic melanoma. Note the grenz zone ➔ separating the tumor from the overlying epidermis.

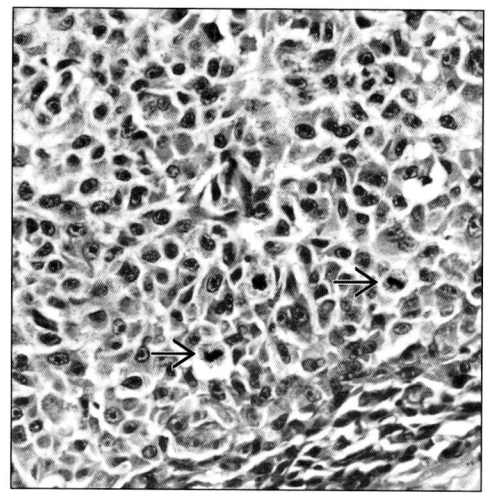

High magnification of PDM typically shows marked cytologic atypia and multiple mitotic figures ➔.

TERMINOLOGY

Abbreviations
- Primary dermal melanoma (PDM)

Synonyms
- Dermal &/or subcutaneous melanoma

Definitions
- Primary melanoma arising in dermis or subcutis, typically mimicking metastatic melanoma (MM)
- Clinically, lack of prior or concurrent melanoma by history and imaging studies
- Histologically, lack of any evidence of epidermal involvement, ulceration, or regression

ETIOLOGY/PATHOGENESIS

Unknown
- Typically arise in sun-damaged skin of elderly, thus may be related to solar damage

CLINICAL ISSUES

Epidemiology
- Incidence
  - Extremely rare (estimated incidence: < 0.1% of all melanoma cases)
- Age
  - Typically occur in older adults (mean age: 70 years)
- Gender
  - More common in males

Presentation
- Dermal mass in sun-damaged skin
  - Often clinically suspected to be a cyst or epithelial tumor
- Amelanotic in most cases

Treatment
- Surgical approaches
  - Complete and wider excision necessary (margins typical for invasive melanoma)
  - Typically, sentinel lymph node biopsy will also be performed for staging purposes

Prognosis
- Relatively good, especially compared to MM of unknown origin and similar depth primary nodular melanomas

Clinical Work-up
- Complete clinical and imaging studies necessary in order to exclude possibility of metastatic melanoma
- Patient cannot have a history of prior invasive melanoma or evidence of melanoma at another site (primary or metastatic)

MACROSCOPIC FEATURES

General Features
- Large, solid to cystic, dermal-based nodule
- Typically not pigmented

MICROSCOPIC PATHOLOGY

Histologic Features
- Atypical nodular dermal-based melanocytic tumor
  - Typically a well-circumscribed, unencapsulated deep dermal &/or subcutaneous mass
  - By definition, no overlying epidermal involvement, ulceration, or evidence of regression can be present
    - Multiple sections should be examined to exclude these features
  - Variable mixture of cell types: Typically epithelioid, but may be spindle-shaped, rhabdoid, or pleomorphic appearing
  - Mitoses are often easily identified

PRIMARY DERMAL MELANOMA

Key Facts

Terminology
- Primary cutaneous melanoma arising in dermis or subcutis, mimicking metastatic melanoma
- By definition, lacks any evidence of epidermal involvement, ulceration, or regression

Clinical Issues
- Often clinically suspected to be a cyst or epithelial tumor
- Complete and wider excision necessary

Microscopic Pathology
- Nodular, well-circumscribed, dermal &/or subcutaneous-based
- Composed of highly atypical melanocytes
- By definition, no overlying epidermal involvement, ulceration, or evidence of regression can be present

Top Differential Diagnoses
- Metastatic melanoma
- Primary nodular melanoma

- ○ Necrosis may be present
- No associated nevus should be present

Cytologic Features
- Cytologic atypia prominent, with enlarged nuclei and prominent nucleoli

ANCILLARY TESTS

Immunohistochemistry
- Strongly positive for melanocytic markers by immunohistochemistry (IHC) including S100, MART-1/Melan-A, and HMB-45 in most cases
- Lower levels of p53, Ki-67, cyclin-D1, and D2-40 (lymphovascular spaces) compared to MM and nodular-type melanomas

DIFFERENTIAL DIAGNOSIS

Metastatic Melanoma
- Ideally, there should be a history of previous or concurrent melanoma
  - ○ If no history, complete clinical examination and imaging studies should be performed
- Well-circumscribed dermal &/or subcutaneous nodular mass, features very similar to PDM
- Epidermal involvement may rarely be seen (epidermotropic metastasis)
- IHC typically shows higher levels of Ki-67, cyclin-D1, p53, and D2-40 compared to PDM

Primary Nodular Melanoma
- Predominantly dermal-based, nodular lesion with deep invasion
- By definition, at least focal overlying epidermal involvement &/or ulceration
- IHC may show higher levels of Ki-67, cyclin-D1, p53, and D2-40 compared to PDM

DIAGNOSTIC CHECKLIST

Pathologic Interpretation Pearls
- Dermal or subcutaneous melanoma lacking overlying in situ component, ulceration, or regression

SELECTED REFERENCES

1. Lee CC et al: Solitary dermal melanoma: beginning or end of the metastatic process? Ann Surg Oncol. 16(3):578-84, 2009
2. Cassarino DS et al: Primary dermal melanoma: distinct immunohistochemical findings and clinical outcome compared with nodular and metastatic melanoma. Arch Dermatol. 144(1):49-56, 2008
3. Swetter SM et al: Primary dermal melanoma: a distinct subtype of melanoma. Arch Dermatol. 140(1):99-103, 2004

IMAGE GALLERY

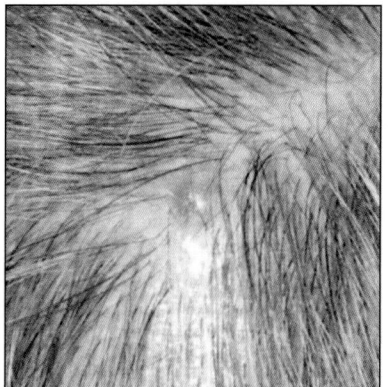 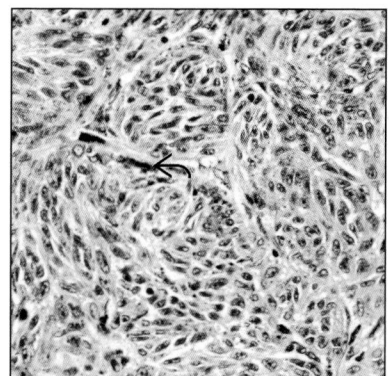 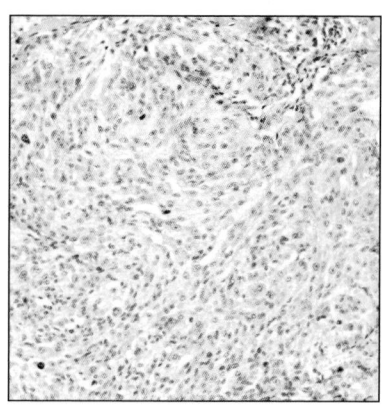

(Left) Clinical photograph shows a nodular-appearing, flesh-colored lesion on the scalp of a patient. Most cases of PDM are not pigmented and are often thought to be a cyst or epithelial tumor clinically. *(Courtesy S. Swetter, MD.)* *(Center)* Most cases of PDM are amelanotic, although a few are pigmented. This case was composed of oval to spindle-shaped cells with scattered cytoplasmic pigmentation and melanophages ➘. *(Right)* Compared to metastatic melanoma, PDM often shows a lower proliferative rate by Ki-67.

OTHER UNUSUAL AND RARE VARIANTS OF MELANOMA

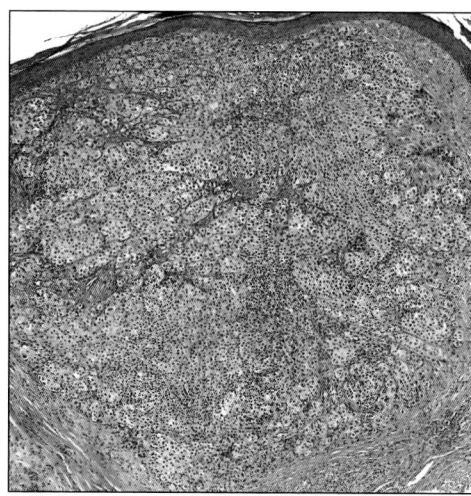

Clear cell melanoma shows a dense nodular to sheet-like dermal proliferation of pale-staining cells. These tumors can mimic clear cell sarcoma, but the superficial location would be highly unusual.

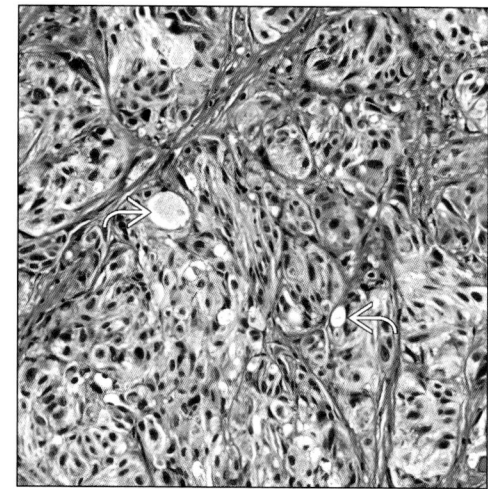

High magnification of clear cell melanoma shows atypical cells with abundant pale to clear-staining cytoplasm and cytoplasmic vacuoles ➦. The nests are surrounded by fibrous bands, mimicking clear cell sarcoma.

TERMINOLOGY

Definitions
- Rare variants of melanoma including clear cell/balloon cell, chondroid, osteoid, myxoid, and rhabdoid melanoma

ETIOLOGY/PATHOGENESIS

Environmental Exposure
- Related to UV exposure in most cases

CLINICAL ISSUES

Epidemiology
- Incidence
  - Very rare tumors
- Age
  - Typically elderly patients

Site
- Sun-damaged skin, typically head and neck region, upper trunk, forearms

Presentation
- Usually presents as papule or nodule with irregular, asymmetric borders

Treatment
- Surgical approaches
  - Complete and wide excision, with clinical margins appropriate for conventional melanoma of similar Breslow depth

Prognosis
- Depends on typical melanoma prognostic features such as Breslow depth, ulceration, mitotic count, and presence of perineural or angiolymphatic invasion

- Rhabdoid melanoma reportedly shows aggressive course in most cases

MICROSCOPIC PATHOLOGY

Histologic Features
- Depends on histologic variant
- Most cases often show areas of conventional-appearing melanoma &/or overlying melanoma in situ
- **Clear cell/balloon cell melanoma**
  - Enlarged cells with abundant clear to vacuolated-appearing cytoplasm
    - May be due to glycogen
  - May appear deceptively bland in some cases
- **Chondroid melanoma**
  - Malignant epithelioid cells associated with myxochondroid-appearing matrix
  - Often shows areas of overlying melanoma in situ or more conventional melanoma with nesting
- **Osteoid melanoma**
  - Malignant epithelioid cells associated with prominent osteoid-appearing material
- **Myxoid melanoma**
  - Atypical epithelioid to spindle-shaped cells scattered in prominent myxoid matrix
- **Rhabdoid melanoma**
  - Proliferation of markedly enlarged and atypical-appearing cells with abundant eosinophilic-staining cytoplasm
  - Peripheral displacement of nucleus by cytoplasmic material (intermediate filaments)
- **Signet ring cell melanoma**
  - Composed of atypical epithelioid cells with pale to clear-staining cytoplasm
    - Likely due to degenerative changes or glycogen
  - Peripheral displacement of nucleus leads to signet ring cell appearance
- **Small cell melanoma**

OTHER UNUSUAL AND RARE VARIANTS OF MELANOMA

Key Facts

Terminology
- Rare variants of melanoma including chondroid and osseous melanoma, myxoid melanoma, rhabdoid melanoma, and balloon cell melanoma

Etiology/Pathogenesis
- Related to UV exposure in most cases

Clinical Issues
- Very rare tumors

Microscopic Pathology
- Most variants often show areas of more conventional-appearing melanoma &/or overlying melanoma in situ
- **Balloon cell/clear cell melanoma**
  - Composed of enlarged cells with abundant clear to vacuolated-appearing cytoplasm

- **Chondroid melanoma**
  - Malignant epithelioid cells associated with prominent myxochondroid-appearing matrix
- **Osteoid melanoma**
  - Malignant epithelioid cells associated with prominent osteoid-appearing material
- **Myxoid melanoma**
  - Atypical epithelioid cells scattered in prominent myxoid matrix
- **Rhabdoid melanoma**
  - Proliferation of markedly enlarged and atypical-appearing melanocytes with abundant eosinophilic-staining cytoplasm
- **Small cell melanoma**
  - Nests and sheets of small, hyperchromatic-staining cells with scant cytoplasm (high N:C ratio)

- Nests and sheets of small, hyperchromatic-staining cells with scant cytoplasm (high N:C ratio)
- Mimics basal cell carcinoma (BCC), Merkel cell carcinoma, or other neuroendocrine carcinomas

Cytologic Features
- Cells are usually enlarged and clearly atypical-appearing with hyperchromatic nuclei, prominent nucleoli
- Cytoplasm is variable: Abundant, clear-staining in balloon cell melanoma; dense, eosinophilic-staining in rhabdoid melanoma

ANCILLARY TESTS

Immunohistochemistry
- All variants are typically positive for melanocytic markers including S100, MART-1/Melan-A, HMB-45, tyrosinase, and MITF

DIFFERENTIAL DIAGNOSIS

Nevi
- Compound nevi may show balloon cell features or rarely show osteoid or chondroid material
- Nevus cells lack significant cytologic atypia, pleomorphism, or mitotic activity

DDx of Chondroid Melanoma
- Chondroma or other tumors with cartilaginous differentiation
  - Benign chondrocytes in myxocollagenous stroma
  - Lack immunohistochemical evidence of melanocytic differentiation

DDx of Osteoid Melanoma
- Osteoma or other tumors with osseous differentiation
  - Benign osteoclastics surrounded by mature-appearing bone
  - IHC negative for melanocytic differentiation

DDx of Myxoid Melanoma
- Benign cutaneous myxoid proliferations
  - Bland-appearing spindle-shaped fibroblasts or myofibroblasts in myoid stroma
  - Often prominent vascularity (e.g., myxoma, angiomyxoma)
- Malignant cutaneous myxoid proliferations
  - Myxofibrosarcoma: Atypical spindle-shaped cells in myxoid stroma with prominent "chicken-wire" pattern of vessels
  - Myxoid liposarcoma (extremely rare in the skin): Also shows "chicken-wire" vascularity

SELECTED REFERENCES

1. Gharpuray-Pandit D et al: Rhabdomyoblastic differentiation in malignant melanoma in adults: report of 2 cases. Int J Surg Pathol. 15(1):20-5, 2007
2. Inoue T et al: Metastatic myxoid melanoma with partial regression of the primary lesion. J Cutan Pathol. 34(6):508-12, 2007
3. Slavik T et al: Primary chondroid melanoma of the nasal skin: a rare melanoma variant at a previously undocumented site. J Cutan Pathol. 34(5):427-30, 2007
4. Rütten A et al: Primary cutaneous signet-ring cell melanoma: a clinico-pathologic and immunohistochemical study of two cases. Am J Dermatopathol. 25(5):418-22, 2003
5. Blessing K et al: Small cell malignant melanoma: a variant of naevoid melanoma. Clinicopathological features and histological differential diagnosis. J Clin Pathol. 53(8):591-5, 2000
6. Lucas DR et al: Osteogenic melanoma. A rare variant of malignant melanoma. Am J Surg Pathol. 17(4):400-9, 1993
7. Kao GF et al: Balloon cell malignant melanoma of the skin. A clinicopathologic study of 34 cases with histochemical, immunohistochemical, and ultrastructural observations. Cancer. 69(12):2942-52, 1992
8. Sarode VR et al: Myxoid variant of primary cutaneous malignant melanoma. Histopathology. 20(2):186-7, 1992
9. Sheibani K et al: Signet-ring cell melanoma. A rare morphologic variant of malignant melanoma. Am J Surg Pathol. 12(1):28-34, 1988
10. Steiner A et al: Verrucous malignant melanoma. Arch Dermatol. 124(10):1534-7, 1988

OTHER UNUSUAL AND RARE VARIANTS OF MELANOMA

Variant Microscopic Features

(Left) Small cell melanoma shows a diffusely invasive tumor extending into the deep dermis ⊃. These cases can be mistaken for BCC or Merkel cell carcinoma at low magnification. However, overlying melanoma in situ component ⊿ is present, providing a clue to the diagnosis, which can be confirmed by immunohistochemistry. (Right) Higher magnification shows infiltrating nests ⊅, cords, and single small blue cells extending into the deep dermis and surrounding adnexal structures ⊿.

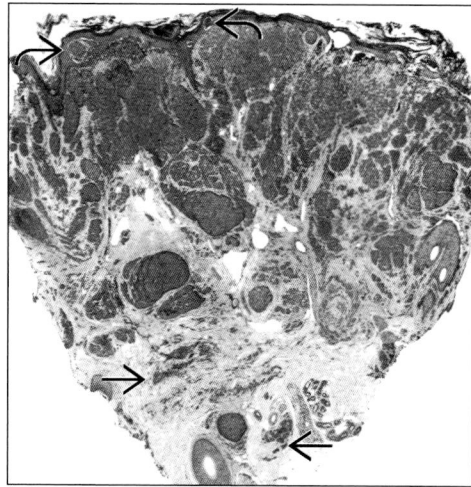
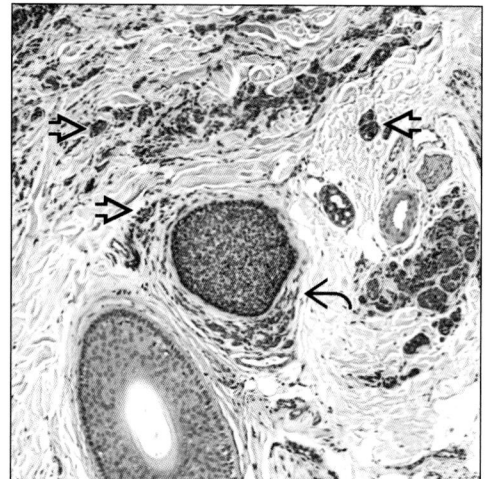

(Left) Small cell melanoma of the sinonasal region shows areas of viable tumor cells clustering around blood vessels ⊅ with intervening edematous stroma. (Right) Small cell melanoma can mimic "small round blue cell tumors." This case shows a proliferation of mostly small, round to oval, hyperchromatic-staining cells, along with a few plasmacytoid and rhabdoid-appearing cells, and scattered enlarged, more pleomorphic-appearing cells ⊅.

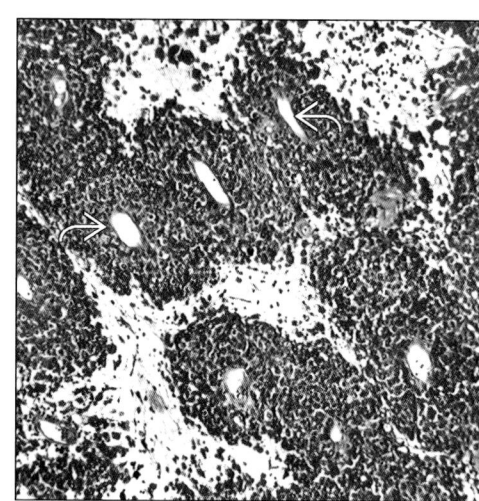
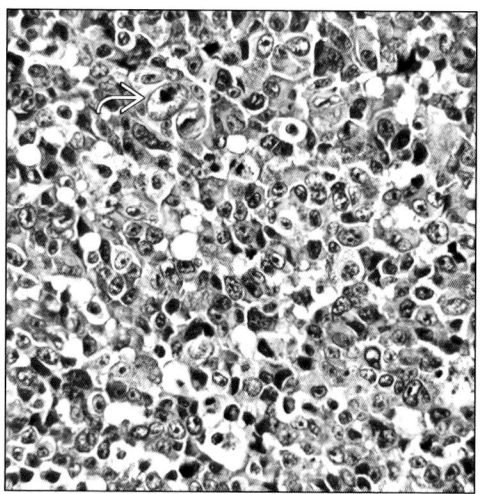

(Left) Plasmacytoid and rhabdoid-appearing melanoma shows cells with peripherally displaced nuclei and eosinophilic to pale-staining cytoplasm, focally mimicking the perinuclear hof ⊅ of plasma cells. A few binucleated, Reed-Sternberg-like cells are also present ⊿. (Right) Rhabdoid melanoma shows a population of rhabdoid-appearing cells with peripherally displaced nuclei and prominent eosinophilic-staining cytoplasm.

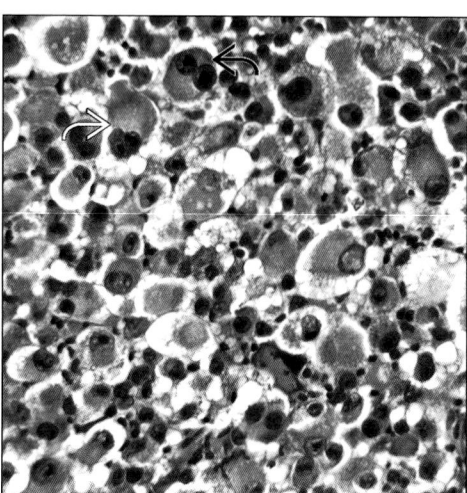
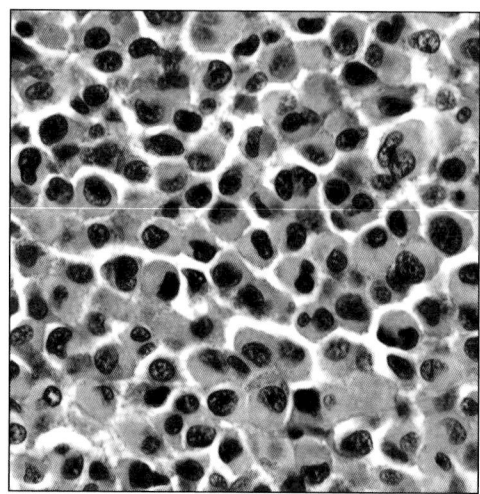

Variant Microscopic Features

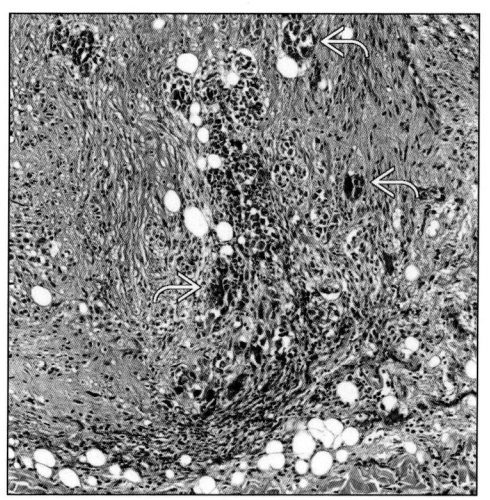

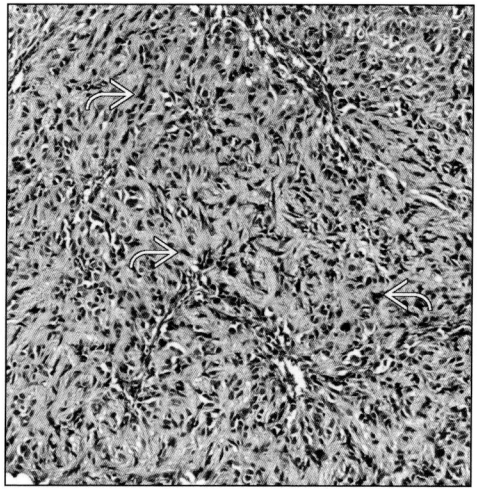

(Left) Myxoid melanoma at low magnification shows a deeply invasive tumor associated with a very prominent mucinous stroma. However, scattered irregular nests ➡ of atypical tumor cells can be identified. (Right) Myxoid melanoma in another area shows a proliferation of markedly atypical-appearing, hyperchromatic-staining, oval to spindle-shaped cells ➡, mimicking a myxoid sarcoma such as a high-grade myxofibrosarcoma.

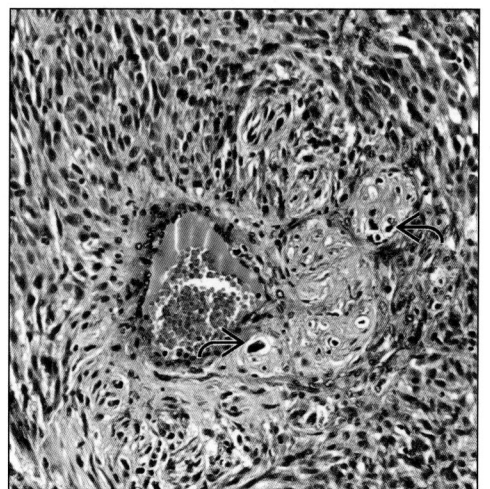

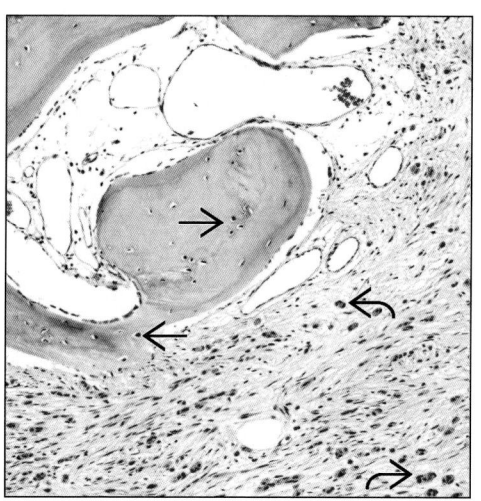

(Left) This spindle cell melanoma shows an area of chondroid differentiation containing small collections of hyperchromatic-staining cells within clear spaces ➡ surrounded by a myxohyalinized stroma. (Right) Osteoid melanoma shows a focus of ossification with atypical-appearing oval to spindle-shaped cells with perinuclear halos ➡ embedded in a dense osseous matrix. Note the mixed spindled and epithelioid cell population with focal nests ➡ in the surrounding stroma.

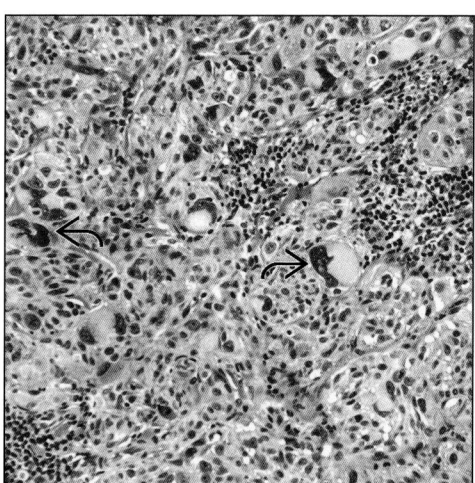

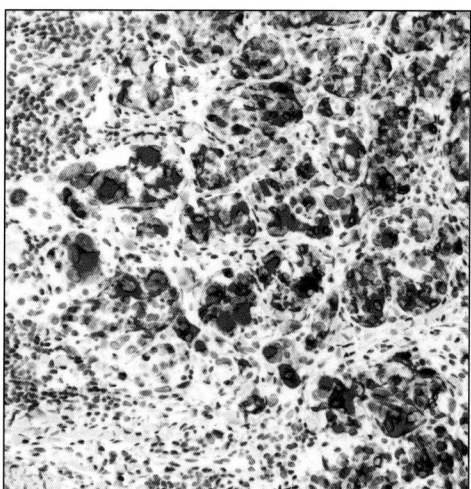

(Left) This is a case of spindle cell/pleomorphic melanoma, which can mimic spindle cell carcinoma, atypical fibroxanthoma, and MFH/pleomorphic sarcoma (as well as other sarcomas). Note the frankly pleomorphic, bizarre-appearing tumor giant cells ➡. (Right) HMB-45 (red chromogen) shows strong and diffuse cytoplasmic staining in this case of spindle cell/pleomorphic melanoma.

PROTOCOL FOR SPECIMENS OF MALIGNANT MELANOMA OF THE SKIN

Melanoma of the Skin

Biopsy, Excision, Reexcision

Procedure (select all that apply)

____ Biopsy, shave

____ Biopsy, punch

____ Biopsy, incisional

____ Excision

____ Reexcision

____ Lymphadenectomy, sentinel node(s)

____ Lymphadenectomy, regional nodes (specify): _____

____ Other (specify): _____

____ Not specified

Specimen Laterality

____ Right

____ Left

____ Midline

____ Not specified

Tumor Site

Specify, if known: _____

____ Not specified

Tumor Size (required only if tumor is grossly present)

Greatest dimension: _____ cm

*Additional dimensions: _____ x _____ cm

____ Indeterminate

Macroscopic Satellite Nodule(s) (required for excision specimens only)

____ Not identified

____ Present

____ Indeterminate

*Macroscopic Pigmentation

*____ Not identified

*____ Present, diffuse

*____ Present, patchy/focal

*____ Indeterminate

Histologic Type

Malignant melanoma

____ Melanoma, not otherwise specified

____ Superficial spreading melanoma

____ Nodular melanoma

____ Lentigo maligna melanoma

____ Acral-lentiginous melanoma

____ Desmoplastic &/or desmoplastic neurotropic melanoma

____ Melanoma arising from blue nevus

____ Melanoma arising in a giant congenital nevus

____ Melanoma of childhood

____ Nevoid melanoma

____ Persistent melanoma

____ Other (specify): _____

Maximum Tumor Thickness

Specify: _____ mm

At least _____ mm

____ Indeterminate

PROTOCOL FOR SPECIMENS OF MALIGNANT MELANOMA OF THE SKIN

*Clark (Anatomic) Level

*____ I (melanoma in situ)

*____ II (melanoma present in, but does not fill and expand, papillary dermis)

*____ III (melanoma fills and expands papillary dermis)

*____ IV (melanoma invades reticular dermis)

*____ V (melanoma invades subcutaneum)

Ulceration

____ Present

____ Not identified

____ Indeterminate

Margins (select all that apply)

Peripheral margins

____ Cannot be assessed

____ Uninvolved by invasive melanoma

Distance of invasive melanoma from closest peripheral margin: _____ mm (required for excisions only)

Specify location(s), if possible: _____

____ Involved by invasive melanoma

Specify location(s), if possible: _____

____ Uninvolved by melanoma in situ

Distance of melanoma in situ from closest margin: _____ mm (required for excisions only)

Specify location(s), if possible: _____

____ Involved by melanoma in situ

Specify location(s), if possible: _____

Deep margin

____ Cannot be assessed

____ Uninvolved by invasive melanoma

Distance of invasive melanoma from margin: _____ mm (required for excisions only)

Specify location(s), if possible: _____

____ Involved by invasive melanoma

Specify location(s), if possible: _____

Mitotic Index

____ < 1/mm²

Specify number/mm²: _____

Microsatellitosis

____ Not identified

____ Present

____ Indeterminate

Lymph-Vascular Invasion

____ Not identified

____ Present

____ Indeterminate

*Perineural Invasion

*____ Not identified

*____ Present

*____ Indeterminate

*Tumor-infiltrating Lymphocytes

*____ Not identified

*____ Present, nonbrisk

*____ Present, brisk

*Tumor Regression

*____ Not identified

PROTOCOL FOR SPECIMENS OF MALIGNANT MELANOMA OF THE SKIN

*____ Present, involving < 75% of lesion

*____ Present, involving ≥ 75% of lesion

*____ Indeterminate

Growth Phase (select all that apply)

*____ Radial

*____ Vertical

*____ Indeterminate

Lymph Nodes (required only if lymph nodes are present in the specimen) (select all that apply)

Number of sentinel nodes examined: _____

Total number of nodes examined (sentinel and nonsentinel): _____

Number of lymph nodes with metastases: _____

*Extranodal tumor extension

    *____ Present

    *____ Not identified

    *____ Indeterminate

*Size of largest metastatic focus: _____ (mm) (for sentinel node)

*Location of metastatic tumor (for sentinel node)

    *____ Subcapsular

    *____ Intramedullary

    *____ Subcapsular and intramedullary

Pathologic Staging (pTNM)

TNM descriptors (required only if applicable) (select all that apply)

____ m (multiple

____ r (recurrent)

____ y (post treatment)

Primary tumor (pT)

____ pTX: Primary tumor cannot be assessed (e.g., shave biopsy or regressed melanoma)

____ pT0: No evidence of primary tumor

____ pTis: Melanoma in situ (i.e., not an invasive tumor: Anatomic level 1)

pT1: Melanoma ≤ 1 mm in thickness, ± ulceration

    ____ pT1a: Melanoma ≤ 1.0 mm in thickness, no ulceration, < 1 mitosis/mm²

    ____ pT1b: Melanoma ≤ 1.0 mm in thickness with ulceration &/or ≥ 1 mitosis/mm²

pT2: Melanoma 1.01-2.0 mm in thickness, ± ulceration

    ____ pT2a: Melanoma 1.01-2.0 mm in thickness, no ulceration

    ____ pT2b: Melanoma 1.01-2.0 mm in thickness, with ulceration

pT3: Melanoma 2.01-4.0 mm in thickness, ± ulceration

    ____ pT3a: Melanoma 2.01-4.0 mm in thickness, no ulceration

    ____ pT3b: Melanoma 2.01-4.0 mm in thickness, with ulceration

pT4: Melanoma > 4.0 mm in thickness, ± ulceration

    ____ pT4a: Melanoma > 4.0 mm in thickness, no ulceration

    ____ pT4b: Melanoma > 4.0 mm in thickness, with ulceration

Regional lymph nodes (pN)

____ pNX: Regional lymph nodes cannot be assessed

____ pN0: No regional lymph node metastasis

pN1: Metastasis in 1 regional lymph node

    ____ pN1a: Clinically occult (microscopic) metastasis

    ____ pN1b: Clinically apparent (macroscopic metastasis

pN2: Metastasis in 2-3 regional lymph nodes or in intralymphatic regional metastasis without nodal metastasis

    ____ pN2a: Clinically occult (microscopic) metastasis

    ____ pN2b: Clinically apparent (macroscopic) metastasis

    ____ pN2c: Satellite or in-transit metastasis without nodal metastasis

____ pN3: Metastasis in ≥ 4 regional lymph nodes, or matted metastatic nodes, or in-transit metastasis or satellite(s) with metastasis in regional node(s)

____ No nodes submitted or found

Number of lymph nodes identified: _____

Number containing metastasis identified macroscopically: _____

Number containing metastases identified microscopically: _____

Matted nodes

    ____ Present

    ____ Not identified

Distant metastasis (pM)

____ Not applicable

____ pM1: Distant metastasis (documented in this specimen)

*____ pM1a: Metastasis in skin, subcutaneous tissues, or distant lymph nodes

*____ pM1b: Metastasis to lung

*____ pM1c: Metastasis to all other visceral sites or distant metastasis at any site associated with an elevated serum lactic dehydrogenase (LDH)

    *Specify site, if known: _____

*Additional Pathologic Findings (select all that apply)

*____ Nevus remnant

*____ Other (specify): _____

*Adapted with permission from College of American Pathologists, "Protocol for the Examination of Specimens from Patients with Melanoma of the Skin." Posting date: November 2011, www.cap.org. *Data elements with asterisks are not required. These elements may be clinically important but are not yet validated or regularly used in patient management.*

Melanoma Staging: Clark Levels

(Left) Clark level I melanoma is a melanoma in situ with no evidence of dermal invasion. *(Right)* Clark level II invasive melanoma focally invades into the papillary dermis ➡️.

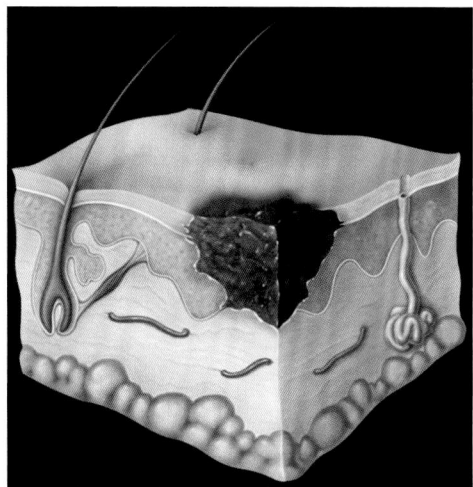 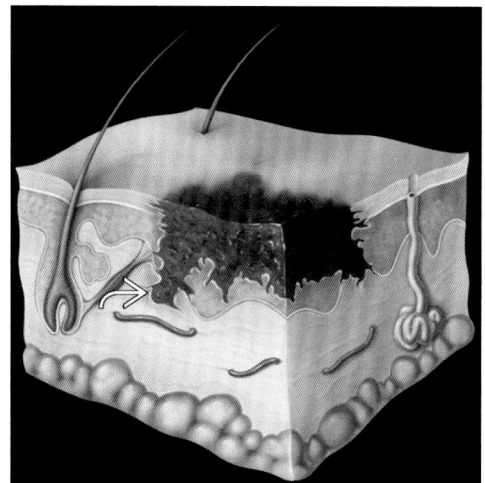

(Left) Clark level III invasive melanoma invades into and expands the papillary dermis ➡️. Note the focal projections extending into the papillary/reticular dermal junction ➡️, a finding that is still compatible with Clark level III. *(Right)* Clark level IV melanoma invades widely and deeply into the reticular dermis ➡️.

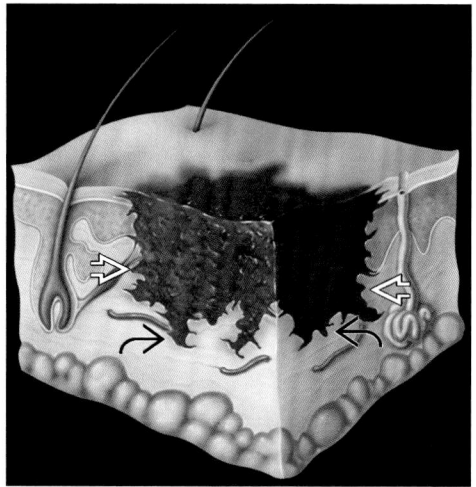 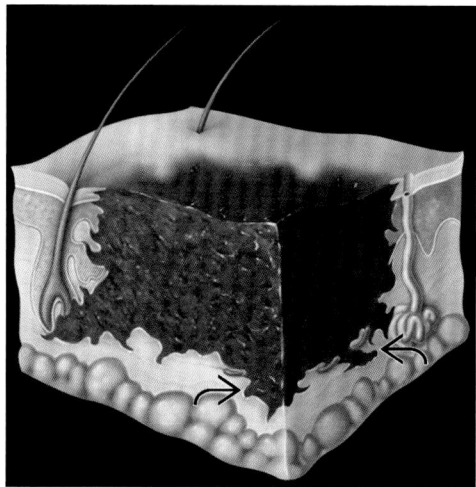

(Left) Graphic demonstrates Clark level IV melanoma with ulceration ➡️ and invasion of the reticular dermis ➡️. *(Right)* Clark level V melanoma invades into the subcutaneous adipose tissue ➡️.

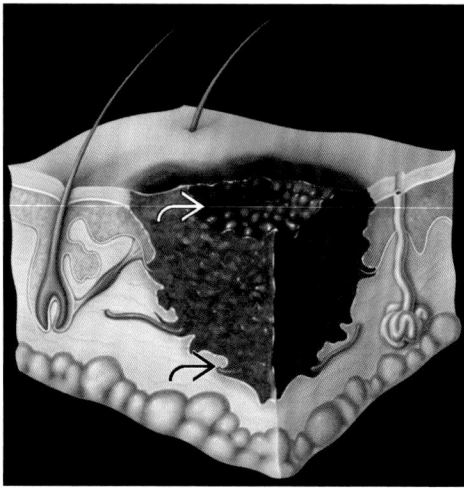 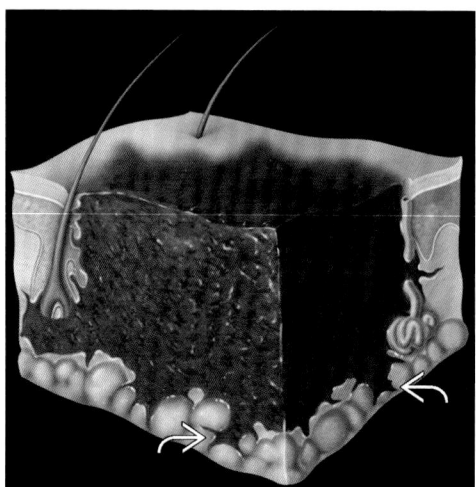

PROTOCOL FOR SPECIMENS OF MALIGNANT MELANOMA OF THE SKIN

Melanoma Tumor Staging

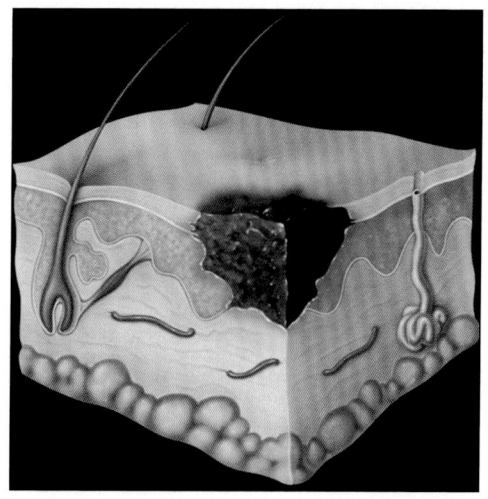
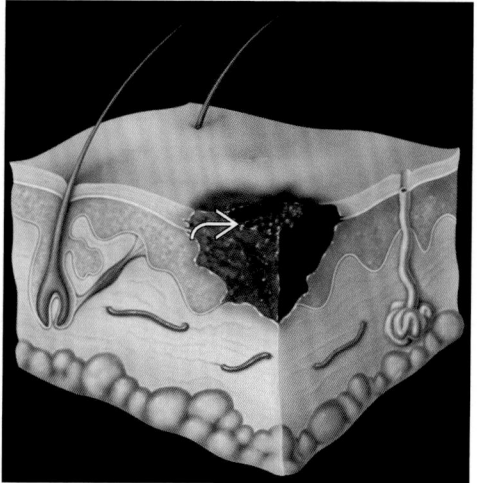

(Left) Tis melanoma is a melanoma in situ with no evidence of dermal invasion. (Right) Tis melanoma is a melanoma in situ with no evidence of dermal invasion. This example shows focal ulceration ➔, but that does not change the stage of in situ melanoma.

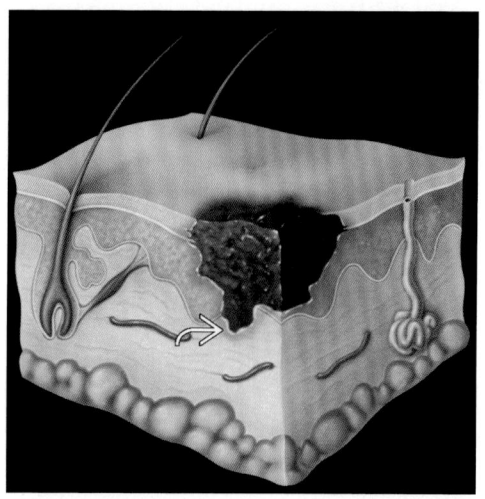
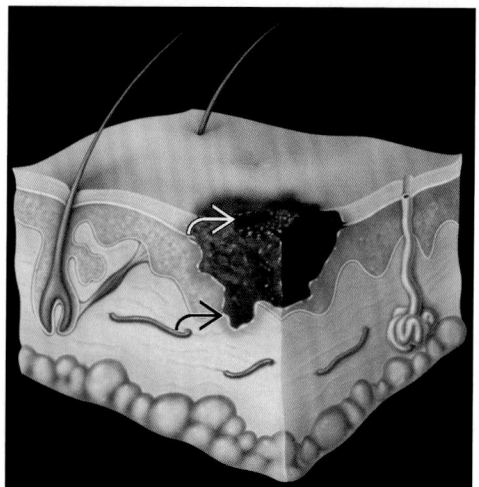

(Left) T1a invasive melanoma shows a tumor with superficial invasion ➔ to less than or equal to 1.0 mm in thickness, without ulceration or evidence of dermal mitotic activity. (Right) T1b invasive melanoma shows a tumor invasive ➔ to less than or equal to 1.0 mm in thickness, with ulceration ➔ &/or evidence of dermal mitotic activity (≥ 1/mm²).

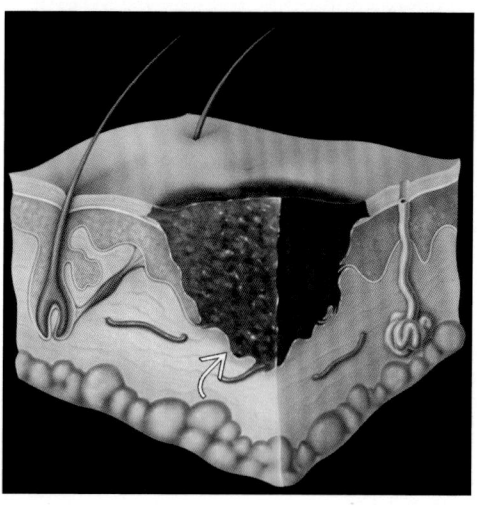
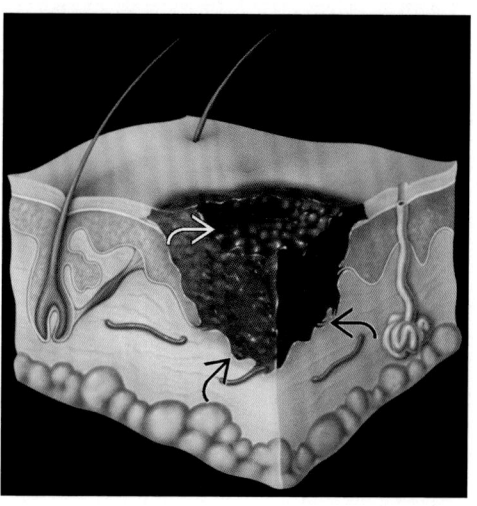

(Left) T2a melanoma invades to greater than 1.0 mm in thickness ➔ but is ≤ 2.0 mm in depth and lacks evidence of ulceration. (Right) T2b melanoma invades to greater than 1.0 mm in thickness ➔ but is ≤ 2.0 mm in depth and shows evidence of ulceration ➔.

PROTOCOL FOR SPECIMENS OF MALIGNANT MELANOMA OF THE SKIN

Melanoma Tumor, Lymph Node, and Metastatic Staging

(Left) T3a melanoma invades to greater than 2.0 mm in thickness but is ≤ 4.0 mm in depth and lacks evidence of ulceration. *(Right)* T3b melanoma invades to greater than 2.0 mm in thickness but is ≤ 4.0 mm in depth and shows evidence of ulceration ➨.

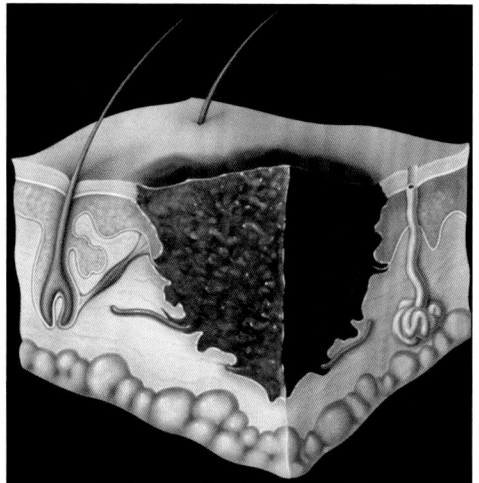
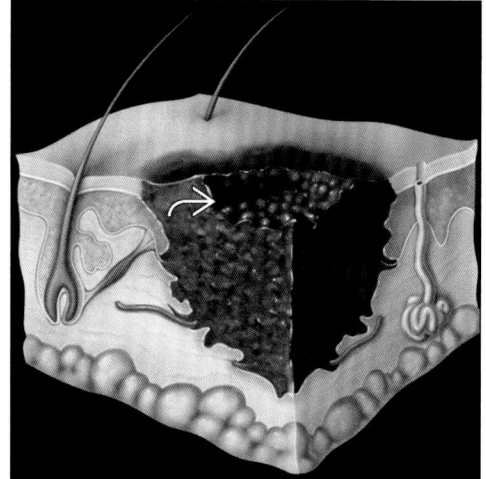

(Left) T4a melanoma invades to greater than 4.0 mm and frequently extends to the dermal/subcutaneous junction ➨. These are often nodular type melanomas. *(Right)* T4b melanoma invades to greater than 4.0 mm and shows overlying ulceration ➨.

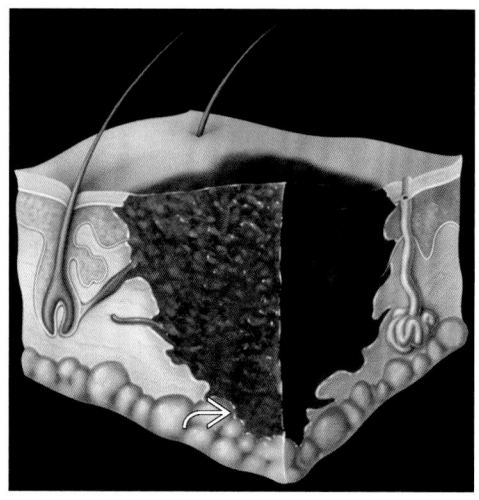
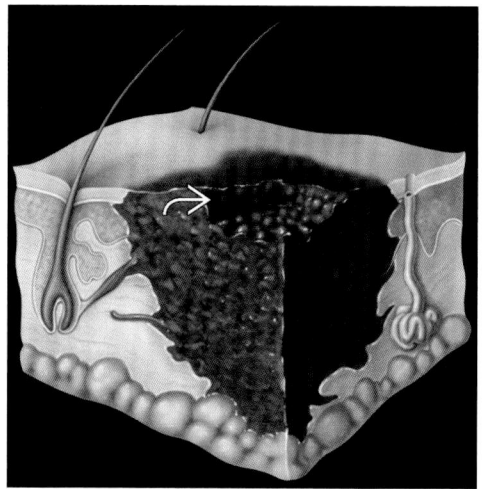

(Left) Nodal metastasis (N stage). N1 disease (left) is defined as metastasis to 1 lymph node ➨. N2 disease (center) is metastasis to 2-3 lymph nodes ➨. N4 disease (right) is 4 or more lymph nodes ➨, matted nodes, or in-transit/satellite metastases with metastatic nodes. *(Right)* In this graphic, a primary cutaneous melanoma of the arm ➨ is associated with proximal skin metastasis ➨ (M1a) and lung metastasis ➨ (M1b).

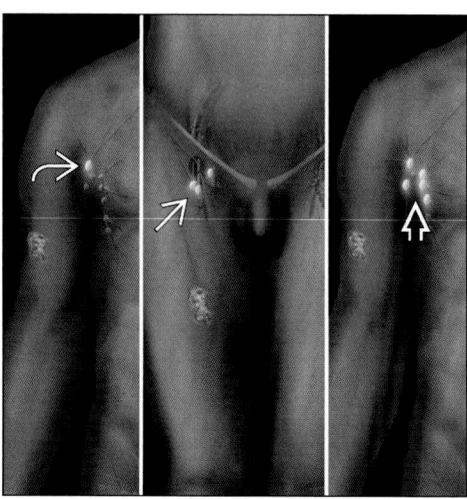
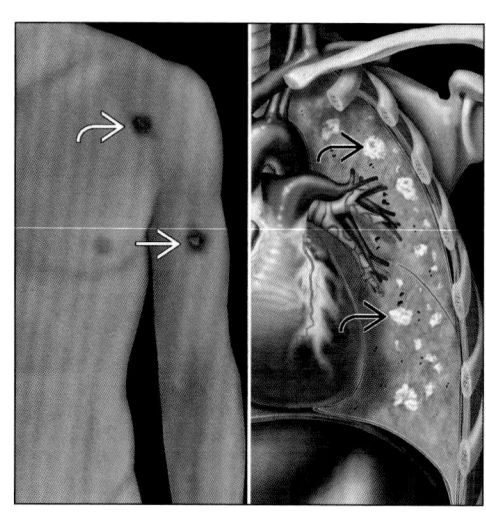

Imaging Features in Metastatic Melanoma

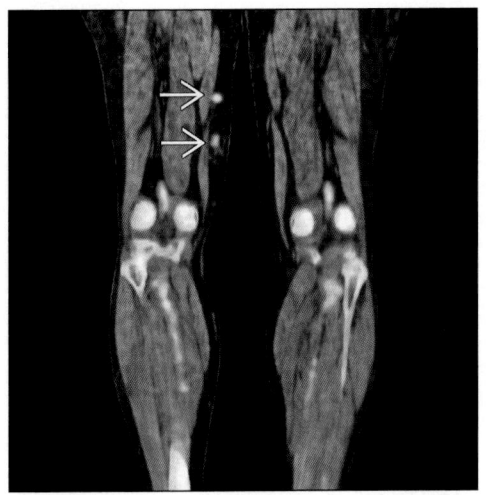 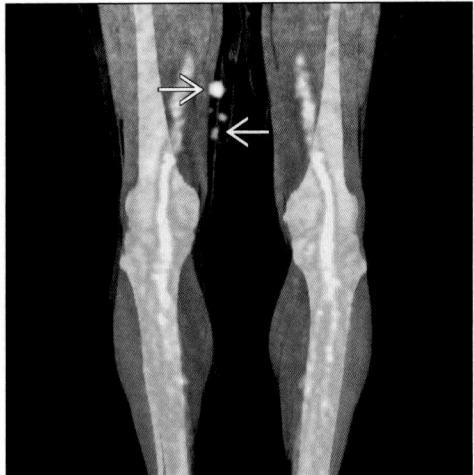

(Left) Coronal fused PET/CT shows multiple intensely FDG-avid subcutaneous nodules ➡ in a patient with T3b melanoma, consistent with in-transit metastases. (Right) Coronal fused PET/CT MIP better shows the multiple subcutaneous nodules ➡, consistent with in-transit metastases in the same patient with T3b melanoma (N2c or N3, if lymph nodes also involved).

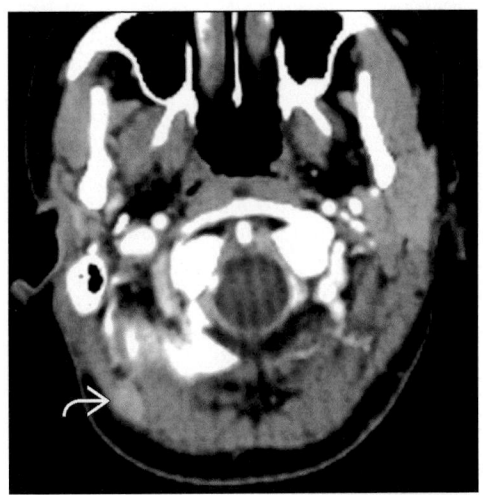 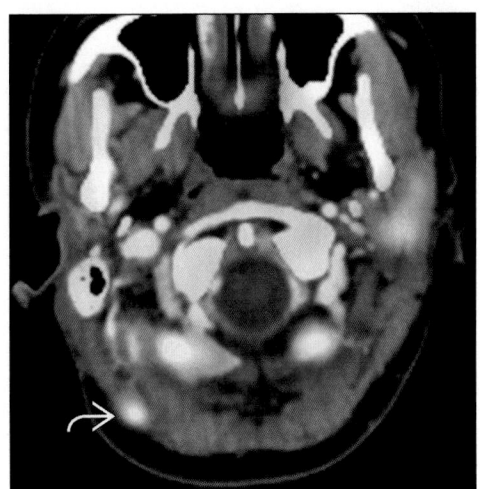

(Left) Axial CECT in a patient with T3a primary melanoma of the upper chest shows a subtle enhancing lesion ➡ of the right posterior neck. (Right) Axial fused PET/CT in the same patient shows intense FDG activity ➡ in the same lesion in the right posterior neck musculature, consistent with metastatic disease (M1a).

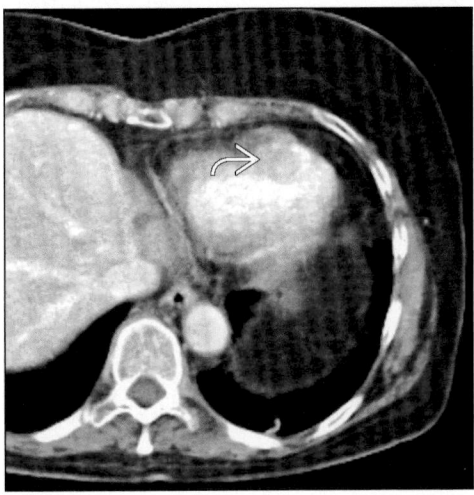 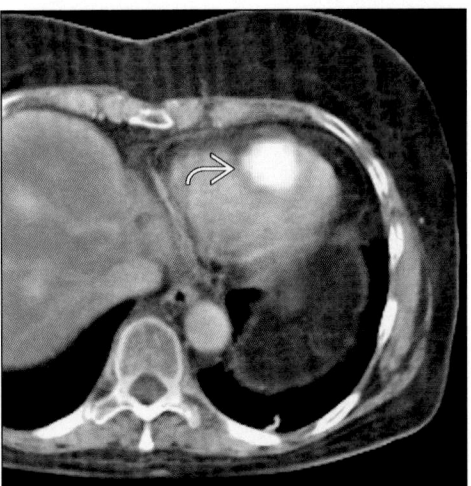

(Left) Axial CECT shows a subtle low-attenuation lesion ➡ in or immediately adjacent to the right ventricle in a patient with a history of metastatic melanoma. (Right) Axial fused PET/CT shows strong FDG activity in the lesion ➡ in or immediately adjacent to the right ventricle, consistent with metastatic melanoma (M1c).

Reference Indices

ANTIBODY INDEX

Antibodies Discussed

Antibody Name/ Symbol	Antibody Description	Clones/Alternative Names	Chapters
α1-antichymotrypsin	alpha 1 antichromotrypsin	A1ACT	Myofibroma and Myofibromatosis; PEComas
α-fetoprotein	alpha 1 fetoprotein	AFP, Z5A06, Clone C3	Metastatic Tumors to the Skin
β-2-microglobulin		B2-microglob	Angioimmunoblastic T-cell Lymphoma; Mycosis Fungoides (and Subtypes)
β-catenin	beta catenin; involved in regulation of cell adhesion and in signal transduction through Wnt pathway	B-catenin, CLONE 14, E-5, RB-9035Po, 17C2, 5H10	Digital Fibromatosis (Infantile Digital Fibromatosis); Ectopic Meningioma; Extranodal NK/T-cell Lymphoma, Nasal Type; Fibromatosis; Fibrosarcoma; Juvenile Hyaline Fibromatosis; Low-Grade Fibromyxoid Sarcoma (Evans Tumor); Myofibroma and Myofibromatosis; Pilomatrixoma and Pilomatrical Carcinoma; Plexiform Fibrohistiocytic Tumor; Pseudosarcomatous Fibroblastic Proliferations
34bE12	cytokeratin, high molecular weight (34bE12- CK 1, 5, 10, 14)	MA-903, CK903	Toker Cell Hyperplasia
Actin-HHF-35	actin, muscle (HHF35)	MSA, HHF-35	Angiomatoid Fibrous Histiocytoma; Myofibroma and Myofibromatosis; PEComas; Sinonasal Melanoma
Actin-sm	actin, smooth muscle	SMA, ASM-1, CGA7, 1A4, HUC1-1	Adenoid Cystic Carcinoma; Angioleiomyoma; Angiomatoid Fibrous Histiocytoma; Angiosarcoma; Atypical Fibroxanthoma; Bronchogenic Cyst; Cellular Neurothekeoma; Congenital Smooth Muscle Hamartoma; Cutaneous Malignant Fibrous Histiocytoma/ Pleomorphic Sarcoma; Dermatofibroma and Fibrous Histiocytoma; Digital Fibromatosis (Infantile Digital Fibromatosis); Distinctive Dermal Clear Cell Mesenchymal Tumor; Epithelioid Hemangioendothelioma; Epithelioid Sarcoma; Glomus Tumors; Infantile Hemangioma; Kaposi Sarcoma; Leiomyosarcoma; Low-Grade Fibromyxoid Sarcoma (Evans Tumor); Myxofibrosarcoma; Neuromas; PEComas; Perineurioma; Pleomorphic Fibroma; Pseudosarcomatous Fibroblastic Proliferations; Sinonasal Melanoma; Spindle Cell Hemangioma; Squamous Cell Carcinoma (and Variants)
Adipophilin	ADFP (adipose differentiation-related protein)	AP125	Hidradenocarcinoma; Hidradenoma
AE1/AE3	mixture of 2 anticytokeratin clones that detect a variety of both high and low molecular weight cytokeratins		Atypical Fibroxanthoma; Congenital Smooth Muscle Hamartoma; Digital Fibromatosis (Infantile Digital Fibromatosis); Epithelioid Sarcoma; Extramammary Paget Disease; Low-Grade Fibromyxoid Sarcoma (Evans Tumor); Median Raphe Cyst; Squamomelanocytic Tumor; Syringocystadenoma Papilliferum
ALK	anaplastic lymphoma kinase 1	ALK1, 5A4, ALKC	Atypical Lipomatous Tumor and Liposarcoma; Histiocytic Sarcoma; Lymphomatoid Papulosis; Primary Cutaneous Anaplastic Large Cell Lymphoma; Systemic T-cell and NK-cell Lymphomas Involving the Skin
ALK1	anaplastic lymphoma kinase 1	5A4, ALKC	Adult T-cell Leukemia/Lymphoma; Cutaneous Malignant Fibrous Histiocytoma/Pleomorphic Sarcoma; Primary Cutaneous Anaplastic Large Cell Lymphoma; Systemic T-cell and NK-cell Lymphomas Involving the Skin
Androgen receptor		AR441, F39.4.1, AR-N20, ANDROGEN RE	Apocrine Carcinoma (Apocrine Adenocarcinoma); Basal Cell Carcinoma; Hidradenoma; Sebaceous Carcinoma; Squamous Cell Carcinoma (and Variants);

			Squamous Cell Carcinoma In Situ (Bowen Disease); Tricholemmal Carcinoma
APC	adenomatous polyposis coliprotein		Fibromatosis; Myofibroma and Myofibromatosis
BAD	Bcl-2-associated agonist of cell death		Mucosal Melanoma (Genital)
BAX	Bcl-2-associated X protein	PU-347-P, B-9, BAX-P, P19, BAX-M	Basal Cell Carcinoma
Bcl-1		Cyclin-D1	Systemic B-cell Lymphomas Involving the Skin
Bcl-2	B-cell lymphoma 2; suppresses apoptosis in a variety of cell systems	ONCL2, BCL2/100/D5, 124, 124.3	Actinic Keratosis; Basal Cell Carcinoma; Cutaneous Marginal Zone B-cell Lymphoma; Diffuse Large B-cell Lymphoma, Leg Type; Digital Fibromatosis (Infantile Digital Fibromatosis); Inverted Follicular Keratosis; Leukemia Cutis; Lymphomatoid Papulosis; Microcystic Adnexal Carcinoma; Nevus Sebaceus and Follicular Hamartomas; Perineurioma; Primary Cutaneous Follicle Center Lymphoma; Primary Neuroendocrine (Merkel Cell) Carcinoma; Sebaceous Carcinoma; Systemic B-cell Lymphomas Involving the Skin; Trichoblastoma; Trichoepithelioma
Bcl-6	B-cell CLL/lymphoma 6	LN22, GI191E/A8, N-3, PG-B6P, P1F6, 3FR-1	Blastic Plasmacytoid Dendritic Cell Neoplasm; Cutaneous Marginal Zone B-cell Lymphoma; Diffuse Large B-cell Lymphoma, Leg Type; Leukemia Cutis; Primary Cutaneous CD4+ Small/Medium Pleomorphic T-cell Lymphoma; Primary Cutaneous Follicle Center Lymphoma
BDCA-2	monoclonal antibody directed toward immature plasmacytoid dendritic cells	CD303	Blastic Plasmacytoid Dendritic Cell Neoplasm
BER-EP4	epithelial cell adhesion molecule	AUA1, VU-1D9, EPCAM, C10, HEA125	Actinic Keratosis; Basal Cell Carcinoma; Hidradenocarcinoma; Hidradenoma; Metastatic Tumors to the Skin; Sebaceoma (Sebaceous Epithelioma); Sebaceous Adenoma; Sebaceous Carcinoma; Squamous Cell Carcinoma (and Variants)
BF1	T-cell receptor antigen	T_Cell_AG_R, Beta-F1, 8A3, TCR	Intravascular Large B-cell Lymphoma
BMI1	B-cell-specific Moloney murine leukemia virus site 1	6C9, F6	Basal Cell Carcinoma
BOB.1	B-cell OCT-binding protein 1	SC955, BOB1	Lymphomatoid Granulomatosis
C-Kit	tyrosine-protein kinase activity	CD117, C-19 (C-KIT), 104D2, 2E4, CKIT, A4502, H300, CMA-767	Cutaneous and Systemic Mastocytosis
c-myc	myelocytomatosis viral oncogene	C-MYC, 9E10, 9E11, 1-262	Atypical Vascular Lesion; Systemic B-cell Lymphomas Involving the Skin
C-reactive protein	Acute phase protein involved in complement activation	CRP	Extranodal NK/T-cell Lymphoma, Nasal Type; Subcutaneous Panniculitis-like T-cell Lymphoma
CA 19-9	related to the Lewis blood group; shown to label multiple types of adenocarcinomas	1116NS19-9	Metastatic Tumors to the Skin
Calcitonin	polypeptide hormone produced by parafollicular cells (C cells) of the thyroid	CALBINDIN28	Metastatic Tumors to the Skin
Caldesmon	actin interacting and calmodulin binding protein found in smooth muscle and other cell types		Digital Fibromatosis (Infantile Digital Fibromatosis); Glomus Tumors; Leiomyosarcoma; Myofibroma and Myofibromatosis; Pseudosarcomatous Fibroblastic Proliferations
Calponin	thin filament-associated protein that is implicated in regulation and modulation of smooth muscle contraction	N3, 26A11, CALP, CNN1, SMCC, Sm Calp	Adenoid Cystic Carcinoma; Angiomatoid Fibrous Histiocytoma; Chondroid Lipoma; Cutaneous Mixed Tumor (Chondroid Syringoma); Cylindroma; Digital Fibromatosis (Infantile Digital Fibromatosis); Fibromatosis; Leiomyoma (Pilar); Leiomyosarcoma; Malignant Mixed Tumor; Myofibroma and Myofibromatosis;

ANTIBODY INDEX

			PEComas; Pseudosarcomatous Fibroblastic Proliferations; Spiradenoma
Calretinin	29 kDa calcium binding protein that is expressed in central and peripheral nervous system and in many normal and pathological tissues	DAK-CALRET, 5A5, CAL 3F5, DC8, AB149	Granular Cell Tumor; Metastatic Tumors to the Skin
Carcinooembryonic antigen		CEA-M, mCEA, CEA-B18, CEA-D14, CEAGOLD 1, T84.6, CEA-GOLD 2, CEA 11, CEA-GOLD 3, CEA 27, CEAGOLD 4, CEA 41, CEA-GOLD 5, T84.1, CEA-M, A5B7, CEJ065, IL-7, T84.66, TF3H8-1, 0062, D14, alpha-7, PARLAM 1, ZC23, CEM010, A115, COL-1, AF4, 12.140.10, 11-7, M773, CEA-M431_31, CEJO65	Clear Cell Papulosis; Cutaneous Mixed Tumor (Chondroid Syringoma); Papillary Eccrine Adenoma
CCND1	protein with important cell cycle regulatory functions	Cyclin-D1, bcl-1 (cyclin D1) A-12, PRAD1, AM29, DCS-6, SP4, 5D4, D1GM, P2D11F11, CCND1, Cyl-1	Systemic B-cell Lymphomas Involving the Skin
CCR4	chemokine receptor 4	CD194	Leukemia Cutis
CD1a	T-cell surface glycoprotein	JPM30, CD1A, O10, NA1/34	Blastic Plasmacytoid Dendritic Cell Neoplasm; Histiocytic Sarcoma; Juvenile and Adult-type Xanthogranuloma; Langerhans Cell Histiocytosis; Leukemia Cutis; Multicentric Reticulohistiocytosis; Non-Langerhans Cell Histiocytoses; Polyvinylpyrrolidone Storage Disease; Reticulohistiocytoma; Rosai-Dorfman Disease
CD2	T-cell surface antigen	271, MT910, AB75, LFA-2	Aggressive Epidermotropic CD8+ Cytotoxic T-cell Lymphoma; Angioimmunoblastic T-cell Lymphoma; Blastic Plasmacytoid Dendritic Cell Neoplasm; Cutaneous and Systemic Mastocytosis; Cutaneous Gamma-Delta T-cell Lymphoma; Histiocytic Sarcoma; Intravascular Large B-cell Lymphoma; Leukemia Cutis; Primary Cutaneous CD4+ Small/Medium Pleomorphic T-cell Lymphoma; Primary Cutaneous Follicle Center Lymphoma; Subcutaneous Panniculitis-like T-cell Lymphoma; Systemic T-cell and NK-cell Lymphomas Involving the Skin
CD3	T-cell receptor	F7238, A0452, CD3-P, CD3-M, SP7, PS1	Adult T-cell Leukemia/Lymphoma; Aggressive Epidermotropic CD8+ Cytotoxic T-cell Lymphoma; Angioimmunoblastic T-cell Lymphoma; Angiosarcoma; Blastic Plasmacytoid Dendritic Cell Neoplasm; Cutaneous Gamma-Delta T-cell Lymphoma; Cutaneous Marginal Zone B-cell Lymphoma; Extramammary Paget Disease; Extranodal NK/T-cell Lymphoma, Nasal Type; Histiocytic Sarcoma; Intravascular Large B-cell Lymphoma; Leukemia Cutis; Lymphomatoid Granulomatosis; Lymphomatoid Papulosis; Non-Langerhans Cell Histiocytoses; Peripheral Neuroepithelioma/Primitive Neuroectodermal Tumor; Primary Cutaneous Anaplastic Large Cell Lymphoma; Primary Cutaneous CD4+ Small/Medium Pleomorphic T-cell Lymphoma; Primary Cutaneous Follicle Center Lymphoma; Reticulohistiocytoma; Subcutaneous Panniculitis-like T-cell Lymphoma; Systemic T-cell and NK-cell Lymphomas Involving the Skin
CD3-ε	T-cell surface antigen T3/Leu-4 epsilon chain	CD3E, CD3e	Extranodal NK/T-cell Lymphoma, Nasal Type
CD4	T-cell surface glycoprotein L3T4	IF6, 1290, 4B12, CD4	Angioimmunoblastic T-cell Lymphoma; Blastic Plasmacytoid Dendritic Cell Neoplasm; Cutaneous Gamma-Delta T-cell Lymphoma; Extramammary Paget Disease; Histiocytic Sarcoma; Leukemia Cutis; Lymphomatoid Granulomatosis; Lymphomatoid Papulosis; Mycosis Fungoides (and Subtypes); Non-Langerhans Cell Histiocytoses; Primary Cutaneous

			Anaplastic Large Cell Lymphoma; Primary Cutaneous CD4+ Small/Medium Pleomorphic T-cell Lymphoma; Subcutaneous Panniculitis-like T-cell Lymphoma; Systemic T-cell and NK-cell Lymphomas Involving the Skin
CD5	T-cell surface glycoprotein Leu1, T1	NCL-CD5, 4C7, 54/B4, 54/F6	Adult T-cell Leukemia/Lymphoma; Aggressive Epidermotropic CD8+ Cytotoxic T-cell Lymphoma; Angioimmunoblastic T-cell Lymphoma; Cutaneous Gamma-Delta T-cell Lymphoma; Intravascular Large B-cell Lymphoma; Leukemia Cutis; Primary Cutaneous CD4+ Small/Medium Pleomorphic T-cell Lymphoma; Subcutaneous Panniculitis-like T-cell Lymphoma; Systemic B-cell Lymphomas Involving the Skin; Systemic T-cell and NK-cell Lymphomas Involving the Skin
CD7	T-cell antigen precursor Leu 9	272, CD7-272	Adult T-cell Leukemia/Lymphoma; Aggressive Epidermotropic CD8+ Cytotoxic T-cell Lymphoma; Angioimmunoblastic T-cell Lymphoma; Blastic Plasmacytoid Dendritic Cell Neoplasm; Cutaneous Gamma-Delta T-cell Lymphoma; Intravascular large B-cell Lymphoma; Leukemia Cutis; Lymphomatoid Granulomatosis; Lymphomatoid Papulosis; Mycosis Fungoides (and Subtypes); Primary Cutaneous Anaplastic Large Cell Lymphoma; Primary Cutaneous CD4+ Small/Medium Pleomorphic T-cell Lymphoma; Primary Cutaneous Follicle Center Lymphoma; Subcutaneous Panniculitis-like T-cell Lymphoma; Systemic T-cell and NK-cell Lymphomas Involving the Skin
CD8	T-cell coreceptor antigen Leu 2, T-cytotoxic cells	M7103, C8/144, C8/144B	Aggressive Epidermotropic CD8+ Cytotoxic T-cell Lymphoma; Angioimmunoblastic T-cell Lymphoma; Cutaneous Gamma-Delta T-cell Lymphoma; Extramammary Paget Disease; Extranodal NK/T-cell Lymphoma, Nasal Type; Intravascular Large B-cell Lymphoma; Leukemia Cutis; Lymphomatoid Papulosis; Mycosis Fungoides (and Subtypes); Primary Cutaneous Anaplastic Large Cell Lymphoma; Primary Cutaneous CD4+ Small/Medium Pleomorphic T-cell Lymphoma; Subcutaneous Panniculitis-like T-cell Lymphoma; Systemic T-cell and NK-cell Lymphomas Involving the Skin
CD9	motility-related protein-1 (MRP-1)	72F16, BA-2	Cutaneous and Systemic Mastocytosis
CD10	neutral endopeptidase	NCL-270, CALLA, neprilysin, neutral endopeptidase, NEP	Adult T-cell Leukemia/Lymphoma; Angioimmunoblastic T-cell Lymphoma; Atypical Fibroxanthoma; Blastic Plasmacytoid Dendritic Cell Neoplasm; Cutaneous Marginal Zone B-cell Lymphoma; Cutaneous Plasmacytoma; Dermatofibroma and Fibrous Histiocytoma; Dermatofibrosarcoma Protuberans; Diffuse Large B-cell Lymphoma, Leg Type; Hidradenocarcinoma; Hidradenoma; Leiomyosarcoma; Leukemia Cutis; Metastatic Tumors to the Skin; PEComas; Pleomorphic Fibroma; Primary Cutaneous Follicle Center Lymphoma; Sebaceous Carcinoma; Squamous Cell Carcinoma (and Variants); Systemic B-cell Lymphomas Involving the Skin; Systemic T-cell and NK-cell Lymphomas Involving the Skin
CD13	plays role in growth of DC/macrophage progenitors and precursors		Extramedullary Hematopoiesis; Histiocytic Sarcoma
CD14	coreceptor for lipopolysaccharide binding protein	FMC32	Cutaneous and Systemic Mastocytosis; Histiocytic Sarcoma; Non-Langerhans Cell Histiocytoses

III

1

ANTIBODY INDEX

CD	Description	Clones	Associated conditions
CD15	reacts with Reed-Sternberg cells of Hodgkin lymphoma and with granulocytes	VIM-2, 3C4, LEU-M1, TU9, VIM-D5, MY1, CBD1, MMA, 3CD1, C3D1, Lewis x, SSEA-1	Cutaneous and Systemic Mastocytosis; Extramedullary Hematopoiesis; Histiocytic Sarcoma; Langerhans Cell Histiocytosis; Lymphomatoid Papulosis; Myxoinflammatory Fibroblastic Sarcoma; Systemic B-cell Lymphomas Involving the Skin
CD16	Fc receptor of IgG found on the surfaces of natural killer cells, neutrophils, monocytes, and macrophages		Cutaneous and Systemic Mastocytosis; Intravascular Large B-cell Lymphoma
CD19	B-cell antigen		Angioimmunoblastic T-cell Lymphoma; Blastic Plasmacytoid Dendritic Cell Neoplasm; Cutaneous Marginal Zone B-cell Lymphoma; Extranodal NK/T-cell Lymphoma, Nasal Type; Intravascular large B-cell Lymphoma; Leukemia Cutis; Primary Cutaneous Anaplastic Large Cell Lymphoma; Primary Cutaneous Follicle Center Lymphoma; Systemic B-cell Lymphomas Involving the Skin
CD20	activated-glycosylated phosphoprotein expressed on the surface of B cells from late pro-B cells through memory B cells	FB1, B1, L26	Angioimmunoblastic T-cell Lymphoma; Blastic Plasmacytoid Dendritic Cell Neoplasm; Cutaneous Gamma-Delta T-cell Lymphoma; Cutaneous Plasmacytoma; Diffuse Large B-cell Lymphoma, Leg Type; Extranodal NK/T-cell Lymphoma, Nasal Type; Histiocytic Sarcoma; Intravascular Large B-cell Lymphoma; Leukemia Cutis; Lymphomatoid Granulomatosis; Lymphomatoid Papulosis; Peripheral Neuroepithelioma/ Primitive Neuroectodermal Tumor; Primary Cutaneous Anaplastic Large Cell Lymphoma; Primary Cutaneous CD4+ Small/Medium Pleomorphic T-cell Lymphoma; Primary Cutaneous Follicle Center Lymphoma; Reticulohistiocytoma; Subcutaneous Panniculitis-like T-cell Lymphoma; Systemic B-cell Lymphomas Involving the Skin; Systemic T-cell and NK-cell Lymphomas Involving the Skin
CD21	CR2, complement component receptor 2, Epstein-Barr virus receptor		Adult T-cell Leukemia/Lymphoma; Angioimmunoblastic T-cell Lymphoma; Cutaneous Marginal Zone B-cell Lymphoma; Cutaneous Plasmacytoma; Diffuse Large B-cell Lymphoma, Leg Type; Histiocytic Sarcoma; Primary Cutaneous Follicle Center Lymphoma; Rosai-Dorfman Disease; Systemic T-cell and NK-cell Lymphomas Involving the Skin
CD22	B-cell receptor	FPC1, LEU 14	Cutaneous Marginal Zone B-cell Lymphoma; Intravascular Large B-cell Lymphoma
CD23	Fc ε RII, low-affinity IgE receptor, IGEBF	1B12, MHM6BU38	Angioimmunoblastic T-cell Lymphoma; Cutaneous Marginal Zone B-cell Lymphoma; Diffuse Large B-cell Lymphoma, Leg Type; Histiocytic Sarcoma; Leukemia Cutis; Primary Cutaneous Follicle Center Lymphoma; Systemic T-cell and NK-cell Lymphomas Involving the Skin
CD25	IL-2 receptor alpha	2A3, 4C9	Adult T-cell Leukemia/Lymphoma; Cutaneous and Systemic Mastocytosis; Leukemia Cutis; Lymphomatoid Papulosis; Mycosis Fungoides (and Subtypes)
CD26	ADA adenosine deaminase complexing protein 2, DPP4	44-4	Leukemia Cutis; Mycosis Fungoides (and Subtypes)
CD29	fibronectin receptor, integrein betaITGB1, 1	29C03, 7F10, HT29_12938	Intravascular Large B-cell Lymphoma
CD30	tumor necrosis factor SF8	BER-H2, KI-1, TNFRSF8	Adult T-cell Leukemia/Lymphoma; Angiomatoid Fibrous Histiocytoma; Angiosarcoma; Cutaneous Malignant Fibrous Histiocytoma/Pleomorphic Sarcoma; Histiocytic Sarcoma; Leukemia Cutis; Lymphomatoid Papulosis;

			Mycosis Fungoides (and Subtypes); Myxoinflammatory Fibroblastic Sarcoma; Primary Cutaneous Anaplastic Large Cell Lymphoma; Systemic B-cell Lymphomas Involving the Skin; Systemic T-cell and NK-cell Lymphomas Involving the Skin
CD31	platelet endothelial cell adhesion molecule	JC/70, JC/70A, PECAM-1	Angiolymphoid Hyperplasia with Eosinophilia; Angiomatoid Fibrous Histiocytoma; Angiosarcoma; Atypical Fibroxanthoma; Dermal Nerve Sheath Myxoma; Dermatofibroma and Fibrous Histiocytoma; Epithelioid Hemangioendothelioma; Epithelioid Sarcoma; Infantile Hemangioma; Kaposi Sarcoma; Kaposiform Hemangioendothelioma; Lymphangioma and Superficial Lymphangioma; Melanoma, Superficial Spreading Type; Multinucleate Cell Angiohistiocytoma; Papillary Intralymphatic Angioendothelioma (Dabska Tumor); Progressive Lymphangioma; Pseudosarcomatous Fibroblastic Proliferations; Retiform Hemangioendothelioma; Spindle Cell and Pleomorphic Lipoma; Superficial Malignant Peripheral Nerve Sheath Tumor; Vascular Hamartomas
CD33	SIGLEC lectin 3	PWS44	Blastic Plasmacytoid Dendritic Cell Neoplasm; Cutaneous and Systemic Mastocytosis; Extramedullary Hematopoiesis; Histiocytic Sarcoma; Leukemia Cutis
CD34	hematopoietic progenitor cell antigen	MY10, IOM34, QBEND10, 8G12, 1309, HPCA-1, NU-4A1, TUK4, clone 581, BI-3c5	Acral Fibrokeratoma; Angiofibroma and Related Lesions; Angioleiomyoma; Angiolymphoid Hyperplasia with Eosinophilia; Angiomatoid Fibrous Histiocytoma; Angiomyofibroblastoma; Angiosarcoma; Atypical Fibroxanthoma; Atypical Lipomatous Tumor and Liposarcoma; Childhood Melanoma; Collagenous Fibroma; Cutaneous Malignant Fibrous Histiocytoma/Pleomorphic Sarcoma; Dermal Nerve Sheath Myxoma; Dermatofibroma and Fibrous Histiocytoma; Dermatofibrosarcoma Protuberans; Dermatomyofibroma; Digital Fibromatosis (Infantile Digital Fibromatosis); Distinctive Dermal Clear Cell Mesenchymal Tumor; Eccrine Hamartomas; Ectopic Meningioma; Epithelioid Hemangioendothelioma; Epithelioid Histiocytoma; Epithelioid Sarcoma; Extramedullary Hematopoiesis; Fibromatosis; Fibrosarcoma; Fibrous Hamartoma of Infancy; Glomus Tumors; Granular Cell Tumor; Hibernoma; Infantile Hemangioma; Kaposi Sarcoma; Kaposiform Hemangioendothelioma; Leiomyosarcoma; Leukemia Cutis; Low-Grade Fibromyxoid Sarcoma (Evans Tumor); Lymphangioma and Superficial Lymphangioma; Multinucleate Cell Angiohistiocytoma; Myofibroma and Myofibromatosis; Myxofibrosarcoma; Myxoinflammatory Fibroblastic Sarcoma; Neurofibroma; Neuromas; Nevus Sebaceus and Follicular Hamartomas; Non-Langerhans Cell Histiocytoses; Papillary Intralymphatic Angioendothelioma (Dabska Tumor); Perineurioma; Pleomorphic Fibroma; Plexiform Fibrohistiocytic Tumor; Progressive Lymphangioma; Pseudosarcomatous Fibroblastic Proliferations; Reticulohistiocytoma; Retiform Hemangioendothelioma; Sclerotic Fibroma; Spindle Cell and Pleomorphic Lipoma; Spindle Cell Hemangioma; Superficial Acral Fibromyxoma; Verrucous Hemangioma

III

ANTIBODY INDEX

CD35	erythrocyte complement receptor 1, CR1, immune adherence receptor, C3b/C4b receptor	BER-MAC-DRC, TO5, CD35, E11	Angioimmunoblastic T-cell Lymphoma; Diffuse Large B-cell Lymphoma, Leg Type; Histiocytic Sarcoma; Primary Cutaneous Follicle Center Lymphoma; Rosai-Dorfman Disease; Systemic T-cell and NK-cell Lymphomas Involving the Skin
CD43	Major sialoglycoprotein on surface of human T lymphocytes, monocytes, granulocytes, and some B lymphocytes	LEU-22, DF-T1, L60, MT1, sialophorin, leukosialin, SPN	Blastic Plasmacytoid Dendritic Cell Neoplasm; Cutaneous Marginal Zone B-cell Lymphoma; Extramedullary Hematopoiesis; Intravascular Large B-cell Lymphoma; Leukemia Cutis; Primary Cutaneous Follicle Center Lymphoma; Systemic B-cell Lymphomas Involving the Skin
CD44	cell adhesion receptor for hyaluronic acid	HCAM, CD44H, B-F24, A3D8, 2C5, CD44S, F10-44.2, 156-3C11, DF1485, BBA10, VFF-14, CD44V10, CD44V3, 3G5, CD44V3-10-P, CD44V3-10, 3D2, CD44V4_5, CD44V5,VFF-8, VFF-7, 2F10, VFF-18, CD44V6, CD44V7, VFF-9, CD44V7_8, VFF-17	Primary Neuroendocrine (Merkel Cell) Carcinoma
CD45	leukocyte common antigen	LCA, PD7/26, 1.22/4.14, T29/33, RP2/18, PD7, 2D1, 2B11+PD7/26	Angiomatoid Fibrous Histiocytoma; Cutaneous and Systemic Mastocytosis; Cutaneous Malignant Fibrous Histiocytoma/Pleomorphic Sarcoma; Extramammary Paget Disease; Giant Cell Tumor of Tendon Sheath; Leukemia Cutis; Multicentric Reticulohistiocytosis; Myxoinflammatory Fibroblastic Sarcoma; Peripheral Neuroepithelioma/Primitive Neuroectodermal Tumor; Primary Neuroendocrine (Merkel Cell) Carcinoma; Spiradenoma; Extramammary Paget Disease; Peripheral Neuroepithelioma/ Primitive Neuroectodermal Tumor
CD45RA	isoform of CD45 expressed by naive T cells	4KB5, MT2, CD45RA, MB1	Blastic Plasmacytoid Dendritic Cell Neoplasm; Leukemia Cutis
CD45RB	isoform of CD45 expressed by naive and memory T cells		Extramedullary Hematopoiesis; Non-Langerhans Cell Histiocytoses; Oral Melanoma; Sinonasal Melanoma
CD45RO	isoform of CD45 located on memory T cells	ICH1-L, low molecular weight isoform LCA	Leukemia Cutis
CD54	ICAM-1 (intracellular adhesion molecule 1)	23G12, CD54-P, ICAM	Intravascular Large B-cell Lymphoma
CD56	NCAM (neutral cellular adhesion molecule)	MAB735, ERIC-1, 25-KD11, 123C3, 24-MB2, BC56C04, 1B6, 14-MAB735, NCC-LU-243, MOC-1, NCAM	Blastic Plasmacytoid Dendritic Cell Neoplasm; Cutaneous Gamma-Delta T-cell Lymphoma; Extranodal NK/T-cell Lymphoma, Nasal Type; Intravascular Large B-cell Lymphoma; Leukemia Cutis; Lymphomatoid Granulomatosis; Lymphomatoid Papulosis; Neuromas; Sinonasal Melanoma; Subcutaneous Panniculitis-like T-cell Lymphoma
CD57	β-1,3-glucuronyl transferase 1 (glucuronosyl transferase P)	LEU-7, NK1, HNK-1, TB01, B3GAT1	Granular Cell Tumor; Intravascular Large B-cell Lymphoma; Peripheral Neuroepithelioma/Primitive Neuroectodermal Tumor; Schwannoma (Neurilemmoma)
CD61	cluster of differentiation found on thrombocytes corresponding to glycoprotein IIb/IIIa	Integrin, beta 3 (platelet glycoprotein IIIa), ITGB3, GP3A, GPIIIa, Y2/5, HPA	Extramedullary Hematopoiesis
CD63	tetraspan intracellular granule protein	NKI/C3, basophil activation test in allergy	Cellular Neurothekeoma; Plexiform Fibrohistiocytic Tumor
CD64	Fc receptor for IgG antibodies, high affinity	HAM56	Reticulohistiocytoma
CD68	cytoplasmic granule protein of monocytes, macrophages	PG-M1, KP-1, LN5	Angiofibroma and Related Lesions; Angiomatoid Fibrous Histiocytoma; Atypical Fibroxanthoma; Atypical Lipomatous Tumor and Liposarcoma; Blastic Plasmacytoid Dendritic Cell Neoplasm; Cellular Neurothekeoma; Chondroid Lipoma; Cutaneous and Systemic Mastocytosis; Dermal Nerve Sheath Myxoma; Dermatofibroma and Fibrous Histiocytoma; Dermatofibrosarcoma Protuberans;

			Distinctive Dermal Clear Cell Mesenchymal Tumor; Epithelioid Histiocytoma; Giant Cell Tumor of Tendon Sheath; Granular Cell Tumor; Histiocytic Sarcoma; Juvenile and Adult-type Xanthogranuloma; Langerhans Cell Histiocytosis; Leiomyosarcoma; Leukemia Cutis; Multicentric Reticulohistiocytosis; Multinucleate Cell Angiohistiocytoma; Myxoinflammatory Fibroblastic Sarcoma; Non-Langerhans Cell Histiocytoses; Pleomorphic Fibroma; Plexiform Fibrohistiocytic Tumor; Polyvinylpyrrolidone Storage Disease; Pseudosarcomatous Fibroblastic Proliferations; Reticulohistiocytoma; Rosai-Dorfman Disease; Squamous Cell Carcinoma (and Variants)
CD79a	immunoglobulin-associated alpha, MB1	MB-1, 11D10, 11E3, CD79A, HM47/A9, HM57, JCB117, CD79-a, CD79-α	Angioimmunoblastic T-cell Lymphoma; Blastic Plasmacytoid Dendritic Cell Neoplasm; Cutaneous Marginal Zone B-cell Lymphoma; Intravascular large B-cell Lymphoma; Leukemia Cutis; Lymphomatoid Granulomatosis; Primary Cutaneous Follicle Center Lymphoma; Sinonasal Melanoma
CD99	cell surface glycoprotein for migration, T-cell adhesion, MIC2	CD99-MEMB, 12E7, HBA71, O13, P30/32MIC2, M3601	Angiomatoid Fibrous Histiocytoma; Atypical Fibroxanthoma; Cutaneous Rhabdomyosarcoma; Digital Fibromatosis (Infantile Digital Fibromatosis); Epithelioid Sarcoma; Leiomyosarcoma; Leukemia Cutis; Metastatic Tumors to the Skin; Perineurioma; Peripheral Neuroepithelioma/Primitive Neuroectodermal Tumor; Pleomorphic Fibroma; Primary Neuroendocrine (Merkel Cell) Carcinoma; Sinonasal Melanoma; Squamous Cell Carcinoma (and Variants)
CD117	C-Kit, tyrosine-protein kinase activity	C-19 (C-KIT), 104D2, 2E4, C-KIT, A4502, H300, CMA-767	Angiosarcoma; Cutaneous and Systemic Mastocytosis; Cutaneous Plasmacytoma; Fibromatosis; Leukemia Cutis; Myxoinflammatory Fibroblastic Sarcoma; Oral Melanoma; PEComas; Sinonasal Melanoma
CD123	receptor for IL-3 (IL-3R)		Blastic Plasmacytoid Dendritic Cell Neoplasm; Leukemia Cutis
CD138	syndecan; a useful marker for plasma cells	B-B4, AM411-10M, MI15	Cutaneous Plasmacytoma; Sinonasal Melanoma; Systemic B-cell Lymphomas Involving the Skin
CD163	macrophage hemoglobin scavenging system	10D6	Dermatofibroma and Fibrous Histiocytoma; Dermatofibrosarcoma Protuberans; Histiocytic Sarcoma; Myxoinflammatory Fibroblastic Sarcoma; Non-Langerhans Cell Histiocytoses; Plexiform Fibrohistiocytic Tumor; Polyvinylpyrrolidone Storage Disease; Reticulohistiocytoma
CD303	monoclonal antibody directed toward immature plasmacytoid dendritic cells	BDCA-2	Leukemia Cutis
CDK4	cyclin dependant kinase 4	C-22, DCS-31	Atypical Lipomatous Tumor and Liposarcoma; Cutaneous Malignant Fibrous Histiocytoma/Pleomorphic Sarcoma; Hibernoma; PEComas; Spindle Cell and Pleomorphic Lipoma
CDX-2	caudal type homeobox transcription factor 2	AMT28, 7C7/D4, CDX-2-88	Extramammary Paget Disease; Lymphoepithelioma-like Carcinoma of the Skin (LELCS); Metastatic Tumors to the Skin; Primary Cutaneous Mucinous Carcinoma
CEA-M	carcinoembryonic antigen, monoclonal	CEA-B18, CEA-D14, CEA-GOLD 1, T84.6, CEA-GOLD 2, CEA 11, CEA-GOLD 3, CEA 27, CEA-GOLD 4, CEA 41, CEA-GOLD 5, T84.1, CEA-M, A5B7, CEJ065, IL-7, T84.66, TF3H8-1, 0062, D14, alpha-7, PARLAM 1, ZC23, CEM010,	Adenoid Cystic Carcinoma; Hidradenocarcinoma; Porocarcinoma; Sebaceous Carcinoma; Squamoid "Eccrine" Ductal Carcinoma

III

ANTIBODY INDEX

		A115, COL-1, AF4, 12.140.10, 11-7, M773, CEA-M431_31, CEJO65, mCEA	
Chromogranin-A	pituitary secretory protein 1	PHE-5, PHE5, E001, DAK-A3	Dermal Nerve Sheath Myxoma; Primary Neuroendocrine (Merkel Cell) Carcinoma; Sinonasal Melanoma
Chymase	serine protease found in mast cells and basophils; acts as a mediator of inflammation		Cutaneous and Systemic Mastocytosis
Chymotrypsin	digestive enzyme synthesized in pancreas, involved in proteolysis		Dermatofibrosarcoma Protuberans
CK-HMW-NOS	cytokeratin high molecular weight, not otherwise specified	CK-HMW, HMWCK, 34bE12, CK903	Atypical Fibroxanthoma; Porocarcinoma; Poroma and Dermal Duct Tumor; Squamous Cell Carcinoma (and Variants)
CK-PAN	cytokeratin-pan (AE1/AE3/LP34); cocktail of high and low molecular weight cytokeratins	keratin pan, MAK-6, K576, LU-5, KL-1, KC-8, MNF 116, pankeratin, pancytokeratin	Angiosarcoma; Atypical Fibroxanthoma; Basal Cell Carcinoma; Cutaneous Rhabdomyosarcoma; Epithelioid Hemangioendothelioma; Epithelioid Sarcoma; Glomus Tumors; Granular Cell Tumor; Leiomyosarcoma; Low-Grade Fibromyxoid Sarcoma (Evans Tumor); Malignant Mixed Tumor; Myofibroma and Myofibromatosis; Neuromas; Oral Melanoma; PEComas; Perineurioma; Primary Neuroendocrine (Merkel Cell) Carcinoma; Sinonasal Melanoma; Squamomelanocytic Tumor; Squamous Cell Carcinoma (and Variants)
CK5/6	cytokeratin 5/6, high molecular weight cytokeratins	D5/16 B4	Atypical Fibroxanthoma; Distinctive Dermal Clear Cell Mesenchymal Tumor; Epithelioid Sarcoma; Extramammary Paget Disease; Leiomyosarcoma; Lymphoepithelioma-like Carcinoma of the Skin (LELCS); Malignant Mixed Tumor; Porocarcinoma; Poroma and Dermal Duct Tumor; Primary Cutaneous Mucinous Carcinoma; Sebaceous Carcinoma; Spiradenoma; Squamoid "Eccrine" Ductal Carcinoma; Squamous Cell Carcinoma (and Variants); Squamous Cell Carcinoma In Situ (Bowen Disease); Syringocystadenoma Papilliferum
CK7	cytokeratin 7, low molecular weight cytokeratin	K72.7, KS7.18, OVTL 12/30, LDS-68, CK 07	Clear Cell Papulosis; Cutaneous Ciliated Cyst; Cylindroma; Epithelioid Sarcoma; Extramammary Paget Disease; Histiocytic Sarcoma; Median Raphe Cyst; Melanoma In Situ, Superficial Spreading Type; Metastatic Tumors to the Skin; Microcystic Adnexal Carcinoma; Mucosal Melanoma (Genital); Primary Cutaneous Mucinous Carcinoma; Primary Neuroendocrine (Merkel Cell) Carcinoma; Sebaceous Carcinoma; Squamoid "Eccrine" Ductal Carcinoma; Squamous Cell Carcinoma In Situ (Bowen Disease); Toker Cell Hyperplasia; Tricholemmal Carcinoma
CK8/18/CAM5.2	cytokeratin 8/18; simple epithelial-type cytokeratins	5D3, Zym5.2, CAM 5.2, KER 10.11, NCL-5D3, cytokeratin LMW	Angiomatoid Fibrous Histiocytoma; Epithelioid Sarcoma; Primary Neuroendocrine (Merkel Cell) Carcinoma
CK10	cytokeratin 10	LHP1, DE-K10, RKSE60	Vellus Hair Cyst
CK13	cytokeratin 13	KS13.1, KS-1A3, AE8, 2D7	Median Raphe Cyst
CK17	cytokeratin 17	E3	Squamoid "Eccrine" Ductal Carcinoma; Vellus Hair Cyst
CK19	cytokeratin 19, low molecular weight cytokeratin	BA17, RCK108, LP2K, B170, A53-BA2, KS19.1, 170.2.14	Cylindroma; Epithelioid Sarcoma
CK20	cytokeratin 20, low molecular weight cytokeratin	KS20.8	Basal Cell Carcinoma; Cutaneous Ciliated Cyst; Cutaneous Rhabdomyosarcoma; Dermatofibroma and Fibrous Histiocytoma; Epithelioid Sarcoma; Extramammary Paget Disease; Leukemia Cutis; Median Raphe Cyst; Metastatic Skin Tumors; Metastatic Tumors to the Skin; Peripheral Neuroepithelioma/Primitive Neuroectodermal Tumor; Primary Cutaneous Mucinous Carcinoma; Primary

			Neuroendocrine (Merkel Cell) Carcinoma; Sebaceous Carcinoma; Spiradenoma; Squamous Cell Carcinoma In Situ (Bowen Disease); Toker Cell Hyperplasia; Trichoblastoma; Trichoepithelioma
CK903	cytokeratin-HMW, not otherwise specified	CK-HMW, CK-HMW-NOS, HMWCK, 34bE12	Atypical Fibroxanthoma; Distinctive Dermal Clear Cell Mesenchymal Tumor; Leiomyosarcoma; Lymphoepithelioma-like Carcinoma of the Skin (LELCS); Squamous Cell Carcinoma (and Variants)
CLA	cutaneous lymphocyte antigen		Blastic Plasmacytoid Dendritic Cell Neoplasm; Leukemia Cutis; Systemic T-cell and NK-cell Lymphomas Involving the Skin
Claudin-1	senescence-associated epithelial membrane protein	JAD.8	Ectopic Meningioma; Low-Grade Fibromyxoid Sarcoma (Evans Tumor); Perineurioma
Clusterin	clusterin, alpha chain specific	41D, E5	Angioimmunoblastic T-cell Lymphoma; Systemic T-cell and NK-cell Lymphomas Involving the Skin
Collagen II	major component of articular and hyaline cartilage	2B1.5	Cutaneous Mixed Tumor (Chondroid Syringoma)
Collagen IV	major constituent of the basement membranes along with laminins, proteoglycans, and enactins	CIV22, COL4A [1-5], collagen α-1(IV) chain	Cutaneous Mixed Tumor (Chondroid Syringoma); Glomus Tumors; Granular Cell Tumor; Perineurioma; Schwannoma (Neurilemmoma)
Cutaneous lymphocyte antigen	skin homing receptor	CLA	Leukemia Cutis; Primary Cutaneous Anaplastic Large Cell Lymphoma; Systemic T-cell and NK-cell Lymphomas Involving the Skin
CXCL13	chemokine CXC ligand 13, B lymphocyte chemoattractant	BCA-1, BLC, BLR1L, ANGIE, CXC chemokine BCL, SCYB13	Adult T-cell Leukemia/Lymphoma; Angioimmunoblastic T-cell Lymphoma; Primary Cutaneous CD4+ Small/Medium Pleomorphic T-cell Lymphoma; Systemic T-cell and NK-cell Lymphomas Involving the Skin
CXCR3	chemokine CXC receptor R3	1C6	Intravascular large B-cell Lymphoma
Cyclin-D1	protein with important cell cycle regulatory functions	bcl-1 (cyclin D1) A-12, PRAD1, AM29, DCS-6, SP4, 5D4, D1GM, P2D11F11, CCND1Cyl-1	Chondroid Lipoma; Epithelioid Sarcoma; Primary Dermal Melanoma; Systemic B-cell Lymphomas Involving the Skin
Cytokeratin			Atypical Fibroxanthoma; Blastic Plasmacytoid Dendritic Cell Neoplasm; Childhood Melanoma; Chondroid Lipoma; Clear Cell Papulosis; Cutaneous Marginal Zone B-cell Lymphoma; Cutaneous Mixed Tumor (Chondroid Syringoma); Cutaneous Rhabdomyosarcoma; Epithelioid Hemangioendothelioma; Epithelioid Sarcoma; Extramammary Paget Disease; Fibromatosis; Glomus Tumors; Hidradenocarcinoma; Histiocytic Sarcoma; Metastatic Skin Tumors; Metastatic Tumors to the Skin; Oral Melanoma; Peripheral Neuroepithelioma/ Primitive Neuroectodermal Tumor; Pilomatrixoma and Pilomatrical Carcinoma; Plexiform Fibrohistiocytic Tumor; Polyvinylpyrrolidone Storage Disease; Porocarcinoma; Sebaceous Adenoma; Squamomelanocytic Tumor; Syringofibroadenoma; Trichoblastoma; Vellus Hair Cyst
Cytokeratin 5/6	high molecular weight cytokeratins	D5/16 B4	Hidradenocarcinoma; Metastatic Tumors to the Skin
Cytokeratin 7	low molecular weight cytokeratin	K72.7, KS7.18, OVTL 12/30, LDS-68, CK 07	Metastatic Tumors to the Skin; Sebaceous Adenoma
Cytokeratin 20	low molecular weight cytokeratin	KS20.8	Metastatic Tumors to the Skin; Pilomatrixoma and Pilomatrical Carcinoma; Trichoblastoma
D2-40	reacts with an O-linked sialoglycoprotein found on lymphatic endothelium	podoplanin, M2A	Lymphangioma and Superficial Lymphangioma; Metastatic Tumors to the Skin; Papillary Intralymphatic Angioendothelioma (Dabska Tumor); Primary Dermal Melanoma;

III

1

ANTIBODY INDEX

			Progressive Lymphangioma; Retiform Hemangioendothelioma; Rosai-Dorfman Disease; Sebaceous Carcinoma; Squamous Cell Carcinoma (and Variants)
Desmin	class III intermediate filaments found in muscle cells	M760, DE-R-11, D33, DE5, DE-U-10, ZC18	Acral Fibrokeratoma; Angioleiomyoma; Angiomatoid Fibrous Histiocytoma; Angiomyofibroblastoma; Angiosarcoma; Atypical Fibroxanthoma; Childhood Melanoma; Collagenous Fibroma; Congenital Smooth Muscle Hamartoma; Cutaneous Malignant Fibrous Histiocytoma/Pleomorphic Sarcoma; Cutaneous Rhabdomyosarcoma; Dermal Nerve Sheath Myxoma; Dermatofibrosarcoma Protuberans; Dermatomyofibroma; Digital Fibromatosis (Infantile Digital Fibromatosis); Distinctive Dermal Clear Cell Mesenchymal Tumor; Epithelioid Sarcoma; Fibromatosis; Fibrous Hamartoma of Infancy; Giant Cell Tumor of Tendon Sheath; Glomus Tumors; Granular Cell Tumor; Hibernoma; Leiomyoma (Pilar); Leiomyosarcoma; Low-Grade Fibromyxoid Sarcoma (Evans Tumor); Myofibroma and Myofibromatosis; Oral Melanoma; Papillary Endothelial Hyperplasia (Masson Tumor); Paraganglioma-like Dermal Melanocytic Tumor; PEComas; Perineurioma; Peripheral Neuroepithelioma/ Primitive Neuroectodermal Tumor; Plexiform Fibrohistiocytic Tumor; Pseudosarcomatous Fibroblastic Proliferations; Reticulohistiocytoma; Rhabdomyoma; Schwannoma (Neurilemmoma); Sinonasal Melanoma; Squamous Cell Carcinoma (and Variants); Superficial Malignant Peripheral Nerve Sheath Tumor
E-cadherin	epithelial calcium dependent adhesion molecule	36B5, ECH-6, ECCD-2, CDH1, 5H9, NCH 38, Clone 36, 4A2 C7, E9, 67A4, HECD-1, SC-8426	Granular Cell Tumor
E2A		Anti-TCF3, TCF3, immunoglobulin enhancer-binding factor E12/E47	Primary Cutaneous Follicle Center Lymphoma
EBER	Epstein-Barr virus encoded RNA		Angioimmunoblastic T-cell Lymphoma; Blastic Plasmacytoid Dendritic Cell Neoplasm; Cutaneous Plasmacytoma; Extranodal NK/T-cell Lymphoma, Nasal Type; Histiocytic Sarcoma; Leiomyosarcoma; Lymphomatoid Granulomatosis; Systemic T-cell and NK-cell Lymphomas Involving the Skin
EGFR	v-erb b1 erythroblastic leukemia viral gene, epidermal growth factor receptor	2-18C9, EGFR1, EGFR PHRMDX, NCL-R1, H11, C-ERBB-1, E30, EGFR.113, 31G73C6, 2-18C9	Myxoinflammatory Fibroblastic Sarcoma
EMA	epithelial membrane antigen	GP1.4, 214D4, MC5, E29, LICRLON- M8, BC3, DF3, VU3D1, MUSEII, RD-1, MA695, MA552, PS2P446, 115D8, MUC1, MAM6, CA15.3, MUC01	Acral Fibrokeratoma; Adenoid Cystic Carcinoma; Angiosarcoma; Apocrine Tubular Adenoma; Atypical Fibroxanthoma; Basal Cell Carcinoma; Cellular Neurothekeoma; Chondroid Lipoma; Cutaneous Ciliated Cyst; Cutaneous Malignant Fibrous Histiocytoma/ Pleomorphic Sarcoma; Cutaneous Mixed Tumor (Chondroid Syringoma); Cutaneous Myxoma and Angiomyxoma; Cutaneous Rhabdomyosarcoma; Cylindroma; Dermal Nerve Sheath Myxoma; Digital Fibromatosis (Infantile Digital Fibromatosis); Eccrine Carcinoma; Eccrine Hamartomas; Ectopic Meningioma; Epithelioid Hemangioendothelioma; Epithelioid Sarcoma; Fibromatosis; Granular Cell Tumor; Hidradenocarcinoma; Hidradenoma; Histiocytic Sarcoma; Low-Grade Fibromyxoid Sarcoma (Evans Tumor); Lymphoepithelioma-like Carcinoma of the Skin (LELCS); Melanoma In Situ, Superficial Spreading

			Type; Microcystic Adnexal Carcinoma; Myxoinflammatory Fibroblastic Sarcoma; Nasal Glial Heterotopia; Neurofibroma; Neuromas; Papillary Eccrine Adenoma; Perineurioma; Peripheral Neuroepithelioma/Primitive Neuroectodermal Tumor; Porocarcinoma; Primary Cutaneous Anaplastic Large Cell Lymphoma; Sebaceoma (Sebaceous Epithelioma); Sebaceous Carcinoma; Sinonasal Melanoma; Spiradenoma; Squamoid "Eccrine" Ductal Carcinoma; Squamous Cell Carcinoma (and Variants); Squamous Cell Carcinoma In Situ (Bowen Disease); Superficial Acral Fibromyxoma; Syringocystadenoma Papilliferum; Syringoma; Systemic T-cell and NK-cell Lymphomas Involving the Skin; Toker Cell Hyperplasia; Trichoblastoma; Tricholemmal Carcinoma
EMA/MUC1	epithelial membrane antigen	EMA, GP1.4, 214D4, MC5, E29, LICRLON-M8, BC3, DF3, VU3D1, MUSEII, RD-1, MA695, MA552, PS2P446, 115D8, MUC1, MAM6, CA15.3, MUC01	Angiomatoid Fibrous Histiocytoma; Congenital Smooth Muscle Hamartoma; Epithelioid Sarcoma; Extramammary Paget Disease; Low-Grade Fibromyxoid Sarcoma (Evans Tumor); Myxofibrosarcoma; Neurofibroma; Perineurioma; Superficial Acral Fibromyxoma
EpCam/BER-EP4/CD326	epithelial cell adhesion molecule	AUA1, VU-1D9, EPCAM, C10, HEA125, BEREP4	Basal Cell Carcinoma; Primary Neuroendocrine (Merkel Cell) Carcinoma
Epithelial membrane antigen		EMA, GP1.4, 214D4, MC5, E29, LICRLON-M8, BC3, DF3, VU3D1, MUSEII, RD-1, MA695, MA552, PS2P446, 115D8, MUC1, MAM6, CA15.3, MUC01	Clear Cell Papulosis; Cutaneous Mixed Tumor (Chondroid Syringoma); Ectopic Meningioma; Fibrolipomatous Hamartoma of Nerve; Oral Melanoma; Papillary Eccrine Adenoma
ER	estrogen receptor protein	1D5, 6F11, SP1, 15D, H222, TE111, ERP, ER1D5, NCLER611, NCL-ER-LH2, PGP-1A6	Angiomyofibroblastoma; Apocrine Carcinoma (Apocrine Adenocarcinoma); Metastatic Tumors to the Skin; Primary Cutaneous Mucinous Carcinoma
ERP	estrogen receptor protein	1D5, 6F11, SP1, 15D, H222, TE111, ER, ER1D5, NCLER611, NCL-ER-LH2, PGP-1A6	Leiomyosarcoma; Primary Cutaneous Mucinous Carcinoma
Factor XIIIa	fibrin stabilizing factor	FXIIIA	Angiofibroma and Related Lesions; Juvenile and Adult-type Xanthogranuloma; Leiomyosarcoma; Non-Langerhans Cell Histiocytoses
FAS	fatty acid synthase	CD95/fas	Cutaneous Marginal Zone B-cell Lymphoma; Extranodal NK/T-cell Lymphoma, Nasal Type
Fascin	marker for Reed-Sternberg cells of Hodgkin disease	55K2	Non-Langerhans Cell Histiocytoses
Fibronectin	extracellular matrix glycoprotein	FN1, A0245, CIG	Cutaneous Mixed Tumor (Chondroid Syringoma)
FLI-1	Friend leukemia virus integration 1	EWSR2, GI146-222, SC356, FLK-1, FLT-1	Angiosarcoma; Epithelioid Hemangioendothelioma; Epithelioid Sarcoma; Kaposi Sarcoma; Kaposiform Hemangioendothelioma; Peripheral Neuroepithelioma/Primitive Neuroectodermal Tumor
FOXP1	forkhead box transcription factor P1	JC12	Diffuse Large B-cell Lymphoma, Leg Type
FOXP3	forkhead box transcription factor P3	FoxP3	Adult T-cell Leukemia/Lymphoma
FVIIIRAg	factor VIII-related antigen	FVIIIRAG, F8/86, von Willebrand factor	Angiolymphoid Hyperplasia with Eosinophilia; Epithelioid Sarcoma; Extramedullary Hematopoiesis; Infantile Hemangioma; Lymphangioma and Superficial Lymphangioma; Papillary Intralymphatic Angioendothelioma (Dabska Tumor); Retiform Hemangioendothelioma; Spindle Cell Hemangioma
FXIIIA	factor XIIIA (fibrin stabilizing factor)	factor XIIIa	Acral Fibrokeratoma; Dermatofibroma and Fibrous Histiocytoma; Dermatofibrosarcoma Protuberans;

ANTIBODY INDEX

			Dermatomyofibroma; Distinctive Dermal Clear Cell Mesenchymal Tumor; Epithelioid Histiocytoma; Juvenile and Adult-type Xanthogranuloma; Multinucleate Cell Angiohistiocytoma; Non-Langerhans Cell Histiocytoses; Pleomorphic Fibroma; Plexiform Fibrohistiocytic Tumor; Reticulohistiocytoma; Sclerotic Fibroma
GCDFP-15	gross cystic fluid protein 15	SABP, GPIP4, Gp17, 23A3, BRST-2, D6 (GROSS CYSTIC DISEASE FLUID PROTEIN)	Apocrine Carcinoma (Apocrine Adenocarcinoma); Apocrine Tubular Adenoma; Clear Cell Papulosis; Cutaneous Ciliated Cyst; Extramammary Paget Disease; Metastatic Tumors to the Skin; Primary Cutaneous Mucinous Carcinoma; Sebaceous Carcinoma; Syringocystadenoma Papilliferum; Toker Cell Hyperplasia
GFAP	glial fibrillary acidic protein	6F2, M761, GA-51, GFP-8A	Dermal Nerve Sheath Myxoma; Granular Cell Tumor; Nasal Glial Heterotopia; Neurofibroma; Neuromas; Perineurioma; Peripheral Neuroepithelioma/Primitive Neuroectodermal Tumor; Schwannoma (Neurilemmoma); Sinonasal Melanoma
Glucose transporter 1		GLUT1	Branchial Cleft Cyst
GLUT1	glucose transporter 1		Infantile Hemangioma; Kaposiform Hemangioendothelioma; Low-Grade Fibromyxoid Sarcoma (Evans Tumor); Perineurioma
GLUT1-cytoplasm	glucose transporter 1-cytoplasmic	GLUT1-CYT	Perineurioma
Glycophorin A	sialoglycoprotein of the human erythrocyte membrane	CD235a, JC159, GYPA, CD235a	Extramedullary Hematopoiesis
Granzyme B	neutral serine protease	GZM-B, 11F1, GR-B7	Subcutaneous Panniculitis-like T-cell Lymphoma
Gross cystic fluid protein 15		GCDPF-15, SABP, GPIP4, Gp17, 23A3, BRST-2, D6 (GROSS CYSTIC DISEASE FLUID PROTEIN)	Clear Cell Papulosis
GZM-B	neutral serine protease	Granzyme B, 11F1, GR-B7	Extranodal NK/T-cell Lymphoma, Nasal Type; Primary Cutaneous CD4+ Small/Medium Pleomorphic T-cell Lymphoma
GZM-M	Serine protease contained by NK cells and some activated lymphocytes		Subcutaneous Panniculitis-like T-cell Lymphoma
H-caldesmon	High molecular weight caldesmon	H-CD	Angiomatoid Fibrous Histiocytoma; Childhood Melanoma; Cutaneous Malignant Fibrous Histiocytoma/Pleomorphic Sarcoma; Cutaneous Rhabdomyosarcoma; Fibromatosis; Glomus Tumors; Granular Cell Tumor; Leiomyoma (Pilar); Plexiform Fibrohistiocytic Tumor;
HCAD	H-caldesmon (high molecular weight caldesmon)	H-CD	Angioleiomyoma; Angiomatoid Fibrous Histiocytoma; Congenital Smooth Muscle Hamartoma; Glomus Tumors; PEComas
Hep-Par1	hepatocyte paraffin 1	OCH1E5.2.10, HEPPAR1	PEComas
HER2	v-erb-b2 erythroblastic leukemia viral gene protein, human epidermal growth factor receptor 2	c-erb-B2, HER2/neu, NEU, HER-2, NCL-CBE1, 10A7, 9G6.10, SP3, 4B5, P185, 9G6.20, A0485, C-ERBB-2, CB11, ERBB-2, 3B5, TAB250, HERCEPTEST, E2-4001, HER-2_NEU	Toker Cell Hyperplasia
HGAL	human germinal center-associated lymphoma		Primary Cutaneous Follicle Center Lymphoma
hHa1	stains specifically human hair keratin expressed starting from the upper part of the hair matrix, lower cortex, and hair cuticle		Pilomatrixoma and Pilomatrical Carcinoma
HHV8	human herpes virus 8	Kaposi sarcoma-associated herpes virus, KSHV, HUMAN HERPESVIRUS-8 LATENT NUCLEAR ANTIGEN-1, 13B10, LNA-1	Angiolipoma; Angiomatoid Fibrous Histiocytoma; Angiosarcoma; Capillary, Venous, and Cavernous Hemangiomas; Dermatofibroma and Fibrous Histiocytoma; Kaposi Sarcoma; Kaposiform Hemangioendothelioma; Multinucleate Cell Angiohistiocytoma; Progressive Lymphangioma; Pseudosarcomatous Fibroblastic Proliferations; Retiform Hemangioendothelioma; Spindle Cell Hemangioma; Venous Lake

ANTIBODY INDEX

HLA-DR	human leukocyte antigen DR	DK22, LN3, TAL.1B5, LK8D3	Blastic Plasmacytoid Dendritic Cell Neoplasm
HMB-45	antigen present in melanocytic tumors such as melanomas	LB39 AA, CMM1, CMM, DNS, FAMMM, Mart1, Melan-A, MLM, tyrosinase	Actinic Keratosis; Angiofibroma and Related Lesions; Angioleiomyoma; Angiolipoma; Atypical Fibroxanthoma; Atypical/Borderline and Malignant Spitz Tumors; Blastic Plasmacytoid Dendritic Cell Neoplasm; Cellular Blue Nevi; Cellular Neurothekeoma; Childhood Melanoma; Conventional Blue Nevi; Dermal Nerve Sheath Myxoma; Distinctive Dermal Clear Cell Mesenchymal Tumor; Epithelioid Histiocytoma; Epithelioid Sarcoma; Extramammary Paget Disease; Fibromatosis; Halo Nevi; Histiocytic Sarcoma; Leiomyosarcoma; Lymphoepithelioma-like Carcinoma of the Skin (LELCS); Melanoma In Situ, NOS; Melanoma, Lentigo Maligna Type; Metastatic Skin Tumors; Neurofibroma; Neuromas; Oral Melanoma; Paraganglioma-like Dermal Melanocytic Tumor; PEComas; Peripheral Neuroepithelioma/Primitive Neuroectodermal Tumor; Pigmented Spindle Cell Nevus (Reed Nevus); Primary Dermal Melanoma; Primary Neuroendocrine (Merkel Cell) Carcinoma; Reticulohistiocytoma; Rhabdomyoma; Schwannoma (Neurilemmoma); Sinonasal Melanoma; Squamous Cell Carcinoma (and Variants); Superficial Malignant Peripheral Nerve Sheath Tumor; Other Unusual and Rare Variants of Melanoma
HPV	human papillomavirus		HPV-related Epidermal Cyst
HTLV-1	p40 tax antibody	Human T-cell Lymphotropic Virus, Human T-lymphotropic virus Type 1 (HTLV-I), Adult T-cell lymphoma virus type 1	Adult T-cell Leukemia/Lymphoma; Aggressive Epidermotropic CD8+ Cytotoxic T-cell Lymphoma; Leukemia Cutis
Human germinal center-associated lymphoma		HGAL	Primary Cutaneous Follicle Center Lymphoma
IgA	immunoglobulin A	IGA	Primary Cutaneous Follicle Center Lymphoma
IgD	immunoglobulin D	IGD	Diffuse Large B-cell Lymphoma, Leg Type; Primary Cutaneous Follicle Center Lymphoma
IgF-2	insulin growth factor-like 2	W2-H1	Infantile Hemangioma
IgG	immunoglobulin G	IGG	Acantholytic and Acantholytic Dyskeratotic Acanthoma; Primary Cutaneous Follicle Center Lymphoma; Prurigo Nodularis; Pseudoepitheliomatous Hyperplasia
IgM	immunoglobulin M	IGM	Diffuse Large B-cell Lymphoma, Leg Type; Primary Cutaneous Follicle Center Lymphoma
IL-15	interleukin 15		Keloid and Cellular Scar
Immunoglobulin A		IgA, IGA	Subcutaneous Panniculitis-like T-cell Lymphoma
Inhibin-α	produced by ovarian granulosa cells; inhibits production or secretion of pituitary gonadotropins, a sensitive marker for majority of sex cord/stromal tumors		Granular Cell Tumor
INI1	member of SWI/SNF chromatin remodeling complex	BAF47/SNF5, SNF5	Angiosarcoma; Epithelioid Sarcoma; Fibromatosis; Myxoinflammatory Fibroblastic Sarcoma
IRF-4	interferon regulatory factor 4	MUM1P, clone MUM1, MUM1-IRF.4, MUM1, M17	Primary Cutaneous Follicle Center Lymphoma
Kappa	kappa light chain	KAPPA, κ light chain	Primary Cutaneous Follicle Center Lymphoma; Systemic B-cell Lymphomas Involving the Skin
KBA62	Anti-melanoma associated antigen KBA6.2		Childhood Melanoma; Desmoplastic Melanoma

ANTIBODY INDEX

Ki-67	Ki-67 (MIB-1); marker of cell proliferation	MMI, KI88, IVAK-2, MIB1	Actinic Cheilitis; Atypical Vascular Lesion; Atypical/Borderline and Malignant Spitz Tumors; Basal Cell Carcinoma; Diffuse Large B-cell Lymphoma, Leg Type; Extranodal NK/T-cell Lymphoma, Nasal Type; Granular Cell Tumor; Halo Nevi; Hidradenocarcinoma; Hidrocystoma (Apocrine and Eccrine); Intravascular Large B-cell Lymphoma; Kaposi Sarcoma; Large Cell Acanthoma; Lymphomatoid Papulosis; Malignant Cellular Blue Nevus (Melanoma Arising in Cellular Blue Nevus); Melanoma In Situ, NOS; Melanoma In Situ, Superficial Spreading Type; Metastatic Skin Tumors; Microcystic Adnexal Carcinoma; Mycosis Fungoides (and Subtypes); Myxoinflammatory Fibroblastic Sarcoma; Nevoid Melanoma; Non-Langerhans Cell Histiocytoses; Peripheral Neuroepithelioma/Primitive Neuroectodermal Tumor; Pigmented Spindle Cell Nevus (Reed Nevus); Poroma and Dermal Duct Tumor; Primary Dermal Melanoma; Sclerotic Fibroma; Sebaceoma (Sebaceous Epithelioma); Sebaceous Carcinoma; Systemic B-cell Lymphomas Involving the Skin; Trichoblastoma; Trichoepithelioma
Lambda	lambda light chain	λ light chain, LAMBDA	Primary Cutaneous Follicle Center Lymphoma; Systemic B-cell Lymphomas Involving the Skin
Laminin	major protein in basal lamina	LAMININ-4C7, 4C12.8, LAM-89	Cutaneous Mixed Tumor (Chondroid Syringoma)
Langerin	CD207 molecule	CD207	Histiocytic Sarcoma; Non-Langerhans Cell Histiocytoses
LCA	leukocyte common antigen	PD7/26, 1.22/4.14, T29/33, CD45RB, RP2/18, CD45, PD7, 2D1, 2B11+PD7/26	Extramammary Paget Disease; Large Cell Acanthoma; Peripheral Neuroepithelioma/Primitive Neuroectodermal Tumor
LEP	leptin		Lipoma
LEU-7	β-1,3-glucuronyltransferase 1 (glucuronosyltransferase P)	CD57, NK1, HNK-1, TB01, B3GAT1	Peripheral Neuroepithelioma/Primitive Neuroectodermal Tumor
LMP1	Epstein-Barr virus latent membrane protein	EBV-LMP, CS 1-4	Aggressive Epidermotropic CD8+ Cytotoxic T-cell Lymphoma; Systemic B-cell Lymphomas Involving the Skin
Lysozyme	1,4-beta N-acetylmuramidase C	Lyz, Lzm, Ec3.2.1.17	Dermatofibrosarcoma Protuberans; Histiocytic Sarcoma; Leukemia Cutis; Multicentric Reticulohistiocytosis; Multinucleate Cell Angiohistiocytoma; Plexiform Fibrohistiocytic Tumor; Reticulohistiocytoma
LYVE-1	lymph vessel endothelial hyaluronan receptor 1		Lymphangioma and Superficial Lymphangioma
MAC387	macrophage antibody		Multicentric Reticulohistiocytosis
Mammaglobin	Breast tissue-specific glycoprotein	304-1A5	Apocrine Carcinoma (Apocrine Adenocarcinoma); Metastatic Tumors to the Skin
Mart-1	mart-1 clone of Melan-A		Mucosal Melanoma (Genital); PEComas
MDM2	murine double minute oncogene (mdm2)	HDM2, IF2, 2A10, 1B10, SMP14, murine double minute 2	Atypical Lipomatous Tumor and Liposarcoma; Cutaneous Malignant Fibrous Histiocytoma/Pleomorphic Sarcoma; Hibernoma; PEComas; Spindle Cell and Pleomorphic Lipoma
Melan-A	melanoma antigen recognized by T cells 1 (MART-1); protein found on melanocytes; melanocyte differentiation antigen	M2-7C10, CK-MM	Angiofibroma and Related Lesions; Atypical/Borderline and Malignant Spitz Tumors; Desmoplastic Melanoma; Fibromatosis; Halo Nevi; Lymphoepithelioma-like Carcinoma of the Skin (LELCS); Metastatic Skin Tumors; Sinonasal Melanoma; Squamomelanocytic Tumor
Melan-A103	clone of Melan-A	A103	Angioleiomyoma; Atypical Fibroxanthoma; Atypical/Borderline and Malignant Spitz Tumors; Cellular Neurothekeoma;

ANTIBODY INDEX

			Desmoplastic Melanoma; Halo Nevi; Metastatic Skin Tumors; Oral Melanoma; Primary Neuroendocrine (Merkel Cell) Carcinoma; Sinonasal Melanoma; Squamomelanocytic Tumor
met	met proto-oncogene	8F11, C-28, C-MET	Cutaneous and Systemic Mastocytosis; Metastatic Tumors to the Skin
MIC2	cell surface glycoprotein for migration, T-cell adhesion	CD99, CD99-MEMB, MIC2, 12E7, HBA71, O13, P30/32MIC2, M3601	Peripheral Neuroepithelioma/Primitive Neuroectodermal Tumor
Micropthalmia transcription factor		MITF, 34CA5, D5, C5+D5	Sinonasal Melanoma
MITF	micropthalmia transcription factor	34CA5, D5, C5+D5	Atypical Fibroxanthoma; Cellular Neurothekeoma; Childhood Melanoma; Metastatic Skin Tumors; Oral Melanoma; PEComas; Plexiform Fibrohistiocytic Tumor; Sinonasal Melanoma; Other Unusual and Rare Variants of Melanoma
MLH1	mutL homolog 1	HMLH1, G168-15, G168-728, MMR family; HNPCC2, COCA2	Sebaceoma (Sebaceous Epithelioma); Sebaceous Adenoma; Sebaceous Carcinoma
MPO	myeloperoxidase		Blastic Plasmacytoid Dendritic Cell Neoplasm; Cutaneous and Systemic Mastocytosis; Extramedullary Hematopoiesis; Histiocytic Sarcoma; Leukemia Cutis
MSA	actin, smooth muscle	actin-sm, ASM-1, CGA7, 1A4, HUC1-1	Adenoid Cystic Carcinoma; Atypical Fibroxanthoma; Childhood Melanoma; Dermatomyofibroma; Leiomyosarcoma; Sinonasal Melanoma
MSH2	mutS homolog 2	FE11	Sebaceoma (Sebaceous Epithelioma); Sebaceous Adenoma; Sebaceous Carcinoma
MSH6	mutS homolog 6	clone 44, GRBP.P1, DNA mismatch repair protein MSH6 antibody, G/T mismatch binding protein antibody, GTBP antibody, GTMBP antibody, HNPCC 5 antibody, HNPCC5 antibody, HSAP antibody, MSH 6 antibody, mutS (*E. coli*) homolog 6 antibody	Sebaceoma (Sebaceous Epithelioma); Sebaceous Carcinoma
MUC4	mucin 4, tracheobronchial	8G7	Low-Grade Fibromyxoid Sarcoma (Evans Tumor)
MUM1	Interferon regulatory factor 4	IRF-4, MUM1P, clone MUM1, MUM1-IRF.4, M17	Blastic Plasmacytoid Dendritic Cell Neoplasm; Diffuse Large B-cell Lymphoma, Leg Type; Leukemia Cutis; Lymphomatoid Papulosis; Primary Cutaneous Follicle Center Lymphoma; Systemic B-cell Lymphomas Involving the Skin
MxA	Protein induced by alpha interferon protein		Blastic Plasmacytoid Dendritic Cell Neoplasm
myc	myelocytomatosis viral oncogene	C-MYC, c-myc, 9E10, 9E11, 1-262	Blastic Plasmacytoid Dendritic Cell Neoplasm; Cutaneous Marginal Zone B-cell Lymphoma; Diffuse Large B-cell Lymphoma, Leg Type
Myeloperoxidase		MPO	Blastic Plasmacytoid Dendritic Cell Neoplasm; Cutaneous and Systemic Mastocytosis; Extramedullary Hematopoiesis; Histiocytic Sarcoma
MYOD1	myogenic differentiation 1	5.8A, 5.2F	Angiomatoid Fibrous Histiocytoma; Congenital Smooth Muscle Hamartoma; Cutaneous Rhabdomyosarcoma; Epithelioid Sarcoma; Pseudosarcomatous Fibroblastic Proliferations; Rhabdomyoma; Sinonasal Melanoma
Myogenin	myogenin	F5D, MYF3, MYF4, MYOGENIN, LO26	Angiomatoid Fibrous Histiocytoma; Angiosarcoma; Congenital Smooth Muscle Hamartoma; Cutaneous Malignant Fibrous Histiocytoma/Pleomorphic Sarcoma; Cutaneous Rhabdomyosarcoma; Epithelioid Sarcoma; Granular Cell Tumor; Hibernoma; Pseudosarcomatous Fibroblastic Proliferations; Rhabdomyoma; Sinonasal Melanoma; Superficial Malignant Peripheral Nerve Sheath Tumor
Myoglobin	iron and oxygen-building protein found in muscle tissue	MG-1	Botryoid Rhabdomyosarcoma; Gingival Granular Cell Tumor of the Newborn;

III

1

			Inflammatory Myofibroblastic Tumor; Rhabdomyoma; Rhabdomyosarcoma
Neurofilament protein	neurofilament H/M phosphorylated protein	NFP, TPNFP-1A3, SMI31, SMI33, NFP, SMI32, TA-51, 2F11	Neurofibroma; Neuromas; Peripheral Neuroepithelioma/Primitive Neuroectodermal Tumor
NFP	neurofilament H/M phosphorylated protein	TPNFP-1A3, SMI31, SMI33, NFP, SMI32, TA-51, 2F11	Neurofibroma; Neuromas; Perineurioma; Peripheral Neuroepithelioma/Primitive Neuroectodermal Tumor
NGFR	nerve growth factor receptor		Granular Cell Tumor
NKI/C3	tetraspan intracellular granule protein	CD63, basophil activation test in allergy	Cellular Neurothekeoma Plexiform Fibrohistiocytic Tumor
NSE	neuron specific enolase	BSS/H14	Blastic Plasmacytoid Dendritic Cell Neoplasm; Cutaneous Mixed Tumor (Chondroid Syringoma); Granular Cell Tumor; Peripheral Neuroepithelioma/ Primitive Neuroectodermal Tumor; Primary Neuroendocrine (Merkel Cell) Carcinoma; Sinonasal Melanoma
Nuclear p53	p53 tumor suppressor gene protein	D07, 21N, BP53-12-1, AB6, CM1, PAB1801, DO1, BP53-11, PAP240, RSP53, MU195, P53	Sebaceoma (Sebaceous Epithelioma); Sebaceous Carcinoma
OCT2	octamer binding transcription factor 2	SC233	Lymphomatoid Granulomatosis
p15	cyclin-dependent kinase 4 inhibitor B	P15-INK4B	Primary Cutaneous Follicle Center Lymphoma
p16	cyclin-dependent kinase 4 inhibitor 2A	P16_INK4A, E6H4, sc1661, JC8, JZ11, P16, G175-405, F-12, DCS-50, 6H12, 16P07, 16P04	Atypical/Borderline and Malignant Spitz Tumors; Childhood Melanoma; Condyloma Acuminatum (Genital Wart); Malignant Cellular Blue Nevus (Melanoma Arising in Cellular Blue Nevus); Melanoma In Situ, NOS; Melanoma In Situ, Superficial Spreading Type; Penile and Vulvar Intraepithelial Neoplasia; Pigmented Spindle Cell Nevus (Reed Nevus); Primary Cutaneous Follicle Center Lymphoma; Sinonasal Melanoma; Syringocystadenoma Papilliferum
p53	p53 tumor suppressor gene protein		Actinic Keratosis; Atypical Vascular Lesion; Basal Cell Carcinoma; Extranodal NK/ T-cell Lymphoma, Nasal Type; Granular Cell Tumor; Hidradenocarcinoma; Microcystic Adnexal Carcinoma; Penile and Vulvar Intraepithelial Neoplasia; Primary Dermal Melanoma; Primary Neuroendocrine (Merkel Cell) Carcinoma; Sebaceoma (Sebaceous Epithelioma); Sebaceous Carcinoma; Superficial Malignant Peripheral Nerve Sheath Tumor; Trichoblastoma; Trichoepithelioma
p63	tumor protein p63	H-137, 7JUL	Adenoid Cystic Carcinoma; Atypical Fibroxanthoma; Basal Cell Carcinoma; Childhood Melanoma; Distinctive Dermal Clear Cell Mesenchymal Tumor; Epithelioid Sarcoma; Extramammary Paget Disease; Hidradenocarcinoma; Histiocytic Sarcoma; Leiomyosarcoma; Lymphoepithelioma-like Carcinoma of the Skin (LELCS); Malignant Mixed Tumor; Median Raphe Cyst; Metastatic Skin Tumors; Metastatic Tumors to the Skin; Papillary Eccrine Adenoma; Porocarcinoma; Primary Cutaneous Mucinous Carcinoma; Proliferating Pilar (Trichilemmal) Cyst/Tumor; Sebaceous Carcinoma; Squamoid "Eccrine" Ductal Carcinoma; Squamous Cell Carcinoma (and Variants); Syringocystadenoma Papilliferum
pax-5	paired box gene 2	Z-RX2, PAX-2	Angioimmunoblastic T-cell Lymphoma; Blastic Plasmacytoid Dendritic Cell Neoplasm; Cutaneous Plasmacytoma; Extranodal NK/T-cell Lymphoma, Nasal Type; Histiocytic Sarcoma; Intravascular Large B-cell Lymphoma; Leukemia Cutis; Primary Cutaneous Anaplastic Large Cell Lymphoma; Primary Cutaneous Follicle Center Lymphoma; Systemic B-cell

			Lymphomas Involving the Skin; Systemic T-cell and NK-cell Lymphomas Involving the Skin
pax-8	paired box gene 8		Sebaceous Carcinoma
PCNA	proliferating cell nuclear antigen	19 A2, PC10	Large Cell Acanthoma; Malignant Cellular Blue Nevus (Melanoma Arising in Cellular Blue Nevus)
PD-1	programmed cell death protein 1	EH12, NAT105, programmed death 1	Angioimmunoblastic T-cell Lymphoma; Primary Cutaneous CD4+ Small/Medium Pleomorphic T-cell Lymphoma
Perforin		P1-8, PE-41-PU, 5B10	Aggressive Epidermotropic CD8+ Cytotoxic T-cell Lymphoma; Blastic Plasmacytoid Dendritic Cell Neoplasm; Cutaneous Gamma-Delta T-cell Lymphoma; Lymphomatoid Papulosis; Primary Cutaneous Anaplastic Large Cell Lymphoma; Primary Cutaneous CD4+ Small/Medium Pleomorphic T-cell Lymphoma; Subcutaneous Panniculitis-like T-cell Lymphoma
PGP9.5	protein gene product 9.5	31A3,13C4	Granular Cell Tumor; Peripheral Neuroepithelioma/Primitive Neuroectodermal Tumor; Plexiform Fibrohistiocytic Tumor
Podoplanin	transmembrane mucoprotein (38 kd) recognized by the D2-40 monoclonal antibody	D2-40, M2A	Angiomatoid Fibrous Histiocytoma; Angiosarcoma; Atypical Vascular Lesion; Cellular Neurothekeoma; Epithelioid Hemangioendothelioma; Kaposi Sarcoma; Kaposiform Hemangioendothelioma; Lymphangioma and Superficial Lymphangioma; Metastatic Tumors to the Skin; Progressive Lymphangioma; Rosai-Dorfman Disease; Sebaceoma (Sebaceous Epithelioma); Sebaceous Carcinoma
PR	progesterone receptor protein	PRP, 10A9, PGR-1A6, KD68, PGR-ICA, PRP-P, PRI, 1A6, 1AR, HPRA3, PGR-636, 636, PR88, NCL-PGR	Aggressive Epidermotropic CD8+ Cytotoxic T-cell Lymphoma; Angiomyofibroblastoma; Apocrine Carcinoma (Apocrine Adenocarcinoma); Cutaneous Gamma-Delta T-cell Lymphoma; Metastatic Tumors to the Skin; Primary Cutaneous Mucinous Carcinoma
PRAD1	protein with important cell cycle regulatory functions	Cyclin-D1, bcl-1 (cyclin D1) A-12, AM29, DCS-6, SP4, 5D4, D1GM, P2D11F11, CCND1Cyl-1	Systemic B-cell Lymphomas Involving the Skin
Prostate specific antigen		PSA, PSA-M, PSA, ER-PR8, PSA-P, F5	Metastatic Tumors to the Skin
PROX1	critical regulator of lymphangiogenesis		Lymphangioma and Superficial Lymphangioma
PSA	prostate specific antigen	PSA-M, PSA, ER-PR8, PSA-P, F5	Lymphoepithelioma-like Carcinoma of the Skin (LELCS); Metastatic Tumors to the Skin; Pilar Sheath Acanthoma
PTEN	phosphatase and tensin homolog	PN37	Fibrolipomatous Hamartoma of Nerve; Mycosis Fungoides (and Subtypes); Tricholemmoma
RCC	renal cell carcinoma antibody	66.4C2, PN-15, RCC MA	Hidradenoma; Metastatic Tumors to the Skin; Sebaceous Carcinoma
S100	low molecular weight protein normally present in cells derived from neural crest (Schwann cells, melanocytes, and glial cells), chondrocytes, adipocytes, myoepithelial cells, macrophages, Langerhans cells, dendritic cells, and keratinocytes	S-100, A6, 15E2E2, Z311, 4C4.9	Actinic Keratosis; Adenoid Cystic Carcinoma; Angiofibroma and Related Lesions; Angioleiomyoma; Angiomyofibroblastoma; Angiosarcoma; Apocrine Tubular Adenoma; Atypical Fibroxanthoma; Atypical Lipomatous Tumor and Liposarcoma; Blastic Plasmacytoid Dendritic Cell Neoplasm; Cellular Neurothekeoma; Childhood Melanoma; Chondroid Lipoma; Collagenous Fibroma; Congenital Smooth Muscle Hamartoma; Cutaneous Malignant Fibrous Histiocytoma/Pleomorphic Sarcoma; Cutaneous Mixed Tumor (Chondroid Syringoma); Cutaneous Myxoma and Angiomyxoma; Cutaneous Rhabdomyosarcoma; Cylindroma;

ANTIBODY INDEX

Dermal Nerve Sheath Myxoma; Dermatofibrosarcoma Protuberans; Dermatomyofibroma; Desmoplastic Melanoma; Digital Fibromatosis (Infantile Digital Fibromatosis); Distinctive Dermal Clear Cell Mesenchymal Tumor; Eccrine Carcinoma; Eccrine Hamartomas; Ectopic Meningioma; Epithelioid Hemangioendothelioma; Epithelioid Histiocytoma; Epithelioid Sarcoma; Extramammary Paget Disease; Fibromatosis; Fibrosarcoma; Glomus Tumors; Granular Cell Tumor; Halo Nevi; Hibernoma; Histiocytic Sarcoma; Juvenile and Adult-type Xanthogranuloma; Keloid and Cellular Scar; Langerhans Cell Histiocytosis; Leiomyosarcoma; Leukemia Cutis; Lipoma; Low-Grade Fibromyxoid Sarcoma (Evans Tumor); Lymphoepithelioma-like Carcinoma of the Skin (LELCS); Malignant Mixed Tumor; Melanoma In Situ, Superficial Spreading Type; Metastatic Skin Tumors; Mucosal Melanoma (Genital); Multicentric Reticulohistiocytosis; Myofibroma and Myofibromatosis; Myxofibrosarcoma; Myxoinflammatory Fibroblastic Sarcoma; Nasal Glial Heterotopia; Neurofibroma; Neuromas; Non-Langerhans Cell Histiocytoses; Oral Melanoma; Other Unusual and Rare Variants of Melanoma; Papillary Eccrine Adenoma; Paraganglioma-like Dermal Melanocytic Tumor; PEComas; Perineurioma; Peripheral Neuroepithelioma/ Primitive Neuroectodermal Tumor; Plexiform Fibrohistiocytic Tumor; Polyvinylpyrrolidone Storage Disease; Primary Dermal Melanoma; Primary Neuroendocrine (Merkel Cell) Carcinoma; Pseudosarcomatous Fibroblastic Proliferations; Reticulohistiocytoma; Rosai-Dorfman Disease; Schwannoma (Neurilemmoma); Sebaceous Carcinoma; Sinonasal Melanoma; Spindle Cell and Pleomorphic Lipoma; Spindle Cell Hemangioma; Spiradenoma; Squamomelanocytic Tumor; Squamous Cell Carcinoma (and Variants); Superficial Acral Fibromyxoma; Superficial Malignant Peripheral Nerve Sheath Tumor; Toker Cell Hyperplasia

S100-A6	S100 calcium binding protein A6	calcyclin, S-100A6, CACY-100	Plexiform Fibrohistiocytic Tumor
S100-pla	S100 placental	S100P, S0084	Angiosarcoma
S100P	S100 placental	S100-pla, S0084	Angiomatoid Fibrous Histiocytoma; Angiosarcoma; Atypical Lipomatous Tumor and Liposarcoma; Congenital Smooth Muscle Hamartoma; Glomus Tumors
SCC	squamous cell carcinoma-related antigen	F2H7C	Basal Cell Carcinoma; Branchial Cleft Cyst; Metastatic Tumors to the Skin; Sebaceous Carcinoma; Squamous Cell Carcinoma (and Variants)
SNF5	member of SWI/SNF chromatin remodeling complex	BAF47/SNF5, INI1	Angiosarcoma
SOX9	SRY (sex-determining region Y)-box 9 protein	CMD1, CMPD1	Basal Cell Carcinoma
SOX10	SRY (sex-determining region Y)-box 10 protein		Childhood Melanoma; Desmoplastic Melanoma
Stem cell factor		SCF	Cutaneous and Systemic Mastocytosis
Surface immunoglobulins		Sig	Primary Cutaneous Follicle Center Lymphoma
Synaptophysin	major synaptic vesicle protein p38 antibody	SVP38, SY38, SNP-88, SYP, SYPH, Sypl, Syn p38	Dermal Nerve Sheath Myxoma; Ectopic Meningioma; Extramammary Paget Disease; Leukemia Cutis; Metastatic Skin Tumors; Peripheral Neuroepithelioma/

			Primitive Neuroectodermal Tumor; Primary Neuroendocrine (Merkel Cell) Carcinoma; Sinonasal Melanoma; Squamous Cell Carcinoma In Situ (Bowen Disease)
TAG72	tumor-associated glycoprotein-72	CC49, B72.3, BRST-3	Metastatic Tumors to the Skin
TARC	thymus and activation regulated chemokine		Leukemia Cutis
TCL1	trophoblast membrane protein 1	NDOG1	Blastic Plasmacytoid Dendritic Cell Neoplasm; Leukemia Cutis
TCR	T-cell receptor antigen	T_Cell_AG_R, Beta-F1, 8A3, BF1	Aggressive Epidermotropic CD8+ Cytotoxic T-cell Lymphoma; Angioimmunoblastic T-cell Lymphoma; Cutaneous Gamma-Delta T-cell Lymphoma; Extranodal NK/T-cell Lymphoma, Nasal Type; Intravascular Large B-cell Lymphoma; Mycosis Fungoides (and Subtypes); Subcutaneous Panniculitis-like T-cell Lymphoma; Systemic T-cell and NK-cell Lymphomas Involving the Skin
TCR-β	Antibody directed toward the beta chain of the TCR-αβ heterodimer		Subcutaneous Panniculitis-like T-cell Lymphoma
TCR-βF1	specific for TCR beta chain constant region	Beta F1	Cutaneous Gamma-Delta T-cell Lymphoma; Subcutaneous Panniculitis-like T-cell Lymphoma
TCR-δ-1	T-cell receptor delta chain 1		Cutaneous Gamma-Delta T-cell Lymphoma
TdT	terminal deoxynucleotidyl transferase	SEN28	Blastic Plasmacytoid Dendritic Cell Neoplasm; Leukemia Cutis
Tenascin	Extracellular matrix glycoprotein	DB7, TN2	Cutaneous Mixed Tumor (Chondroid Syringoma)
Thyroglobulin	dimetric protein specific to thyroid gland	DAK-TG6	Metastatic Tumors to the Skin
TIA	T-cell intracellular antigen 1	NS/1-AG4, 2G9, TIA-1	Cutaneous Gamma-Delta T-cell Lymphoma; Extranodal NK/T-cell Lymphoma, Nasal Type; Primary Cutaneous Anaplastic Large Cell Lymphoma; Primary Cutaneous CD4+ Small/Medium Pleomorphic T-cell Lymphoma; Subcutaneous Panniculitis-like T-cell Lymphoma
TIA-1	T-cell intracellular antigen 1	NS/1-AG4, 2G9, TIA	Adult T-cell Leukemia/Lymphoma; Blastic Plasmacytoid Dendritic Cell Neoplasm; Cutaneous Gamma-Delta T-cell Lymphoma; Extranodal NK/T-cell Lymphoma, Nasal Type; Leukemia Cutis; Lymphomatoid Papulosis; Subcutaneous Panniculitis-like T-cell Lymphoma
TRAP	tartrate-resistant acid phosphatase	26E5, 9C5	Giant Cell Tumor of Tendon Sheath; Neurofibroma; Nevoid Melanoma
Tryptase	serine proteinase contained in mast cells		Cutaneous and Systemic Mastocytosis
TTF-1	transcription termination factor	8G7G3/1, SPT-24, SC-13040	Lymphoepithelioma-like Carcinoma of the Skin (LELCS); Metastatic Skin Tumors; Metastatic Tumors to the Skin; Primary Neuroendocrine (Merkel Cell) Carcinoma; Sebaceous Carcinoma
TTF-1 cytoplasmic	transcription termination factor-cytoplasmic	SC-13040_CP, 8G7G3/1_CP, TTF-1 CYTOP	Metastatic Skin Tumors
Tyrosinase	catalyzes production of melanin	NCL-TYROS, T311	Actinic Keratosis; Atypical Fibroxanthoma; Blastic Plasmacytoid Dendritic Cell Neoplasm; Childhood Melanoma; Desmoplastic Melanoma; Distinctive Dermal Clear Cell Mesenchymal Tumor; Extramammary Paget Disease; Halo Nevi; Histiocytic Sarcoma; Melanoma In Situ, NOS; Oral Melanoma; PEComas; Sinonasal Melanoma; Superficial Malignant Peripheral Nerve Sheath Tumor; Other Unusual and Rare Variants of Melanoma
Uroplakin-3		AU 1, Uroplakin III	Extramammary Paget Disease
VEGF	vascular endothelial growth factor	JH121, 26503.11, VPF, VPF/VEGF, VEGFA, VEGF-C, RP 077, VEGFR-1, RP 076, VEGFR-2, 9D9, VEGFR-3, FLT-4	Infantile Hemangioma

ANTIBODY INDEX

VEGFR-3	vascular endothelial growth factor	JH121, 26503.11, VPF, VPF/VEGF, VEGFA, VEGF-C, RP 077, VEGFR-1, RP 076, VEGFR-2, 9D9, VEGF, FLT-4	Lymphangioma and Superficial Lymphangioma; Papillary Intralymphatic Angioendothelioma (Dabska Tumor); Retiform Hemangioendothelioma
Vimentin	major subunit protein of the intermediate filaments of mesenchymal cells	43BE8, 3B4, V10, V9, VIM-3B4, VIM	Atypical Fibroxanthoma; Cutaneous Mixed Tumor (Chondroid Syringoma); Dermatofibroma and Fibrous Histiocytoma; Distinctive Dermal Clear Cell Mesenchymal Tumor; Epithelioid Sarcoma; Fibrosarcoma; Fibrous Hamartoma of Infancy; Malignant Mixed Tumor; Multinucleate Cell Angiohistiocytoma; Myofibroma and Myofibromatosis; Neurofibroma; Oral Melanoma; Peripheral Neuroepithelioma/ Primitive Neuroectodermal Tumor; Pleomorphic Fibroma; Sclerotic Fibroma; Sinonasal Melanoma; Squamous Cell Carcinoma (and Variants)
WT1	Wilms tumor gene-1	6F-H2, C-19	Metastatic Tumors to the Skin; Vascular Hamartomas; Verrucous Hemangioma

Molecular Factors Discussed

Molecular Factor	Chromosomal Location	Definition/Alternative Names	Chapters
β-catenin (see CTNNB1)			
10p, loss of	10p		Childhood Melanoma
10q, loss of	10q		Childhood Melanoma; Perineurioma
11p, gain of	11p		Atypical/Borderline and Malignant Spitz Tumors; Childhood Melanoma; Peripheral Neuroepithelioma/Primitive Neuroectodermal Tumor
11p15.5	11p15.5		Cutaneous Rhabdomyosarcoma
11q, loss of	11q		Childhood Melanoma
11q12	11q12		Collagenous Fibroma
11q13-21	11q13-21		Hibernoma
12p, loss of	12p		Blastic Plasmacytoid Dendritic Cell Neoplasm
12q13-15	12q13-15		Lipoma; Atypical Lipomatous Tumor and Liposarcoma
13q, loss of	13q		Blastic Plasmacytoid Dendritic Cell Neoplasm; Lipoma; Spindle Cell and Pleomorphic Lipoma
13q14	13q14		Angiomyofibroblastoma
15q, loss of	15q		Blastic Plasmacytoid Dendritic Cell Neoplasm
16p13.3	16p13.3	TSC2	PEComas
16q, loss of	16q		Spindle Cell and Pleomorphic Lipoma
17q, gain of	17q		Childhood Melanoma
17q11	17q11	NF1	Superficial Malignant Peripheral Nerve Sheath Tumor
17q11.2	17q11.2		Neurofibroma
17q13	17q13	P53	Superficial Malignant Peripheral Nerve Sheath Tumor
18q11	18q11		Epithelioid Sarcoma
18q21.31-33	18q21.31-33		Diffuse Large B-cell Lymphoma, Leg Type
1p, alterations of	1p		Angioimmunoblastic T-cell Lymphoma
1p13	1p13	CSF1	Giant Cell Tumor of Tendon Sheath
1p21-22	1p21-22		Glomus Tumors
1p36	1p36		Primary Neuroendocrine (Merkel Cell) Carcinoma
1q, gain of	1q		Childhood Melanoma; Sinonasal Melanoma
20q, gain of	20q		Childhood Melanoma
22q, alterations of	22q		Epithelioid Sarcoma
2p23	2p23	ALK	Primary Cutaneous Anaplastic Large Cell Lymphoma; Systemic T-cell and NK-cell Lymphomas Involving the Skin
3p11-12	3p11-12		Myxoinflammatory Fibroblastic Sarcoma
5q, loss of	5q		Blastic Plasmacytoid Dendritic Cell Neoplasm
6p, gain of	6p, gain of		Childhood Melanoma; Sinonasal Melanoma
6p21-23	6p21-23		Lipoma
6q, loss of	6q		Angioimmunoblastic T-cell Lymphoma; Blastic Plasmacytoid Dendritic Cell Neoplasm; Childhood Melanoma; Systemic T-cell and NK-cell Lymphomas Involving the Skin
7p, gain of	7p		Childhood Melanoma
7q, gain of	7q		Childhood Melanoma
7q, isochromosome	i(7q)		Intravascular large B-cell Lymphoma; Systemic T-cell and NK-cell Lymphomas Involving the Skin
7q22-36	7q22-36		Intravascular large B-cell Lymphoma
8q, gain of	8q, gain of		Childhood Melanoma; Sinonasal Melanoma
9p, loss of	9p, loss of		Childhood Melanoma
9q, loss of	9q, loss of		Childhood Melanoma
9q34	9q34	TSC1	PEComas; Systemic T-cell and NK-cell Lymphomas Involving the Skin

MOLECULAR FACTORS INDEX

ALK	2p23		Histiocytic Sarcoma; Lymphomatoid Papulosis; Primary Cutaneous Anaplastic Large Cell Lymphoma; Systemic T-cell and NK-cell Lymphomas Involving the Skin
ANTXR2	4q21.21	anthrax toxin receptor 2	Juvenile Hyaline Fibromatosis
AP12/MLT	t(11;18)(q21;q21)		Cutaneous Marginal Zone B-cell Lymphoma
APC	5q21	adenomatosis polyposis coli	Fibromatosis; Myofibroma and Myofibromatosis
API2	11q22	apoptosis inhibitor 2; BIRC3	Systemic B-cell Lymphomas Involving the Skin
ATF1	12q13	activating transcription factor 1	Myxoinflammatory Fibroblastic Sarcoma
ATIC	2q35	5-aminoimidazole-4-carboxamide ribonucleotide formyltransferase/IMP cyclohydrolase	Primary Cutaneous Anaplastic Large Cell Lymphoma
BAX	19q13.3-q13.4	BCL2-associated X protein	Basal Cell Carcinoma
BCL10	1p22	B-cell CLL/lymphoma 10	Systemic B-cell Lymphomas Involving the Skin
BCL2	18q21.3	B-cell CLL/lymphoma 2	Diffuse Large B-cell Lymphoma, Leg Type; Histiocytic Sarcoma; Primary Cutaneous Follicle Center Lymphoma; Systemic B-cell Lymphomas Involving the Skin
BCL6	3q27	B-cell CLL/lymphoma 6	Cutaneous Marginal Zone B-cell Lymphoma; Diffuse Large B-cell Lymphoma, Leg Type
BMI1	10p11.23	polycomb ring finger oncogene	Basal Cell Carcinoma
BRAF	7q34	v-raf murine sarcoma viral oncogene homolog B1	Common Acquired Melanocytic Nevi
C11orf95-MKL2	16p13.12	myocardin-like 2	Chondroid Lipoma
CCND1	11q13	cyclin D1; BCL1	Systemic B-cell Lymphomas Involving the Skin
CDK4	12q14	cyclin-dependent kinase 4	Atypical Lipomatous Tumor and Liposarcoma; Cutaneous Malignant Fibrous Histiocytoma/ Pleomorphic Sarcoma
CDKN2A	9p21	cyclin-dependent kinase inhibitor 2A;p16INK4A	Childhood Melanoma; Diffuse Large B-cell Lymphoma, Leg Type; Mycosis Fungoides (and Subtypes)
CDKN2B	9p21	cyclin-dependent kinase inhibitor 2B;p15INK4b	Diffuse Large B-cell Lymphoma, Leg Type
CHOP			Cutaneous Gamma-Delta T-cell Lymphoma
Chromosome 1, alterations of	1		Peripheral Neuroepithelioma/Primitive Neuroectodermal Tumor; Primary Neuroendocrine (Merkel Cell) Carcinoma;
Chromosome 10, alterations of	10		Perineurioma
Chromosome 11, alterations of	11		Peripheral Neuroepithelioma/Primitive Neuroectodermal Tumor
Chromosome 12, gain of	12		Cutaneous Rhabdomyosarcoma; Systemic B-cell Lymphomas Involving the Skin
Chromosome 13, gain of	13		Cutaneous Rhabdomyosarcoma
Chromosome 17, alterations of	17		Peripheral Neuroepithelioma/Primitive Neuroectodermal Tumor
Chromosome 18, gain of	18		Systemic B-cell Lymphomas Involving the Skin
Chromosome 2, alterations of	2		Primary Cutaneous Anaplastic Large Cell Lymphoma
Chromosome 2, gain of	2		Cutaneous Rhabdomyosarcoma;
Chromosome 22, alterations of	22		Perineurioma; Schwannoma (Neurilemmoma)
Chromosome 3, gain of	3		Systemic B-cell Lymphomas Involving the Skin
Chromosome 6, alterations of	6		Peripheral Neuroepithelioma/Primitive Neuroectodermal Tumor
Chromosome 8, alterations of	8		Leukemia Cutis
Chromosome 8, gain of	8		Cutaneous Rhabdomyosarcoma; Systemic B-cell Lymphomas Involving the Skin
c-KIT (see KIT)			
CLTC	17q11-qter	clathrin, heavy chain	Primary Cutaneous Anaplastic Large Cell Lymphoma
c-MYC (see MYC)			
COL1A1-PDGFB	t(17;22)(q22;q13)	COL1A1-PDGFβ	Fibrosarcoma; Superficial Malignant Peripheral Nerve Sheath Tumor
CREB3L1	11p11.2	cAMP responsive element binding protein 3-like 1	Low-Grade Fibromyxoid Sarcoma (Evans Tumor)

MOLECULAR FACTORS INDEX

CREB3L2	7q34	cAMP responsive element binding protein 3-like 2	Low-Grade Fibromyxoid Sarcoma (Evans Tumor)
CSF1	1p21-p13	colony stimulating factor 1	Giant Cell Tumor of Tendon Sheath
CTNNB1	3p21	β-catenin; beta-catenin	Extranodal NK/T-cell Lymphoma, Nasal Type; Fibromatosis; Myofibroma and Myofibromatosis; Pilomatrixoma and Pilomatrical Carcinoma
CYLD	16q12.1	cylindromatosis (turban tumor syndrome)	Cylindroma
del(11q)	11q		Systemic B-cell Lymphomas Involving the Skin
del(13q)	13q		Systemic B-cell Lymphomas Involving the Skin
del(17p)	17p		Systemic B-cell Lymphomas Involving the Skin
del(6)	6		Systemic B-cell Lymphomas Involving the Skin
del(6)(q21q25)	6q21-25		Extranodal NK/T-cell Lymphoma, Nasal Type
del(6q21)	6q21		Systemic B-cell Lymphomas Involving the Skin
EBER		EBV-encoded small nuclear RNA	Blastic Plasmacytoid Dendritic Cell Neoplasm; Cutaneous Gamma-Delta T-cell Lymphoma; Diffuse Large B-cell Lymphoma, Leg Type; Extranodal NK/T-cell Lymphoma, Nasal Type; Histiocytic Sarcoma; Lymphomatoid Papulosis; Primary Cutaneous CD4+ Small/Medium Pleomorphic T-cell Lymphoma; Subcutaneous Panniculitis-like T-cell Lymphoma
ETV6-NTRK3	t(12;15)(p13;q26)		Fibrosarcoma
EVER1/TMC6	17q25.3	transmembrane channel-like 6; epidermodysplasia verruciformis 1	Epidermodysplasia Verruciformis (EDV)
EVER2/TMC8	17q25.3	transmembrane channel-like 8; epidermodysplasia verruciformis 2	Epidermodysplasia Verruciformis (EDV)
EWS	22q12.2	Ewing sarcoma	Myxoinflammatory Fibroblastic Sarcoma
EWS-ATF1	t(12;22)(q13;q12)		Epithelioid Sarcoma; Fibromatosis; Myxoinflammatory Fibroblastic Sarcoma; PEComas; Superficial Malignant Peripheral Nerve Sheath Tumor
EWS-CREB1	t(2;22)(q33;q12)		Myxoinflammatory Fibroblastic Sarcoma; PEComas; Superficial Malignant Peripheral Nerve Sheath Tumor
EWS-FLI1	t(11;22)(q24;q12)		Peripheral Neuroepithelioma/Primitive Neuroectodermal Tumor
EWSR1-CREB1	t(2;22)(q33;q12)		Angiomatoid Fibrous Histiocytoma
FAS	10q24.1	TNF receptor superfamily, member 6; CD95	Cutaneous Marginal Zone B-cell Lymphoma; Extranodal NK/T-cell Lymphoma, Nasal Type
FIP1L1-PDGFRA	4q12	FIP1L1-PDGFRα; del(4)(q12)	Cutaneous and Systemic Mastocytosis
FOXC2	16q24.1	forkhead box C2; MFH1	Lymphangioma and Superficial Lymphangioma
FOXO1	13q14.1	forkhead box O1; FKHR; FOXO1A	Angiomatoid Fibrous Histiocytoma; Cutaneous Rhabdomyosarcoma
FOXP1	3p14.1	forkhead box P1	Diffuse Large B-cell Lymphoma, Leg Type
FUS	16p11.2	fused in sarcoma	Low-Grade Fibromyxoid Sarcoma (Evans Tumor)
FUS-ATF1	t(12;16)(q13;p11)		Angiomatoid Fibrous Histiocytoma
FUS-CREB3L2	t(7;16)(q34;p11)		Fibromatosis
GNA11	19p13.3	guanine nucleotide binding protein (G protein), alpha 1	Malignant Cellular Blue Nevus (Melanoma Arising in Cellular Blue Nevus)
GNAQ	9q21	guanine nucleotide binding protein (G protein), q polypeptide	Malignant Cellular Blue Nevus (Melanoma Arising in Cellular Blue Nevus)
i(6)(p10)	i(6)(p10)		Extranodal NK/T-cell Lymphoma, Nasal Type
i(8)(q10)	i(8)(q10)		Systemic T-cell and NK-cell Lymphomas Involving the Skin
IGH	14q32.33	Immunoglobulin heavy chain gene	Angioimmunoblastic T-cell Lymphoma; Blastic Plasmacytoid Dendritic Cell Neoplasm; Cutaneous Marginal Zone B-cell Lymphoma; Cutaneous Plasmacytoma; Diffuse Large B-cell Lymphoma, Leg Type; Extranodal NK/T-cell Lymphoma, Nasal Type; Histiocytic Sarcoma; Intravascular large B-cell Lymphoma; Lymphomatoid Granulomatosis; Primary Cutaneous CD4+ Small/Medium Pleomorphic T-cell Lymphoma; Primary Cutaneous Follicle Center Lymphoma; Systemic B-cell Lymphomas Involving the Skin

III

1

MOLECULAR FACTORS INDEX

IGH-BCL2	t(14;18)(q32;q21)		Diffuse Large B-cell Lymphoma, Leg Type
IGHV	14q32.33	Immunoglobulin heavy chain variable region	Diffuse Large B-cell Lymphoma, Leg Type
immunoglobulin heavy chain gene	14q32.33	IGH	Cutaneous Gamma-Delta T-cell Lymphoma; Primary Cutaneous Follicle Center Lymphoma; Subcutaneous Panniculitis-like T-cell Lymphoma
INK4A	9p21	p16INK4A; CDKN2A	Superficial Malignant Peripheral Nerve Sheath Tumor
inv(14)(q11q32)	inv(14)(q11q32)		Systemic T-cell and NK-cell Lymphomas Involving the Skin
inv(2)(p23;q35)	inv(2)(p23;q35)		Primary Cutaneous Anaplastic Large Cell Lymphoma
IRF4	6p25-p23	interferon regulatory factor 4	Systemic T-cell and NK-cell Lymphomas Involving the Skin
Isochromosome 12	i(12)		Histiocytic Sarcoma
Ki-67	10q26.2	MKI67	Diffuse Large B-cell Lymphoma, Leg Type; Kaposi Sarcoma; Systemic B-cell Lymphomas Involving the Skin
KIT	4q11-q12	v-kit Hardy-Zuckerman 4 feline sarcoma viral oncogene homolog; CD117	Cutaneous and Systemic Mastocytosis; Cutaneous and Systemic Mastocytosis; Extranodal NK/T-cell Lymphoma, Nasal Type; Fibromatosis; Mucosal Melanoma (Genital); Oral Melanoma; PEComas
KRAS	12p12.1	v-Ki-ras2 Kirsten rat sarcoma viral oncogene homolog	Extranodal NK/T-cell Lymphoma, Nasal Type
MALT1	18q21	mucosa associated lymphoid tissue lymphoma translocation gene 1	Diffuse Large B-cell Lymphoma, Leg Type; Systemic B-cell Lymphomas Involving the Skin
MDM2	12q15	p53 binding protein homolog (mouse)	Atypical Lipomatous Tumor and Liposarcoma; Cutaneous Malignant Fibrous Histiocytoma/Pleomorphic Sarcoma
MET	7q31	proto-oncogene (hepatocyte growth factor receptor); c-MET	Cutaneous and Systemic Mastocytosis
MIC2	Xp22.32 & Yp11.3	CD99	Peripheral Neuroepithelioma/Primitive Neuroectodermal Tumor
MLH1	3p21.3	mutL homolog 1	Sebaceoma (Sebaceous Epithelioma); Sebaceous Carcinoma
MLT1 (see MALT1)			
Monosomy 10	10		Perineurioma
Monosomy 9	9		Blastic Plasmacytoid Dendritic Cell Neoplasm
MSH2	2p21	mutS homolog 2	Sebaceoma (Sebaceous Epithelioma); Sebaceous Carcinoma
MSH6	2p16	mutS homolog 6	Sebaceoma (Sebaceous Epithelioma); Sebaceous Carcinoma
MSI		Microsatellite Instability	Sebaceous Carcinoma
MSN	Xq11.1	moesin	Primary Cutaneous Anaplastic Large Cell Lymphoma
MUM1	6p25-p23	multiple myeloma oncogene 1; IRF4	Blastic Plasmacytoid Dendritic Cell Neoplasm; Diffuse Large B-cell Lymphoma, Leg Type; Systemic B-cell Lymphomas Involving the Skin
MYC	8q24	v-myc myelocytomatosis viral oncogene homolog;c-MYC	Atypical Vascular Lesion; Atypical Vascular Lesion; Blastic Plasmacytoid Dendritic Cell Neoplasm; Blastic Plasmacytoid Dendritic Cell Neoplasm; Cutaneous Marginal Zone B-cell Lymphoma; Diffuse Large B-cell Lymphoma, Leg Type; Systemic B-cell Lymphomas Involving the Skin
MYH9	22q13.1	myosin, heavy chain 9, non-muscle	Primary Cutaneous Anaplastic Large Cell Lymphoma
ND			Primary Cutaneous Anaplastic Large Cell Lymphoma
NF1	17q11.2	neurofibromin 1	Neurofibroma; Schwannoma (Neurilemmoma); Superficial Malignant Peripheral Nerve Sheath Tumor
NF2	22q12.2	neurofibromin 2	Perineurioma; Schwannoma (Neurilemmoma)
NPM	5q35	Nucleophosmin	Primary Cutaneous Anaplastic Large Cell Lymphoma
NRAS	1p13.2	neuroblastoma RAS viral (v-ras) oncogene homolog	Mucosal Melanoma (Genital); Oral Melanoma
P15	9p21	CDKN2B	Primary Cutaneous Follicle Center Lymphoma;
P16	9p21	CDKN2A	Mycosis Fungoides (and Subtypes); Penile and Vulvar Intraepithelial Neoplasia; Primary Cutaneous

MOLECULAR FACTORS INDEX

			Follicle Center Lymphoma; Syringocystadenoma Papilliferum
P53	17p13.1	TP53	Actinic Keratosis; Basal Cell Carcinoma; Extranodal NK/T-cell Lymphoma, Nasal Type; Penile and Vulvar Intraepithelial Neoplasia; Superficial Malignant Peripheral Nerve Sheath Tumor; Superficial Malignant Peripheral Nerve Sheath Tumor
PAX3	2q35	paired box 3	Cutaneous Rhabdomyosarcoma
PAX3/7	2q35 & 1p36.13	paired box 3/7	Angiomatoid Fibrous Histiocytoma
PAX5	9p13	paired box 5	Systemic B-cell Lymphomas Involving the Skin
PAX7	1p36.13	paired box 7	Cutaneous Rhabdomyosarcoma
PROX1	1q41	prospero homeobox 1	Lymphangioma and Superficial Lymphangioma
PTCH (see PTCH1)			
PTCH1	9q22.3	patched 1	Basal Cell Carcinoma; Cutaneous Keratocyst; Nevus Sebaceus and Follicular Hamartomas; Rhabdomyoma; Syringocystadenoma Papilliferum
PTEN	10q23.31	phosphatase and tensin homolog	Fibrolipomatous Hamartoma of Nerve; Mycosis Fungoides (and Subtypes); Tricholemmoma
REL	2p13-p12	v-rel reticuloendotheliosis viral oncogene homolog; c-REL	Primary Cutaneous Follicle Center Lymphoma
RMRP	9p21-p12	RNA component of mitochondrial RNA processing endoribonuclease	Basal Cell Carcinoma
SAS	12q13.3	sarcoma-amplified sequence	Atypical Lipomatous Tumor and Liposarcoma
SOX18	20q13.33	SRY (sex determining region Y)-box 18	Lymphangioma and Superficial Lymphangioma
SOX9	17q23	SRY (sex-determining region Y)-box 9 protein	Basal Cell Carcinoma
t(1;10)	t(1;10)		Myxoinflammatory Fibroblastic Sarcoma
t(1;13)	t(1;13)		Peripheral Neuroepithelioma/Primitive Neuroectodermal Tumor
t(1;13)(p36;q14)	t(1;13)(p36;q14)		Cutaneous Rhabdomyosarcoma
t(1;14)(p22;q32)	t(1;14)(p22;q32)	IGH-BCL10	Systemic B-cell Lymphomas Involving the Skin
t(1;2)(q25;p23)	t(1;2)(q25;p23)		Primary Cutaneous Anaplastic Large Cell Lymphoma
t(10;22)	t(10;22)		Epithelioid Sarcoma
t(11;14)	t(11;14)		Primary Cutaneous Follicle Center Lymphoma
t(11;14)(q13;q32)	t(11;14)(q13;q32)	IGH-CCND1	Systemic B-cell Lymphomas Involving the Skin
t(11;16)	t(11;16)		Collagenous Fibroma
t(11;16)(p11;p11)	t(11;16)(p11;p11)	FUS-CREB3L1	Low-Grade Fibromyxoid Sarcoma (Evans Tumor)
t(11;16)(q13;p12-13)	t(11;16)(q13;p12-13)		Chondroid Lipoma
t(11;18)	t(11;18)		Cutaneous Marginal Zone B-cell Lymphoma
t(11;18)(q21;q32)	t(11;18)(q21;q32)	API2-MLT1	Systemic B-cell Lymphomas Involving the Skin
t(11;22)	t(11;22)		Epithelioid Sarcoma
t(11;22)(q24;q12)	t(11;22)(q24;q12)	EWS-FLI1	Peripheral Neuroepithelioma/Primitive Neuroectodermal Tumor
t(12;22)	t(12;22)		Superficial Malignant Peripheral Nerve Sheath Tumor
t(12;15)(p13;q26)	t(12;15)(p13;q26)	ETV6-NTRK3	Fibrosarcoma
t(12;16)	t(12;16)		Chondroid Lipoma; Hibernoma
t(12;16)(q13;p11)	t(12;16)(q13;p11)	FUS-ATF1	Epithelioid Hemangioendothelioma
t(12;22)	t(12;22)		Chondroid Lipoma; Hibernoma
t(14;14)(q11;q32)	t(14;14)(q11;q32)		Systemic T-cell and NK-cell Lymphomas Involving the Skin
t(14;18)	t(14;18)		Blastic Plasmacytoid Dendritic Cell Neoplasm; Cutaneous Marginal Zone B-cell Lymphoma; Diffuse Large B-cell Lymphoma, Leg Type; Histiocytic Sarcoma; Primary Cutaneous Follicle Center Lymphoma; Systemic B-cell Lymphomas Involving the Skin
t(14;18)(q32;q21)	t(14;18)(q32;q21)	IGH-MLT1	Cutaneous Marginal Zone B-cell Lymphoma; Diffuse Large B-cell Lymphoma, Leg Type; Histiocytic Sarcoma; Primary Cutaneous Follicle Center

MOLECULAR FACTORS INDEX

			Lymphoma; Systemic B-cell Lymphomas Involving the Skin
t(17;22)(q22;q13)	t(17;22)(q22;q13)	COL1A1-PDGFβ	Superficial Malignant Peripheral Nerve Sheath Tumor
t(2;10)(p23;q24)	t(2;10)(p23;q24)		Perineurioma
t(2;11)(q31;q12)	t(2;11)(q31;q12)		Collagenous Fibroma
t(2;13)	t(2;13)		Peripheral Neuroepithelioma/Primitive Neuroectodermal Tumor
t(2;13)(q35;q14)	t(2;13)(q35;q14)	PAX3-FKHR	Cutaneous Rhabdomyosarcoma
t(2;17)(p23;q23)	t(2;17)(p23;q23)		Primary Cutaneous Anaplastic Large Cell Lymphoma
t(2;17)(p23;q25)	t(2;17)(p23;q25)		Primary Cutaneous Anaplastic Large Cell Lymphoma
t(2;19)(p23;p13.1)	t(2;19)(p23;p13.1)		Primary Cutaneous Anaplastic Large Cell Lymphoma
t(2;22)(p23;q11.2)	t(2;22)(p23;q11.2)		Primary Cutaneous Anaplastic Large Cell Lymphoma
t(2;3)(p23;q12)	t(2;3)(p23;q12)		Primary Cutaneous Anaplastic Large Cell Lymphoma
t(2;5)	t(2;5)		Systemic T-cell and NK-cell Lymphomas Involving the Skin
t(2;5)(p23;q35)	t(2;5)(p23;q35)	ALK-NPM	Lymphomatoid Papulosis; Primary Cutaneous Anaplastic Large Cell Lymphoma; Systemic T-cell and NK-cell Lymphomas Involving the Skin
t(2;6)(q31;p21.3)	t(2;6)(q31;p21.3)		Myxoinflammatory Fibroblastic Sarcoma
t(2;8)	t(2;8)	MYC-kappa	Systemic B-cell Lymphomas Involving the Skin
t(7;16)	t(7;16)		Collagenous Fibroma
t(7;16)(q32-34;p11)	t(7;16)(q32-34;p11)	FUS-CREB3L2	Low-Grade Fibromyxoid Sarcoma (Evans Tumor); Fibrosarcoma
t(8;14)	t(8;14)		Blastic Plasmacytoid Dendritic Cell Neoplasm
t(8;14)(q22.3;q13)	t(8;14)(q22.3;q13)		Vascular Hamartomas
t(8;22)	t(8;22)	MYC-lambda	Systemic B-cell Lymphomas Involving the Skin
t(8;22)(q22;q11)	t(8;22)(q22;q11)		Epithelioid Sarcoma
t(8;8)(p12;q11)	t(8;8)(p12;q11)		Systemic T-cell and NK-cell Lymphomas Involving the Skin
t(9;11)(q34;q13)	t(9;11)(q34;q13)		Hibernoma
t(9;17)	t(9;17)		Chondroid Lipoma
t(9;17)(q22;q11)	t(9;17)(q22;q11)	NR4A3-TAF2N	Epithelioid Hemangioendothelioma
t(9;22)	t(9;22)		Chondroid Lipoma
t(9;22)(q22;q12)	t(9;22)(q22;q12)	EWSR1-NR4A3	Epithelioid Hemangioendothelioma
t(X;14)(q28;q11)	t(X;14)(q28;q11)		Systemic T-cell and NK-cell Lymphomas Involving the Skin
t(X;18)(p11;q11)	t(X;18)(p11;q11)		Fibrosarcoma
t(X;2)(q11-12;p23)	t(X;2)(q11-12;p23)	MSN-ALK	Primary Cutaneous Anaplastic Large Cell Lymphoma
T-cell receptor gamma gene	7p14	TCRγ	Aggressive Epidermotropic CD8+ Cytotoxic T-cell Lymphoma; Blastic Plasmacytoid Dendritic Cell Neoplasm; Subcutaneous Panniculitis-like T-cell Lymphoma
T-cell receptor gene		TCR	Lymphomatoid Granulomatosis; Lymphomatoid Papulosis
TCL1A	14q32.1	T-cell leukemia/lymphoma 1A	Systemic T-cell and NK-cell Lymphomas Involving the Skin
TCR		T-cell receptor gene	Angioimmunoblastic T-cell Lymphoma; Extranodal NK/T-cell Lymphoma, Nasal Type; Intravascular large B-cell Lymphoma; Mycosis Fungoides (and Subtypes); Primary Cutaneous CD4+ Small/Medium Pleomorphic T-cell Lymphoma; Subcutaneous Panniculitis-like T-cell Lymphoma; Systemic T-cell and NK-cell Lymphomas Involving the Skin
TCRβ	7q34	T-cell receptor beta gene	Cutaneous Gamma-Delta T-cell Lymphoma
TCRγ	7p14	T-cell receptor gamma gene	Cutaneous Gamma-Delta T-cell Lymphoma
TCRδ	4q11.2	T-cell receptor delta gene	Cutaneous Gamma-Delta T-cell Lymphoma
TET2	4q24	tet methylcytosine dioxygenase 2	Cutaneous and Systemic Mastocytosis
TFG	3q12.2	TRK-fused gene	Primary Cutaneous Anaplastic Large Cell Lymphoma
TPM3	1q21.2	tropomyosin 3	Primary Cutaneous Anaplastic Large Cell Lymphoma
TPM4	19p13.1	tropomyosin 4	Primary Cutaneous Anaplastic Large Cell Lymphoma

MOLECULAR FACTORS INDEX

Trisomy 21	21		Angioimmunoblastic T-cell Lymphoma
Trisomy 3	3		Angioimmunoblastic T-cell Lymphoma
Trisomy 5	5		Angioimmunoblastic T-cell Lymphoma
Trisomy 6	6		Primary Neuroendocrine (Merkel Cell) Carcinoma
TSC1	9q34	tuberous sclerosis 1	Acral Fibrokeratoma; Angiofibroma and Related Lesions; PEComas
TSC2	16p13.3	tuberous sclerosis 2	Acral Fibrokeratoma; Angiofibroma and Related Lesions; PEComas
VEGFR3	5q35.3	FLT4	Lymphangioma and Superficial Lymphangioma
X, gain of	X		Angioimmunoblastic T-cell Lymphoma; Systemic T-cell and NK-cell Lymphomas Involving the Skin
X, inactivation of	X		Neurofibroma

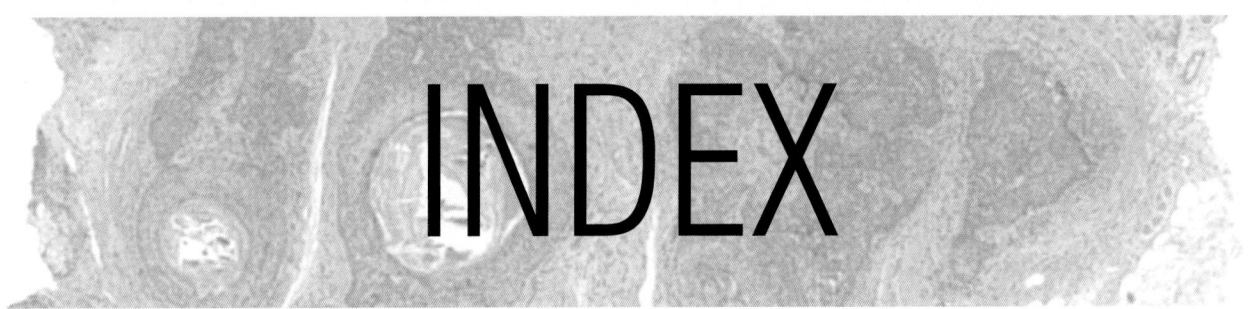

INDEX

A

INDEX

INDEX

INDEX

INDEX

INDEX

INDEX

INDEX

INDEX

INDEX

INDEX

INDEX

INDEX

INDEX

INDEX

INDEX

INDEX

INDEX

INDEX

INDEX

INDEX

INDEX

INDEX

INDEX

INDEX

INDEX

INDEX

INDEX

INDEX

INDEX

INDEX

INDEX

INDEX

INDEX

INDEX

INDEX

INDEX

INDEX

INDEX

INDEX

INDEX

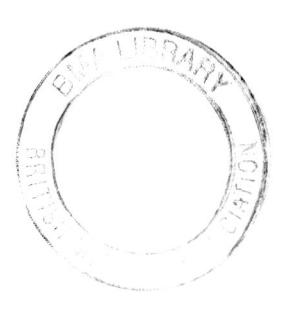